Thrombosis and Bleeding Disorders

Theory and Methods

Edited by

Nils U. Bang
Fritz K. Beller
Erwin Deutsch
Eberhard F. Mammen

95 Illustrations

1971

Georg Thieme Verlag · Stuttgart
Academic Press · New York · London

Academic Press, Inc.
111 Fifth Avenue, New York, New York 10003

Georg Thieme Verlag
Herdweg 63, 7000 Stuttgart 1

Library of Congress Catalog Card Number: 75 141604
Academic Press Inc.: ISBN 0 12 077750 9
Georg Thieme Verlag: ISBN 3 13 459201 0

Preface

This volume represents an international effort to bring together the most recent information on the laboratory and research aspects of thrombosis and hemorrhagic disorders in man. We have attempted in this text to provide not only a detailed description of the most widely-used laboratory assays but also to bring this technical information into its proper perspective by presenting reviews of the underlying theory, the physiology and biochemistry of hemostasis and thrombosis, the enzymology of blood coagulation and fibrinolysis.

The last 50 years have taught us the complexity of the physical-chemical phenomena resulting in the conversion of the soluble plasma protein fibrinogen into the insoluble network gel fibrin; more recently, we have also taken great strides to improve our knowledge of the biochemistry of the platelet aggregation phenomenon, a necessary prerequisite for normal hemostasis as well as thrombosis. The complexity of the systems under investigation has resulted in the development of a multitude of assays which often have lacked the specificity and reproducibility required for a sound and exacting enzyme kinetic analysis of the systems under investigation. The lack of such specific and quantitative techniques, the lack of the precise tools which must be at hand for the accurate analysis of any biological phenomenon has lead, in turn, to the development of a confusing number of conflicting or only partly compatible theories of the basic mechanisms involved in blood coagulation. And yet, the wide variety of semiquantitative test systems developed over the years have been of indisputable value and have helped to advance our knowledge in important clinical areas. The battery of laboratory tests currently available has made it possible to establish with great accuracy the differential diagnoses between the hemophilias and hemophilia-like syndromes. On the other hand, it can be argued whether these widely-used laboratory assays and the clinical knowledge which has emerged as a consequence of their wide-spread use has contributed in any lasting way to the fundamental theories of underlying mechanisms. We must also at this point ask ourselves whether the laboratory methodology which has contributed so significantly to the understanding of clinical problems of hemorrhagic states, whether all this progress has brought us any closer to a truer understanding of thrombosis in vivo.

It appears to most serious workers in the field today that the final classification of the coagulation mechanism can be achieved only when all the procoagulants alleged to be parts of the system on the basis of clinical observations of the hemophilias, when all of these procoagulants can be made available as purified homogeneous proteins possessing the theoretically maximum specific activities. Only the future will tell whether the understanding of the exact enzymic mechanisms making these systems operative will in turn provide the key to the many unresolved questions of thrombogenesis in man.

It is on this background that we chose to organize this textbook at three levels for three specific purposes. First, it has been our intention to compile the most reliable, most widely-accepted laboratory assays of undisputed diagnostic clinical value to provide the newcomer in the field as well as the more experienced worker in the coagulation laboratory with a reference manual as a guide to his everyday work in a clinically-oriented environment.

Secondly, we hope with the theoretical sections focusing on mechanisms to give our readership inside and outside the field an up-to-date review of the current state of the art, to sketch in outline the appearance of these systems as they present themselves today on the basis of the best currently available biochemical tools and assay systems. We are clearly aware of the deficiencies in these presentations and the magnitude of future achievements necessary to fill the gaps in our basic comprehension of blood coagulation.

Thirdly, we decided to include a systematic review of the most modern and successful purification techniques for individual coagulation factors and moieties of the fibrinolytic enzyme system, hoping thereby to provide the serious student of human blood coagulation with a reference list of the tools which he must develop to further advance our knowledge in the field.

This book will see the light of day only because of the unstinted efforts of and serious dedication to the job at hand from all of our contributors. We wish to take this opportunity to extend to all contributors our grateful appreciation for their generosity with their time and efforts, their patience and courtesy in spite of the delays and problems which we encountered in the course of preparing this volume.

July, 1970

The Editors

Contributors

AMBRUS, CLARA, M., M. D., Ph. D.
Associate Research Prof. of Pediatrics
State University of New York at Buffalo
Principle Cancer Research Scientist,
Roswell Park Memorial Institute
666 Elm Street
Buffalo, New Qork 14203, USA

ASTRUP, TAGE, Ph. D.
Director of Research
The James F. Mitchell Foundation
Institute for Medical Research
5401 Western Avenue N. W.
Washington D. C. 20015, USA

BANG, NILS, U., M. D.
Associate Professor of Medicine
Lilly Laboratory for Clinical Research
Marion County General Hospital and
Indiana University Medical Center
Indianapolis, Indiana 46202 USA

BARNHART, MARION I., Ph. D.
Professor of Physiology and Pharmacology
Wayne State University School of Medicine
1400 Chrysler Freeway
Detroit, Michigan 48207, USA

BELLER, FRITZ K., M. D., Med. Sci. D.
Professor of Obstetrics and Cynecology
New York University School of Medicine
Career Scientist of the Health
Research Council of the City of New York (I 296)
New York, New York 10016, USA

BENEKE, GUENTHER, M. D.
Professor of Pathology
Leiter der Abteilung für Pathologie II der
Universität Ulm
Head, Department of Pathology II,
University of Ulm
79 Ulm/Donau
Steinhoevelstr. 9, Germany

BETTEX-GALLAND, M., Ph. D.
Research Associate
Anatomisches Institut der Universität
Department of Normal Anatomy,
University of Berne
Buehstr. 26
3000 Bern, Switzerland

BORCHGREVINK, K. CHRISTIAN, M. D.
Professor, Institute of General Practice
Fr. Stangs gt 11/13
Oslo 2, Norway

BRAKMAN, PIETER, M. D., Ph. D.
Senior Investigator
The James F. Mitchell Foundation
Institute for Medical Research
5401 Western Avenue N. W.
Washington, D. C. 20015, USA

DEUTSCH, ERWIN, M. D.
Professor,
Head of the First Department of Medicine
University of Vienna
Lazarettgasse 14
A 1090 Vienna, Austria

DOUGLAS, A. S., BSC, M. D., FRCP, F. C. Path.
Professor of Medicine
University of Glasgow
Royal Infirmary
86 Castle Street
Glasgow C 4, Scotland

DUCKERT, F., PD, Ph. D.
Head of the Coagulation and Fibrinolysis
Laboratories
Department of Internal Medicine
University of Basel
Bürgerspital
Medizinische Universitäts-Klinik
4000 Basel, Switzerland

FISCHBACHER, WALTER, M. D.
Chief of Service
Bürgerspital St. Gallen
9000 St. Gallen, Switzerland

FORBES, CHARLES, D., M. B., CLB, MRCP
Registrar in Medicine
Glasgow Royal Infirmary
86 Castle Street
Glasgow C 4, Scotland

GLAS, PIA, M. D.
James F. Mitchell Foundation
Institute for Medical Research
5401 Western Avenue N. W.
Washington, D. C. 20015, USA

GORMSEN, JOHS, M. D.
Co-chairman
Medical Department
Sundby Hospital
2300 Copenhagen S, Denmark

GRAEFF, HENNER, M. D., P. D.
I. Department of Obstetrics and Gynecology
Maistr. 11,
8 München, Germany

Grammens, Jary, L., Ph. D.
Department of Physiology and Pharmacology
Wayne State University School of Medicine
1400 Chrysler Freeway
Detroit, Michigan 48207, USA

Halberstadt, M. D., PD
Assistant
Department of Obstetrics and Gynecology
Ludwig-Rehn-Str.
Frankfurt/Main, Germany

Hartert, Helmut, M. D.
Chief of Service, City Hospital Kaiserslautern
Clinical Professor of Medicine
Saar University
Turmstr. 45
Kaiserslautern, Germany

Heberlein, P. J., Ph. D. Deceased 1969
Research Associate
Department of Physiology and Pharmacology
Wayne State University School of Medicine
1400 Chrysler Freeway
Detroit, Michigan 48207, USA

Henry, L. Raymond, Ph. D.
Associate Professor
Department of Physiology and Pharmacology
Wayne State University School of Medicine
1400 Chrysler Freeway
Detroit, Michigan 48207, USA

Horowitz, Herbert I., M. D.
Hematologist
Bronx-Lebanon Hospital Center
Clinical Assistant Professor of Medicine
Cornell Medical College
1276 Fulton Avenue
Bronx, New York 10456, USA

Husby, Rolf M., Ph. D.
Senior Biochemist
Lilly Laboratory for Clinical Research,
Eli Lilly and Co.
Indianapolis Ind. 46206, USA

Jorpes, Erik J., M. D.
Emeritus Professor of Biochemistry
Karolinska Institutet
Stockholm 60,
Torsgatan 8
11123 Stockholm, Sweden

Kline, Daniel L., Ph. D.
Professor and Chairman
Department of Physiology
University of Cincinnati
College of Medicine
Eden & Bethesda Avenues
Cincinnati, Ohio 45219, USA

Kok, Preben, M. Sc.
Investigator
James F. Mitchell Foundation
Institute for Medical Research
5401 Western Avenu N. W.
Washington, D. C. 20015, USA

Langdell, Robert D., M. D.
Professor of Pathology
School of Medicine
University of North Carolina
Chapel Hill, N. C. 27514, USA

Lechner, Klaus, M. D.
Assistant
First Department of Medicine
University of Vienna
1090 Vienna, Austria
Lazarettgasse 14

Maki, Masahiro, M. D., Ph. D.
Associate Professor
Department of Obstetrics and Gynecology
Hirosaki University School of Medicine
2 Sagara-cho
Hirosaki, Japan

Latallo, Z. S., M. D.
Associate Professor
Instytut Bodań Jadrowich
Osrodek Zerań
Ulica Dorodna 16
Warszawa 9, Poland

Mammen, Eberhard F., M. D.
Professor of Pathology, Physiology and Pharmacology
Wayne State University School of Medicine
1400 Chrysler Freeway
Detroit, Michigan 48207, USA

McCoy, Lowell E., Ph. D.
Assistant Professor
Department of Physiology and Pharmacology
Wayne State University School of Medicine
1400 Chrysler Freeway
Detroit, Michigan 48207, USA

McMillan, Campbell W., M. D.
Associate Professor of Pediatrics
Associate Director Clinical Research Unit
University of North Carolina School of Medicine
Chapel Hill, North Carolina 27514, USA

Mozen, Milton M., Ph. D.
Director Biochemical Research Cutter Laboratories
Fourth and Parker Streets
Berkeley, California 94710, USA

Murano, Genesio, Ph. D.
Research Associate
Department of Physiology and Pharmacology
Wayne State University School of Medicine
1400 Chrysler Freeway
Detroit, Michigan 48207, USA

O'Brien, J. R., MA, DM. MRCS, LRCP, F. C. Path.
Consultant Hematologist
Portsmouth and Isle of Wight Area Pathology Service
Central Laboratory
St. Mary's General Hospital
(East Wing)
Milton Road, Portsmouth, England

PENICK, GEORGE D., M. D.
Professor of Pathology
University of North Carolina School of Medicine
Chapel Hill, North Carolina 27514, USA

RATNOFF, OSCAR D., M. D.
Professor of Medicine
Career Investigator of the American Heart Association
Case Western Reserve University School of Medicine
University Hospitals of Cleveland
Cleveland, Ohio 44106, USA

RIZZA, CHARLES, R. C., M. D., MRCP
Consultant Physician
Oxford Hemophilia Centre
Clinical Lecturer in Hematology at the University of Oxford
Oxford Haemophilia Centre
Churchill Hospital
Headington, Oxford, England

ROBERTS, HAROLD R., M. D.
Associate Professor of Medicine and Pathology
University of North Carolina School of Medicine
Chapel Hill, North Carolina 27514, USA

SCHRÖER, HEINZ, M. D.
Scientific Advisor and Professor
Physiologisches Institut
Universität Würzburg
Department of Physiology
University of Würzburg
Roentgenring 9
8700 Würzburg, Germany

SCHWICK, GERHARD H., Ph. D.
Director of Research, Behring Werke
Dozent, University of Marburg
355 Marburg/Lahn
Georg-Voigt-Str. 69
Germany

SIXMA, J. J., M. D., Ph. D.
Head of the Division of Haemostasis
Consulting Physician in Internal Medicine
Interne Klinik
Akademisches Krankenhaus
Utrecht, Holland

SHULMAN, RAPHAEL N., M. D.
Chief Clinical Hematology Branch
National Institute of Arthritis and Metabolic Diseases
National Institutes of Health
Clinical Center
NIH
10-9N250
Bethesda, Maryland 20014, USA

SPIELVOGEL, ARTHUR RALPH, M. D.
Associate Hematologist
The Bronx-Lebanon Hospital
Instructor in Medicine
New York College of Medicine
1650 Grand Concourse
Bronx, New York, USA

STEHBENS, WILLIAM E., M. D., Ph. D.
Professor of Pathology
Director of Electron Microscopy Unit
Veterans Administration Hospital
Albany, New York 12208, USA

TRIANTAPHYLLOPOULOS, DEMETRIOS C., M. D.
Senior Research Scientist
The American National Red Cross
Blood Research Laboratory
9312 Old Georgetown Road
Bethesda, Maryland 20014, USA

TRIANTAPHYLLOPOULOS, EUGENIE, M. D., Ph. D.
Chief Coagulation Research
Department of Hematology
Washington, D. C. 20010, USA

TROLL, WALTER, Ph. D.
Professor Environmental Medicine
New York University School of Medicine
550 First Avenue
New York, New York 10016, USA

WALKER, WILLIAM, MB, FRCP (ed)
Physician
City Hospital Aberdeen, Scotland
Clinical Lecturer in Medicine University of Aberdeen
City Hospital
Urquhart Road
Aberdeen, Scotland

WESSLER, STANFORD, M. D.
Professor of Medicine
Washington University School of Medicine
Physician-in-Chief
The Jewish Hospital of St. Louis
216 South Kings Highway
St. Louis, Missouri 63110, USA

Table of Contents

Partial Thromboplastin Time Techniques
by R. D. Langdell

Prothrombin Consumption Tests
by N. R. Shulman

Thrombin and Thromboplastin Generation Techniques
by Ch. D. Forbes and A. S. Douglas

One-Stage Prothrombin Time Techniques
by Ch. R. Rizza and W. Walker

Chapter IV

Purification of Prothrombin
by G. Murano

Purification of Prethrombin "Modified Zymogen"
by G. Murano

Purification of Thrombin
by G. Murano

Chapter 1

Physiology and Biochemistry of Blood Coagulation

Eberhard F. Mammen

I. Introduction

Blood coagulation is an important part of hemostasis in the mammalian system. Hemostasis is accomplished by the harmonious interplay of the blood vessel walls with some cellular elements of the blood, especially the platelets, and some of the plasma proteins (blood coagulation factors). The vessel walls contract at and near the site of injury, while the blood platelets adhere and aggregate at this site. The initial adhesion and aggregation of the platelets leads to the formation of a first hemostatic plug. Lower forms of life use local vasoconstriction and cell aggregation as the only means of hemostasis. However, most vertebrates have one more safety factor added to their mechanism of hemostasis. This is the solidification of the blood plasma by the activation of the blood coagulation mechanism. The fluid plasma is transformed to a gel by the conversion of fibrinogen to fibrin. The resulting fibrin clot can be regarded as the second and final hemostatic plug. After fibrin formation, the polymerized fibrin monomers are stabilized by the enzymic action of a fibrin stabilizing factor (Factor XIII). The crosslinking enzyme has been identified as a transglutaminase (Matacic and Loewy, 1966). Next, the fibrin clot will retract, and in this process of clot retraction platelets are of considerable importance. In the subsequent process of wound healing the fibrin clot is slowly dissolved while fibroblasts grow into the clot.

This chapter will be limited to a description of the physiology and biochemistry of prothrombin activation. The initial phase of the hemostasis mechanism involving platelets is described in Chapter IX, p. 412; the biochemistry and physiology of the fibrinogen to fibrin conversion is covered in Chapter VI, p. 222, and finally the physiology and biochemistry of fibrinolysis is outlined in Chapter VIII, p. 292.

II. Historical Aspects of Blood Coagulation

One of the earliest blood coagulation theories was proposed by Morawitz (1904, 1905) and involved the postulated existence of four coagulation factors, fibrinogen, prothrombin, tissue thrombokinase, and calcium ions. These factors were subsequently termed factors I, II, III and IV. Morawitz (1905) postulated that prothrombin was converted to thrombin by tissue thrombokinase (thromboplastin) and calcium ions. Thrombin was believed to be the enzyme which converted fibrinogen to fibrin. Already in 1911, Addis accumulated evidence for the existence of another coagulation factor in plasma when he prepared and studied a globulin fraction which would correct the coagulation defect in hemophilic plasma in vitro. Addis assumed that the globulin fraction contained prothrombin, and consequently postulated that hemophilia might be caused by an abnormal prothrombin molecule. This assumption was disputed by Howell (1914) and Howell and Cekade (1926) when they established that prothrombin in hemophilic plasma was normal in quantity and quality. Howell (1914) held the view that hemophilia was caused by a qualitative platelet defect. This assumption was challenged when Feissly and Fried (1924) and Govaertz and Gratia (1931) pointed out that platelet-free normal plasma would correct the coagulation defect in hemophilic blood. Patek and Stetson (1936) then demonstrated that the "antihemophilic globulin" was not removed from plasma by Berkefeld filtration, and that it could be found in the globulin fraction originally prepared by Addis (1914). Finally, Quick and Stefanini (1948) concluded that normal and hemophilic platelets were equally active. Brinkhous (1939) investigated the delayed thrombin formation in hemophilic plasma and observed that the addition of tissue thromboplastin would normalize thrombin formation. These observations established the existence of yet another blood clotting factor in addition to the factors postulated by Morawitz (1905). The factor was subsequently called "antihemophilic factor", "antihemophilic globulin" or "factor VIII". Brinkhous' work provided the early evidence for a pathway in coagulation not involving tissue thromboplastin. This concept had already been introduced by Bordet and Gengou (1901) and Morawitz (1905) who independently established that blood may clot in the *absence* of tissue thromboplastin when brought into contact with glass. These experiments were basic to our present concept of prothrombin activation via two pathways, an *extrinsic* one, involving tissue thromboplastin, and an *intrinsic* one, involving only plasma constitutents and platelets. Additional coagulation factors, at present believed to be involved in the extrinsic and intrinsic pathways of prothrombin activation, have been recognized mainly, although not entirely, from clinically oriented research work. In 1947, Owren (1947a, b) discovered a patient with a coagulation disturbance which differed from classical hemophilia. The patient had normal prothrombin and fibrinogen levels, but, in contrast to classical hemophilia, the addition of tissue thromboplastin did not correct the clotting abnormality. Owren (1947a, b) called the disease "parahemophilia" and implied that a hitherto unrecognized coagulation factor necessary for prothrombin activation was absent in the patient's plasma. Since normal plasma corrected the patient's abnormal clotting mechanism, the factor was considered to be present in normal plasma. The activity was termed "factor V". Soon it became apparent that factor V possessed the same activity as a plasma fraction already recognized in 1938 by Seegers et al. (1938a), later referred to as "Ac-globulin" by Ware et al. (1947a, b). Quick (1943) had termed this activity "labile factor".

The following years were marked by the additional recognition of further "prothrombin activation accelerators", such as "factor VII" also termed serum prothrombin conversion accelerator (SPCA), Proconvertin or stable factor (Alexander et al. 1949a; DeVries et al. 1949; Alexander et al. 1951; Koller et al. 1951, 1952); "factor IX" also called plasma thromboplastin component (PTC), Christmas factor or antihemophilic factor B (Pavlovsky, 1947; Koller et al. 1950; Aggeler et al. 1952; Biggs et al. 1952; Schulman and Smith, 1952); "factor X" also known as Stuart factor, Prower factor or Stuart-Prower factor (Telfer et al. 1956; Hougie et al. 1957); "factor XI" originally described as plasma thromboplastin antecedent (PTA) (Rosenthal et al. 1953); and "factor XII" also termed Hageman factor (Ratnoff and Colopy, 1955). In most instances, a patient with a bleeding tendency and an impaired prothrombin conversion was observed. When the defect seemed to be different from any one previously recognized, the defect was attributed to the absence of a hitherto unknown coagulation factor. In many instances the patient's name was attached to the supposedly missing factor. Since normal plasma would correct the patient's clotting defect, normal plasma was assumed to contain the factor in question. Such reasoning is acceptable as long as it is clearly understood that it is only a working hypothesis. Rather than assuming the complete absence of a factor, the factor may be present in a biochemically modified form. The resulting pathology would be the same in either case. From the hemoglobinopathies it is well recognized that the exchange of one amino acid in the molecular structure of the hemoglobin molecule produces severe functional changes in the molecule. Recently, the same observation has been made in a family with an abnormal fibrinogen molecule (Blombäck et al. 1968, Mammen et al. 1969). The exchange of one amino acid caused an impaired polymerization of the fibrinogen molecules and a severe hemorrhagic tendency. Such abnormalities could underlie other deficiency states, resulting in congenital bleeding disorders, and would be fully compatible with the established pattern of heredity. It also must be kept in mind that the correction of a "deficiency" plasma by normal plasma does not necessarily imply the existence of a separate clotting factor. The existence of individual clotting factors is ultimately proven by the isolation of the factor from plasma and by appropriate characterization of its properties.

Brinkhous (1959) wrote in his review, "Today it is realized generally that detailed chemical studies will be required before hypotheses (which include all coagulation reactions) of lasting value can be developed. Such chemical studies are beginning to appear, but many uncontrolled and at present seemingly uncontrollable variables still plague the investigator". Kline (1965) pointed out that investigators have not been content to wait for detailed chemical studies and have proposed comprehensive blood coagulation schemes. "Since his (the investigator's) hypotheses are not on firm ground, constant revision is the price the imaginative scientist must pay in exchange for exhilerating leaps into the partially known" (Kline, 1965). This statement indeed finds its reflection in the number of coagulation schemes proposed in the last 15–20 years. Obviously, it will not be possible to discuss all of them in this chapter. This outline will be limited to a discussion of basically *two* theories which have emerged over the last few years to explain the events leading to the activation of prothrombin.

The first theory is the "cascade" or "waterfall" hypothesis of prothrombin activation originally proposed by Davie and Ratnoff (1964) and by Macfarlane (1964a). It was subsequently reviewed and expanded by Macfarlane (1965, 1966) and Davie and Ratnoff (1965). This hypothesis states that all clotting factors are distinct entities in plasma, synthesized independently, and present in plasma as inactive precursors. Each coagulation factor is activated by the preceeding one in a chain of events that ultimately leads to the conversion of prothrombin to thrombin. Inherited coagulopathies are believed to be due to absence of specific coagulation factors.

The second concept of prothrombin activation has been proposed over the last 20 years by Seegers and his associates and is found in a number of books and review articles (Seegers, 1962; 1964; 1965; 1967; 1968; 1969; Seegers et al. 1967a; Mammen, 1968). Seegers' basic approach to blood coagulation consists of the purification and biochemical characterization of the coagulation constituents in question and of a study of the kinetics of their interaction. Seegers was the first to purify prothrombin from plasma (Seegers et al. 1938b; Seegers, 1940; Seegers and Smith, 1941; Seegers, 1952; Ware and Seegers, 1948a). He placed the original concept of blood coagulation proposed by Morawitz (1905) on a firm basis. His studies of the prothrombin molecule suggested that prothrombin may be a multifunctional entity that not only can be converted into thrombin, but which can also dissociate to produce other derivates, termed "autoprothrombins".

At a superficial glance these two theories seem to have very little in common. This would mean that prothrombin is activated in one way for one group of investigators and in another way for another group. Obviously, there is only *one* way, in vivo. Assuming that the immense number of experiments performed by the supporters of both theories are correct, there must be some kind of a common denominator that ultimately indicates the most likely mechanism by which prothrombin is activated. In this review, an attempt will be made to correlate both concepts. It will not be possible to cite each one of the several thousand articles that have been written on this subject but an attempt will be made to highlight the most important contributions. Therefore, the bibliography will be selective rather than complete.

III. Nomenclature

A serious problem in understanding blood coagulation has been and still is, to a certain extent, the conflicting nomenclature used for the description of the various coagulation constitutents. This has rendered communication difficult among experienced research workers in the field. The uninitiated investigator who starts working in this area is especially handicapped by this state of semantic confusion. The confusion commenced when different names were employed for the same activity, and when identical names were used for different activities. Part of this is due to the almost simultaneous discovery of similar bleeding disorders in different laboratories, as discussed in the historical outline above. An International Committee on Blood Clotting Factors was formed in 1954 and given the task to design a common symbolic language for the unequivocal identification of blood coagulation factors. The Committee has met almost annually and Roman numerals have been assigned to activities, the "absence" of which results in clinical abnormalities of blood coagulation. The reports of the Committee, published since 1959 as Supplements to Thrombosis et Diathesis Haemorrhagica, include some biochemical and physicochemical properties of preparations containing the activity in question, but it must be recognized that the chemical identity of a number of these activities remains uncertain.

In the symbolic description established by the nomenclature committee, a Roman Numeral refers to the inactive precursor state of the clotting factor in question; the corresponding active form of the clotting factor is denoted by the Roman Numeral followed by the letter "a". Since numerals in themselves are principally meaningless, a table is composed (Table 1) in which the Roman Numerals are correlated with the most common synonyms that are or were used in the literature.

Table 1

Roman Numerals	Synonyms
Factor I	Fibrinogen
Factor II	Prothrombin
Factor III	Tissue Thromboplastin, Tissue Thrombokinase, Extrinsic Thromboplastin
Factor IV	Calcium ions
Factor V	Plasma Accelerator Globulin, Plasma Ac-Globulin, Proaccelerin, Labile Factor
Factor VI	Not Assigned
Factor VII	Serum Prothrombin Conversion Accelerator (SPCA), Proconvertin, Stable Factor, Autoprothrombin I
Factor VIII	Antihemophilic Factor (AHF), Antihemophilic Globulin (AHG), Antihemophilic Globulin A, Platelet Cofactor I, Thromboplastinogen A, Facteur Antihemophilique A
Factor IX	Plasma Thromboplastin Component (PTC), Christmas Factor, Antihemophilic Factor B, Antihemophilic Globulin B, Platelet Cofactor II, Thromboplastinogen B, Facteur Antihemophilique B, Autoprothrombin II
Factor X	Stuart Factor, Prower Factor, Stuart-Prower Factor, Prephase Accelerator (PPA)*, Plasma Thromboplastin*, Coagulation Product I*, Autoprothrombin III, Autoprothrombin C*
Factor XI	Plasma Thromboplastin Antecedent (PTA), Antihemophilic Factor C
Factor XII	Hageman Factor, Surface Factor, Contact Factor, Clot-Promoting Factor
Factor XIII	Fibrin Stabilizing Factor (FSF), Fibrin Stabilizing Enzyme, Laki-Lorand Factor, Fibrinase, Plasma Transglutaminase

* Most likely activited Factor X

IV. Physicochemical Properties of Coagulation Constituents

In recent years, it has become increasingly evident that biochemical procedures have to be applied to the study of blood coagulation in order to better understand this physiological mechanism. In biochemistry, a first order requirement is the isolation of the substance in question in the purest possible form. Once isolated, the component can be characterized in terms of its structure and function. This approach has been difficult in the case of a number of coagulation constituents because of the inherent lability of these components. In spite of these difficulties, a number of coagulation factors have been purified and characterized to a certain extent. In the following, we will examine the physical-chemical properties of coagulation constitutents involved in prothrombin activation. Procedures for the purification of individual factors are found in Chapter IV.

A. Prothrombin

Prothrombin was one of the earliest coagulation proteins isolated from bovine plasma, in the pioneering work of Seegers and his associates (Seegers et al. 1938b; Seegers, 1940; Seegers and Smith, 1941; Seegers et al. 1945a; Ware and Seegers, 1948a; Seegers, 1952; 1962). Other procedures for the isolation of bovine prothrombin have been described by Goldstein et al. (1959), Moore et al. (1965) and Tishkoff et al. (1968). Prothrombin from human plasma has been isolated by a number of investigators (Lanchantin et al. 1963; Lanchantin and Friedmann, 1963; Magnusson, 1965a; Shapiro and Waugh, 1966; Aronson (1966).

Plasma of other animal species has also been the source of purified prothrombin. These procedures include those of Anderson and Barnhart (1964) for the isolation of canine prothrombin, the method of Miller and Phelan (1967) and Miller and McGarrahan (1958) for the purification of equine prothrombin, and the procedure of Li and Olson (1967) for the preparation of purified rat prothrombin. The preparations from the various animal plasmas vary considerably in their activity and purity. Probably the best prothrombin preparations have been obtained from bovine plasma; consequently, most of the physico-chemical studies have been performed on bovine prothrombin. According to available comparative studies, bovine and human prothrombin are similar in most respects (Lanchantin et al. 1968a, b).

The concentration of prothrombin in bovine plasma was found to be 0.1–0.15 mg/ml (Seegers, 1962); it may be lower in the human.

In both bovine and human plasma the prothrombin activity migrated electrophoretically with the α_2-globulin fraction (Owen and McKenzie, 1954; Seegers, 1962). Purified bovine prothrombin preparations migrated in the area of the α_1-globulins (Seegers et al. 1950). Purified *human* prothrombin had the mobility of an α_2-globulin. By means of moving boundary electrophoresis bovine prothrombin complex had an isoelectric point of pH 4.25 in a buffer of ionic strength 0.2 (Seegers et al. 1966a); in buffers of ionic strength 0.1 an isoelectric point of pH 4.1 was found (Tishkoff et al. 1968).

Purified bovine prothrombin preparations with a specific activity of 2,200 Iowa units/mg protein were homogeneous in the analytical ultracentrifuge. In free electrophoresis experiments, the same products also displayed a single symmetrical peak at pH's below 7.0; above pH 7.0 the prothrombin tended to dissociate (Seegers et al. 1966a). Despite the apparent physical homogeneity, these prothrombin preparations contain factor X, VII and IX activities. These activities can be removed by chromatography on DEAE-cellulose. In the following, the chromatographed prothrombin preparations will be referred to as "prothrombin" or "DEAE-prothrombin", while the non-chromatographed preparations will be termed "prothrombin complex". The sedimentation rate for bovine prothrombin complex ($S^o_{20,w}$) was 5.22 Svedberg units (Harmison et al. 1961), the partial specific volume ($\bar{v}$) was 0.70 ml/gm, and the diffusion coefficient ($D_{20,w}$) was 6.25×10^{-7} cm²/sec (Lamy and Waugh, 1953). From these biophysical measurements, a molecular weight of 68,000 to 68,500 has been calculated (Lamy and Waugh, 1958; Harmison et al. 1961). Using sedimentation equilibrium analysis a molecular weight of 70,500 was obtained for bovine prothrombin complex (Tishkoff et al. 1968). Molecular weight determinations on thin-layer gel filtration gave an average value of 68,000 ± 4,000 (Murano, 1968). The sedimentation constant for DEAE-prothrombin was also 5.3 S (Seegers et al. 1969). The molecular weight by physical analysis, as reported by Tishkoff et al. (1968), was 65,500 ± 1,247. Murano (1968) found by thin-layer gel filtration a molecular weight of 66,500 ± 3,000. The molecular weight of human prothrombin was reported as 68,700 (Lanchantin et al. 1968a). Equine prothrombin complex had a sedimentation coefficient of 5.35 Svedberg units, a diffusion coefficient of 3.8×10^{-7} cm^2/sec, and a molecular weight of about 130,000 (Miller and McGarrahan, 1958). It is apparently twice as large as bovine prothrombin complex.

The bovine prothrombin complex possessed the apparent shape of an ellipsoid with a length of 119 Å and a width of 34 Å (Lamy and Waugh, 1953) when calculated by the method of Flory and Fox (1950), and a length of 134 Å and width of 35 Å when calculated on the basis of its molecular weight (Harmison et al. 1961). In the electron microscope, prothrombin complex displayed a rather uniform globular appearance with a height of 105 Å (Riddle et al. 1963). Allowing for loss of internal hydration, these dimensions would agree with the values derived from studies of its hydrodynamic behaviour.

The amino acid composition of the bovine prothrombin complex has been determined by several investigators (Laki et al. 1954; Magnusson, 1965b; Seegers et al. 1967b). All values are in fair agreement and the most recent one (Seegers et al. 1967b), is listed in Table 2. The prothrombin complex contained 526 amino acid residues. This value may not represent the accurate number of residues in prothrombin, since the prothrombin complex contains variable quantities of factors X, VII and IX. Using the procedure of Brand (1946), a molecular weight of 58,800 has been calculated on the basis of the amino acid composition (Seegers et al. 1967b). This value is slightly below the one previously calculated on the basis of a different amino acid composition (Harmison and Mammen, 1967). If allowance was made for the carbohydrate content of prothrombin complex, a carbohydrate weight of approximately 8,000 had to be added to the molecular weight based on the amino acid composition. The molecular weight for the entire glycoprotein would then be about 66,800 which is in close approximation with the molecular weight calculated from biophysical measurements. Seegers et al. (1969) determined the amino acid composition of prothrombin chromatographed on DEAE cellulose (Table 2).

The amino acid composition of human prothrombin (Table 2) is similar to that of bovine prothrombin, with the exception of the values for threonine and tryptophan. A total of 556–559 amino acid residues were found for the protein moiety of human prothrombin (Lanchantin et al. 1968a).

In 8 molar urea solution, 8 moles of disulfide were found per mole of bovine prothrombin complex (Carter and Warner, 1954, 1956).

The terminal amino acids of prothrombin complex have been studied by several investigators and the N-terminal amino acid is alanine (Magnusson, 1958; 1965b; Miller, 1958; Thomas and Seegers, 1960; Murano, 1968). Prothrombins prepared by a variety of different procedures had identical N-terminal residues. Two C-terminal amino acids, tyrosine and glycine, were found in non-chromatographed and on IRC-50 chromatographed bovine prothrombin complex (Thomas and Seegers, 1960) using the ammonium thiocyanate method (Tibbs, 1951). With the carboxypeptidase method no C-terminal amino acids could be determined (Miller and Van Vunakis, 1956a; Magnusson and Steele, 1965). Apparently, the C-terminal residues of prothrombin are not available for carboxypeptidase action (Magnusson, 1965c).

The total carbohydrate content of bovine prothrombin complex was 11.2 % (Schwick and Schultze, 1959), respectively 11.6 % (Magnusson, 1965d). Galactose, mannose and fucose were 3.06, 1.53, and 0.09 %, respectively; hexosamine was 2.3 % and sialic acid was 4.2 % (Schwick and Schultze, 1959; Magnusson, 1965b). Tishkoff et al. (1968) reported similar values. The total carbohydrate content of human prothrombin was found to be around 10 % (Lanchantin et al. 1968a).

From the empirical data it is apparent that prothrombin complex and DEAE-prothrombin are very similar. This indicates that the associated activities (factors X, VII and IX) in the prothrombin complex constitute such a slight "contamination" as to not influence physical measurements.

B. Prethrombin

When prothrombin complex is converted to thrombin, a dissociation of the complex takes place which precedes the actual development of thrombin activity (Lorand et al. 1953; Seegers and Alkjaersig, 1956). This dissociation has been observed in the analytical ultracentrifuge (Lamy and Waugh, 1954; 1958), in moving boundary electrophoresis (Seegers et al. 1950), and by N-terminal amino acid determinations (Magnusson, 1958, 1964; Murano, 1968). At the time of dissociation, 60–80 % of the carbohydrate and approximately 40 % of the protein became soluble in trichloroacetic acid (Lorand et al. 1953; Seegers and Alkjaersig, 1956). Since at the time of dissociation no thrombin activity could be measured, it had to be assumed that thrombin was present in an inactive fragment which had to be different from the original prothrombin. This fragment has been isolated in purified form and was termed *prethrombin* (Seegers and Marciniak, 1965; Marciniak and Seegers, 1965; Seegers et al. 1965a; 1967b). Similar "inert" degradation products of bovine and human prothrombin have been described and studied by other investigators (Asada et al. 1961; Magnusson, 1965f; Lanchantin et al. 1965a; 1967; 1968b; Aronson, 1966; Aronson and Ménache, 1966; Tishkoff et al. 1968).

In contrast to prothrombin, prethrombin could neither be converted to thrombin in 25 % sodium citrate solution (Seegers et al. 1967b) nor by tissue thromboplastin under the conditions of the two-stage analytical procedure, described by Ware and Seegers (1949) (Seegers and Marciniak, 1965). Only when autoprothrombin C (activated factor X) was added, thrombin would form from prethrombin. Basically, autoprothrombin C alone activated the substrate (Seegers and Marciniak, 1965; Marciniak and Seegers, 1966a; 1966b; Seegers et al. 1967b). Prethrombin, in contrast to prothrombin, could not be activated in the presence of platelet factor 3 and factor VIII (Marciniak and Seegers, 1966a). While purified prothrombin complex readily corrected the clotting defect of factor VII, IX and X deficient plasmas, purified prethrombin was inactive in this respect (Marciniak and Seegers, 1965; 1966a).

Prethrombin has been isolated from purified bovine prothrombin complex which had been dissociated with thrombin at pH 7.0 (Seegers and Marciniak, 1965; Marciniak and Seegers, 1965; Seegers et al. 1967b). The actual procedure is described in Chapter IV. When assayed with a modified two-stage analytical procedure (Marciniak and Seegers, 1965), specific activities as high as 40,000–45,000 Iowa units/mg tyrosine were obtained. These activities are near the specific activity of purified thrombin (Seegers et al. 1958).

In the analytical ultracentrifuge and by cellulose acetate electrophoresis, purified prethrombin displayed homogeneity (Seegers et al. 1967b). A sedimentation coefficient ($S^{o}_{20,w}$) of 3.93 Svedberg units was found. The regression line relating sedimentation rate to concentration had a small positive slope (Seegers et al. 1967b). It resembled in this respect, to a certain extent, the positive slope obtained with thrombin. The sedimentation coefficient of prethrombin was smaller than that of prothrombin, but still larger than that of thrombin (3.76 Svedberg units). Diffusion coefficient and partial specific volume have not been determined for prethrombin so that no molecular weight has been calculated on the basis of physical measurements. On the basis of thin-layer gel filtration, prethrombin had a molecular weight of 52,000 ± 9,000 (Murano, 1968). Tishkoff et al. (1968) used sedimentation equilibrium centrifugation and found a molecular weight of 52,395 ± 3,449 for their "modified zymogen" which is apparently identical with prethrombin.

The isoelectric point of prethrombin in acetate buffer of ionic strength 0.1 was pH 5.5 (Seegers et al. 1967b) which again is markedly different from prothrombin complex (pH 4.1), but only slightly different from thrombin (pH 5.75).

The amino acid composition of prethrombin was determined by Seegers et al. (1967b) and is listed in Table 2.

The N-terminal amino acids were determined by Murano (1968). Prethrombin had two N-terminal amino acids, lysine and threonine. The average recovery of lysine was 1.03 M/52,000 gm, the average recovery of threonine 0.97 M/52,000 gm.

These findings place the prethrombin fragment as an intermediate between prothrombin and thrombin. Based on molecular weight, prethrombin is smaller than prothrombin but still larger than thrombin. Prothrombin has 1 mole N-terminal alanine per 65,000 to 70,000 gm, indicating that it is a single chain molecule. Prethrombin has two N-terminal amino acids, lysine and threonine (1 mole of each per 52,000 gm), indicating that it is a two-chain molecule. These findings indicate that the activation of prothrombin to prethrombin by thrombin involves the N-terminal end of the prothrombin molecule; apparently a peptide containing the alanine N-terminal portion in prothrombin is cleaved and discarded. However, one additional cleavage point must occur in order to form a two-chain molecule from a one-chain molecule. This cleavage most likely occurs between an intra-chain disulfide bridge. Thereby, prethrombin becomes a two-chain molecule, like thrombin. Moreover, one of the N-terminal amino acids (threonine) is the same as in thrombin. However, the active site of the thrombin molecule must still be masked in prethrombin since prethrombin possesses no proteolytic activity against fibrinogen. The conversion of prethrombin to thrombin with generation of proteolytic activity can not be achieved by thrombin. Autoprothrombin C (activated factor X, thrombokinase) is necessary for this final activation.

C. Thrombin

Thrombin can be obtained by activating purified prothrombin or prothrombin complex in different ways, and again a number of investigators have attempted its isolation (Seegers et al. 1958; Magnusson, 1965c; Miller and Copeland, 1965; Berg et al. 1966; Baughman and Waugh, 1967; Hussain and Newcomb, 1964). Bovine preparations containing 45,000 to 52,000 Iowa units/mg tyrosine or 4,100 Iowa units/mg protein were homogeneous in the ultracentrifuge and in moving boundary electrophoresis(Seegers et al. 1958; 1966a). The sedimentation constant for bovine thrombin ($S^o_{20,w}$) was 3.76 Svedberg units, the diffusion coefficient ($D_{20,w}$) was 8.70×10^{-7} cm²/sec, and the partial specific volume ($\bar{v}$) was 0.69 ml/gm (Harmison et al. 1961). From these biophysical measurements a molecular weight of 33,700 was calculated (Harmison et al. 1961). This value is in agreement with figures described by Magnusson (1965e) and by Baughman and Waugh (1967), obtained by different methods. When the molecular weight was calculated on the basis of specific activitites, a value of 33,600 was obtained (Harmison et al. 1961). Using thin-layer gel filtration Murano (1968) determined a molecular weight of $32,000 \pm 2,500$ for bovine thrombin. Lanchantin et al. (1965a) estimated the molecular weight of human thrombin, using exclusion chromatography on Sephadex G-100 and found a value of 35,000. On the basis of kinetic studies, Kezdy et al. (1965) calculated a maximal value of 32,600, while Magnusson (1965e) found on the basis of the N-terminal amino acid content a molecular weight of 26,000 to 32,000 for human thrombin. Miller et al. (1965) reported a value of 26,200. Based on its hydrodynamic characteristics the length of the bovine thrombin molecule was calculated with 84 Å, the width being 30 Å (Harmison et al. 1961). This is in fair agreement with measurements obtained by electron microscopy, where the mean particle height was measured at 91 to 92 Å (Riddle et al. 1963). The particles displayed remarkable homogeneity.

The isoelectric point of bovine thrombin was calculated at pH 5.6 when measured by paper electrophoresis (Levine and Neuhaus, 1959) and pH 5.75 when determined by moving boundary electrophoresis (Seegers et al. 1966a). The amino acid composition of bovine thrombin has been determined by several investigators (Miller et al. 1959; Schrier et al. 1962; Laki and Gladner, 1964; Seegers et al. 1967b) and remarkable agreement was obtained. The latest reported amino acid composition (Seegers et al. 1967b) is listed in Table 2. The 3.7 S thrombin molecule very likely contains 258 amino acid residues.

The molecular weight based on the amino acid composition using the method of Brand (1946) was found to be 28,400 (Seegers et al. 1969). Correcting this figure for the carbohydrate content of bovine thrombin gives a value which is in good agreement with the molecular weight calculated from physical measurements and specific activities.

Carter and Warner (1956) titrated 2.15 moles of disulfide per mole of thrombin. On the basis of the amino acid composition 3 moles per mole have to be assumed.

The bovine thrombin molecule had 2 N-terminal amino acids, isoleucine and threonine (Magnusson, 1965c; Murano, 1968). One mole of each was found per 33,000 gm (Murano, 1968). This indicates that thrombin is a two-chain molecule. Magnusson (1968) has identified an A-chain and a B-chain in bovine thrombin, held together through disulfide linkage. The N-terminal amino acid of the A-chain was threonine. The chain consisted of 49 amino acids. The N-terminal amino acid of the B-chain was isoleucine and at present the sequence of the first four amino acids of this chain has been reported (Magnusson, 1965e). These were Ileu-Val-Glu-Gly. For human thrombin this sequence was Ileu-Val-Gly-Gly (Magnusson, 1965e).

The total carbohydrate content of thrombin has been estimated at 9.68 % (Schwick and Schultze, 1959), with 2.34 % galactose, 1.17 % mannose, 0.07 % fucose, 2.2 % hexosamine and 3.9 % sialic acid.

Thrombin is a proteolytic enzyme that introduces the conversion of fibrinogen to fibrin by splitting arginyl-glycyl bonds at the N-terminal end of the fibrinogen molecule. Details of this action are outlined in Chapter VI, p. 224. Thrombin, furthermore, dissociates prothrombin to yield prethrombin, autoprothrombin III and an inhibitor (Marciniak and Seegers, 1965; Seegers and Marciniak, 1965; Seegers et al. 1967a; Seegers, 1968, 1969).

The esterolytic activity of thrombin was first described by Sherry and Troll (1954), and a pronounced effect was noted on tosyl-L-arginine methyl ester (TAMe). In addition to TAMe, benzoylarginine methyl ester (BAMe), tosyl-L-lysine methyl ester (TLMe), benzoylarginine-p-nitroanilide, and other acyl- and peptidyl-arginyl amides, as well as certain beta-naphthylamides are split (Sherry and Troll, 1954; Ehrenpreis et al. 1957; Ronwin, 1959; Martin et al. 1959; Lorand et al. 1962; Ratnoff, 1962; Deutsch et al. 1962; Elmore and Curragh, 1963; Lanchantin et al. 1965b; Magnusson, 1965c). Apparently, acytelated arginine and lysine esters are rapidly hydrolized by thrombin, whereas tosyl substrates with glycine and tyrosine are not split (Sherry et al. 1954).

By acetylation of thrombin with acetic anhydride most of the clotting power of the enzyme was destroyed. However, the esterolytic activity was maintained (Landaburu and Seegers, 1959). This esterase-thrombin or "thrombin-E" has been isolated, it was homogeneous in the ultracentrifuge, and had a sedimentation coefficient of 3.2 Svedberg units (Seegers et al. 1960a). The infusion of esterase-thrombin in dogs resulted in an activation of the fibrinolytic system (Seegers et al. 1960b; Seegers, 1961). The fibrinolytic action of thrombin had already been noted previously (Nolf, 1908; Guest and Ware, 1950).

Active center studies on thrombin have revealed that DFP (Diisopropylfluorophosphate) destroyed the clotting and esterolytic activity of the enzyme (Gladner and Laki, 1956; Miller and Van Vanukis, 1956b). Since DFP combines with a single serine amino acid residue (Gladner and Laki, 1958) it can be assumed that serine constitutes a part of the active center of the thrombin molecule. The thrombin activity was also inhibited by 1-chloro-3-tosyl-amido-7-amino-2-heptanone (TLCK) (Shaw et al. 1965; Marciniak and Seegers, 1966a), indicating that histidine is also a part of the active center of thrombin. TPCK (tosylphenylalanine chloromethyl ketone) did not inhibit thrombin activity (Seegers et al. 1965b). In contrast to this, phenylmethanesulfonyl fluoride (PMSF) destroyed thrombin activity (Seegers et al. 1965b). Also oxidizing agents, especially potassium permanganate, and amino group reagents, such as S-acetyl mercaptosuccinic anhydride and formaldehyde, inhibited the activity of thrombin (Caldwell and Seegers, 1965).

Recently, Seegers et al. (1968) rechromatographed 3.76 S thrombin on Amberlite IRC-50 and thereby raised the specific activity from about 4,200 U/mg protein to 8,200 U/mg protein. This compares favorably with the high specific activities found for human thrombin (Miller and Copeland, 1962, 1965). In the analytical ultracentrifuge this rechromatographed thrombin had a sedimentation coefficient of 3.2 S Svedberg units (Seegers et al. 1968) with the usual negative slope, when protein concentration was plotted against sedimentation rate. The amino acid composition of this thrombin is listed in Table 2. Upon calculation, it becomes apparent that 75 amino acid residues have been removed from the 3.76 S thrombin. The total number of residues (predominantly glutamic and aspartic acid) for the 3.2 S thrombin was 183, instead of 258 for the 3.76 S thrombin. Cystine and tryptophan residues remained unchanged. This seems to indicate that acidic peptides were removed which normally adhered to the 3.76 S thrombin (Seegers et al. 1968). The removal of these peptides resulted in a shift of the isoelectric point from pH 5.75 for the 3.76 S thrombin to pH 6.2 for the 3.2 S thrombin (phosphate buffer, ionic strength 0.1).

Based on the amino acid composition, a molecular weight of 21,100 was calculated for the protein moiety (Seegers et al. 1969). Corrected for the carbohydrate content, the 3.2 S thrombin had a molecular weight of 22,800 (Seegers et al. 1968). Using thin-layer gel filtration Murano (1968) found a molecular weight of $23{,}000 \pm 1{,}000$.

The orcinol reactive carbohydrate content of the 3.2 S thrombin was 5.02 %, with 1.7 % sialic acid, 0.69 % glucosamine and 0.46 % galactosamine (Seegers et al. 1968).

The N-terminal amino acids of rechromatographed thrombin (3.2 S) were also threonine and isoleucine in a ratio of 1 mole of each per 23,000 gm (Seegers et al. 1968; Murano, 1968). In this respect, they are not different from the 3.76 S thrombin. Therefore, one can assume that the 75 amino acid residues were not removed from the N-terminal end of the molecule.

Since the removal of the 75 amino acid residues (29 % of the total protein) resulted in a doubling of the specific activity, one must assume that the acidic peptides had inhibitory properties (Seegers et al. 1968). This interpretation would be consistent with the findings of Landaburu et al. (1965) who found inhibitory material associated with the 3.76 S thrombin. When 3.2 S thrombin was acetylated with acetic anhydride, as described by Landaburu and Seegers (1959), the clotting activity was reduced to less than 1 %, but no change was observed in the sedimentation coefficient (Seegers et al. 1968). When 3.76 S thrombin was acetylated, the sedimentation constant was reduced to 3.2 Svedberg units (Seegers et al. 1960a). Upon determination of the amino acid composition of the acetylated 3.76 S thrombin and the acetylated 3.2 S thrombin (Table 2) it became apparent that both acetylated thrombins exhibited identical amino acid compositions (Seegers et al. 1968). Moreover, the amino acid composition of the acetylated 3.76 S thrombin and the acetylated 3.2 S thrombin was, within the limits of error, identical with the one of non-acetylated 3.2 S thrombin (Seegers et al. 1968). It appears that the identical 75 amino acids residues were removed by acetylation of the 3.76 S thrombin and by rechromatography on Amberlite IRC-50. In the latter procedure, however, the clotting power is retained.

Seegers et al. (1968) determined the Michaelis Constant for these three types of thrombin, using p-toluenesulfonyl-L-arginine methyl ester (TAMe) as substrate. They found $K_m = 2.97 \times 10^{-4}$ M for 3.76 S thrombin, $K_m = 9.5 \times 10^{-5}$ M for 3.2 S thrombin and $K_m = 4.85 \times 10^{-4}$ M for acetylated 3.76 S thrombin.

The physical-chemical data at present available for thrombin clearly indicate that thrombin has about half the molecular weight of prothrombin. These findings have led Seegers and coworkers to hypothesize that the other half of the prothrombin might be composed of autoprothrombin III (inactive factor X). In view of more recent findings which will be discussed later, this hypothesis can no longer be upheld. Newer investigations by Murano (1968) and Seegers et al. (1968) seem to open the possibility that prothrombin might be a dimer of two thrombin molecules. This interesting assumption is at present under investigation.

Table 2: Amino Acid Composition

Amino Acids	Ratio of appearance using methionine as reference						
	Prothrombin complex bovine[1]	Prothrombin complex human[2]	Prothrombin bovine[3]	Prethrombin bovine[4]	3.7 S thrombin bovine[5]	3.2 S thrombin bovine[6]	Acetylated 3.7 S thrombin bovine[7]
Asp	9.0	7.9–8.0	9.0	9.0	7.0	5.3	5.7
Thr	4.5	5.4	5.0	4.0	3.2	2.7	2.7
Ser	6.0	5.3–5.4	6.2	5.0	3.5	3.3	3.0
Glu	11.0	9.9	12.8	10.0	7.2	6.7	6.3
Pro	5.3	4.4	5.8	5.2	3.5	3.0	3.3
Gly	7.8	6.1	8.3	7.2	5.2	5.0	5.0
Ala	5.3	4.9	6.0	5.0	3.0	3.0	3.0
Cys/2	2.7	3.3	2.0	2.0	1.5	2.0	2.0
Val	5.7	4.1	6.2	5.2	4.0	2.7	3.0
Met	1.0	1.0	1.0	1.0	1.0	1.0	1.0
Ile	3.0	3.0	3.3	2.7	2.7	2.7	2.7
Leu	6.8	5.4	7.6	6.7	6.0	5.3	5.3
Tyr	3.2	3.0	4.2	3.2	2.5	2.3	2.3
Phe	3.2	2.9	3.8	3.2	2.5	2.7	2.7
Lys	4.3	3.7	5.8	5.0	4.5	3.7	3.7
His	1.7	1.3	1.6	1.5	1.3	1.3	1.3
Arg	5.3	5.0–5.1	8.2	5.8	4.2	4.3	4.3
Try	1.8	2.9	1.8	2.5	1.5	2.0	2.0

[1] Seegers et al. (1967b)
[2] Lanchantin et al. (1968a)
[3] Seegers et al. (1969)
[4] Seegers et al. (1967b)
[5] Seegers et al. (1967b)
[6] Seegers et al. (1968)
[7] Seegers et al. (1968)

D. Factor X

Morawitz (1905) observed that blood, carefully collected without contamination with tissue material, would yield thrombokinase when brought into contact with glass. This thrombokinase was thought to activate prothrombin to thrombin. It was believed to have similar properties to thrombokinase from tissues. Mellanby (1909) indicated that a prothrombin activator could be obtained from plasma globulins. In 1912, Collingwood and McMahon suggested that thrombokinase existed in an inactive form in blood and suggested that this precursor of thrombokinase comes from platelets. The authors termed this precursor "prothrombokinase". Subsequently, Dale and Walpole (1916) established that thrombokinase comes from plasma and not from platelets. Several years later Lenggenhager (1936, 1940) and Widenbauer and Reichel (1942) supported the concept that thrombokinase is present in plasma in an inactive precursor form. Milstone (1942, 1947, 1948, 1949, 1951, 1952a, 1952b, 1952c, 1955, 1959a, 1959b) confirmed that thrombokinase is the activator of prothrombin; he isolated thrombokinase from plasma (Milstone, 1960a, 1960b) and gave an elaborate description of its functional properties (Milstone, 1962, 1964; Milstone et al. 1963).

In 1953, Biggs et al. (1953a) indicated that blood contained all of the components necessary for "blood" or "intrinsic" thromboplastin formation, and described a test system which measured the rate of plasma thromboplastin formation (Biggs and Douglas, 1953). This test is the so-called plasma thromboplastin generation test. Biggs et al. (1953b, 1953c) suggested that the formation of thromboplastin may progress in a stepwise fashion.

In 1956, Bergsagel and Hougie (1956) reported that the incubation of factors VIII, IX and X together with calcium ions results in the formation of a powerful procoagulant which together with factor V and platelets forms blood thromboplastin. They termed this procoagulant "product I". Subsequently, product I was partially purified and its functional properties investigated (Bergsagel, 1956; Zucker-Franklin et al. 1961, Spaet and Cintron 1959, 1960, 1961, 1963; Horowitz and Spaet, 1961, Spaet, 1962, 1964).

Further interest in factor X was generated when Telfer et al. (1956), Hougie (1956) and Hougie et al. (1957) described patients with a bleeding disorder and impaired prothrombin activation. This disease was closely related to the so-called factor VII deficiency previously described by Alexander et al. (1949a, 1951), De Vries et al. (1949) and Koller et al. (1951, 1952). The new disease was later called Stuart-Prower factor deficiency or factor X deficiency. Several years later, Macfarlane (1961) and Esnouf and Williams (1961) presented evidence that factor X was the substrate for the clotting action of Russel's Viper Venom, and Esnouf and Williams (1962a) studied this interaction after purifying the venom. At the same time, they isolated the substrate (factor X) from plasma and serum and described some of its physicochemical properties (Esnouf and Williams, 1962b, 1962c).

During the same year, Marciniak and Seegers (1962) discovered that besides thrombin, a second enzyme would form when prothrombin complex, prepared by the method of Seegers (1952), was activated in 25 % sodium citrate solution. They referred to this enzyme as autoprothrombin C, and hypothesized that the enzyme might be a part of the prothrombin molecule and not an independent plasma protein. The term autoprothrombin C had been introduced by Kowarzyk and Marciniak (1961) and Marciniak (1961) when it was noted that thrombin products differed in their ability to promote prothrombin consumption in hemophilic plasma. Autoprothrombin C was subsequently isolated (Seegers et al. 1963a, 1966b) and its functional and physicochemical properties have been described in detail (Seegers and Marciniak, 1962a, 1962b; Seegers et al. 1962a, 1962b, 1962c, 1963a, 1963b, 1963c, 1965a, 1965b, 1966b, 1967a, 1967b; Marciniak et al. 1962a, 1962b, 1962c; Seegers, 1964, 1965, 1967, 1968; Cole et al. 1962; Seegers and Kagami, 1964; Caldwell and Seegers, 1965; Marciniak and Seegers, 1965; Harmison and Mammen, 1967).

The inactive precursor of autoprothrombin C was termed autoprothrombin III when conditions were found where purified prothrombin complex could be activated without generating autoprothrombin C activity (Seegers et al. 1962a, 1964b). Autoprothrombin III has also been isolated and some of its properties have been described (Seegers et al. 1964b, 1967a, 1967b; Seegers and Marciniak, 1965; Harmison and Mammen, 1967; Seegers, 1964, 1965, 1967, 1968).

It is now apparent that autoprothrombin C, activated factor X, thrombokinase and intermediate coagulation product I are one and the same substance (Spaet, 1964, Kline, 1965; Lechner and Deutsch, 1965; Marciniak and Seegers, 1965; Seegers, 1967, 1968; Harmison and Mammen, 1967). It follows then that autoprothrombin III and inactive factor X are also identical entities.

1. Molecular Characteristics of Inactive Factor X

Inactive factor X (autoprothrombin III) has been isolated from bovine plasma (Esnouf and Williams, 1962b); Papahadjopoulos et al. 1964a; Lechner and Deutsch, 1965) and from purified prothrombin complex preparations (Seegers et al. 1964b; Seegers and Marciniak, 1965; Lechner and Deutsch, 1965). Details of the procedure are described in Chapter IV, p. 151. In cellulose acetate electrophoresis purified factor X samples from plasma migrated in the area of the α_1-globulins (Papahadjopoulos et al. 1964a). The electrophoretic mobility in 0.08 M NaCl buffered with 0.01 M tris: HCl buffer was 7.26×10^{-5} cm²/V/sec (Esnouf, 1965). The isoelectric point of autoprothrombin III in either phosphate or acetate buffer at 0.1 ionic strength was found to be pH 4.75 (Seegers et al. 1967b).

Esnouf and Williams (1962b, 1962c) obtained for their factor X preparation a sedimentation coefficient ($S^{o}_{20,w}$) of 4.23 Svedberg units, a diffusion coefficient (D_{20}) of 4.57×10^{-7} cm²/sec and a partial specific volume ($\bar{v}$) of 0.738. On the basis of these data a molecular weight of 87,000 was calculated. Ultracentrifuge analysis revealed a molecular weight of $84{,}800 \pm 7{,}000$. Autoprothrombin III had a sedimentation coefficient ($S^{o}_{20,w}$) of 3.4 Svedberg units (Seegers et al. 1967b), a figure which is lower than that obtained by Esnouf and Williams (1962b). However, diffusion coefficient and partial specific volume have not as yet been determined for autoprothrombin III, and hence no molecular weight estimates have been feasable. Murano (1968) using thin-layer gel filtration, estimated a molecular weight of 74,000 ± 9,000 for autoprothrombin III. Jackson and Hanahan (1968) described a molecular weight of 55,000 for factor X.

The amino acid composition of autoprothrombin III (Table 3) was determined by Seegers et al. (1967b, 1969). On the basis of the amino acid composition a molecular weight of 52,600 was calculated (Seegers et al. 1969). The molecule might be composed of 472 amino acid residues (Seegers et al. 1969).

Esnouf and Williams (1962b) using the DNP-procedure of Sanger (1945) determined the N-terminal amino acids of factor X as alanine and glycine. Högenauer et al. (1968), in a preliminary report, found glycine and serine as the N-terminal amino acids of factor X, using the procedure of Gray and Hartley (1963). Murano (1968) determined the N-terminal amino acids of autoprothrombin III using the Edman procedure (Edman, 1950; Edman and Sjöquist, 1956) and found glycine, alanine and serine. No quantitative data were given.

Using the carboxypeptidase method, Högenauer et al. (1968) established glycine and serine as the C-terminal amino acids fo factor X but no quantitative values were stated. These data suggest that factor X is a two chain molecule. From these data it becomes apparent that inactive factor X (autoprothrombin III) has a molecular weight similar to that of prothrombin. This rules out that autoprothrombin III is a part of the prothrombin molecule as suggested by Seegers and his associates. It seems to be evident that the prothrombin preparations originally prepared by Seegers were contaminated with inactive factor X which, due to its low concentration and due to its similar physical properties, escaped physical detection. Chromatography of these prothrombin preparations on DEAE-cellulose removes these impurities.

Table 3: Amino Acid Composition

Ratio of appearance using methionine as reference

Amino Acids	Inactive factor X bovine[1]	Active factor X bovine[2]	Active factor X bovine[3]	Factor VII bovine[4]	Factor IX bovine[5]	Factor V bovine[6]	Factor V bovine[7]	Factor XII human[8]	Factor XII bovine[9]
Asp	7.8	7.0	7.3	15.0	7.7	5.8	7.4	9.0	9.0
Thr	4.5	3.7	5.5	6.9	2.7	3.3	5.0	8.0	11.0
Ser	5.5	4.3	5.5	9.6	3.5	3.7	6.6	11.0	14.0
Glu	10.2	7.3	11.3	15.1	8.0	6.0	9.2	11.0	10.0
Pro	4.3	3.3	3.5	7.5	4.0	2.6	5.6	6.0	7.0
Gly	6.7	5.0	7.5	12.1	6.2	4.1	5.8	13.0	8.0
Ala	5.3	3.7	5.7	9.3	4.5	3.7	4.4	8.0	6.0
Cys/2	3.2	2.7	4.0	5.0	1.0	1.0	2.3	1.0	3.0
Val	4.7	4.3	4.7	8.1	4.2	4.3	4.5	5.0	11.0
Met	1.0	1.0	1.0	1.0	1.0	1.0	1.0	1.0	1.0
Ile	2.3	2.0	2.2	2.6	2.2	2.6	3.2	4.0	3.0
Leu	5.8	5.0	5.5	9.5	5.2	5.0	5.0	7.0	8.0
Tyr	2.7	2.3	1.7	4.3	1.7	1.7	2.8	2.0	4.0
Phe	3.8	3.0	3.8	4.9	2.2	2.5	2.7	3.0	3.0
Lys	4.0	4.2	3.5	4.4	4.3	3.4	–	6.0	6.0
His	1.5	1.3	1.7	1.9	1.0	1.2	3.0	2.0	2.0
Arg	3.8	2.7	4.3	7.7	4.3	2.2	2.6	3.0	4.0
Try	1.7	1.7	2.2	1.0	1.5	–	1.4	–	–

[1] Seegers et al. (1969)
[2] Seegers et al. (1969)
[3] Jackson et al. (1968)
[4] Harmison et al. (1965)
[5] Harmison and Seegers (1962)
[6] Aoki et al. (1963)
[7] Esnouf and Jobin (1967)
[8] Speer et al. (1965)
[9] Mammen and Grammens (1967a, b)

2. Molecular Characteristics of Activated Factor X

Activated factor X (autoprothrombin C, thrombokinase, intermediate coagulation product I) has been isolated by Esnouf and Williams (1962b) and Seegers et al. (1963a, 1966b). The procedures are described in Chapter IV, p. 151.

Esnouf and Williams (1962b, 1962c) found a sedimentation coefficient of 2.8 Svedberg units, but observed variations. Using the sedimentation coefficient of 2.8 Svedberg units and assuming the partial specific volume ($\bar{v}$) not to be different from the inactive form of the enzyme, a diffusion coefficient of 6.2×10^{-7} cm²/sec was determined. The molecular weight was calculated at 36,000.

Seegers et al. (1963a) found a sedimentation constant of 2.27 Svedberg units, a partial specific volume of 0.695 ml/gm and a diffusion coefficient of 8.4×10^{-7} cm²/sec for autoprothrombin C. When these values were used in the Svedberg equation, a molecular weight of 21,500 was obtained. The dimensions of the molecule were calculated to be 126 Å by 21 Å (Seegers et al. 1963a).

The amino acid composition of autoprothrombin C (Table 3) was determined by Seegers et al. (1963a, 1969) and Jackson et al. (1968). The molecule is very likely composed of 195 amino acid residues (Seegers et al. 1969). Using the procedure of Brand (1946) and five reference amino acids, Seegers et al. (1963a) calculated an average molecular weight of 24,000 on the basis of the amino acid composition. This figure was recently revised to 21,900 (Seegers et al. 1969). Correcting for 7 % carbohydrate (orcinol) and 3.8 % hexosamine, a molecular weight of 25,000–27,000 can be obtained for the glycoprotein.

Recently, Tishkoff et al. (1968) obtained factor X from purified prothrombin and found in sedimentation equilibrium studies, using 6 M guanidine HCl and 0.5 % mercaptoethanol as solvent, an average molecular weight of $37{,}772 \pm 1{,}234$ for factor X. Since evidence of partial activation was found one might assume that the factor X was in its activated form.

The N-terminal amino acids of activated factor X were found to be alanine, glycine and either leucine or isoleucine (Esnouf and Williams, 1962b). Murano (1968) found alanine, glycine and serine in autoprothrombin C. Murano (1968) thus found no difference in N-terminal amino acids between autoprothrombin III and autoprothrombin C.

Besides its clot-promoting activity, activated factor X had esterolytic activity when measured on TAMe (p-toluene-sulfonyl-arginine methyl ester) (Milstone, 1959b, 1964; Esnouf and Williams, 1962b; Marciniak and Seegers, 1962; Seegers et al. 1962c; Lechner and Deutsch, 1965). The K_m for this substrate was 2.5×10^{-2} M (Esnouf, 1965). No esterase activity was found when lysine ethyl ester was used as a substrate (Esnouf and Williams, 1962b).

The activity of the enzyme was not inhibited by diisopropylfluorophosphate (DFP) (Seegers et al. 1962c; Esnouf, 1965) or 1-chloro-3-tosylamido-7-amino-2-heptanone (TLCK) (Marciniak and Seegers, 1966a), indicating that neither serine nor histidine are a part of the active center of the autoprothrombin C molecule. Also tosylphenylalanine chloromethyl ketone (TPCK), phenylmethanesulfonyl fluoride (PMSF) (Seegers et al. 1965b), pancreatic inhibitor (Esnouf, 1965) and hirudin (Markwardt et al. 1964) failed to inhibit autoprothrombin C activity. In contrast, soybean trypsin inhibitor did block thrombokinase activity (Milstone, 1960a, 1962).

The effect of chemical enzyme inhibitors on autoprothrombin C activity has been studied by Caldwell and Seegers (1965). Reducing agents, oxidizing agents and carbonyl group reagents destroyed the activity, whereas sulfhydryl-blocking agents and amino group reagents did not destroy its biological activity. Interestingly, it was also found that antithrombin quantitatively inactivated autoprothrombin C (Seegers and Marciniak, 1962a; Seegers et al. 1964a).

Based on the molecular weight and the amino acid composition, activated factor X seems to have about half the size of its precursor form (inactive factor X). This raises the question: What is the other half of the molecule? Seegers et al. (1969) have speculated that inactive factor X could be like prothrombin, a dimer of two active factor X molecules. This hypothesis is at present under investigation.

E. Factor VII

The greater clot promoting activity of serum over plasma was already noted by Bordet and Gengou (1904) and Bordet (1919) and again emphasized by Nolf (1945). This activity in serum is now known as factor VII, proconvertin, SPCA, or autoprothrombin I. Extensive studies have revealed that this coagulation entity is of importance in the conversion of prothrombin to thrombin in the presence of tissue thromboplastin (extrinsic pathway). It is reduced in liver disorders and under coumarin drugs and its activity levels are low in newborn infants (Alexander, 1952, 1955, 1959, 1961; Alexander et al. 1948, 1949b, 1950, 1951; DeVries et al. 1949; Owen and Bollman, 1948; Owen et al. 1951; Owren, 1951, 1953; Koller et al. 1951, 1952; Biggs et al. 1953c; Mann and Hurn, 1950, 1951, 1953; Hardisty, 1955; Gray et al. 1956; Hougie et al. 1957; Hougie, 1959; Hjort, 1957; Witte and Dirnberger, 1953; Douglas, 1952, 1955). A number of patients with bleeding disorders associated with factor VII deficiency have subsequently been described, details of which were recently summarized by Mammen (1967a). Over the last years evidence has been accumulated that factor VII together with tissue thromboplastin and calcium ions converts inactive factor X to activated factor X (Hougie, 1959; Straub and Duckert, 1961; Nemerson and Spaet, 1964; Williams, 1964), and Williams and Norris (1966), Nemerson (1966, 1968) and Barton (1967) presented evidence that factor VII, tissue thromboplastin and calcium ions form a complex which activates factor X. It has been suggested that factor VII occurs in plasma in a precursor form and that it is activated during coagulation (Alexander, 1952; Alexander et al. 1954; De Vries et al. 1949; Pechet and Alexander, 1961; Alexander and Pechet, 1962).

In 1952, McClaughry and Seegers first noted an accelerator of prothrombin activation arising from purified prothrombin complex, a finding later elaborated on by Seegers et al. (1955) and Alkjaersig et al. (1955a). It was found that this procoagulant would develop from purified prothrombin complex preparations in the presence of platelet factor 3 and calcium ions (Seegers et al. 1955; Penner and Seegers, 1956). This prothrombin derivative was termed autoprothrombin I (Penner and Seegers, 1956). The accelerator developed during coagulation. In addition to platelet factor 3, tissue thromboplastin was found to facilitate its formation from prothrombin complex (Seegers et al. 1956). The experimental conditions for obtaining autoprothrombin I from purified prothrombin complex were further investigated by Mammen et al. (1960a) and concentrates were obtained from purified prothrombin complex and serum. The coagulation defect in factor VII deficient plasma could be corrected with autoprothrombin I (Johnson and Seegers, 1953; Seegers and Alkjaersig, 1955).

In 1962, Seegers et al. (1962b) described another condition by which autoprothrombin I could be generated from purified prothrombin complex. The activation was brought about by the addition of autoprothrombin C (activated factor X) to purified prothrombin complex preparations. Since this derivative had different solubility properties from the one obtained by activating purified prothrombin complex with platelet factor 3 and calcium ions, the former was termed autoprothrombin I_c and the latter autoprothrombin I_p. (I_c indicated its formation with autoprothrombin C, I_p its formation with platelet factor 3). It was interesting to note that both autoprothrombin I_p and I_c were inactivated by plasma antithrombin and purified antithrombin (Seegers et al. 1964c).

Factor VII (proconvertin, SPCA, autoprothrombin I_p, autoprothrombin I_c) has been purified from serum (Deutsch and Schaden, 1953; Alexander, 1959; Fisch, 1958; Straub, 1960; Duckert et al. 1953, 1961; Soulier et al. 1962; Prydz, 1964; Osborn, 1965; Shaw et al. 1966; Mammen et al. 1960a), plasma (Duckert et al. 1953; Tishkoff et al. 1960; Williams and Norris, 1966; Deutsch et al. 1966; Lewis et al. 1958; Pechet et al. 1960; Högenauer et al. 1968) and from activated purified prothrombin complex (Mammen et al. 1960a; Seegers et al. 1962b; Seegers and Kagami, 1964; Tishkoff et al. 1968).

Factor VII from serum migrated in the electrophoretic field between the α and β-globulins (Fisch, 1958; Lewis et al. 1958). The sedimentation coefficient for autoprothrombin I_c was found to be 3.34 Svedberg units (Harmison et al. 1965; Harmison and Mammen, 1967). Harmison et al. (1965) determined the molecular weight for autoprothrombin I_c, using the approach to equilibrium method of van Holde and Baldwin (1958). They found an average molecular weight of 34,300. The molecular weight on the basis of the amino acid composition (Table 3) using the method of simultaneous equations described by Brand (1946) and four reference amino acids was found to be 34,300 (Harmison et al. 1965). Prydz (1965) used Sephadex G-200 for the molecular weight of factor VII from serum and found approximately 48,000. Tishkoff et al. (1968) using the sedimentation equilibrium analysis of Yphantis (1964), and a dissociating solvent consisting of 6 M guanidine HCl and 0.5 % mercaptoethanol, found a molecular weight of $33{,}900 \pm 3{,}390$ for factor VII, obtained from the prothrombin complex.

This is in good agreement with the findings of Harmison et al. (1965). Factor VII obtained from plasma had an estimated molecular weight of 55,000 using Sephadex G-200 (Deutsch et al. 1966), while Prydz (1965) also using Sephadex G-200 estimated 63,000.

The amino acid composition of factor VII is listed in Table 3. Based on a molecular weight of about 34,000, the factor VII molecule was estimated to consist of 221 amino acid residues.

Deutsch et al. (1966) using the procedure of Gray and Hartley (1963) determined the N-terminal amino acids of factor VII from plasma to be either threonine or glycine. Recently, the same group of investigators found glycine and serine (Högenauer et al. 1968). The C-terminal amino acids of factor VII were also glycine and serine when the carboxypeptidase method was employed (Högenauer et al. 1968). No quantitative values were given for either C-terminal and N-terminal amino acids. The C-terminal and N-terminal amino acids of factor VII and factor X are apparently identical. Moreover, fingerprints of the trypsin digest of both factors using the procedure of Schmer and Kreil (1967), were not significantly different (Högenauer et al. 1968). These observations are of interest. Factor VII from plasma seems to be considerably larger than factor VII from serum or activated prothrombin complex. Moreover, the molecular weights of factor VII from plasma and inactive factor X are fairly similar. These observations and the ones reported by Högenauer et al. (1968) raise the question: Could factor VII be one chain of the inactive factor X molecule, while active factor X is the other? If this were true, inactive factor X could not be a dimer of two active factor X molecules. This speculation, if true, would certainly explain the genetic identity of both deficiency diseases. The findings on factor VII also seem to indicate that it is not a part of the prothrombin molecule as suggested by Seegers and coworkers. Factor VII activity can be separated from the prothrombin complex by chromatography on DEAE-cellulose.

Prydz (1965) determined the carbohydrates in factor VII and found a total content of about 51 %. Of these, 1 % was methyl-pentose and 1.2 % hexosamines. No sialic acid could be found. The unusually high content of carbohydrate, if correct, seems to be largely hexoses.

Sulfhydryl blocking reagents, such as para-hydroxymercuribenzoate (PMB), 5,5′-dithiobis-(2-nitrobenzoic acid) and iodoacetic acid greatly reduced factor VII activity, PMB being the most effective one (Prydz, 1965).

F. Factor IX

In 1947, Pavlovsky made the observation that the blood of two hemophiliacs, when mixed, clotted in shorter times than either one alone. A similar finding was reported by Koller et al. (1950). In 1952, three groups of investigators (Aggeler et al. 1952; Biggs et al. 1952; Schulman and Smith, 1952) described patients with a congenital bleeding disorder which were clinically indistinguishable from classical hemophilia. The disease was termed plasma thromboplastin component (PTC) deficiency, Christmas disease or hemophilia B. The coagulation factor in question was called plasma thromboplastin component (PTC), Christmas factor, antihemophilic factor B, autoprothrombin II, or factor IX. Unlike the antihemophilic globulin (factor VIII), this new coagulation factor seemed to be present in serum as well as in plasma. It was fairly stable upon storage, did not precipitate in Cohn's Fraction I and could be adsorbed by all previously known prothrombin adsorbents. The factor could be eluted from the adsorbents in the same manner as prothrombin (Aggeler et al. 1952; White et al. 1953a; Biggs et al. 1953a; Soulier and Larrieu, 1953).

Soulier et al. (1958), Waaler (1959) and Soulier (1960) first indicated that factor IX would participate in the early phases of intrinsic prothrombin activation. It was postulated that factor IX would be changed to its active form by plasma thromboplastin antecedent (PTA). Further evidence for this was more recently reported by Ratnoff and Davie (1962a), Schiffman et al. (1963), Nossel (1964a, 1964b), Cattan and Denson (1964), Kingdon et al. (1964), Davie and Ratnoff (1964, 1965), and Macfarlane (1964a, 1965, 1966).

The generation of factor IX activity from purified prothrombin complex was already recognized by Mertz et al. (1939) and Seegers and McClaughry (1949), but its procoagulant properties in the intrinsic coagulation mechanism were first described by Seegers and Johnson (1956). They referred to this prothrombin activator as "autoprothrombin II". Autoprothrombin II activity could be generated from purified prothrombin complex preparations when thrombin was added (Seegers and Johnson, 1956; Penner et al. 1956; Mammen et al. 1960a). This activation was greatly enhanced by the presence of lipids (Penner et al. 1956). In plasma of dicumarol treated animals and patients, the autoprothrombin II activity was markedly decreased (Johnson and Seegers, 1956; Johnson et al. 1957). Autoprothrombin II would also correct the coagulation defect in hemophilia B plasma (Christmas disease) (Mammen et al. 1960a). Therefore, it was reasonable to assume that autoprothrombin II corresponded to factor IX (Mammen et al. 1960a).

Attempts have been made to concentrate factor IX from plasma (Biggs et al. 1952; White et al. 1953b; Aggeler et al. 1954b; Blatrix and Soulier, 1959; Blatrix et al. 1959; Didisheim et al. 1959a; Biggs et al. 1961; Yin and Duckert, 1961; Bidwell, 1962; Schiffman et al. 1963; Hink and Johnson, 1964; Tullis et al. 1965; Bidwell et al. 1967), but the degree of purity of these preparations is still unsatisfactory for physicochemical characterization. Some of these fractions have been used therapeutically in the treatment of patients with hemophilia B (Christmas disease).

Factor IX fractions have also been purified from serum (White et al. 1953a; Aggeler et al. 1954a; Mammen et al. 1960a; Soulier et al. 1962), but again the degree of purity is too low for molecular studies.

The only factor IX preparation of reasonable purity was obtained from activated purified prothrombin complex (Mammen et al 1960a). In plasma and serum factor IX migrated electrophoretically with the α_1 and α_2-globulins (Lewis et al. 1958), whereas purified fractions migrated in the β_2 region (Aggeler et al. 1954a, b). Some biophysical properties of autoprothrombin II have been described by Harmison and Seegers (1962). The preparations were obtained from activated bovine prothrombin complex using the procedure of Mammen et al. (1960a). Similar preparations were also produced from activated human prothrombin complex (Ulutin et al. 1961).

The sedimentation coefficient for autoprothrombin II was found to be 4.33 Svedberg units. The diffusion coefficient was 7.45×10^{-7} cm^2/sec, and the partial specific volume was 0.708 ml/gm. Using the Svedberg equation, a molecular weight of 49,900 was calculated (Harmison and Seegers, 1962). On the basis of the amino acid composition (Table 3), using the method of Brand (1946), a molecular weight of 39,500 was obtained for the protein moiety (Harmison and Seegers, 1962). Corrected for 20 % carbohydrate (Mammen et al. 1960a), the molecular weight for the entire glycoprotein was found to be 51,200 (Mammen, 1964a). The length of the molecule was calculated to be 93 Å, the width 35 Å (Harmison and Seegers, 1962). From the amino acid composition it appears that the molecule consists of 262 amino acid residues.

The N-terminal amino acid of autoprothrombin II was found to be proline, the C-terminal amino acid was tyrosine (Mammen et al.

1960a). No quantitative data were made available.

The effect of chemical enzyme inhibitors on autoprothrombin II activity was studied by Marshall (1965). Oxidizing agents, sulfhydryl-blocking agents and carbonyl group reagents readily destroyed autoprothrombin II activity, while reducing agents and amino group reagents had little effect.

From the presently available data it is difficult to decide whether factor IX is a prothrombin derivative as suggested by Seegers and coworkers or whether it is a protein different from prothrombin. There are a number of arguments that could be presented to support either one of the two concepts. A final decision on this question can only be made after further studies.

G. Factor VIII

Factor VIII (antihemophilic factor) is a plasma protein which will correct the coagulation defect of patients with classical hemophilia (hemophilia A). Classical hemophilia is not only one of the oldest but also one of the most frequently occurring congenital coagulopathies. Its medical history related to coagulation, recently reviewed by Hecht (1966a), apparently dates back to 1839 when Liston described the delayed clotting of hemophilic blood.

Factor VIII is intimately related to the activation of prothrombin to thrombin in the intrinsic pathway. This has been described by numerous investigators since it was first clearly demonstrated almost three decades ago by Brinkhous (1939).

The amount of factor VIII in plasma varies greatly from one species to another (Brinkhous and Wagner, 1959; Thelin and Wagner, 1961) and its concentration in human plasma seems to be around 0.02–0.05 mg/ml (Brinkhous, 1958; Pool and Robinson, 1959). The site of synthesis of factor VIII is not clearly established but spleen, liver and leucocytes have been found to contain factor VIII activity (Pool, 1966; Webster et al. 1967; Norman et al. 1967; Zacharski et al. 1968). The author and Dr. M. I. Barnhart (unpublished observation) have found factor VIII in plasma cells using fluorescent antibody techniques.

The clinical finding that small amounts of normal plasma added to hemophilic plasma would correct the coagulation defect, has generated great interest in the purification of factor VIII from plasma. Probably the first concentration was prepared by Addis (1911) using isoelectric precipitation which was later employed by other investigators as well (Bendien and van Creveld, 1936; Patek and Stetson, 1936; Alexander and Landwehr, 1948). Salting-out procedures also have been used (Bidwell, 1955a, b; Brinkhous and Wagner, 1959; Spaet and Kinsell, 1953), besides fractionation of factor VIII from plasma by alcohol. Under these conditions the activity precipitates together with fibrinogen in Cohn's fraction I (Achenbach et al. 1959; Baumgarten et al. 1963; Kalinke and Egli, 1967). Ether has also been employed for precipitating factor VIII (Kekwick and Wolf, 1957; Holman and Wolf, 1963). Recently, cryoprecipitation was introduced to obtain factor VIII preparations for clinical use (Pool et al. 1964; Pool and Shannon, 1965; Hershgold et al. 1966; Simson et al. 1966; Brown et al. 1967; Alexander and Odake, 1967). A number of investigators have utilized more complex purification procedures and efforts have been made to separate fibrinogen from factor VIII (van Creveld et al. 1956, 1959, 1960, 1961, 1966; Wagner et al. 1957, 1964a, b; Soulier et al. 1957; Seegers et al. 1957, 1959; Shinowara, 1957a, 1964; Blombäck, 1958; Niemetz et al. 1961; Simonetti et al. 1961, 1964; Janiak and Soulier, 1962; Pavlovsky et al. 1962; Langdell, 1962; Michael and Tunnah, 1963, 1966; Mammen, 1963; Nour-Eldin, 1963; Kekwick and Walton, 1965; Rizza et al. 1965; Veder, 1966; Bidwell et al. 1966; Hurt et al. 1966a, b; Barrow et al. 1966a; Gugler, 1966, Morrison, 1966; Weaver et al. 1966, 1967; Johnson et al. 1967; Brinkhous et al. 1968). The separation of fibrinogen from factor VIII not only results in a decreased stability of the biological activity but also in different precipitation properties (van Creveld et al. 1959, 1960, 1961; Michael and Tunnah, 1963; Barrow et al. 1966b). Gobbi (1960) noted this when factor VIII was purified from plasma of a patient with congenital afibrinogenemia, while Mammen (1964b) described these differences in factor VIII fractions obtained from serum.

The extreme lability of the biological activity of factor VIII has made purification for physicochemical characterization very difficult and only limited information is available.

Mammen and Harmison (addendum to Shulman et al. 1960) and Mammen (1964c) have determined the sedimentation coefficient for bovine factor VIII and found a $S^{o}_{20,w}$ of 6.65 Svedberg units. Shinowara (1964) found a sedimentation constant of 6.0–6.5 Svedberg units. Hershgold and Sprawls (1966) reported $S^{o}_{20,w}$ values of 19 and 12 for human, bovine and porcine factor VIII. This discrepancy is apparently due to aggregation (Hershgold and Sprawls, 1966; Mammen, 1964c). A diffusion coefficient of 3.30×10^{-7} cm²/sec was calculated by Shulman et al (1960). Using the Svedberg equation, Shulman et al. (1960) calculated a molecular weight of 196,000 for bovine factor VIII. This figure is in close agreement with a molecular weight of 180,000 determined by electron irradiation (Aronson et al. 1962). Hershgold et al. (1967) recently reported a molecular weight of 2.8×10^{6}, but again aggregation is obviously responsible for such findings.

Using moving boundary electrophoresis an isoelectric point of pH 6.4 was determined by Seegers et al. (1957). The electrophoretic mobility was 3.0×10^{-5} cm²/V/sec which would identify factor VIII as a β-globulin of plasma. These findings are in agreement with those reported by van Creveld et al. (1956), Spaet and Kinsell (1953), Shinowara (1964) and Hershgold and Sprawls (1966). Using continuous flow curtain electrophoresis Lewis et al. (1958) found factor VIII activity associated with α_1 and α_2 globulins.

Amino acid composition and terminal amino acids have as yet not been reported. The question has been raised whether factor VIII might be a lipoprotein rather than a protein (Blombäck et al. 1962; Simonetti et al. 1964). Shinowara (1964) reported only 0.4 % of cholesterol in his still heterogeneous preparations while Mammen (1964c) found less than 1 % lipid phosphorus and esterified fatty acids in factor VIII preparations purified by the procedure described by Seegers et al. (1959).

A total carbohydrate content of 3.6 % was found in factor VIII by Seegers et al. (1957). Shinowara (1964) determined 0.9 % hexose in his preparations.

A major problem in purification and standardization of factor VIII concentrates is the great lability which increases as purification progresses (Mammen, 1964c; Blombäck, 1964). Numerous attempts have been made to find suitable stabilizing agents. Glycerol, albumin and glycine ethyl ester seem to improve the stability (Seegers et al. 1957; Michael and Tunnah, 1963; Kekwick and Walton, 1962; Goulian and Beck, 1966; Kisker, 1967).

No esterolytic activity was found in human factor VIII preparations (van Creveld et al. 1967).

H. Factor V

Factor V (Ac-globulin) is a plasma protein which is necessary for prothrombin conversion to thrombin in both the extrinsic and intrinsic pathways (Owren, 1961). Its existence was first recognized by Seegers et al. (1938b) and was termed Ac-globulin by Ware et al. (1947a). Further interest in factor V was generated when Owren (1947a, b) described a patient with a bleeding disorder in whom this factor was absent. The disorder was termed parahemophilia. In patients with severe liver disorder factor V levels may be found decreased indicating that this protein is synthesized in the liver. Hepatic damage by chloroform will also decrease its plasma levels (Sykes et al. 1948). Using fluorescent antibody techniques, Barnhart et al. (1963) demonstrated the hepatocyte as the site of synthesis for factor V.

Ac-globulin is a fairly labile coagulation constituent and the type of anticoagulant used to collect the plasma, storage temperature and pH all have to be considered carefully. The activity decreases more rapidly when potassium oxalate is used as the anticoagulant than when trisodium citrate is used (Surgenor et al. 1961). In bank blood its activity is greatly diminished within one week of storage (Stefanini, 1950; Rapaport et al. 1959). In addition, species differences have been observed in relation to stability, and bovine factor V seems to be most stable (Murphy et al. 1947; Fahey et al. 1948; Seegers, 1962). In human plasma, factor V is consumed when clotting occurs, whereas in bovine serum factor V activity is well presented (Seegers, 1962). Factor V in plasma is not adsorbed by Seitz filtration or barium sulfate, is only partially adsorbed on aluminum hydroxide, magnesium hydroxide, aluminum oxide and tricalcium phosphate, but is markedly adsorbed by Asolectin (soybean lecithin) (Owren, 1961). On the basis of purification, Aoki et al. (1963) calculated its concentration in human plasma at about 0.01 mg/ml, in bovine plasma at around 0.09 mg/ml.

A partial purification of factor V from plasma was attempted as early as 1948 (Owren, 1948; Ware and Seegers, 1948b) and more recently by several other investigators (Lewis and Ware, 1953; Cox et al. 1956; Surgenor et al. 1961; Fenichel and Rose, 1961; Landaburu and Seegers, 1961; Korsan-Bengtsen and Ygge, 1961; Blombäck and Blombäck, 1963; Aoki et al. 1963; Esnouf et al. 1963; Urayama and Asada, 1964; Barton and Hanahan, 1967; Esnouf and Jobin, 1967; White et al. 1968).

Esnouf and Jobin (1965, 1967) prepared bovine factor V which was homogeneous in the analytical ultracentrifuge and by immunoelectrophoresis. They determined a sedimentation coefficient of 8.68 Svedberg units for bovine factor V. The partial specific volume was 0.73 ml/gm. From these data a molecular weight of approximately 290,000 was calculated. Lewis (1964) using gel filtration established a molecular weight of greater than 200,000, and Papahadjopoulos et al. (1964b) came to a similar conclusion. This figure stands in contrast to the molecular weight of 180,000 reported by Hussain and Newcomb (1963). Aoki et al. (1963) determined a *minimal* molecular weight of 97,000 for bovine factor V on the basis of the amino acid composition using the method of Brand (1946).

An electrophoretic mobility of 3.3×10^{-5} cm^2/V/sec was determined in moving-boundary electrophoresis at pH 7.0 (Esnouf and Jobin, 1967). On paper electrophoresis factor V migrated between the β and α-globulins (Owen and McKenzie, 1954). In continuous flow electrophoresis of human plasma, factor V was found in the albumin fraction (Lewis et al. 1958; Johnston et al. 1959a, b).

The amino acid composition was determined by Aoki et al. (1963), Urayama and Asada (1964) and Esnouf and Jobin (1967) but several differences were noted in the preparations. Urayama and Asada (1964) only determined 15 amino acids on a qualitative basis while Aoki et al. (1963) and Esnouf and Jobin (1967) gave quantitative data. Even these show great differences (Table 3) which may be due to different degrees of purity.

The terminal amino acids have as yet not been described. Oxidizing agents, SH blocking agents and monoiodoacetate destroyed the activity of purified factor V preparations while reducing agents did not have an effect (Aoki et al. 1963). Free SH groups were apparently necessary for factor V activity but sulfhydryl-containing substances, such as cysteine and reduced glutathione did not prevent the loss of factor V activity (Aoki et al. 1963). This indicates that the labile nature of factor V cannot be attributed solely to the oxidation of SH groups. It has been reported that the removal of divalent cations, particularly of the alkaline earths, greatly decrease the stability during purification (Blombäck and Blombäck, 1963; Zucker and Borelli, 1958). This may indicate that the structural integrity of factor V depends on the presence of divalent metal ions (Esnouf and Jobin, 1967). The instability of factor V has led to the search for stabilizing agents. Storage in 50% glycerol in water (Aoki et al. 1963; Esnouf and Jobin, 1967) and in 0.02 M tris-hydrochloric acid buffer, pH 7.5 (Esnouf and Jobin, 1967) have been found to be suitable. Dialysis of freshly prepared concentrates against distilled water or 0.02 M sodium phosphate buffer, pH 7.0 was also found to stabilize the activity (Esnouf and Jobin 1967), but Aoki et al. (1963) had only partial success with dialysis against water. Drying from frozen state preserves the activity (Aoki et al. 1963).

In some of the earlier papers on Ac-globulin, it was reported that thrombin would enhance factor V activity (Ware et al. 1947b; Ware and Seegers, 1948b; Lewis and Ware, 1953; Cox et al. 1956). This observation was again made using purified factor V preparations (Aoki et al. 1963; Barton and Hanahan, 1967), and the calculation was made that this activation involves 1 thrombin molecule for every 10 factor V molecules (Aoki et al. 1963). Thrombin ultimately destroys human factor V activity after the initial phase of potentiation. In contrast, trypsin destroys the factor V activity immediately and no potentiation of activity can be demonstrated in the incubation mixture. Thrombin does not destroy bovine factor V activity.

I. Factor XII

In 1954, Ratnoff and Ratnoff and Colopy (1955) described a coagulation abnormality which was not associated with a bleeding tendency. They termed the disorder "Hageman trait". The factor assumed to be missing in the patient's plasma was called Hageman factor (Factor XII). Hageman factor is a glycoprotein which is found in plasma in an inactive form. Its concentration in plasma has been estimated as less than 0.01 mg/ml (Davie and Ratnoff, 1965). It can be found in blood of mammalian and many amphibian species, but is absent in birds and reptiles (Ratnoff and Rosenblum, 1957; Didisheim et al. 1959b; Hackett and LePage, 1961; Didisheim, 1962). Hageman factor changes to its active form upon contact with glass, kaolin, diatomaceous earth, barium carbonate, celite, super-cel, bentonite, silicic acid, carboxymethyl cellulose and asbestos (Rapaport et al. 1955; Margolis, 1957, 1958a, b; Ratnoff and Rosenblum, 1957, 1958; Johnston et al. 1958; Soulier et al. 1959, Waaler, 1959; Ratnoff, Chapter V, p. 214), is activated by long-chain fatty acids (Margolis, 1962; Didisheim and Mibashan, 1963; Speer and Ridgway, 1967), ellagic acid (Ratnoff and Crum, 1963, 1964; Iatridis, 1966; Cliffton, 1967), skin contact (Nossel, 1966), collagen and elastin (Niewiarowski et al. 1964, 1965; Wilner et al. 1968) and sodium urate crystals (Kellermeyer and Breckenridge, 1965). Margolis (1962, 1963) and Speer and Ridgway (1967) have suggested that the factor XII molecule unfolds during activation or changes its molecular configuration to expose active enzymatic sites. It was also found that activated factor XII reversed to inactive factor XII. This process of activation and inactivation could be repeated several times, indicating that the unfolded activated molecule might, dependent upon the environment, refold to its inactive form (Speer and Ridgway, 1967). These suggested conformational changes are difficult to reconcile with the accepted thermodynamic laws applying to proteins in solution.

Hageman factor will shorten the prolonged coagulation times of plasma collected under siliconized conditions. This seems to be due to its effect on plasma thromboplastin antecedent (PTA). Hardisty and Margolis (1959), Soulier et al. (1959), Waaler (1959), and Ratnoff et al. (1961) have presented evidence that Hageman factor might convert PTA from an inactive form into an active form. Hageman factor is also supposed to have an effect on the fibrinolytic system (Niewiarowski and Prou-Wartelle, 1959; Iatridis and Ferguson, 1962; Holemans and Roberts, 1964; Holemans et al. 1966). The author has not observed any changes in the fibrinolytic system after infusion of large quantities of purified Hageman factor (unpublished data).

It has also been proposed that Hageman factor has an influence on platelet aggregation and that it is adsorbed on platelet surfaces (Sharp, 1958; Waaler, 1959; Jürgens, 1962; Iatrides and Ferguson, 1965). Barth et al. (1966) failed to find an effect of Hageman factor on platelet aggregation. However, Mammen and Grammens (1967a, b) using purified Hageman factor found it to have platelet aggregation properties in vitro and in vivo. Hageman factor acted like ADP. In addition to its role in hemostasis, Hageman factor seems to activate plasma kallikreinogen to kallikrein and subsequently to biologically active polypeptide kinins (Kallidin II and I; Bradikinin) (Margolis, 1958a, b, 1959, 1960; Ratnoff and Miles, 1964; Habermann, 1966, Shigeharu et al. 1968). This observation seems to be related to the findings that activated Hageman factor increases vascular permeability (Margolis, 1958c, 1963; Ratnoff and Miles, 1964; Graham et al. 1965; Johnston and Barrow, 1965; Kellermeyer, 1967; Donaldson, 1968), dilates blood vessels (Webster and Ratnoff, 1961), contracts smooth muscle (Margolis, 1958b) and induces leucocyte migration through blood vessel walls (Graham et al. 1965). Donaldson (1968) has found that factor XII changes the first component of complement to its biologically active form, c'l-esterase.

The exact site of synthesis of Hageman factor is unknown. However, decreased plasma levels have been observed in association with liver disorders (Jürgens, 1962).

Several investigators have attempted to purify this glycoprotein from bovine and human plasma (Schiffman et al. 1960; Haanen et al. 1961; Ratnoff et al. 1961; Ratnoff and Davie, 1962b; Schoenmakers et al. 1963, 1965; Speer et al. 1965; Mammen and Grammens, 1967a, b) and some of the procedures are described in Chapter IV, p. 160. Several of these preparations were homogeneous by a number of physicochemical criteria. Schoenmakers et al. (1965) determined a sedimentation coefficient of 7.08 S which is in close agreement with a value of 7.04 reported by Mammen and Grammens (1967a, b). Donaldson and Ratnoff (1965) reported a sedimentation coefficient of approximately 4.5 for purified human Hageman factor and 6.0 for Hageman factor in citrated plasma. The diffusion coefficient at infinite dilution was 7.14×10^{-7} cm²/sec (Schoenmakers et al. 1965). On the basis of these data and assuming a partial specific volume of 0.7 ml/gm, Schoenmakers et al. (1965) calculated a molecular weight of 82,000. Mammen and Grammens (1967a, b) calculated a molecular weight of 79,000. Both figures are in agreement with a molecular weight of 60,000–100,000, obtained by Haanen et al. (1965) with ionizing radiation. These data stand in contrast to molecular weights reported by Speer et al. (1965) who found 20,000 using the sedimentation-equilibrium method, but greater than 100,000 using gel filtration techniques. Together with A. S. Prasad and G. L. Grammens, the author (unpublished) has recently recalculated the molecular weight and found an average molecular weight of 142,000 for bovine Hageman factor using equilibrium ultracentrifugation (Yphantis, 1964). Using thin-layer gel filtration a molecular weight of 140,000 was obtained. A partial specific volume of 0.724 ml/gm was determined. Treatment of the Hageman factor preparations with 5 M guanidine hydrochloride did not change the sedimentation characteristics of the molecule. However, subsequent cleavage with sodium sulfite resulted in the formation of subunits with an average molecular weight of 24,000. The sedimentation coefficient for these sulfitolized sub-units was 1.97 Svedberg units.

Davie and Ratnoff (1965) reported the electrophoretic mobility of Hageman factor in the β-region, while Speer et al. (1965) and Mammen and Grammens (1967a, b) found Hageman factor in the γ-region. Lewis et al. (1958) also found it in the γ-region when using plasma. An isoelectric point of pH 8.0 was found using cellulose acetate as the supporting medium (Mammen and Grammens, 1967a, b), but more recently a value of pH 7.8 was determined using the more accurate electrofocusing method.

The amino acid composition of Hageman factor was determined by Speer et al. (1965) for human preparations and by Mammen and Grammens (1967a, b) (see Harmison and Mammen, 1967 for exact data) for bovine Hageman factor. Both are listed in Table 3 and good agreement seems to exist in 11 amino acids. In particular, the same high values for serine and glutamic acid were found. Grammens and Mammen (1967a, b) calculated the minimal molecular weight for Hageman factor on the basis of the amino acid composition and found a value of 14,500.

Speer et al. (1965) determined arginine as the N-terminal amino acid and methionine as the C-terminal amino acid for human Hageman factor. Grammens and Mammen (unpublished) found glycine and valine as the N-terminal amino acids for bovine Hageman factor.

The carbohydrate content of bovine factor XII was determined by Schoenmakers et al. (1965) and a total content of 5.9 % was found. Galactose was 3.6 %, mannose was 1.8 % and fucose 0.5 %. The total amount of hexosamines was 4.8 %, and glucosamine (3.2 %) and galactosamine (1.6 %) were identified. The sialic acid content was 4.4 %. These data stand in considerable contrast to the ones obtained on bovine factor XII prepared by Mammen and Grammens (1967a, b). The total hexosamine content was only 0.87 %, the amount of protein bound hexose 1.95 %, and only 0.20 % of fucose was found. The sialic acid content was only 0.37 %.

In contrast to Becker (1960) and Schoenmakers et al. (1964), Ratnoff and Davie (1962b) found that DFP (diisopropyl fluorophosphate) failed to destroy the activity of purified Hageman factor. Speer et al. (1965) reported that chemicals altering sulfhydryl, disulfide, amino, carboxyl and aliphatic hydroxyl groups, as well as hydrogen and ionic bonds would destroy Hageman factor activity.

Niewiarowski et al. (1962) and Schoenmakers et al. (1965) reported that Hageman factor possessed esterolytic activity. Becker (1960), Ratnoff and Davie (1962a), Speer et al. (1965) and Mammen and Grammens (1967a, b) found no esterolytic activity in highly purified Hageman factor preparations. Sherry et al. (1966) studied the effect of human plasma on several arginine and lysine esters and found that the developing esterolytic activity was not due to Hageman factor itself, but due to another enzyme not yet identified which becomes activated by Hageman factor. This finding might explain the differing reports in the literature.

Nossel and Niemetz (1965) and Nossel et al. (1968) described an inhibitor against Hageman factor in plasma. Mammen and Grammens (1967a, b) found that purified bovine Hageman factor added to normal human and bovine plasma was stable for several hours. No loss in activity was encountered.

J. Factor XI

The existence of factor XI (plasma thromboplastin antecedent, PTA) and its importance in the conversion of prothrombin to thrombin became apparent when Rosenthal et al. (1953) described a family with a mild bleeding tendency in whom the coagulation defect was different from all the others known at that time. It was assumed that this factor was absent in the plasma of the patients with this disorder. Since normal plasma or serum corrected the defective prothrombin activation, the factor was assumed to be present in both plasma and serum. This factor seems to differ from factor XII in a number of properties (Rosenthal, 1961). Electrophoretically factor XI migrated in the area of β_2-globulins (Rosenthal, 1955; Lewis et al. 1958). Like Hageman factor, factor XI is not completely adsorbed from plasma or serum on barium salts (Rosenthal, 1955), and loses very little activity upon heating for 30 min at 56° C (Biggs et al. 1958; Waaler, 1959; Soulier and Larrieu, 1958). Rosenthal (1955) and Ramot et al. (1955) precipitated factor XI from plasma by ammonium sulfate fractionation at 33 % saturation. Biggs et al. (1958) and Soulier and Larrieu (1958) similarly found activity in fractions obtained at 30–50 % saturation. Using the Cohn fractionation scheme of plasma (Cohn et al. 1946), Rosenthal (1955) found activity in Cohn Fraction IV-1 and III. A partial separation of factor XI and XII from plasma was achieved by adsorbing with low concentrations of celite (10–15 mg/ml) whereas higher concentrations (3 mg/ml) absorbed both factors (Soulier and Prou-Wartelle, 1960).

The site of biosynthesis of factor XI is not known. Attempts have been made to purify factor XI from plasma and serum but its association with Hageman factor and its spontaneous activation has made procedures difficult (Ratnoff et al. 1961). Schiffman et al. (1960) separated factor XI and XII by means of DEAE-cellulose chromatography, but no information regarding the grade of purity or physicochemical properties of the product was given.

Ratnoff et al. (1961) purified factor XI from Hageman deficient plasma (technique see Chapter IV, p. 167). The preparations were 10–20 fold purified over plasma. Ratnoff and Davie (1962a) and Kingdon et al. (1964) purified factor XI from human serum (technical details in Chapter IV, p. 168) and achieved a 150-fold purification, but these preparations were still impure (Kingdon et al. 1964).

The factor XI preparations had esterolytic activity on p-toluene-sulfonyl-L-arginine methyl ester (TAMe) and benzoyl-L-arginine ethyl ester (BAEe) (Ratnoff and Davie, 1962a). Factor XI activity was destroyed by DFP (Kingdon et al. 1964, Cattan and Denson,

1964). Physicochemical data have not been reported for these factor XI preparations either.

K. Lipids as Clotting Accelerators

The effect of lipids on blood coagulation has been the subject of intense research and the problems involved have been extensively reviewed in a monograph by Hecht (1965). In both the intrinsic and extrinsic pathways of prothrombin activation lipids play an important role. During prothrombin activation via the extrinsic pathway, lipids and/or enzymes from tissue (tissue thromboplastins) are intimately involved, while during activation via the intrinsic pathway phospholipids from platelets or erythrocytes (platelet factor 3, partial thromboplastins) are of importance.

1. Tissue Thromboplastins

Extracts from almost all mammalian tissues have procoagulant activity in the conversion of prothrombin to thrombin. Hecht et al. (1958) suggested to use the term tissue thromboplastin to describe just one of the procoagulants which may vary in preparation and species specificity. For example, "lung extract thromboplastin (bovine)" indicates a preparation from bovine lung tissue and the word "extract" implies its heterogeneous composition. These types of tissue extracts cannot be considered as chemical entities. They invariably contain procoagulants and anticoagulants, as well as various other substances not essential to blood coagulation. The qualitative and quantitative composition of these extracts determines their individual properties and specifity.

When lung extract thromboplastin (bovine) is further purified, preparations are obtained that are termed "lung thromboplastin (bovine)". This material is a lipoprotein and has a high molecular weight. Cohen and Chargaff (1941a, b), Chargaff et al. (1942), Chargaff and Bendich (1944) and more recently Williams (1964) have studied lung thromboplastin. The preparations consisted on the average of 7.7 % nitrogen and 1.6 % phosphorus (Chargaff et al. 1944). The sedimentation coefficient was 330 Svedberg units, the diffusion constant was 0.38×10^{-7} cm²/sec, and the partial specific volume was 0.87 gm/ml. From these data Chargaff et al. (1944) calculated a molecular weight of 167,000,000. The electrophoretic mobility was 8.4×10^{-5} cm²/V/sec. On the basis of these data lung thromboplastin (bovine) was classified as a lipoprotein (Chargaff, 1945). When this lung thromboplastin was extracted with an alcohol-ether solution, about 50 % of the original weight was removed. From this 50 % of material, 40–45 % was recovered as lipids with the following chemical composition: 19 % cholesterol, 18 % fat and 63 % phospholipids. The phospholipids were composed of 25 % lecithin, 25 % cephalin, and 12 % sphingomyelin (Chargaff et al. 1944). The material remaining after lipid extraction consisted of protein and carbohydrate. Besides phospholipids Williams (1964) found potent enzymatic activity in specific clotting assays.

Extracts from brain tissue are also frequently employed in blood coagulation studies. For example, "brain extract thromboplastin (rabbit)" is an acetone extract from rabbit brain (Quick, 1940), but extracts from brain of other species have also been prepared (Fischer and Hecht, 1934). According to Thies (1957) the gray substance of human brain is more active than the white substance. Brain extract thromboplastins are crude preparations. They can be further purified, and in the case of rabbit brain "brain thromboplastin (rabbit)" is obtained (Hecht et al. 1958). According to Hecht et al. (1958), this material is a complex lipid consisting of sterol, glutamic acid, serine, ethanolamine, and probably sphingosine. This material rapidly activates prothrombin to thrombin via the extrinsic pathway. Boiling the material with alcohol destroys its capability to function as an extrinsic activator and the remaining material now acts like phosphatides in the intrinsic pathway of prothrombin activation (partial thromboplastin). Nemerson and Spaet (1964), Irsigler (1964) and Deutsch et al. (1964) separated a protein portion from the lipid moiety and found that, for full activity, both had to be present. The lipid by itself served as a partial thromboplastin in the intrinsic system while the protein portion was inert (Irsigler, 1964; Deutsch et al. 1964). Nemerson and Spaet (1964) described enzymatic activity, similar to the one obtained from lung thromboplastin. Irsigler (1964) and Deutsch et al. (1964) upon recombination of the lipid and protein portions, obtained full thromboplastin activity. Analysis of the protein portion revealed the presence of 15 amino acids, while the lipid portion was composed of phosphatidyl ethanolamine, phosphatidyl choline, phosphatidyl serine, phosphatidyl inositol, lysophosphatidyl ethanolamine, and sphingomyelin. Irsigler (1964) and Deutsch et al. (1964) stated that brain thromboplastin is a lipoprotein and not a complex lipid as suggested by Hecht et al. (1958). In contrast, Hecht (1966b) and Hecht and Oosterbaan van Lit (1967) could not separate brain thromboplastin into distinct protein and lipid moieties. They found the 15 amino acids described by Irsigler (1964) and Deutsch et al. (1964) also in the lipid portion and therefore concluded that the amino acids in these preparations were contaminants rather than a constituent of a specific phospholipoprotein.

Phospholipids

It was pointed out that neither the lipid portion of lung thromboplastin nor the alcohol boiled brain thromboplastin function in the extrinsic prothrombin activation pathway. However, both preparations can serve as activators in the intrinsic pathway (partial thromboplastins). They thus display the same features as platelet factor 3. The altered thromboplastins had cholesterol, sphingomyelins and various phosphatides as common constituents. Cholesterol had only weak clotting activity which disappeared when it was repeatedly crystallized. This effect may have been due to contamination (Fischer and Hecht, 1934; Hecht, 1965). Sphingomyelins in pure form possessed no clotting activity (Hecht, 1953; Rouser et al. 1958), and sphingosine, a part of the sphingomyelin molecule, had anticoagulant activity (Hecht, 1965). This leaves the various phosphatides as possible clot promoting agents.

The effect of phospholipids on blood coagulation has been extensively investigated and a number of conflicting reports have been published. For example, phosphatidyl serine has been described as a platelet substitute (Troup and Reed, 1958; Marcus and Spaet, 1958; Marcus et al. 1962), but also as an inhibitor in the thromboplastin generation test (Turner and Silver, 1963; Barkhan et al. 1958), and as an anticoagulant when infused (Silver et al. 1957; Mustard et al. 1962). Phosphatidyl ethanolamine was described as an accelerator of coagulation (O'Brien, 1956; Hoelzl-Wallach et al. 1959; Rouser et al. 1958; Robinson and Poole, 1956; Turner et al. 1963; Poole and Robinson, 1956). Rapport (1956) found the combination of phosphatidyl ethanolamine and phosphatidyl choline most active, while Therriault et al. (1958) and Troup et al. (1960) found the combination of phosphatidyl choline and phosphatidyl serine most effective. Slotta (1960) and Hecht and Slotta (1962) reported a mixture of phosphatidyl ethanolamine and phosphatidyl serine as most active, but found also some activity when phosphatidyl serine and phosphatidyl choline were mixed. These conflicting results may be due to differences in test systems (Mustard et al. 1962); differences in the colloidal state of the phospholipid particles; differences in pH or ionic strength (Hoelzl-Wallach et al. 1959); the state of purity or rate of decomposition of the various phospholipids (Daemen et al. 1965). The degree of unsaturation and the localization of the fatty acid constituents on the phospholipids may also have contributed to these discrepancies (Rouser and Schloredt, 1958).

Daemen et al. (1965) used pure synthetic phospholipids and found that the combination of phosphatidyl ethanolamine and phosphatidyl serine was most effective in the conversion of prothrombin to thrombin. Only phospholipid suspensions that contained one acidic or negatively charged phospholipid were significantly active. These findings support the view that the procoagulant activity of phospholipids is related to the surface charge of the lipid micelles and that apparently a certain negative Zeta potential is a prerequisite (Bangham, 1961; Papahadjopoulos et al. 1962; Silver et al. 1963).

The major source of phospholipids in the circulating blood are the platelets. Phosphatidyl ethanolamine and phosphatidyl serine have been found in abundant quantities in platelets

(Troup et al. 1960; Marcus et al. 1962; Barkhan et al. 1961; Ferguson et al. 1963; Woodside et al. 1964). The platelet factor 3 activity was first located in the cytoplasmic granules of the platelets (Johnson et al. 1959; Schulz and Hiepler, 1959; Maupin, 1959). Later, more activity was found in the platelet membranes (Marcus and Spaet, 1964; Marcus and Zucker, 1965). Apparently intact platelet membranes can furnish the proper surface for interaction with coagulation proteins. However, this may not be due to phospholipids since the outer and inner surface of the platelet membranes is covered by a layer of protein. The exact mechanisms by which the coagulation factors interact with the platelet membrane are not known.

Marcus and Zucker (1965) hypothesized that a protein which may either be an inherent part of the platelet membrane or an adsorbed plasma protein, as suggested by Rodman et al. (1962), might be removed from the platelets during the early steps of coagulation. The removal of this protein might enable the platelet membranes to interact with certain coagulation factors. Another possibility is that Hageman factor (factor XII) which is apparently adsorbed on the platelet surface (Sharp, 1958; Waaler, 1959; Jürgens, 1962; Iatridis and Ferguson, 1965) becomes activated. Since activated factor XII has a positive electrical charge at physiological pH (Mammen and Grammens, 1967a, b) its activation on the platelet surface might lead to considerable changes in surface potentials. These might provide the means for interaction with more negatively charged proteins from the plasma. These ideas are at present only speculative and have to be investigated.

When platelets undergo morphological changes, and their membranes disintegrate, the above mentioned phosphatides become available. They in turn can facilitate prothrombin activation. It appears then that two mechanisms are operative, one related to "intact" platelet membranes and one related to the phospholipids, the former very likely preceding the latter.

Erythrocyte stroma has the same clot promoting properties as platelet factor 3 (Shinowara, 1957b; 1961) and apparently the same phosphatides (phosphatidyl ethanolamine and phosphatidyl serine) can be found in the stroma (Troup et al. 1960; Barkhan et al. 1961). The author (unpublished data) applied the procedure for the purification of platelet factor 3 as described by Alkjaersig et al. (1955b) to erythrocyte stroma and obtained a product with a biological activity identical to that of platelet factor 3. These data suggest that erythrocyte membranes can furnish the same combination of phosphatides that are usually derived from platelets, thereby making procoagulants available for coagulation.

L. Inhibitors

The existence of a clot-inhibiting principle was first discussed by Alexander Schmidt (1892, 1895) and has since been the subject of continuing interest. Alexander Schmidt considered anticoagulants to be intimately related to the maintenance of the fluidity of blood in vivo.

It has been suggested that under physiological conditions the clotting system of the living organism is in a steady state of subliminal activation. This implies that the formed fibrin must be removed by a steady state of subliminal activation of the fibrinolytic system. Such a state of limited activation of both the clotting and fibrinolytic systems in vivo can only be maintained as long as the reactions promoting clotting are largely or completely inhibited. Activated clotting reactions must therefore exist in a state of dynamic equilibrium with inhibitory, anticoagulant substances. The physiological inhibitors of the coagulation mechanism are designed in such a manner that they inhibit a variety of activation steps at strategically important points in the complex process. In vivo, some of the inhibitors regulate the conversion of prothrombin to thrombin, while others are directly concerned with the neutralization of activated factor X (autoprothrombin C) and thrombin (antithrombins). Substances which prevent coagulation in vitro, such as decalcifying agents, adsorbents, synthetic chemical inhibitors, hirudin and snake venoms will not be discussed here. They were recently reviewed by Mammen (1967b). The physiology and biochemistry of antithrombin has been discussed in Chapter VII

(p. 268). Jorpes elaborated on heparin in the same Chapter on p. 277. The effect of the fibrinogen split products on coagulation has been discussed in Chapter VI, p. 247. This leaves predominantly those inhibitors which regulate the conversion of prothrombin to thrombin.

1. Inhibitor Source Material

When blood clots, factor VIII activity disappears from plasma and cannot be found in serum (Graham et al. 1951; Johnson et al. 1952). Thrombin was found to be responsible for this inactivation (Penick, 1957; Rizza and Walker, 1957), and the assumption has been made that thrombin in its capacity as a proteolytic enzyme digests factor VIII (Brinkhous and Wagner, 1959).

Johnson and Seegers (1954) and Mammen et al. (1960b) found that factor VIII activity could be recovered from serum following ether treatment. This observation suggested that the factor VIII is not inactivated by thrombin, instead, it was suggested that factor VIII activity is lost as factor VIII during coagulation combines with "inhibitor source material", extractable by ether. This contention was supported by the later observation that thrombin does not destroy the activity of purified factor VIII. Later, factor VIII was purified from serum (Mammen, 1964b), again indicating that factor VIII is not destroyed when blood clots.

Inhibitor source material has been isolated from plasma and was identified as a lipid. It is very likely a glyceride (Mammen, 1965). This lipid when added to plasma, prolonged the coagulation times of plasma and inhibited prothrombin activation in both the intrinsic and extrinsic pathways (Mammen et al. 1960b; Mammen, 1965). Inhibitor source material is thus a physiological inhibitor of prothrombin activation. During coagulation, the inhibitor forms a complex with factor VIII. This complex formation is mediated by thrombin only; activated factor X (autoprothrombin C) and plasmin do not produce this complex formation (Mammen, 1965). The complex formation between factor VIII and inhibitor source material accounts for the disappearance of factor VIII during clotting.

2. Antithromboplastins

Antithromboplastins have been defined as substances that interfere with the prothrombin conversion to thrombin. In general, substances that interfere with the intrinsic activation mechanism, as measured by the thromboplastin generation test, have been termed "antiplasma thromboplastins". Substances that inhibit prothrombin conversion by tissue thromboplastins, as measured by one-stage prothrombin time tests, have been called "antitissue thromboplastins".

a) Antiplasma thromboplastins: The instability of the activity obtained in the thromboplastin generation test has been studied by several investigators (Spaet and Garner, 1955; Egli et al. 1957; Deutsch and Fuchs, 1958; Deutsch and Mammen, 1958). Two fractions of plasma were found to inhibit plasma thromboplastin activity, one with an immediate effect, and one with a progressive type of action (Deutsch and Mammen, 1958). These two activities also differed in their precipitation characteristics and in some of their physical properties (Deutsch and Mammen, 1958). Schimpf et al. (1962) found two different antiplasma thromboplastins by preparative ultracentrifugation of serum. Very likely these two are identical to those described by Deutsch and Mammen (1958). Both migrate in electrophoresis with the α_2-globulins (Deutsch and Mammen, 1958). Of interest is the increase in activity during coagulation, and the fact that serum contains more antiplasma thromboplastin activity than plasma (Klesper and Egli, 1957; Schimpf et al. 1960, 1964; Schimpf, 1963). Patients undergoing dicumarol therapy, on the other hand, have less activity in their serum than in their plasma (Schimpf, 1963). These findings have led to the speculation that antiplasma thromboplastin might be part of the prothrombin complex and develop when the prothrombin complex is dissociating (Schimpf, 1963; Schimpf et al. 1960, 1962). A possible close relationship to factor IX has also been suggested (Egli et al. 1957; Schimpf and Osamo, 1963; Schimpf et al. 1964).

In 1960, Mammen et al. (1960b) described the development of an inhibitor from the prothrombin complex when the latter was dissociated by thrombin. Its close relationship to factor IX (autoprothrombin II) was noted and the term autoprothrombin II-A was proposed for this anticoagulant. Autoprothrombin II-A inhibited prothrombin activation by both pathways, intrinsic and extrinsic. Seegers and Marciniak (1965) described a similar anticoagulant activity arising from activated prothrombin and separated the inhibitor from the activation mixture (Seegers and Marciniak, 1965; Seegers et al. 1965a). Murano (1966) and Marciniak et al. (1967) subsequently found that this inhibitor competitively inhibits autoprothrombin C (activated factor X). It has been suggested that the inhibitor might arise from the prethrombin portion of the prothrombin complex (Marciniak et al. 1967). Recent work has suggested that the inhibitor is an intermediate product between prothrombin and prethrombin, the dissociation going from prothrombin to inhibitor to prethrombin to thrombin (Murano, 1969).

Autoprothrombin II-A and the inhibitor described by Seegers and Marciniak (1965) seem to be identical entities. They may also be identical with antiplasma thromboplastins.

b) Antitissue thromboplastins: In plasma and serum there are substances which can inhibit the prothrombin activation via the extrinsic pathway. The substances have been studied by Schneider (1947), Thomas (1947), Lanchantin and Ware (1953), Berry (1957), and Deutsch and Fuchs (1958). Usually one-stage prothrombin time tests were used to study these substances. Unfortunately the data are too scarce to make valid comparisons between this group of inhibitors and the antiplasma thromboplastins discussed above. All that can be stated with fair certainty at present is that the antitissue thromboplastins are proteins which are adsorbed on barium salts. It is possible that the antitissue thromboplastins are identical with autoprothrombin II-A since this inhibitor also blocked prothrombin activation via the extrinsic pathway. This is not surprising since the inhibitor is a competitive blocker of activated factor X.

3. Lipids as Inhibitors

It was pointed out earlier that lipids can function in blood clotting as accelerators and inhibitors. The most important lipids considered here are sphingosine and certain other phospholipids.

a. Sphingosine: The clot-delaying action of sphingomyelin was first noted by Chargaff (1937). Hecht (1951a, b, 1953) later discovered that sphingosine inhibited the activation of prothrombin to thrombin. Hecht et al. (1957a, b) subsequently found that sphingosine inhibited prothrombin activation via the intrinsic as well as the extrinsic pathways.

The development of thrombin from prothrombin decreased proportionally to the amount of sphingosine added. When added in very low concentration sphingosine exhibited clot promoting rather than inhibiting activity. This activity was demonstrated only when prothrombin was activated via the intrinsic pathway. Hecht and Shapiro (1957a, b) studied the structure-activity relationships of several synthetic derivatives of sphingosine. The double bond in the molecule in addition to free functional hydroxyl and amino groups were found to be essential for the inhibitor effect of sphingosine. Sphingosine is a constituent of brain tissue and it can be assigned a physiological function in blood clotting only if it can be found in circulating blood. Analysis by gas-liquid chromatography revealed small amounts to be present in plasma (Hecht, 1965).

b. Other phospholipids: The phospholipids have clot promoting activity when they are present in micellar form, as was outlined before. Their effect seems to be related to the surface charge of the micelles and a certain negative Zeta potential seems to be prerequisite, and three phospholipids have been extensively studied; phosphatidyl ethanolamine, phosphatidyl choline and phosphatidyl serine. Of these, only phosphatidyl serine can exhibit anticoagulant properties. Its inhibitory properties can, however, only be observed when phosphatidyl serine is solubilized (Barkhan and Silver, 1962). In its micellar form it has procoagulant activity (Kazal, 1965). The solubilization of phosphatidyl serine by lipoproteins was reported by Kazal et al. (1962) and Kazal (1965). Besides α_1-lipoproteins, also β-lipoproteins and albumin had a solubilizing effect on phosphatidyl serine (Barkhan and Silver, 1962; Kazal, 1965). According to Kazal (1965) phosphatidyl serine is first accepted by lipoproteins and only secondarily by albumin. The nature of these phosphatidyl serine-lipoprotein complexes is not known. They displayed antithromboplastic effects in the thromboplastin generation test (Kazal et al. 1962) and in prothrombin activation (Holburn and Silver, 1964). In vivo, phosphatidyl serine also displayed anticoagulant activity (Mustard et al. 1962).

This work is relevant to the anticephalins or antithromboplastins first suggested by Tocantins (1943a). This group of inhibitors was found to be present in normal plasma and elevated in hemophilia A plasma (Tocantins, 1943b, 1944, 1945, 1954). Kazal (1965) suggested that the anticephalin activity resulted from the interaction of plasma lipoproteins with phosphatidyl serine. According to Mulder (1961), these phospholipid-lipoprotein interactions may also account for other antithromboplastin effects, such as for example the Bridge-anticoagulant effect described by Nour-Eldin and Wilkinson (1958a, b).

4. Inhibitor Against Factor XI

Normal plasma and serum contains an inhibitor against activated factor XI (Margolis, 1957; Ratnoff and Rosenblum, 1958; Ratnoff et al. 1961; Nossel, 1964a; Iatrides et al. 1964a, b; Nossel and Niemetz, 1965). This inhibitor progressively inactivates factor XI. The inhibitor was recently purified from plasma (Niemetz and Nossel, 1967) and a 100-fold purification was achieved. Electrophoretically the inhibitor migrated with the α-globulins, was stable over a pH range from approximately pH 5 to 10, was stable upon heating up to 56° C and had a sedimentation constant ($S^{o}_{20,w}$) of 3.69. The inhibitor was not consumed during the interaction with factor XI and it specifically blocked factor XI activity.

V. Activation of Prothrombin

The formation of thrombin from prothrombin is a complex mechanism in which several plasma coagulation factors, phospholipids and/or extracts from tissue cells participate. The sequence in which these constituents become involved has been the subject of considerable controversy. It was pointed out earlier in this review that basically two theories have emerged to explain this event, the cascade or waterfall theory, originally proposed by Davie and

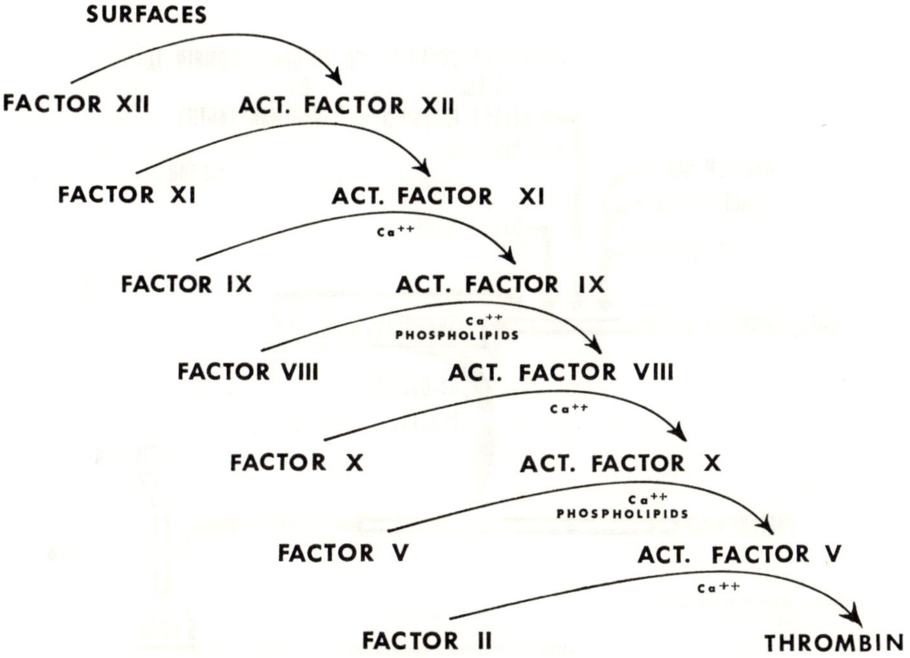

Fig. 1. Cascade or waterfall concept of prothrombin activation (intrinsic pathway) as postulated by Davie and Ratnoff (1964) and Macfarlane (1964a).

Ratnoff (1964) and by Macfarlane (1964a) (Fig. 1), and the concept of Seegers and his associates (Fig. 2) (Seegers, 1962, 1964, 1965, 1967, 1968, 1969; Seegers et al. 1967a). Rather than discuss each one of the views separately, an attempt is made to correlate both schools of thought.

A. Formation of Thrombin

The concept that thrombin is generated from a precursor, called prothrombin was proposed by Morawitz as early as 1904, 1905. This hypothesis was substantiated by Seegers and coworkers after the purification of the zymogen from plasma (Seegers et al. 1938a; Seegers, 1940; Seegers and Smith, 1941). This proenzyme would yield thrombin under appropriate conditions. When prothrombin was converted to thrombin a dissociation of the complex was noted (Seegers et al. 1950; Lorand et al. 1953; Seegers and Alkjaersig, 1956; Lamy and Waugh, 1954, 1958; Magnusson, 1958, 1964). Since the dissociation preceded the actual development of thrombin activity, it was assumed that during the initial phase of dissociation the enzyme was in a physical state different from the original prothrombin (Asada et al. 1961; Magnusson, 1965f; Lanchantin et al. 1965a; 1967, 1968b; Aronson, 1966; Aronson and Ménaché, 1966; Tishkoff et al. 1968). This inactive prothrombin fragment was isolated and termed "prethrombin" (Seegers and Marciniak, 1965; Marciniak and Seegers, 1965; Seegers et al. 1965a, 1967b). Tishkoff et al. (1968) called this fragment "modified zymogen". Prethrombin is smaller than prothrombin (see p. 7) and has two N-terminal amino acids, lysine and threonine (1 mole of each per 52,000 gm) (Murano, 1968). Prothrombin has only 1 mole of alanine per 65,000 gm (see p. 6). This indicates that during the initial dissociation of prothrombin, two peptide bonds are cleaved: one close to the N-terminal end of the molecule and one located somewhere under an intra-chain disulfide bridge (Murano, 1968). This would explain the formation of a two chain molecule from a one chain molecule with the loss of a fragment having alanine as the N-terminus. Although the active site of the enzyme thrombin is as yet not exposed, prethrombin has already the two chain configuration of the thrombin molecule. Moreover, already one of the N-terminal amino acids of thrombin, threonine is exposed.

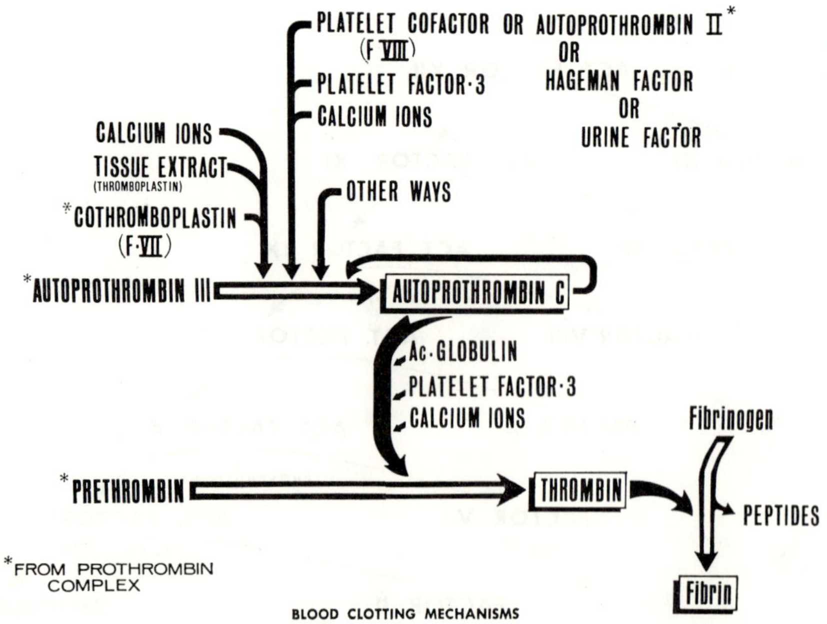

Fig. 2. Activation of prothrombin to thrombin according to Seegers and coworkers.

The dissociation of prothrombin to prethrombin is facilitated only by thrombin; activated factor X (autoprothrombin C) has no effect (Seegers et al. 1967a). This activation reaction is shown in Eq. 1.

$$\text{Prothrombin} \xrightarrow{\text{Thrombin}} \text{Prethrombin} \quad (1)$$

The further dissociation of prethrombin to thrombin was extensively studied after prethrombin was isolated and characterized (Marciniak and Seegers, 1966a). Prethrombin could not be activated in strong salt solutions (25 % sodium citrate solution). However, when activated factor X (autoprothrombin C) was added, thrombin formed by a first order reaction with respect to the substrate (Seegers and Marciniak, 1965; Seegers et al. 1965a, 1967a, 1967b). Prethrombin also yielded thrombin with trypsin, but thrombin itself, Russel's viper venom, tissue thromboplastin, and the reagents used in the two-stage analytical prothrombin assay failed to produce thrombin from prethrombin (Seegers et al. 1965a, 1967a, 1967b). These experiments clearly indicate that *activated factor X* (autoprothrombin C) is the enzyme which facilitates the ultimate formation of thrombin (Eq. 2).

$$\text{Prethrombin} \xrightarrow{\text{Activated factor X}} \text{Thrombin} \quad (2)$$

The conversion of prethrombin to thrombin by activated factor X alone is a slow process (Seegers and Marciniak, 1965). Nevertheless, the conversion is complete when the proper enzyme to substrate ratio is maintained. If cephalin, phospholipids from platelets (platelet factor 3) or lipids from tissue thromboplastin were added, together with Ac-globulin (factor V) and calcium ions, the conversion of prethrombin to thrombin by activated factor X was completed within minutes (Seegers et al. 1967a, 1967b). These data indicated that these constituents greatly *accelerate* the effect of activated factor X on prethrombin. Baker and Seegers (1967) have studied the relationship of the individual constituents to each other and found that reducing activated factor X, factor V or phospholipids toward zero concentration decreased the rate of formation and yield of thrombin. Highest yields of thrombin were formed most rapidly when factor V and activated factor X were in a 1:1 molar ratio. These data clearly demonstrated that factor X is the enzyme which catalyzes the formation of thrombin, and that factor V, phospholipids and calcium ions function synergistically (Eq. 3).

$$\text{Prethrombin} \xrightarrow{\substack{\text{Activated factor X} \\ \text{Factor V} \\ \text{Phospholipids} \\ \text{Calcium ions}}} \text{Thrombin} \quad (3)$$

These findings stand in contrast to the cascade or waterfall concept of prothrombin activation (Fig. 1), as originally proposed by Davie and Ratnoff (1964) and by Macfarlane (1964a). According to Davie and Ratnoff (1964), activated factor X is converting factor V in the presence of phospholipids and calcium ions to activated factor V which in turn converts prothrombin to thrombin. In view of Seegers' findings one would have to imply that it is prethrombin rather than prothrombin which is converted to thrombin by activated factor V. The view that factor V is activated and converts prothrombin to thrombin is controversial. Macfarlane (1964a) states in his presentation on the cascade hypothesis: "Each stage represented is fairly well supported by evidence, with the exception of the supposed activation of Factor V, which is included for completeness despite lack of information".

The precise function of factor V in the formation of thrombin has been the subject of controversy. The close relationship between factor V and activated factor X has been acknowledged by several investigators and most of them seem to agree that activated factor X does not function efficiently in the absence of factor V (Douglas, 1956; Bergsagel and Hougie, 1956; Hougie, 1957; Macfarlane, 1961; Kowarzyk et al. 1961; Seegers and Marciniak, 1962a; Spaet and Cintron, 1963; Seegers, 1964, 1965, 1967). While Surgenor et al. (1961) assigned a catalytic role to factor V in the prothrombin conversion, Owren (1953), Jensen et al. (1955), and Gray et al. (1956) have expressed the view that factor V and activated factor X act together, a concept shared by Seegers and his associates. In contrast, Hardisty

(1955), Straub and Duckert (1961), Breckenridge and Ratnoff (1963, 1964, 1965), and Davie and Ratnoff (1964, 1965) concluded that activated factor V is the ultimate enzyme which forms thrombin from prothrombin and that activated factor X functions in activating factor V. Seegers and coworkers who have investigated the interrelationship between factor V and activated factor X (autoprothrombin C), have not been able to demonstrate that autoprothrombin C activates factor V. Only thrombin seems to change the reactivity of factor V. Moreover, they clearly established that activated factor X is the enzyme which by itself can form thrombin from prethrombin (Seegers and Marciniak, 1965; Seegers et al. 1965a, 1967a, 1967b; Baker and Seegers, 1967). Factor V alone does not activate prethrombin. However, optimum generation of thrombin is only achieved when activated factor X, factor V, phospholipids and calcium ions are functioning together. This view has also been expressed by several other investigators (Esnouf and Williams, 1962b; Milstone, 1962; Jobin and Esnouf, 1967; Barton, 1967; Barton et al. 1967; Hemker et al. 1967; Prentice et al. 1967). In addition, elaborate kinetic studies of the cascade concept of prothrombin activation indicated that standard methods of enzyme kinetics were not applicable (Hemker et al. 1965). On the other hand, enzyme kinetical analysis was suitable when applied to conditions where activated factor X functioned together with factor V, phospholipids and calcium ions (Hemker and Kahn, 1967). This still leaves open the question; how do these constituents inter-react together? Hougie (1957) presented evidence that activated factor X forms a complex with phospholipids (intermediate product II). Moreover, several investigators have shown that activated factor X and factor V are adsorbed to phospholipid micelles and that calcium ions favor the binding of activated factor X (Papahadjopoulos and Hanahan, 1964; Cole et al. 1964, 1965; Esnouf and Jobin, 1965; Jobin and Esnouf, 1967). Phosphatidyl ethanolamine together with phosphatidyl serine seem to be the most active combination of phospholipids (Therriault et al. 1958; Troup et al. 1960; Slotta, 1960; Hecht and Slotta, 1962; Daemen et al. 1965). As mentioned, evidence has been presented that the clot promoting effect of these phospholipids is related to the surface charge of the micelles, and that a certain negative Zeta potential is a prerequisite for this effect (Bangham, 1961; Papahadjopoulos et al. 1962; Silver et al. 1963).

The major source of the two phospholipids during clotting are platelets (Troup et al. 1960; Barkhan et al. 1961; Marcus et al. 1962; Ferguson et al. 1963; Woodside et al. 1964), but as was pointed out earlier, erythrocyte stroma can also furnish these phospholipids (Shinowara, 1957b, 1961; Barkhan et al. 1961). Baker and Seegers (1967) found that the lipid portion of tissue thromboplastin (partial thromboplastin) also functioned together with activated factor X, factor V and calcium ions in the conversion of prethrombin to thrombin. In this connection it is of interest to note that the lipid portion of lung thromboplastin and brain thromboplastin seems to contain the same phospholipids besides a wide and varying spectrum of other lipids (Chargaff et al. 1944; Hecht et al. 1958; Hecht, 1965).

In view of these recently accumulated experimental data, it seems likely that the formation of thrombin from prothrombin, or more accurately from prethrombin, is facilitated by a complex consisting of phospholipids (phosphatidyl ethanolamine and phosphatidyl serine), activated factor X, factor V and calcium ions (Eq. 4).

$$\underbrace{\text{Activated factor X} + \text{Factor V} + \text{Phospholipids} + \text{Calcium ions}}_{\text{Complex}}$$
$$\text{Prethrombin} \longrightarrow \text{Thrombin} \qquad (4)$$

This concept is compatable with recent data obtained with purified reagents and synthetic substrates, and meets the criteria of standard enzyme kinetics (Hemker and Kahn, 1967). Whereas calcium ions seem to favor the binding of activated factor X into this complex, the actual function of factor V remains obscure. Although its function is similar to that of a coenzyme (Esnouf, 1968), by definition it is not a coenzyme. It is a protein with a substantial molecular weight. Since as yet no substrate for factor V has been discovered, factor V may control the rate constant of the enzyme substrate complex formation. Alternatively, it may modify the conformation of the substrate, rendering it more susceptible to the enzyme (Esnouf, 1968). Further work is required to elucidate the exact role of Ac-globulin in the formation of thrombin from its zymogen.

B. Formation of Activated Factor X (Autoprothrombin C)

The formation of the prethrombin activating complex (Eq. 4) is dependent upon the formation of active factor X from its zymogen. This activation can be achieved in two ways, extrinsically and intrinsically.

1. The Extrinsic Pathway

The term "extrinsic pathway" is used to denote activation of the clotting mechanism with the aid of tissue substances, not normally present in the circulating blood. More specifically, it implies the participation of tissue factors in the generation of thrombin. The powerful procoagulant action of tissue extracts in vivo and in vitro was already recognized around the turn of this century (Rauschenbach, 1882; Wooldridge, 1893; Morawitz, 1904). These authors postulated that tissue extracts would be the prime activator of prothrombin. The activity of tissue extracts on prothrombin was termed "tissue thrombokinase" or "tissue thromboplastin", the latter term being widely adopted following the work of Quick (1935, 1936).

Early studies on the extrinsic pathway of thrombin formation revealed that the incubation of serum with factor V and brain tissue extracts resulted in a potent prothrombin converting activity (Flynn and Coon, 1953; Biggs et al. 1953c; Mann and Hurn, 1953; Hardisty, 1955; Gray et al. 1956; Hjort, 1957). The active component in serum was believed to be factor VII. After factor X was discovered, it became apparent that this coagulation factor was also involved in the extrinsic pathway of prothrombin activation, and Hougie (1959) suggested that tissue extracts reacted with factors V, VII, X and calcium ions to form a prothrombin converting principle. Hougie (1959) indicated that the concentration of factor VII influenced the rate of thrombin formation, while the factor X concentration affected the yield of thrombin formation. Similar conclusions were drawn by Straub and Duckert (1961) who called the activity "extrinsic reaction product". They suggested that factor X was the substrate in this reaction and factor VII in combination with tissue extracts the enzyme.

Johnston et al. (1959b) and Johnston and Hjort (1961) found that the level of factor VII activity was higher in serum than in plasma. This finding and the work of Pechet and Alexander (1961) and Alexander and Pechet (1962) was later interpreted as evidence that factor VII occurred in plasma in an inactive form and that is would be activated during clotting in the presence of tissue extracts.

Nemerson and Spaet (1964) made the interesting observation that a lipid poor fraction of brain thromboplastin activated factor X in the presence of factor VII, but that this reaction did not yield thrombin from prothrombin unless phospholipids were added. These phospholipids were provided by crude tissue extracts. Williams (1964, 1966) found that microsomal preparations from lung, brain and placenta reacted with a mixture of factor VII and X to produce activated factor X. However, Williams was unable to determine the exact relationship between the "tissue factor" and factor VII. Williams and Norris (1966) presented some indirect evidence that factor VII might slowly activate factor X in the absence of tissue extracts, but no product corresponding to "activated factor VII" could be separated from such mixtures. Davie and Ratnoff (1965) postulated that factor VII would be converted by tissue thromboplastin to active factor VII which in turn would activate factor X (Fig. 3). This postulated sequence is in conflict with recent findings by Williams and Norris (1966), and Nemerson (1966) who presented evidence that factor VII forms a complex with tissue thromboplastin and calcium ions. Attempts to separate "activated factor VII" from the lipoprotein complex were unsuccessful. The dis-

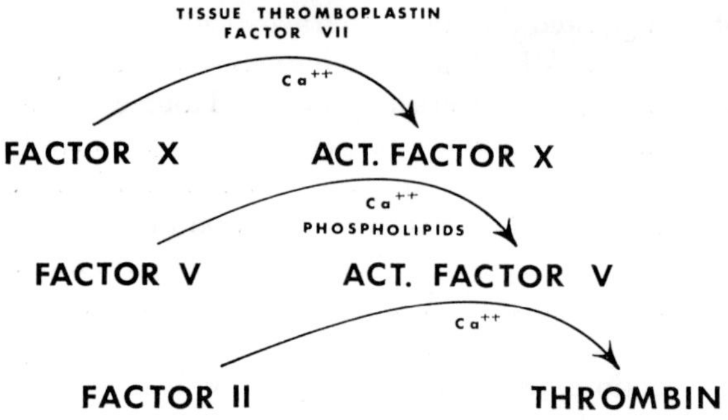

Fig. 3. Extrinsic pathway of prothrombin activation according to Davie and Ratnoff (1965).

ruption of the complex by a variety of reagents either failed to dissociate the complex or resulted in the loss of its ability to form activated factor X. Barton (1967) and Nemerson (1968) have supported this view and Eq. 5 might present the *tentative* extrinsic pathway for the conversion of factor X into its enzymatic form (activated factor X, autoprothrombin C).

$$\underbrace{\text{Tissue thromboplastin} + \text{Factor VII} + \text{Calcium ions}}_{\text{Complex}}$$
$$\text{Inactive factor X} \longrightarrow \text{Active factor X} \qquad (5)$$

Although most recent experimental work seems to support this concept, the details of this equation remain uncertain. In particular, the exact role of tissue thromboplastin and factor VII in this complex remains to be elucidated. Seegers et al. (1967a, b) studied the conversion of highly purified autoprothrombin III (inactive factor X) to autoprothrombin C (activated factor X) and found that sedimentable brain thromboplastin together with calcium ions would facilitate the conversion (Fig. 2). However, when the thromboplastin was mixed with serum, the conversion was enhanced, indicating that something in serum (very likely factor VII) accelerated the autoprothrombin III conversion. Best results were obtained when serum and thromboplastin were of the same species. These findings and those reported by Williams and Norris (1966) and Nemerson (1966) seem to indicate that the actual enzyme which converts factor X might reside in the tissue thromboplastin and that factor VII may have a function similar to that of factor V in the prethrombin converting complex (Eq. 4). Factor VII possibly controls the rate constant of the enzyme substrate complex, or it might modify the conformation of the substrate to render it more susceptible to the enzyme. So far, no synthetic substrate is recognized for this "enzyme" and very little is known about specific enzyme inhibitors. Most inhibitors of "antithromboplastin" activity are inhibitors of activated factor X rather than inhibitors of earlier reactions.

The enzymic action of tissue thromboplastin is supported by the observation that cathepsin produced autoprothrombin C (activated factor X) from prothrombin complex (Purcell and Barnhart, 1963). Most of the other evidence for the enzymic action of tissue thromboplastin is more indirect. Williams and Norris (1966) indicated that the product of "tissue factor" and factor VII resembled in its reaction with factor X the activity produced by the coagulant protein of Russel's viper venom. The observation of Williams (1964) and Nemerson and Spaet (1964) support this concept more directly and provide some evidence that the "protein portion" of tissue thromboplastin (brain and lung tissue) has enzymic function. It is well known that the extracted "lipid portion" of tissue thromboplastin no longer has full thromboplastin activity, i. e. it only supports thrombin formation in the intrinsic pathway (partial thromboplastin) (Hecht et al. 1958; Hecht, 1965; Irsigler, 1964; Deutsch et al. 1964). When the "lipid portion" of brain thromboplastin was recombined with the "protein portion" which by itself was inactive, full thromboplastin activity was obtained (Irsigler, 1964; Deutsch et al. 1964). Hecht (1966b) and Hecht and Oosterbaan van Lit (1967) have reinvestigated this concept by elaborate chemical procedures and found no evidence that the extracted "protein portion" was indeed a protein. Although they found all amino acids present in both the "lipid" and "protein" portion, they regarded them as contaminations rather than part of the structure of the phospholipid molecules. Nevertheless, the amino acid or peptide constituents seem to be of real importance in the biological function of tissue thromboplastins. Nemerson (1968) has recently separated the phospholipids from tissue thromboplastin and found that the "extracted tissue factor" (i. e. the non-phospholipid portion, only containing 2 % phospholipids) had by itself in the presence of factor VII and calcium ions very little activity in converting inactive factor X to active factor X. However, recombination with the extracted phospholipids or with purified phospholipids from other sources reestablished full activation.

On the basis of these data one can slightly modify Eq. 5 in order to incorporate these findings (Eq. 6).

$$\underbrace{\text{“Tissue factor”} + \text{Phospholipids} + \text{Factor VII} + \text{Calcium ions}}_{\text{Complex}}$$
$$\text{Inactive factor X} \longrightarrow \text{Active factor X} \qquad (6)$$

2. The Intrinsic Pathway

The activation of factor X via the intrinsic activation pathway involves the participation of Hageman factor (factor XII), plasma thromboplastin antecedent (PTA, factor XI), factor IX, factor VIII, phospholipids and calcium ions. Furthermore, the release of the phospholipids from various sources is necessary. Compared to the extrinsic pathway, entirely different constituents react together in the intrinsic pathway. It will be noted that factor VII does not participate in the intrinsic pathway, whereas factors XII, XI, IX and VIII do not participate in the extrinsic pathway.

Once again, the exact mechanism of interaction of these constituents in the intrinsic pathway is a matter of considerable uncertainty. One of the major problems is the lack of satisfactory purification of the participating coagulation factors. This has rendered kinetic studies rather difficult, and as a result, much of the evidence to be presented for their interaction is indirect.

a) Contact activation in vitro: The fact that blood remains fluid within the vessels, but coagulates when shed, has been recognized for many centuries. Lister (1863) was the first to indicate that the clotting of shed blood might be related to the surface of the container in which it was collected. Lister made special reference to glass surfaces. Subsequently, Freund (1888) and Bordet and Gengou (1901) reported that coating of glass surfaces with petroleum jelly or paraffin kept the blood fluid for several hours. Lampert (1931) studied the effect of several different surfaces on coagulation and concluded that wettability by water would be an important factor. These findings led Lenggenhager (1936) to speculate that glass affected a substance in plasma which he called "prothrombokinin". About 15 years later, it was proposed that glass exerted its action on a "plasma thromboplastin precursor" (Hartmann et al. 1949; Conley et al. 1949; Ratnoff and Conley, 1951).

Biggs et al. (1953b) were the first to suggest that factor IX and platelets probably participated in the early stages of clotting. Later, an activation of factor IX by glass contact was suggested (Rapaport et al. 1955). Shafrir and De Vries (1956) subsequently demonstrated that a clot-promoting effect could also be obtained from plasma *free* of platelets and factor IX. Margolis (1956, 1957) then indicated that a contact factor would be formed from a precursor in plasma. This contact factor was supposed to act on factor XI. In 1958 and 1959, several investigators found that this contact factor was intimately related to factor XII (Hageman factor) which Ratnoff and Colopy (1955) had described as being absent in a patient with a coagulation disturbance. The findings indicated that factor XII might be activated by glass contact (Biggs et al. 1958; Johnston et al. 1958; Lewis and Merchant, 1958; Ratnoff and Rosenbluhm, 1958; Vroman, 1958; Didisheim, 1959; Hardisty and Margolis,

1959; Soulier et al. 1959; Waaler, 1959; Soulier and Prou-Wartelle, 1960). These observations found their reflection in the cascade or waterfall concept of intrinsic prothrombin activation (Fig. 1). The activation of factor XII is the first step in the postulated sequence of events.

In the meantime it has been found that factor XII is also activated by a number of other materials, such as kaolin, diatomaceous earth, barium carbonate, asbestos, celite, Super-Cel, bentonite, sodium urate, long chain fatty acids, collagen, elastin, skin contact and possibly many more inorganic and organic substances (see p. 21 for references). However, the efficiency of these various materials to activate Hageman factor seems to vary, as was pointed out by Davie and Ratnoff (1965).

The molecular changes occurring during the activation of factor XII on surfaces are poorly understood. When Hageman factor comes into contact with wettable surfaces, it becomes firmly adsorbed (Margolis, 1963; Vroman, 1963, 1965, 1967, 1968). It is known from purification procedures that it can only be desorbed from these surfaces by strong salt solutions. Vroman (1963, 1967, 1968) has indicated that Hageman factor adsorbs so readily to wettable surfaces because of its hydrophilic characteristics. In the process of adsorption a molecular reorientation is postulated and Vroman (1963, 1967, 1968) has speculated that more hydrophobic sites of the molecule are exposed as a consequence of this molecular reorientation. This concept finds support by the observation that factor XII solubility decreases with activation (Donaldson and Ratnoff, 1965). Margolis (1962, 1963) has suggested that the factor XII molecule unfolds on adsorption and thereby exposes the active site of the enzyme. Recently, as mentioned, Speer and Ridgway (1967) have proposed that the unfolded active molecule can refold to its original inactive structure. Esnouf and Macfarlane (1968) proposed that activated Hageman factor consisted of a tetramer of subunits with a molecular weight of 20,000 which would associate in the presence of suitable surfaces. The assumption was based on molecular weight measurements of 82,000 for activated factor XII (Schoenmakers et al. 1965) and 20,000 as reported by Speer et al. (1965). In our recent studies we have confirmed that Hageman factor indeed consists of subunits with a molecular weight of 24,000, but they can only be obtained through cleavage of disulfide bridges. In view of this, Esnouf and Macfarlane's assumption becomes open to question, since it is difficult to conceive of disulfide bond formation through surface contact.

Several investigators have presented indirect evidence that adsorbed Hageman factor activates factor XI (Margolis, 1958b; Hardisty and Margolis, 1959; Soulier et al. 1958, 1959; Waaler, 1959; Ratnoff, 1960). The implication is that adsorbed factor XII acts as an enzyme which in turn converts factor XI to its active form. However, Hageman factor only activates factor XI as long as both are adsorbed to the appropriate surfaces (Hardisty and Margolis, 1959). The first direct evidence for the enzymic nature of Hageman factor and its effect on factor XI was presented by Ratnoff et al. (1961). The authors obtained crude Hageman factor from factor XI deficient plasma and crude factor XI from Hageman deficient plasma. Upon incubation of both crude preparations together in siliconized test tubes, a powerful clot-promoting activity was generated. The magnitude of this activity depended upon the concentration of factor XI, and the rate of its formation on the concentration of Hageman factor. The effect of Hageman factor on factor XI, and the activity of factor XI itself was inhibited by DFP. These data indeed support the view that both activated factors act as enzymes. Additional evidence was presented when Schoenmakers et al. (1965) who found that their purified Hageman factor preparations digested chymotrypsinogen and possessed esterolytic activity, in addition to their clot-promoting effect. Both clotting and esterolytic activity were inhibited by DFP and Lima bean trypsin inhibitor. In contrast to this, Becker (1960), Ratnoff and Davie (1962a), Speer et al. (1965) and Mammen and Grammens (1967a, b) did not find esterolytic activity in their purified preparations, although all of them corrected the clotting abnormality in Hageman deficient plasma. However, Ratnoff and Davie (1962a) and Davie and Ratnoff (1965) described esterolytic activity in factor

XI concentrates. Moreover, Sherry et al. (1966) presented evidence that the esterolytic activity in plasma was due not to Hageman factor itself, but to an enzyme activated by Hageman factor. This created the possibility that the preparations of Schoenmakers et al. (1964) contain some factor XI, despite the fact that the preparations did not correct a factor XI deficient plasma. In addition, Schoenmakers' preparations have different physical characteristics (see p. 22), and an entirely different carbohydrate content than those described by Mammen and Grammens (1967a, b). This discrepancy in physicochemical properties is at present puzzling but will, hopefully be resolved in the near future. In this connection, it is of interest that Schoenmakers' preparations have kallikreinogen activating properties, whereas our preparations do not (Habermann, 1968). A parallelism seems to exist between esterolytic activity and kallikreinogen converting activity. If the esterolytic activity in Schoenmakers' preparations is due to factor XI, then the kallikreinogen converting activity might be due to factor XI rather than factor XII. The failure of a Hageman factor deficient plasma to activate kallikreinogens does not contradict this assumption because in such a plasma factor XI would not be activated very readily. Earlier preparations of purified Hageman factor apparently were frequently contaminated with factor XI (Davie and Ratnoff, 1965).

The inhibiting effect of DFP on Hageman factor activity, as originally described by Schoenmakers et al. (1964), Becker (1960) and Ratnoff et al. (1961) has been disputed by Ratnoff and Davie (1962b) and Davie and Ratnoff (1965). The authors felt that the earlier reported DFP effect was due to a contamination of their original factor XII preparations with factor XI. Later preparations were more purified. However, in view of the findings of Speer et al. (1965) that reagents interfering with aliphatic hydroxyl groups destroy Hageman factor activity, the failure of DFP to inactivate Hageman activity is difficult to understand. Esnouf and Macfarlane (1968) suggested that the findings of Ratnoff and Davie (1962b) could be accounted for if the concentration of enzyme incubated with DFP had been too low. In an attempt to further study the possible enzymic role of factor XII, Speer et al. (1965) tested their purified preparations not only for esterolytic activity on TAMe, but also against appropriate substrates for acid and alkaline phosphatase, hyaluronidase, sulfatase, G-O and G-P transaminases, leucine amino peptidase, creatine phosphokinase, isocitric dehydrogenase, lactic dehydrogenase, amylase, lipase and aldolase, but failed to demonstrate activity of factor XII in any of these assay systems. However, reagents interfering with sulfhydryl, disulfide, amino, carboxyl and aliphatic hydroxyl groups destroyed factor XII activity. Destruction of hydrogen and ionic bonds proved equally lethal.

These conflicting reports have complicated the understanding of the role of factor XII in blood coagulation and especially its interaction with factor XI. At present, only hypotheses can be formulated. In our view, the best assumption precludes that both factor XII and XI are zymogens in "intact" plasma and that their interaction follows the Michaelis-Menten theory:

$$\text{Enzyme} + \text{Substrate} \rightleftharpoons \text{Enzyme-Substrate-Complex} \longrightarrow \text{Enzyme} + \text{Product} \qquad (6)$$

Translated in specific "glass contact activation" terms this would mean:

$$\text{Factor XII}_a + \text{Factor XI} \rightleftharpoons \text{Factor XII}_a\text{-XI-Complex} \longrightarrow \text{Factor XII}_a + \text{Enzymic factor XI} \qquad (7)$$

The complex formation would be initiated by factor XII being adsorbed onto suitable surfaces due to its hydrophilic characteristics. This could lead to a molecular reorientation or "activation" in which relatively more hydrophobic sites are exposed, as suggested by Vroman (1963, 1967, 1968). This in turn could provide a favorable hydrophobic bonding arrangement for factor XI which is a protein with hydrophobic characteristics (Vroman, 1963, 1967, 1968). The actual attachment of a factor XI molecule next or close to an adsorbed activated factor XII molecule could be aided by electrical charges since activated factor XII must be positively charged (the isoelectric point of activated Hageman factor is 7.8). During participation in this complex formation, factor XI zymogen could be activated by active factor XII, producing activated factor XI. Haanen et al. (1967) suggested that Hageman factor complexed with other factor XI molecules would no longer be able to react with other factor XI molecules. This would explain why the amount of active complex is proportional to the area of available surface. The adsorption of Hageman factor on surfaces, its activation and the subsequent activation of factor XI do not require the presence of calcium ions (Soulier and Prou-Wartelle, 1960; Ratnoff et al. 1961; Egli and Buscha, 1959; Davie and Ratnoff, 1965). Such a complex formation between factors XII and XI on suitable surfaces has been postulated by Hardisty and Margolis (1959), Soulier et al. (1958, 1959), Waaler (1959), Nossel (1964a) and more recently by Haanen et al. (1967). This concept is compatible with enzyme chemistry. Nevertheless, final proof of this hypothesis employing highly purified factor XII and XI preparations, is still pending.

Activated factor XI is supposed to activate factor IX and from kinetic studies it was concluded that factor XI was the enzyme acting on factor IX (see later). This raises the question whether factor XI is dissociated from the factor XII_a-XI complex before it acts on factor IX, or whether the entire complex is desorbed from the surface. Of course, the third possibility that they remain complexed on the surface cannot be excluded.

It has been recognized that the clot-promoting activity of contact activated plasma is unstable (Margolis, 1957; Ratnoff, 1958; Waaler, 1959; Nossel, 1964a). This cannot be attributed to lability of Hageman factor, since Schoenmakers et al. (1964), Haanen et al. (1967) and Mammen and Grammens (1967a, b) found their activated preparations to be very stable. No evidence is at present available for an inhibitor against activated factor XII (Ratnoff et al. 1961; Haanen et al. 1967; Mammen and Grammens, 1967a, b). Margolis (1958), Ratnoff and Rosenbluhm (1958), Ratnoff et al. (1961), Nossel (1964a), Iatridis et al. (1964a, b) and Nossel and Niemetz (1965) have presented evidence that activated factor XI is inhibited by an antifactor XI in plasma. The amount of factor XI left in serum was inversely proportional to the amount of activation product initially formed (Nossel, 1964a; Haanen et al. 1967). The factor XI inhibitor was recently purified from plasma (Niemetz and Nossel, 1967), and this purified inhibitor specifically inhibited factor XI activity. If activated factor XI is dissociated from the factor XII_a-XI complex, it would be inactivated by this inhibitor and new factor XI molecules would have the opportunity to complex with the already activated factor XII. This would lead to a continuous formation and deterioration of activated factor XI, ending in a complete consumption of factor XI during clotting. This is apparently not the case since factor XI is present in serum, indicating only a limited activation and consumption. Haanen et al. (1967) have demonstrated that factor XI is consumed only when factor XII and the contact surface are present simultaneously. Factor XII itself remains unaltered. These findings strongly suggest that the factor XII_a-XI complex exists after factor XI is inactivated. Keeping the inactivated factor XI in complex with factor XII would not only explain the limited activation of factor XI during clotting, but also its limited consumption. However, this interpretation does not take into account the simple experiment that contact activated plasma transferred to a siliconized test tube clots as fast upon recalcification as if it had been recalcified in the first place in a glass tube. This experiment seems to indicate that either activated factor XI dissociated from the complex, or the entire complex was desorbed, as suggested by many investigators. If all of the initially bound factor XII_a-XI complexes are desorbed, new factor XII molecules are adsorbed to the just vacated surface, leading to new complex formation. This in turn implies that in time all of the factor XII and XI would be consumed during clotting in a glass tube which is not the case, as pointed out. The answer to this problem very likely lies in the findings reported by Vroman (1967, 1968) that not only factor XII has an affinity to glass surfaces but that many other clotting and non-clotting proteins have the same characteristics. There is competition among the plasma proteins for any available wettable surface. This in turn suggests that only a limited number of factor XII molecules are adsorbed when plasma is exposed to glass surfaces, and that after desorption of some of the factor XII_a-XI complexes, the "vacant" surface area is occupied by proteins, other than factor XII. This would leave inactive Hageman factor molecules and also inactive factor XI molecules in plasma. This hypothesis, suggested by Haanen et al. (1961, 1967), would provide an explanation for most of the phenomena reported in association with glass contact activation.

Esnouf (1968) has recently offered another suggestion and indicated that factor XI might act like factor V in the prothrombin converting complex. This would mean that factor XI is not an enzyme, but rather a substance that aids factor XII in its enzymic function ("coenzyme-like"). This is certainly a possibility, but the implication is that the reported enzymic properties of factor XI arise from a contaminant which could be a hitherto unrecognized clotting factor. This difference in opinion can be only resolved when factor XI is isolated from plasma or serum in highly purified form.

b) Contact activation in vivo: The hypothetical mechanisms for contact activation, outlined above, apply a priori only to clotting in vitro, unless surface characteristics similar to glass can be demonstrated in vivo. The observation that ellagic acid produces "hypercoagulability" by activating Hageman factor (Ratnoff and Crum, 1963, 1964; Ratnoff et al. 1965; Botti and Ratnoff, 1963; Iatridis, 1966; Cliffton, 1967) is of some interest in this connection. Also, the findings that sodium urate crystals activate factor XII (Kellermeyer and Breckenridge, 1965), and that fatty acids, especially long chain fatty acids act similarly (Margolis, 1962; Didisheim and Mibashan, 1963; Nossel, 1964a; Connor et al. 1963) are of interest. For physiological considerations, the findings that collagen and elastin activate factor XII (Niewiarowski et al. 1964, 1965; Wilner et al. 1968) are of greatest interest. It will be remembered that collagen not only induces platelet adhesion and aggregation but also viscous metamorphosis (Zucker and Borelli, 1962; Spaet et al. 1962); it thereby facilitates the formation of the first hemostatic plug (see Chapter IX, p. 412). In view of our own findings that activated Hageman factor powerfully aggregates platelets (Mammen and Grammens, 1967a, b), the possibility must be considered that the collagen effect on platelet aggregation is mediated by activated Hageman factor. It is of further interest that Hageman factor is apparently adsorbed on platelet surfaces (Sharp, 1958; Waaler, 1959; Jürgens, 1962; Iatridis and Ferguson, 1965). If platelets adhere to collagen, the Hageman factor on the platelet surface would become activated. Thereby, platelet aggregation would be promoted. Undoubtedly, the positive electrical charges displayed by the activated factor XII could influence the adhesion of the negatively charged platelets. This is not to imply that other mechanisms of platelet adhesion and aggregation are not important. The factor XII mediated mechanism of platelet adhesion and aggregation on collagen might just be another pathway that apparently can be conveniently by-passed, since most patients with Hageman factor deficiency have normal platelet adhesiveness and aggregation (Salzman, 1963). Viscous metamorphosis leads to the release of platelet factor 3 (see Chapter IX, p. 412), a phospholipid which also has been found to activate Hageman factor (Lüscher, 1968). Quick (1960), Quick et al. (1961) had already indicated that erythrocyte stroma could induce contact activation. Since erythrocyte stroma and platelet factor 3 seem to contain the same phospholipids (Shinowara, 1957b, 1961; Barkhan et al. 1961; Troup et al. 1960), the contact activation effect of platelet factor 3 is not surprising. Ollendorff (1961, 1962) had already stressed the important dependence of contact activation on the presence of platelets. The close interrelationship of platelet factor 3 release and contact activation was demonstrated by Castaldi et al. (1965), who found that in thrombasthenic patients, the delayed platelet factor 3 release coincided with a slow contact activation.

These interesting observations clearly indicate that factor XII can adsorb and activate on collagen as well as on phospholipids from platelets and red cell stroma, and thereby initiate the intrinsic pathway of thrombin formation. This implies that factor XI is equally readily available for the subsequent interaction with activated factor XII. Taking into consideration the in vivo possibilities of contact activation, the formation of enzymic factor XI could occur as outlined in the following equation (Eq. 8):

$$\text{Phospholipids} + \text{Factor XII} \rightarrow \text{Phospholipid-Factor XII}_a\text{-Complex} + \text{Factor XI} \rightleftharpoons \text{Phospholipid-Factor XII}_a\text{-Factor XI-Complex} \rightarrow \text{Phospholipid-Factor XII}_a + \text{Activated Factor XI} \quad (8)$$

It must be kept in mind that the complex (Eq. 8) may not necessarily dissociate, and that the phospholipids can apparently be replaced by collagen.

This hypothesis must now be critically analysed in view of the findings that patients with a deficiency of Hageman factor have no clinically apparent bleeding disorder, while patients with factor XI deficiency have a bleeding problem. This seems to indicate that patients without Hageman factor are able to initiate the activation of factor XI by other pathways. As judged by in vitro experiments, these alternate pathways are certainly not as efficient as the pathway in persons *with* Hageman factor. Nevertheless, in vivo, this alternate mechanism must be adequate since these patients do not bleed. The efficiency of this alternate mechanism is born out by the fact that Mr. Hageman, after whom the disorder was named, recently died of pulmonary embolism (Ratnoff et al. 1968). Two patients with this disorder have been reported as having suffered from myocardial infarctions (Glueck and Roehill, 1966; Hoak et al. 1966), and Botti and Ratnoff (1964) have reported thrombophlebitis.

Since Connor et al. (1963) have suggested that long chain fatty acids in their salt form might activate factor XI directly, thus bypassing factor XII, it has been speculated that collagen or phospholipids may act similarly in vivo (Rapaport, 1959). However, this raises the question: How can surfaces convert a proenzyme to an enzyme, especially in view of the fact that factor XI apparently is a protein with entirely different surface characteristics than factor XII? One would almost have to postulate another enzyme which can substitute for factor XII and even if this were so, the real function of Hageman factor would have to be justified. The activation of the intrinsic thrombin forming potential in glass tubes can hardly be considered a reasonable explanation.

It has also been suggested that in vivo tissue thromboplastins might serve to bypass factor XII. Dilute tissue thromboplastins were found to correct the coagulation defect not only in factor XII but also in factor XI deficient plasmas, while plasmas deficient in other coagulation factors were not influenced (Biggs and Nossel, 1961; Josso and Prou-Wartelle, 1965). This finding suggests that both factors might be bypassed in vivo. This immediately raises another question: Why do patients with factor XI deficiency bleed when those with Hageman factor deficiency do not?

P. G. Iatridis et al. (1964) have indicated that only very small amounts of Hageman factor could liberate phospholipids from platelets and that patients with Hageman factor deficiency might have these small amounts available. This brings us back to my statement in the beginning of this review that we only *assume* that patients with coagulation defects have a *deficiency* in one or another factor. It is quite conceivable that patients with Hageman trait might have an abnormal factor XII molecule. Due to an abnormality in the molecular structure its function might be delayed but not totally absent. This hypothesis is certainly supported by the findings that plasma of patients with Hageman trait does not clot promptly in vitro, but in time it *will* clot. An analogous situation is represented in patients with "Fibrinogen Detroit" in which a single amino acid replacement was identified in the alpha (A) chain of the fibrinogen molecule (Blombäck et al. 1968). This fibrinogen is initially not clottable but in time it will clot (Mammen et al. 1969). Similar molecular aberrations may explain other coagulation defects.

c) Interaction of activated factor XI and factor IX: The possible interrelationship between contact activation and factor IX was first suggested by Rapaport et al. (1955) who found that glass contact led to the appearance of factor IX activity. Subsequently, several groups of investigators have presented additional evidence supporting this concept (Soulier et al. 1958; Caen and Bernard, 1958; Fisch, 1958; Fisch and Duckert, 1959; Waaler, 1959; Soulier and Prou-Wartelle, 1960; Ratnoff, 1960; Yin and Duckert, 1961; Duckert, 1961). The work of Ratnoff and Davie (1962a), Schiffman et al. (1963), Nossel (1964a, c) and Cattan and Denson (1964) indicated that activated factor XI was the enzyme which acted on factor IX as a substrate, converting the latter to activated factor IX. Factor XI required for its action the presence of divalent metal ions. Calcium ions were most effective (Kingdon et al. 1964; Kingdon and Davie, 1965). The enzymic action of factor XI on factor IX was inhibited by DFP (Ratnoff and Davie, 1962a), whereas factor IX activity itself was not inhibited by this compound. Kingdon et al. (1964) presented evidence that DFP reacted with the hydroxyl group of serine in the factor XI molecule.

The activation of factor IX by active factor XI was also inhibited by heparin and heparin analogs (Ratnoff and Davie, 1962a; Kingdon et al. 1964), the effect of which could be neutralized by protamine sulfate and Polybrene (Kingdon and Davie, 1965). Soybean trypsin inhibitor had no effect on the activation of factor IX (Ratnoff and Davie, 1962a).

The actual evidence that factor IX is activated in this way is only indirect since the chemical events are unknown, and an identification and separation of an inactive factor IX from an active factor IX has not been achieved. However, it is recognized that the amount of factor IX activity in serum is greater than in plasma (Benney and Lewis, 1959; Duckert, 1961; Lewis and Nour-Eldin, 1962). The addition of "contact product" (factor XI) or Celite will further increase the activity of factor IX in serum (Sen et al. 1967; Nossel, 1967).

Factor IX in plasma is a part of the prothrombin complex, and its complete separation from prothrombin has not been possible (Tishkoff et al. 1968). The generation of factor IX activity from the prothrombin complex has been studied by Mammen et al. (1960a) and here again the importance of contact has been recognized (Schröer et al. 1965). These data seem to indicate that the factor IX formation during clotting is intimately related to the contact phase.

d) Role of activated factor IX in the conversion of factor X: Early investigations of the intrinsic thrombin forming mechanism suggested that factors VIII and IX might interact with each other (Biggs et al. 1953a, b). Bergsagel and Hougie (1965), Hougie et al. (1957), Fisch and Duckert (1959), Biggs and Bidwell (1959) and Spaet and Cintron (1963) subsequently reported that these factors would act together with factor X and calcium ions to form "product I". Product I in turn was supposed to form together with platelet phospholipids and factor V a prothrombin converting activity, called product II. From the work of Macfarlane et al. (1964) it became apparent that factors VIII and IX interacted with each other to form a factor X converting activity. This activator reached its maximum activity within 2–4 minutes and then declined very rapidly. The activity could be regenerated by the addition of factor VIII, but not by adding factor IX, activated by contact product. Calcium ions were required for this reaction and phospholipids potentiated the factor X converting activity (Macfarlane, 1964). Similar results were obtained by Lundblad and Davie (1964). The implication was that the activity would derive from factor VIII upon its interaction by activated factor IX. Factor VIII was thought to be converted to its active form by activated factor IX in the presence of phospholipids and calcium ions (Lundblad and Davie, 1964). The activation of factor VIII could be blocked by heparin and heparin analogs, but neither DFP, nor soybean trypsin inhibitor affected this reaction (Lundblad and Davie, 1965). Rapaport et al. (1963) and Biggs et al. (1965) reported that thrombin had a powerful accelerating effect on the reaction between activated factor IX and factor VIII. The effect of thrombin was thought to be on factor VIII. It was speculated that factor VIII becomes "activated" by thrombin, possibly by dissociation from a protective association with fibrinogen. Thrombin in turn would destroy factor VIII activity. The effect of thrombin on factor VIII is thus very similar to its effect on factor V, as outlined before.

These experimental data led Macfarlane (1964a) and Davie and Ratnoff (1964) to propose that activated factor IX would activate factor VIII which in turn would convert inactive factor X to active factor X. Davie and Ratnoff (1964) added into their cascade (Fig. 1) the phospholipid and calcium ion requirement for activated factor IX. The postulate that factor VIII activates factor X was supported by experiments performed by Macfarlane (1963), Marfarlane and Ash (1964) and Lundblad and Davie (1965).

Apart from this sequence of indirect evidence, there is no further support that factor VIII is converted from an inactive to an active form. Activated factor VIII has not been isolated, and attempts to separate active factor IX and VIII from mixtures has resulted in the loss of activity (Hougie, 1966). No natural substrate for the enzymic form of factor VIII has been found as yet, and van Creveld et al. (1967) have found no evidence of enzymic activity on synthetic substrates. It must also be kept in mind that neither factor IX nor factor VIII have been purified sufficiently to meet stringent biochemical criteria for purity.

Recently, Seegers and Marciniak (1969) have found that purified autoprothrombin III (inactive factor X) could be converted to autoprothrombin C (active factor X) by factor VIII in the presence of phospholipids from platelets and calcium ions (Fig. 2). A large amount of factor VIII was needed, and on a weight basis, more than fifteen times the amount of factor VIII than autoprothrombin III was required to obtain activation. This relationship is very unusual for an enzyme substrate reaction and tends to favor the view that factor VIII is *not* an enzyme.

Hemker and Kahn (1967) and Barton (1967) have recently hypothesized that inactive factor X is converted to active factor X by a complex composed of activated factor IX, factor VIII, phospholipids and calcium ions. Both, factor VIII and factor IX were adsorbed on the surfaces of phospholipid micelles, and calcium ions were required for the binding of these two factors. Such a complex formation had already been suggested by Hougie (1966) using gel filtration techniques. Barton (1967) found that if this complex was rechromatographed in the absence of calcium ions, factor VIII and activated IX could be recovered unchanged, and no additional factor X activating activity could be eluted from the Sephadex columns. These findings strongly support the view that the function of factor VIII in this complex is analogous to that of factor V in the factor X complex (Eq. 4). According to this analogy, activated factor IX is the enzyme, calcium ions mediate the binding of the enzyme to the phospholipids, and factor VIII either controls the rate constant of the enzyme substrate complex or renders the substrate more susceptible to the enzyme. This sequence of events is represented in the following equation (Eq. 9):

$$\underbrace{\text{Activated factor IX} + \text{Factor VIII} + \text{Phospholipids} + \text{Calcium ions}}_{\text{Complex}}$$
$$\text{Factor X} \longrightarrow \text{Active factor X} \qquad (9)$$

This concept greatly unifies and simplifies the entire aspect of intrinsic and extrinsic thrombin formation and indicates that the generation of thrombin is facilitated by a number of complexes formed between phospholipids and various coagulation factors (Fig. 4). Some of these factors act as enzymes, while others have a "coenzyme-like" function.

C. Inhibitory Mechanisms

Like all physiological reactions, the thrombin forming mechanisms are counteracted by several inhibitor devices. The inhibitors are either directed against thrombin itself or against various reactions which lead to its formation. The first inhibitor device in the *intrinsic* pathway seems to be an anti-factor XI which can be found in plasma and serum (Margolis, 1957; Ratnoff and Rosenblum, 1958; Ratnoff et al. 1961; Nossel, 1964a; Iatridis et al. 1964a, b; Nossel and Niemetz, 1965). This inhibitor specifically blocks the enzymic action of factor XI (Niemetz and Nossel, 1967). This means that the activation of factor IX and consequently the complex formation between active factor IX, factor VIII, phospholipids and calcium ions (Eq. 9) can be kept under control by this inhibitor.

The second inhibitor mechanism in the *intrinsic* pathway is established at the level of the complex formed between activated factor IX, factor VIII, phospholipids and calcium ions (Eq. 9). It consists of the ability of factor VIII to complex with inhibitor source material. Inhibitor source material is a lipid, and very likely a glyceride which is normally present in plasma and serum (Johnson and Seegers, 1954; Mammen et al. 1960b; Mammen, 1965). This lipid forms a complex with factor VIII in the presence of thrombin. Factor VIII activity becomes neutralized during this complex formation. This results in its absence in serum, as described by Graham et al. (1951), Johnson et al. (1952), Penick (1957) and Rizza and Walker (1957). Removing factor VIII from plasma deprives activated factor IX of its "coenzyme" which will subsequently lead to a disturbed function of the factor IX-VIII-phospholipid-calcium complex. This in turn results in a controlled formation of activated factor X. Since thrombin is required for the initiation of this regulating device, this reaction can be regarded as a negative feedback mechanism.

The third inhibitor device consists of an inhibitor acting on activated factor X itself (antiplasma thromboplastin). There are strong indications that this inhibitor arises during the dissociation of the prothrombin complex (Schimpf, 1963; Schimpf et al. 1960, 1962; Mammen et al. 1960b; Seegers and Marciniak, 1965; Seegers et al. 1965a; Murano, 1966; Marciniak et al. 1967). The inhibitor competitively inhibits factor X activity (Murano, 1966; Marciniak et al. 1967). Since thrombin is the enzyme which leads to the dissociation of the prothrombin complex (Seegers et al. 1967a), this inhibitor device can also be considered a negative feedback mechanism. Once thrombin is formed, the inhibitor will counteract its further formation by blocking factor X activity.

The fourth line of defense is located at the level of the complex formed between activated factor X, factor V, phospholipids and calcium ions (Eq. 4). This time it is directed against factor V, the "coenzyme" to activated factor X and is mediated through the ability of thrombin to ultimately destroy human factor V, as reported by Ware et al. (1947b), Owren (1953), Lanchantin and Ware (1955), Hjort (1957), Johnston and Jensen (1958), Seegers (1962, 1967, 1968a), Rapaport et al. (1963), and Bergsagel and Nockolds (1965). The destruction of factor V, probably due to the proteolytic action of thrombin, results in the inability of the activated factor X-V-phospholipid-calcium-complex to form and thereby convert further prethrombin to thrombin. Again, this is a negative feedback mechanism.

The fifth and probably final inhibitor device is directed against thrombin itself and its inactivation by antithrombin. Several antithrombins have been recognized which specifically or nonspecifically inactivate thrombin. As outlined in Chapter VII, p. 268, the term antithrombin should be restricted to the native power of plasma or serum to neutralize thrombin. This antithrombin, also termed antithrombin III (Seegers et al. 1954), has been concentrated from plasma and serum (Monkhouse et al. 1955; Shinowara and Buckley, 1960; Monkhouse and Milojewic, 1963; Hensen and Loeliger, 1963) and some of its physicochemical characteristics have been described (Monkhouse and Clarke, 1957; Seegers et al., 1964a). From recent investigations it has become apparent that the so-called antithrombin II (heparin cofactor) is identical with antithrombin III (Lyttleton, 1954; Burstein, 1955; Burstein and Loeb, 1956; Monkhouse et al. 1955; Monkhouse and Clarke, 1957; Monkhouse, 1967), and that antithrombin IV (Seegers et al. 1954) is also identical with antithrombin III (Sokal, 1955; Seegers et al. 1964a; Monkhouse and Milojewic, 1965; Seegers, 1962). Antithrombin III destroys thrombin enzymatically, and in this process the antithrombin itself is apparently inactivated (Monkhouse, 1967). It has been found that the amount of antithrombin remaining in serum after clotting is inversely proportional to the amount of thrombin formed, indicating that antithrombin has indeed a protective function against the sudden appearance of thrombin in vivo (Monkhouse, 1967).

Although the initial destruction of some of the thrombin by antithrombin is rapid, the overall process of neutralization is progressive with time, and even under optimal conditions traces of thrombin remain active (Klein and Seegers, 1950).

It is of further interest that antithrombin III can neutralize activated factor X (autoprothrombin C).

Some of the thrombin may also be adsorbed on fibrin (antithrombin I effect), as originally described by Seegers et al. (1945b). This may account for the final removal of the last traces of thrombin at the site of fibrin formation. This antithrombin I effect is non-specific. The antithrombin VI effect, or the capability of fibrinogen split products to neutralize thrombin is also non-specific, as described by Triantaphyllopoulos (1957), Niewiarowski and Kowalski (1957) and Stormorken (1957). Although small amounts of fibrinogen split products are normally found in plasma and serum, their role in neutralizing thrombin under physiological conditions is not clearly understood. For details the reader is referred to Chapter VI, p. 247.

Some of the inhibitor mechanisms operative in the *extrinsic* pathway of thrombin formation are the same as the ones for the intrinsic pathway. These are the inhibitors against active factor X, the destruction of factor V by thrombin and the effect of antithrombin on thrombin. Whether the initial extrinsic complex ("tissue factor"-factor VII-phospholipids-calcium, Eq. 6) is controlled by special inhibitors remains obscure. The existence of "antitissue thromboplastins" has been described by several investigators (Schneider, 1947; Thomas, 1947; Lanchantin and Ware, 1953; Berry, 1957; Deutsch and Fuchs, 1958). From the few physicochemical properties known, this inhibitor could be identical with the inhibitor against activated factor X, derived during the dissociation of the prothrombin complex. On the other hand, the findings of Seegers et al. (1964c) that antithrombin also neutralizes factor VII (autoprothrombin I) might have some bearing on the physiological control of the early stage of the extrinsic system. It would indicate that the "coenzyme" for the "tissue factor" can be eliminated, thus rendering the complex (Eq. 6) less effective in the formation of activated factor X. It is conceivable that the amount of tissue thromboplastin released locally is limited because it is determined by the degree of tissue damage at the site of injury. Moreover, as long as blood flows by the site of injury, some tissue thromboplastin will be carried away from the site of later fibrin formation. This by itself might serve as some kind of a control device in the early stage of extrinsic thrombin formation.

This leaves sphingosine and phosphatidyl serine as additional possible inhibitors of thrombin formation, as outlined above. According to Hecht et al. (1957a, b) sphingosine blocked the development of thrombin from its precursor in vitro, via the intrinsic and extrinsic pathways. Although sphingosine is basically a constituent of brain tissue, small amounts may be present in plasma (Hecht, 1965). Whether these small amounts have any physiological significance in inhibiting thrombin formation is not known at present.

Whereas phosphatidyl serine in the micellar form has procoagulant activity (Kazal, 1965), it has anticoagulant properties in its solubilized form (Barkhan and Silver, 1962). Even if it should be released from platelets during viscous metamorphosis in the insoluble form, it can become solubilized by α_1-lipoproteins, β-lipoproteins and albumin (Kazal et al. 1962; Barkhan and Silver, 1962; Kazal, 1965). Such solubilized phosphatidyl serine-lipoprotein complexes had antithromboplastic (intrinsic) properties in the thromboplastin generation test and blocked the conversion of purified prothrombin to thrombin (Kazal et al. 1962; Holburn and Silver, 1964). The same anticoagulant effect was found in vivo (Mustard et al. 1962). The exact mechanism of action of phosphatidyl serine during clotting is not known, but it is conceivable that it has some regulatory control function in determining the rate of thrombin formation in vivo.

VI. Conclusions and Summary

The formation of thrombin from its zymogen is a complex mechanism in which several plasma coagulation factors participate together with phospholipids and calcium ions. It appears that several complexes are formed between phospholipids and certain coagulation proteins. In the absence of tissue breakdown products (tissue thromboplastin) the phospholipids seem to originate mainly from the platelets. However, erythrocyte stroma may also serve as a source of these phospholipids. Among the platelet or erythrocyte phospholipids, phosphatidyl ethanolamine and phosphatidyl serine are two phosphatides which participate in the formation of these complexes. To be effective they must be in the micellar form and they must possess a negative Zeta potential. In all instances, two coagulation proteins seem to be involved in each one of the complexes formed. One of these proteins may be an enzyme (activated factor X, factor IX, "tissue factor") which was generated from its proenzymic form by a preceding complex. The second protein seems to have no enzymic effect (factor V, factor VIII, factor VII) and its exact function remains obscure. Nevertheless, its presence is mandatory and it is assumed that this protein either controls the rate constant of the enzyme substrate complex formation or that it modifies the conformation of the substrate to render it more susceptible to the enzyme. Calcium ions seem to be necessary in the formation of these complexes because they favor the binding of the respective enzymes into the complex. The indication that these enzymic reactions leading to thrombin formation occur on phospholipid surfaces is unusual in terms of the common concepts of enzyme chemistry, but this mechanism apparently contributes to keep coagulation localized at sites of phospholipid availability. Coagulation in vivo is almost always preceded by platelet adhesion and aggregation, and platelets almost always accumulate first at a local site of injury. They attach themselves more or less to the injured vessel wall and as they undergo viscous metamorphosis, exposed phospholipids become available at sites for the various enzymic reactions leading to thrombin formation. Since almost all of the plasma coagulation factors are loosely adsorbed on the platelet surface, they are immediately available for use in these complexes. Without these provisions it would be very difficult to keep coagulation localized, and as long as blood flows by the site of injury, non-bound enzymes would be readily carried away.

Theoretically, local thrombin formation can be initiated in vivo by the release of tissue extracts (extrinsic pathway) or by the release of phosphatides from platelets or erythrocytes (intrinsic pathway). Even if coagulation is primarily initiated via the extrinsic pathway, the intrinsic pathway will be activated simultaneously. The first traces of thrombin induce viscous metamorphosis of the platelets and release of the platelet phosphatides. In contrast, the activation of the intrinsic pathway could proceed *without* the simultaneous participation of the extrinsic pathway. This reasoning is probably irrelevant for most *local* in vivo coagulation processes since local hemostasis or local thrombosis is accomplished by some kind of tissue damage in almost all instances. This, in turn, produces the release of tissue thromboplastin and the activation of the extrinsic pathway.

The entire concept of thrombin formation via both the extrinsic and intrinsic pathways, as outlined in this review, is schematically represented in Fig. 4. The actual formation of thrombin from prothrombin apparently proceeds through an intermediate, called prethrombin. The prothrombin molecule dissociates first to prethrombin. Prethrombin has as yet no enzymic activity, it is smaller than prothrombin and is, in contrast to prothrombin, already a two-chain molecule. One of the N-terminal amino acids is already identical to one later found in thrombin. The dissociation of prothrombin to prethrombin is apparently facilitated by thrombin only. This raises the question: Where does this initial thrombin come from? The answer remains at present uncertain. This reaction can be explained only by assuming that prothrombin could be converted directly to thrombin without going through the intermediate prethrombin. There is at present no experimental evidence to support this assumption, but such a possibility cannot be excluded. Prethrombin could be a laboratory artifact, and it is also possible that additional intermediates might be found.

The formation of thrombin from either prethrombin or prothrombin requires the presence

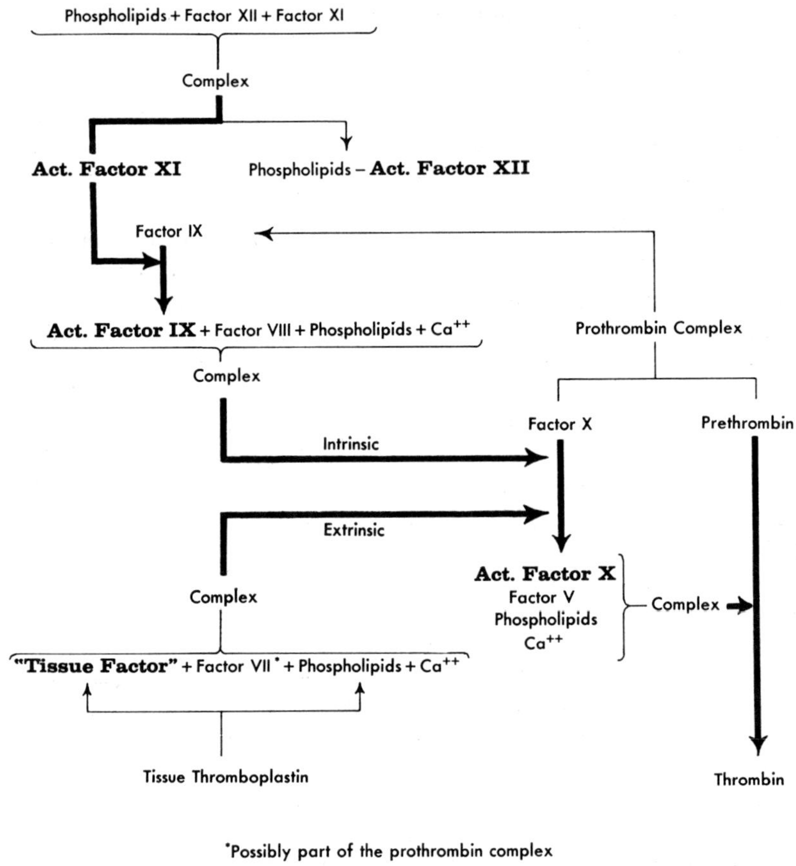

Fig. 4. Activation of prothrombin to thrombin via the intrinsic and extrinsic pathways. This concept incorporates the most recent findings and promotes the idea that several complexes, formed between phospholipids, certain coagulation factors and calcium ions, are involved in the formation of thrombin from prothrombin.

of activated factor X (autoprothrombin C). For optimal effect, activated factor X must be complexed with phospholipids and factor V (Fig. 4). Calcium ions favor the binding of activated factor X into the complex. The role of factor V remains somewhat uncertain. Most of the experimental evidence indicates that factor V is not an enzyme. Current evidence rather suggests that factor V is a protein which controls the rate constant of the enzyme-substrate complex formation or introduces conformational changes of the substrate. Factor V becomes more reactive when acted upon by thrombin, but the molecular changes produced by thrombin are unknown. It is also unknown whether this thrombin contact is a prerequisite for the proper action of factor V. All of these findings await further experimental studies once factor V can be obtained from plasma as a single molecular entity. In human plasma, factor V is ultimately destroyed by thrombin. This can be regarded as a negative feedback mechanism, and could be one important steering device in the mechanism of thrombin formation. The neutralization of activated factor X activity may represent a second steering device. Both the inactivation of factor X and the destruction of factor V would control the effect of the complex on the formation of thrombin. Activated factor X activity is competitively blocked by an inhibitor which apparently arises from the prothrombin complex during its dissociation. This mechanism of inactivation corresponds to the antiplasma thromboplastin concept. This inhibitor is at present only recognized as an activity, its purification has still to be accomplished. Activated factor X can also be inactivated by antithrombin, a substance present in plasma and serum. Before this thrombin forming complex can become operative, factor X must be activated into its enzymic form. This can be accomplished in two ways, the extrinsic pathway or the intrinsic pathway. Factor X seems to be a plasma protein which is closely related to prothrombin. It is, therefore, considered a part of the prothrombin complex. Recent evidence seems to indicate that it is not a part of the prothrombin molecule, as originally suggested by Seegers. It only shares several physicochemical properties with prothrombin.

The extrinsic pathway of factor X activation requires the release of tissue thromboplastin from tissues and cells. On the basis of recent experimental data, tissue thromboplastin seems to contain enzymic activity besides the various lipid constituents. The chemical nature of the enzymic activity is unknown, but some data indicate that it is an integral part of the chemical structure of tissue thromboplastin. It is possible that additional cell bound proteolytic enzymes participate in this reaction and cathepsins have been identified as prothrombin activators. In view of this uncertainty, the term "tissue factor" has been used to somehow characterize this enzymic activity (Fig. 4). Of the various lipids present in tissue thromboplastin, the phospholipids are again of greatest importance in the formation of active factor X. Whether these are identical to the phospholipids originating from platelets or erythrocytes remains to be elucidated. These phosphatides from tissue thromboplastin can also serve in the activated factor X-factor V-calcium complex. It is assumed that the "tissue factor" is the actual enzyme which converts factor X to enzymic factor X, and that factor VII acts like factor V in either controlling the rate constant of the enzyme substrate complex formation or in introducing conformational changes on inactive factor X. Calcium ions would probably favor the binding of the enzyme to the phospholipids. This complex concept also awaits further experimental proof, once the "tissue factor" and factor VII have been isolated. From biochemical point of view, factor VII seems to be closely related to factor X, as more recent investigations have revealed. This probably accounts for the great similarity of the clinical symptoms of factor VII and factor X "deficiencies". It is at present unknown whether there is an inhibitor mechanism which controls the effect of this complex on factor X. The information available on the so-called antitissue thromboplastins does not exclude with certainty that this effect might be directed against active factor X.

The formation of activated factor X by the intrinsic pathway is facilitated by a complex formed between activated factor IX, factor VIII, phospholipids from platelets or erythrocytes and calcium ions (Fig. 4). Activated factor IX might be the enzyme in this complex. It is apparently formed from a precursor which may be a part of the prothrombin complex. Factor IX is in many respects closely related to prothrombin, but it is not known with certainty whether it is a part of the prothrombin molecule, possibly a derivative, or a protein completely different from prothrombin. No separation of inactive and active factor IX has as yet been accomplished, and it remains to be seen whether the *purified* factor IX (autoprothrombin II) represents the active or the inactive form. The evidence indicating that activated factor IX is an enzyme is only indirect and awaits further study. Calcium ions might again favor the binding of activated factor IX onto the phospholipids. Factor VIII is a normal plasma constituent which has not been completely purified either, but so far no evidence has been found that it is an enzyme. It shares many properties with factor V, and it is assumed that its biological function might also be similar to that of factor V. It would thus be the protein in this particular complex which either controls the rate constant of the enzyme substrate complex formation or induces conformational changes on factor X. However, this assumption requires further proof and awaits the isolation and final purification of factor VIII. There is some indication that thrombin increases the reactivity of factor VIII and this has been interpreted as "activation". Ultimately, thrombin also catalyses the inactivation of factor VIII. But in contrast to factor V which seems to be digested by thrombin, factor VIII is complexed with a plasma lipid, called inhibitor source material. This lipid has some anticoagulant activity which disappears once it combines with factor VIII. The inactivation of factor VIII by thrombin again represents a negative feedback mechanism which controls the effectiveness of this complex on the activation of factor X. No anti-factor IX has as yet been identified.

The activation of factor IX from its precursor seems to be facilitated by activated factor XI. Factor XI in turn is activated by factor XII. This sequence of activation is also closely related to surfaces, and extensive studies in vitro have been performed using glass or similar inorganic surfaces. The sequence of events seems to begin with the adsorption of factor XII onto these surfaces. Factor XII has hydrophilic characteristics and its adsorption on wettable surfaces apparently produces a molecular reorientation. It is speculated that during the molecular change more hydrophobic sites of the protein are exposed. Factor XI has basically hydrophobic characteristics which could favor its attachment to the reorientated factor XII molecule. It is known that the reorientation of the factor XII molecule is associated with a shift in the isoelectric point toward the alkaline side, suggesting a positive surface charge. This positive charge could further favor the binding of factor XI. Factor XI has so far only been concentrated from plasma, but its enzymic function seems to be fairly well established. Nothing is as yet known about inactive factor XI or inactive factor XII. In contrast to active factor XI, the "enzymic" form of factor XII has been isolated from plasma of various species, but some controversy still exists with regard to various physicochemical properties.

In vivo, factor XII is readily adsorbed on phospholipids and collagen. Very likely these two establish the proper surface for factor XII and XI adsorption and interaction. It is not known with certainty whether the two factors, once activated, dissociate from their initial complex with the surfaces or whether they remain attached. There is some evidence that some of the activity which acts on factor IX is indeed detached. These reactions await further experimental study and confirmation. Most of the evidence supporting this assumption is at present indirect.

In as much as the fine details of the presented concept of thrombin formation remain to be elaborated on, the overall concept seems to be feasable, attractive and practical. It would establish a certain basic pattern for all reactions leading to thrombin formation. The concept is compatible with all physiological principles called upon to maintain homeostasis. The concept is not only in accordance with kinetic studies, but it also seems to account for most of the experimental evidence accumulated by supporters of the cascade or waterfall concept as well as by the supporters of the Seegers concept. It becomes evident that the emphasis for future work in this interesting field of human physiology must be placed on *biochemical* studies, and it is hoped that more biochemists will find blood coagulation as attractive and challenging as DNA and RNA.

References

Achenbach, W., Egli, H., Kesseler, K. H., and Overkamp, H. (1959). *Deut. Med. Wochschr. 84,* 675.

Addis, T. (1911). *J. Pathol. Bacteriol. 15,* 427.

Aggeler, P. M., White, S. G., Glendenning, M. B., Page, E. W., Leake, T. B., and Bates, G. (1952). *Proc. Soc. Exptl. Biol. Med. 79,* 692.

Aggeler, P. M., Spaet, T. H., and Emery, B. E. (1954a). *Science 119,* 806.

Aggeler, P. M., Spaet, T. H., White, S. G., Fowell, A., and Johnson, F. (1954b). *Rev. Hématol. 9,* 447.

Alexander, B. (1952). *Rev. Hématol. 7,* 168.

Alexander, B. (1955). *New Engl. J. Med. 252,* 423, 484, 526.

Alexander, B. (1959). *Proc. 4th Intern. Congr. Biochem., Vienna,* 1958. *10,* 37.

Alexander, B. (1961). *Thromb. Diath. Haemorrhag. Suppl. 3,* 392.

Alexander, B., and Landwehr, G. (1948). *J. Clin. Invest. 27,* 98.

Alexander, B., and Odake, K. (1967). *Federation Proc. 26,* 487.

Alexander, B., and Pechet, L. (1962). *Proc. 8th Congr. Eur. Soc. Haematol. Vienna,* 1961. Paper No. 404. Karger, Basel.

Alexander, B., De Vries, A., and Goldstein, R. (1948). *J. Clin. Invest. 27,* 523.

Alexander, B., De Vries, A., Goldstein, R., and Landwehr, G. (1949a). *Science 109,* 545.

Alexander, B., De Vries, A., and Goldstein, R. (1949b). *Blood, 4,* 739.

Alexander, B., Goldstein, R., and Landwehr, G. (1950). *J. Clin. Invest. 29,* 881.

Alexander, B., Goldstein, R., Landwehr, G., and Cook, C. D. (1951). *J. Clin. Invest. 30,* 596.

Alexander, B., Goldstein, R., Rich, L., Le Bolloch, A. G., Diamond, L. K., and Borges, W. (1954). *Blood 9,* 843

Alkjaersig, N., Abe, T., Johnson, S. A., and Seegers, W. H. (1955a). *Am. J. Physiol. 182,* 443.

Alkjaersig, N., Abe, T., and Seegers, W. H. (1955b). *Am. J. Physiol. 181,* 304.

Anderson, G. F., and Barnhart, M. I. (1964). *Am. J. Physiol. 206,* 929.

Aoki, N., Harmison, C. R., and Seegers, W. H. (1963). *Can. J. Biochem. Physiol. 41,* 2409.
Aronson, D. L. (1966). *Thromb. Diath. Haemorrhag. 16,* 491.
Aronson, D. L., and Ménache, D. (1966). *Biochemistry 5,* 2635.
Aronson, D. L., Preiss, J. W., and Mosesson, M. W. (1962). *Thromb. Diath. Haemorrhag. 8,* 270.
Asada, T., Masaki, Y., Kitahara, K., Nagayama, R., Hatashita, T., and Yanagisawa, I. (1961). *J. Biochem. 49,* 721.
Baker, W. J., and Seegers, W. H. (1967). *Thromb. Diath. Haemorrhag. 17,* 205.
Bangham, A. D. (1961). *Nature 192,* 1197.
Barkhan, P., and Silver, M. J. (1962). *Prog. Hematol. 3,* 170.
Barkhan, P., Silver, M. J., Da Costa, P. B., and Tocantins, L. M (1958). *Nature 182,* 1031.
Barkhan, P., Silver, M. J., and O'Keefe, L. M. (1961). In *"Blood Platelets"* (S. A. Johnson, R. W. Monto, J. W. Rebuck, and R. C. Horn, Eds.) pp. 303—318. Little, Brown and Co., Boston.
Barnhart, M. I., Ferar, J., and Aoki, N. (1963). *Federation Proc. 22,* 164.
Barrow, E. M., Amos, S. M., Heindel, C., and Graham, J. B. (1966a). *Proc. Soc. Exptl. Biol. Med. 121,* 1001.
Barrow, E. M., Amos, S., and Graham, J. B. (1966b). *J. Lab. Clin. Med. 68,* 803.
Barth, P., Kommerell, B., and Pfleiderer, T. (1966). *Thromb. Diath. Haemorrhag. 16,* 378.
Barton, P. G. (1967). *Nature 215,* 1508.
Barton, P. G., and Hanahan, D. J. (1967). *Biochim. Biophys. Acta 133,* 506.
Barton, P. G., Jackson, C. M., and Hanahan, D. J. (1967). *Nature 214,* 923.
Baughman, D. J., and Waugh, D. F. (1967). *J. Biol. Chem. 242,* 5252.
Baumgarten, W., Sanders, B. E., Belkin, B. D., Pagenkemper, F. F., Albers, W. G., and Ciminera, J. L. (1963). *Thromb. Diath. Haemorrhag. 9,* 354.
Becker, E. L. (1960). *J. Lab. Clin. Med. 56* 136.
Bendien, W. M., and Van Creveld, S. (1936). *Maandschr. Kindergeneesk. 6,* 179.
Benney, W. E., and Lewis, F. J. W. (1959). *J. Clin. Pathol. 12,* 551.
Berg, W., Korsan-Bengtsen, K., and Igge, J. (1966). *Thromb. Diath. Haemorrhag. 15,* 501.
Bergsagel, D. E. (1956). *Brit. J. Haematol. 2,* 130
Bergsagel, D. E., and Hougie, C. (1956). *Brit. J. Haematol. 2,* 113.
Bergsagel, D. E., and Nockolds, E. R. (1965). *Brit. J. Haematol. 11,* 395.
Berry, C. G. (1957). *J. Clin. Pathol. 10,* 342.
Bidwell, E. (1955a). *Brit. J. Haematol. 1,* 35.
Bidwell, E. (1955b). *Brit. J. Haematol. 1,* 386.
Bidwell, E. (1962). *Thromb. Diath. Haemorrhag. Suppl. 5,* 205.
Bidwell, E., Dike, G. W., and Denson, K. W. (1966). *Brit. J. Haematol. 12,* 583.
Bidwell, E., Booth, J. M., Dike, G. W., and Denson, K. W. E. (1967). *Brit. J. Haematol. 13,* 568.
Biggs, R., and Bidwell, E. (1959). *Proc. 4th. Intern. Congr. Biochem., Vienna,* 1958, *10,* 172.
Biggs, R., and Douglas, A. S. (1953). *J. Clin. Pathol. 6,* 23.
Biggs, R., and Nossel, H. L. (1961). *Thromb. Diath. Haemorrhag. 6,* 1.
Biggs, R., Douglas, A. S., Macfarlane, R. G., Dacie, J. V., Pitney, W. R., Merskey, C., and O'Brien, J. R. (1952). *Brit. Med. J. II,* 1378.
Biggs, R., Douglas, A. S., and Macfarlane, R. G. (1953a). *J. Physiol. 119,* 89.
Biggs, R., Douglas, A. S., and Macfarlane, R. G. (1953b). *J. Physiol. 122,* 538.
Biggs, R., Douglas, A. S., and Macfarlane, R. G. (1953c). *J. Physiol. 122,* 554.
Biggs, R., Sharp, A. A., Margolis, J., Hardisty, R. M., Stewart, J., and Davidson, W. M. (1958). *Brit. J. Haematol. 4,* 177.
Biggs, R., Bidwell, E., Handley, D. A., Macfarlane, R. G., Trueta, J., Elliot-Smith, A., Dike, G. W., and Ash, B. J. (1961). *Brit. J. Haematol. 7,* 349.
Biggs, R., Macfarlane, R. G., Denson, K. W., and Ash, B. J. (1965). *Brit. J. Haematol. 11,* 276.
Blatrix, C., and Soulier, J. P. (1959). *Pathol. et Biol. 7,* 2477.
Blatrix, C., Steinbuch, M., and Soulier, J. P. (1959). *Pathol. et Biol. 7,* 2487.
Blombäck, B. (1964). *In* "The Hemophilias" (K. M. Brinkhous, Ed.). pp. 118—128. University of North Carolina Press, Chapel Hill.
Blombäck, B., and Blombäck, M. (1963). *Nature 198,* 886.
Blombäck, B., Blombäck, M., and Struwe, I. (1962). *Thromb. Diath. Haemorrhag. Suppl. 5,* 172.
Blombäck, M. (1958). *Arkiv Kemi 12,* 387.
Blombäck, M., Blombäck, B., Mammen, E. F., and Prasad, A. S. (1968). *Nature 218,* 134.
Bordet, J. (1919). *C. R. Soc. Biol. 82,* 896.
Bordet, J., and Gengou, O. (1901). *Ann. Inst. Pasteur 15,* 129.
Bordet, J., and Gengou, O. (1904). *Ann. Inst. Pasteur 18,* 98.
Botti, R. E., and Ratnoff, O. D. (1964). *J. Lab. Clin. Med. 64,* 385.
Brand, E. (1946). *Ann. N. Y. Acad. Sci. 47,* 187.
Breckenridge, R. T., and Ratnoff, O. D. (1963). *Am. J. Med. 35,* 813.
Breckenridge, R. T., and Ratnoff, O. D. (1964). *Clin. Research 12,* 221
Breckenridge, R. T., and Ratnoff, O. D. (1965). *Thromb. Diath. Haemorrhag. 17,* 217.
Brinkhous, K. M. (1939). *Am. J. Med. Sci. 198,* 509.
Brinkhous, K. M. (1958). *Proc. 6th Congr. Intern. Soc. Hematol., Boston, 1956,* p. 463, Grune and Stratton, New York.
Brinkhous, K. M. (1959). *Ann. Rev. Physiol. 21,* 271.
Brinkhous, K. M., and Wagner, R. H. (1959). *Proc. 4th Intern. Congr. Biochem. Vienna, 1958,* Vol. 10, pp. 1—12. Pergamon, New York.
Brinkhous, K. M., Shanbrom, E., Roberts, H. R., Webster, W. P., Fekete, L., and Wagner, R. H. (1968). *J. Am. Med. Assoc. 205,* 613.
Brown, D. L., Hardisty, R. M., Kosoy, M. H., and Bracken, C. (1967). *Brit. med. J. 2,* 79.
Burstein, M. (1955). *Arch. Intern. Pharmacodynam. 101,* 285.
Burstein, M., and Loeb, J. (1956). *Rev. Franc. études Clin. Biol. 1,* 752.
Caen, J., and Bernard, J. (1958). *Rev. Hématol. 13,* 154.
Caldwell, M. J., and Seegers, W. H. (1965). *Thromb. Diath. Haemorrhag. 13,* 373.
Carter, J. R., and Warner, E. D. (1954). *Am. J Physiol.* 179, 549
Carter, J. R., and Warner, E. D. (1956). *Am. J. Physiol. 184,* 195.
Castaldi, P. A., Larrieu, M. J., and Caen, J. (1965). *Nature 207,* 422.
Cattan, A. D., and Denson, K. W. E. (1964). *Thromb. Diath. Haemorrhag. 11,* 155.
Chargaff, E. (1937). *J. Biol. Chem. 121,* 175.
Chargaff, E. (1945). *Advan. Enzymol. 5,* 31.
Chargaff, E., and Bendich, A. (1944). *Science 99,* 147.
Chargaff, E., Moore, D. H., and Bendich, A. (1942). *J. Biol. Chem. 145,* 593.
Chargaff, E., Bendich, A., and Cohen, S. S. (1944). *J. Biol. Chem. 156,* 161.
Cliffton, E. E. (1967). *Am. J. Med. Sci. 254,* 483.
Cohen, S. S., and Chargaff, E. (1941a). *J. Biol. Chem. 139,* 741.
Cohen, S. S., and Chargaff, E. (1941b). *J. Biol. Chem. 140,* 689.
Cohn, E. J., Strong, L. E., Hughes, W. L., Mulford, D. J., Ashworth, D. J., Melin, M., and Taylor, H. L. (1946). *J. Am. Chem. Soc. 68,* 459.
Cole, E. R., Marciniak, E., and Seegers, W. H. (1962). *Thromb. Diath. Haemorrhag. 8,* 434.
Cole, E. R., Koppel, J. L., and Olwin, J. H. (1964). *Can. J. Biochem. 42,* 1595.
Cole, E. R., Koppel, J. L., and Olwin, J. H. (1965). *Thromb. Diath. Haemorrhag. 14,* 431.
Collingwood, B. J., and MacMahon, M. T. (1912). *J. Physiol. 45,* 119.
Conley, C. L., Hartmann, R. C., and Morse, W. I. (1949). *J. Clin. Invest. 28,* 340.
Connor, W. E., Hoak, J. C., and Warner, E. D. (1963). *J. Clin Invest. 42,* 860.
Cox, F. M., Lanchantin, G. F., and Ware, A. G. (1956). *J. Clin Invest. 35,* 106.
Daemen, F. J. M., Van Arkel, C., Hart, H. C., Van der Drift, C., and Van Deenen, L. L. M. (1965). *Thromb. Diath. Haemorrhag. 13,* 194.

Dale, H. H., and Walpole, G. S. (1916). *Biochem. J. 10,* 331.
Davie, E. W., and Ratnoff, O. D. (1964). *Science 145,* 1310.
Davie, E. W., and Ratnoff, O. D. (1965). *In:* "The Proteins" (H. Neurath, ed.) 2. Edition, Vol. III, pp. 359—443. Academic Press, New York.
Deutsch, E., and Fuchs, H. (1958). *Acta Haematol. 20,* 97.
Deutsch, E., and Mammen, E. (1958). *Thromb. Diath. Haemorrhag. 2,* 324.
Deutsch, E., and Schaden, W. (1953). *Biochem. Ztschr. 324,* 266.
Deutsch, E., Köbele, B., and Nesvadba, H. (1962). *Wiener Ztschr. Inn. Med. 43,* 248.
Deutsch, E., Irsigler, K., and Lomoschitz, H. (1964). *Thromb. Diath. Haemorrhag. 12,* 12.
Deutsch, E., Lechner, K., and Schmer, G. (1966). *Thromb. Diath. Haemorrhag. Suppl. 20,* 275.
De Vries, A., Alexander, B., and Goldstein, R. (1949). *Blood 4,* 247.
Didisheim, P. (1959). *Federation Proc. 18,* 474.
Didisheim, P. (1962). *Arch. Int. Med. 110,* 170.
Didisheim, P., and Mibashan, R. S. (1963). *Thromb. Diath. Haemorrhag. 9,* 346.
Didisheim, P., Loeb, J., Blatrix, C., and Soulier, J. P. (1959a). *J. Lab. Clin. Med. 53,* 322.
Didisheim, P., Hattori, K., and Lewis, J. H. (1959b). *J. Lab. Clin. Med. 53,* 866.
Donaldson, V. H. (1968). *J. Exptl. Med. 127,* 411.
Donaldson, V. H., and Ratnoff, O. D. (1965). *Science 150,* 754.
Douglas, A. S. (1952). *Lancet 2,* 761.
Douglas, A. S. (1955). *Brit. Med. Bull. 11,* 39.
Douglas, A. S. (1956). *J. Clin. Invest. 35,* 533.
Duckert, F. (1961). *Thromb. Diath. Haemorrhag. 6,* 254.
Duckert, F., Koller, F., and Matter, M. (1953). *Proc. Soc. Exptl. Biol. Med. 82,* 259.
Duckert, F., Yin, E. T., and Straub, W. (1961). *In* "Protides of the Biological Fluids" (H. Peeters, Ed.) pp. 41—45. Elsevier, Amsterdam.
Edman, P. (1950). *Acta Chem. Scand. 4,* 277, 283.
Edman, P., and Sjöquist, J. (1956). *Acta Chem. Scand. 10,* 1507.
Egli, H., and Buscha, H. (1959). *Thromb. Diath. Haemorrhag. 3,* 604.
Egli, H., Kesseler, K., and Klesper, R. (1957). *Acta Haematol. 17,* 338.
Ehrenpreis, S., Leach, S. J., and Sheraga, H. A. (1957). *J. Am. Chem. Soc. 79,* 6086.
Elmore, D. T., and Curragh, E. F. (1963). *Biochem. J. 86,* 9.
Esnouf, M. P. (1965), *Bibliotheca Haematol. 23,* 1337.
Esnouf, M. P. (1968). *Plenary Session Papers, 12th Intern. Soc. Hematol., New York,* 315.
Esnouf, M. P., and Jobin, F. (1965). *Thromb. Diath. Haemorrhag. Suppl. 17,* 103.
Esnouf, M. P., and Jobin, F. (1967). *Biochem. J. 102,* 660.
Esnouf, M. P., and Macfarlane, R. G. (1968). *Advances Enzymol. 30,* 255.
Esnouf, M. P., and Williams, W. J. (1962a). *Biochem. J. 84,* 52.
Esnouf, M. P., and Williams, W. J. (1962b). *Biochem. J. 84,* 62.
Esnouf, M. P., and Williams, W. J. (1962c). *Thromb. Diath. Haemorrhag. Suppl. 5,* 213.
Esnouf, M. P., Jobin, F., and Peden, J. C. (1963). *Biochem. J. 89,* 44.
Fahey, J. L., Ware, A. G., and Seegers, W. H. (1948). *Am. J. Physiol. 154,* 122.
Feissly, R., and Fried., A. (1924). *Klin. Wochschr. 3,* 831.
Fenichel, R. L., and Rose, L. (1961). *Thromb. Diath. Haemorrhag. 5,* 601.
Ferguson, J. H., Marcus, A. J., and Robinson, A. J. (1963). *Blood 22,* 19.
Fisch, U. (1958). *Thromb. Diath. Haemorrhag. 2,* 60.
Fisch, U., and Duckert, F. (1959). *Thromb. Diath. Haemorrhag. 3,* 98.
Fischer, A., and Hecht, E. (1934). *Biochem. Z. 269,* 115.
Flory, P. J., and Fox, T. G. (1950). *J. Polymer. Sci. 5,* 745.
Flynn, J. E., and Coon, R. W. (1953). *Am. J. Physiol. 175,* 289.
Freund, E. (1888). *Wien. Med. Jahrbuch 3,* 259.
Gladner, J. A., and Laki, K. (1956). *Arch. Biochem. Biophys. 62,* 501.
Gladner, J. A., and Laki, K. (1958). *J. Am. Chem. Soc. 80,* 1263.
Glueck, H. I., and Roehill, W. (1966). *Ann. Int. Med. 64,* 390.
Gobbi, F. (1960). *Thromb. Diath. Haemorrhag. 4,* 253.
Goldstein, R., LeBolloch, A., Alexander, B., and Zonderman, E. (1959). *J. Biol. Chem. 234,* 2857.
Goulian, M., and Beck, W. S. (1966). *Nature 211,* 74.
Govaertz, P., and Gratia, A. (1931). *Rev. Belge Sci. Med. 3,* 689.
Graham, J. B., Penick, G. D., and Brinkhous, K. M. (1951). *Am. J. Physiol. 164,* 710.
Graham, R. C., Ebert, R. H., Ratnoff, O. D., and Moses, J. M. (1965). *J. Exptl. Med. 121,* 807.
Gray, E. J., Schaefer, E. H., and Jensen, H. (1956). *Acta Haematol. 15,* 314.
Gray, W. R., and Hartley, B. S. (1963). *Biochem. J. 89,* 59.
Guest, M. M., and Ware, A. G. (1950). *Science 112,* 21.
Gugler, E. (1966). *Thromb. Diath. Haemorrhag. Suppl. 19,* 119.
Haanen, C., Hommes, F., Benraad, H., and Morselt, G. (1961). *Thromb. Diath. Haemorrhag. 5,* 201.
Haanen, C., Morselt, G., Schoenmakers, J., Maters, M., and Braams, M. (1965). *Scand. J. Haematol. 2,* 248.
Haanen, C., Morselt, G., and Schoenmakers, J. (1967). *Thromb. Diath. Haemorrhag. 17,* 307.
Habermann, E. (1966). *In* "Neue Aspekte der Trasylol Therapie" (R. Gross and G. Kroneberg, Eds.) pp. 126—134. Schattauer Verlag, Stuttgart.
Habermann, E. (1968). Personal Communication.
Hackett, E., and LePage, R. (1961). *Australian J. Exptl. Biol. Med. Sci. 39,* 67.
Hardisty, R. M. (1955). *Brit. J. Haematol. 1,* 323.
Hardisty, R. M., and Margolis, J. (1959). *Brit. J. Haematol. 5,* 203.
Harmison, C. R., and Mammen, E. F. (1967). *In* "Blood Clotting Enzymology" (W. H. Seegers, Ed.) pp. 23—101. Academic Press, New York.
Harmison, C. R., and Seegers, W. H. (1962). *J. Biol. Chem. 237,* 3074.
Harmison, C. R., Landaburu, R. H., and Seegers, W. H. (1961). *J. Biol. Chem. 236,* 1693.
Harmison, C. R., Schröer, H., and Seegers, W. H. (1965). *Thromb. Diath. Haemorrhag. 13,* 587.
Hartmann, R. C., Conley, C. L., and Lalley, J. S. (1949). *Bull. John Hopkins Hosp. 85,* 231.
Hecht, E. (1951a). *Nature 161,* 279, 633.
Hecht, E. (1951b). *Ned. Tijdschr. Geneesk. 95,* 2371.
Hecht, E. (1953). *Acta Haematol. 9,* 237.
Hecht, E. (1965). "Lipids in Blood Clotting". Charles C. Thomas, Springfield, Illinois.
Hecht, E. (1966a). *Med. Welt 40,* 2139.
Hecht, E. (1966b). *Thromb. Diath. Haemorrhag. Suppl. 19,* 149.
Hecht, E., and Oosterbaan Van Lit, W. L. (1967). *Thromb. Diath. Haemorrhag. 18,* 223.
Hecht, E., and Shapiro, D. (1957a). *Thromb. Diath. Haemorrhag. 1,* 359.
Hecht, E., and Shapiro, D. (1957b). *Science 125,* 1041.
Hecht, E., and Slotta, K. H. (1962). *Am. J. Clin. Pathol. 37,* 126.
Hecht, E., Landaburu, R. H., Cho, M. H., and Seegers, W. H. (1957a). *Z. Physiol. Chem. Hoppe-Seyler's 307,* 263.
Hecht, E., Landaburu, R. H., and Seegers, W. H. (1957b). *Am. J. Physiol. 189,* 203.
Hecht, E., Cho, M. H., and Seegers, W. H. (1958). *Am. J. Physiol 193,* 584.
Hemker, H. C., and Kahn, M. J. P. (1967). *Nature 215,* 1201.
Hemker, H. C., Hemker, P. W., and Loeliger, E. A. (1965). *Thromb. Diath. Haemorrhag. 13,* 155.
Hemker, H. C., Esnouf, M. P., Hemker, P. W., Swart, A. C. W., and Marfarlane, R. G. (1967). *Nature 215,* 248.
Hensen, A., and Loeliger, E. A. (1963). *Thromb. Diath. Haemorrhag. Suppl. 10,* 3—84.
Hershgold, E. J., and Sprawls, S. (1966). *Federation Proc. 25,* 317.
Hershgold, E. J., Pool, J. G., and Pappenhagen, A. R. (1966). *J. Lab. Clin. Med. 67,* 23.
Hershgold, E., Silverman, L., Davidson, A., and Janszen, M. (1967). *Federation Proc. 26,* 488.
Hink, J. H., and Johnson, F. F. (1964). *In* "The Hemophilias" (K. M. Brinkhous, Ed.) pp. 156—158. University of North Carolina Press, Chapel Hill.
Hjort, P. F. (1957). *Scand. J. Clin. Lab. Invest. 9, Suppl. 27,* 1.
Hoak, J. C., Swanson, L. W., Warner, E. D., and Connor, W. E. (1966). *Lancet 2,* 884.

Högenauer, E., Lechner, K., and Deutsch, E. (1968). *Thromb. Diath. Haemorrhag. 19,* 304.
Hoelzl-Wallach, D. F., Maurice, P. A., Steele, B. B., and Surgenor, D. M. (1959). *J. Biol. Chem. 234,* 2829.
Holburn, R. R., and Silver, M. J. (1964). *Thromb. Diath. Haemorrhag. 11,* 283.
Holemans, R., and Roberts, H. R. (1964). *J. Lab. Clin. Med. 64,* 778.
Holemans, R., McConnell, D., and Johnston, J. G. (1966). *Am. J. Med. Sci. 251,* 557.
Holman, C. A., and Wolf, P. (1963). *Lancet II,* 4.
Horowitz, H. I., and Spaet, T. H. (1961). *J. Appl. Physiol. 16,* 112.
Hougie, C. (1956). *Proc. Soc. Exptl. Biol. Med. 93,* 570.
Hougie, C. (1957). *J. Lab. Clin. Med. 50,* 61.
Hougie, C. (1959). *Proc. Soc. Exptl. Biol. Med. 101,* 132.
Hougie, C. (1966). *Federation Proc. 25,* 193.
Hougie, C., Barrow, E. M., and Graham, J. B. (1957). *J. Clin. Invest. 36,* 485.
Howell, W. H. (1914). *Arch. Int. Med. 13,* 76.
Howell, W. H., and Cekade, E. B. (1926). *Am. J. Physiol. 78,* 500.
Hurt, J. P., Wagner, R. H., and Brinkhous, K. M. (1966a). *Thromb. Diath. Haemorrhag. 15,* 327.
Hurt, J. P., Wagner, R. H., and Brinkhous, K. M. (1966b). *Federation Proc. 25,* 317.
Hussain, Q. Z., and Newcomb, T. F. (1963). *Ann. Biochem. 23,* 569.
Hussain, Q. Z., and Newcomb, T. F. (1964). *Proc. Soc. Exptl. Biol. Med. 115,* 301.
Iatridis, P. G., and Ferguson, J. H. (1965). *Thromb. Diath. Haemorrhag. 13,* 114.
Iatridis, P. G., Ferguson, J. H., and Iatridis, S. G. (1964). *Thromb. Diath. Haemorrhag. 11,* 355.
Iatridis, S. G. (1966). *Hemostase 6,* 363.
Iatridis, S. G., and Ferguson, J. H. (1962). *J. Clin. Invest. 41,* 1277.
Iatridis, S. G., Ferguson, J. H., Iatridis, P. G., and Mauldin, R. (1964a). *Thromb. Diath. Haemorrhag. 12,* 35.
Iatridis, S. G., Iatridis, P. G., and Ferguson, J. H. (1964b). *Thromb. Diath. Haemorrhag. 12,* 489.
Irsigler, K. (1964). *Thromb. Diath. Haemorrhag. Suppl. 13,* 433.
Jackson, C. M., and Hanahan, D. J. (1968). *Biochemistry 7,* 4506.
Janiak, A., and Soulier, J. P. (1962). *Thromb. Diath. Haemorrhag. 8,* 406.
Jensen, H., Gray, E. J., and Schaefer, E. H. (1955). *Acta Haematol. 13,* 377.
Jobin, F., and Esnouf, M. P. (1967). *Biochem. J. 102,* 666.
Johnson, A. J., Newman, J., Howell, M. B., and Puszkin, S. (1967). *Thromb. Diath. Haemorrhag. Suppl. 26,* 377.
Johnson, S. A., and Seegers, W. H. (1953). *Mich. State Med. J. 52,* 537.
Johnson, S. A., and Seegers, W. H. (1954). *Rev. Hématol. 9,* 529.
Johnson, S. A., and Seegers, W. H. (1956). *Circulation Res. 4,* 182.
Johnson, S. A., Rutzky, J., Schneider, C. L., and Seegers, W. H. (1952). *Proc. 4th Congr. Intern. Hematol., Mar Del Plata, 1952,* 373.
Johnson, S. A., Seegers, W. H., Koppel, J. L., and Olwin, J. H. (1957). *Thromb. Diath. Haemorrhag. 1,* 158.
Johnson, S. A., Sturrock, R. M., and Rebuck, J. W. (1959). *Proc. 4th Intern. Congr. Biochem., Vienna, 1958, 10,* 105.
Johnston, B. R., and Jensen, H. (1958). *Am. J. Physiol. 194,* 1.
Johnston, C. L., and Barrow, E. S. (1965). *Scand. J. Clin. Lab. Invest. 17, Suppl. 84,* 52.
Johnston, C. L., and Hjort, P. F. (1961). *J. Clin. Invest. 40,* 743.
Johnston, C. L., Ferguson, J. H., and O'Hanlon, F. A. (1958). *Proc. Soc. Exptl. Biol. Med. 99,* 197.
Johnston, C. L., Ferguson, J. H., O'Hanlon, F. A., and Payne, R. B. (1959a). *Proc. Soc. Exptl. Biol. Med. 101,* 747.
Johnston, C. L., Ferguson, J. H., O'Hanlon, F. A., and Black, W. L. (1959b). *Thromb. Diath. Haemorrhag. 3,* 367.
Josso, F., and Prou-Wartelle, O. (1965). *Thromb. Diath. Haemorrhag. Suppl. 17,* 35.
Jürgens, J. (1962). *Thromb. Diath. Haemorrhag. 7,* 48.
Kalinke, H., and Egli, H. (1967). *Thromb. Diath. Haemorrhag. 18,* 389.
Kazal, L. A. (1965). *Trans. N. Y. Acad. Sci. 27,* 613.
Kazal, L. A., Miller, O. P., Turner, D. L., and Tocantins, L. M. (1962). *Federation Proc. 21,* 59.
Kekwick, R. A., and Walton, P. L. (1962). *Nature 194,* 878.
Kekwick, R. A., and Walton, P. L. (1965). *Brit. J. Haematol. 11,* 537.
Kekwick, R. A., and Wolf, P. (1957). *Lancet 272,* 647.
Kellermeyer, R. W. (1967). *J. Lab. Clin. Med. 70,* 372.
Kellermeyer, R. W., and Breckenridge, R. T. (1965). *J. Lab. Clin. Med. 65,* 307.
Kezdy, F. J., Lorand, L., and Miller, K. D. (1965). *Biochemistry 4,* 2302.
Kingdon, H. S., and Davie, E. W. (1965). *Thromb. Diath. Haemorrhag. Suppl. 17,* 15.
Kingdon, H. S., Davie, E. W., and Ratnoff, O. D. (1964). *Biochemistry 3,* 166.
Kisker, C. T. (1967). *Thromb. Diath. Haemorrhag. 17,* 381.
Klein, P. D., and Seegers, W. H. (1950). *Blood 5,* 742.
Klesper, R., and Egli, H. (1957). *Proc. 6th Congr. Europ. Soc. Hematol. Copenhagen, 1957,* 529.
Kline, D. L. (1965). *Ann. Rev. Physiol. 27,* 285.
Koller, F., Krüsi, G., and Luchsinger, G. (1950). *Schweiz. Med. Wochschr. 80,* 1101.
Koller, F., Loeliger, A., and Duckert, F. (1951). *Acta Haematol. 6,* 1.
Koller, F., Loeliger, A., and Duckert, F. (1952). *Rev. Hématol. 7,* 156.
Korsan-Bengtsen, K., and Ygge, J. (1961). *Scand. J. Clin. Lab. Invest. 13,* 604.
Kowarzyk, H., and Marciniak, E. (1961). *Polski Tygod. Lekar. 16,* 1641.
Kowarzyk, H., Marciniak, E., and Czerwinska, B. (1961). *Arch. Immunol. Terap. Doswiadczalne 9,* 719.
Laki, K., and Gladner, J. A. (1964). *Physiol. Rev. 44,* 127.
Laki, K., Kominz, D. R., Symonds, P., Lorand, L., and Seegers, W. H. (1954). *Arch. Biochem. Biophys. 49,* 276.
Lampert, H. (1931). "Die Physikalische Seite des Blutgerinnungsproblems". Thieme, Leipzig.
Lamy, F., and Waugh, D. F. (1953). *J. Biol. Chem. 203,* 489.
Lamy, F., and Waugh, D. F. (1954). *Physiol. Rev. 34,* 722.
Lamy, F., and Waugh, D. F. (1958). *Thromb. Diath. Haemorrhag. 2,* 188.
Lanchantin, G. F., and Friedmann, J. A. (1963). *Proc. Soc. Exptl. Biol. Med. 114,* 584.
Lanchantin, G. F., and Ware, A. G. (1953). *J. Clin. Invest. 32,* 381.
Lanchantin, G. F., and Ware, A. G. (1955). *Biochim. Biophys. Acta 18,* 288.
Lanchantin, G. F., Friedmann, J. A., DeGroot, J., and Mehl, J. W. (1963). *J. Biol. Chem. 238,* 238.
Lanchantin, G. F., Friedmann, J. A., and Hart, D. W. (1965a). *J. Biol. Chem. 240,* 3276.
Lanchantin, G. F., Presant, C. A., Hart, D. W., and Friedmann, J. A. (1965b). *Thromb. Diath. Haemorrhag. 14,* 159.
Lanchantin, G. F., Friedmann, J. A., and Hart, D. W. (1967). *J. Biol. Chem. 242,* 2491.
Lanchantin, G. F., Hart, D. W., Friedmann, J. A., Saavedra, N. V., and Mehl, J. W. (1968a). *J. Biol. Chem. 243,* 5479.
Lanchantin, G. F., Friedmann, J. A., and Hart, D. W. (1968b). *J. Biol. Chem. 243,* 476.
Landaburu, R. H., and Seegers, W. H. (1959). *Can. J. Biochem. Physiol. 37,* 1361.
Landaburu, R. H., and Seegers, W. H. (1961). *Thromb. Diath. Haemorrhag. 6,* 435.
Landaburu, R. H., Abdala, O. E., and Morrone, M. J. (1965). *Science 148,* 380.
Langdell, R. D. (1962). *Thromb. Diath. Haemorrhag. Suppl. 5, 192.*
Lechner, K., and Deutsch, E. (1965). *Thromb. Diath. Haemorrhag. 13,* 314.
Lenggenhager, K. (1936). *Klin. Wochschr. 15,* 1835.
Lenggenhager, K. (1940). *Helv. Med. Acta 7,* 262.
Levine, W. G., and Neuhaus, O. W. (1959). *Proc. Soc. Exptl. Biol. Med. 101,* 64.
Lewis, F. J., and Nour-Eldin, F. (1962). *Blood 20,* 41.
Lewis, J. H. (1964). *Proc. Soc. Exptl. Biol. Med. 116,* 120.

Lewis, J. H., and Merchant, W. R. (1958), *J. Clin. Invest. 37,* 911.
Lewis, J. H., Walters, D., Didisheim, P., and Merchant, W. R. (1958). *J. Clin. Invest. 37,* 1323.
Lewis, M. L., and Ware, A. G. (1953). *Proc. Soc. Exptl. Biol. Med. 84.* 636.
Lewis, M. L., and Ware, A. G. (1954). *Blood 9,* 520.
Li, L. F., and Olson, R. E. (1967). *J. Biol. Chem. 242,* 5611.
Lister, J. (1863). *Proc. Roy. Soc. (London) 12,* 580.
Liston, R. (1839). *Lancet II,* 137.
Lorand, L., Alkjaersig, N., and Seegers, W. H. (1953). *Arch. Biochem. Biophys. 45,* 312.
Lorand, L., Brannen, W. T., and Rule, N. G. (1962). *Arch Biochem. Biophys. 96,* 147.
Lüscher, E. F. (1968). *Thromb. Diath. Haemorrhag. Suppl. 25,* 79.
Lundblad, R. L., and Davie, E. W. (1964). *Biochemistry 3,* 1720.
Lundblad, R. L., and Davie, E. W. (1965). *Biochemistry 4,* 113.
Lyttleton, J. W. (1954). *Biochem. J. 58,* 8.
Macfarlane, R. G. (1961). *Brit. J. Haematol. 7,* 496.
Macfarlane, R. G. (1963). *Thromb. Diath. Haemorrhag. Suppl. 11,* 221.
Macfarlane, R. G. (1964a). *Nature 202,* 498.
Macfarlane, R. G. (1964b). *In* "Metabolism and Physiological Significance of Lipids" (R. M. C. Dawson and D. N. Rhodes, Eds.) pp. 325—335, Wiley, London-New York.
Macfarlane, R. G. (1965). *Thromb. Diath. Haemorrhag. Suppl. 17,* 45.
Macfarlane, R. G. (1966). *Thromb. Diath. Haemorrhag. 15,* 591.
Macfarlane, R. G., and Ash, B. J. (1964). *Brit. J. Haematol. 10,* 217.
Macfarlane, R. G., Biggs, R., Ash, B. J., and Denson, K. W. (1964). *Brit. J. Haematol. 10,* 530.
Magnusson, S. (1958). *Acta Chem. Scand. 12,* 355.
Magnusson, S. (1964). *Arkiv Kemi 23,* 271.
Magnusson, S. (1965a). *Arkiv Kemi 24,* 367.
Magnusson, S. (1965b). *Arkiv Kemi 23,* 271.
Magnusson, S. (1065c). *Arkiv Kemi 24,* 349.
Magnusson, S. (1965d). *Arkiv Kemi 23,* 285.
Magnusson, S. (1965e). *Arkiv Kemi 24,* 375.
Magnusson, S. (1965f). *Arkiv Kemi 24,* 217.
Magnusson, S. (1968). Personal Communication.
Magnusson, S., and Steele, B. (1965). *Arkiv Kemi 24,* 359.
Mammen, E. F. (1963a). *Vox Sang. 8,* 474.
Mammen, E. F. (1963b). *Thromb. Diath. Haemorrhag. 9,* 30.
Mammen, E. F. (1964a). *In* "The Hemophilias" (K. M. Brinkhous, Ed.), pp. 174—176. University of North Carolina Press, Chapel Hill.
Mammen, E. F. (1964b). *Thromb. Diath. Haemorrhag. 11,* 127.
Mammen, E. F. (1964c). *Thromb. Diath. Haemorrhag. Suppl. 14,* 89.
Mammen, E. F. (1965). *Federation Proc. 24,* 452.
Mammen, E. F. (1967a). *In* "Blood Clotting Enzymology" (W. H. Seegers, Ed.) pp. 421—485. Academic Press, New York.
Mammen, E. F. (1967b). *In* "Blood Clotting Enzymology" (W. H. Seegers, Ed.) pp. 345—377. Academic Press, New York.
Mammen, E. F. (1968). *Thromb. Diath. Haemorrhag. Suppl. 25,* 15.
Mammen, E. F., and Grammens, G. L. (1967a). *Federation Proc. 26,* 760.
Mammen, E. F., and Grammens, G. L. (1967b). *Thromb. Diath. Haemorrhag. 18,* 306.
Mammen, E. F., Thomas, W. R., and Seegers, W. H. (1960a). *Thromb. Diath. Haemorrhag. 5,* 218.
Mammen, E. F., Yoshinari, M., and Seegers, W. H. (1960b). *Thromb. Diath. Haemorrhag. 5,* 38.
Mammen, E. F., Prasad, A. S., Barnhart, M. I., and Au, C. C. (1969). *J. Clin. Invest. 48,* 235.
Mann, F. D., and Hurn, M. (1950). *Am. J. Clin. Pathol. 20,* 225.
Mann, F. D., and Hurn, M. (1951). *Am. J. Physiol. 164,* 105.
Mann, F. D., and Hurn, M. M. (1953). *Am. J. Physiol. 175,* 65.
Marciniak, E. (1961). *Bull. Acad. Polon. Sci. Ser. Sci. Biol. 9,* 381.
Marciniak, E., and Seegers, W. H. (1962). *Can. J. Biochem. Physiol. 40,* 597.
Marciniak, E., and Seegers, W. H. (1965). *New Istanbul Contrib. Clin. Sci. 8,* 117.
Marciniak, E., and Seegers, W. H. (1966a). *Thromb. Diath. Haemorrhag. 15,* 633.
Marciniak, E., and Seegers, W. H. (1966b). *Nature 209,* 621.
Marciniak, E., Rodriguez-Erdmann, F., and Seegers, W. H. (1962a). *Science 137,* 421.
Marciniak, E., Cole, E. R., and Seegers, W. H. (1962b). *Nature 195,* 1305.
Marciniak, E., Cole, E. R., and Seegers, W. H. (1962c). *Thromb. Diath. Haemorrhag. 8,* 425.
Marciniak, E., Murano, G., and Seegers, W. H. (1967). *Thromb. Diath. Haemorrhag. 18,* 161.
Marcus, A. J., and Spaet, T. H. (1958). *J. Clin. Invest. 37,* 1836.
Marcus, A. J., and Zucker-Franklin, D. (1964). *J. Clin. Invest. 43,* 1241.
Marcus, A. J., and Zucker, M. B. (1965). "The Physiology of Blood Platelets". Grune and Stratton, New York.
Marcus, A. J., Ullman, H. L., Safier, L. B. and Ballard, H. S. (1962). *J. Clin. Invest. 41,* 2198.
Margolis, J. (1956). *Nature 178,* 805.
Margolis, J. (1957). *J. Physiol. 137,* 95.
Margolis, J. (1958a). *Nature 182,* 1102.
Margolis, J. (1958b). *J. Physiol. 144,* 1.
Margolis, J. (1958c). *Nature 181,* 635.
Margolis, J. (1959). *Australian J. Exptl. Biol. Med. Sci. 37,* 239.
Margolis, J. (1960). *J. Physiol. 151,* 238.
Margolis, J. (1962). *Australian J. Exptl. Biol. Med. Sci. 40,* 505.
Margolis, J. (1963). *Ann. N. Y. Acad. Sci. 104,* 133.
Markwardt, F., Hoffmann, A., and Landmann, H. (1964). *Thromb. Diath. Haemorrhag. 11,* 230.
Marshall, C. G. (1965). M. Sc. Thesis, Wayne State Univ.. Detroit, Michigan.
Martin, C. J., Golubow, J., and Axelrod, A. E. (1959). *J. Biol. Chem. 234,* 1718.
Matačić, S., and Loewy, A. G. (1966). *Biochem. Biophys. Res. Commun. 24,* 858.
Maupin, B. (1959). *Sang. 30,* 114.
McClaughry, R. I., and Seegers, W. H. (1952). *Proc. Soc. Exptl. Biol. Med. 80,* 372.
Mellanby, J. (1909). *J. Physiol. 38,* 28.
Mertz, E. T., Seegers, W. H., and Smith, H. P. (1939). *Proc. Soc. Exptl. Biol. Med. 41,* 657.
Michael, S. E., and Tunnah, G. W. (1963). *Brit. J. Haematol. 9,* 236.
Michael, S. E., and Tunnah, G. W. (1966). *Brit. J. Haematol. 12,* 115.
Miller, K. D. (1958). *J. Biol. Chem. 231,* 987.
Miller, K. D., and Copeland, W. H. (1962). *Proc. Soc. Exptl. Biol. Med. 111,* 512.
Miller, K. D., and Copeland. W. H. (1965). *Exptl. Mol. Pathol. 4,* 431.
Miller, K. D., and MacGarrahan, J. F. (1958). *N. Y. State Dept. Health, Ann. Rept. Div. Lab. Res., 1958.* 69.
Miller, K. D., and Phelan, A. W. (1967). *Biochem. Biophys. Res. Commun. 27,* 505.
Miller, K. D., and Van Vunakis, H. (1956a). *J. Michigan State Med. Soc. 55,* 967.
Miller, K. D., and Van Vunakis, H. (1956b). *J. Biol. Chem. 223,* 227.
Miller, K. D., Brown, R. K., Casillas, G., and Seegers, W. H. (1959). *Thromb. Diath. Haemorrhag. 3,* 362.
Miller, K. D., Copeland, W. H., and Lawson, W. B. (1965). *Thromb. Diath. Haemorrhag. 8,* 575.
Milstone, J. H. (1942). *J. Gen. Physiol. 25,* 679.
Milstone, J. H. (1947). *Science 106,* 546.
Milstone, J. H. (1948). *Proc. Soc. Exptl. Biol. Med. 68,* 225.
Milstone, J. H. (1949). *Proc. Soc. Exptl. Biol. Med. 72,* 315.
Milstone, J. H. (1951). *J. Gen. Physiol. 35,* 67.
Milstone, J. H. (1952a). *Yale J. Biol. Med. 25,* 19.
Milstone, J. H. (1952b). *Yale J. Biol. Med. 25,* 173.
Milstone, J. H. (1952c). *Medicine 31,* 411.
Milstone, J. H. (1955). *J. Gen. Physiol. 38,* 757.
Milstone, J. H. (1959a). *J. Gen. Physiol. 42,* 665.
Milstone, J. H. (1959b). *Proc. Soc. Exptl. Biol. Med. 101,* 660.
Milstone, J. H. (1960a). *Nature 187,* 1127.

Milstone, J. H. (1960b). *Proc. Soc. Exptl. Biol. Med. 103,* 361.

Milstone, J. H. (1962). *J. Gen. Physiol. 45, No. 4, Part 2 (Suppl.),* 103.

Milstone, J. H. (1964). *Federation Proc. 23,* 742.

Milstone, J. H., Oulianoff, N., and Milstone, V. K. (1963). *J. Gen. Physiol. 47,* 315.

Monkhouse, F. C. (1967). *In* "Blood Clotting Enzymology". (W. H. Seegers, Ed.) pp. 323—344. Academic Press, New York.

Monkhouse, F. C., and Clarke, D. W. (1957). *Can. J. Biochem. Physiol. 35,* 373.

Monkhouse, F. C., and Milojevic, S. (1963). *Thromb. Diath. Haemorrhag. 9,* 221.

Monkhouse, F. C., and Milojevic, S. (1965). *Can. J. Physiol. Pharmacol. 43,* 819.

Monkhouse, F. C., France, E. S., and Seegers, W. H. (1955). *Circulation Res. 3,* 397.

Moore, H. C., Lux, S. E., Malhorta, O. P., Bakerman, S., and Carter, F. R. (1965). *Biochem. Biophys. Acta 111,* 174.

Morawitz, P. (1904). *Deut. Arch. Klin. Med. 79,* 1.

Morawitz, P. (1905). *Ergeb. Physiol. 4,* 307.

Morrison, F. S. (1966). *Blood 28,* 479.

Mulder, E. (1961). *Thromb. Diath. Haemorrhag. 6,* 160.

Murano, G. (1966). "Prothrombin Derivate As An Anticoagulant". M. Sc. Thesis, Wayne State University, Detroit, Michigan.

Murano, G. (1968). "Some Biochemical Aspects of the Prothrombin Complex". Ph. D. Dissertation, Wayne State University, Detroit.

Murano, G. (1969). Personal Communication.

Murphy, R. C., Ware, A. G., and Seegers, W. H. (1947). *Am. J. Physiol. 151,* 338.

Mustard, J. F., Medway, W., Downie, H. G., and Roswell, H. C. (1962). *Nature 196,* 1063.

Nemerson, Y. (1966). *Biochemistry 5,* 601.

Nemerson, Y. (1968). *J. Clin. Invest. 47,* 72.

Nemerson, Y., and Spaet, T. H. (1964). *Blood 23,* 657.

Niemetz, J., and Nossel, H. L. (1967). *Thromb. Diath. Haemorrhag. 17,* 335.

Niemetz, J., Weilland, C., and Soulier, J. P. (1961). *Nouvelle Rev. Franc. Hématol. 1,* 880.

Niewiarowski, S., and Kowalski, E. (1957). *Bull. Acad. Polon. Sci. Classe II 5,* 169.

Niewiarowski, S., and Prou-Wartelle, O. (1959). *Thromb. Diath. Haemorrhag. 3,* 593.

Niewiarowski, S., Stachurska, J., and Wegrzynowicz, Z. (1962). *Thromb. Diath. Haemorrhag. 7,* 514.

Niewiarowski, S., Bańkowski, E., and Fiedoruk, T. (1964), *Experentia 20,* 367.

Niewiarowski, S., Bańkowski, E., and Rogowicka, I. (1965). *Thromb. Diath. Haemorrhag. 14,* 387.

Nolf, P., (1908). *Arch. Intern. Physiol. 6,* 306.

Nolf, P. (1945). *Schweiz. Med. Wochschr. 75,* 110.

Norman, J. C., Lambilliotte, J. P., Kojima, Y., and Sise, H. S. (1967). *Science 158,* 1060.

Nossel, H. L. (1964a). "The Contact Phase of Blood Coagulation". Blackwell, Oxford.

Nossel, H. L. (1964b). *In* "The Hemophilias". (K. M. Brinkhous, Ed.), pp. 166—172. University of North Carolina Press, Chapel Hill.

Nossel, H. L. (1964c). *Thromb. Diath. Haemorrhag. 12,* 505.

Nossel, H. L. (1966). *Proc. Soc. Exptl. Biol. Med. 122,* 16.

Nossel, H. L. (1967). *Blood 29,* 331.

Nossel, H. L., and Niemetz, J. (1965), *Blood 25,* 712.

Nossel, H. L., Rubin, H., Drillings, M., and Hsieh, R. (1968). *J. Clin. Invest. 47,* 1172.

Nour-Eldin, F. (1963). *Nature 199,* 187.

Nour-Eldin, F., and Wilkinson, J. F. (1958a). *Brit. J. Haematol. 4,* 38.

Nour-Eldin, F., and Wilkinson, J. F. (1958b). *Brit. J. Haematol. 4,* 292.

O'Brien, J. R. (1956). *J. Clin. Pathol. 9,* 47.

Ollendorff, P. (1961). *Thromb. Diath. Haemorrhag. 6,* 104.

Ollendorff, P. (1962). *Scand. J. Clin. Lab. Invest. 14,* 641.

Osborn, E. C. (1965). *Clin. Chim. Acta 12,* 415.

Owen, C. A., and Bollman, J. L. (1948). *Proc. Soc. Exptl. Biol. Med. 67.* 231.

Owen, C. A., and McKenzie, B. F. (1954). *J. Appl. Physiol. 6,* 696.

Owen, C. A., Magath, T. B., and Bollman, J. L. (1951). *Am. J. Physiol. 166,* 1.

Owren, P. A. (1947a). *Acta Med. Scand. 128, Suppl. 194,* 1.

Owren, P. A. (1947b). *Lancet I,* 446.

Owren, P. A. (1948). *Biochem. J. 43,* 136.

Owren, P. A. (1951). *Scand. J. Clin. Lab. Invest. 3,* 168.

Owren, P. A. (1953). *Am. J. Med. 14,* 201.

Owren, P. A. (1961). *Thromb. Diath. Haemorrhag. Suppl. 3,* 387.

Papahadjopoulos, D., and Hanahan, D. J. (1964). *Biochim. Biophys. Acta 90,* 436.

Papahadjopoulos, D., Hougie, C., and Hanahan, D. J. (1962). *Proc. Soc. Exptl. Biol. Med. 111,* 412.

Papahadjopoulos, D., Yin, E. T., and Hanahan, D. J. (1964a). *Biochemistry 3,* 1931.

Papahadjopoulos, D., Hougie, C., and Hanahan, D. J. (1964b). *Biochemistry 3,* 264.

Patek, A. J., and Stetson, R. P. (1936). *J. Clin. Invest. 15,* 531.

Pavlovsky, A. (1947). *Blood 2,* 185.

Pavlovsky, A., Peterson, H., Casillas, G., Simonetti, C., and Canaveri, A. M. (1962). *Thromb. Diath. Haemorrhag. Suppl. 5,* 197.

Pechet, L., and Alexander, B. (1961). *Federation Proc. 20,* 57.

Pechet, L., Alexander, B. and Tishkoff, G. H. (1960), *Thromb. Diath. Haemorrhag. Suppl. 1,* 47.

Penick, G. D. (1957). *Proc. Soc. Exptl. Biol. Med. 96,* 277.

Penner, J. A., and Seegers, W. H. (1956). *Am. J. Physiol. 186,* 343.

Penner, J. A. , Duckert, F., Johnson, S. A., and Seegers, W. H. (1956). *Can. J. Biochem. Physiol. 34,* 1199.

Pool, J. G. (1966). *Federation Proc. 25,* 317.

Pool, J. G., and Robinson, J. (1959). *Brit. J. Haematol. 5,* 17.

Pool, J. G., and Shannon, A. E. (1965). *Federation Proc. 24,* 512.

Pool, J. G., Hershgold, E. J., and Pappenhagen, A. R. (1964). *Nature 203,* 312.

Poole, J. C. F., and Robinson, D. S. (1956). *Quart. J. Exptl. Physiol. 41,* 295.

Prentice, C. R. M., Ratnoff, O. D., and Breckenridge, R. T. (1967). *Brit. J. Haematol. 13,* 898.

Prydz, H. (1964). *Scand. J. Clin. Lab. Invest. 16,* 101.

Prydz, H. (1965). *Scand. J. Clin. Lab. Invest. 17, Suppl. 84,* 78.

Purcell, G. M., and Barnhart, M. I. (1963). *Biochim. Biophys. Acta 78,* 800.

Quick, A. J. (1935). *J. Biol. Chem. 109,* 73.

Quick, A. J. (1936). *Am. J. Physiol. 114,* 282.

Quick, A. J. (1940). *Science 92,* 113.

Quick, A. J. (1943). *Am. J. Physiol. 140,* 212.

Quick, A. J. (1960). *Am. J. Med. Sci. 239,* 51.

Quick, A. J., and Stefanini, M. (1948). *Proc. Soc. Exptl. Biol. Med. 67,* 111.

Quick, A. J., Inglis, J. A., and Halliday, J. W. (1961). *Nature 192,* 882.

Ramot, B., Angelopoulos, B., and Singer, K. (1955). *Arch. Internal Med. 95,* 705.

Rapaport, S. I. (1959). *Angiology 10,* 391.

Rapaport, S. I., Aas, K., and Owren, P. A. (1955). *J. Clin. Invest. 34,* 9.

Rapaport, S. I., Ames, S. B., and Mikkelsen, S. (1959). *Am. J. Clin. Pathol. 31,* 297.

Rapaport, S. I., Schiffman, S., Patch, M. J., and Ames, S. B. (1963). *Blood 21,* 221.

Rapport, M. M. (1956). *Nature 178,* 591.

Ratnoff, O. D. (1954), *J. Lab. Clin. Med. 44,* 915.

Ratnoff, O. D. (1958). *J. Clin. Invest. 37,* 923.

Ratnoff, O. D. (1960). *Thromb. Diath. Haemorrhag. Suppl. 1,* 116.

Ratnoff, O. D. (1962). Cited by Davie, E. W., and Ratnoff, O. D., *In* "The Proteins" (H. Neurath, Ed.) Vol. III, p. 359. Academic Press, New York.

Ratnoff, O. D., and Colopy, J. E. (1955). *J. Clin. Invest. 34,* 602.

Ratnoff, O. D., and Conley, C. L. (1951). *Bull. John Hopkins Hosp. 89,* 245.

Ratnoff, O. D., and Crum, J. D. (1963). *J. Lab. Clin. Med. 62,* 1006.

Ratnoff, O. D., and Crum, J. D. (1964). *J. Lab. Clin. Med. 63,* 359.
Ratnoff, O. D., and Davie, E. W. (1962a). *Biochemistry 1,* 677.
Ratnoff, O. D., and Davie, E. W. (1962b). *Biochemistry 1,* 967.
Ratnoff, O. D., and Miles, A. A. (1964). *Brit. J. Exptl. Pathol. 45,* 328.
Ratnoff, O. D., and Rosenblum, J. M. (1957). *J. Lab. Clin. Med. 50,* 941.
Ratnoff, O. D., and Rosenblum, J. M. (1958). *Am. J. Med. 25,* 160.
Ratnoff, O. D., Davie, E. W., and Mallett, D. L. (1961). *J. Clin. Invest. 40.* 803.
Ratnoff, O. D., Botti, R. E., Crum, J. D., and Donaldson, V. H. (1965). *Thromb. Diath. Haemorrhag. Suppl. 17,* 7.
Ratnoff, O. D., Busse, R. J., and Sheon, R. P. (1968). *New Engl. J. Med. 279,* 760.
Rauschenbach, F. (1882). "Über die Wechselwirkung zwischen Protoplasma und Blutplasma mit einem Anhang betreffend die Blutplättchen von Bizzozero." Laakmann, Dorpat.
Riddle, J. M., Bernstein, M. H., and Seegers, W. H. (1963). *Thromb. Diath. Haemorrhag. 9,* 12.
Rizza, C., and Walker, W. (1957). *Nature 180,* 143.
Rizza, C. R., Chan, K. E., and Henderson, M. P. (1965). *Nature* 207, 90.
Robinson, D. S., and Poole, J. C. F. (1956). *Quart. J. Exptl. Physiol. 41,* 36.
Rodman, N. F., Mason, R. G., McDevitt, N. B., and Brinkhous, K. M. (1962). *Am. J. Pathol. 40,* 271.
Ronwin, E. (1959). *Biochim. Biophys. Acta 33,* 326.
Rosenthal, R. L. (1955). *J. Lab. Clin. Med. 45,* 123.
Rosenthal, R. L. (1961). *Thromb. Diath. Haemorrhag. Suppl. 3,* 379.
Rosenthal, R. L., Dreskin, O. H., and Rosenthal, N. (1953), *Proc. Soc. Exptl. Biol. Med. 82,* 171.
Rouser, G., and Schloredt, D. (1958). *Biochim. Biophys. Acta 28,* 81.
Rouser, G., White, S. G., and Schloredt, D. (1958). *Biochim. Biophys. Acta 28,* 71.
Salzman, E. W. (1963). *J. Lab. Clin. Med. 62,* 724.
Sanger, F. (1945). *Biochem. J. 39,* 507.
Schiffman, S., Rapaport, S. I., Ware, A. G., and Mehl, J. W. (1960). *Proc. Soc. Exptl. Biol. Med. 105,* 453.
Schiffman, S., Rapaport, S. I., and Patch, M. J. (1963). *Blood 22,* 733.
Schimpf, K. (1963). *Klin. Wochschr. 41,* 283.
Schimpf, K., and Osamo, N. O. (1963). *Klin. Wochschr. 41,* 1066.
Schimpf, K., Gramlich, H., and Türk, A. (1960). *Z. Ges. Exptl. Med. 133,* 123.
Schimpf, K., Brierger, G., Mühlhäusler, W., Teupel, R., and Türk, A. (1962). *Acta Haematol. 28,* 359.
Schimpf, K., Brieger, G., and Osamo, N. O. (1964). *Klin. Wochschr. 42,* 134.
Schmer, G., and Kreil, G. (1967). *J. Chromatogr. 28,* 458.
Schmidt, A. (1892). "Zur Blutlehre". Vogel, Leipzig.
Schmidt, A. (1895). "Weitere Beiträge zur Blutlehre". Springer (Bergmann), Wiesbaden.
Schneider, C. L. (1947). *Am. J. Physiol. 149,* 123.
Schoenmakers, J. G. G., Kurstjens, R. M., Haanen, C., and Zilliken, F. (1963). *Thromb. Diath. Haemorrhag. 9,* 546.
Schoenmakers, J. G. G., Matze, R., Haanen, C., and Zilliken, F. (1964). *Biochim. Biophys. Acta 93,* 433.
Schoenmakers, J. G. G., Matze, R., Haanen, C., and Zilliken, F. (1965). *Biochim. Biophys. Acta 101,* 166.
Schrier, E. E., Broomfield, C. A., and Scheraga, H. A. (1962). *Arch. Biochem. Biophys. 99, Suppl. 1,* 309.
Schröer, H., Heene, D. L., and Seegers, W. H. (1965). *Thromb. Diath. Haemorrhag. 13,* 187.
Schulman, I., and Smith, C. H. (1952). *Blood 7,* 794.
Schulz, H., and Hiepler, E. (1959). *Klin. Wochschr. 37,* 273.
Schwick, G., and Schultze, H. E. (1959). *Clin. Chim. Acta 4,* 26.
Seegers, W. H. (1940). *J. Biol. Chem. 136,* 103.
Seegers, W. H. (1952). *Record Chem. Progress 13,* 143.
Seegers, W. H. (1961). *Thromb. Diath. Haemorrhag. Suppl. 3,* 101.
Seegers, W. H. (1962) "Prothrombin". Harvard University Press, Cambridge, Mass.
Seegers, W. H. (1964). *Federation Proc. 23,* 749.
Seegers, W. H. (1965). *Thromb. Diath. Haemorrhag. 14,* 213.
Seegers, W. H. (1967). "Prothrombin in Enzymology, Thrombosis and Hemophilia". Thomas, Springfield, Ill.
Seegers, W. H. (1968). *Pflügers Arch. Ges. Physiol. 299,* 226.
Seegers, W. H. (1969). *Ann. Rev. Physiol. 31,* 269.
Seegers, W. H., and Alkjaersig, N. (1955). *Circulation Res. 3,* 514.
Seegers, W. H., and Alkjaersig, N. (1956). *Arch. Biochem. Biophys. 61,* 1.
Seegers, W. H., and Johnson, S. A. (1956). *Am. J. Physiol. 184,* 259.
Seegers, W. H., and Kagami, M. (1964). *Can. J. Biochem. 42,* 1249.
Seegers, W. H., and Marciniak, E. (1962a). *Nature 193,* 1188.
Seegers, W. H., and Marciniak, E. (1962b). *Thromb. Diath. Haemorrhag. 8,* 1.
Seegers, W. H., and Marciniak, E. (1965). *Life Sci. 4,* 1721.
Seegers, W. H., and Marciniak, E. (1969). *In* "Recent Advances in Hemophilia and Hemophiloid Diseases". (K. M. Brinkhouse, Ed.), University of North Carolina Press. Chapel Hill, N. C.
Seegers, W. H., and McClaughry, R. I. (1949). *Proc. Soc. Exptl. Biol. Med. 72,* 247.
Seegers, W. H., and Smith, H. P. (1941). *J. Biol. Chem. 140,* 677.
Seegers, W. H., Brinkhous, K. M., Smith, H. P., and Warner, E. D. (1938a). *J. Biol. Chem. 126,* 91.
Seegers, W. H., Smith, H. P., Warner, E. D., and Brinkhous, K. M. (1938b). *J. Biol. Chem. 123,* 751.
Seegers, W. H., Loomis, E. C., and Vandenbelt, J. M. (1945a). *Arch. Biochem. 6,* 85.
Seegers, W. H., Nieft, M. L., and Loomis, E. C. (1945b). *Science 101,* 520.
Seegers, W. H., McClaughry, R. I., and Fahey, J. L. (1950). *Blood 5,* 421.
Seegers, W. H., Johnson, J. F., and Fell, C. (1954). *Am. J. Physiol. 176,* 97.
Seegers, W. H., Alkjaersig, N., and Johnson, S. A. (1955). *Am. J. Physiol. 181,* 589.
Seegers, W. H., Johnson, S. A., and Penner, J. A. (1956). *Can. J. Biochem. Physiol. 34,* 887.
Seegers, W. H., Landaburu, R. H., and Fenichel, R. L. (1957). *Am. J. Physiol. 190,* 1.
Seegers, W. H., Levine, G., and Shepard, R. S. (1958). *Canad. J. Biochem. Physiol. 36,* 603.
Seegers, W. H., Mammen, E., Lee, J. M., Landaburu, R. H., Cho, M. H., Baker, W. J., and Shepard, R. S. (1959). *In* "Hemophilia and Other Hemorrhagic States" (K. M. Brinkhous, Ed. pp. 38—46, University of North Carolina Press, Chapel Hill.
Seegers, W. H., Shepard, R. S., and Landaburu, R. H. (1960a). *Thromb. Diath. Haemorrhag. 4,* 299.
Seegers, W. H., Landaburu, R. H., and Johnson, J. F. (1960b). *Science 131,* 726.
Seegers, W. H., Aoki, N., and Marciniak, E. (1962a). *New Istanbul Contrib. Clin. Sci. 5,* 170.
Seegers, W. H., Cole, E. R., and Marciniak, E. (1962b). *Thromb. Diath. Haemorrhag. 7,* 239.
Seegers, W. H., Marciniak, E., and Cole, E. R. (1962c). *Am. J. Physiol. 203,* 397.
Seegers, W. H., Cole, E. R., Harmison, C. R., and Marciniak, E. (1963a). *Can. J. Biochem. Physiol. 41,* 1047.
Seegers, W. H., Cole, E. R., and Aoki, N. (1963b). *Can. J. Biochem. Physiol. 41,* 2441.
Seegers, W. H., Cole, E. R., Aoki, N., and Oliveira, A. (1963c). *Nature 200,* 1014.
Seegers, W. H., Cole, E. R., Harmison, C. R., and Monkhouse, F. C. (1964a). *Can. J. Biochem. 42,* 359.
Seegers, W. H., Cole, E. R., Aoki, N., and Harmison, C. R. (1964b). *Can. J. Biochem. 42,* 229.
Seegers, W. H., Schröer, H., and Kagami, M. (1964c). *Can. J. Biochem. 42,* 1425.
Seegers, W. H., Marciniak, E., and Heene, D. (1965a). *Texas Rept. Biol. Med. 23,* 675.
Seegers, W. H., Heene, D., Marciniak, E., Ivanovic, N., and Caldwell, M. J. (1965b). *Life Sci. 4,* 425.
Seegers, W. H., Harmison, C. R., Ivanovic, N., and Heene, D. L. (1966a). *Thromb. Diath. Haemorrhag. 15,* 343.
Seegers, W. H., Heene, D. L., and Marciniak, E. (1966b). *Thromb. Diath. Haemorrhag. 15,* 1.

Seegers, W. H., Schröer, H., and Marciniak, E. (1967a). In "Blood Clotting Enzymology" (W. H. Seegers, Ed.) pp. 103—142. Academic Press, New York.

Seegers, W. H., Marciniak, E., Kipfer, R. K., and Yasunaga, K. (1967b). *Arch. Biochem. Biophys. 121,* 372.

Seegers, W. H., McCoy, L., Kipfer, R. K., and Murano, G. (1968). *Arch. Biochem. Biophys. 128,* 194.

Seegers, W. H., Murano, G., McCoy, L., and Marciniak, E. (1969). *Life Sci. 8,* 925.

Sen, N. N., Sen, R., Denson, K. W. E., and Biggs, R. (1967). *Thromb. Diath. Haemorrhag. 18,* 241.

Shafrir, E., and De Vries, A. (1956). *J. Clin. Invest. 35,* 1183.

Shapiro, S. S., and Waugh, D. F. (1966). *Thromb. Diath. Haemorrhag. 16,* 469.

Sharp, A. A. (1958). *Brit. J. Haematol. 4,* 28.

Shaw, E., Mares-Guia, M., and Cohen, W. (1965). *Biochemistry 4,* 2219.

Shaw, S., Pegrum, G. D., Farthing, C. P., and Wolff, S. (1966). *Thromb. Diath. Haemorrhag. 15,* 294.

Sherry, S., and Troll, W. (1954). *J. Biol. Chem. 208,* 95.

Sherry, S., Troll, W., and Glueck, H. (1954). *Physiol. Rev. 34,* 736.

Sherry, S., Alkjaersig, N., and Fletscher, A. P. (1966). *Thromb. Diath. Haemorrhag. Suppl. 20,* 244.

Shigeharu, N., Takahashi, H., Koida, M., and Suzuki, T. (1968). *Biochem. Biophys. Res. Comm. 32,* 644.

Shinowara, G. Y. (1957a). *Am. J. Med. Sci. 233,* 528.

Shinowara, G. Y. (1957b). *J. Biol. Chem. 225,* 63.

Shinowara, G. Y. (1961). *In* "Blood Platelets" (S. A. Johnson, R. W. Monto, J. W. Rebuck, and R. C. Horn, Eds.), pp. 347—356. Little, Brown and Co., Boston.

Shinowara, G. Y. (1964). *In* "The Hemophilias" (K. M. Brinkhous, Ed.) pp. 87—99. University of North Carolina Press, Chapel Hill.

Shinowara, G. Y., and Buckley, D. J. (1960). *Thromb. Diath. Haemorrhag. 4,* 17.

Shulman, S., Landaburu, R. H., and Seegers, W. H. (1960). *Thromb. Diath. Haemorrhag. 4,* 336.

Silver, M. J., Turner, D. L., and Tocantins, L. M. (1957). *Am. J. Physiol. 190,* 8.

Silver, M. J., Turner, D. L. Rodalewicz, I., Giordano, N., Holburn, R., Herb, S. F., and Luddy, F. E. (1963). *Thromb. Diath. Haemorrhag. 10,* 164.

Simonetti, C., Casillas, G., and Pavlovsky, A. (1961), *Hémostase 1,* 57.

Simonetti, C., Casillas, G., and Pavlovsky, A. (1964). *In* "The Hemophilias" (K. M. Brinkhouse, Ed.) pp. 100—105. University of North Carolina Press. Chapel Hill.

Simson, L. R., Oberman, H. A., Penner, J. A., Lien, D. M., and Warner, C. L. (1966). *Am. J. Clin. Pathol. 45,* 373.

Slotta, K. H. (1960). *Proc. Soc. Exptl. Biol. Med. 103,* 53.

Sokal, B. (1955). *Acta Haematol. 14,* 34.

Soulier, J. P. (1960). *Thromb. Diath. Haemorrhag. Suppl. 1,* 123.

Soulier, J. P., and Larrieu, M. J. (1953). *New Engl. J. Med. 249,* 547.

Soulier, J. P., and Larrieu, M. J. (1958). *Thromb. Diath. Haemorrhag. 2,* 1.

Soulier, J. P., and Prou-Wartelle, O. (1960). *Brit. J. Haematol. 6,* 88.

Soulier, J. P., Gobbi, F., and Larrieu, M. J. (1957). *Rev. Hématol. 12,* 481.

Soulier, J. P., Wartelle, O., and Ménaché, D. (1958). *Rev. Franc. Études Clin. Et Biol. 3,* 263.

Soulier, J. P., Wartelle, O., and Ménaché, D. (1959). *Brit. J. Haematol. 5,* 121.

Soulier, J. P., Blatrix, C., Prou-Wartelle, O., and Vignal, A. (1962). *Nouvelle Rev. Franc. Hématol. 2,* 27.

Spaet, T. H. (1962). *Thromb. Diath. Haemorrhag. 8,* 276.

Spaet, T. H. (1964). *Federation Proc. 23,* 757.

Spaet, T. H., and Cintron, J. (1959). *Proc. Soc. Exptl. Biol. Med. 101,* 799.

Spaet, T. H., and Cintron, J. (1960). *Proc. Soc. Exptl. Biol. Med. 104,* 498.

Spaet, T. H., and Cintron, J. (1961). *Thromb. Diath. Haemorrhag. 5,* 447.

Spaet, T. H., and Cintron, J. (1963). *Blood 21,* 745.

Spaet, T. H., and Garner, E. S. (1955). *J. Clin. Invest. 34,* 1807.

Spaet, T. H., and Kinsell, B. G. (1953). *Proc. Soc. Exptl. Biol. Med. 84,* 314.

Spaet, T. H., Cintron, J., and Spivack, M. (1962). *Proc. Soc. Exptl. Biol. Med. 111,* 292.

Speer, R. J., and Ridgway, H. (1967). *Thromb. Diath. Haemorrhag. 18,* 259.

Speer, R. J., Ridgway, H., and Hill, J. M. (1965). *Thromb. Diath. Haemorrhag. 14,* 1.

Stefanini, M. (1950). *Am. J. Clin. Pathol. 20,* 233.

Stormorken, H. (1957). *Brit. J. Haematol. 3,* 299.

Straub, W. (1960). *Thromb. Diath. Haemorrhag. 4,* 451.

Straub, W., and Duckert, F. (1961). *Thromb. Diath. Haemorrhag. 5,* 402.

Surgenor, D. M., Wilson, N. A., and Henry, A. S. (1961). *Thromb. Diath. Haemorrhag. 5,* 1.

Sykes, E. M., Seegers, W. H., and Ware, A. G. (1948). *Proc. Soc. Exptl. Biol. Med. 67,* 506.

Telfer, T. P., Denson, K. W., and Wright, D. R. (1956). *Brit. J. Haematol. 2,* 308.

Thelin, G. M., and Wagner, R. H. (1961). *Arch. Biochem. Biophys. 95,* 70.

Therriault, D., Nichols, T., and Jensen, H. (1958). *J. Biol. Chem. 233,* 1061.

Thies, H. A. (1957). "Menschliche und tierische Gewebethrombokinasen. Ihre Eigenschaften und ihre Bedeutung für die Anwendung von Antikoagulantien." Thieme, Stuttgart.

Thomas, L. (1947). *Bull. John Hopkins Hosp. 81,* 1.

Thomas, W. R., and Seegers, W. H. (1960). *Biochim. Biophys. Acta 42,* 556.

Tibbs, J. (1951). *Nature 168,* 910.

Tishkoff, G. H., Pechet, L., and Alexander, B. (1960). *Blood 15,* 778.

Tishkoff, G. H., Williams, L. C., and Brown, D. M. (1968). *J. Biol. Chem. 243,* 4151.

Tocantins, L. M. (1943a). *Proc. Soc. Exptl. Biol. Med. 54,* 94.

Tocantins, L. M. (1943b). *Am. J. Physiol. 139,* 265.

Tocantins, L. M. (1944). *Proc. Soc. Exptl. Biol. Med. 55,* 291.

Tocantins, L. M. (1945). *Am. J. Physiol. 143,* 67.

Tocantins, L. M. (1954). *Blood 9,* 281.

Triantaphyllopoulos, D. C., (1957). *Proc. Western Group Div. Med. Res. Natl. Council Can. 11,* 21.

Troup, S. B., and Reed, C. F. (1958). *J. Clin. Invest. 37,* 937.

Troup, S. B., Reed, C. F., Marinetti, G. V., and Swisher, S. N. (1960). *J. Clin. Invest. 39,* 342.

Tullis, J. L., Melin, M., and Jurigian, P. (1965). *New Engl. J. Med. 273,* 667.

Turner, D. L., and Silver, M. J. (1963). *Nature 200,* 370.

Turner, D. L., Holburn, R. R., DeSipin, M., Silver, M. J., and Tocantins, L. M. (1963). *J. Lipid. Res. 4,* 52.

Ulutin, O. N., and Seegers, W. H. (1962). *Thromb. Diath. Haemorrhag. Suppl. 1,* 256.

Ulutin, O. N., Johnson, J. F., and Seegers, W. H. (1961). *Am. J. Physiol. 201,* 660.

Urayama, T., and Asada, T. (1964). *Biochim. Biophys. Acta 93,* 683.

Van Creveld, S., Hoorweg, P. G., Ottolander, G. J. H., and Veder, H. A. (1956). *Acta Haematol. 15,* 1.

Van Creveld, S., Veder, H. A., Pascha, C. N., and Kroeze, W. F. (1959). *Thromb. Diath. Haemorrhag. 3,* 572.

Van Creveld, S., Veder, H. A., and Pascha, C. N. (1960). *Thromb. Diath. Haemorrhag. 4,* 211.

Van Creveld, S., Pascha, C. N., and Veder, H. A. (1961). *Thromb. Diath. Haemorrhag. 6,* 282.

Van Creveld, S., Mochtar, I. A., and Pascha, C. N. (1966). *Thromb. Diath. Haemorrhag. 15,* 338.

Van Creveld, S., Mochtar, I. A., and Pascha, C. N. (1967). *Thromb. Diath. Haemorrhag. 17,* 188.

Van Holde, K. E., and Baldwin, R. L. (1958). *J. Phys. Chem. 62, 734.*

Veder, H. A. (1966). *Thromb. Diath. Haemorrhag. 16,* 738.

Vroman, L. (1958). Ph. D. Thesis, Univ. of Utrecht, Netherlands.

Vroman, L. (1963). *Thromb. Diath. Haemorrhag. 10,* 455.

Vroman, L. (1965). *In* "Biophysical Mechanisms in Vascular Homeostasis and Intravascular Thrombosis" (P. N. Sawyer, Ed.) pp. 81—96. Appleton, New York.

Vroman, L. (1967). *In* "Blood Clotting Enzymology" (W. H. Seegers, Ed.), pp. 279—322. Academic Press, New York.

Vroman, L. (1968). *Thromb. Diath. Haemorrhag. Suppl. 25,* 89.

Waaler, B. A. (1959). *Scand. J. Clin. Lab. Invest. Suppl. 37,* 1.
Wagner, R. H., Richardson, B. A., and Brinkhous, K. M. (1957). *Thromb. Diath. Haemorrhag. 1,* 1.
Wagner, R. H., McLester, W. D., Smith, M., and Brinkhous, K. M. (1964a). *Thromb. Diath. Haemorrhag. 11,* 64.
Wagner, R. H., Smith, M., and McLester, W. (1964b). *In* "The Hemophilias" (K. M. Brinkhous, Ed.), pp. 81—86. University of North Carolina Press, Chapel Hill.
Ware, A. G., and Seegers, W. H. (1948a). *J. Biol. Chem. 174,* 565.
Ware, A. G., and Seegers, W. H. (1948b). *Am. J. Physiol. 152,* 567.
Ware, A. G., and Seegers, W. H. (1949). *Am. J. Clin. Pathol. 19,* 471.
Ware, A. G., Guest, M. M., and Seegers, W. H. (1947a). *Science 106,* 41.
Ware, A. G., Murphy, R. C., and Seegers, W. H. (1947b). *Science 106,* 618.
Weaver, R. A., Gabriel, D. A., and Langdell, R. D. (1966). *Federation Proc. 25,* 317.
Weaver, R. A., Gabriel, D. A., and Langdell, R. D. (1967). *Transfusion 7,* 168.
Webster, M. E., and Ratnoff, O. D. (1961). *Nature 192,* 180.
Webster, W. P., Reedick, R. L., Roberts, H. R., and Penick, G. D. (1967). *Nature 213,* 1146.
White, N. B., Ferguson, J. H., and Hitsumoto, S. (1968). *Am. J. Med. Sci. 255,* 143.
White, S. G., Aggeler, P. M., and Glendening, M. B. (1953a). *Blood 8,* 101.
White, S. G., Aggeler, P. M., and Emery, B. E. (1953b). *Proc. Soc. Exptl. Med. 83,* 69.
Widenbauer, F., and Reichel, C. (1942). *Biochem. Z. 311,* 307.
Williams, W. J. (1964). *J. Biol. Chem. 239,* 933.
Williams, W. J. (1966). *J. Biol. Chem. 241,* 1840.
Williams, W. J., and Norris, D. G. (1966). *J. Biol. Chem. 241,* 1847.
Wilner, G. D., Nossel, H. L., and LeRoy, E. C. (1968). *J. Clin. Invest. 47,* 2608.
Witte, S., and Dirnberger, P. (1953). *Klin. Wochschr. 31,* 781.
Woodside, E. E., Therriault, D. G., and Kocholaty, W. (1964). *Blood 24,* 76.
Wooldridge, L. C. (1893). "Chemistry of the Blood". Kegan, Trench, Trübner and Co., London.
Yin, E. T., and Duckert, F. (1961). *Thromb. Diath. Haemorrhag. 6,* 215.
Yphantis, D. A. (1964). *Biochemistry 3,* 297.
Zacharski, L. R., Bowie, E. J. W., Titus, J. L., and Owen, C. A. (1968). *Mayo Clinic Proc. 43,* 617.
Zucker, M. B., and Borreli, J. (1958). *J. Appl. Physiol. 12,* 453.
Zucker, M. B., and Borrelli, J. (1962). *Proc. Soc. Exptl. Biol. Med. 109,* 779.
Zucker-Franklin, D., Javid, J., and Spaet, T. H. (1961). *Federation Proc. 20,* 53.

CHAPTER 2

Equipment and General Requirements for the Coagulation Laboratory

FRITZ K. BELLER and HENNER GRAEFF

I. Introduction

Although the work in a modern day coagulation laboratory has come to resemble closely work in general protein chemistry, a number of largely traditional and empirical ground rules are still important to follow.

In the following an outline will be provided for selected procedures which apply specifically to coagulation work and which have been found to be useful and necessary for optimum results in the author's laboratory.

II. Equipment

Most coagulation studies are performed at constant temperatures and water baths supplied with a thermostat accurate enough to maintain a water temperature of $37 \pm 1^\circ$ C are widely used. Glass or plastic straight-walled containers are preferable to round containers since they allow observation and magnification without removing tubes. A good light source placed at the side or the bottom of the container is helpful. Water baths designed specifically for coagulation work have been described (Juergens and Beller, 1959) and are commercially available from Buehler Company, Tuebingen, Germany (Fig. 1) or Phipps and Bird Inc., Richmond, Va. (Fig. 2). A water bath built into the laboratory table as used by Astrup (personal communication) is shown in Fig. 3.

Stop watches are essential in the coagulation laboratories; some investigators find foot switch devices convenient. For large scale routine prothrombin time assays mechanical equipment has been designed. Two instruments developed in recent years were found by us to be reliable and mechanically dependable. One model developed by Schnitger and Gross (1954) performed well in the authors' experience. This apparatus is equipped to handle four assays simultaneously (Fig. 4). The apparatus is distributed by Hch. Amelung. 4922 Brake ueber Lemgo, Germany, and in the U. S. by Becton, Dickinson and Co., Rutherford, N. J. Another similar instrument (Fig. 5) is the Mechrolab clot timer (Heller-Laboratories, San Mateo, Calif.). The smaller model is capable of handling two samples, the larger model handles four samples simultaneously. The standard error is less than ± 0.2 seconds. Assays like prothrombin time, thromboplastin generation test, thrombin test, etc. can be adequately performed using such mechanical devices*.

Miale (1965) compared the Fibrometer (Baltimore Biological Laboratory, Becton, Dickinson Co., Rutherford, N. J.), another semiautomated device, with conventional manual techniques, and found excellent correlation between the two. A number of photo-optical devices for the continuous registration of clotting and fibrinolysis have been described in the literature (Lackner and Goosen, 1959; Kuhnke and Gill, 1960, 1963). However, with the exception of the thrombelastograph (see Chapter III, page 70) such automated devices have not found wide acceptance.

---

* After this manuscript was finished, Hyland, Division of Travenol Laboratories Inc. Los Angeles, invented a new automatic clot timer (CLOTEK®) which was found reliable and helpful.

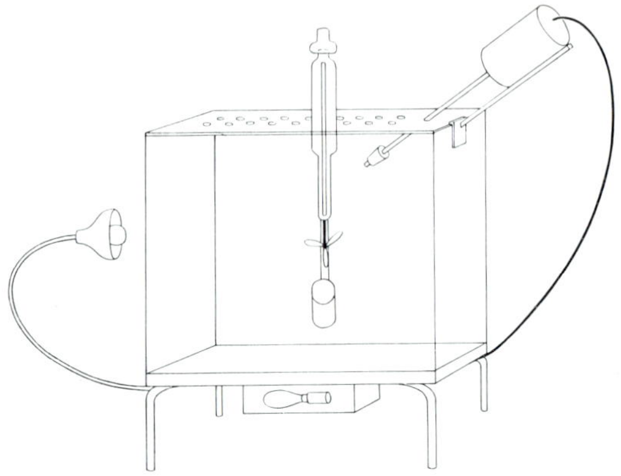

Fig. 1. Water bath designed for coagulation studies according to Jürgens and Beller (1959), manufactured by Buehler, G. M. B. H. Tübingen Germany.

III. Collection of Blood

The prerequisite for reproducable and quantitative results in blood coagulation tests is a clean venipuncture. Minimal contamination with tissue thromboplastin, or contact of the blood with human skin (Nossel, 1966) or dirty glassware are factors which invariably produce serious errors. Agitation of the blood sample, air bubbles, foaming and hemolysis are additional sources of error. The widely used vacutainer systems are not recommended for this work.

A. Collection of Human Blood

Blood from an antecubital vein is preferred. Minimal stasis (20–40 mm Hg) should be applied since excessive and prolonged venous stasis results in local fibrinolytic activity which may interfere with the results of a number of clotting assays. The skin overlaying the vein is cleaned with an alcohol or ether soaked swab and dried. An inside polished V 2 A steel canula of the largest width possible is preferred; however, disposable needles are adequate in most instances. Free flow is best achieved by a coneless needle. A special needle allowing free flow as well as the attachment to a syringe was designed by Hartert (1951) (Fig. 6). In the U.S., the two syringe technique is usually recommended. Two to three ml of blood are withdrawn and the syringe is then replaced by another one which contains the anticoagulant. The syringe is tilted gently to achieve adequate mixing. At least 10 ml of blood should be discarded prior to sampling if an indwelling polyethylene catheter is used. Clean venipunctures

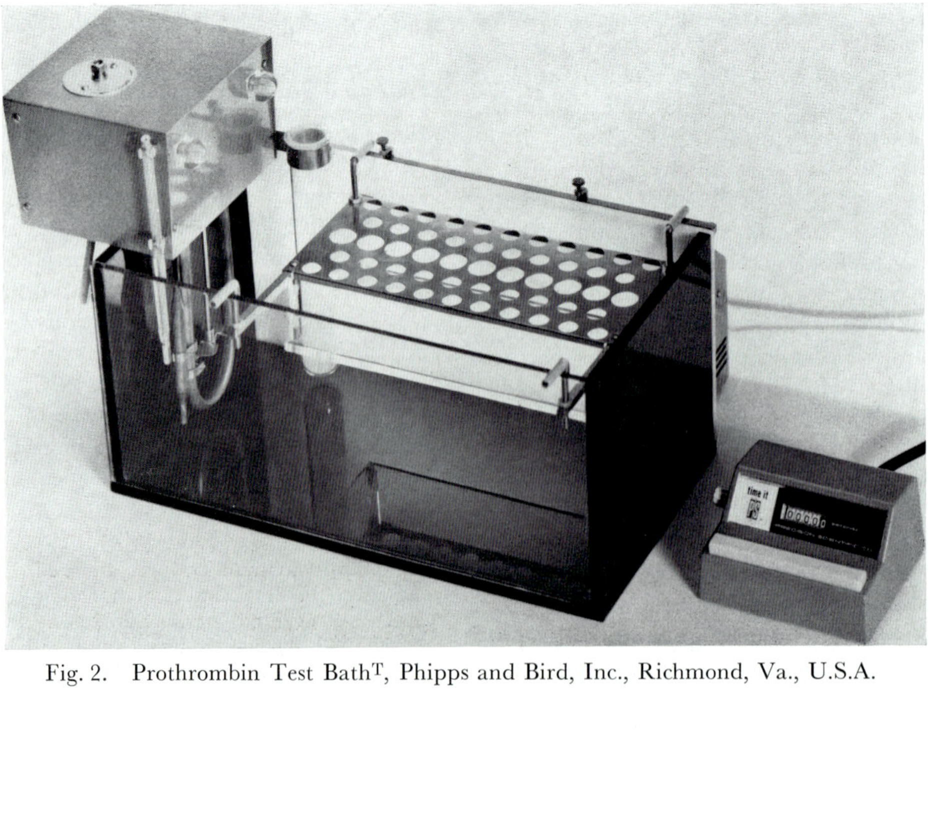

Fig. 2. Prothrombin Test Bath[T], Phipps and Bird, Inc., Richmond, Va., U.S.A.

from the cubital vein, femoral vein or subclavian vein do not substantially influence the results of the coagulation studies.

B. Collection of Animal Blood

In the rabbit either the marginal vein or the central artery at the base of the ear is accessible after prewarming. Longer lasting infusions and repeated collections of blood are best done by an insertion of a polyethylene tubing (Rodriguez-Erdmann, 1959). The vein at the base of the ear (dorsal surface) is dissected free under local anesthesia and two ligatures passed under it. The vein is approached near the base of the ear proximal to the bifurcation of its lateral branch. The vessel is punctured by a 14 gauge needle and a polyethylene catheter (Intramedic, Clay Adams, Inc., New York; Becton, Dickinson, Rutherford, N. J., polyethylene tubing; i. d. 0.030″ o. d. 0.048″) is passed through the lumen of the needle (Fig. 7). It is sufficient to insert the needle only partially if the diameter of the vessel is small. The catheter tip is bevelled and is inserted up to a prefixed mark. In grown rabbits, it is most likely located in the superior vena cava if the catheter is inserted 4–5 inches. The central venous pressure may be determined. Movements of the fluid level synchronically with respiration and a pressure of 2–5 cm of water indicates proper adjustment. If the pressure exceeds 10 cm of water, the catheter tip may be in the right ventricle or in the pulmonary artery. Withdrawal of a few centimeters brings the tip back to proper position.

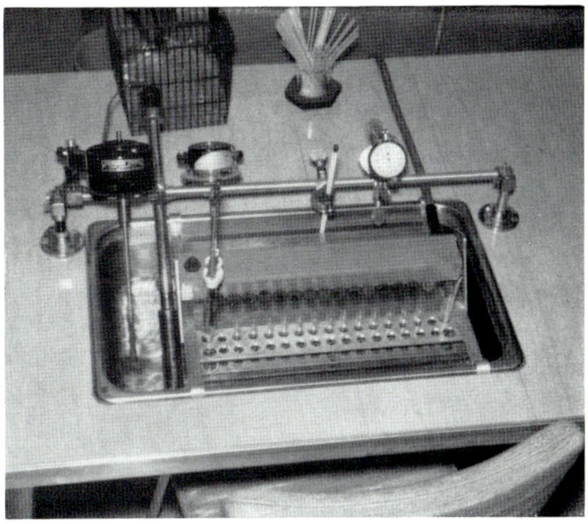

Fig. 3. Water bath built into laboratory bench.

In the dog, the radial, femoral, saphenous, or jugular veins are easily accessible. The preferred site in puppies and rats is the jugular vein. In the pig the superior vena cava or major vessels in the neck may be entered with a catheter (Rowsell and Mustard, 1963). Ducks' blood may be drawn from a vein located along the medial aspect of the shank of the duck's leg (Murdock and Lewis, 1964). Sampling of blood by the methods of passive drip from a lateral ear vein in the rabbit, from clipped toe nails in the dog, by cardiac puncture in the rabbit, by orbital sinus bleeding in the mouse or rat, by tail vein and penis vein bleeding in the mouse, is less suitable for coagulation methods since the blood may be contaminated with tissue juice (Riley, 1960; Pettit, 1913; Sanders, 1966; Stone, 1954; Lehnert, 1967). A reliable method of obtaining samples of ar-

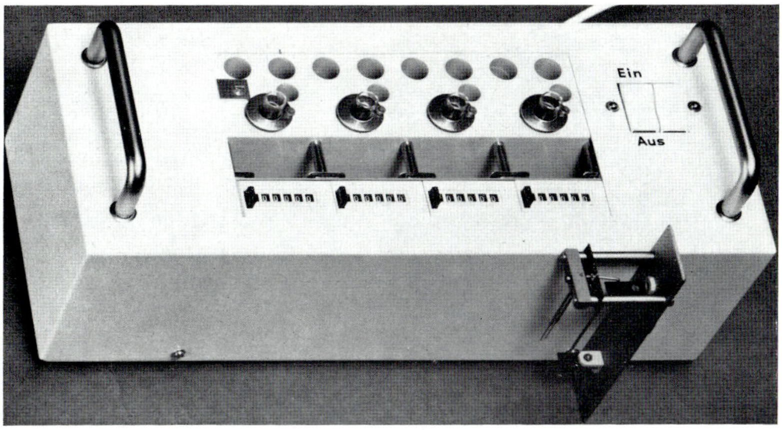

Fig. 4. Automatic clot timer according to Schnitger and Gross (1954).

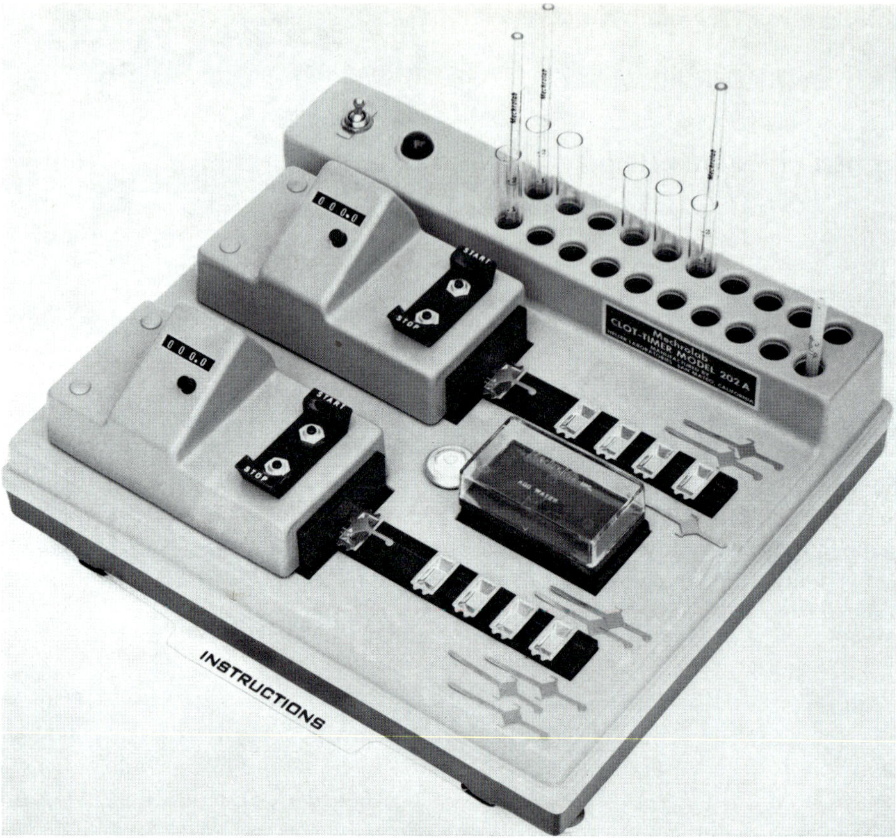

Fig. 5. Mechrolab model 202 A dual channel clottimer (Heller Laboratories, San Mateo, Calif.).

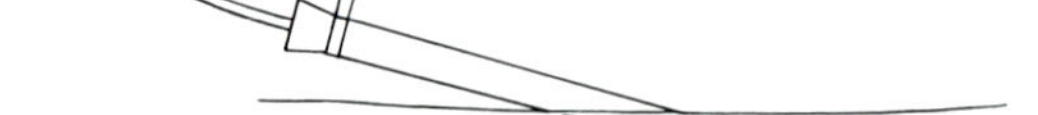

Fig. 6. Special canulla as designed by Hartert allowing free flow of blood and attachment of a syringe as well.

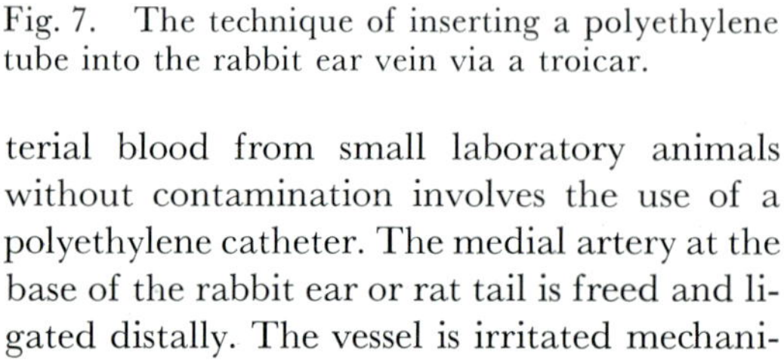

Fig. 7. The technique of inserting a polyethylene tube into the rabbit ear vein via a troicar.

terial blood from small laboratory animals without contamination involves the use of a polyethylene catheter. The medial artery at the base of the rabbit ear or rat tail is freed and ligated distally. The vessel is irritated mechanically until it is swollen and then temporarily clamped proximally. A small incision is made and the bevelled catheter tip inserted for 1 cm and fixed by a ligature. The clamp is opened, whereupon blood will flow freely from the catheter.

When native blood is to be tested immediately as for instance thrombelastography, the blood should be transported at 37° C (see Chapter 3, p. 72).

In general, it is advisable to keep anticoagulated blood samples in ice water. Subsequent centrifugation and storing should be done at a temperature of about 4° C (refrigerated centrifuge) and if the assay procedure is not performed within the next 2 hours, the plasma samples should be frozen at –20° C. The preparation of serum for special test purposes, i. e. prothrombin consumption tests and thromboplastin generation tests, is outlined in the appropriate sections in this book.

IV. Cleaning and Preparation of Glassware

A. Treatment of Unsiliconized Glassware

Soaking overnight in a detergent or washing with soap and water are the best cleaning procedures. Chromic sulphuric acid, chromic nitric acid or treatment with 40 % NaOH are frequently used. However, these techniques have certain disadvantages in that chromium adheres strongly to the glass surfaces and may destroy enzymes even in trace amounts when not properly rinsed. After any such treatments, the glassware must be rinsed several times with tap water and distilled water. Etched, scratched or cracked glassware should be discarded. Pipettes are soaked in detergent or tap water, treated with nitric sulphuric acid or an equivalent, and rinsed with tap water overnight in an automatic rinsing device. Then they are rinsed with distilled water. The glassware is finally dried in an oven at 120° C for about 60–90 minutes.

B. Treatment of Siliconized Glassware

Silicone coated and non coated glassware has to be stored separately. The removal of silicone is rather difficult to achieve and is done by thoroughly scrubbing with soap or detergent and water, or by soaking the coated glassware in saturated solution of NaOH in 95 % alcohol or water. Tocantins (1964) suggested a mixture containing technical grade acetone (2 liters), H_2O (2 liters), and NaOH solid (200 gm). Glassware coated with dichlordimethylsilane in toluol is cleaned with a detergent or by soaking in nitric sulphuric acid.

C. Coating of Glassware, Syringes and Needles

To coat glassware and other laboratory equipment polymers derived from organic silicone compounds are used (Jaques et al. 1946). For this purpose methylchlorosilane in liquid form (Reagent General Electric Dri-Film No. 9987) or a solution of 1 part dri film and 4 parts of petroleum ether is poured from one tube to the next. Individual tubes or other pieces of glassware are rinsed with distilled water. The glassware is then dried in the oven at 120° C for 60–90 minutes. When "Silicone Oel" (Bayer Leverkusen, Germany) is used the tubes are baked at 350° C for 2 hours. An easy and preferred method for obtaining a thin unimolecular film involves using dichlordimethylsilane as 5 % solution in toluol. The glassware is brought into contact with the substance for 5 minutes, rinsed twice with methanol and then with distilled water, and dried at room temperature. The polymer coats the surface with a thin unimolecular film. Volumetric differences are negligible, pipettes are well coated and changes in volume capacity are insignificant for practical purposes. The thin film, renewed after each use, has no disadvantages compared to thicker and baked silicone films (Graeff and Kuhn, 1966). Additional silicones recommended are DC 110 1,5 % in carbon tetrachloride (Dow Corning Corp., Midland, Mich.; Hopkin and Williams Ltd., Chadwell Heath Essex). MS 550 (Savory and Moore, Ltd., Lawrence Road, London N. 15) Dow Corning "Z 4141" Dow Corning Corp., Midland Mich.; Silikonölemulsion Wacker).

V. Buffer Solutions

Reactions involved in blood coagulation are all enzymatic in nature and hence due consideration should be paid establishing optimum conditions in terms of pH and ionic strength whenever an assay procedure in this area is developed.

Most routine assays are performed in buffer systems covering the physiologic pH range of the blood (pH 7.34–7.43), a figure which is arrived at by inference since the pH optimum for a number of the enzyme systems involved in blood coagulation is unknown. Moreover, the buffer salts which are routinely utilized have been established empirically and no systematic evaluation of the influence different buffer systems on the enzymes of different phases of blood clotting has been carried out.

In the following section the buffer systems most frequently used, will be discussed. Reference to special buffers may be found in the appropriate sections of this book.

A. Preparations

Stock solutions and buffers should be prepared from pyrogen free distilled water. Buffer solutions should be stored at 4° C and discarded when clouded, precipitated or flocculated. Merthiolate can be added in an end concentration of 1:10,000. Its high absorbance at 275 mμ should be kept in mind.

1. Sodium Barbital Buffers "Michaelis Buffer" (Michaelis, 1930)

Stock solution A is prepared by dissolving 20.6 gm sodium diethylbarbiturate in distilled water adjusting final volume to 1 liter (A = 0.1 M sodium diethylbarbiturate (MW – 206.18)). Stock solution B = 0.1 M hydrochloric acid. To prepare Michaelis Buffer to a given pH, the following outline can be utilized:

pH	Stock Solution (ml to be added) A	B	Sodium Chloride (gm to be added)
7.0	268	232	7.43
7.2	277	223	7.38
7.4	290	210	7.30
7.6	307	193	7.18
7.8	331	149	7.07
8.0	359	141	6.89

Adjust to final volume of 1,000 ml with distilled water.

Sodium barbital buffer is widely used in coagulation and fibrinolysis studies. With a pK^1 of 7.43 the range of pH near the physiological value is well covered. This buffer system may be utilized for the preparation of a buffered isotonic calcium chloride solution as follows: 25 mM $CaCl_2$, 290 ml A, 210 ml B, 2.9 ml NaCl, distilled water to final volume of 1,000 ml.

2. Imidazole Buffers

Stock solution A is prepared by dissolving 6.8 gm of Imidazole powder (Eastman Kodak, Rochester, N. Y.) in 1 liter of distilled water (A = 0.1 M Imidazole solution (MW 68.08)). Stock solution B is 0.1 M hydrochloric acid. The ionic strength can be considered equal to the total mEq/l hydrochloric acid added. To prepare this buffer to a given pH, the following outline can be utilized:

pH	Stock Solution (ml to be added) A	B	Sodium Chloride (gm to be added)
6.4	500	398	6.67
6.6	500	355	6.92
6.8	500	304	7.22
7.0	500	243	7.59
7.2	500	186	7.91
7.4	500	136	8.20

Adjust to final volume of 1,000 ml with distilled water.

Imidazole buffer was recommended by Mertz and Owen (1940) and is preferred by Seegers (1962). Witw pK^1 of 6.95 (Kirby and Neuberger, 1938) its buffering capacity is adequate for a pH range between 6.2 and 7.8.

3. Sodium Phosphate Buffers (Miller and Golder, 1950)

Stock solution A is prepared by dissolving 17.8 gm of disodium phosphate ($Na_2HPO_4 \cdot 2H_2O$, MW 178.01) in water adjusting final volume to 1 liter. Prepare stock solution B by dissolving 13.8 gm mono sodium phosphate ($NaH_2PO_4 \cdot H_2O$, MW 138.01) in water adjusted to final volume of 1 liter. The ionic strength is calculated assuming total dissociation of A to 2 Na+ and HPO_4– and of B to Na+ and H_2PO_4–. To prepare this buffer to a given pH the following outline can be utilized:

pH	Stock Solution (ml to be added) A	B	Sodium Chloride (gm to be added)
6.0	23	132	7.82
6.5	41.5	74	7.84
7.0	56.7	32	7.82
7.5	60.7	10	7.86

Adjust to final volume of 1,000 ml with distilled water.

Phosphate buffer was widely used since its description by Soerensen in 1912. In the given preparation, the pH is scarcely temperature dependent. An increase of temperature by 1° C leads to an approximate decrease of 0.004 pH units. Phosphate buffers of a higher phosphate salt concentration and/or a combination of sodium and potassium phosphate are also widely recommended (for instance: $Na_2HPO_4 \cdot 2H_2O$: 7.156 gm; KH_2PO_4: 1.306 gm; NaCl: 1.40 gm; dissolve in 900 ml distilled water, adjust pH to 7.5 with 1 M sodium hydroxyde and adjust to a final volume of 1 liter, $\mu = 0.154$). The pK[1] values for HPO_4- and H_2PO_4- are 2 and 6.8 at this ionic strength. Phosphate ions may enhance fibrinolysis (Brakman, 1967). It should be remembered that addition of calcium chloride to phosphate buffer solutions results in precipitation of insoluble calcium phosphate salts.

4. Tris Buffer (THAM, Tris Hydroxymethyl Aminomethane) (Gomori, 1946)

Stock solution A is prepared by dissolving 12.1 gm of Tris (MW 121.14) in water adjusted to 1 liter of final volume (A = 0.1 M tris solution). Stock solution B = 0.1 M hydrochloric acid.

The ionic strength is given by the total mEq/l HCl added. To prepare this buffer to a given pH, the following outline can be utilized:

pH	Stock Solution (ml to be added) A	B	Sodium Chloride (gm to be added)
7.2	500	442	6.41
7.4	500	414	6.58
7.6	500	384	6.76
7.8	500	326	7.00
8.0	500	268	7.43
8.2	500	220	7.71
8.4	500	166	8.03
8.6	500	122	8.28

Adjust to final volume of 1,000 ml with distilled water.

With a pK[1] value of 8.07 (West et al. 1966) the buffer capacity in the prescribed concentration is diminishing but still adequate in the range of pH 7.4. The temperature dependency of pH for tris buffers is greater than for phosphate buffers. An increase in temperature by 1° C leads to an approximate decrease of 0.02–0.03 pH units.

5. Tes Buffer (N-Tris (Hydroxymethyl) methyl-2-Aminomethanesulfonic Acid) (Good et al. 1966)

Good et al. (1966) described several new hydrogen buffers. One of these is N-Tris (hydroxymethyl) methyl-2-aminomethanesulfonic acid. It is an amino acid zwitterion. The buffer solution is prepared by adding 60 mM Tes (Calbiochem, N. Y. Inc. P. O. Box 331, Spring Valley, N. Y. 10977) and 90 mM sodium chloride solution to 1 liter buffer.

Prepare 13.75 mg (MW 229.24) and 5.25 gm of sodium chloride, adjust volume to 900 ml with distilled water, adjust to pH 7.5 at working temperature with 1/10 N NaOH and adjust to final volume of 1 liter with distilled water.

Tes has negligible metal binding properties for Mg^{++}, Ca^{++} and Mn^{++} (weak for Cu^{++}). Apparent pK[1] values when 0.1 M at 0° C: 7.92; at 20° C: 7.50; at 37° C: 7.14. The effect of concentration on pK[1] is weak between 0.2 M and 0.01 M. Compared to Tris or Phosphate buffer the Tes buffer has a higher buffer capacity in the range desired with no side effects in different biological test systems. The temperature dependence is moderate.

VI. Anticoagulants

The use of compounds capable of binding ionized calcium is indispensable in coagulation work. Trisodium citrate, sodium oxalate and disodium ethylenediamine tetracetate (EDTA) are all highly effective. Heparin, of course, has no place in coagulation tests. Each anticoagulant substance possesses certain disadvantages. Oxalate is a microcristalline insoluble salt, which on centrifugation destroys platelets with a release of platelet factors. For ill understood reasons labile procoagulants (factors V and VIII) are more labile in oxalate than in citrate or EDTA. The activities of factors II, VII and X for equally poorly understood reasons are enhanced with storage in citrate. EDTA is well suited for most coagulation assays but cannot be used for platelet function tests.

Disodium Ethylenediamine Tetracetate Na_2 (EDTA) is prepared as a 1% (1 gm/100 ml H_2O) solution; at this concentration 1 part of anticoagulant is mixed with 9 parts of blood.

Trisodium Citrate ($Na_3C_6H_5O_7 \cdot 2H_2O$) is prepared as a 3.8% (3.8 gm/100 ml H_2O) solution and usually 1 part of anticoagulant are mixed with 9 parts of blood.

Potassium Oxalate is prepared as a 1.4% (1.4 gm/100 ml H_2O) solution and also usually 1 part of anticoagulant is used with 9 parts of blood.

Lately, evacuated glass test tubes (Vacutainers) containing various anticoagulants are coming into clinical use. The anticoagulant is indicated by the color of the stopper (blue for citrate, black for oxalate, lavender for EDTA) (Becton Dickerson and Co., Columbus, Ne. and Rutherford, N. J.). Their application for blood coagulant assays cannot be recommended because the ratio of anticoagulant to blood is difficult to standardize and because the foaming induced when blood is aspirated into a vacuum may denature labile clotting factors (factors I, V and VIII).

The following anticoagulants are used for special purposes:

Potassium oxalate
(1.4 gm/100 ml H_2O; 1 and 9).
Lithium oxalate
(1.4 gm/100 ml H_2O; 1 and 9).
Ammonium oxalate
(1.4 gm/100 ml H_2O; 1 and 9).
Sodium fluoride
(40 gm/100 ml H_2O; 1 and 99).
ACD solution
(0.44 gm citric acid, 1.32 gm tri sodium citrate, 1.47 gm dextrose/100 ml H_2O; 1 and 4) (Holburn, 1964).

VII. Ion Exchange Resins

Cationic exchange resins such as Dowex 50 or Amberlite IRC-50 can be used to remove ionized calcium from blood. The preparation and equilibration of these materials in their sodium cycle at a desired pH differs in no way from the procedures numerated in many textbooks for general biochemistry. It is assumed that removal of ionized calcium by ion exchange methods does not effect any other blood constituents (Stefanini and Dameshek, 1962).

References

Brakman, P. (1967). "Fibrinolysis", Scheltema and Holkema, Amsterdam.

Gomori, G. (1946). *Proc. Soc. exp. Biol. 62*, 33.

Good, N. E., Winget, G. D., Winter, W., Connolly, Th. N., Izawa, S. and Singh, R. M. M. (1966). *Biochemistry 5*, 467.

Graeff, H. and Kuhn, W. (1966). *Klin. Wschr. 44*, 646.

Hartert, H. (1951). *Zschr. exp. Med. 117*, 189.

Holburn, R. R. (1964). *In:* "Blood Coagulation, Hemorrhage and Thrombosis" (L. M. Tocantins and L. A. Kazal, eds.), p. II, Grune and Stratton, New York.

Jaques, L. B., Lidlar, E., Feldsted, E. T. and MacDonald, A. G. (1946). *Can. Med. Assoc. J. 55*, 26.

Juergens, J. and Beller, F. K. (1959). "Klinische Methoden der Blutgerinnungsanalyse", Thieme, Stuttgart.

Kirby, A. H. and Neuberger, A. (1938). *Biochem. J. 32*, 1146.

Kuhnke, E. and Gill, I. S. (1960). *Pfluegers Arch. Exptl. Pathol. 272*, 191.

Kuhnke, E. and Gill, I. S. (1963). *Thromb. Diath. Haemorrhag 10*, 247.

Lackner, H. and Goosen, C. G. (1959). *Acta Haematol. 22*, 58.

Lehnert, J. P. (1967). *Amer. J. Clin. Pathol. 47*, 416.

Mertz, E. T. and Owen, G. A. (1940). *Proc. Soc. Exptl. Biol. 43*, 204.

Miale, J. B. (1965). *Amer. J. Clin. Pathol. 43*, 475.

Michaelis, L. (1930). *J. Biol. Chem. 87*, 33.

Miller, G. L. and Golder, R. H. (1950). *Arch. Biochem. 29*, 420.

Murdock, H. R. and Lewis, J. O. (1964). *Proc. Soc. Exptl. Biol. Med. 116*, 51.

Nossel, H. L. (1966). *Proc. Soc. Exptl. Biol. Med. 122*, 16.

Pettit, A. (1913). *Compt. Rend. Soc. Biol. 74*, 11.

Riley, V. (1960). *Proc. Soc. Exptl. Biol. and Med. 104*, 751.

Rodriguez-Erdmann, F. (1959). *Pfluegers Arch. Ges. Physiol. 269*, 306.

Roswell, H. C. and Mustard, J. F. (1963). *Laboratory Animal Care 13*, 752.

Sanders, B. J. (1960). *Am. J. Clin. Pathol. 40*, 46.

Schnitger, H. and Gross, R. (1954). *Klin. Wschr. 32*, 1011.

Seegers, W. H. (1962). "Prothrombin". Harvard University Press, Cambridge, Massachusetts.

Soerensen, S. P. L. (1912). *Ergebn. Physiol. 12*, 393.

Stefanini, M., Dameshek, W. (1962). "The Hemorrhagic Disorders". Grune and Stratton, London.

Stone, S. H. (1954). *Science 119*, 100.

Tocantins, L. M. (1964). *In:* "Blood Coagulation, Hemorrhage and Thrombosis" (L. M. Tocantins and A. K. Kazal eds.), pp. 9—10, Grune and Stratton, New York.

West, E. St., Todd. W. R., Mason, H. S. and van Bruggen, J. T. (1966). "Textbook of Biochemistry", Macmillan Co., New York.

CHAPTER 3

Clotting Time Techniques

F. K. BELLER and H. GRAEFF

I. Introduction

The technique of whole blood clotting described by Lee and White (1913) was the first attempt at a standardized coagulation assay. The recalcification time was a somewhat more sophisticated technique described by Howell (1916) to detect clotting abnormalities, specifically hemophilia. When the significance of surface activation was realized, it became obvious that the recalcification time was influenced by contact activation. For this reason, several authors have attempted to make the test more sensitive by reducing surface activation through the use of either siliconized glass or plasticware. In other laboratories, techniques for more improved standardization of the test were developed. In most instances this was accomplished by introducing glass beads and agents with similar surface characteristics to insure consistent maximal surface activation.

The activation of Hageman factor takes place in the presence of substances not present in the vascular system, e. g. silica particles. Activation is also achieved by fatty acids, ellagic acid and collagen (Margolis, 1957; Waaler, 1959; Nossel, 1964; Niewirarowski et al. 1966; Botti and Ratnoff, 1964; Hoak et al. 1967; and Vroman, 1967).

II. Whole Blood Coagulation Time

Principle of the method: Blood taken by venipuncture is allowed to clot in the test tubes.

Material: Disposable needles (18 or 20 gauge), disposable plastic syringes, 5 and 10 ml. Glass, siliconized or plastic test tubes (11 mm × 75 mm). Constant temperature water bath (37° C). Special tubes, evacuated to draw 2 ml and containing 12 mg diatomite, are supplied by Becton Dickinson & Co., Rutherford, N. J. (see 59).

Assays are carried out as follows:

A. Using Glass Tubes (Lee and White, 1913)

Blood is collected by a clean venipuncture, using the two syringe technique. One ml of blood is introduced into each of 3 prewarmed glass tubes (tubes 1, 2 and 3) and the tubes are placed in the 37° C water bath. Tube 1 is tilted every 30 seconds until flow of blood stops, leaving tubes 2 and 3 untouched. Next, tube 2 is tilted every 30 seconds until completely clotted. At that point, the tilting of tube 3 is started. The endpoint for the test is the time when the blood is clotted in tube 3. Clotting time is the total time elapsed from the start of withdrawal of the blood from the vein until completion of clotting in tube 3. Normal values range from 10 to 15 min.

B. Using Siliconized Tubes (Margulies and Barker, 1949)

The technique is exactly as outlined under A, only siliconized glass tubes and syringes are used. Reproducible results depend on attention to detail and careful technique in siliconizing and rinsing glassware (see Section 61). Normal values range from 35 to 55 min.

C. Using Glass Tubes With Diatomite (Hattersley, 1966)

Blood is drawn as above and allowed to flow into each of three vacuum tubes. The tubes are inverted a few times to achieve effective contact activation. Coagulation is observed as described under A. Normal values range from 1 min 20 sec to 2 min 20 sec.

D. Comment

Reliability and reproducibility of the results depend entirely on strict adherence to details of procedure. As a screening test, the method is of value; 1) in the detection of moderate to severe coagulopathies, 2) for control of heparin treatment, and 3) as a rapid test for hypofibrinogenemia in obstetrical cases (Hattersley, 1966; Didisheim, 1967; Quick et al. 1948; Beller, 1964). Further modifications of the technique include the use of capillary tubes, and dilution of the blood (Menghini, 1950).

III. Recalcification Time

Principle of the Method: Platelet rich plasma is recalcified and the time measured until clotting occurs.

Material: Disposable needles (18 or 20 gauge), disposable plastic syringes, 5 and 10 ml. Test tubes, 11×75 mm, glass, siliconized or plastic. Water bath of 37° C. Isotonic, buffered calcium chloride solution (25 mM $CaCl_2$) (see Chapter 2), Kaolin or celite powder ("J. M. Hyflo-Super-Cel 101-3", Johns Mansville).

A. Using Siliconized Tubes

Procedure: Citrated blood is collected by the two syringe technique (9 parts of blood and 1 part of 3.8 % Trisodium citrate solution (see Chapter 2). Platelet rich plasma is prepared as previously described (see Chapter 9). A tube with 0.2 ml of plasma is placed in a 37° C water bath and prewarmed for 2–3 min and 0.2 ml of prewarmed calcium chloride solution is added and a stopwatch started. Clotting may be observed by tilting the tube or by determining the end point with a platinum wire loop. Triple determinations are recommended. Normal range: 160 to 260 sec.

B. Using Celite Activation (Voss, 1964)

Procedure: Platelet rich plasma is prepared, and a 0.2 ml aliquot is pipetted into a glass tube containing 18 mg Celite. The tube is placed in a water bath at 37° C and agitated occassionally for 6 min. Calcium chloride solution (0.2 ml) is added and a stop watch started. Clotting is observed by tilting or by the platinum wire loop technique. Triple determinations are recommended. Normal range: 16 to 47 sec.

C. Comment

The recalcification time is found prolonged in most congenital and acquired coagulopathies, in the presence of endogenous inhibitors, and under heparin treatment. The latter technique of standardized contact activation can be modified to include Kaolin etc. (Margolis, 1958; Voss, 1964; Nossel, 1964). Citrated plasma is preferred to oxalated plasma because large amounts of platelets are trapped in the buffy coat of oxalated plasma during centrifugation even at low speeds (Barkhan, 1957).

References

Barkhan, P. (1957). *J. Clin. Pathol. 10*, 26.

Beller, F. K. (1964). *Clin. Obstet. Gynecol. 7*, 372.

Botti, R. E., and Ratnoff, O. D. (1964). *J. Lab. Clin. Med. 64*, 385.

Didisheim, P. (1967). *Am. J. Clin. Pathol. 47*, 622.

Hattersley, P. G. (1966). *J. Am. Med. Assoc. 196*, 436.

Hoak, J. C., Warner, E. D., and Connor, W. E. (1967). *Circulation Res. 20*, 11.

Howell, W. H. (1916). *Am. J. Physiol. 40*, 526.

Lee, R. I., and White, P. D. (1913). *Am. J. Med. Sci. 145*, 495.

Margolis, J. (1967). *J. Physiol. 137*, 95.

Margolis, J. (1958). *J. Clin. Pathol. 11*, 406.

Margulies, H., and Barker, N. W. (1949). *Am. J. Med. Sci. 218*, 42.

Menghini, G. (1950). *Schweiz. Med. Wochschr. 6*, 139.

Niewiarowski, St., Stuart, R. K., and Thomas, D. P. (1966). *Proc. Soc. Exptl. Biol. Med. 123*, 196.

Nossel, H. L. (1964). "The Contact Phase of Blood Coagulation". Scientific Publications, Oxford.

Quick, A. J., Honoratio, R., and Stefanini, M. (1948). *Blood 3*, 1120.

Voss, D. (1964). *Thromb. Diath. Haemorrhag. 12*, 295.

Vroman, L. (1967). *In:* "Blood Clotting Enzymology" (W. H. Seegers, ed.), pp. 279—322, Academic Press, New York.

Waaler, B. A. (1959). *Scand. J. Clin. Lab. Invest. 11, Suppl. 37*, 1.

Heparin Sensitized Clotting Time

Johs. Gormsen

I. Introduction

The in vitro heparin sensitized clotting time was introduced by Waugh and Ruddick (1944) who intended to obtain "a controlled deacceleration, a slow-motion registration of the coagulation with a magnification of finer changes" especially regarding increase in overall coagulability.

The various models of the test were designed for the diagnosis of hypercoagulable states and later applied as a guide in determining dosage of antiprothrombinic drugs as they were suggested to offer a better measure of total coagulability than the prothrombin complex methods of Quick (1957) and Owren and Aas (1951).

From the biochemical viewpoint, it is noteworthy that the "sensitization" of the clotting time technique depends on multiple sites of action of heparin; its inhibition of thrombin, prothrombin activation as well as platelet function and tissue thromboplastin.

II. Description of Methods

The in vitro methods require the addition of heparin to venous whole blood, oxalated or citrated plasma. The principle of in vivo methods is to measure the clotting time of blood or plasma before and after intravenous injection of heparin. Capillary blood has also been used.

A. In Vitro Methods

1. Whole Blood

In the original method described by Waugh and Ruddick (1944) 1 ml of venous blood was added to each of 8 tubes containing increasing amounts of heparin in saline (0.1 to 1 U/0.5 ml). The tubes were placed in a rack mechanically tilted 70°–80° every 2 min. at room temperature. The clotting time was defined as the time when blood no longer flowed down the side of the tube. The normal range using 0.1 U/0.5 ml was 10–25 min. No statistical evaluation was given. This technique has not gained wide acceptance.

Fitzgerald Peel (1953) simplifying the above test used a single tube test adding 1.0 ml of venous blood to 0.1 ml heparin solution at 37° C. Rosenbaum and Barker (1948), using plasma rather than whole blood, tried to eliminate the difficulties in reading the end point by means of a photocell system, a method unsuitable for routine use. Although a number of investigators prefer the use of whole blood because it is more physiological, this technique is impossible to standardize.

According to Marbet and Winterstein (1950) citrated whole blood (1 part 3.8 % trisodium citrate plus nine parts of blood) is admixed with a heparin test solution (Hoffmann La-Roche, Basle, Switzerland). A 0.2 ml aliquot of the heparin test solution is diluted with 9.8 ml of a 1/40 M calcium chloride solution. Citrated blood (0.5 ml) is mixed with 0.5 ml of the heparin-calcium chloride mixture. The tube is left for 1 min in the water bath, and subsequently tilted every 15 sec. until clotting is completed. Normal values lie around 180 sec.

2. Platelet Rich Plasma

Silverman (1948) first introduced the use of platelet rich plasma. A number of authors have subsequently modified this technique.

According to Poller (1954) 4.5 ml of venous blood is admixed with 0.5 ml of a 1 % solution of potassium oxalate. Platelet rich plasma is obtained by slow centrifugation (see Chapter 9) and 0.5 ml of the plasma is admixed with 0.5 ml of a 0.25 % solution of calcium chloride and 0.1 ml of heparin solution (1 U/0.1 ml). The clotting time is read at the appearance of a distinct fibrin web or film. The tubes are not reversed, only tilted carefully. The normal range (100 normal heatlhy adults of both sexes and all age groups) was between 6.5 and 13 min, with an experimental error of around 10%. The heparin solution used (Pularin®, 10 U/ml) could be stored for months at 4° C. Beaumont and Lenegre (1952), Soulier (1955) and Soulier and LeBolloch (1950) have collected extensive experience with their modification of the heparin sensitized clotting time (heparin tolerance test). Systematic studies of potential errors in methodology were carried out by these authors. Incorrect venipuncture, too frequent tilting of the tubes, hemolysis, and more than 4 hours delay before testing will simulate an increase in heparin resistance. Too rapid centrifugation, the use of citrated instead of oxalated plasma, and the use of insufficiently cleaned acid washed glassware will result in an apparent decrease in heparin resistance. The heparin solution (in calcium chloride) is stable only for 6 days (4° C).

According to Soulier (1955), 4.5 ml of venous blood is admixed with 0.5 ml of Wintrobes oxalate. After centrifugation, a series of tubes containing 0.5 ml of platelet rich plasma is recalcified at 37° C with 0.5 ml of a 0.025 M calcium chloride solution containing 0, 0.3, 0.5, 0.7 and 1.0 U of heparin/0.5 ml. The tubes are left in the water bath and tilted very little. The clotting time is read when the tube can be inverted without escape of the clot. Normal range for 1 U of heparin in the system is 8–12 min. A normal control subject is tested with each patient. According to Soulier (1955), the test is very useful for the control of anticoagulant therapy, and apparently better suited than the one-stage prothrombin time. Some objections have been raised to Soulier's technique, particularly the difficulties in establishing an accurate endpoint.

Gormsen (1959, 1960) recommends the use of citrated plasma because an inhibitor might be neutralized by recalcification of oxalated plasma (Nilsson and Wenchert, 1954). Venous blood is collected directly into standardized, chilled siliconized centrifuge tubes. The tubes are immediately centrifuged at room temperature for 3 min. at 200 x g. This generally produces at least 1 ml of platelet rich plasma containing no erythrocytes unless the hematocrit is very high. The platelets are counted in all plasma samples and the presence of spontaneous aggregation is noted. A low count and/or significant aggregation might indicate an unsuccessful venipuncture. A 0.5 ml aliquot of plasma is prewarmed for 1 min. at 37° C in a standardized test tube (internal diameter 8 mm) and next recalcified with 0.5 ml of 0.025 M solution of calcium chloride containing 1 U/ml heparin (Leo). The heparin-$CaCl_2$ mixture should be prepared at least 24 hrs before testing and should not be older than 6 days. The tubes are stoppered, inverted once, left stoppered in the water bath for 3 min., once more, and again left in the water bath. From there on they are inspected every minute until a change in opalescence indicates the beginning of clotting. At that point the tubes are inspected every 30 sec. and tilted very slightly. Clotting time is read when a significant fibrin web is seen. In plasma exhibiting increased heparin resistance this is followed quickly by formation of a firm clot. In 90% of 350 normal healthy adults of both sexes and all age groups, the clotting time was between 10 and 15 min. The standard error for repeated tests on plasma pools or from 10 consecutive plasma samples obtained from one and the same individuals was about 10% for clotting times at 10 min. and about 20% for clotting times at 15 min. All tests were carried out within one hour after withdrawal. Plasma exhibiting significant increase in heparin resistance could be left in stoppered, siliconized tubes for 2–3 hrs. at 4° C without change.

B. In Vivo Methods

An in vivo method was first introduced by De Takats (1943). He injected 10 mg of heparin intravenously and measured the clotting time of capillary blood before and 10, 20, 30, 40 and 50 min. after the injection.

Koller (1945), measured the thrombin time of oxalated plasma before and 30 minutes after injection of 40 mg of heparin. Hagedorn and Barker (1948) estimated whole blood clotting times before and 10 min. after injection of 25 mg heparin. All authors have found significant differences in the individual reaction to heparin. In vivo methods provide interesting results but are not very practical. Problems such as rate of elimination and effect of clearing factor etc., complicate interpretation of the results.

C. Plasma Thrombin Times

Increase in heparin resistance as identified by a recalcification time might also, in some instances, be demonstrated by a heparin sensitized thrombin time (Gormsen, 1960, 1961) (for technical detail see section VII).

III. General Discussion

The final diagnostic value of these tests are not firmly established since the parameters measured are largely unknown. It is known that heparin interferes with thromboplastic, thrombin and some platelet functions. Platelets contain an antiheparin factor. Defects in any of these activities are associated with a decreased heparin resistance.

Increase in heparin resistance is particularly marked in patients suffering from thromboembolic disorders, but a large number of patients show an equally marked increase without any clinically evident thrombotic complication (Gormsen and Haxholdt, 1960).

Godal (1961) suggested that increase in heparin resistance is caused by some proteins generally found in patients suffering from malignant disease, acute or chronic inflammatory, and degenerative diseases, proteins without any known influence on the clotting system. Holger-Madsen (1962) transferred protein fractions containing no clotting factors from plasma with increased heparin resistance to normal plasma, which afterwards showed increase in resistance.

Heparin resistance generally decreases during hypoprothrombinic treatment. However, there are patients who do not react (Gormsen, 1960). It may develop post-operatively in patients receiving hypoprothrombinic agents even at times when no change has occured in prothrombin time measurements (Gormsen and Haxholdt, 1961). Increase in heparin resistance has also been described in patients developing thromboembolic complications while adequately controlled by thrombin time measurements while on anticoagulant therapy.

Because of its pronounced electron-negative charge, heparin may combine with any net-positively charged protein molecule (Fisher, 1935; Jaques, 1943; Jorpes, 1935). It is therefore possible that an increase in heparin resistance depends on proteins which have no influence on the clotting mechanism.

References

Beaumont, J. P., and Lenegre, J. (1952). *Rev. Hematol. 7,* 228.

Fisher, A. (1935). *Biochem. Z. 278,* 133.

Fitzgerald Peel, A. A. (1953). *Brit. Heart J. 15,* 8.

Godal, H. C. (1961). *Scand. J. Clin. Lab. Invest. 13,* 314.

Gormsen, J. (1959). *Brit. J. Haematol. 5,* 257.

Gormsen, J. (1960). *Acta Haematol. 24,* 213.

Gormsen, J. (1961). *Thromb. Diath. Haemorrhag. 6,* 144.

Gormsen, J., and Haxholdt, B. F. (1960). *Acta Chir. Scand. 120,* 121.

Gormsen, J., and Haxholdt, B. F. (1961). *Acta Chir. Scand. 121,* 367.

Hagedorn, A. B., and Barker, N. V. (1948). *Amer. Heart J. 35,* 603.

Holger-Madsen, T. (1962). *Acta Haematol. 27,* 294.

Jaques, L. B. (1943). *Biochem. J. 37,* 189.

Jorpes, E. (1935). *Biochem. J. 29,* 1817.

Koller, F. (1945). *Schweiz. Med. Wochschr. 75,* 290.

Marbet, R., and Winterstein, A. (1950). *Aerztl. Forsch. 10,* 460.

Nilsson, J. M., and Wenckert, A. (1954). *Acta Med. Scand. 150, Suppl. 297.*

Owren, P. A., and Aas, K. (1951). *Scand. J. Clin. Lab. Invest. 3,* 201.

Poller, L. (1954). *Angiology 5,* 21.

Quick, A. J. (1957). "Haemorrhagic Diseases". Lea & Febiger, Philadelphia.

Rosenbaum, E. E., and Barker, N. W. (1948). *J. Lab. Clin. Med. 33,* 1342.

Silverman, S. B. (1948). *Blood 3,* 147.

Soulier, J. P. (1955). 1st Inter. Conf. Thrombosis and Embolism, Basel, 1954. B. Schwabe & Co., p. 793.

Soulier, J. P., and LeBolloch, A. G. (1950). *Rev. Hematol. 5,* 148.

De Takats, G. (1943). *Surg. Gynecol. Obstet. 77,* 31.

Waugh, T. R., and Ruddick, D. W. (1944). *Can. Med. Assoc. J. 50,* 547.

Thrombelastography

HELLMUT HARTERT

I. Introduction

During the conversion of fibrinogen to fibrin a number of plasma constituents contribute not only to the formation of fibrin, but also to the proper firmness of the formed clot. This is documented by the fact that a clot obtained from purified fibrinogen by the addition of thrombin lacks several physical properties, in particular proper firmness, which a fibrin clot formed in plasma possesses. Thrombeblastography (Hartert, 1948, 1949, 1950, 1951, 1960; Hartert and Schaeder, 1962), also called thrombodynamography (Leroux, 1957), basically measures the firmness of a clot, or more precisely, the modulus of shear elasticity. A blood clot has been referred to as a Maxwell body (Scott-Blair, 1960), indicating that it has viscous as well as elastic properties. Whereas the viscosity of the blood as a whole has no influence on thrombelastography, the viscosity of the fibrin has to some extent. This can be measured directly as an individual parameter.

The thrombelastograph (TEGraph)* allows the continuous visual and photo-kymographic observation of a blood or plasma sample during all phases of coagulation, and the resulting recording is termed a thrombelastogram (TEG).

II. Basic Description of Apparatus and Principle

A blood or plasma sample is placed in a cylindrical cuvette of stainless steel (18/8 chromium nickel steel of the quality of Krupp's V2A steel) which is thermostatically maintained at a temperature of 37° C. The cylinder is connected to a moving device by means of which it is periodically rotated back and forth over an angle of 4°45′ ($^1/_{12}$ radian) around the vertical axis. A cylindrical rod of stainless steel is lowered into the cuvette to a distance of 1 mm from the bottom and the walls of the cuvette. The rod which carries a small mirror is suspended on a steel torsion wire with an established elastic momentum while the other end of the wire is fixed (Fig. 1). The mirror reflects

* Fa. Hellige, Freiburg, Germany; U.S.A. distributor: Haemoscope Corp. 866 Willis Ave., Albertson, L. I., N. Y.; Canada Distributor: Oxyjector Company, 80 Coe Hill Drive, Toronto 3, Ont.

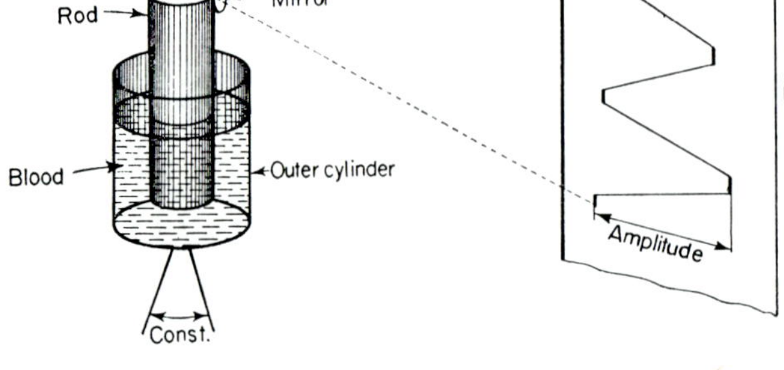

Fig. 1. Schematic drawing of the basic unit of a thrombelastograph and its principle of action.

the light from a slit lamp on a scale of opaque glass, allowing direct readings of the movements of the rod, but also reflects the light onto photographic paper (width 100 mm) which moves at a rate of 2 mm/min. As long as the blood or plasma sample is not clotted, the suspended rod will remain motionless, and it will only begin to turn after coagulation has started. This time span represents the coagulation time (Fig. 1). The transfer of the periodical movement of the cuvette onto the suspended rod is caused by the network of elastic fibrin forming between cell wall and rod. As fibrin formation and solidification of the coagulum progresses, the rotations of the rod increase proportionally, resulting in a progressive increase in positive and negative deflections of the light ray from the mirror. The motion of the cuvette takes 3.5 sec for one 4°45′ turn in either one direction, after which the cuvette stands still for 1 sec in either one of the end-positions. An entire cycle lasts a total of 9 sec. The light of the slit lamp is so attenuated that the photographic paper is blackened only during the stationary periods of the cuvette in the end-positions, resulting in the typical thrombelastographic tracing (Fig. 2). One full range motion of the cuvette theoretically equals a deflection (amplitude) of exactly 100 mm. A TEG of such an amplitude does not occur in practice, since it would require a clot of infinitely high shear modulus (elasticity). The mechanical constants of the TEGraph are standardized in such a way that the shear modulus (elasticity) of a normal plasma clot from recalcified platelet-rich citrated plasma results in a deflection (amplitude) of 50 mm. The correlation between shear modulus (elasticity) and amplitude is not linear in the TEG which has the advantage of a high sensitivity for even markedly decreased shear moduli. An amplitude (a) of 50 mm was assigned an elasticity modulus (ε) of 100 arbitrary units which equals approximately 5,000 dynes/cm^2. The corresponding equation is:

$$= \frac{100\,a}{100 - a} \qquad (1)$$

Based on this equation, a table was made which allows the conversion of any amplitude (a), measured in mm, into its elasticity (ε) units (Table 1). In normal thrombelastograms the amplitudes will very gradually decrease after having reached a maximal amplitude (m a). This slow but gradual decrease in amplitude seems to be the result of a growing flaccidity of the clot. It has, therefore, become customary to measure the greatest amplitude of the tracing (maximal amplitude) and convert it with the use of Table 1 into maximal elasticity (m ε) units.

III. Techniques of Measurement

The blood for thrombelastographic measurements should, as a matter of principle, always be venous blood and not capillary blood, and should be obtained from a clean venipuncture. Contamination of the blood with tissue fluid no longer gives proper and reproducable measurements. More over, it is of considerable importance to establish a certain mode of operation when using the thrombelastograph and strictly adhere to this pattern. Every modification may influence the results. For example, the measurements are greatly influenced by temperature and, therefore, it is imperative to allow for proper pre-heating of the thrombelastograph and the cuvettes.

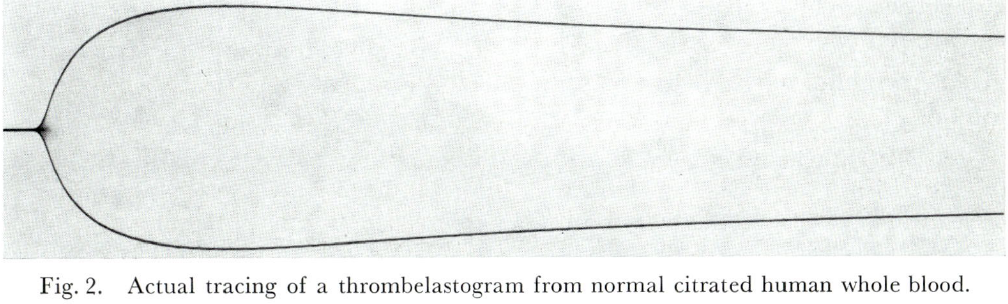

Fig. 2. Actual tracing of a thrombelastogram from normal citrated human whole blood.

Table 1: Conversion of Amplitudes (a) in millimeters into Elasticity Units (ε)

a	ε	a	ε	a	ε	a	ε
1	1 (r)	39	64	63	170	82	455
2	2	40	67		174		471
3	3	41	69	64	178	83	488
4	4	42	72		182		506
5	5	43	75	65	186	84	525
6	6	44	79		190		545
7	8	45	82	66	194	85	567
8	9	46	85		199		587
9	10	47	89	67	203	86	614
10	11	48	92		207		641
11	12	49	96	68	212	87	668
12	13	50	100		217		700
13	15		102	69	222	88	733
14	16	51	104		228		770
15	18		106	70	233	89	808
16	19	52	108		239		852
17	20		110	71	245	90	900
18	22	53	113		251		958
19	23		115	72	257	91	1011
20	25 (k)	54	117		264		1076
21	27		119	73	270	92	1150
22	28	55	122		277		1233
23	30		125	74	284	93	1328
24	32	56	127		292		1438
25	33		130	75	300	94	1566
26	35	57	133		308		1718
27	37		135	76	317	95	1900
28	39	58	138		326		2122
29	41		141	77	335	96	2400
30	43	59	144		344		2751
31	45		147	78	355	97	3233
32	47	60	150		365		3900
33	49		153	79	377	98	4900
34	52	61	156		388		6566
35	54		160	80	400	99	9900
36	56	62	163		413		19900
37	59		167	81	426		
38	61				440		

The thrombelastographic measurements can be carried out in native whole blood, in recalcified citrated whole blood, and in recalcified citrated plasma. The values obtained for each of the three types of measurement are different and cannot be directly compared.

A. Measurements with Native Whole Blood

Measurements with native whole blood precludes the patient's presence in the laboratory or at least in a very close distance from the laboratory. If the patient is in the laboratory the blood may directly run from the needle into the cuvette placed in a portable container thermostatically maintaining a cuvette temperature of 37° C ("Thermophor"T) (Petersen et al. 1954). The cuvette is then immediately transferred into the TEGraph. The cuvette should be filled up to approximately 2/3 of its volume or 0.36 ml. The blood may also be collected in a siliconized tube at 37° C, following which 0.36 ml of blood is pipetted by means of a siliconized pipette into the cuvette preheated to 37° C for at least 5 min in the TEGraph. If the patient is located at a close distance from the laboratory, the blood is run directly from the needle into the cuvette which is placed in the thermophor, and then immediately transported in the thermophor to the laboratory. There it is promptly transferred into the TEGraph. Obviously all of these manipulations have to be done before coagulation begins and, therefore, time is the limiting factor when working with native whole blood. The time elapsed from the beginning of withdrawal of the blood from the vein until the beginning of the thrombelastographic recording has to be accurately measured by means of a stopwatch, and later on added to the recorded coagulation time. In practice, a stopwatch is put into action as soon as the first drop of blood enters the cuvette or the siliconized glass tube.

As the cuvettes are placed into the TEGraph, the rods are lowered into the cuvettes. The surface of the blood should be about 1/2 mm from the upper end of the cuvette after the rod is lowered into position. Excess of blood may quickly be removed by a dry syringe. Actually, overfilling affects the accuracy of the measurements much less than incomplete filling. The surface of the blood is then covered over with paraffin oil to avoid evaporation and the recording is started.

B. Measurements with Citrated Whole Blood

More convenient and in many instances more accurate are measurements with citrated whole blood. Blood is withdrawn into a 5 ml siliconized glass or plastic syringe containing 3.8 % sodium citrate (0.5 ml citrate plus 4.5 ml blood). The blood is immediately transferred into a siliconized glass tube at 37 °C. By carefully tilting the tube twice or three times a thorough mixing of citrate and blood is guaranteed. The citrated blood should be used as promptly as possible but not later than within two to four hours after its withdrawal. Before use the blood has to be recalcified. With a siliconized pipette 0.6 ml of citrated whole blood is transferred to a small siliconized serological test tube which contains 0.4 ml m/40 $CaCl_2$ solution. The $CaCl_2$ solution is mixed with the blood by once tilting the tube. Immediately thereafter, 0.36 ml of the recalcified blood is pipetted with a siliconized pipette into a cuvette preheated in the TEGraph at 37 °C for at least 5 min. Foaming has to be avoided. The rod is lowered into position, the surface of the blood covered with paraffin oil and the recording started. Again the time which elapsed from the addition of the citrated blood to the $CaCl_2$ solution until the beginning of the recording is accurately measured by means of a stopwatch and later on added to the recorded coagulation times.

C. Measurements with Citrated Plasma

Thrombelastographic recordings may also be obtained from citrated plasma, but the measurements are greatly dependent upon the number of platelets in the plasma. Therefore, platelet rich plasma should always be used. Blood is collected in 3.8 % sodium citrate as described above and centrifuged in a siliconized tube for 3 min at 800 x g at room temperature (Marchal et al. 1961). The plasma is separated by means of a siliconized pipette and collected in a siliconized glass tube, kept at 37 °C. Care must be exercised not to contaminate the plasma with leucocytes or erythrocytes. The thrombelastographic measurements should be performed as soon as possible and no later than two hours after collection of the blood. For recalcification 0.36 ml of plasma are transferred by means of a siliconized pipette to a siliconized serological test tube containing 0.36 ml m/40 $CaCl_2$ solution. Proper mixing is achieved by tilting the tube carefully once. Immediately thereafter 0.36 ml of the recalcified plasma is transferred with a siliconized pipette into the cuvette, avoiding foaming, and the rod is lowered into position. The plasma is immediately covered by paraffin oil and the recording is started. As for citrated whole blood, the time from adding the plasma to the $CaCl_2$ solution until the beginning of recording is accurately measured by means of a stopwatch. This time has to be added to the recorded coagulation time.

IV. Evaluation of the Thrombelastogram

A. Evaluation Technique

The distance from the beginning of the recording to the point where the amplitude has reached 1 mm (measured from the outer edge of the upper branch to the inner edge of the lower branch) is termed "r" time (reaction time) (Fig. 3) and is equivalent to the coagulation time of the specimen. Since the photographic paper moves at a speed of 2 mm/min, the measured distance in mm is divided by 2 in order to get the conversion of mm to minutes and seconds. In the case of whole blood measurements, the time from the withdrawal of the blood from the vein until the beginning of recording on the photographic paper has to be added to the measured r-time, in order to get the accurate coagulation times of the blood. In the case of the citrated whole blood or citrated plasma, the time elapsed from the beginning of recalcification until beginning of the actual recording on the TEGraph is added.

The time elapsed from the end of the r-time to a point where an amplitude of 20 mm is attained, is termed "k" time or thrombus formation time (Fig. 3). The k-time is a measure of

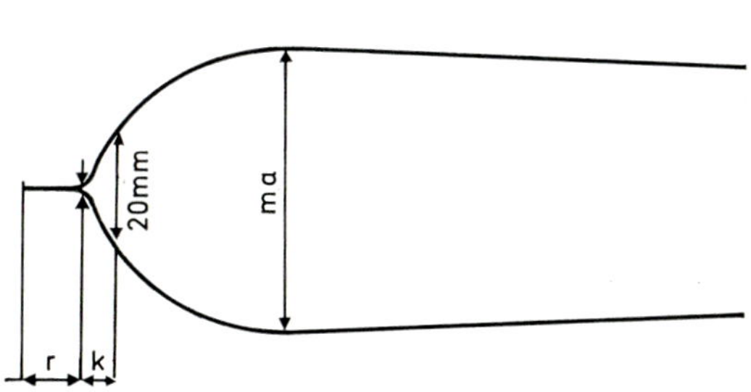

Fig. 3. Thrombelastographic tracing with a description of r-time, k-time and maximal amplitude (m a).

the speed with which a clot of a certain solidity is developed, or the time which elapses until the clot has reached an elasticity modulus (ε) of 25 (Table 1). Therefore, the distance between the two lines is measured in mm, and by division with 2 the actual time in minutes and seconds is obtained.

As coagulation progresses and the clot reaches an increasing solidity, the positive and negative deflections will reach a maximum. After that the deflections decrease slightly, due to an increased flaccidity of the clot. This phenomenon can, therefore, be envisioned as the relaxation (also referred to as "softening") of the clot and is entirely different from fibrinolysis. The point of the TEG where the amplitude (measured from the outer edge of the upper branch to the inner edge of the lower branch) is greatest, is termed "maximal amplitude" (m a) (Fig. 3). The amplitude (a) measured in mm is then converted to elasticity (ε) units by means of table 1 to give the maximal elasticity (m ε).

B. Mean Values

The thrombelastographic measurements not only depend upon the type of blood used (whole blood, citrated whole blood, citrated plasma), but also upon the techniques used. The amount of surface contact which a specimen makes before the actual recording is of considerable influence on the measurements. Therefore, one has to adopt a certain working technique and strictly adhere to this procedure in order to obtain reproducable and comparable results. The measurements may even be influenced by microscopical scratches on the cuvettes and rods, and it is of importance to strictly adhere to the cleaning techniques described in the manual accompanying the apparatus. In order to minimize this, Loeliger (1958) introduced disposable cuvettes made from polystyrole. However, the rod is not disposable. The disadvantage of the disposable type cuvettes is that they need a considerably longer time to reach a temperature of 37° C, so that temperature differences might influence the measurements.

Several investigators have calculated mean values for the various types of thrombelastographic measurements and these are summarized in table 2. The differences in measurements comparing whole blood with citrated whole blood and citrated plasma are evident. The differences noted in the measurements by different investigators for the *same* type of blood are due to slight differences in the technique used, such as withdrawal of blood or recalcification.

V. Abnormal Thrombelastographic Measurements

A number of changes have been observed in thrombelastographic recordings when abnormal blood clotting states were investigated.

Table 2: Normal Values for Thrombelastographic Measurements of Whole Blood, Citrated Whole Blood and Citrated Plasma. The Data are Compiled from Several Publications.

Authors	Type of Blood	r-time	k-time	Maximal Elasticity (m ε)
Hartert (1951)	Whole Blood	12′	6′	90–150
Hartert and Schaeder (1962)	Citrated Whole Blood	4″	2′	100
Hartert (1951)	Citrated Plasma	8′ 40″	3′ 20″	122
Walther and Volhard (1951)	Whole Blood	12′ 18″ ± 2′ 36″	6′ 6″ ± 1′ 12″	105 ± 17
Beller et al. (1956)	Whole Blood	9′–14′	5′–8′	80–180
Beller et al. (1956)	Citrated Plasma	4′–6′ 30″	1′–2′ 30″	150–350
Leroux (1957)	Citrated Plasma	7′ 30″– 10′ 45″	2′ 15″–4′ 15″	85.5–167
Schneider et al. (1962)	Whole Blood	12′ 36″ ± 1′ 34″	5′ 53″ ± 1′ 1″	108 ± 17.7
Schneider et al. (1962)	Citrated Whole Blood	8′ 25″ ± 1′ 2″	4′ 4″ ± 47″	109 ± 17.3

Fig. 4. Thrombelastographic patterns for fibrinolysis. The series on the left side was obtained by adding plasmin in increasing concentrations to plasma. The plasmin concentrations were as follows (from top): 0.49, 0.74, 0.97, 1.23, 1.47 casein units. Bottom record is the control. The series of thrombelastograms on the right side was obtained by adding urokinase to plasma. The final urokinase concentrations were as follows (from top): 1.38, 2.75, 5.50, 11.0 and 22.0 Ploug units. The bottom record is again the control. (Astrup and Egeblad, 1967).

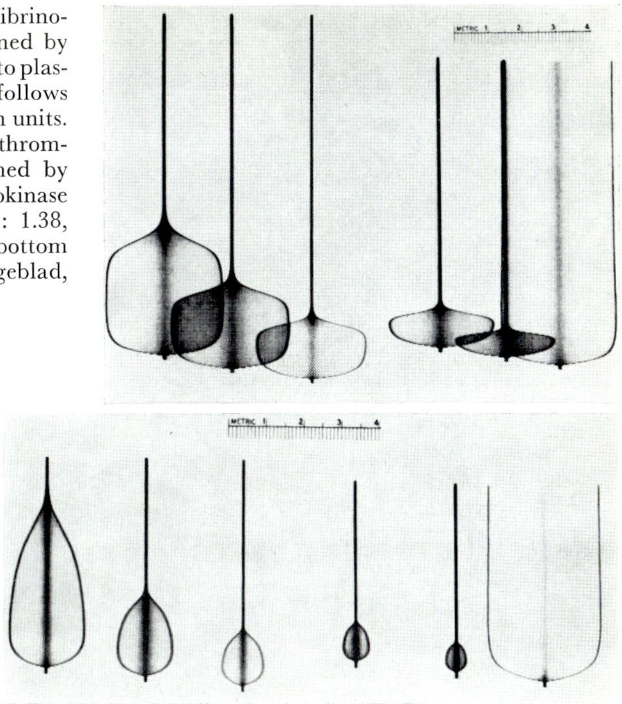

The r-times and k-times are considerably prolonged in the blood of patients with both types of hemophilia whereas very little changes are observed in patients with congenital factor V and factor VII deficiency (Beller et al., 1956). Patients with so-called factor X deficiency display prolonged r-times and k-times (Beller et al., 1956). The same changes are observed in patients with Hageman deficiency, in the course of heparin treatment, and in the presence of fibrinogen breakdown products. Changes in the maximal amplitudes are usually related to decreased concentrations of fibrinogen or platelets, and TEGs' of patients with hypofibrinogenemia and/or thrombocytopenia display a considerable decrease in maximal amplitudes. The r-times are usually normal in these disease states. Prolonged r-times and decreased maximal amplitudes are associated with some types of dysfibrinogenemia (Mammen et al., 1968). The presence of fibrinogen split products also causes a decrease in maximal amplitudes.

Shortening of r-times and k-times has been associated with "hypercoagulable" states (Beller, 1957; Marchal et al., 1961).

Fibrinolysis produces a sudden sharp decline in the amplitudes and in most instances they reach values of zero, indicating that the initially formed clot was completely dissolved. A number of thrombelastographic patterns typical for fibrinolysis are shown in Fig. 4. The pattern differs depending on the degree of lysis. Astrup and Egeblad (1967) have noted that the lysis pattern changed greatly with the addition of either plasmin or urokinase (Fig. 4). The time of lysis can be established by measuring the distance from the beginning of the k-times until the point where the amplitude reaches zero again.

The continuous regular decrease in maximal amplitude, as seen in fibrinolysis, should not be confused with a phenomenon which is characterized by an *irregular* decline in amplitude. This pattern is caused as first observed by Beller (1957) by a detachment of the clot from the wall of the cuvette and has been observed in patients with uremia, leukemia, hemolytic anemia and thrombocytosis, but was also observed during pregnancy and in the puerperium (Beller, 1957). This phenomenon has no relationship to fibrinolysis.

References

Astrup, T. and Egeblad, K. (1967). *Am. J. Physiol. 209,* 84.
Beller, F. K. (1957). "Die Gerinnungsverhaeltnisse bei den Schwangeren und beim Neugeborenen". Barth, Leipzig.
Beller, F. K., Koch, F. and Mammen, E. (1956). *Blut 2,* 112.
Hartert, H. (1948). *Klin. Wochschr. 26,* 577.
Hartert, H. (1949). *Klin. Wochschr. 27,* 789.
Hartert, H. (1950). *Klin. Wochschr. 28,* 77.
Hartert, H. (1951). *Z. Exptl. Med. 117,* 189.
Hartert, H. (1960). In: "Flow Properties of Blood and Other Biological Systems". (A. L. Copley and G. Stainsby, Ed.) pp. 188—189, Pergamon, Oxford.
Hartert, H. and Schaeder, J. A. (1962). *Biorheology 1,* 31.
Leroux, M. E. (1957). La thrombélastographie (thrombodynamographie). Etudes théoriques, techniques, expérimentales et cliniques sur la thrombélastographie et sur quelques problèmes connexes liés à la Thèse Doct. Médicine, Paris.
Loeliger, E. A. (1958). *Thromb. Diath. Haemorrhag. 2,* 441.
Mammen, E. F., Prasad, A. S., Barnhart, M. I. and Au, C. C. (1969). *J. Clin. Invest. 48,* 235.
Marchal, G., Leroux, M. E. et Samama, M. (1961). Atlas de la Thrombodynamographie, Pise, Paris.
Petersen, H., Breddin, K. and Roettger, K. (1954). *Klin. Wochschr. 32,* 328.
Schneider, W., Rodermund, O. E. and Egli, H. (1962). *Thromb. Diath. Haemorrhag. 7,* 35.
Scott-Blair, G. W. (1960). In: "Flow Properties of Blood and Other Biological Systems". (A. L. Copley and G. Stainsby, Ed.) pp. 63—83, Pergamon, Oxford.
Walther, G. and Volhard, E. (1951). *Medizinische 17,* 651.

Partial Thromboplastin Time Techniques

Robert D. Langdell

I. Introduction

The partial thromboplastin time has been used extensively in studies of plasma coagulation disorders. It is sensitive to a deficiency of any of several plasma procoagulants and to the presence of certain coagulation inhibitors. It has been found to be an effective method for screening patients with a bleeding tendency, for evaluating the effect of therapy in procoagulant disorders, and as the basis for several specific assay procedures.

Plasma from patients with hemophilia was found to clot as rapidly as did plasma from normal individuals in the presence of potent tissue thromboplastin by Quick et al. (1935). It was shown by Langdell et al. (1953) that this potent tissue thromboplastin when appropriately diluted no longer had the ability to compensate for the plasma defect of hemophilia. A number of thromboplastins were found to be similar to the dilute tissue thromboplastin in that they failed to compensate for the hemophilic defect. The term "complete thromboplastin" is used for those materials which have the ability to compensate completely for the hemophilic defect in one-stage clotting systems. Those materials which, in similar systems, do not appear to compensate completely for the hemophilic defect were termed "partial thromboplastins". One-stage type clotting tests using partial thromboplastin were termed "partial thromboplastin time". It was shown by Brinkhous et al. (1954) that other plasma procoagulant deficiencies also were not compensated for by partial thromboplastin in one-stage type clotting tests. The method has been found to be a measure of a deficiency of any of the plasma procoagulants other than factor VII.

II. Reagents

A. Partial Thromboplastin Suspension

A number of materials have been found to have partial thromboplastin activity. These include platelet suspensions, appropriately dilute tissue thromboplastin, vegetable phospholipids, and animal cephalins. Results appear more consistent with laboratory prepared animal cephalins or with commercially prepared partial thromboplastins. At least five preparations are now available from commercial sources: Thrombofax, Ortho; Platelin, Warner-Chilcott; Hyland Partial Thromboplastin, Hyland Labs; Cephaloplastin, Dade Reagents; and Tachostyptest, Hormonchemie, Munich, Germany.

An acetone insoluble, ether soluble crude animal cephalin can be prepared from brain tissue of various animals.

1. Wash the brain with tap water and remove the meninges, accessible blood vessels, brain stem and cerebellum.

2. The amount of tissue to be processed is not critical. About 100 gm of wet tissue is a convenient amount with which to work. This is cut into small pieces and placed in a mortar.

3. Add sufficient acetone to cover the tissue. Mash the tissue under acetone with a pestle. When the solution becomes cloudy, the acetone should be discarded and replaced with fresh acetone. After this procedure has been repeated several times, the acetone will remain clear and the tissue will be dry and flaky.

4. The acetone dehydrated tissue is then ground with clean sand. The sand and ground tissue are placed in a flask that can be stoppered. Sufficient ether is added to cover the solid material. After mixing, the flask is stoppered and allowed to stand overnight (about 12 hours) at room temperature. It is important that the solid material remains well covered by ether throughout this period.

5. The solid material is removed by filtration and discarded. The fluid portion is evaporated to dryness, preferably under vacuum. The waxy residue is washed twice with boiling acetone and then air dried.

6. The waxy residue is then suspended in isotonic saline to make a 3 % suspension. This is stored in 0.1 ml lots below −20° C.

7. The working suspension of 0.3 % is prepared by adding sufficient isotonic saline. It is important that a uniform suspension by prepared.

B. Anticoagulant Reagents

Blood is obtained by venipuncture and mixed immediately with anticoagulant solution. Either sodium oxalate (0.1 M) or sodium citrate (0.11 M) may be used (1 part of anticoagulant plus 9 parts of blood). Each has some advantages and disadvantages. Oxalate forms a cloudy suspension of calcium oxalate when calcium chloride is added to the mixture. The end point is quite sharp and distinct as the fibrin clot incorporates the suspension and the fluid becomes clear at the time of clotting. Citrate forms a soluble complex with calcium so that the end point is a fibrin web in the clear fluid. It is generally believed that citrate has a stabilizing influence on the labile procoagulants. It is of importance that the test and control samples be handled in exactly the same manner. Plasma samples may be kept at room temperature for a short time. If more than 30 min will elapse before testing, it is best to keep plasma samples in an ice water bath.

III. Steps in procedure

1. In separate tubes place partial thromboplastin reagent and calcium chloride (0.02 M) in a 37° C water bath. About 0.3 ml of each reagent will be needed for each plasma sample to be tested.

2. Into a clean dry test tube (10×75 mm) add 0.1 ml plasma and place in 37° C water bath.

3. Allow plasma to reach water bath temperature (a standard time should be selected. Thirty seconds is usually a convenient time). In rapid succession add 0.1 ml partial thromboplastin suspension and 0.1 ml 0.02 m $CaCl_2$.

4. Start a timer as soon as calcium solution has been added. Mix contents of tube thoroughly.

5. While constantly agitating the tube, observe the contents with a good light source.

6. Stop the timer as soon as the first evidence of a visible clot forms. Record the elapsed time between the addition of $CaCl_2$ and visible clotting. Repeat the procedure to obtain at least duplicate results. Triplicate determinations will increase the accuracy of the method.

IV. Interpretation of Results

With a satisfactory partial thromboplastin normal human plasma will clot in about 60–70 second. Any results 10 seconds greater than the control time are to be considered as abnormal. Plasmas with severe deficiencies will usually require 120 seconds or more to clot. Additional studies are necessary to characterize the abnormality.

V. Modifications

A. Test for Clotting Inhibitors

Mix equal volumes of test plasma with normal control plasma. Determine the partial thromboplastin time of the mixture. If the clotting time of the mixture is not within 10 seconds of the control, an inhibitor is probably present.

B. Presumptive Diagnostic Method

A long partial thromboplastin time indicates a significant defect in at least one of the plasma procoagulants. When the partial thromboplastin time is used in combination with the prothrombin time, most procoagulant disorders can be classified. The prothrombin time is abnormal with deficiencies of prothrombin, factor V, factor VII, and factor X. The partial thromboplastin time is abnormal with deficiencies of prothrombin, factor V, factor VIII, factor IX, factor X, factor XI, and factor XII.

1. A plasma with a long prothrombin time and a normal partial thromboplastin time is probably deficient in factor VII.
2. If both the prothrombin time and the partial thromboplastin time are long, the plasma is deficient in prothrombin, factor V, or factor X, provided an afibrinogenemia or dysfibrinogenemia has been excluded.
3. If the prothrombin time is normal but the partial thromboplastin time is long, the plasma is deficient in factor VIII, factor IX, factor XI or factor XII.

The use of barium sulfate adsorbed normal plasma in the test system will allow further classification. Barium sulfate treated plasma contains factor V and factor VIII, but is deficient in prothrombin, factor VII, factor IX and factor X. Barium sulfate treated normal plasma will correct the prothrombin time and partial thromboplastin time abnormality due to factor V deficiency but will not correct for factor X deficiency. Barium sulfate treated normal plasma will correct the long partial thromboplastin time due to factor VIII deficiency but will not correct for factor IX deficiency.

Definitive diagnosis depends upon the failure of correction of the defective plasma under investigation by a plasma known to be deficient in a specific factor. When done on a simple 1:1 mixing basis, this serves as a qualitative diagnostic procedure. When quantitative amounts of test plasma are added to a plasma substrate of known deficiency, this is the basis as a quantitative assay procedure.

C. Additive Reagents

It was noted in the original description of the method that various unrelated materials could accelerate the partial thromboplastin time of both normal and abnormal plasma. The effect of these materials was similar to that produced by increasing the concentration of tissue thromboplastin. That is, the clotting time decreased and the time interval separating the clotting time of normal plasma from hemophilic plasma decreased. Although duplicability is improved with the faster clotting time, the differential between normal and abnormal approaches zero.

One must make a choice between sensitivity and duplicability. Sensitivity is usually of more importance when the procedure is used as a diagnostic screening test while duplicability is of more importance when the procedure is used to assay for a specific factor.

Insoluble materials containing silica have been added to activate the plasma used in the test (Procter and Rapaport, 1961). The use of these materials was reviewed by Nye et al. (1962). Some commercial preparations contain these activator materials. If such partial thromboplastins are used, the directions supplied by the manufacturer must be followed.

D. Micro Method

A method using capillary blood rather than venous blood has been described (Miale, 1962). A specially calibrated glass tube is recommended. This is calibrated to hold 0.015 ml sodium citrate and 0.15 ml blood. Blood is obtained by a capillary puncture. After mixing, the tube is sealed and centrifuged. The plasma is obtained by breaking the tube.

All reagents are warmed to 37° C, then 0.05 ml partial thromboplastin reagent and 0.05 ml $CaCl_2$ (0.02 M) are pipetted into a clean dry glass tube (10×75 mm). After mixing the calcium and thromboplastin, 0.05 ml of plasma is blown into the tube and a timer started. The first appearance of a fibrin clot is the end point. The results are interpreted as in the standard method.

VI. Precautions

The partial thromboplastin time is simple to perform but to achieve meaningful results strict adherence to good technique is essential. The glassware must be chemically clean. Pipetting must be done with accuracy. Many minor modifications are possible and may be of convenience. However, a standard system must be developed and done exactly the same each time a test is done.

If plasma is tested at intervals during the first 30–45 minutes after collection, the partial thromboplastin time gradually decreases. When the sample is allowed to stand as whole blood in a glass tube for 45 minutes prior to centrifugation, the partial thromboplastin time of the plasma is relatively constant. The use of silicone treated glassware will delay this acceleration phenomenon but gradual shortening of the clotting time still occurs.

Best results are obtained with reasonable fresh plasma. If testing is to be delayed for more than 1–2 hours, the plasma should be frozen. A control sample should be handled in exactly the same manner.

References

Brinkhous, K. M., Langdell, R. D., Penick, G. D., Graham, J. B. and Wagner R. H. (1954). *J. Am. Med. Assoc. 154,* 481.

Langdell, R. D., Wagner, R. H. and Brinkhous, K. M. (1953). *J. Lab. Clin. Med. 41,* 637.

Miale, J. B. (1962). "Laboratory Medicine-Hematology" Ed. 2, Mosby, St. Louis.

Nye, S. W., Graham, J. B., and Brinkhous, K. M. (1962). *Am. J. Med. Sci. 243,* 279.

Procter, R. R. and Rapaport, S. I. (1961). *Am. J. Clin. Pathol. 36,* 212.

Quick, A. J., Stanley-Brown, M., and Bancroft, F. W. (1935). *Am. J. Med. Sci. 190,* 501.

Prothrombin Consumption Tests

N. Raphael Shulman

I. Introduction

Prothrombin consumption tests are designed to measure the rate at which prothrombin disappears as blood clots. If all of the prothrombin that disappears from plasma during coagulation became thrombin and remained active, then the amount of thrombin generated would accurately reflect the amount of prothrombin consumed. However, as discussed (see Chapter 2), thrombin is rapidly inactivated by high levels of antithrombin in plasma or serum and little or no thrombin activity is detectable shortly after blood clots. Using a technique in which the effect of antithrombin is neutralized by dilution, prothrombin consumed during clotting can be determined by comparing the amount of prothrombin present initially in plasma with amounts remaining at intervals during the clotting process.

This section concerns a description of the types of information that can be obtained by determining the amount of prothrombin consumed when blood clots.

The most accurate method of measuring prothrombin in plasma or serum is the so-called "two-stage" procedure, which has been developed by several groups of investigators (Soulier, 1948; Ware and Seegers, 1949; Warner et al. 1936). The principles of the two-stage prothrombin assay form the foundation for the methods of determining prothrombin consumption rates as outlined in the following.

II. Measurement of Prothrombin Consumption

A. In Normal Blood

Figure 1 shows the rate at which prothrombin disappears from whole blood in glass tubes incubated at 37° C under conditions of the Lee-White clotting time (see Chapter III). The prothrombin consumption technique used to obtain this information (Shulman et al. 1964) is a modification of previously described techniques (Dick et al. 1954; Graham et al. 1955). Specifically, blood is obtained by the two-syringe technique. Three ml aliquots of blood from fasting subjects are placed in 10×75 mm acid cleaned glass tubes and incubated at 37° C. At desired intervals prothrombin conversion is stopped by mixing the blood thoroughly with 0.03 ml of 1.36 M trisodium citrate, using a glass rod for breaking clots to assure admixture. Each prothrombin consumption value is based on the average prothrombin content of three tubes of incubated blood, compared to the prothrombin content of citrated plasma from the same donor. The interval of incubation is measured from the time blood enters the second syringe. For the first 5 to 7 min of incubation, blood remains fluid and there is no detectable prothrombin consumption because the factor that converts prothrombin to thrombin has not yet become activated through the complex biochemical sequence of the "intrinsic" and "extrinsic" clotting systems (see Chapter I). At the time that blood clots (7 to 14 min, in Fig. 1), there is a rapid burst of prothrombin conversion and free thrombin is measurable in blood (see Chapter I). Approximately 10 to 30 % of prothrombin is consumed at the time that the third tube of the Lee-White test clots. After blood clots and all fibrinogen is converted to fibrin, prothrombin consumption continues until at the end of approximately 1 hr, in normal blood, more than 90 % of prothrombin is consumed. In the usual test for prothrombin consumption, residual prothrombin is measured in blood that has been incubated at 37° C for 60 min from the time blood enters the second syringe. The three tubes of the Lee-White clotting time further incubated after clotting are suitable for this purpose, even though they have been "tipped" (Shulman et al. 1964).

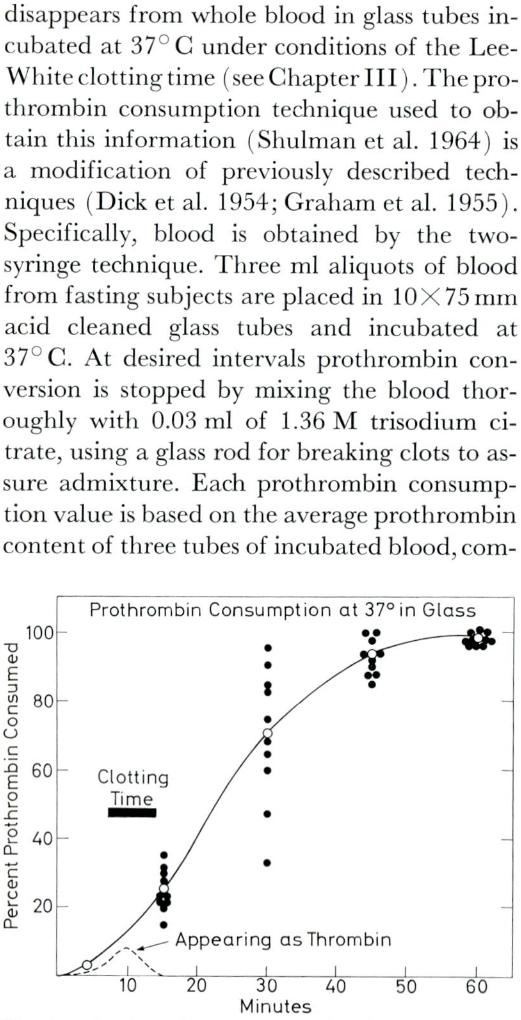

Fig. 1. *Prothrombin consumption in ten normal individuals*
Each solid dot represents the average prothrombin consumption value obtained from three separate tubes of blood on each of 10 individuals (see text). The mean value is shown by open circles. The dashed line indicates the amount of active thrombin that can be measured in blood at about the time blood clots.

The original prothrombin consumption tests that were described were "one-stage" procedures, i. e., essentially prothrombin times with a source of fibrinogen added to serum. In the one-stage tests the actual amount of prothrombin consumed cannot be measured because marked accelerator activity develops early in the course of blood coagulation and makes the prothrombin time of serum shorter than that of plasma until almost all prothrombin is consumed (DeVries et al. 1949; Langdell et al. 1950). A recent review of the one-stage prothrombin consumption time test is found in Quick (1965). In the past, this test was used frequently as a diagnostic aid, but is now superseded by more specific and precise techniques.

B. In Abnormal Blood

Any abnormality of blood that decreases the rate of activation of the clotting system slows the rate of prothrombin conversion. The abnormalities that delay prothrombin conversion

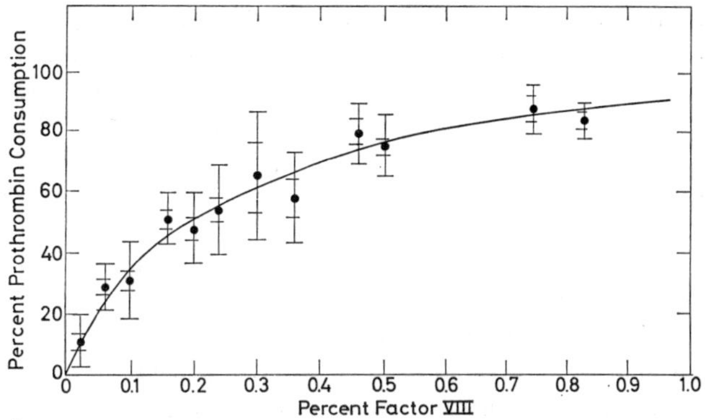

Fig. 2. *Values for 60-minute prothrombin consumption of hemophilic blood containing various concentrations of Factor VIII*
These in vivo levels were obtained by infusing plasma from normal individuals into hemophiliacs. The estimation of concentration is based on dilution of small amounts of donor plasma in the recipient's plasma volume. All recipients had a clotting time in glass > 60 minutes before normal plasma was infused. The points represent the mean of 6 to 8 prothrombin consumption values for each concentration of Factor VIII, the inner brackets the standard deviation of the mean, and the outer brackets the standard deviation of individual determinations. (This figure is reproduced from Shulman et al. 1964.)

include deficiency of an antihemophilic factor, i. e., of Factor XII, XI, IX, or VIII, which activate the "intrinsic" clotting system; deficiency of Factor X, the pivotal enzyme involved in prothrombin activation; or a severe deficiency of platelets or Factor V, both of which accelerate the "extrinsic" clotting system.

Not only deficiency of clotting factors but also changes in the conditions of clotting tests affect prothrombin consumption. Marked inhibition of prothrombin consumption occurs when the "contact phase" of clotting is prevented by use of siliconized or plastic surfaces. Even partial siliconization of glassware through slight contamination decreases prothrombin consumption. Lower temperatures retard the over-all enzymatic process of blood clotting and decrease the rate of prothrombin conversion, as do suboptimal or above-optimal Ca^{++} concentrations, or pH values on either side of the 7.1 to 7.5 range.

The 60-min prothrombin consumption values of blood completely deficient in Factor VIII (or other antihemophilic factors) is close to 0 %. If increasing amounts of Factor VIII are added to the deficient blood either in vivo or in vitro, prothrombin consumption increases as shown in Fig. 2. Prothrombin consumption is almost normal, i. e., 90 % or more, when Factor VIII concentration is 1 to 2 % of normal. The relationship between prothrombin consumption and clotting time values of partially corrected Factor VIII deficient blood is shown in Fig. 3. The data of Figs. 2 and 3 are typical of data obtained for other antihemophilic factors, but the concentration producing

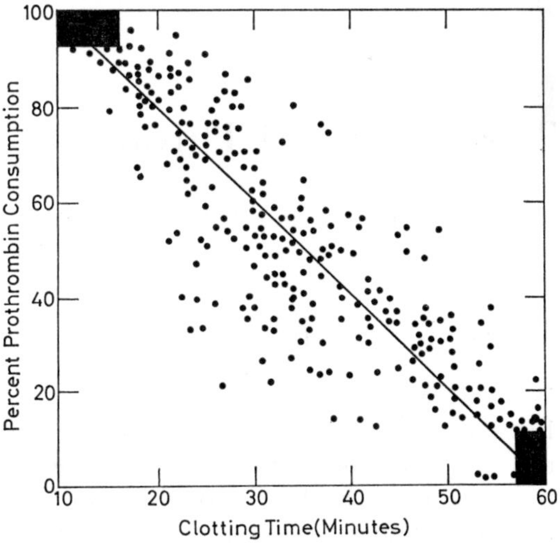

Fig. 3. *Relationship between the three-tube clotting time in plain glass and percent prothrombin consumption*
Each point represents the average of 3 prothrombin consumption determinations done on the separate tubes used to measure the clotting time. There was no statistical difference in the prothrombin consumption measured in the first and third tubes used. Clotting time and prothrombin consumption were measured from the time that blood entered the second syringe. (This figure is reproduced from Shulman et al. 1964.)

a given effect varies for each factor. Generally a deficiency of a clotting factor or of platelets that is severe enough to decrease prothrombin consumption also prolongs the clotting time. This circumstance occurs only when the level of the clotting factor or platelets is less than 2% of normal. The rate of prothrombin conversion in glass, like the clotting time, does not reflect in vivo hemostatic effectiveness, for clotting factor concentrations in the range of 15 to 30% of normal are necessary to prevent hemorrhage. Prothrombin consumption measurements are therefore not helpful in diagnosing mild deficiency states, and the more serious deficiency states can be detected with simpler tests. Prothrombin consumption tests, however, do afford a means of assaying certain clotting factors at levels too low to be detected by other techniques. Research applications of this method of measuring Factor VIII in distribution and survival studies and in studies of circulating anticoagulants have been described (Langdell et al. 1955; Shulman et al. 1964).

References

DeVries, A., Alexander, B., and Goldstein, R. (1949). *Blood 4,* 247.

Dick, F. W., Jackson, D. P., and Conley, C. L. (1954). *J. Clin. Invest. 33,* 1423.

Graham, J. B., Penick, G. D., and Brinkhous, K. M. (1955). *In:* "The Coagulation of Blood" (Tocantins, L. M., ed.), pp. 77—80, Grune and Stratton, New York.

Herz, N., DeVries, A., and Heiman-Hollander, E. (1950). *Acta Med. Scand. 138,* 211.

Langdell, R. D., Graham, J. B., and Brinkhous, K. M. (1950). *Proc. Soc. Exptl. Biol. Med. 74,* 424.

Langdell, R. D., Wagner, R. H., and Brinkhous, K. M. (1955). *Proc. Soc. Exptl. Biol. Med. 88,* 212.

Quick, A. J. (1965). *Tech. Bull. of Regis. Med. Technol. 35,* 217.

Shulman, N. R., Marder, V. J., and Hiller, M. C. (1964). *In:* "The Hemophilias" (Brinkhous, K. M., ed.), pp. 29—43. Univ. of North Carolina Press, Chapel Hill, N. C.

Soulier, J. P. (1948). *Rev. Hematol. 3,* 302.

Ware, A. G., and Seegers, W. H. (1949). *Am. J. Clin. Pathol. 19,* 471.

Warner, E. D., Brinkhous, K. M., and Smith, H. P. (1936). *Am. J. Physiol. 114,* 667.

Thrombin and Thromboplastin Generation Techniques

Charles D. Forbes and A. Stuart Douglas

I. Introduction

When a clean venepuncture is performed and half the blood is delivered to a plain glass tube and half to a tube containing some tissue extract, the blood in the empty glass tube may take ten minutes to clot whereas that in the tissue extract tube takes ten seconds to coagulate. Since such tissue is outwith the vascular endothelium and not in contact with blood, this mechanism for prothrombin conversion is called the extrinsic prothrombin converting system. The blood in the plain glass tube is clotting under the influence of a prothrombin converting principle formed from reagents contained in normal blood and not requiring the presence of any tissue extract. This intrinsic prothrombin converting principle has also been called blood or plasma thromboplastin or intrinsic prothrombin activator. Some authorities have objected to the use of the term thromboplastin in this context because this was used originally to describe tissue extract in the classical theory of blood coagulation as postulated by Morawitz (1905) at the beginning of this century. The tests described in this chapter include the thromboplastin generation test; since this term has been in common usage in this context for fifteen years, it would be confusing now to make a change in descriptive terminology. The tests described in this chapter are designed to study the intrinsic prothrombin converting principle and are not concerned with the extrinsic system. These techniques test the ability of the blood to react to surface contact and thereafter, as a result, to form blood thromboplastin. In a sense these tests are all non-specific, in that, no one specific aspect of the complex reactions leading to prothrombin conversion is studied. The tests can, however, be modified to make them more specific.

A. Thrombin Generation

In the thrombin generation test the appearance of thrombin in the test sample (whole blood or recalcified plasma) is detected by subsampling into fibrinogen, the clotting time of which is determined. As the fibrinogen preparation is relatively free from prothrombin, this indicator system is a measure of thrombin in the incubation tube. The clotting time of the fibrinogen samples can be related to incubation time and a curve representing the appearance and disappearance of thrombin can be drawn. When samples are removed from whole blood and tested for thrombin activity by transferring into fibrinogen, no thrombin activity can be detected for some time. When coagulation starts, much thrombin is suddenly released and continues to be formed even after fibrin formation is complete. Thrombin formation occurs because of the development of a powerful prothrombin converting substance. There is, however, a delay phase before this prothrombin converting principle is formed. When there is a failure of formation of the prothrombin converting principle, thrombin generation may be delayed or suboptimal. Prothrombin conversion may also be incomplete. This latter point can be tested after thrombin disappearance is complete by adding brain extract to the incubation tube and determining whether any further thrombin is formed.

B. Thromboplastin Generation

The thromboplastin generation test was devised in 1952; at that time it was known that in two conditions-thrombocytopenia and hemophilia – there was defective prothrombin consumption as a consequence of failure of formation of the prothrombin converting principle. It seemed probable, therefore, that platelets and the plasma factor missing in haemophilia were two of the components of blood thromboplastin. A crude preparation of the plasma factor missing in haemophilia could be made by adsorbing normal plasma with an inorganic precipitate such as aluminium hydroxide, which was removed by centrifugation. The adsorbed normal plasma was relatively free from prothrombin which was removed on the inorganic precipitate. Platelets were prepared by differential centrifugation of plasma and then washed. Adsorbed normal plasma and platelets were incubated together in the presence of calcium, and this incubation mixture was then used in place of brain in a one-stage "prothrombin" time technique by addition to normal plasma, which was simultaneously recalcified. No significant thromboplastin activity, however, was developed in the mixture of adsorbed normal plasma, platelets and calcium. It was concluded therefore that this incubation mixture did not contain all the constituents required to make blood thromboplastin. When coagulated normal blood is incubated for an hour at 37° C there is minimal residual prothrombin in the serum. If such serum is added to the mixture containing adsorbed normal plasma, platelets and calcium and the mixture tested as before on plasma in a one-stage technique, then in this incubation mixture there develops a very powerful prothrombin converting principle. As the time of incubation increases, the substrate clotting times are reduced and ultimately reach a minimum. This reduction indicates the formation of a prothrombin activator in the incubation mixture. It is now appreciated that this incubation mixture of adsorbed normal plasma, normal serum, platelets and calcium contains many factors required for blood thromboplastin formation (factor V, factor VIII, factor IX, factor X, factor XI, factor XII and the lipid from the platelets). In subsequent modifications of the test other lipids have been used in lieu of platelets, e. g. phospholipid from human brain (Bell and Alton, 1954) or inosithin, a commercial soy-bean phospholipid. When obtained from normal subjects these reagents (adsorbed plasma, serum and platelets) are relatively free from prothrombin; however, the incubation mixture usually coagulates, indicating some thrombin formation in the incubation tube from residual traces of prothrombin. The clotting times of the substrate plasma are therefore a measure, in the main, of prothrombin converting principle and to a very minor degree of thrombin. When the serum in the test system is derived from a patient with a defect in the blood thromboplastin system with, in consequence, defective prothrombin consumption there may be more thrombin present in the incubation tube.

All the reagents used in this test have been exposed to contact with glass and thus the earliest stages of clotting are not taken into account.

Normal serum which has been incubated for at least two hours at 37° C contains traces of prothrombin, no factor V and no factor VIII, as all of these are utilized or consumed in the coagulation of normal blood. The serum contains factors IX and X but no significant amounts of factors II, V or VIII. The serum also contains factors XI and XII, which are involved in blood thromboplastin formation, and in addition factor VII, which is not concerned with blood thromboplastin formation. The serum also contains no thrombin and no significant amounts of blood thromboplastin. The adsorbed normal plasma contains factors V, VIII, XI and XII, but no prothrombin, or factors VII, IX and X. Adsorbed plasma, serum and platelets are prepared from control blood and from the patient's blood. The test is usually used to study patients who have a normal one-stage prothrombin time, i. e. they have no deficiency of factors V, VII or X.

The main abnormalities which can be demonstrated with the thromboplastin generation test are shown in Table 1. Mixture 2 in this table would also be abnormal in factor V deficiency, especially if a platelet substitute is used (human platelets have factor V activity). This abnormality, however, would have been detected in the one-stage prothrombin time which would have been carried out before the thromboplastin generation test. Similarly, factor X deficiency would also be detected in mixture 3, but again this would have been suspected from the abnormal one-stage test.

If mixtures 2 and 3 both give grossly abnormal results then the probability is that the disorder is due to a circulating anticoagulant. If the abnormality in mixtures 2 and 3 is only slight then the explanation may be deficiencies of factor XI or factor XII, and a more definitely abnormal result will then be found in mixture 4; the same pattern of abnormality in mixtures 2, 3 and 4 will occur in combined deficiency of factors VIII and IX.

It is probable that in some patients with certain forms of thrombocytopathy substitution of patient's platelets in lieu of normal platelets will give an abnormal result.

C. Thrombin-Thromboplastin Generation (Thromboplastin "Screening" Test)

The third test described in this section is the thromboplastin screening test. When dilute platelet-poor plasma is recalcified in the presence of platelet substitute, intrinsic blood thromboplastin is formed and in consequence thrombin formation from prothrombin occurs progressively from the time of recalcification. The development of thrombin and thromboplastin can be followed by transferring aliquots of the reacting mixture to normal platelet-poor plasma, which is simultaneously recalcified. The clotting time of this indicator plasma re-

Table 1: Practical Application of the Thromboplastin Generation Test.

Mixture	Source of reagents			Coagulation disorder giving abnormal result
	$Al(OH)_3$ treated plasma	Serum	Platelets	
1	normal	normal	normal	Control – done in all experiments
2	patient	normal	normal	Factor VIII deficiency (Haemophilia)
3	normal	patient	normal	Factor IX deficiency (Christmas disease)
4	patient	patient	normal	Circulating anticoagulant Factor XI or XII deficiency

flects the thrombin plus thromboplastin activity in the incubation tube at the time of transfer of the aliquot. Reproducibility of the test can be enhanced by pre-incubating the test plasma with an optimal amount of kaolin immediately before recalcification; by this method variations due to degrees of contact activation can be eliminated.

II. Thrombin Generation Test

A. Methods

1. Whole Blood (Macfarlane and Biggs, 1953)

After clean venepuncture 2 ml of venous blood is delivered to a graduated glass centrifuge tube of standard size and shape. The tube contains 0.2 ml. of 0.85% saline. Immediately after delivery of the blood a wooden swab stick (with the end split) is placed in the tube, which is then incubated in a waterbath at 37° C. At two-minute intervals until clotting is seen in the incubation tube, 0.1 ml. samples are withdrawn and added to 0.4 ml. amounts of fibrinogen previously placed in the waterbath. The fibrinogen is prepared by a phosphate buffer method as described by Biggs and Macfarlane (1962). The clotting times of the fibrinogen specimens are recorded. The transferred samples consist of whole blood, i.e. they contain red cells. Using a thrombin-fibrinogen dilution curve, constructed as described by Biggs and Macfarlane (1962) the clotting times can be interpreted as thrombin units. The only technically difficult part of the test is the removal of the fibrin and this should be wound onto the swab stick as soon as it starts to form. Unless fibrin is removed as it forms the transfer of the aliquots may become difficult, as fibrin blocks the end of the pipette. Furthermore, if fibrin is transferred to the indicator tube, this may distort the clotting time. In the study of patients with blood thromboplastin defects fibrin formation is slow and the successful removal of the fibrin in these circumstances may require some practice. As soon as clotting starts in the incubation tube, the aliquots should be removed at one-minute intervals. Several stop watches are required in order to perform the test.

As thrombin forms, the clotting times in the fibrinogen tubes shorten and then progressively lengthen. When thrombin in significant amounts has ceased to be present (fibrinogen clotting times over 3 minutes), an addition of 0.1 ml. of brain thromboplastin is made and the presence of thrombin tested again at minute intervals for a further three minutes. A renewed generation of thrombin will occur if the blood thromboplastin system has been so defective as to leave unconverted prothrombin in the incubation tube.

In experimental circumstances the 0.2 ml. of saline can be replaced by reagents under test, e. g. serum. The test can be modified by carrying it out in silicone-coated glassware, in order to study the first stages of blood coagulation.

In Table 2, the results of this technique are given on blood taken from a control, a patient with mild haemophilia and a patient with moderate but not severe haemophilia. In blood from a patient with severe haemophilia no thrombin was generated during the incubation period shown in the table.

2. Plasma (Pitney and Dacie, 1953)

In order that this test provide reliable data, the plasma under test must be compared with a control specimen handled in an identical way. For example, the amount and duration of glass contact should be the same in the two specimens (control and test) and the platelet content should also be similar. The control and test specimens should therefore both be collected by clean venepuncture, using the same size needle and same type and size of syringe. The blood specimens should be collected at about the same time and delivered into identical tubes containing 1 volume of trisodium citrate (3.8%) per nine volumes of blood. The blood samples should be centrifuged together at about 800 x g for 5 minutes to avoid differences in platelet levels in the two samples. To carry out the test 0.25 ml. of test plasma is mixed with 0.25 ml saline and recalcified with 0.25 ml. of M/40 calcium chloride. At one-minute intervals 0.1 ml. of the reaction mixture is transferred to 0.4 ml. fibrinogen solution and the clotting time recorded. The clot which forms in the incubation tube can easily

Table 2: Thrombin Generation Test

Incubation time in mins.	2	3	4	5	6	7	8	9
Normal blood	180″+	180″+	57″	20″	14″	19″	28″	46″
Mild haemophilia	180″+	–	180″+	–	180″+	90″	52″	19″
Moderate haemophilia	180″+	–	180″+	–	180″+	–	180″+	–

Incubation time in mins.	10	11	12	13	14	15	16
Normal blood	63″	80″	130″	180″+	–	–	–
Mild haemophilia	21″	24″	24″	65″	180″+	–	–
Moderate haemophilia	180″+	–	100″	87″	54″	46″	45″

be removed by winding onto a wooden applicator stick.

B. Comments

This test may give abnormal results when there is a defective formation of blood thromboplastin or when there is a deficiency of prothrombin. Deficiency of prothrombin may be found in coumarin drug therapy or as one of the features of the coagulation inhibitor complicating systemic lupus erythematosus. When prothrombin is deficient thrombin appears at the normal time in the test but is reduced in amount. In blood thromboplastin defects, thrombin formation is delayed in its appearance and may be reduced in its amount. Deficiency of any of the components of blood thromboplastin (factors V, VIII, IX, X, XI and XII) may give an abnormal result. Inhibitors of blood thromboplastin formation (e.g. acquired anticoagulants or heparin administration) may also give abnormal results. In very severe defects there may be no thrombin formation during the period of incubation of the blood. In less severe defects there will be delayed and limited thrombin formation. After the addition of brain extract to the incubation tube in such patients more thrombin may then be generated. In mild blood thromboplastin defects the test may give a result which falls within the normal range.

This technique has been responsible for major advances in our understanding of blood thromboplastin (Biggs, 1952; Macfarlane and Biggs, 1953). Though the technique still has a place in the research approach to coagulation problems, its place as a routine test has been superseded. Some mild blood thromboplastin defects with normal whole blood clotting times will give a normal result in the thrombin generation test. Relatively mild blood thromboplastin defects with normal results in the thrombin generation tests may have abnormal results in the prothrombin consumption test. The thrombin generation test is therefore less sensitive than the prothrombin consumption test, which in turn is less sensitive than the kaolin cephalin clotting time in the screening of patients for blood thromboplastin defects. It is also more time consuming and more complex to carry out. Though the test may suggest deficiency of prothrombin, this factor requires to be assayed by techniques for this purpose (see Chapter V, p. 175). The test is also non-specific and if a blood thromboplastin defect is suspected then specific factor assays must be carried out to establish this. The test also has the disadvantage that the results cannot readily be expressed quantitatively.

III. Thromboplastin Generation Test

A. Methods

Aluminium hydroxide can be made in the individual laboratory (the method of Bertho and Grassman (1938) as described by Biggs and Macfarlane (1962). Alternatively, aluminium hydroxide moist gel (British Drug Houses or Behringwerke, Marburg, Germany) may be used; 3 gm. are suspended in 4 ml. distilled water to form a stock suspension. For use, this is diluted about 1 in 6. Due precautions should be taken to avoid admixing or contamination of the stock suspension with other components of the test system. Instead of aluminium hydroxide, barium salts ($BaSO_4$, $BaCO_3$) may be utilized; the latter preferably when oxalated plasma is used. Usually 100 mg/ml. plasma are sufficient.

1. Adsorbed Plasma

Blood is obtained from the patient and the control at approximately the same time and withdrawn using the same size of needle and syringe. Clean venepuncture is essential. Nine ml. of blood is delivered into a standard graduated centrifuge tube containing 1 ml. of 3.8 % sodium citrate. The two citrated bloods are centrifuged at 2,000 x g for 15 minutes and the plasmas separated into identical containers. A 0.1 ml. aliquot of aluminium hydroxide is added to 1 ml. of citrated plasma and incubated with gentle stirring at 37° C for 1–2 minutes. The aluminium hydroxide adsorption of the plasma should be tested by performing the one-stage prothrombin time; this should be greater than 60 seconds. The adsorbed plasma is diluted 1 in 5 in physiological saline.

2. Serum

Approximately 10 ml. of blood is delivered into another plain glass centrifuge tube and incubated for two hours at 37° C. Again similar specimens are obtained from control and patient. There is a tendency for the activity of diluted serum to increase with time and therefore the dilutions of serum should be made immediately prior to use in the test. The serum is diluted 1 in 10 in physiological saline.

3. Platelets or Platelet Substitutes

Platelet-rich normal plasma is prepared by centrifugation of citrated blood at 600 x g for 5 minutes. Plasma thus obtained is separated and spun at 2,000 x g for 30 minutes and the platelets are deposited as a pellet at the bottom of the tube. The residual plasma is suitable as substrate in the test. The pellet is washed three times with 0.85 % saline and the platelets are resuspended in a volume of saline equivalent to one-third to one-half of the original plasma volume. This platelet suspension can be used fresh or maintained frozen at –20° C. It is reasonably stable and can be frozen and thawed on several occasions and still remain suitable for use in the test with only slightly limited potency.

An alternative is the use of platelet substitutes available commercially, e. g. chloroform extract of brain as described by Bell and Alton (1954) (Stayne Laboratories Ltd.) used at a concentration of 1 in 150 in saline or inosithin-soy a bean phospholipid (Associated Concentrates Inc., N. J., obtained in Britain through V. A. Howe and Co., Ltd., platelet substitute, Behring-Werke, Marburg, Germany; Tachostyptest, Hormonchemie, München, Germany; Platelin, Warner-Chilcott, Morris Plains, New Jersey).

4. Substrate or Indicator Plasma

This is normal citrate plasma which has been "high-spun" to remove platelets. This may be the plasma from which the platelets have been prepared. This can be used fresh or stored frozen at –20° C for 2–3 weeks but should not be refrozen and used on a subsequent occasion.

All the reagents should be kept at the temperature of melting ice for the duration of the test. The glassware used in carrying out the test should be of standard size i.e. for the incubation tube and for substrate clotting times. Substrate plasma in 0.1 ml. amounts are pipetted into each of 6 tubes which are then placed in a waterbath at 37° C. The incubation mixture is made by adding together 0.3 ml. adsorbed plasma diluted 1 in 5, 0.3 ml. serum diluted 1 in 10, 0.3 ml. platelet suspension and recalcifying with 0.3 ml. M/40 calcium chloride. At one minute intervals 0.1 ml. of the incubation mixture is pipetted simultaneously with 0.1 ml. of M/40 calcium chloride into the substrate plasma, the clotting time of which is recorded. The small fibrin clot which forms in the incubation mixture is removed by means of a wooden applicator stick. Care should be taken to avoid transfer of any fragments of fibrin to the substrate tube. The simultaneous manipulation of the two pipettes requires practice before adequate expertise is established.

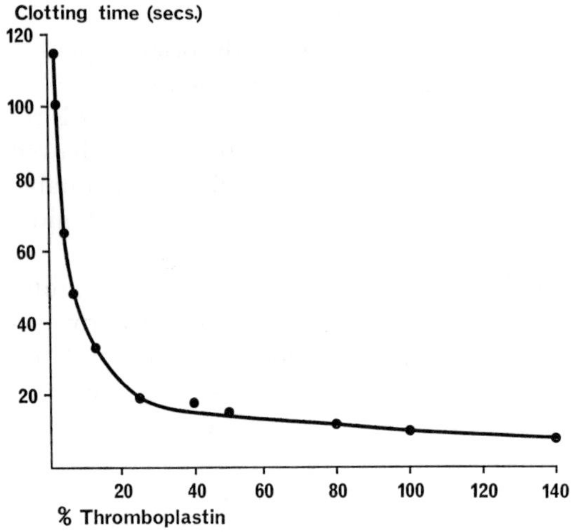

Fig. 1. This figure shows the thromboplastin dilution curve constructed from clotting times of substrate plasma obtained from various dilutions of blood thromboplastin.

Several stop watches are required to carry out the tests. An example of results if given in Table 3.

The amount of thromboplastin can be assessed from a thromboplastin dilution curve which is prepared as follows. Blood thromboplastin is prepared from the diluted adsorbed normal plasma, diluted normal serum, platelets and M/40 calcium chloride. When a minimum substrate clotting time is obtained the incubation mixture is placed at the temperature of melting ice. Dilutions from 1 in 2 to 1 in 32 are made with 0.85 % saline. The dilutions are kept on melting ice and are tested with normal substrate plasma as already described. A curve relating clotting time and thromboplastin concentration can then be drawn (Fig. 1). The data, e.g. in Table 3 from the patient with haemophilia, can then be expressed graphically was shown in Fig. 2.

The test should be performed with the following mixtures:

	Adsorbed Plasma	*Serum*
(1)	Control	Control
(2)	Patient	Patient
(3)	Patient	Control
(4)	Control	Patient
(5)	Control	Control

The repeat of line (1) in position (5) provides a check on the stability of the system. Line (2) is likely to demonstrate whether there is abnormality. If line (3) is abnormal but (4) is normal, the defect is haemophilia (factor VIII deficiency). If line (4) is abnormal but line (3) is normal, the disorder is Christmas Disease (factor IX deficiency). If there is a gross abnormality in both (3) and (4), the most likely explanation is the presence of a circulating anticoagulant. As already explained, abnormalities in both (3) and (4) can be due to deficiencies of factors XI or XII, or to double deficiencies (factors VIII and IX), or possibly factors V and X if the one-stage prothrombin time test is prolonged. The presence of a circulating anticoagulant can be detected by minor modification of the test. The control line is repeated with an addition of 0.3 ml of saline in the incubation tube prior to recalcification.

Table 3: Results Using the Thromboplastin Generation Test

Condition tested	Source of Reagents			Incubation time in minutes					
	$Al(OH)_3$ adsorbed plasma	Serum	Platelets	1	2	3	4	5	6
				Clotting time in seconds					
Normal	Normal	Normal	Normal	61	50	32	11	10	10
Haemophilia	Patient	Normal	Normal	65	62	59	55	50	48
(Factor VIII deficiency)	Normal	Patient	Normal	55	49	20	11	10	10
Christmas disease	Normal	Patient	Normal	69	59	60	49	47	47
(Factor IX deficiency)	Patient	Normal	Normal	55	45	31	10	10	10
Circulating anticoagulant	Normal	Patient	Normal	79	75	72	69	61	55
	Patient	Normal	Normal	75	75	70	70	65	57
PTA deficiency	Normal	Patient	Normal	61	51	38	13	12	12
(Factor XI deficiency)	Patient	Normal	Normal	59	53	37	14	12	12
	Patient	Patient	Normal	61	58	42	33	26	20

This will make little difference to the amount of thromboplastin recorded in the indicator plasma. If 0.3 ml. of patient's diluted adsorbed plasma or diluted serum is added to the incubation tube in place of saline then the inhibitor will be readily demonstrated.

B. Comments

The technique as described above is very similar to the original technique of Biggs and Douglass (1953) and is that used by the authors. Many modifications have been made and these have been satisfactory in the hands of individual workers. The most important issue is that the person carrying out the technique is experienced in the particular modification of the test being used. Some authors use higher dilutions of the adsorbed plasma and normal serum. Others make the dilutions in buffer instead of saline. Some advise collection of the serum on the day before the test and that the diluted serum should be stored at +4° C overnight; this is because there is some increase in activity of the serum, which occurs over the first few hours when serum is diluted and allowed to stand. Other laboratory workers have modified the indicator system; in the method used by Biggs and Macfarlane (1962) 0.1 ml. of the incubation mixture is added at minute intervals to 0.2 ml. of M/40 calcium chloride; a few seconds later 0.2 ml. of normal plasma is added; the clotting time is recorded from the time of addition of the plasma. Others have used a different adsorbing agent such as barium sulphate. The test is best recorded as the clotting time data, though this may be converted to percentages of thromboplastin from the thromboplastin dilution curve and the data recorded graphically. The disadvantage of the latter is that a two-seconds difference (from 10 sec to 8 sec) at the higher level of the scale may represent a large difference on the percentage scale (100% to 140%). In a technique of this kind the recording of a genuine two seconds difference is extremely difficult.

The thromboplastin generation technique has been widely used in coagulation studies and has been modified particularly to assay factors VIII and IX (Biggs and MacFarlane, 1962). The test is still a useful method for the study of blood thromboplastin defects. Its routine use, however, has largely been superseded by other techniques. In the detection of blood thromboplastin defects most laboratories rely for initial screening on the kaolin-cephalin clotting time combined with specific assays of factors VIII and IX. Many laboratories add in one further screening procedure; some use the prothrombin consumption test, others the thromboplastin screening technique (see below); in this laboratory the thromboplastin generation test is still used as the additional screening procedure. It undoubtedly lacks sensitivity in comparison with the kaolin-cephalin clotting time of the specific assays for factors VIII and IX. Patients with mild haemophilia or mild Christmas Disease may not be detected. When levels of factor VIII or factor IX are above 10% they are unlikely to be detected in the thromboplastin generation test. Since patients may have excessive bleeding with levels below 30% of either of these factors, the specific assays are required to detect these patients. The technique involving the preparation of two of the reagents (adsorbed plasma and serum) has potentially large technical variation, but with major coagulation defects the differences from normal obtained with pathological specimens are so large that this technical variation is not important. A disadvantage is that the preparation of the various reagents is time consuming.

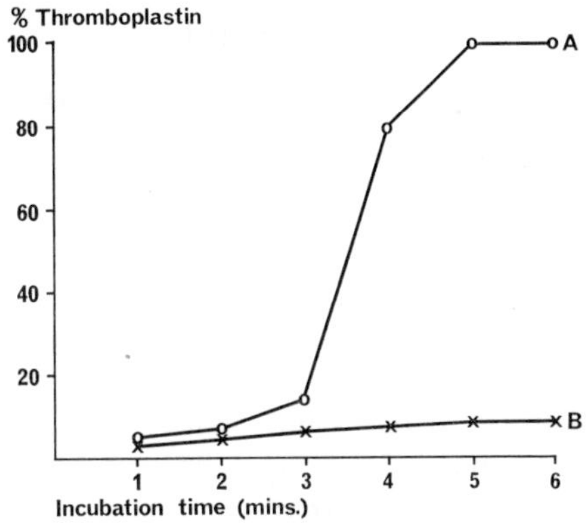

Fig. 2. This figure shows the results of the thromboplastin generation test expressed in percentage thromboplastin from normal reagents (curve A) (normal adsorbed plasma, normal serum) and from a patient with haemophilia (curve B) (patient adsorbed plasma, normal serum).

IV. Thromboplastin "Screening" Test (Thrombin-Thromboplastin Generation Test

A. Methods

The technique recorded here is based on the methods of Hicks and Pitney (1957) and MacPherson and Hardisty (1961) and is described by Hardisty and Ingram (1965).

Suspension of light kaolin. Light kaolin (B.D.H.) is suspended in "tris" buffer (0.05 M. in 0.05 % saline, pH 7.35)–0.5 gm per 100 ml. This is further diluted in 1 in 5 in tris buffer for use in the thromboplastin screening test. The reagent is stored at 4° C and the bottle should contain a few glass beads to aid resuspension.

Inosithin. This is a commercial soy-bean phospholipid which forms a convenient platelet substitute (Associated Concentrates, Inc., N. J., obtainable in Britain through V. A. Howe & Co. Ltd). This material comes as waxy granules forming colloidal solutions in water; a stock is prepared at a concentration of 1 mg. per 100 ml buffer; the preparation of this colloidal solution requires prolonged agitation. When made, this should be frozen in 1 ml. amounts. For use, the reagent is thawed and diluted approximately 1 in 50. Additional details on the preparation of inosithin for use in clotting test systems is given by Hardisty and Ingram (1965).

Substrate or indicator plasma — as described above under thromboplastin generation test.

Platelet-poor (high spun) plasma (control and patient) is diluted with 9 volumes of buffered isotonic saline. A 0.1 ml. aliquot of the kaolin suspension is measured into a 12 mm tube and placed in a waterbath at 37° C; 0.2 ml. of patient (or control) diluted plasma is then added and a stop watch started. The tube is maintained at 37° C with occasional shaking, until the time on the watch is approaching 5 minutes, when 0.2 ml. of inosithin is added followed by 0.2 ml. of M/40 calcium chloride at exactly 5 minutes.

As the time approaches 7 minutes, 0.1 ml. of M/40 calcium chloride is pipetted into the first of a series of four clotting tubes, each containing 0.1 ml. of substrate plasma, previously warmed to 37° C. At exactly 7 minutes, 0.1 ml. of the reacting mixture is pipetted into the same tube. A second stop watch is started at this time and the clotting time of the substrate plasma is recorded. Further 0.1 ml. samples of the incubation mixture are transferred to the substrate tubes immediately after recalcification at 9, 11 and 13 minutes as shown on the master stop watch (i.e. at 4, 6, and 8 minutes after recalcification of the incubation mixture).

With experience, both patient and control plasma can be tested concurrently by recalcification of the incubation tubes one minute apart and transferring subsamples from each incubation tube alternately to the substrate plasma tubes.

The shortest clotting time of the substrate plasma should be between 7 and 12 seconds and this should be reached not later than 4 minutes after recalcification of the incubation mixture. Differences of 3 (or more) seconds between the shortest clotting times obtained from patient and control plasma, or a delay of 2 (or more) minutes in reaching the minimum time, provide evidence of an abnormality in blood thromboplastin formation. This may be due to a deficiency of factors V, VIII, IX, X, XI, or XII or to a circulating anticoagulant.

An example of the application of this test is given in Table IV.

B. Comments

This test will not distinguish between the different defects but is often sufficiently sensitive to detect mild deficiencies (e. g. plasmas with 20 % factor VIII or factor IX). Platelet abnormalities cannot be detected. Hardisty and Ingram (1965) report on the use of capillary bloods samples obtained from babies. Plasma derived from a 1 in 10 dilution of whole blood is tested from both patient and control. The slightly higher dilution resulting from the use of whole blood makes little difference to the normal range of clotting or incubation times. In the original method described by Hicks and Pitney (1957) there can be a wide range in the clotting times of the indicator plasma if duplicate estimations are made on the same sample. This is due to variations in the degree of contact activation by glass tubes. MacPherson and Hardisty (1961), (in the technique as described above) have overcome this problem by incubating the diluted plasma with an optimal amount of kaolin before recalcification. This increases the reproducibility of the test and enables minor degrees of abnormality in blood thromboplastin formation to be detected with greater certainty.

V. Thromboplastin Activation Test

This test procedure was described by Astrup and Ollendorf (1961).

A. Method

1. Reagents

a. Platelet Poor Substrate Plasma: Human blood is collected in siliconized tubes using 3.8 % trisodium citrate as anticoagulant (1 part citrate plus 9 parts blood). The blood is centrifuged for 30 min at xg at 4° C and the plasma is collected in siliconized tubes using siliconized pipettes and stored in icewater.

b. Platelet Rich Patient's Plasma: Blood is drawn as described above but only centrifuged for 10 min at 600 x g. The plasma is also kept in icewater.

c. Calcium Chloride Solutions: An 0.025 M calcium chloride solution in water is used for the first stage of the test and an 0.0083 M calcium chloride solution for the second stage. The latter is obtained by diluting the 0.025 M calcium chloride solution with two volumes of buffer, described below.

d. Saline-Barbital Buffer: An 0.05 M Diethylbarbital buffer, pH 7.75 containing 0.1 M NaCl is prepared. The total ionic strength should be 0.15.

2. Procedure

The platelet poor substrate plasma is diluted with two volumes of saline-barbital buffer and 0.1 ml. aliquots are placed in 15 non-siliconized test tubes (80×10 mm) and placed in a 37° C waterbath.

In another test tube (100×14 mm) 2.0 ml. saline-barbital buffer are mixed with 0.25 ml of 0.025 M calcium chloride solution. The tube is placed in the 37° C waterbath and after reaching the temperature of the bath, 0.25 ml. of the platelet-rich patient's plasma is added, and a stopwatch started.

At 1 min. intervals, 0.1 ml. of the above mixture is pipetted into one of the above listed 15 tubes containing the diluted substrate plasma. At the same time, 0.1 ml. of the 0.0083 M calcium chloride solution is added and the clotting times are recorded.

3. Evaluation

The clotting times of each of the 15 tubes are plotted on semilogarithmic paper (logarithm of clotting times in seconds against incubation times in minutes). The curve thus obtained is the activation curve.

B. Comments

The clotting times obtained with this procedure are longer than with the thromboplastin generation test because no serum is added. Since serum is an endproduct of coagulation the thromboplastin activation test is probably more "physiological".

Caution must be exercised in the use of the platelet poor substrate plasma. It suitability must be tested before use by recalcification (0.1 ml. diluted substrate plasma plus 0.1 ml. saline-barbital buffer plus 0.1 ml. 0.0083 M calcium chloride solution). The clotting times

Table 4: Thromboplastin Screening Test

Incubation time in minutes from recalcification	4	6	8
Control	10	10	11
Mild Christmas Disease	15	13	10

Clotting times in seconds

should be greater than 4 min. Substrate plasma which clots in a shorter time than 4 min. is not suitable.

The clot which forms in the incubation mixture should be removed as it forms using a wooden applicator stick.

The test reveals abnormal results in patients with hemophilia A and B, as well as thrombocytopenia and should also be useful in diagnosing PTA-deficiency. The test does not allow a differentiation between these bleeding disorders.

References

Astrup, T., and Ollendorf, P. (1961). *Scand. J. Lab. Invest. 13*, 377.

Bertho, A. and Grassman, W. (1938). Laboratory Methods of Biochemistry. MacMillan, London.

Bell, W. N. and Alton, H. G. (1954). *Nature 174*, 880.

Biggs, R. (1952). *Nature 170*, 280.

Biggs, R. and Douglas, A. S. (1953). *J. Clin. Path. 6*, 15.

Biggs, R. and MacFarlane, R. G. (1962). Human Blood Coagulation and Its Disorders. Blackwell Scientific Publications, Oxford.

Hardisty, R. M. and Ingram, G. I. C. (1965). Bleeding Disorders-Investigation and Management. Blackwell Scientific Publications, Oxford.

Hicks, N. D. and Pitney, W. R. (1957). *Brit. J. Haemat. 3*, 227.

MacFarlane, R. G. and Biggs, R. (1953). *J. Clin. Path. 6*, 3.

MacPherson, J. C. and Hardisty, R. M. (1961). *Thromb. Diath. Haemorrh. 6*, 492.

Morawitz, P. (1905). *Ergebn. Physiol. 4*, 307.

Pitney, W. R. and Dacie, J. V. (1953). *J. Clin. Path. 6*, 9.

One-Stage Prothrombin Time Techniques

Charles R. Rizza and William Walker

I. Introduction

That the name of this procedure remains and is likely to remain "prothrombin time" is a testimonial to the significance of the contribution to coagulation studies made by its originator, Armand J. Quick (1935). The central landmark in coagulation techniques, it was originally designed to indicate and measure deficiency of prothrombin in plasma when the other requirements in the classical theory of coagulation, thromboplastin (tissue extract) and calcium, were supplied in optimal concentrations. The requirement of tissue thromboplastin in this test is the basis for the alternate term "thromboplastin time" which is used occasionally in Europe. Quick found that mixtures of normal recalcified human plasma and rabbit brain extract consistently gave clotting times of twelve seconds. Plasmas giving longer clotting times were considered to be deficient in prothrombin, and this deficiency could be measured by reference to a saline dilution curve of normal plasma.

It is now known that a prolonged prothrombin time may be due to deficiency not only of prothrombin (Factor II) and fibrinogen (Factor I) but also of Factors V, VII and X, whether occurring singly or in combination. In vitamin K deficiency and coumarin therapy, it reflects a variable depression of Factors II, VII and X. The test is the cornerstone in our knowledge of the extrinsic pathway of blood coagulation and the only means of recognizing Factor VII deficiency. It also facilitates the study of an intermediate stage in the series of enzymatic reactions leading to the intrinsic prothrombin-converting substance in blood. It is an essential tool in the diagnosis of coagulation disorders and the only feasible means of controlling treatment with coumarin-type drugs.

Superficially a simple test because its technique is straightforward and applicable almost anywhere, it is in fact potentially misleading unless certain basic conditions of its performance and reporting, often ignored or overlooked, are observed and obeyed.

II. Practical Applications

A. Diagnostic

A prothrombin time prolonged by only a few seconds but usually much more will be found in deficiency, congenital or acquired, of the following coagulation factors: I (fibrinogen), II (prothrombin), V, VII and X. If the deficient factor or factors can be added to the test plasma the prothrombin time becomes normal or nearly so. Factors VII and X are present in normal serum but absent from normal plasma adsorbed with barium sulphate or aluminium hydroxide, whereas Factor V and fibrinogen are absent from normal serum but present in adsorbed plasma. Adsorbed stored plasma contains fibrinogen only. Factor II is present only in normal plasma, being absent in both adsorbed plasma and serum. Repetition of the test, with the addition in low concentration of serum, adsorbed plasma, adsorbed stored plasma and whole plasma in turn to the test plasma is a simple modification which, read in conjunction with other screening procedures such as the thromboplastin generation test, may give a provisional diagnosis to be confirmed as necessary by more definitive procedures such as specific factor assays (Table 1). Circulating anticoagulants may cause a prolonged prothrombin time. In this case the addition of normal plasma to the test plasma has no effect.

Table 1: The One-Stage Prothrombin Time as a Diagnostic Tool.

Normalization with 1/5 vol. of	Deficiency of
Normal plasma	I, II, V, VII, X
Absorbed normal plasma	I, V
Absorbed stored plasma	I
Normal serum	VII, X
No normalization with normal plasma	Circulating anticoagulant

In Vitamin K deficiency from faulty diet, intestinal malabsorption or obstructive jaundice the prothrombin time, prolonged because of the deficiency of Factors II, VII and X, will return to normal within eight hours after parenteral administration of 1 mg Vitamin K_1 or methylnaphthoquinone. Vitamin K_1 has no effect in severe hepatocellular disease (Koller's Test, 1941) and in cases with congenital deficiency of factors II, V, VII, X.

B. Control of Anticoagulant Therapy

This is currently the commonest use made of this test, and the one most subject to error. It is still insufficiently appreciated how poorly comparable are the results of the test done under conditions often widely and importantly different, especially between different centres of treatment but often in the one laboratory, and how greatly the "therapeutic range" and hence the dosage of anticoagulant drugs are affected by the choice and preparation of thromboplastic agent, the method of reporting, and the nature of the diluent (saline or adsorbed plasma) for the dilution curve.

III. The Unmodified One-Stage Test

A. Reagents

1. Anticoagulants

0.1 M trisodium citrate, or 0.1 M sodium oxalate.

2. Test Material

Whole blood or plasma may be used. One part of anticoagulant solution and 9 parts of blood are mixed in a syringe or are allowed to run from the needle into a graduated siliconized glass or plastic tube after a clean venepuncture. If plasma is used, the blood is centrifuged (speed is not critical). If the hematocrit is over 50 % and plasma is used for the test the amount of anticoagulant is adapted according to the table of Hellem (1960) (Fig. 1) to keep the calcium concentration optimal. Capillary blood should not be used in this test system.

3. Thromboplastin

a. Acetone Dried Rabbit Brain (Quick, 1938): The blood vessels are carefully removed with the pia. The brain is macerated in a mortar and extracted with acetone. The solvent is poured off and this is repeated until a granular powder is obtained. The powder is dried and stored in a refrigerator.

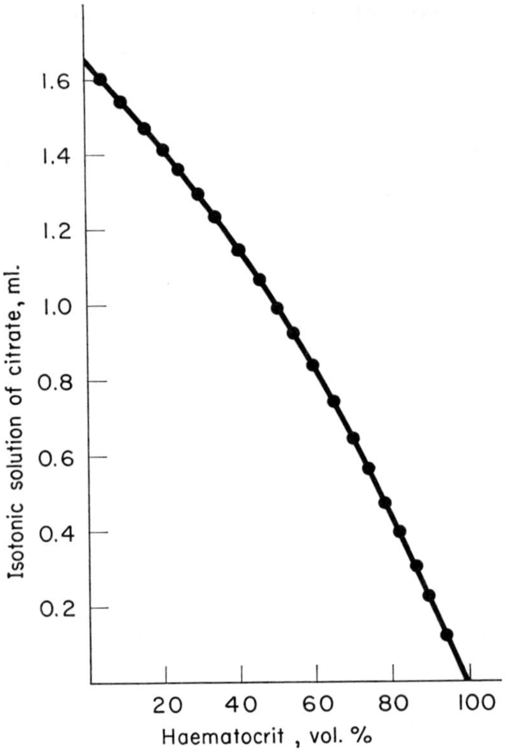

Fig. 1. Graph used to obtain a constant concentration of trisodium citrate in plasma at any hematocrit. Place correct amount of citrate in tube and add blood to a final volume of 10 ml. (According to Hellem, 1960.)

Dehydrated rabbit brain (0.3 g) is extracted with 5 ml normal saline containing 0.1 ml oxalate, incubated at 45° C for 10 minutes, slowly centrifuged. The milky supernatant is used.

b. Acetone Dried Human Brain: A fresh human brain is cleaned and freed from all meninges and blood vessels. The gray material is roughly separated from the white substance and ground in a mortar with 2–3 volumes of acetone. The acetone is decanted and the procedure repeated with new acetone until a fine easily sedimented brain powder is formed. The powder is dried in vacuo and stored at –20° C. It is stable for at least 6 months. If stored in vacuo or under nitrogen it is stable even at room temperature.

The working solution is prepared by extracting 3.0 g brain powder with 50 ml saline for 30 min at 37° C. The particulate matter is precipitated by slow centrifugation. The sediment is again extracted with 25 ml saline for 60 min and slowly centrifuged. The activity of the extract is tested, and the extraction procedure is repeated until there is no more activity. The supernatants are mixed, quick frozen and stored in small portions at –20° C for about 1 month.

c. Saline Extract of Human Brain (Owren, 1949): A fresh human brain (obtained less than 6 hours after death) is freed from all meninges and blood vessels under a stream of cold water. The whole brain is emulsified for 2–3 min in 1,500 ml of 0.85 % saline at 37° C. This process of emulsifying can be carried out in one of the many "blenders" available. The saline-brain emulsion is then centrifuged at 700 x g for 30 min and the sediment discarded. The supernatant is tested undiluted and diluted $^1/_2$, $^1/_4$, $^1/_8$ in 0.85 % saline in the one-stage prothrombin test. The dilution giving the shortest clotting time is ascertained, the rest of the supernatant is similarly diluted in saline and 10 % of Owren's veronal buffer (see p. 62) is added. The diluted extract of brain is then dispensed in 2–5 ml aliquots into containers and stored at –20° C for several months.

d. Commercial Thromboplastins.

4. 0.025 M $CaCl_2$

5. Oxalated Buffer

1.5 g sodium oxalate are dissolved in 1,000 ml of Owren's buffer.

6. Adsorbed Plasma

Human oxalated plasma is adsorbed with 100 mg/ml $BaSO_4$ or citrated plasma with $^1/_{10}$ volume of 2 % aluminium hydroxide suspension for 10 minutes and centrifuged.

B. Technique

Tubes containing the saline extract of brain and the 0.025 M calcium chloride are placed in a water bath to warm to 37° C. A 0.1 ml. pipette is placed in each of these reagents. Similar pipettes are used for each of the plasma samples to be tested. The test is carried out by mixing 0.1 ml. of plasma with 0.1 ml. of the brain extract in a glass tube in the water bath. After incubating for $^1/_2$–1 min to allow the mixture to reach 37° C, 0.1 ml of the warmed 0.025 M $CaCl_2$ is added and a stop watch started. The tube is tilted gently at frequent intervals until a solid clot forms, the stop watch is stopped and the clotting time noted. It is important to return the tube to the water bath after each tilt in order to keep the temperature of the reaction mixture at 37° C, or the tubes remain in the water bath and a platinum wire is immersed and withdrawn at short intervals until the first fibrin strands have formed. The test is carried out in duplicate on the control plasma and on the test plasma.

C. Comments

The original method of Quick (1938) uses oxalated plasma, acetone dried rabbit brain, and tilting of the tubes. Anticoagulation with citrate is now preferred because factor V is more stable in citrate than in oxalate. If citrated blood or plasma is stored in glass tubes at 4° C until tested a slight shortening of the coagulation time may occur. The citrated blood or plasma should, therefore, be placed in siliconized or plastic tubes. The test should be performed within 4–5 hours after drawing the blood. The determination of the test in plasma is more reliable than in whole blood. Depending on the use of whole blood or plasma for the test the normal control value and the calibration curve must be prepared from whole blood or plasma, respectively. Commercial thromboplastins differ very much in their sensitivity to factors VII and X. This influences the results of the tests and makes the comparison between laboratories difficult.

D. Method of Reporting

1. Diagnostic Test

The clotting time of the test plasma is simply given together with the clotting time of the control, or the activity read from the dilution curve. This will suffice for most purposes, for example liver disease and intestinal malabsorption or multiple coagulation defects in which a prolonged prothrombin time plays a subsidiary part. When a congenital deficiency of a factor is in question or the diagnosis is obscure, specific determinations of the factors II, V, VII or X should be made.

2. Control of Anticoagulant Therapy

Several methods have been used, the method itself being important as it may introduce confusing variables in the expression of the "therapeutic ratio" over and above those inherent in the choice of thromboplastin and technique.

a. Prothrombin Index. For Example:

$$\frac{13 \text{ (control plasma clotting time)}}{26 \text{ (test plasma clotting time)}} = 50\,\%$$

The therapeutic range is reckoned to be 40–65 % using saline extract of brain. This method greatly exaggerates variations arising from other sources, and is easily confused with percentage results from dilution curves. It is the least satisfactory method.

b. Prothrombin Ratio: As in diagnostic reporting, the clotting times may simply be given for control and test plasmas, and a "therapeutic range" of $1^1/_2$ to $2^1/_2$ times the control figure accepted. These clotting times may be expressed as a "prothrombin ratio", and ratios from 1.5 to 2.5 regarded as being within the therapeutic range. The results are influenced to a great extent by the thromboplastin used and by minor technical differences. The ratios are not comparable from one laboratory to another.

Although this method of reporting has the apparent advantage of simplicity and directness, it gives a very rough and inadequate reflection of the extent to which coagulability is depressed.

c. Percentage "Prothrombin" Activity From Dilution Curves: This is the most practical method for reporting the results of diagnostic tests and for the control of anticoagulant therapy. The results are in good agreement for one laboratory from day to day, and reduce the discrepancies between laboratories although they do not completely eliminate the influence of the thromboplastins used. These dilution curves were first prepared by making a series of dilutions of normal whole blood or plasma, preferably pooled, in oxalated saline. A suitable range of dilutions would contain 10, 20, 30, 40 and 60 % of normal plasma. A straight

line is obtained if log. clotting time is plotted against log. of dilution or reciprocals of clotting time against dilutions. The therapeutic range is between 15 and 25 %.
The use of saline as diluent has the disadvantage that fibrinogen and factor V are diluted in addition to the coumarin dependent factors. This is avoided by the use of adsorbed plasma as diluent. However, these dilution curves are very flat, the error in reading the results is greater and the advantage over the saline dilution curve is negligible. The therapeutic range is lower (5–15 %).

E. Standardization

The main source of the discrepancies is the use of different thromboplastin preparations which differ even between batches of the same preparation in clotting times, in the slope of the dilution curve, in stability and in sensitivity to single clotting factors, especially to factor VII (Table 2) (from Biggs and Denson, 1967).

This influences predominantly the results during initiation of the therapy.
Two approaches to standardize the one-stage prothrombin time have been investigated:

Table 2: One-stage prothrombin times on a normal plasma sample and three plasma samples from persons receiving anticoagulants. Six different techniques were employed. The clotting times were expressed in seconds. The clotting time ration was obtained by dividing the clotting times for the abnormal plasma by those of the normal. (Biggs and Denson, 1967). C = Clotting Times; R = Ratio.

Sample	Method 1		Method 2		Method 3		Method 4		Method 5		Method 6	
	C.	R.	C.	R.	C.	R.	C.	R.	C.	R.	C.	R.
Normal	45	1.0	44	1.0	13.2	1.0	19	1.0	19.7	1.0	14	1.0
Patient 1	56	1.25	50	1.13	14	1.08	21	1.1	22.5	1.24	15.7	1.12
Patient 2	120	2.65	96	2.2	19	1.44	35	1.85	38	1.94	21.5	1.54
Patient 3	106	2.35	82	1.87	18.8	1.42	38	2.0	33	1.68	24	1.72

Table 3: Calibration Table for use with the One-stage Prothrombin-time Methods of Varying Sensitivity to the Coumarin Defect.

%	Ratio Equivalent to Standard Ratio of 2												
	1.3	1.4	1.5	1.6	1.7	1.8	1.9	2.0	2.1	2.2	2.3	2.4	2.5
5	2.4	2.87	3.35	3.84	4.33	4.79	5.27	5.72	6.23	6.68	7.15	7.63	8.1
6	2.16	2.55	2.94	3.34	3.74	4.1	4.5	4.93	5.28	5.67	6.06	6.45	6.84
7	2.0	2.32	2.66	2.99	3.34	3.65	3.98	4.34	4.66	4.98	5.33	5.64	5.98
8	1.85	2.14	2.43	2.73	3.03	3.29	3.57	3.88	4.17	4.44	4.73	5.03	5.32
9	1.77	2.0	2.25	2.52	2.77	3.00	3.26	3.54	3.78	4.03	4.28	4.53	4.8
10	1.68	1.88	2.12	2.34	2.57	2.78	3.02	3.25	3.47	3.69	3.92	4.14	4.37
11	1.6	1.8	2.0	2.23	2.42	2.61	2.83	3.02	3.23	3.43	3.63	3.82	4.04
12	1.55	1.73	1.92	2.09	2.28	2.45	2.64	2.82	3.0	3.18	3.38	3.55	3.73
13	1.5	1.67	1.83	2.0	2.18	2.33	2.5	2.67	2.84	3.0	3.18	3.34	3.52
14	1.47	1.62	1.77	1.93	2.09	2.24	2.39	2.54	2.7	2.85	3.0	3.15	3.32
15	1.43	1.57	1.71	1.85	2.0	2.14	2.28	2.44	2.57	2.7	2.85	2.99	3.14
16	1.39	1.52	1.65	1.78	1.93	2.05	2.18	2.32	2.44	2.56	2.7	2.84	2.98
17	1.37	1.48	1.62	1.74	1.87	1.98	2.1	2.23	2.35	2.47	2.59	2.72	2.85
18	1.34	1.45	1.57	1.68	1.8	1.92	2.02	2.14	2.25	2.37	2.48	2.59	2.72
19	1.32	1.42	1.53	1.63	1.74	1.85	1.95	2.08	2.17	2.28	2.38	2.48	2.58
20	1.3	1.4	1.5	1.6	1.7	1.8	1.9	2.0	2.1	2.2	2.3	2.4	2.5
25	1.23	1.3	1.37	1.45	1.54	1.6	1.69	1.76	1.83	1.9	1.98	2.05	2.14
30	1.17	1.23	1.29	1.34	1.41	1.47	1.53	1.59	1.64	1.69	1.75	1.83	1.87
40	1.12	1.15	1.18	1.23	1.27	1.3	1.34	1.37	1.42	1.45	1.49	1.53	1.57
50	1.07	1.1	1.12	1.15	1.18	1.2	1.23	1.25	1.28	1.3	1.33	1.35	1.37
100	1.0	1.0	1.0	1.0	1.0	1.0	1.0	1.0	1.0	1.0	1.0	1.0	1.0

1. Standardization of Methodology and Reagents

a. The Subcommittee on Coagulation Reagents of the American College of Pathologists (Miale and LaFond, 1967) has recommended the use of undiluted citrated plasma, neutral pH of reagents, $37.5 \pm 0.2°$ C and an automatic end-point reading apparatus, but they have not yet succeeded in finding stable reference plasmas and uniform thromboplastin preparations.

b. Poller (1967) has managed to supply a large area in England with a stable and well standardized saline extract of human brain for general use or at least as a reference standard for comparison with the locally used thromboplastins.

c. The thrombotest method (Owren, 1959) (see below). The manufacturer (Nyegaard, Nycovenen, Oslo, Norway) supplies a well standardized and reproducible reagent and a reliable dilution curve for the calculation of activity which provides identical results in all laboratories.

2. Mathematical Approach

Biggs and Denson (1967) found linearity between clotting time ratio

$$\text{Quotient} = \frac{\text{abnormal clotting time}}{\text{normal clotting time}}$$

and reciprocal of concentration (Fig. 2), and between clotting time ratios obtained with different methods (Fig. 3). This makes it easily possible to compare the results of an individual method with a standard method, and to transform the percent result obtained with the individual method to the standard values (Fig. 4). One determines the ratio of 10–20 patients on anticoagulant treatment with the individual and the standard thromboplastin preparation and plots the regression line; one calculates then the ratio equivalent to the ratio of 2.0 of the standard preparation graphically. By means of Table 3 (taken from Biggs and Denson, 1967) it is easily possible to calculate percent values of activity which are comparable to the results obtained anywhere with the same method of calculation. Thrombotest could be used as the standard method.

IV. The "P and P" Method (Owren and Aas, 1951)

A. Principle

The test system of the one-stage prothrombin time is supplemented by adsorbed bovine plasma to keep factor V (and fibrinogen) constant. Barium sulfate adsorbed plasma is used instead of the originally recommended Seitz-

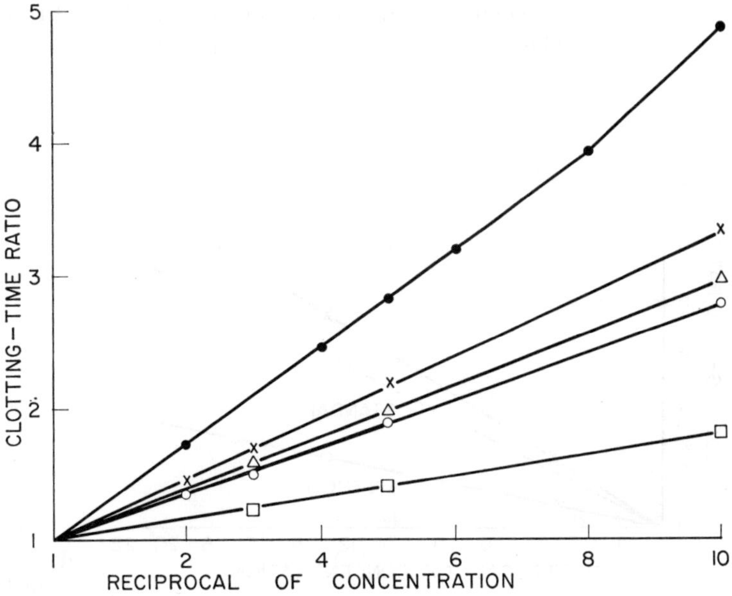

Fig. 2. Dilution curves for a variety of methods. Reciprocal of normal plasma concentration plotted against clotting time ratio. Lowest curve represents a normal plasma diluted with plasma from a patient with severe vitamin K deficiency, using human brain extract thromboplastin. The other curves were obtained using commercial reagents. (Biggs and Denson, 1967.)

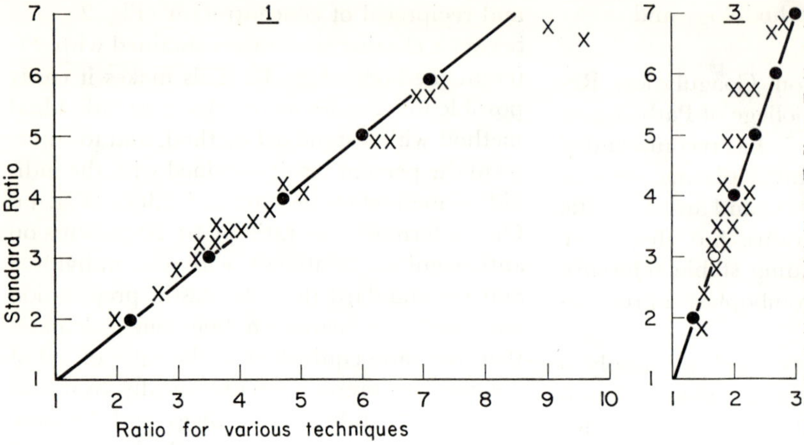

Fig. 3. Prothrombin time determination on 20 pa- receiving anticoagulant therapy using two different test method (1 and 3) and a standard procedure. Clotting time ratios were determined, and for each of the methods the ratio was plotted against the ratio obtained with the standard procedure. The full circles represent the ratios likely to give the best results in comparing the two methods. (Biggs and Denson, 1967.)

filtered plasma for reasons of convenience in preparation.

B. Reagents

1. Anticoagulants (see III, A, 1)

If the sample should be mailed to the laboratory, 25 mg heparin (100 U/ml) and 25 mg merthiolate are added to 250 ml anticoagulant solution.

2. Test Sample: see III, A, 2.

3. Thromboplastin

Saline extract of human brain; see III, A, 3, c.

4. Adsorbed Bovine Plasma

Oxalated (1:10) bovine blood is centrifuged at 2,000 x g. The plasma is adsorbed with 100 mg/ml $BaSO_4$ for 30 min. at room temperature with mechanical stirring, centrifuged and stored in aliquots at –20° C. It is stable for at least half a year.

5. 0.025–0.035 M $CaCl_2$

Optimal concentration must be determined for each batch of bovine plasma.

6. Dilution Fluids

a. 240 ml 0.1 M trisodium citrate are diluted with 760 ml distilled water.

b. 200 ml Owren's barbital buffer are mixed with 200 ml solution *a* and 600 ml normal saline are added.

c. 100 ml 0.1 M sodium citrate are diluted with 600 ml 0.9 % saline.

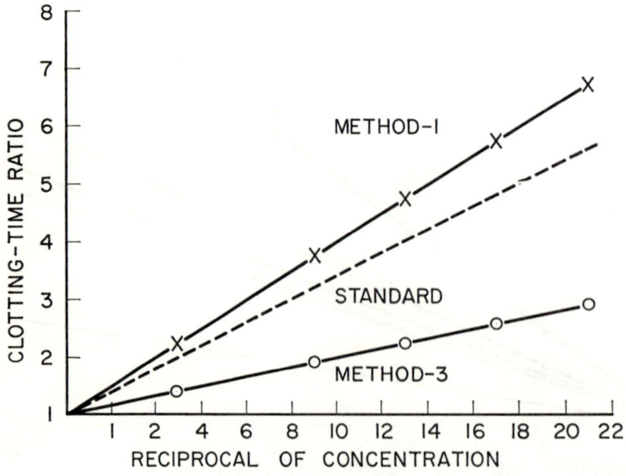

Fig. 4. Calibration graphs for the standard procedure and methods 1 and 3 from Fig. 3.

C. Technique

The reagents are prewarmed to 37° C and 0.1 ml test plasma is mixed with 0.9 ml dilution fluid *b*, diluted plasma (0.1 ml), adsorbed bovine plasma (0.1 ml) and thromboplastin solution (0.1 ml) are mixed in a small glass tube and recalcified with 0.1 ml $CaCl_2$. The end point is determined by tilting or with a platinum loop as described in section III, B.

D. Preparation of the Calibration Curve

Cooled normal plasma is diluted 1:2, 1:4, 1:8, 1:16 in dilution fluid c. Undiluted plasma and these dilutions are further diluted in the test 1:10 with dilution fluid b, and the test is performed as described in section C. Log. clotting times plotted against log. plasma concentrations should give a straight line.

E. Comments

The method may only be used for control of anticoagulant therapy. Samples mailed in plastic tubes to the laboratory may be used even 24 to 36 hours after drawing the blood. The method is not suitable for diagnosis of hemorrhagic diseases.

V. The Thrombotest Method (Owren, 1959)

A. Principle

All necessary reagents are combined in one reagent containing calcium in optimal concentration and absorbed bovine plasma as source of factor V and fibrinogen. A mixture of crude cephalin from human brain or soybeans and an animal thromboplastin from bovine or equine brain. This reagent gives longer coagulation times than recorded with the one-stage prothrombin time tests and according to Owren (1959) reflects sensitivity to intrinsic system factors particularly factor IX. The reagent is very sensitive to the concentration of factors VII and X. It can be used with whole blood, plasma and capillary blood. A similar preparation is the 2/7/10 reagent of Denson (1961).

B. Reagents

1. Thrombotest Reagent (Nyegaard & Co., Nycoven, Oslo, Norway)

If capillary blood is used, the thrombotest reagent is dissolved in 2.2 ml distilled water; if whole blood and plasma method is used, in 2.2 ml calcium chloride.

2. 3.2 mM $CaCl_2$

Provided by the manufacturer.

3. 0.1 M Trisodium Cirtrate.

C. Technique

A 0.25 ml aliquot of reagent is prewarmed to 37° C in a small test tube (diameter 7–8 mm) and subsequently, 0.05 ml capillary blood, citrated whole blood or 3:2 in saline diluted plasma is mixed with the reagent. The time elapsed between addition of the blood to the reagent and the formation of a solid clot is recorded. The clotting time is converted to coagulation activity in percent of normal using the reference curve supplied with the reagent. An incision of sufficient depth to produce free flow of capillary blood is necessary for reliable results.

If the result is above 50 % and an exact value is required, the test must be repeated with 0.5 ml reagent and 0.02 ml blood. The activity is read from the reference curve and the result multiplied with the factor 4.3.
The final result is corrected for very abnormal hematocrit values with the aid of a graph supplied by the manufacturer.

D. Comments

The method is designed for the control of anticoagulant therapy, not for diagnosis of bleeding disorders. Its accuracy is highest with activity values below 50 %. In the normal range, a higher dilution of the blood in the reagent has to be used. The therapeutic range for anticoagulant therapy is 5–15 %. It should be emphasized that blood must be handled in siliconized or plastic equipment to avoid surface activation, leading to erroneously short clotting times by activation of the intrinsic clotting system. Heparin interferes with the test. The test may be used as a reference standard for comparison of the results obtained with different modifications of the one-stage prothrombin time in different laboratories according to the calculations of Biggs and Denson (1967).

References

Biggs, R. and Denson, K. W. E. (1967). *Brit. Med. J. 1,* 84.
Denson, K. W. E. (1961). *J. Med. Lab. Tech. 18,* 257.
Hellem, A. J. (1960). *Scand. J. Clin. Lab. Invest.* Suppl. to vol. *12.*
Koller, F. (1941). Das Vitamin K und seine klinische Bedeutung. Thieme, Leipzig.
Miale, J. B. and LaFond, D. (1967). Trans Conf. Int. Com. Haemostasis an Thrombosis.
Owren, P. A. (1949). *Scand. J. Clin. Lab. Invest. 1,* 131.
Owren, P. A. (1959). *Lancet* 2, 754.
Owren, P. A. and Aas, K. (1951). *Scand. J. Clin. Lab. Invest. 3,* 201.
Poller, L. (1967). Trans. Conf. Int. Comm. Haemostasis and Thrombosis.
Quick, A. J. (1935). *J. Biol. Chem. 109,* 73.
Quick, A. J. (1938). *J. Am. Med. Ass. 110,* 1658.

CHAPTER 4

Purification of Prothrombin

GENESIO MURANO

I. Introduction

At the beginning of the century, Morowitz set up an equation to illustrate his view on blood coagulation.

$$\begin{array}{c} \text{Prothrombin} \\ \downarrow \leftarrow \text{Calcium} \\ \downarrow \leftarrow \text{Thrombokinase} \\ \text{Thrombin} \\ \downarrow \\ \text{Fibrinogen} \longrightarrow \text{Fibrin} \end{array}$$

Since that time, this system has been elaborated upon rather extensively. Of primary interest has been the isolation of the zymogen prothrombin. The pioneering work of Seegers et al. (1938); Seegers (1940); Seegers et al. (1945), resulted in the first high quality prothrombin isolated from bovine plasma (Seegers, 1952; 1964).

Modifications of the Seegers Method (Magnuson, 1965a, 1965b; Goldstein et al. 1959; Moore et al. 1965) have produced preparations of high activity. Prothrombin has been isolated from other species as well:

a. Equine prothrombin (Miller and Phelan, 1967).

b. Canine prothrombin (Anderson and Barnhart, 1964).

c. Rat prothrombin (Li and Olson, 1967).

d. Human prothrombin (Magnuson, 1965b; Shapiro and Waugh, 1966; Lanchantin et al. 1963).

In all procedures, principles of isoelectric precipitation, adsorption and elution, salt and alcohol fractionation and chromatography are applied.

II. Methods of Purification

A. Bovine Prothrombin – Method of Seegers (1952)

The method described is a two day procedure. Six liters of plasma can be processed with great ease. By overlapping, four products can be made in five days. This is accomplished by commencing the second product while finishing the first on the second day.

The following principles are applied: Blood is mixed with a special anticoagulant, designed to keep the salt concentration of plasma low. The formed elements are removed by centrifugation. The zymogen is precipitated isoelectrically from diluted plasma, adsorbed selectively on magnesium hydroxide, and subsequently liberated by decomposition with CO_2 under pressure. The magnesium is removed by dialysis, and the prothrombin further concentrated by isoelectric precipitation and ammonium sulfate fractionation (Seegers, 1952; Seegers, 1964).

1. Materials

a. Plasma: The blood is collected in a special anticoagulant: 1.85 % potassium oxalate ($K_2C_2O_4 \cdot 2H_2O$) and 0.5 % oxalic acid ($H_2C_2O_4 \cdot 2H_2O$). One part anticoagulant to 9 parts of blood is used. The plasma is obtained as soon as possible by centrifugation in a Sharples centrifuge. At this point it may be stored at –20° C if necessary until ready to be used. Alternatively, it is possible to obtain plasma commercially in batches of several liters. It is advisable to allow the material to thaw overnight, and transfer it in 3 liter portions in polyethylene containers which may be stored until ready to be used.

b. Oxalated Saline: 0.75 gm $K_2C_2O_4 \cdot 2H_2O$ is mixed with 0.85 gm NaCl and dissolved in 100 ml H_2O. This reagent may be prepared in larger quantities and stored at refrigerator temperature.

c. Magnesium Hydroxide Cream: To 20 liters of 20 % $MgCl_2$ are slowly added 5 liters of concentrated NH_4OH with constant stirring. The precipitate is allowed to settle and washed several times with water until there is no detectable ammonium odor. Five hundred grams of the packed $Mg(OH)_2$ paste are suspended in one liter of water. A commercially prepared paste "Hydro-Magma Paste" (Dow Chemical Co.) may be used instead of the preparation described. It is used in the proportion of 1.4 kilo/2.8 liters of H_2O.

d. Ammonium Sulfate: This is a 4 M solution and is saturated at 0° C.

2. Procedure

a. Isoelectric Precipitation:

1. Two large Pflaundler tanks or large metal containers of the type that usually find service in commercial kitchens, are partially filled with approximately 40 liters of cold tap water.
2. Cracked ice is added and the water agitated with a metal (aluminum) paddle until a temperature of 0° C is achieved.
3. The excess ice is removed with a strainer.
4. Three liters of plasma that has been strained through several layers of saline (0.9 %) washed gauze are added to each tank. This gives a fluid plasma-water ratio of 1:15.
5. The contents in the tank are thoroughly mixed with the metal paddle by gentle agitation in an upward-downward motion. To minimize surface denaturation, excessive foaming should be avoided.
6. The pH of the solution is adjusted to 5.15 by slowly adding cold 1 % acetic acid simultaneously stirring with the paddle to avoid local superconcentration. The pH of the solution may be monitored by removing a sample from the tank in a 50 ml beaker and analyzed on a pH-meter.
7. When the desired pH is obtained, the tanks are covered and allowed to stand for three to four hours at ambient temperature. The prothrombin and other proteins will settle to the bottom.
8. At the end of the settling period, the supernatant is removed by suction. A suction pump will speed up this process although a faucet aspirator will suffice. Caution is to be exercised, since the protein layer may become easily dislodged and sucked off. It is recommended that the tanks be gently tilted to a 30 to 45° angle for removal of the last 3 inches of supernatant.
9. The precipitate is drawn from the base of the tank into a 2 liter metal container. The last of the precipitate may be collected with the aid of rubber spatula and subsequent mixing with a few ml of saline or distilled water.
10. The precipitate is centrifuged in the cold at 3,100 g for 10 min. This may be accomplished in 100 ml centrifuge tubes or preferably in 600 ml swinging buckets.
11. The supernatant is discarded and the precipitate transferred into a Waring blender. The transfer is facilitated with the use of a large soup spoon machined in such a fashion that the tip, and one of the sides, make a 90° angle.
12. The centrifuge buckets are rinsed with oxalated saline which is transferred to the precipitate already in the blender.
13. Enough oxalated saline (at 37° C) is added to the blender to obtain adequate mixing. The blender is used to procure complete mixing, avoiding frothing as much as possible.
14. The suspension is transferred to a 2 liter beaker.

Steps 12 to 14 may have to be repeated, depending on the capacity of the blender. A minimal amount of oxalated saline is used to rinse out the blender and this wash is added to the beaker. The total volume of oxalated saline used is 1 liter.

15. A mechanical stirrer is placed in the beaker and a pH electrode immersed into the solution. The pH at this point is about 5.1 to 5.3.
16. With stirring, 0.1 N NaOH is added slowly until the pH is raised to above 6.4, usually 7.0. The alkali must be added slowly to prevent local denaturation. It is recommended that the mechanical stirrer be turned off while reading the pH.

17. The neutralized solution is placed in 600 ml centrifuge cups and centrifuged in the cold at 3,100 g for 10 min.
18. The supernatant is transferred into a large beaker and stirred mechanically.

b. Adsorption on Magnesium Hydroxide:

1. To the stirring solution are added 400 ml of $Mg(OH)_2$ previously prepared and stored in the refrigerator. Thorough mixing (25 minutes) is essential since it is at this point that the prothrombin is adsorbed on the $Mg(OH)_2$.
2. The suspension is centrifuged at 3,100 g for 25 min in the swinging buckets.
3. The supernatant is discarded. It may be easily decanted since the $Mg(OH)_2$ will adhere to the bottom of the cups.
4. The precipitate is washed with 1 liter of 0.85 % cold saline. This is accomplished by adding the saline in small aliquots and mixing the pasty precipitate with a pestel. This tool may be easily procured in the laboratory by securing a No. 12 rubber stopper to the end of a 12″ metal rod. The narrow end of the stopper faces the handle. With graceful circular motion, the paste is suspended in the saline. It is important that no particulate (lumpy) matter remains.
5. When an adequate particulate-free suspension is obtained, the cups are placed in the centrifuge and spun at 3,100 g for 20 min.
6. The supernatant is discarded. Then with the aid of the customized spoon, the precipitate is dislodged and transferred to the Waring blender. If caution is exercised, the precipitate may be removed in one or two pieces.
7. The cups are washed with a portion of a total volume of 300 ml of cold 0.85 % NaCl and it is added to the Waring blender.
8. The pasty suspension is blended for approximately one minute.

c. Liberation of Prothrombin from Magnesium:

1. When a complete suspension is obtained, the mixture is transferred to a special pressure bottle. This is a heavy walled metal container, fitted with a pressure cap which can be screwed in place and tightened. The cap is attached to a tank of CO_2 by pressure tubing.
2. After flushing the bottle with CO_2 to insure that all atmospheric air is removed, the cap is secured and the CO_2 pressure is raised to 40 p. s. i. The bottle is placed in a metal jacket, secured tightly with wooden wedges, and mechanically agitated for 25 to 30 min. The metal jacket is actually secured and is a part of the shaker.
3. After this time, the valve on the CO_2 tank is shut off. The pressure bottle is removed from the shaker and placed in an ice bath. The pressure is maintained until the apparatus has cooled, at which time, the pressure cap is unscrewed slowly to prevent excessive foaming.
4. The mixture is removed from the pressure bottle and placed in a metal beaker. The inside of the bottle may be rinsed with a few ml of 0.85 % NaCl and added to the beaker.
5. The beaker is placed in a refrigerator and allowed to stand overnight. In most instances, a gelatinous material is observed in the morning. Storage for one week is possible.
6. The contents are strained through 6 layers of gauze previously washed with cold oxalated saline. Gentle manual squeezing is recommended. The eluate is collected in a 500 ml graduated cylinder. Usual volume is approximately 350 ml. The solution is acidified to pH 6.1 with 1.0 N HCl while stirring. About 75 ml are required.
7. The solution is centrifuged in 100 ml tubes at 3,500 g for 10 min.
8. The supernatant is transferred into a 2 liter beaker immersed in a salt-ice bath. Constant mechanical stirring will prevent the solution from freezing.

At this point, one can select from several possibilities to make useful products (Seegers et al. 1945). The procedure of preference is described.

d. Precipitation with Ammonium Sulfate:

1. When the temperature of the solution has reached 0° C, a volume of saturated ammonium sulfate equal to the volume of the eluate (50 % v/v) is added slowly, so that the temperature does not rise.
2. The beaker is transferred to an ordinary ice bath and the contents transferred into 100 ml centrifuge tubes precooled in an ice bath.
3. Centrifugation is carried out for 15 min at 3,500 g.

4. The supernatant is transferred into a 2 liter metal beaker. The beaker is again placed in a salt-ice bath and the contents mechanically stirred.
5. When 0° C is reached, more ammonium sulfate equal to the original volume of the eluate is added slowly. This should give a final concentration of 67 % $(NH_4)_2SO_4$.
6. The mixture is transferred into a precooled glass beaker in an ice bath, and allowed to stand for 20 min. Crystals of magnesium salts are formed, and settle on the bottom.
7. The liquid is decanted into 100 ml centrifuge tubes, avoiding transferring the salt crystals as much as possible.
8. The tubes are centrifuged in the cold at 3,500 g for 15 min. The supernatant is discarded. Steps 7 and 8 may have to be repeated more than once depending on the centrifuge capacity.
9. At this point, it is important to wash the sides of the tubes with cold distilled water, but the water must not touch the precipitate. This may be accomplished by keeping the tubes inverted at all times after the supernatant has been poured off (Step 8), and directing a stream of water from a rinse bottle up the sides of the tubes.
10. The tubes are placed in an ice bath. The precipitate in the first tube is broken up with a glass rod and 10 ml of distilled water are added. With gentle manipulation, the protein will dissolve. This is transferred to the second tube and the process repeated until all the tubes have been rinsed.
11. The material from the last tube may be removed with a hypodermic syringe fitted with a 15 gauge hypodermic needle or a similar implement.
12. The rinsing procedure with 3 to 5 ml of distilled water is repeated several times in a serial fashion and the final volume collected in the same manner.

e. Dialysis against Distilled Water:

1. The product is dialyzed against cold distilled water. A most convenient apparatus consists of two disks of DuPont cellophane sandwiched by a cast aluminum frame. An accurate description of this apparatus may be found in Seegers' (1952) original text. Dialysis is carried out for 3 hours, with water changes at 15 min intervals.
2. A specific resistance of 1,700 Ohms or higher should have been reached at the end of three hours. If this value is not obtained, the process should be continued until the desired resistance is reached.

f. Isoelectric Precipitation:

1. The dialyzed product is transferred into a small beaker in an ice bath. This is the first step of isoelectric precipitation.
2. Into the solution is immersed a pH electrode. Dropwise, 0.1 N HCl is added from a micropipette with constant stirring, until a pH of 5.4 is reached.
3. The cloudy solution is placed in a 100 ml tube and centrifuged at 3,500 g for 10 min.
4. The supernatant is returned to a small beaker and the pH adjusted to 4.6 by dropwise addition of 0.1 N HCl.
5. The milky white suspension is centrifuged for 5 min at 3,500 g.
6. The supernatant is discarded. The precipitate is broken up with a stirring rod and 5 ml of distilled water are added slowly.
7. The suspension is transferred with a pipette to a 25 ml beaker in an ice bath. The tube is washed two more times with 2 ml of distilled water or less and added to the beaker.
8. With constant mechanical stirring, 0.1 N NaOH is added dropwise until the pH is raised to 7.0. After neutralization the product should be completely in solution.
9. The neutralized product is transferred with a 5 ml pipette to a storage bottle (screw cap). A few ml of distilled water are used to rinse the pH electrode and the beaker.
10. The final volume is recorded and 0.5 ml removed for immediate analysis by the two stage analytical procedure (Ware & Seegers, 1949). The product can be frozen at –60° C or lyophilized for storage in a dessicator.

3. Analysis and Improvements

This method yields 40 to 60 % of the original prothrombin in plasma. In bovine plasma the concentration is about 10 to 15 mg% (Seegers et al. 1962). Careful work usually results in a product with a specific activity of 23,000 to 30,000 Iowa Units/mg of Tyrosine (Folin

& Ciocalteau, 1927). The usual end volume is 15 to 20 ml. Variations of these values may be ascribed to technical errors or to use of different lots of plasma.

Should a product of poor quality be obtained, it is possible to raise the specific activity by several methods.

a. Barium Carbonate Adsorption: 20 ml of prothrombin solution is agitated with 1 gm of barium carbonate which will adsorb impurities. The barium carbonate is removed by slow speed centrifugation. This process will usually raise the specific activity from 26,000 to 29,000 or higher but decreases slightly the total numbers of units.

Products with a specific activity of not less than 20,000 may be improved by chromatography.

b. Chromatography with Amberlite IRC-50 (XE-64) (Miller, 1958):

1. A column 2.2×80 cm is equilibrated with 0.1 M phosphate buffer at pH 5.95 at room temperature.
2. One hundred mg of prothrombin are dissolved in 5 ml 0.1 M phosphate buffer adjusted to pH 5.6 with 0.1 N HCl.
3. Sample is placed on the column and the flow rate is adjusted to 3 to 12 ml/hour.
4. Phosphate buffer 0.1 M pH 5.95 is the eluent.
5. The sample is collected in 5 to 10 ml aliquots.

By this chromatography, one of the associated substances removed is trans-α glucosylase.

c. Chromatography on DEAE-cellulose (Seegers & Landaburu, 1960):

This technique utilizes an interrupted phosphate buffer elution system.

Buffers: A. 0.3 M pH 8.0
2.194 gm $NaH_2PO_4 \cdot H_2O$
40.333 gm Na_2HPO_4
B. 0.05 M pH 7.0
2.691 gm $NaH_2PO_4 \cdot H_2O$
4.331 gm Na_2HPO_4
C. 0.075 M pH 7.2
1 part buffer A
9 parts buffer B
D. 0.175 M pH 7.45
5 parts buffer A
5 parts buffer B

1. The cellulose is conditioned by washing several times with buffer B. The nonsedimenting material is removed by decantation.
2. The slurry is poured in a column and allowed to settle by gravity. Light pressure may be applied to hasten the process (10 p.s.i.). Column size 0.9×25 cm.
3. About 10,000 units are taken up in 4 to 5 ml of 0.05 M pH 7.0 buffer and applied to the top of the column.
4. The sample is allowed to enter the column, followed with buffer B.
5. Drop rate is adjusted to 3 per min.
6. About 40 ml of buffer B are allowed to pass through the column, then buffer C is applied (70 to 100 ml).
7. Buffer D is applied. This buffer will elute the prothrombin which will begin to elute after 30 or 40 ml of buffer have passed through the column.
8. The sample is collected in 10 ml aliquots, at refrigerator temperature.

Caution is to be exercised in this technique, since the prothrombin molecule will dissociate with great ease when subject to DEAE-cellulose.

d. Chromatography by Gel-filtration (Mammen & Ramien, 1962):

A column 0.9×60 cm is used. Sephadex G-75 (medium) is equilibrated with 0.9% NaCl at pH 7.0. A sample no larger than 12% of the column volume is applied. The flow-rate is 5 ml per hour. The prothrombin is eluted as one symmetrical peak, with an average increase in specific activity of 36%.

e. Chromatography on TEAE-cellulose (Magnusson, 1965a):

1. Three grams of TEAE-cellulose are suspended in 0.01 M sodium acetate pH 5.5 buffer, and allowed to sediment for 20 min.
2. The supernatant is removed by suction and the process repeated.
3. The sediment is suspended in buffer and poured portionwise into a glass column 0.9× 25 cm, with a sintered glass filter (D-1) to support the ion exchanger, allowed to sediment and then compressed by means of a glass rod fitting tightly into the column. During the packing procedure, the bottom of the column

is immersed in a beaker containing 0.01 M buffer, up to 2 cm above the level of the sintered glass filter, in order to avoid the formation of air bubles in the column. The final column length ranges from 14 to 19 cm.

4. The column is equilibrated with 0.01 M sodium acetate buffer pH 5.5 in a cold room at 1–5° C, with a hydrostatic pressure of 50–100 cm giving flow-rates of 5–9 ml/hr.

5. 40–150 mg of prothrombin are dissolved in 2.0 ml of 0.01 M buffer and applied to the column. Compressed air may be used to hasten the inflow.

6. Gradient elution may be started immediately or it may be preceded by 2–16 hours elution with 0.01 M buffer. The gradient equipment consists of a glass vessel open to the atmosphere, connected to a closed glass vessel equipped with a magnetic stirrer; the latter vessel is connected to the top of the column. The ionic strength gradient is obtained by letting 0.5–1.0 M buffer from the open vessel flow into the constant volume (closed) vessel which, at the start, contains 50–300 ml of 0.01 M buffer.

7. The effluent may be monitored by standard chromatographic technology.

8. All fractions belonging to one protein peak are pooled, dialyzed and freeze-dried.

This entire procedure is also applicable to DEAE-cellulose.

4. Evaluation

Nonchromatographed bovine prothrombin prepared by the above procedure when analyzed in the ultra-centrifuge, displays a Schlieren pattern consistent with homogeneity (Lamy and Waugh, 1953). In free boundary electrophoresis, one symmetrical peak is observed at pH values below 7.0. Above pH 7.0, two major peaks are noticeable. This phenomenon is attributed to the dissociation of the molecule into subunits (Seegers et al. 1966). The specific activity ranges between 2,000 and 6,000 Units/mg protein.

Bovine prothrombin chromatographed on IRC-50 (Miller, 1958) also is homogeneous in the ultracentrifuge and in electrophoresis. Immunochemical tests confirm the presence of one molecular species.

Bovine prothrombin chromatographed on DEAE-cellulose (Seegers and Landaburu, 1960), also displays homogeneity by the aforementioned parameters. The sedimentation constant of this product is the same as the constant for the non-chromatographed prothrombin (Seegers, 1952), but it displays different activation characteristics. Depending on the quality of the starting material, the specific activity may be increased by as much as 50 % or better. When bovine prothrombin is chromatographed on TEAE-cellulose (Magnuson, 1965a), two main peaks are obtained. 1.5–24.8 % of the protein appears in peak I and 62.0 to 94.1 % of the protein appears in peak II. The prothrombin activity by the two-stage analytical procedure (Ware and Seegers, 1949) resides in peak II. Bioactivation is slow, and it does not activate in sodium citrate solution. Peak I may be activated to thrombin in the presence of serum. Unusual as it may appear, the specific activity of peak II is consistently lower than the starting material.

This TEAE-cellulose chromatographed prothrombin (peak II) behaves like the material prepared after filtration of plasma through an asbestos pad (Goldstein et al. 1959), and also like prothrombin prepared according to Seegers and Landaburu (1960). It is an "altered zymogen" free of autoprothrombin III activity.

B. Bovine Prothrombin – Method of Goldstein et al. (1959)

This procedure utilizes principles of Seitz filtration, to remove "Factor VII" activity, adsorption of prothrombin on barium sulfate, elution with citrate, ammonium sulfate fractionation and isoelectric precipitation.

The technique is applicable to both bovine and human plasma, although the human material is "contaminated" with a plethora of coagulation factors (Goldstein et al. 1959).

1. Procedure

a. Collection of Blood:

1. Bovine blood is collected at the slaughter house into 0.15 M sodium or potassium oxalate (9 volumes of blood to 1 volume of oxalate).

2. The cellular elements are removed by centrifugation for 30 min at 1,500 g, at room temperature.
3. The plasma is recentrifuged at 4,000 g for 40 min at 5° C.

b. Filtration on Asbestos:
1. The plasma is passed through 20 % asbestos Seitz filter pads (14 cm diameter, Carlson Ltd., London) at 45 to 60 drops per min.
2. The first 75 ml of filtrate are discarded.
3. The next 150 to 200 ml are collected in 25 ml portions. 60 to 70 % of the original prothrombin and less than 1 % "Factor VII" appear in this fraction.
4. Each portion is tested separately for Factor VII activity, and those aliquots, in which this is sufficiently low, are combined.

c. Advice: The authors advise that no more than 300 ml of plasma be filtered through a single pad. They maintain that continued filtration through the same pad results in progressively increasing amounts of Factor VII activity in the filtrate.

d. Adsorption on $BaSO_4$:
1. The combined portions are cooled to 0–5° C.
2. $BaSO_4$ (35 mg/ml) is added to the plasma under stirring.
3. Stirring is continued for 1 hour.
4. The mixture is centrifuged at 1,500 g for 20 min.
5. The supernatant is discarded. The sediment is washed twice with one-half plasma volume of cold 0.1 M potassium oxalate in 0.15 M sodium chloride solution.
6. The sediment is washed a third time with one-half plasma volume of 0.15 M sodium chloride.

e. Elution from $BaSO_4$:
1. Cold 0.17 M sodium critrate (one-twentieth plasma volume) is added to the $BaSO_4$ sediment.
2. The suspension is agitated for 30 min.
3. The suspension is centrifuged in the cold. The supernatant is recovered.
4. Steps 1, 2 and 3 are repeated. About 70 to 90 % of the adsorbed prothrombin is recovered.

f. Dialysis:
1. The combined eluates are dialyzed against running tap water, or approximately 50 liters of distilled water, at 5–10° C for 12 hours.
2. The material, now increased in volume by about 30 %, is centrifuged at 3,000 to 4,000 g to remove any inert particulate matter which often appears.

g. Removal of "Factor VII" and Ac-G activity with $BaSO_4$:
1. To the dialyzed material, solid NaCl is added to a final concentration of 0.05 %.
2. $BaSO_4$ (25 mg/ml) is added. The readsorption is carried out a 0–5° C for 30 min.
3. The suspension is centrifuged and the precipitate discarded. At this ionic strength, $BaSO_4$ will selectively adsorb "Factor VII" and Ac-G.

h. Ammonium Sulfate Fractionation:
1. The supernatant from the repeat $BaSO_4$ adsorption is cooled to 0–3° C.
2. Saturated ammonium sulfate, adjusted to pH 7.2 to 7.3 with 1 N ammonium hydroxide, is added dropwise with constant stirring.
3. At 50 % saturation, the precipitate is promptly removed by centrifugation at 4,000 g for 15 min at 0–5° C.
4. To the supernatant, more of the same saturated ammonium sulfate is added until a 66 % saturation is reached.
5. The suspension is allowed to stand in the cold for 20 min.
6. The suspension is centrifuged at 4,000 g for 30 min at 0–5° C.

i. Dialysis:
1. The sediment is dissolved in 3 to 5 ml of cold distilled water.
2. The solution is placed in a 6 inch diameter rotating dialysis apparatus, and dialyzed against 16 liters of cold distilled water for 12 hours.

j. Isoelectric Precipitation: This process results in an improvement of the specific activity, but with a considerable loss in yield.
1. To the dialyzed material 0.01 N HCl is added dropwise, with constant stirring at 0° C until the pH is reduced to 5.2–5.4.

2. The precipitate is removed by centrifugation at 4,000 g for 15 min and discarded.
3. To the supernatant 0.01 N HCl is added until a pH of 4.6 is reached.
4. The precipitate is collected by centrifugation, as before. The supernatant is discarded.
5. The sediment is dissolved in a few ml of cold distilled water and the pH adjusted to 7.0–7.5 with NaOH.

2. Evaluation

The best preparations of bovine prothrombin are obtained by the method described above, up to isoelectric precipitation. The specific activity ranges from 1,250 to 1,520 units per mg protein depending on whether Seitz filtration is utilized or not. This activity can be further ameliorated by the isoelectric precipitation step.

The product can be stored in the frozen state or lyophilized – under the latter condition maintaining full activity for at least six months. In the frozen state, it is less stable. At refrigeration temperature stability is variable.

No physico-chemical analysis is available on this product, but the authors assure us that the material is free from thrombin, fibrinogen, antihemophilic factor, and Ac-G. The Seitz filtration, of course, insures the removal of "Factor VII".

In the preparation of human prothrombin, the Seitz filtration step is omitted since it has proved to be relatively ineffective in the removal of "Factor VII".

The authors discourage any attempts at isolation of prothrombin from ACD plasma, or outdated Red Cross lyophilized material.

C. Bovine Prothrombin – Method of Moore et al. (1965)

The purification procedure described below, is applicable to both bovine and canine plasma. The technology is comprised primarily of principles employed in the Lanchantin (1958) and Seegers (1952) method. The authors have exercised maximal precautions in each step to prevent denaturation and to obtain products of highest purity with adequate yields. The entire procedure is performed at 1–2° C.

1. Procedure

a. Collection of Blood: Approximately 2.8 liters of fresh, non-lipemic blood is collected in 2.85 % sodium citrate (1:8 dilution) by a non-traumatic rapid venipuncture from the jugular vein of live animals, previously starved for 24 hours. The blood is centrifuged. About 1.8 liters of plasma is obtained.

b. Adsorption of Prothrombin on Barium Citrate:

1. To the gently stirring plasma, 1 M $BaCl_2 \cdot 2H_2O$ (10 ml per 125 ml of plasma) is added slowly (one drop per second) to the side of the beaker.
2. Following addition of the $BaCl_2$, the solution is stirred for an additional 10 min.
3. The suspension is centrifuged at 3,600 g for 25 min in 80 ml tubes. The supernatant is discarded.
4. The barium citrate-prothrombin precipitate is triturated in each tube with 10 to 15 ml aliquots of a 1:10 dilution of stock citrate-saline (9.0 % NaCl and 0.2 M $Na_3C_6H_5O_7 \cdot 2H_2O$) until a uniform suspension is obtained.
5. The suspension is transferred to a beaker. The tubes are rinsed with diluted citrate-saline, the total volume employed being 600 ml.
6. The suspension is stirred for 10 min, after which time, the beaker is covered with parafilm and allowed to stand for 1 hour.
7. For a second time, the same total volume of $BaCl_2$ (10 ml per 125 ml of suspension) is added dropwise to the stirring suspension, from the side of the breaker. Stirring is continued for an additional 10 min.
8. The beaker is covered with parafilm and allowed to stand overnight.
9. The suspension is centrifuged for 25 min at 3,600 g. The supernatant is discarded. The sides of the tubes are wiped with filter paper to remove residual supernatant.
10. For a second time, the precipitate is suspended in citrate-saline, stirred for 10 min, and allowed to stand for 1 hour.
11. For a third time, $BaCl_2$ (10 ml per 125 ml of suspension) is added dropwise and the solution allowed to stir for an additional 10 min.
12. The suspension is allowed to stand for 1 hour; it is then centrifuged at 3,600 g for

25 min, the supernatant discarded and the sides of the tubes wiped with filter paper.

c. Elution and Dialysis:

1. Approximately 8 ml of 0.2 M EDTA (adjusted to pH 7.40 with 10 N NaOH) are added to each tube, and the precipitate triturated until a uniform suspension is achieved.
2. The suspension is placed in equal proportions in six dialysis bags (14 inch segments of Visking Casing), previously soaked in hot EDTA for 10 min and then soaked and stored at 1–2° C in redistilled water, with frequent changes for 1 week prior to use.
3. The tubes are rinsed in sequence with a total volume of 114 ml of EDTA and the rinse is added to each of the bags in equal volumes.
4. The contents are mixed gently. The precipitate, in each bag, is thusly suspended in 35 ml of EDTA which frees the prothrombin by removing the barium from the complex.
5. The contents are dialyzed against a mixture consisting of 360 ml of 0.2 M EDTA, 360 ml of stock citrate-saline, and 2,880 ml of redistilled water. The process is carried out for 30 min with the aid of a magnetic stirrer.
6. At the end of this time, dialysis against 360 ml of stock citrate-saline made up to 3.6 liters with redistilled water, is continued for an additional three hours, with changes of the dialysate at 30 min intervals. It is advisable to gently tilt the bags, each time the dialysate is changed. This will insure complete mixing. Dialysis is continued overnight.

d. Fractionation with Ammonium Sulfate:

1. The contents of the dialysis bags are transferred to a beaker.
2. With constant stirring, with a magnetic stirrer, a volume of saturated $(NH_4)_2SO_4$ (adjusted to pH 7.0 with concentrated NH_4OH) equal to the total volume of the viscous solution is added (one drop per second) to the side of the beaker.
3. After all of the $(NH_4)_2SO_4$ has been added, stirring is continued for an additional 5 min.
4. The suspension is placed in four 290 ml polycarbonate bottles and centrifuged for 30 min at 3,300 g. The precipitate is discarded.
5. Steps 2 and 3 are repeated. This should give a final concentration of 67 % $(NH_4)_2SO_4$.
6. The solution is allowed to stand for 30 min.
7. The opaque solution is again centrifuged in the polycarbonate bottles and the supernatant discarded. The sides of the bottles are wiped with filter paper to remove the residual supernatant.

e. Ammonium Sulfate Wash and Dialysis Against Water:

1. To each bottle, 15 ml aliquots of 67 % saturated $(NH_4)_2SO_4$ are added, and the precipitate triturated very carefully until a uniform suspension is obtained.
2. The suspension is centrifuged at 3,300 g for 20 min. The supernatant is discarded and the sides of the bottles wiped with filter paper.
3. The precipitate is dissolved in 30–40 ml of cold redistilled water and then transferred to a dialysis bag with two additional 5 ml rinses.
4. Dialysis is continued against 4 liters of redistilled water for 20 hours with 3–4 changes of dialysate.

f. Isoelectric Precipitation:

1. Following testing for traces of SO_4^{2-} with 1 N $BaCl_2$, the prothrombin solution is adjusted to pH 5.35–5.40 with 0.25 % (v/v) HCl.
2. The suspension is centrifuged at 2,500 g for 30 min. The precipitate consisting of non-prothrombin material varies in amount from one preparation to another and is discarded.
3. The pH of the supernatant is adjusted to 4.6 with the same HCl and allowed to stand for 10–15 min.
4. The suspension is centrifuged for 10 min at 650 g. The supernatant is discarded. The precipitate should contain the prothrombin.

g. Dialysis Against Phosphate Buffer:

1. The prothrombin precipitate is triturated gently with 5 ml of phosphate buffer (0.05 M in 0.1 NaCl, pH 6.86 ± 0.02) until all is solubilized.
2. The solution is transferred to a dialysis bag to which is added a 3–5 ml phosphate buffer rinse.
3. Dialysis is carried out for 5 hours against 4 liters of phosphate buffer with dialysate changes after 2 and 4 hours.

h. Adsorption with Kaolin and Bentonite:
1. The volume of prothrombin solution is measured accurately (8–9 ml) and the protein concentration determined (approx. 20 mg/ml).
2. The prothrombin solution is diluted with phosphate buffer to a concentration of approximately 15 mg/ml.
3. Kaolin (acid-washed, American Standard, Fisher Scientific Co.) is added (125 mg/ml) and the vessel covered with parafilm.
4. The tube containing the prothrombin and the adsorbant is fixed to the platform of an Eberbach Rotator at an angle of 5–10°.
5. The rotator is oscillated for 15 min at a rate of 120 per min with an amplitude of 20 mm.
6. The contents are centrifuged for 15 min at 3,600 g.
7. The supernatant is decanted into a centrifuge tube and the centrifugation and decantation repeated.
8. Bentonite, standardized according to Ido and Grisolia (1959) is added to the supernatant at a concentration of 10 mg/ml.
9. Steps 4 to 7 are repeated.
10. The supernatant is now ready for quick freezing in dry ice and acetone and stored in a deep freeze at –85° C.

2. Evaluation

Bovine prothrombin prepared precisely as outlined above, consistently yields approximately 50–60 % of the prothrombin in the starting plasma, with a specific activity of 2,400 to 3,000 Iowa Units per mg of protein. Products of high specific activity (2,800–3,000 Units per mg of protein) show a single symmetrical peak in the ultracentrifuge and in moving boundary electrophoresis at pH 6.86.

The authors maintain that due to the high purity of the preparations, it is necessary to modify the two stage analytical procedure of Ware and Seegers (1949) and the N α-p-toluenesulfonyl-L-arginine methyl ester assay procedure (Glueck, 1958; Hough et al. 1964). According to the authors this is due to their product being free of factor VII–X complex. They do not indicate the modifications of the assay. It appears, however, that bovine prothrombin isolated by this five day method is identical to the product obtained by the two day procedure of Seegers and Landaburu (1960).

D. Canine Prothrombin – Method of Anderson and Barnhart (1964)

The two day purification schedule herein described involves the adsorption of prothrombin from fresh dog plasma on barium citrate, followed by ammonium sulfate and isoelectric precipitation. Borate buffer is used as the solvent for the final product.

1. Procedure

a. Collection of Blood:
1. A dog is anesthetized intravenously with pentobarbital (30 mg/kg).
2. The blood is permitted to flow from a canulated carotid artery into a beaker containing 2.85 % sodium citrate (45 ml of citrate/300 ml of blood).
3. The blood is centrifuged in a refrigerated centrifuge for 20 min at 2,750 g. Generally, 600 ml of plasma can be obtained from a medium size dog.

b. Adsorption on Barium Citrate:
1. To the citrated plasma at 0° C, 1.0 M $BaCl_2$ is added dropwise (40 ml/600 ml of plasma) with constant stirring.
2. The suspension is centrifuged at 5,860 g for 20 min, at 4° C.
3. The precipitate is resuspended in 600 ml of citrate-saline solution (a 1:10 dilution of 0.2 M $Na_3C_6H_5O_7$ in 9.0 % NaCl).
4. $BaCl_2$ (40 ml/600 ml) is added dropwise at 0° C with constant stirring.
5. The suspension is allowed to stand for 30 min at 4° C.
6. The precipitate is collected by centrifugation at 5,860 g for 20 min.
7. The precipitate is suspended in 100 ml of 0.2 M EDTA previously adjusted to pH 7.4 with 1 N NaOH.

c. Dialysis:
1. The suspension is placed in dialysis casings and dialyzed at 1–4° C for 30 min against 3 liters of a mixture of buffered saline (150 ml 0.2 M EDTA, 150 ml undiluted citrate-saline and 1,200 ml distilled water).
2. Dialysis is continued for four more hours, against a mixture of 600 ml of stock citrate-

saline in 6 liters of phosphate buffered distilled water at pH 7.2. The dialysis fluid is changed every hour.
The stock citrate-saline is prepared by dissolving 360 gm of sodium citrate and 235.2 gm of sodium chloride in four liters of distilled water.
3. The dialyzed material is stored overnight at 1–4° C.

d. Ammonium Sulfate Fractionation:

1. The dialysate is chilled to 0° C.
2. An equal volume of saturated ammonium sulfate is added dropwise with constant stirring with a magnetic stirrer for 10 min.
3. The suspension is centrifuged at 5,860 g for 15 min at 4° C. The precipitate is discarded.
4. To the supernatant, the same volume (step 2) of ammonium sulfate is added dropwise, at 0° C and stirred slowly for 10 min. This gives a final $(NH_4)_2SO_4$ concentration of 66.6 %.
5. The suspension is centrifuged at 5,860 g for 15 min at 4° C. The supernatant is discarded.
6. The precipitate is dissolved in distilled water.

e. Rapid Dialysis:

The product is placed in a rapid dialyzer (Seegers, 1952) and dialyzed against 6 liters of phosphate buffered distilled water at pH 7.2, 0.01 M, for 4 hours with hourly changes of fluid.

f. Isoelectric Precipitation:

1. The dialyzed opaque solution is placed in an ice bath.
2. 0.01 N HCl is added slowly until pH 5.4 is achieved.
3. The precipitation is removed by centrifugation at 755 g for 5 min and discarded.
4. To the supernatant, in an ice bath, 0.01 N HCl is added slowly until pH 4.6 is reached.
5. The precipitate is collected by centrifugation at 4,340 g for 10 min. The supernatant is discarded.
6. The precipitate (prothrombin) is suspended in 1–3 ml of borate buffer solution (11.25 gm H_3BO_3, 4 gm $Na_2B_4O_7 \cdot 12H_2O$, and 2.25 gm NaCl per liter) adjusted to pH 7.45.
Alternatively, prothrombin can be dissolved in either 0.9 % NaCl or distilled water.
7. The product is assayed immediately by the method of Ware and Seegers (1949).

2. Evaluation

Canine prothrombin prepared as outlined above is relatively stable in the deep freeze. The products range in specific activity from 18,000 to 38,000 Units/mg Tyrosine (Folin and Ciocalteau, 1927). According to immunologic tests, products with high specific activity display homogeneity.
This technique may also be applied to human plasma, providing that the centrifugation after ammonium sulfate fractionation and isoelectric precipitation be carried out at 9,000 g or higher.

E. Equine Prothrombin – Method of Miller and Phelan (1967)

Crystalline preparations of horse prothrombin have been obtained by Miller and Phelan (1967). Prothrombin from this species can be obtained in high yields with great ease. Principles of repetitive adsorption on barium citrate (Lewis and Ware, 1953), isoelectric precipitation and chromatography are employed. Crystallization is easily achieved in a chloroform-methanol medium.

1. Procedure

a. Collection of Blood:

1. Horse blood (17 parts) is collected into 1 part of 0.165 M sodium citrate.
2. The formed elements are removed in the usual manner by centrifugation and the plasma decanted. For very large volumes, the formed elements are allowed to settle for 4–24 hours at 3° C. Then the plasma is siphoned off.

b. Adsorption on Barium Citrate:

1. To the cold (2–5° C) citrated plasma is added 1.0 M $BaCl_2$, dropwise until a final concentration of 0.10 M is achieved. Constant stirring is necessary.
2. The solution is stirred for an additional 10 min. The barium citrate-prothrombin complex will precipitate.
3. The precipitate is recovered by centrifugation.

4. The supernatant is discarded. To the precipitate is added a minimum amount of cold water and transferred to a Waring Blender.
5. The suspension is gently stirred in the Blender maintained at low speed by a Variac.
6. The suspension is then diluted to one-half the original plasma volume with cold water and stirred.

c. Decomposition of Complex:

1. To the stirring solution, dry Amberlite IRF-97 (Na^+) (Rohm and Haas, Philadelphia) is added in increments (3–15 grams of resin per 100 ml of suspension). The weak carboxylic exchange IRF-97, in the sodium cycle, serves to decompose the barium citrate and absorb impurities.
2. After stirring for 10 min, the supernatant will clear upon standing for 1–2 min. This is an indication of complete dissolution of the barium citrate. The pH of the clear supernatant should be in the range of 7.0–9.0.
3. The resin is removed by filtration on fluted Schleicher and Schuell No. 520-B-1/2 papers, or their equivalent.

d. Second Adsorption on Barium Citrate:

1. To the filtrate, which contains about 70% of the original prothrombin, is added dropwise 1.0 M $BaCl_2$ until a 0.1 M concentration is achieved.
2. After stirring for 10 min at 2–5° C, the barium citrate is recovered by centrifugation.
3. The supernatant is discarded. The precipitate is blended with cold water and again diluted with water to one-half the original plasma volume.

e. Second Decomposition of Complex:

1. Dissolution of the barium citrate is carried out as described above using one-half the original amount of IRF-97 (Na^+).
2. The second barium citrate eluate should contain 60–65% of the original plasma prothrombin. This eluate is adjusted to pH 4.7–4.9 by dropwise addition of 0.5 N HCl with stirring at 3–5° C.
3. The solution is allowed to stand for 30 min at 2–5° C.
4. The solution is centrifuged at 1,200 g for 20 min.
5. The supernatant is discarded. The prothrombin precipitate is suspended in cold water and stirred with either 0.1 N NaOH or dry IRF-97 (Na^+) sufficient to raise the pH to 6.0–6.5. Fifty to sixty per cent of the original horse plasma prothrombin should be recovered in this final product.

At this point, the zymogen can be crystallized or chromatographed and then crystallized.

f. Chromatography:

Gel Filtration.

Column size:	100 to 190 cm
Gel:	Sephadex G-200 (63–88 Mesh)
Developer:	0.10 M Borate Buffer pH 8.0 at 3° C

Ion Exchange.

Column size:	60 cm
Resin:	Amberlite IRC-50 (200–400 Mesh)
Developer:	0.10 M Phosphate Buffer pH 5.9 at 3° C

Standard equilibration and development procedures are applied in both systems.

g. Crystallization:

1. The prothrombin is dialyzed against at least 8 changes of distilled water, each water volume being at least 150 times that of the prothrombin solution.
2. Subsequent to dialysis, the prothrombin is lyophilized by standard procedures.
3. The dry protein is suspended in cold (–10° C) chloroform-methanol (2:1) or chloroform-ethanol (2:1). A sheen appears in 5–10 min of stirring. The suspension is composed predominantly of microscopic needles.
4. An equal volume of cold (–10° C) ethanol is added and the crystals are harvested by centrifugation in glass tubes or a sintered glass or paper filter.
5. The crystals are washed three times with cold (–10° C) ethanol to remove excess chloroform, and dried in vacuo.

The entire procedure can be carried out with cold (–10° C) n-butanol instead of the chloroform-methanol mixture.

An alternative crystallization procedure is the following:

1. A 1 % aqueous solution of horse prothrombin at pH 6.0–7.0 is prepared.
2. The solution is partially lyophilized to $^1/_5$–$^1/_{10}$ the original volumes.
3. The lyophilization flask and contents are then placed at 2–5° C before the remaining frozen material thaws completely, and seed crystals are added. Further crystallization occurs overnight.

2. Evaluation

Evidence that the crystals are prothrombin is provided by constant specific activity on recrystallization from aqueous medium and on partial and complete solution of the crystals. Horse prothrombin is remarkably susceptible to purification by these methods, in contradistinction to other species. The crystalline properties in the aforementioned media also appear to be unique to this species. Human Cohn fraction IV (Cohn et al. 1946) is stable to cold chloroform-methanol treatment; bovine prothrombin (Seegers, 1952) responded to the same treatment in one instance only, (personal communications). The crystalline barium-prothrombin complex reported by Tishkoff et al. 1966) does not correspond to the analogous horse barium-prothrombin complex.

Disc electrophoresis, by the method of Hjerten et al. (1965), of the Sephadex G-200 chromatographed crystallized horse prothrombin demonstrates a sharp major component with a slowly migrating contaminant comprising less than 1 % of the total protein.

Crystalline or lyophilized preparations of horse prothrombin, stored at pH 6.0–6.5 at –20° C, are stable for at least 18 months.

The horse prothrombin isolated by Miller and McGarrahan (1958) is reported to have a specific activity of 1,000–1,100 units per mg of dry weight.

The technique described above yields products with a specific activity of 1,300 units/mg of dry weight.

F. Rat Prothrombin – Method of Li and Olson (1967)

Preparations of rat prothrombin have been obtained by Li and Olson (1967). The authors have combined and modified the procedure for preparation of human prothrombin by Lanchantin et al. (1963) and the procedure for preparation of bovine prothrombin by Goldstein et al. (1959). The technology consists of barium sulfate adsorption, desalting by ion exchange resin, and subsequent chromatography on DEAE-cellulose.

1. Procedure

a. Collection of Plasma:

1. Male and female rats of the Edward Doisy Colony at St. Louis University, originally of the Wistar strain, ranging in weight from 300 to 500 gm are used.
2. Blood is drawn by heart puncture and mixed with 0.15 M potassium oxalate (9 volumes of blood to 1 volume of oxalate).
3. Cellular elements are removed by centrifugation at 2,000 g for 30 min at 4° C. All steps are carried out at 0–4° C.

b. Adsorption on Barium Sulfate:

1. Powdered $BaSO_4$ (Baker) is added to the oxalated plasma (35 mg/ml).
2. The mixture is stirred slowly with a magnetic stirrer for 1 hour.
3. The mixture is centrifuged at 1,500 g for 20 min. The supernatant is discarded.
4. The $BaSO_4$ sediment is washed twice with 0.50 plasma volume of cold 0.1 M potassium oxalate in 0.15 M sodium chloride solution.
5. The precipitate is washed a third time with 0.50 plasma volume of cold 0.15 M sodium chloride.

c. Elution of Prothrombin from $BaSO_4$:

1. To the precipitate are added 0.067 plasma volumes of cold 0.17 M sodium citrate, pH 8.0.
2. The solution is stirred for 30 min, and then centrifuged.
3. The citrate eluate is decanted.
4. Steps 1, 2, and 3 are repeated, and the eluate is combined with the first eluate. This is designated as $BaSO_4$ citrate eluate.

d. Removal of Barium from the Mixture:

1. Dowex 50 (Na^+), (AG 50 W-X4, 200 to 400 mesh, total capacity 1.2 meq/ml of resin bed, Bio-Rad), is mixed with the $BaSO_4$ citrate eluate in a 1:10 volume.
2. The suspension is stirred for 1 hour.

3. The resin is removed by centrifugation at 1,500 g for 20 min.
4. The pH of the supernatant solution is adjusted to 7.0 by addition of 0.05 M sodium phosphate buffer.
5. The final phosphate concentration is made to 0.005 M by addition of cold distilled water.

e. Adsorption on DEAE-cellulose: The cellulose is conditioned in the following fashion prior to use: DEAE-cellulose powder (Cellex-D, exchange capacity 0.8 meq/gm, Bio-Rad) is first washed with 0.5 M NaOH until the washings are clear, then with distilled water until the pH of the washings drops below 8.0, then briefly with 0.1 N HCl. The excess acid absorbed by the cellulose is removed by repeated washings with distilled water. The washed DEAE-cellulose is equilibrated with 0.005 M sodium phosphate buffer, pH 7.0, by suspending it in three changes of the buffer for 24 hours. The excess buffer is removed by filtration through Whatman 1 filter paper.
1. DEAE-cellulose is added to the prothrombin solution in the ratio of 40 mg dry weight to 1 ml of solution.
2. The mixture is stirred for 1 hour.
3. The mixture is centrifuged at 2,000 g for 20 min.
4. To the sediment is added a mixture of 0.1 M NaCl – 0.05 M sodium phosphate buffer, pH 4.5, until the pH is lowered to 5.2.
5. The mixture is stirred for 30 min.
6. The mixture is centrifuged at 2,000 g for 20 min.
7. More phosphate buffer (pH 4.5) is added to the sediment until pH 4.9 is reached.
8. The mixture is stirred for 30 min.
9. The supernatant is removed by filtration through Whatman 42 filter paper and discarded.
10. The DEAE-cellulose cake is washed with approximately 2 liters of cold distilled water.

f. Elution of Prothrombin from DEAE-cellulose:
1. The DEAE-cellulose prothrombin complex is suspended in a volume of 0.2 M sodium citrate, equal to the original barium sulfate-citrate eluate (section c).
2. The suspension is stirred for 1 hour.
3. The eluate is collected by filtration and designated as DEAE-cellulose-citrate eluate.

A sample of this solution is assayed immediately for its prothrombin activity, by the two-stage procedure of Ware and Seegers (1949) with slight modifications (Li and Olson, 1967). The product may be stored at –10° C or desalted by gel filtration through a column of Sephadex G-25 (Pharmacia).

The product is then lyophilized and stored at –10° C in a vacuum dessicator.

2. Evaluation

Prothrombin isolated by this procedure results in a 1,500 to 1,900 fold purification over rat plasma. The specific activity is in the range of 2,000 to 2,400 NIH units per mg of protein. The total recovery represents 59 % of the total rat plasma prothrombin. In the ultracentrifuge, the product is homogeneous. On Acrylamide gel disc electrophoresis, a major band with two minor bands are observed. This prothrombin displays unusual activation characteristics when compared to Seegers' bovine prothrombin (Seegers, 1952).

Human Prothrombin

Human prothrombin has been prepared in several laboratories (Seegers and Andrews, 1952; Alexander, 1959; Lanchantin, 1958; Goldstein et al. 1959; Streuli, 1959; Asada et al. 1961; Miller and Copeland, 1962, 1964, 1965; Hemker et al. 1964; Magnusson, 1965a, 1965b, Lanchantin et al. 1963 and Shapiro and Waugh, 1966).

The merits of these authors' pensive nights and laborious days are unquestionable, but unfortunately in no case has "final" purification been achieved. The greatest degree of purity has been obtained by Magnusson (1965b), Lanchantin et al. (1963), Shapiro and Waugh (1966).

G. Method of Magnusson (1965b)

1. Procedure

a. Plasma Fractionation:

1. Blood is drawn from donors in citrate. Six liters of citrated plasma are fractionated by method 6 of Cohn et al. (1946).

2. Supernatant I is treated to obtain fractions II and III.
3. The material is stored overnight at –5° C.
4. In the morning, the material is centrifuged at 1,250 g for 30 min at –5° C.

b. Adsorption on Barium Citrate:

1. The precipitate of II and III are quickly dissolved in 0.25 plasma volumes of 0.02 M trisodium citrate at 0° C, and 0.025 plasma volumes of 1 M $BaCl_2$, added slowly during stirring with a vibrating mixer.
2. The barium citrate adsorbed prothrombin precipitate is collected by centrifugation at 1,250 g at 0° C for 20 min.
3. The precipitate is suspended in 0.025 plasma volumes of 1 M $BaCl_2$ by stirring for 10 min with the vibrating mixer.
4. The suspension is centrifuged at 1,250 g at 0° C for 20 min.

c. First Elution with XE-64 (Na^+):

1. The sediment is suspended in 0.125 plasma volumes of deionized water at 0° C.
2. Enough XE-64 (Na^+) is added with constant stirring with the vibrating mixer to raise the pH to 8.5. The precipitate dissolves.
3. The resin (XE-64) is removed by centrifugation at 1,250 g for 15 min at 0° C or by filtration through Whatman 42 paper.

d. Second Adsorption on Barium Citrate:

1. 0.0125 plasma volumes of 1 M $BaCl_2$ is added to the supernatant and stirred.
2. The barium citrate precipitate is collected by centrifugation, same as before.
3. The sediment is suspended in 0.025 plasma volumes of deionized water, at 0° C.

e. Second Elution with XE-64 (Na^+):

The same as steps 2 and 3 in the first elution.

f. Alcohol Precipitation:

1. The solution is diluted with two volumes of water.
2. The pH is adjusted to 4.7 with 0.1 M HCl.
3. Ethanol is added to a concentration of 15–20 %.
4. The resulting precipitate is collected by centrifugation at 1,250 g for 15 min at 0°–3° C.
5. The sediment is suspended in 0.025 plasma volumes of deionized water.
6. The pH is adjusted to 6.5–7.0 with 0.1 M NaOH. The prothrombin will solubilize.
7. The material is lyophilized.

2. Analysis and Improvements

The average yield of prothrombin activity from plasma is 42 %. The specific activity ranges from 860–1,220 NIH Units/mg protein. The wide variation depending to some extent on varying salt content.
The material is stored at –20° C and is used as starting material for further purification.

Chromatography on Sephadex G-200:

1. Approximately 100 mg of the freeze-dried material is dissolved at 0°–4° C in 2-3 ml of 0.15 M calcium chloride and applied to a Sephadex G-200 column, previously washed with 2–3 bed volumes of the 0.15 M $CaCl_2$ and equilibrated accordingly.
2. Elution is performed in a cold room at 0°—4° C at a flow-rate of 4–8 ml per hour, using a hydrostatic pressure of 80–100 cm and collecting 3–5 ml fractions. The protein peaks are dialyzed and lyophilized.

3. Evaluation

Two peaks are obtained. Peak I contains only traces of prothrombin activity. The prothrombin activity applied on the column is obtained almost quantitatively in peak II. The degree of purification, based on protein content is 1.3 to 2.8 times.

H. Method of Shapiro and Waugh (1966)

The following procedure is described for plasma from a single 500 ml unit of blood (approximately 250 ml of plasma). The same technology can be applied to larger or smaller quantities, using proportionate amounts of reagents and suitably scaled columns. The plasma is processed within two hours after collection.

1. Procedure

a. Preparation of DEAE-cellulose:

1. 100 grams of DEAE-cellulose (0.60–0.62 meq/gm) (Bio-Rad Laboratories) are suspended in distilled water in a 2 liter cylinder.
2. The slurry is allowed to settle for one hour, and the supernatant discarded.
3. The cellulose is suspended in 2 liters of 95 % ethanol, stirred for 1 hour at 50° C and then transferred to a Buchner-type funnel with a coarse fitted glass disc, and washed extensively with distilled water with the aid of suction.
4. The filter cake is treated with 1 liter of a solution 0.5 M NaOH and 0.5 M NaCl, then with a solution 0.5 M HCl and 0.5 M NaCl.
5. The base-acid cycle is repeated once more.
6. The cake is finally washed with 8 liters of distilled water and aspirated to remove all the water.
7. The DEAE-cellulose is suspended in distilled water and stored at 4° C. After exposure to plasma, the cellulose must be completely recycled.

b. Collection of Blood:

1. Human blood is collected in ACD anticoagulant (acid-citrate-dextose solution A) in plastic bags.
2. The formed elements are removed by centrifugation at 2° C for 25 min.

c. Adsorption of Prothrombin on DEAE-cellulose:

During blood centrifugation, the stored DEAE-cellulose is prepared as follows:

1. A filter cake equivalent to 10 grams of dry cellulose is again treated with alkali and acid as described above. The final wash with distilled water is continued, however, until the effluent pH is 4.1 or higher. This requires 8–10 liters of water.
2. The filter cake is aspirated as dry as possible, finely divided with a spatula, and added to the cold plasma in a polyethylene beaker.
3. The slurry is stirred for 5 min, then it is poured into a sintered glass Buchner funnel 8.5 cm in diameter, previously siliconized with GE dri-film SE 87 (General Electric Co., Schenectady, N. Y.).
4. With the aid of gentle suction, the entrapped plasma is removed.
5. Without allowing the filter cake to become dry, four successive 250 ml aliquots of 0.154 M NaCl, previously cooled to 4° C, are passed through.

d. Elution from DEAE-cellulose:

1. The prothrombin is eluted by washing the DEAE cake with about 150 ml of cold 0.5 M NaCl.
2. The initial 45 ml of filtrate (prothrombin free) are discarded. The following 105 ml are collected in a siliconized flask. Mild suction may be applied, but care must be taken to avoid foaming. The actual temperature during this step is 12°–14° C.

e. Barium Citrate Precipitation:

1. The eluate is placed in a 600 ml, wide-mouth, polyethylene centrifuge bottle, at room temperature.
2. 200 ml of distilled water and 50 ml of 0.109 M trisodium citrate are added.
3. With constant stirring, 15 grams of $BaCl_2 \cdot 2H_2O$ are added. Stirring is continued for an additional 3 min.
4. The barium-citrate-prothrombin precipitate is centrifuged for 30 min at 4° C at 2,400 rpm (I.E.C. rotor 276). The supernatant is discarded.
5. The precipitate is suspended in a total of 40 ml cold (4° C) distilled water and transferred to a 50 ml polyethylene centrifuge tube.
6. The tube is centrifuged for 10 min at 4° C at 3,500 rpm (I.E.C. rotor 833). The supernatant is discarded.
7. The precipitate is washed twice more, each time with 10 ml of cold distilled water.
8. The precipitate is suspended in 10 ml of 0.17 M trisodium citrate at 0–2° C, eluting the prothrombin.

f. Ammonium Sulfate Fractionation:

1. The suspension is cooled in an ice bath, and 5 ml of ammonium sulfate (Enzyme Grade, Mann Biochemicals) saturated at 0° C are added with constant stirring.
2. The tube is allowed to stand for 5 min.
3. The $BaSO_4$ precipitate, formed by decomposition of barium citrate, is removed by cen-

trifugation for 10 min at 0° C at 3,500 rpm (I.E.C. rotor 833).

4. The supernatant is decanted into a fresh 50 ml polyethylene centrifuge tube, and 15 ml of the same ammonium sulfate are added.

5. The tube is allowed to stand for 5 min and once again centrifuged as in step 3.

6. The supernatant is decanted without disturbing the prothrombin precipitate and, while inverted, the inner wall of the tube is wiped dry.

7. The precipitate is dissolved by adding 1 ml of 0.17 M trisodium citrate (or any other suitable buffer) at room temperature. Ocassionally, the solution will contain a small amount of fine precipitate, apparently $BaSO_4$, which can be removed by centrifugation.

g. Chromatography on Sephadex G-100:

1. The sample is applied to a Sephadex G-100 column, 0.9 cm × 90 cm, previously equilibrated with buffer containing 0.25 M NaCl and 0.01 M trisodium citrate, adjusted to pH 7.0 with concentrated HCl.

2. The column is developed at room temperature with the same buffer at a flow-rate of 8–10 ml per hour. One ml fractions are collected.

3. The initial, small, non-prothrombin peak is discarded. Only the peak tubes of the prothrombin peak are collected.

h. Dialysis:

1. The peak tubes are pooled (12 ml total volume) and placed in a dialysis sac.

2. The solution is dialyzed against 100 ml of a 10% solution of polyethylene glycol in a suitable buffer for 15–18 hours.

3. The final volume in the dialysis sac will be about 1 ml.

4. Dialysis is continued against pure buffer for an additional several hours. The choice of buffer will depend upon the subsequent use to be made of the prothrombin.

2. Evaluation

The specific activity of this material ranges from 1,120–1,180 two-stage units per optical density unit of protein (extinction coefficient of prothrombin E'_{280} is 13.6). Development of the Sephadex column with 0.15 M $CaCl_2$ produces similar results. The total recovery is 50–55% of the original prothrombin in human plasma.

I. Method of Lanchantin et al. (1963)

1. Procedure

a. Collection of Blood:

1. Human blood is collected in ACD anticoagulant solution B, in siliconized bottles or plastic bags and processed within 3 hours after collection.

b. Barium Citrate Adsorption:

(Lewis and Ware, 1953)

1. One hundred ml of cold citrated plasma (citrate concentration approximately 0.02 M) are placed in a centrifuge cup of 125 ml capacity.

2. Ten ml of 1 M barium chloride are added dropwise with shaking and the mixture inverted once or twice to mix.

3. The tube is allowed to stand in the cold for 10–15 min and then centrifuged in a refrigerated centrifuge at 3,000 g for 25–30 min.

4. The supernatant is discarded. The precipitate is dissolved at room temperature in sufficient 0.02 M sodium citrate in saline to give a volume of 100 ml. A small amount of insoluble residue remains. It is removed by centrifugation at low speed for a few min.

5. The supernant is transferred to another centrifuge tube.

6. Ten ml of 1 M barium chloride are added dropwise.

7. The suspension is allowed to stand in the cold for 10–15 min and then centrifuged for 25–30 min at top speed.

8. The supernatant is discarded. The precipitate is suspended in sufficient 0.02 M sodium citrate in saline at room temperature to give a final volume of 50 ml.

c. Elution from Barium Citrate:

(Goldstein and Zonderman, 1958)

A description of this procedure may be found on page 115.

d. Adsorption on DEAE-cellulose:

All operations are performed at room temperature.

1. The eluate, 200 ml, is adjusted to pH 7.0 and the final phosphate concentration adjusted to 0.005 M with the addition of 0.05 M phosphate buffer.
2. Thoroughly washed DEAE-cellulose, 0.64 meq per gram, is added to a concentration of 40 mg per ml of eluate and triturated on a magnetic stirrer for 60 min.
3. The suspension is centrifuged. The supernatant is discarded.
4. The DEAE-cellulose is suspended in 400 ml of 0.1 M NaCl, 0.05 M phosphate buffer, pH 4.5 and again triturated for 30 min. The resulting pH is approximately 5.15.
5. The suspension is centrifuged. The supernatant is discarded.
6. To the sediment, 50 ml of the same buffer (step 4) are added to obtain an adequate suspension.
7. Additional buffer is added until a pH of 4.9 is obtained.
8. The mixture is stirred for 30 min, and then filtered on Whatman 42 paper.
9. Several 1,000 ml washes with water, serve to remove remaining traces of buffer.

e. Elution from DEAE-cellulose:

1. The cellulose is suspended in 250 ml of 0.2 M sodium citrate.
2. The suspension is triturated for 60 min.
3. The suspension is filtered through Whatman 42 paper. The eluate containing the prothrombin is collected.

f. Fractionation with Ammonium Sulfate: (Lewis and Ware, 1953)

1. The beaker containing the eluate is placed in an ice-salt bath.
2. Cold saturated ammonium sulfate solution is added dropwise, with constant stirring, to a concentration of 50 % saturation.
3. The mixture is centrifuged in the cold for 30 min at about 3,000 g. The precipitate is discarded.
4. The supernatant is decanted into a beaker in an ice-salt bath, and cold saturated ammonium sulfate is added dropwise, with constant stirring, to a concentration of 66 % saturation.
5. The suspension is centrifuged in the cold for 30 min at top speed. The supernatant is discarded.
6. The precipitate is washed in 66 % ammonium sulfate and recovered by high speed centrifugation.

g. Sephadex Chromatography:

1. The precipitate is dissolved in 5 ml distilled water and placed on a column of Sephadex G-25 medium, 2×40 cm, prepared according to Flodin (1961).
2. With water as the eluent, 3 ml aliquots are collected in a GME automatic fraction collector equipped with a 280 mμ scanning device and recorder.
3. Separation from ammonium ions is detected by a sensitive indophenol reaction (Chaney and Marback, 1962).
4. Prothrombin is eluted as a single component with a void volume of approximately 65 ml.
5. The salt-free prothrombin peak is pooled, lyophilized and stored at –20° C. Prothrombin is assayed according to Ware and Seegers (1949).

2. Analysis and Improvements

The average yield of human prothrombin by the above procedure is 30 to 40 %. The product is electrophoretically homogeneous from pH 7.0 to 9.0 and devoid of extraneous plasma proteins by immuno-electrophoresis. The specific activity ranges from 1,010 to 2,325 Units/mg protein. Zonal centrifugation in a density gradient indicates that the homogeneity of the preparation is questionable. To improve the specific activity of the above preparation, Sephadex G-200 filtration is warranted (Lanchantin and Friedmann, 1963).

Gel Filtration on Sephadex G-200

This procedure is performed at room temperature.

1. A Sephadex column (1.3 × 30 or 1.3 × 60 cm) is equilibrated with low ionic strength phosphate buffer at pH 6.0 ($\mu = 0.15$).
2. A prothrombin sample, 5–20 mg/ml (2 ml) is applied on the column and the flow-rate adjusted to 4 ml/hr.
3. Elution is performed with the same buffer.
4. The effluent is collected in 1 ml aliquots.

3. Evaluation

Although the chromatographic pattern appears rather disperse, the peak tubes show an increase in specific activity by a factor of 2 or greater, when compared to the starting material.

III. Discussion

As is apparent from the methodology, the prothrombin products obtained by the different procedures, vary considerably in activity. This variability may be expected in the case of species differences but it seems difficult to reconcile the fact that so many ramifications of the two-stage analytical procedure of Ware and Seegers (1949) are necessary to assay the activity of prothrombin. In several instances, the authors point out that this or that modification of the two-stage analysis was necessary, in order to assay the particular product in question.

In most cases, the modification consists of the addition of plasma or serum under the assumption that it in turn is supplying a "Factor" (primarily VII and/or X) which will aid in the activation of prothrombin to thrombin. This postulate is not uncommon in the literature and it has found a way to perpetuate itself in many circles.

The physical homogeneity of the prothrombin complex isolated by the method of Seegers (1952) is unquestionable. It has the ability to be activated to thrombin in the absence of added "Factors VII or X". The ability of this product to generate thrombin may be altered by various chromatographic procedures.

Indications are that the alteration involves the removal not of a contaminant, rather of an integral portion of what is referred to as "prothrombin complex". Seegers and coworkers have elaborated on this hypothesis (Seegers et al. 1969).

It appears then, that the modifications of the two-stage analytical procedure are truly justified, but the reasons are false. In other words, the "Factors" supplied by plasma or serum may be non other than that portion of the prothrombin complex which was removed during the isolation procedure.

Contrarywise, one may question the homogeneity of the prothrombin isolated by Seegers, in terms of stoicheometry, e. g. that the contained factor X activity of the molecule, on a dry weight basis, consists of no more than 10 % of the total weight. This discrepancy is difficult to reconcile at first, but if one were to assume that the population of prothrombin molecules need not be homogeneous chemically, then the problem is simplified.

This latter hypothesis is not so absurd. Singer and Doolittle (1966) have summarized the evidence for chemical heterogeneity of a single population of antibodies having one specific activity.

In view of the aforementioned parameters, it seems incorrect to compare the quality of products prepared by the various methods. From a technical standpoint, the method of Seegers is by far the most efficient.

References

Alexander, B. (1959). *Proc. 4th Intern. Congr. Biochem., Vienna, 1958, 10,* 37.

Anderson, G. F., and Barnhart, M. I. (1964). *Am. J. Physiol. 206,* 929.

Asada, T., Masaki, Y., Kitahara, K., Nagayama, R., Hatashita, T., and Yanagisawa, I. (1961). *J. Biochem. (Tokyo) 49,* 721.

Chaney, A. L., and Marback, E.P. (1962). *Clin. Chem. 8,* 130.

Cohn, E. J., Strong, L. E., Hughes, W. L. Jr., Mulford, D. J., Ashworth, J. M., Melin, M., and Taylor, H. L. (1946). *J. Am. Chem. Soc. 68,* 459.

Flodin, P. F. (1961). *Chromatog. 5,* 103.

Folin, O., and Ciocalteau, U. (1927). *J. Biol. Chem. 73,* 627.

Glueck, H. I. (1958). *Am. J. Physiol. 194,* 285.

Goldstein, R., and Zonderman, E. B. (1958). *Proc. Xth. Intern. Congr. Intern. Soc. Hematol., Rome 1958,* 1006.

Goldstein, R., LeBolloch, A., Alexander, B., and Zonderman, E. (1959). *J. Biol. Chem. 234,* 2857.

Hemker, H. C., Ménaché, D., and Soulier, J. P. (1964). *Abstr. Federation European Biochem. Soc. Symp.* 1st, London 1964.

Hjerten, S., Jerstedt, S., and Tiselius, A. (1965). *Anal. Biochem. 11,* 219.

Hough, D. A., Lyons, L. V., Koppel, J. L., and Olwin, J. H. (1964). *J. Am. Med. Assoc. 188,* 207.

Ito, N., and Grisolia, J. (1959). *J. Biol. Chem. 234,* 242.

Lamy, F., and Waugh, D. F. (1953). *J. Biol. Chem. 203,* 489.

Lanchantin, G. F. (1958). *Am. J. Physiol. 194,* 7.

Lanchantin, G. F., and Friedman, J. A. (1963). *Proc. Soc. Exptl. Biol. Med. 114,* 584.

Lanchantin, G. F., Friedman, J. A., DeGroot, J., and Mehl, J. W. (1963). *J. Biol. Chem. 238,* 238.

Lewis, M. L., and Ware, A. G. (1953). *Proc. Soc. Exptl. Biol. Med. 84,* 636.
Li, L. F., and Olson, R. E. (1967). *J. Biol. Chem. 242,* 5611.
Magnusson, S. (1965a). *Arkiv Kemi 24,* 217.
Magnusson, S. (1965b). *Arkiv Kemi 24,* 367.
Mammen, E. F., and Ramien, A. (1962). *Thromb. Diath. Haemorrhag. 8,* 37.
Miller, K. D. (1958). *J. Biol. Chem. 231,* 987.
Miller, K. D., and Copeland, W. H. (1962). *Proc. Soc. Exptl. Biol. Med. 111,* 512.
Miller, K. D., and Copeland, W. H. (1964). *Vox Sanguinis 9,* 231.
Miller, K. D., and Copeland, W. H. (1965). *Exptl. Mol. Pathol. 4,* 431.
Miller, K. D., and McGarrahan, J. F. (1958). *N. Y. State Dept. Health. Ann. Rept. Div. Lab. Res.,* 69.
Miller, K. D., and Phelan, A. W. (1967). *Biochem. Biophys. Res. Commun. 27,* 505.
Moore, H. C., Lux, S. E., Malhotra, O. P., Bakerman, S., and Carter, J. R. (1965). *Biochem. Biophys. Acta 111,* 174.
Seegers, W. H. (1940). *J. Biol. Chem. 136,* 103.
Seegers, W. H. (1952). *Record Chem. Progress 13,* 143.
Seegers, W. H. (1964). In: "Blood Coagulation, Hemorrhage and Thrombosis" (L. M. Tocantis and C. A. Kazal Eds.), pp. 174—181, Grune and Stratton, New York.
Seegers, W. H., and Andrews, E. B. (1952). *Proc. Soc. Exptl. Biol. Med. 79,* 112.
Seegers, W. H., and Landaburu, R. H. (1960). *Canad. J. Biochem. Physiol. 38,* 1405.
Seegers, W. H., Smith, H. P., Warner, E. D., and Brinkhous, K. M. (1938). *J. Biol. Chem. 123,* 751.
Seegers, W. H., Loomis, E. C., and Vandenbelt, J. M. (1945). *Arch. Biochem. 6,* 85.
Seegers, W. H., Aoki, N., and Marciniak, E. (1962). *New Istanbul Contrib. Clin. Sci. 5,* 170.
Seegers, W. H., Harmison, C. R., Ivanovic, N., and Heene, D. L. (1966). *Thromb. Diath. Haemorrhag. 15,* 343.
Seegers, W. H., Murano, G., McCoy, L., and Marciniak, E. (1969). *Life Sciences 8,* 925.
Shapiro, S. S., and Waugh, D. F. (1966). *Thromb. Diath. Haemorrhag. 16,* 469.
Singer, S. J., and Doolittle, R. F. (1966). *Science 153,* 3731.
Streuli, F. (1959). *Thromb. Diath. Haemorrhag. 3,* 194.
Tishkoff, G. H., Williams, C. M., and Jacobstein, J. (1966). *Federation Proc. 25,* 318.
Ware, A. G., and Seegers, W. H. (1949). *Am. J. Clin. Pathol. 19,* 471.

Purification of Prethrombin "Modified Zymogen"

Genesio Murano

I. Introduction

The sequential activation of a zymogen via intermediates to the active enzyme is not an uncommon occurrence in protein chemistry. Prethrombin, the immediate thrombin precursor, falls in the catogory of an intermediate in the activation sequence of the prothrombin complex to thrombin.

Prothrombin ⟶ Prethrombin ⟶ Thrombin.
The existence of such an intermediate has been implied for many years (Seegers et al. 1950; Lorand et al. 1953; Lamy and Waugh, 1954; Asada et al. 1961; Lanchantin et al. 1965; Magnusson, 1965).

The term *prethrombin* was introduced when it was first isolated in Seegers' laboratory (Seegers and Marciniak, 1965; Marciniak and Seegers, 1965; Seegers et al. 1965; Marciniak and Seegers, 1966).

Recently, Tishkoff et al. (1968) have described the isolation and properties of a "modified zymogen" which, in all probability, is analogous to prethrombin.

II. Methods of Purification

A. Bovine Prethrombin – Method of Seegers and Marciniak (1965)

This method involves the activation of purified prothrombin with thrombin at neutral pH, followed by chromatography on DEAE-Cellulose with an interrupted buffer system.

1. Procedure

a. Prothrombin Activation

1. About 250,000 units of purified bovine prothrombin (Seegers, 1952) are diluted 1:2 with 0.025 M sodium phosphate buffer, pH 7.0.
2. Purified bovine thrombin (Seegers et al. 1958; Seegers et al. 1968) is added to a concentration of 45 units/1000 units of prothrombin.
3. The mixture is incubated at 28° C for 90 min. The disappearance of prothrombin is followed by the two stage analytical procedure of Ware and Seegers (1949).

b. Chromatography on DEAE-Cellulose (Seegers and Landaburu, 1960)

The chromatography is performed at room temperature.

1. DEAE-Cellulose is equilibrated in 0.025 M sodium phosphate buffer at pH 7.0.
2. A gravity packed column 40 x 1–2 cm is prepared.
3. The activated prothrombin mixture is applied.
4. Once the sample has entered the cellulose bed, 0.025–M pH 7.0 phosphate buffer is applied. The flow rate is adjusted to 2 ml/min. One column volume of this buffer is eluted. It is relatively protein free.
5. Phosphate buffer (0.05 M pH 7.0) is applied to the column. A small protein peak is eluted. It consists mainly of inactive protein with traces of prothrombin and prethrombin.
6. Phosphate buffer (0.075 M pH 7.2) is applied. Prethrombin is eluted with this buffer. Ten to 15 ml fractions are collected.

At this point the chromatography may be terminated. However, in the interest of the curious investigator, the column may be further treated with 0.175M pH 7.4 phosphate buffer to elute a fraction displaying competitive inhibitory activity in the activation of prothrombin (Marciniak et al. 1967). Further elution with 0.4 M pH 8.2 phosphate yields a fraction containing autoprothrombin III (see p. 153).

c. Removal of Salts

1. The peak tubes are pooled. Ammonium sulfate (0.5 gm/ml) is added with constant stirring in an ice bath.
2. The suspension is centrifuged for 45 min at 4,000 g at 4° C.
3. The supernatant is decanted. The precipitate is suspended in 25 ml of cold distilled water.
4. An equal volume (25 ml) of cold (–60° C) acetone is added.
5. The resulting precipitate is collected by centrifugation at 4,080 g for 10 min at 4° C.
6. The prethrombin may be suspended in a minimum amount of either distilled water or imidazole buffered saline (0.9 %). Alternatively, the acetone precipitation step may be substituted by rapid dialysis against cold distilled water as described by Seegers (1952).

d. Gel Filtration

1. Sephadex G-100 (Pharmacia Fine Chemicals Piscataway, N. J.) is swollen by standard technology.
2. A column of adequate dimensions to accomodate the sample volume is prepared (usually 1.5×95 cm is adequate).
3. The column is equilibrated at a flow-rate of 5 ml/hr with either distilled water or 0.9 % NaCl.
4. The sample is applied. 2 ml fractions are collected. The chromatogram does not show a homogeneous symmetrical peak. Rather, it usually displays a small heavier peak which is partially masked by the main peak. The prethrombin activity resides exclusively in the main peak.
5. The peak tubes are pooled and subjected to ammonium sulfate and acetone fractionation as previously described.

2. Evaluation

The specific activity of this product is in the vicinity of 40,000 units/mg tyrosine (Marciniak and Seegers, 1965). The assay procedure is a modification of the two-stage analysis of Ware and Seegers (1949). This involves the activation of prethrombin to thrombin by substituting purified autoprothrombin C and lipids in lieu of thromboplastin (Marciniak and Seegers, 1965). In 25 % sodium citrate solution, without autoprothrombin C, prethrombin does not activate to thrombin.

In the ultracentrifuge, a single symmetrical peak is observed (Seegers et al. 1967).

B. Preparation of "Modified Zymogen" – Method of Tishkoff et al. (1968)

This procedure consists of the preparation of "prothrombin", and subsequent chromatography of the complex on DEAE-Sephadex.

1. Procedure

Bovine blood is collected into siliconized plastic buckets containing sodium citrate (0.11 M) as anticoagulant, in a ratio of 9:1. The blood is processed within two hours after collection.

a. Barium Citrate Adsorption and Elution

1. To 1.7 liters of centrifuged plasma are added 170 ml of 1.0 M barium chloride.
2. The suspension is stirred gently for 60 min and centrifuged for 30 min at 2,500 g. The supernatant is discarded.
3. The yellowish precipitate is suspended in 850 ml of distilled water and stirred gently with 35 gm of Dowex 50W-X8 resin (Na^+ form, 20–50 mesh) to elute the prothrombin.
4. The resin is removed by filtration through a coarse, sintered glass filter, and washed with 25 ml of 0.11 M sodium citrate. The total volume of the combined filtrates is about 290 ml. The solution appears cloudy.
5. "Prothrombin" is readsorbed by adding 92 ml of 1.0 M barium chloride, stirring for 20 min, and collecting the precipitate by centrifugation as before.
6. The slightly yellowish sediment is suspended in 225 ml of distilled water and stirred, once again, with 20 gm of Dowex 50W-X8 resin.
7. The resin is removed by filtration and washed as in step 4.

b. Dialysis

1. The combined filtrates are placed in Visking casing and dialyzed against running tap water for 16–18 hours.
2. The insoluble globulins are removed by centrifugation for 40 min at 2,500 g.

Total volume of the supernatant is about 295 ml. The protein concentration ranges from 1–18 mg/ml, and the barium 0.6 mg/ml; the pH is about 8.2; the specific activity is 1,070 U/mg protein; the yield of prothrombin is 100 %.

c. Crystallization

The solution is divided into 50 ml aliquots and frozen at –20° C. On thawing, a well defined crystalline sheen is evident. The crystals are insoluble in water and isotonic NaCl. They are soluble in 0.11 M sodium citrate; the specific activity is 1,940 U/mg protein; the yield of prothrombin is 64 %.

d. Recrystallization

1. The suspension of crystals from each aliquot is centrifuged and the supernatant discarded.
2. The precipitate is dissolved in 12.5 ml of 0.11 M sodium citrate. Any insoluble residue is discarded.
3. The supernatant is dialyzed with stirring against 1 liter of a freshly prepared solution of barium citrate, at room temperature for 4–5 hours.
4. A heavy cloudiness appears. The solution is subsequently dialyzed against 2 liters of distilled water for 22 hours at 4° C.
5. The solution is centrifuged at 2,500 g for 30 min, and the supernatant frozen at –20° C.
6. On thawing, crystals appear. The specific activity of this product is 2,460 U/mg protein; yield of prothrombin is 42 %. Further recrystallization is unsuccessful.

e. Gel Filtration

For this purpose, singly crystallized products are employed.

1. The crystals from a single aliquot (30–45 mg of protein) are collected by centrifugation for 30 min at 2,500 g, and dissolved in 12.5 ml of 0.11 M sodium citrate.
2. The solution is centrifuged to remove insoluble material. The sediment is discarded.
3. The supernatant is passed through a column (0.9×4.6 cm) of AG-50W-resin (Na^+ form, 100 to 200 mesh), followed by 5 ml of distilled water.
4. The eluate (18 ml) is concentrated by ultrafiltration to 2 or 3 ml against phosphate-NaCl buffer pH 6.0 (0.015 M phosphate containing 0.127 M NaCl). (The specific activity of this material increases).
5. The concentrated eluate is applied to a Sephadex G-100 column equilibrated with 0.42 M phosphate buffer, pH 5.9.
6. The elution is carried out with the same buffer.
7. The peak tubes (46 % of activity), are pooled, dialyzed against phosphate-NaCl buffer, pH 6.0, and concentrated by ultrafiltration as in step 4.

This material is referred to as "purified prothrombin". All preparations evidence significant factor VII, IX, and X activities.

f. Chromatography on DEAE-Sephadex

1. A column of DEAE-Sephadex A 50 (2.5 × 40 cm) is prepared and equilibrated with 0.05 M phosphate buffer at pH 5.92.

2. The ultrafiltered "purified prothrombin" is diluted to 10 ml with 0.05 M phosphate buffer, pH 5.92.

3. About 18 mg are applied to the column.

4. Elution is carried out with an exponential gradient produced with 250 ml of 0.05 M phosphate buffer, pH 5.92, in a constant volume mixing chamber, and 0.05 M phosphate-1.0 M NaCl buffer, pH 6.61 in the reservoir.

5. The flow rate is adjusted to 10–20 ml per hour. Fractions of 3 ml are collected for the first 100 tubes, then the volume is reduced to 1.5 ml. At least 200 tubes are collected.

The protein profile is characterized by six major protein peaks labeled A-F. The modified zymogen activity resides exclusively in the second peak (fraction B). Incidentally, fraction C contains prothrombin and factor IX activity. From one experiment to another, an inverse relationship exists between the amount of protein in fraction B and fraction C. Fractions D, E, F, contain factor VII and X activity.

The "modified zymogen" may be concentrated by ultrafiltration.

2. Evaluation

Fraction B constitutes about 28 % of the total protein, and is devoid of coagulant activity. In 25 % sodium citrate, for 96 hours at 25° C, this fraction does not activate to thrombin. However, if fraction F (factor X) is added to the incubation mixture, prompt generation of thrombin occurs. Physical analysis of this component shows that its molecular size is less than that of "prothrombin", but greater than that of thrombin.

III. Discussion

Prethrombin is apparently an intermediate in the prothrombin activation sequence. Physically, the molecule is smaller than prothrombin, but larger than thrombin. It is reasonably certain that prethrombin is the immediate precursor of the enzyme thrombin (Seegers and Marciniak, 1965; Marciniak and Seegers, 1965; Marciniak and Seegers, 1966).

In 25 % sodium citrate, prethrombin or "modified zymogen" (Tishkoff et al. 1968) is activated to thrombin only very slowly, if at all. The addition of thrombin does not accelerate this reaction, but the addition of autoprothrombin C (factor Xa) or trypsin results in a rapid activation of prethrombin to thrombin (Seegers and Marciniak, 1965; Marciniak and Seegers, 1966; Tishkoff et al. 1968). The zymogen may also be activated with the autoprothrombin C precursor, autoprothrombin III, but more slowly (Seegers and Marciniak, 1965). As might be expected, soybean trypsin inhibitor blocks these activations.

In physiologic saline solutions trypsin or autoprothrombin C also convert prethrombin to thrombin very rapidly (Seegers and Marciniak, 1965).

In the presence of Ac-globulin (prepared according to Aoki et al. [1963]) calcium ions and cephalin, the reactions outlined above are appreciably accelerated (Marciniak and Seegers, 1966).

It appears then, that prothrombin is acted upon by thrombin to yield the intermediate prethrombin or "modified zymogen". It is the function of the enzyme autoprothrombin C (factor X_a) to carry out the ultimate proteolysis in the conversion of prethrombin to the enzyme thrombin.

The appearance of "modified zymogen" in the chromatographic procedure of Tishkoff et al. (1968) is not at all startling, since traces of thrombin in the "prothrombin" preparation are sufficient to trigger the limited proteolysis. It may be noted that this phenomenon may coincide with the "two stage refractoriness" of prothrombin first described by Seegers et al. (1951).

References

Aoki, N., Harmison, C. R., and Seegers, W. H. (1963). *Can. J Biochem. Physiol. 41,* 2409.
Asada, T., Masaki, Y., Kitahara, K., Nagayama, R., Hatashita, T., and Yanagisawa, I. (1961). *J. Biochem. (Tokyo) 49,* 721.
Lamy, F., and Waugh, D. F. (1954). *Physiol. Rev. 34,* 722.
Landhantin, G. F., Friedman, J. A., and Hart, D. W. (1965). *J. Biol. Chem. 240,* 3276.
Lorand, L., Alkjaersig, N., and Seegers, W. H. (1953). *Arch. Biochem. Biophys. 45,* 312.
Magnusson, S. (1965). *Arkiv Kemi 24,* 217.
Marciniak, E., and Seegers, W. H. (1965). *New Istanbul Contrib. Clin. Sci. 8,* 117.
Marciniak, E., and Seegers, W. H. (1966). *Nature 209,* 621.
Marciniak, E., Murano, G., and Seegers, W. H. (1967). *Thromb Diath. Haemorrhag. 18,* 161.
Seegers, W. H. (1952). *Record Chem. Progr. 13,* 143.
Seegers, W. H., and Landaburu, R. H. (1960). *Can. J. Biochem. Physiol. 38,* 1405.
Seegers, W. H., and Marciniak, E. (1965). *Life Sci. 4,* 1721.
Seegers, W. H., McClaughry, R. I., and Fahey, J. L. (1950) *Blood 5,* 421.
Seegers, W. H., Andrews, E. B., and McClaughry, R. I. (1951). *Am. J. Physiol. 164,* 722.
Seegers, W. H., Levine, W. G., and Shepard, R. S. (1958). *Canad. J. Biochem. Physiol. 36,* 603.
Seegers, W. H., Marciniak, E., and Heene, D. (1965). *Texas Rept. Biol. Med. 52,* 449.
Seegers, W. H., Marciniak, E., Kipfer, R. K., and Yasunaga, K. (1967). *Arch. Biochem. Biophys. 121,* 372.
Seegers, W. H., McCoy, L., Kipfer, R. K., Murano, G. (1968). *Arch. Biochem. Biophys. 128,* 194
Tishkoff, G. H., Williams, L. C., Brown, D. M. (1968). *J. Biol. Chem. 243,* 4151.
Ware, A. G., and Seegers, W. H. (1949). *Am. J. Clin. Pathol. 19,* 471.

Purification of Thrombin

Genesio Murano

I. Introduction

The activation of purified prothrombin in strong salt solutions was discovered when an attempt was made to block the development of trace quantities of thrombin (Seegers, 1949). Thrombin of excellent quality can be obtained by the autocatalytic activation of purified prothrombin in 25 per cent sodium citrate solution.

Bioactivation of prothrombin to thrombin is an alternate route by which good quality thrombin can be obtained.

In most purification procedures, principles of ion exchange chromatography are applied. The earliest of these was introduced by Rasmussen (1955) and Seegers et al. (1958), using Amberlite IRC-50.

In 1961, highly purified human thrombin was obtained by Korsan-Bengsten and Igge, with carboxymethyl cellulose. In 1962, Schrier et al. made use of Duolite to obtain thrombin in purified form. In the same year, Miller and Copeland (1962) purified human thrombin with adsorption to barium citrate, precipitation with ethanol and rivanol and finally chromatography on an IRC-50 rivanol column.

Magnusson (1965) prepared highly purified bovine thrombin by means of ethanol fractionation and chromatography on Amberlite IRC-50. Berg et al. (1966) have employed gel filtration and CM-Sephadex as a means of purification. This procedure insures the removal of plasminogen.

Recently, Seegers et al. (1968) have improved on the original procedure of 1958 by incorporating a second chromatography on Amberlite IRC-50.

II. Methods of Purification

A. Bovine Thrombin – Method of Seegers et al. (1958)

Thrombin of good quality may be obtained by the autocatalytic activation of purified prothrombin in 25 per cent sodium citrate or by bioactivation with calcium ions, tissue extracts and Ac-globulin (Factor V).

1. Procedures

a. Sodium Citrate Activation

1. Purified bovine prothrombin (Seegers, 1952) is dissolved in 25 % sodium citrate solution so that the final concentration of prothrombin is about 1–1.5 %.
2. To start the autocatalytic reaction, thrombin may be added (4 units per 100 units of prothrombin).
3. The solution is allowed to stand at room temperature and the thrombin titer monitored. The reaction should be complete within 6 to 8 hours. The end volume of the reaction mixture is approximately 25 ml.
4. The thrombin in citrate solution is precipitated by increasing the concentration of sodium citrate to 40 %. This is accomplished by adding crystalline sodium citrate.
5. The precipitate is collected by centrifugation in the cold at 3,800 g for 45 min and dissolved in water up to the original volume.
6. The suspension is cooled to 0° C and an equal volume of cold acetone (–80° C) is added, while the solution is gently stirred.
7. The suspension is centrifuged in the cold at 3,800 g for 5 min, the supernatant discarded, the precipitate dissolved in water and the acetone precipitation repeated. After the last centrifugation, the remaining acetone is removed by handwarming the tube while passing a stream of air over it.
8. The sediment is suspended in a minimum amount of appropriate buffer, depending on the chromatographic procedure to be applied.

Alternatively, prothrombin may be activated to thrombin by bioactivation.

b. Bioactivation

1. About 500,000 units of prothrombin (15–25 ml) are diluted 1:2 with physiologic saline solution buffered at pH 7.2 with imidazole.
2. The reaction vessel (100 ml beaker) is placed in a water bath at 28° C.
3. Thromboplastin ("Hecht Material", Hecht et al. 1958) 20 γ per 1,000 units of prothrombin are suspended in 5 ml of physiologic saline solution and shaken for 5 min.
4. 0.25 M $CaCl_2$ is added to the thromboplastin while stirring (1 ml/25 ml of final reaction mixture).
5. The calcium-thromboplastin mixture is added to the prothrombin.
6. Ac-globulin (Aoki et al. 1963), 20 units/1,000 units of prothrombin, is added.
7. A total of 10,000 units of thrombin may be added to prime the reaction.
8. The activation is monitored by the thrombin assay every 15 min. Within 90 min, the reaction should be complete. If not, more Ac-globulin should be added (5,000 units).
9. The reaction mixture is centrifuged for 90 min at 30,000 rpm in a N° 30 rotor (Beckman Model L Centrifuge) in order to remove the thromboplastin.
10. The acetone procedure described above is applied once to the supernatant.

c. Chromatography on IRC-50 (XE-64): An interrupted buffer system is utilized in the technique.

1. The resin is equilibrated at pH 7.0 with 0.05 M sodium phosphate buffer (2.691 gm $NaH_2PO_4 \cdot H_2O$ and 4.331 gm Na_2HPO_4 in distilled water up to 1 liter).
2. A column 2.5 × 25 cm is poured.
3. About 200,000 to 250,000 units of thrombin are dissolved in 2.5 ml of 0.05 M sodium phosphate buffer, pH 7.0 and applied to the column.
4. As soon as the sample has entered the resin, 1 ml of the same buffer is placed on the column, and allowed to enter the resin bed.
5. The resin bed is layered with buffer in large quantities, and a pressure head established so that the effluent rate is about 2 drops/min.
6. Five to fifteen ml of buffer are allowed to pass through the column. This effluent contains mostly inert protein and autoprothrombin C. The buffer is removed from the surface of the resin by aspiration.
7. Sodium phosphate buffer at pH 8.0, 0.3 M is applied to the column (2.195 gm $NaH_2PO_4 \cdot H_2O$ and 40.333 gm Na_2HPO_4 in distilled water up to 1 liter).
8. The flow rate is adjusted once again to 2 drops/min. The thrombin is eluted in the range of 160 to 260 ml of effluent (10 ml samples are collected). The effluent is monitored by standard techniques.

d. Removal of Salts

1. The thrombin-containing tubes are pooled, and the protein precipitated in the cold (0° C) by the addition of ammonium sulfate powder to 75 per cent saturation. The sodium phosphate is soluble under these conditions.
Alternatively, the pooled sample is cooled to 0° C until phosphate crystals form. The crystallization is hastened by seeding with phosphate crystals. Centrifugation for 5 min at 3,800 g removes the crystals. Then, ammonium sulfate (0.5 g/ml) is added.
2. The suspension is centrifuged in the cold for 45 min at 3,800 g. The supernatant is discarded. The sides of the tube are rinsed with cold distilled water, with the tube in an inverted position.
3. The thrombin sediment is dissolved in 30 ml of cold distilled water and precipitated by adding an equal volume of acetone previously cooled at –80° C.
4. The suspension is again centrifuged for 5 min at 3,800 g and the supernatant discarded.
5. The acetone precipitation is repeated several times to insure the removal of all ammonium sulfate. Last traces of acetone are removed as previously described. The precipitate is suspended in a few ml of buffered saline, assayed and stored at –60° C.

Note: Judging from personal experience, it is advisable that the acetone precipitations be carried out as quickly as possible and the pH not allowed to drop below 6.0 during the procedure.
Alternatively, the incubation mixture may be chromatographed on phosphate cellulose (P. W.) (California Co. for Biochemical Research, Los Angeles). This is an anionic exchanger.

e. Chromatography on Phosphate Cellulose

1. Preparation of buffers:

Buffer A: 0.01 M, pH 7.0
0.538 gm $NaH_2PO_4 \cdot H_2O$
0.866 gm Na_2HPO_4

Buffer B: 0.05 M, pH 7.0
2.691 gm $NaH_2PO_4 \cdot H_2O$
4.331 gm Na_2HPO_4

Buffer C: 0.15 M, pH 8.0
1.097 gm $NaH_2PO_4 \cdot H_2O$
20.166 gm Na_2HPO_4

2. PW cellulose (1 meq phosphorus/g) is equilibrated with buffer A.
3. A column 2 × 13 cm is poured and packed under gravity.
4. About 150,000 units of bovine thrombin (12,000 units/mg tyrosine) are applied on the column. The total volume does not usually exceed 3 ml.
5. The thrombin adsorbs on the cellulose. Buffer A is applied and the flow-rate adjusted to 6–8 drops/min. 10 ml aliquots are collected.
6. About 100 ml of buffer A are collected. This eluate contains mostly impurities and very little thrombin.
7. Buffer B is applied and 60 ml are eluted. This eluate consists of non-thrombin protein.
8. Buffer C is applied. The thrombin elutes rapidly after 60 to 80 ml of this buffer have passed through the resin.
9. The thrombin peak is pooled and freed from salts in the same manner as described above.

2. Evaluation

Purified thrombin, by the method described herein, is referred to as "resin thrombin" and has a specific activity of 4,100 units/mg of dry weight, or 45,000 units/mg of tyrosine. In 0.3 M pH 8.0 phosphate buffer, the thrombin is stable at room temperature for five days. At 4° C, about 70 % of activity remains after 20 weeks. Resin thrombin can lose clotting power while retaining the esterase activity. Contrarywise, the esterase activity can be depressed without diminishing the clotting activity.
Resin thrombin is unstable to lyophilization.

B. Bovine Thrombin – Method of Seegers et al. (1968)

This procedure is similar to the one previously described (Seegers et al. 1958), with slight modifications. In addition, a second chromatography has been introduced.

1. Procedure

a. Sodium citrate activation

1. Purified bovine prothrombin (500,000 units) is activated at 37° C in 25 % (w/v) sodium citrate with autoprothrombin C or thrombin

added at zero time. The final concentrations are as follows:

prothrombin	8000 U/ml
thrombin	40 U/ml
or	
autoprothrombin C	20 U/ml

2. The activation is complete in about 4 hours.
3. The sample is diluted into 4 volumes of cold distilled water and cooled to 4° C.
4. Ammonium sulfate (crystalline) is added to 3.5 M concentration (constant stirring).
5. The precipitate is collected by centrifugation in the cold at 3,800 g for 45 min.
6. The sediment is suspended in 20 ml of 0.05 M phosphate buffer at pH 7.0.

b. First chromatography

1. The protein solution is added to a packed 200–325 mesh Amberlite IRC-50 cation-exchange resin at a level of 1 ml of packed resin per 2,500 units of thrombin. (The resin has been previously equilibrated with 0.05 M, pH 7.0 potassium phosphate buffer).
2. The mixture is stirred in the cold for 30 min. Upon settling of the resin-thrombin complex, the supernatant is tested for thrombin activity. If more than 100 units/ml remain unadsorbed, more resin may be added until the thrombin concentration in the supernatant does not exceed 100 units/ml.
3. The resin-thrombin complex is centrifuged. (The supernatant may be retained for the isolation of autoprothrombin C – factor X section – otherwise it is discarded).
4. The packed resin-thrombin complex is washed with 3 volumes of 0.05 M, pH 7.0, phosphate buffer. Washing is continued until the fluid is protein free.
5. The washed, packed, resin-thrombin complex is suspended in ½ volume of 0.05 M, pH 7.0 buffer and poured on top of a thrombin-free IRC-50 bed, 2.5 × 25 cm. This is done at refrigerator temperature.
6. The resin-thrombin complex is allowed to settle. The buffer on top is removed by aspiration.
7. Potassium phosphate buffer (0.3 M, pH 8.0) is applied. The pressure head is regulated to establish a flow rate of 0.5 ml/min.
8. The chromatography is carried out for 2 days.
9. Tubes containing peak activity (about 45,000 units/mg tyrosine) are pooled.
10. The protein is precipitated out of solution with ammonium sulfate as previously described.
11. The sediment is dissolved in about 8 ml of 0.05 M, pH 7.0 potassium phosphate buffer.

This thrombin product is essentially analogous to the thrombin product obtained in the 1958 procedure of Seegers et al.

c. Second chromatography

The thrombin obtained in step b-11 (above) is readsorbed on IRC-50 resin and rechromatographed. The manipulations are the same as those for the first chromatography beginning with step b-1, up to step b-10.

d. Desalting

Thrombin may be freed of salts either by dialysis against distilled water in the cold, or by chromatography on Sephadex G-25.

2. Evaluation

Thrombin obtained by the first chromatography is referred to as "3.7S Thrombin" and the product obtained by the second chromatography is referred to as "3.2S Thrombin". In each instance, the numbers are derived from the S^{o}_{20w} values.

3.7S thrombin has a specific activity of about 45,000 units/mg tyrosine, whereas the 3.2S thrombin ranges from 75,000 to 90,000 units/mg tyrosine. The doubling in specific activity is concomitant with the removal of an inhibitory fraction. The final yield is about 25 % of that in the original prothrombin sample.

The physical properties of this "super thrombin" are described in Chapter I, page 10.

C. Bovine Thrombin – Method of Magnusson (1965)

1. Procedure

a. Prothrombin preparation: Bovine prothrombin is prepared according to Seegers (1952) as previously described through those steps (p. 101) which include euglobulin precipitation, extraction of prothrombin, adsorption on magnesium hydroxide, and elution with carbon di-

oxide. The eluate (approximately 800 ml from 20 liters of plasma) is cleared by centrifugation (10 min, 1,250 g) and dialyzed against deionized water overnight. The pH during and after dialysis is 7.5 to 7.9.
The volume of the dialysate is measured and $^1/_{30}$ volume of 3 M sodium acetate is added. The pH is adjusted to 7.2–7.5 with 1.0 M acetic acid. The entire procedure described above is performed at 0–4° C.

b. Prothrombin activation

1. To determine the optimum activation conditions, pilot experiments are performed. Thus: 2 ml of the prothrombin solution +0.2, 0.4, and 0.8 ml of thromboplastin suspension + 0.2 ml of 0.18 M calcium chloride are incubated at 37° C, and samples taken at 5 min intervals and tested for thrombin activity. Maximal thrombin titer usually develops in 20–40 min.
2. The optinum conditions are used for the full-scale activation of the entire batch which is carried out with constant stirring at 37° C. The prothrombin solution, the thromboplastin suspension, and calcium chloride are prewarmed to 37° prior to incubation.
3. The activation mixture is centrifuged at 0° C for 10 min at 1,250 g. The thromboplastin material sediments.

c. Alcohol Precipitation

1. Maintaining the temperature of the supernatant at 0–1° C, 135 ml of 53.3% aqueous ethanol (precooled at –5° C) is added per 1,000 ml supernatant with stirring, and lowering of the temperature to –4° C.
2. The precipitate is separated by centrifugation at –4° C (10 min, 1,250 g) and discarded.
3. The pH of the supernatant is adjusted to 5.5–6.0 with 1.0 M acetic acid.
4. One volume of 65% (v/v) cold (–10° C) aqueous ethanol is added with stirring and further lowering the temperature to –6° C.
5. Stirring is continued for 30 min.
6. The thrombin is collected by centrifugation at –6° C for 30 min at 1,250 g.
7. The thrombin precipitate is dissolved in 90 to 120 ml of deionized water.

d. Dialysis and Drying

1. The material is dialyzed overnight against ten liters of deinonized water at 0–2° C.
2. The suspension is clarified by centrifugation (20 min, 0° C, 25,000 g, angle head), and freeze-dried.

2. Analysis and Improvements

This material has a greyish-white appearance. The yield from 20 liters of plasma is 900–1400 mg with a specific activity of 240–290 NIH units/mg. In the freeze-dried state, in vacuo, at –15° to –20° C all of the activity remains after 6 years. A solution (3.2 mg/ml in deionized water) can be sterile filtered through cellulose nitrate membranes (Membranfilter No. 6, Sartorius-Werke A. G., Göttingen, Germany) and freeze-dried without change in specific activity.

a. Chromatography on Amberlite IRC-50 (XE-64)

1. Amberlite IRC-50 (XE-64) (200–400 mesh) is washed with acetone, 2 M NaOH and 4 M HCl. The finest particles are removed by sedimentation as described by Hirs (1955).
2. The resin is equilibrated batchwise with 0.05 M sodium orthophosphate buffer pH 7.0.
3. The suspended resin is poured into a glass column 2.0–2.2 cm in diameter, with a coarse sintered glass filter (D-1) to support the ion exchanger. Either a 60 cm or a 20 cm column may be used. The disadvantage of using the longer column is the 2–3 days required to elute the thrombin. The 20 cm column is a preferred system.
4. The column is packed at a hydrostatic pressure of 50–100 cm and equilibrated at pH 7.0 ± 0.1 with 0.05 M phosphate buffer.
5. 300 mg (or less) of crude bovine thrombin are dissolved in 2–6 ml of 0.05 M phosphate buffer pH 7.0.
6. The sample is applied to the column.
7. Elution with 0.05 M sodium phosphate pH 7.0 is carried out until the absorbancy of the effluent at 280 mμ is decreased to 0.05 or less (~430 ml of effluent).
8. 0.3 M sodium phosphate pH 8.0 is applied and the flow rate adjusted to 4 drops/min.

9. The sample is collected in 10–13 ml aliquots. A typical chromatogram will result in three peaks.

b. Recovery of Thrombin from the Column Effluent

1. All tubes from the thrombin peak (III) having an absorbancy at 280 mμ greater than 0.25 are pooled.
2. After cooling to 0° C, 0.70 gm of solid ammonium sulfate are added per ml of effluent.
3. The mixture is stirred for 1 hour, then left overnight at –4° C.
4. The precipitate is collected by centrifugation at 25,000 g for 10 min at –4° C, in 25 ml polypropylene tubes.
5. The sediment is dissolved in 10 ml deionized water at 0° C and transferred to one tube.
6. 10 ml of acetone (pro-Analysi, Merk), precooled to –55° C is rapidly added with stirring.
7. The mixture is quickly centrifuged for 15–30 sec at 15,000 g at –5° C to –8° C.
8. The precipitate may be recovered either as a sediment or as a cake floating between the upper and lower liquid phases of the systems.
9. The sediment is resuspended in deionized water and reprecipitation from 50 % acetone performed two more times. During acetone precipitation, extreme care must be exercised in maintaining the low temperature. The pH is maintained at 6.0 to 6.5 by addition of 0.1 M NaOH, otherwise it will drop to 3–4 with ensuing protein denaturation. The entire process of acetone precipitation is performed as quickly as possible (20–30 min).
10. The material is finally dissolved in 20 ml of deionized water and freeze-dried.

3. Evaluation

The thrombin yield ranges from 68.2 to 81.2 mg with a specific activity of 2098 ± 134 NIH units/mg dry weight. This material is not as stable in the freeze-dried state as the non-chromatographed material. Some preparations will retain 50–60 % of their activity for a period of 18 months, whereas others will completely loose activity and solubility. In starch gel electrophoresis, thrombin prepared as described above behaves as a homogeneous protein. In the ultracentrifuge, no sign of heterogeneity is apparent.

D. Human Thrombin Method of Miller and Copeland (1965)

1. Procedure

a. Reagents and Materials

1. Human plasma fraction III is either prepared by the method of Oncley et al. (1949) or obtained from E. R. Squibb and Sons, New Brunswick, N. J., or the American National Red Cross.

2. Thromboplastin is prepared from human, equine, or bovine brain after removal of gross blood vessels and meninges. The tissue is ground in 0.15 N NaCl and washed four times with cold 0.15 N NaCl (each wash being centrifuged for 15 min at 17,000 g). The solid material is heated for 15 min in a boiling water bath, washed twice with 0.15 N NaCl, suspended in 10 times its volume of 0.15 N NaCl and stored frozen. For every 100 ml of prothrombin to be activated, 2 ml of this suspension are used. The required volume is centrifuged at 17,000 g for 15 min. The pellet is suspended in a volume of bovine serum equal to the volume of suspension used. The suspension is placed in an ice bath for 15 min with occasional stirring. The mixture is centrifuged at 17,000 g and washed twice with cold 0.15 N NaCl. The washed thromboplastin (with adsorbed factors) is suspended in a solvent consisting of 0.15 M $CaCl_2$ und 0.1 M Tris or cacodylate buffer, pH 7.2–7.4. The volume of this solvent is one fifth that of the prothrombin solution to be activated.

3. All reagents are analytical reagent grade.

4. Sephadex G-100 and G-200 are swollen 3–4 days in 0.15 N NaCl containing 2 % n-butanol.

5. Sephadex columns are supported by two layers of glass wool sandwitched between two 16 mesh stainless steel screens. These units, held together by cotton thread stitches, are cut to fit the adaptors in chromaphlex column systems (Kontes Glass Co.). Thus supported, 4 × 40 cm G-200 column flow at 35–65 ml per hour with reservior levels 15–40 cm above the level of the column bottom.

6. IRC-50 Na^+ (XE-64) is routinely cycled through the H^+ to the Na^+ form before use.

7. CG-50 Na^+ (Mallinckrodt) (100–200 or 200–400 mesh) is equilibrated with 0.1 M cacodylate or Tris buffer pH 7.0.
8. Prothrombin and thrombin are measured according to Ware and Seegers (1949).

b. Extraction of Fraction III
1. Human lyophilized fraction III is extracted 3 times with cold chloroform methanol (2:1) at a temperature below 0° C. Each extraction is stirred for 15 min and filtered through Whatman No. 3 paper on a Buchner funnel.
2. To remove the residual chloroform, the protein is stirred for 15 min with cold (–10° C) acetone and filtered on a Buchner funnel. Aspiration is continued until the protein has a dry, sandy consistency.
3. A suspension of the extracted powder is prepared in 0.02 M sodium citrate at room temperature (5 gm per 100 ml).
4. The pH is adjusted to 8.0–8.5 and stirred for no longer than 30–60 min.
5. The undissolved material is allowed to settle.
6. The supernatant is decanted into fluted Schleicher and Schuell No. 520-Bl/2,40 cm filter papers, or their equivalent. The residue is poured onto the same papers, and with gently squeezing, most of the fluid is expressed.

c. Adsorption on Barium Citrate
1. The extract, termed the "original extract", is cooled to 0–5° C and stirred.
2. To the stirring solution, 1.0 M $BaCl_2$ is added dropwise to a final concentration of 0.10 M.
3. Stirring is continued for an additional 15 min.
4. The suspension is centrifuged at 0–5° C. The sediment consists of the barium citrate-prothrombin complex. For large lots, a Sharpless Super Centrifuge may be used.
5. The precipitate is suspended in a volume of water at 3–5° C, equal to one-half the original extract volumes. This is done in a Waring Blendor at a low speed (maintained by a Variac) to avoid excessive aeration.

d. Elution from Barium Citrate
1. To the stirring suspension, IRC-50 Na^+ (XE-64), 3 gm/100 ml of suspension is added.
2. The mixture is stirred until, when permitted to stand for 60 sec, a clear supernatant appears on top of the settling resin. The degradation should be complete in 10 min and the pH of the supernatant should be in the range 7.0–9.0.
3. The suspension is filtered through the fluted Schleicher and Schuell No. 520-Bl/2 papers as described above. The filtrate contains the prothrombin and is referred to as the "1st eluate".

e. Second Adsorption and Elution: 1.0 M $BaCl_2$ is added dropwise to the first eluate with stirring to 0.1 M at 0–5° C. After centrifugation, the precipitate is suspended in one tenth the original eluate volume of cold water in the Waring Blendor, at low speed. IRC-50 Na^+ (XE-64), 3 gm/100 ml of suspension is added, and stirred, until the barium citrate is dissolved (as tested for above). The suspension is filtered as above. This is the "2nd eluate".

f. Solvent Change: The pH of the second eluate is adjusted to 6.0 and either dialyzed or chromatographed to remove the citrate.
a. Dialysis is carried out against 0.15 M NaCl.
b. Sephadex G-100 equilibrated with 0.15 N NaCl is employed for chromatography. Dialysis is the method of choice, particularly for the larger volumes.

g. Activation of Prothrombin
1. The pH of the prothrombin is adjusted to 7.2–7.4 at room temperature.
2. One-fifth volume of a suspension of washed brain thromboplastin (with adsorbed factors) in 0.15 M $CaCl_2$ is added.
3. The mixture is stirred gently and the thrombin titer monitored at room temperature. Activation should be complete in 30 min or less.
4. The incubation mixture is cooled to 0–5° C and centrifuged at 17,000 g or more. The precipitate is discarded.
5. The pH of the supernatant is adjusted to 6.0 with 0.1 N HCl.
6. Butramidine or Benzamidine is added to a concentration of about 0.1 M.
7. The mixture is dialyzed against cold 0.15 N NaCl.
Alternatively, the thrombin may be concentrated by addition of two volumes of cold (–10° C) acetone dropwise at pH 6.0. The sus-

pension is centrifuged. The precipitate is dissolved in 0.1 N NaCl and dialyzed against 0.15 N NaCl.

h. Ion Exchange Chromatography

1. A (G-50 Na^+, 100–200 or 200–400 mesh) column 4 × 10 cm is equilibrated with 0.10 M cacodylate or tris buffer at pH 7.5. (This size column will retain 1×10^6 Iowa units of dialyzed human thrombin.)

2. The sample is placed on the column and allowed to adsorb at room temperature.

3. After adsorption of the thrombin, the column is washed with 5–column volumes of 0.1 M cacodylate or Tris buffer, pH 7.0.

4. The thrombin is eluted with 0.2 M $CaCl_2$.

5. The thrombin eluates are cooled to 0–5° C, and the pH adjusted to 6.0 with 0.1 N HCl.

6. Two volumes of cold acetone (–10° C) are added dropwise, with stirring, maintaining the temperature below 5° C.

7. The precipitate is recovered by centrifugation, and dissolved in sufficient 0.15 N NaCl to give 30,000 to 50,000 Iowa units/ml.

If the specific activity of the thrombin at this stage does not approximate 10,000 Iowa units/mg of protein, gel filtration is warranted.

i. Gel Filtration: A column of Sephadex G-200 is prepared and developed with 0.15 N NaCl that is 0.05 M with respect to acetate buffer (pH 5.5–6.0) and 2 % n-butanol. The thrombin activity will appear in one of the several peaks in the chromatogram.

The peak containing the activity is dialyzed against either cold distilled water or 0.15 N NaCl. Alternatively, it may be rechromatographed on Sephadex G-75 with 0.15 N NaCl as a developer. The final product is lyophylized.

2. Evaluation

Human thrombin isolated by the method described will retain all of its activity after 3 months storage at –10° C. Lyophilization does not reduce its activity. The average yield is 50–66 % of the starting prothrombin titer. The average specific activity is 10,000 Iowa units/mg of protein.

E. Human and Bovine Thrombin – Method of Berg et al. (1966)

1. Procedure

a. Preparation of Human Crude Thrombin

1. Fresh oxalated human plasma is stirred with $BaSO_4$ (100 mg/ml of plasma) at 37° C for 15 min.

2. The $BaSO_4$ is collected by centrifugation.

3. The precipitate is washed three times with physiologic saline solution.

4. The adsorbed protein is eluted from the $BaSO_4$ by washing the sediment with 6 % (w/v) trisodium citrate (10 % of the original plasma volume).

5. Tissue thromboplastin (prepared according to Owren (1947), centrifuged at 19,000 g, resuspended in physiologic saline solution and again centrifuged three times) is added (1 ml/100 ml of eluate).

6. $CaCl_2$, 1 M (2 ml/100 ml of eluate) is added.

7. The solution is dialyzed against running tap water for 24 hours.

8. The tissue thromboplastin is removed by centrifugation at 19,000 g for 6 min.

b. Preparation of Bovine Crude Thrombin: The procedure is the same as described above except that fresh oxalated bovine plasma is used and the source of thromboplastin is calf brain instead of human brain.

c. Commercial Bovine Crude Thrombin (Topostasin): This crude thrombin preparation is obtained from Hoffmann LaRoche & Co., Basel, Switzerland.

d. Gel Filtration: Gel filtration is performed according to Flodin (1962). The inner surface of the column is coated with silicone and the entire unit is jacketed for cooling purposes. The effluent is collected in plastic tubes.

1. A column 6 × 120 cm of Sephadex G-75 is prepared, and equilibrated with NaCl-Tris buffer pH 8.0. This buffer is prepared by mixing 0.1 M Tris-HCl pH 8.0 and 0.5 M NaCl in a 1:4 ratio.

2. Forty ml of crude thrombin are applied to the column.

3. The column is cooled with running tap water at about 4° C. The effluent is placed in a refrigerator until ready for analysis.

2. Analysis and Improvements

The bulk of inert protein appears as a major peak in the first 800 ml of effluent. The clotting activity is well separated from this major peak. Except in the case of Topostasin, as the crude thrombin starting sample, no plasminogen activity is found in the thrombin containing fraction.

a. Chromatography on CM-Sephadex

1. The bulk of the thrombin from the gel filtration on Sephadex G-75 (200–250 ml) is dialysed against 0.1 M Tris-HCl (pH 7.5).
2. A CM-Sephadex A-50 (medium) resin bed 1.5 × 30 cm is prepared in a column coated with silicone and cooled with running tap water. Equilibration is achieved with 0.1 M Tris-HCl pH 7.5 buffer.
3. The dialyzed sample is percolated through the column at a flow-rate of 2 ml/min. A small amount of inert protein is not adsorbed and filters through the resin, but all the thrombin is adsorbed to the CM-Sephadex.
4. After washing with 0.1 M Tris-HCl pH 7.5, the buffer is changed to 0.3 M Tris-HCl (pH 8.0). A small amount of inert protein is eluted but no thrombin.
5. 0.5 M NaCl-Tris pH 8.0 buffer (prepared as described above) is applied.
6. The thrombin is eluted as a sharp peak.

3. Evaluation

Chromatography on CM-Sephadex concentrates the thrombin from gel filtration about 20 times. The elution diagram is similar for bovine, human and "Topostasin" thrombin. The activity of this product is about 30,000 NIH units/mg of tyrosine. All preparations are free of plasminogen, except "Topostasin" which contains traces of this contaminant even after chromatography on CM-Sephadex.

F. Bovine Thrombin – Method of Baughman and Waugh (1967)

Thrombin of constant specific activity may be obtained by this procedure. Principles of ion exchange chromatography and gel filtration are applied to commercial preparations of crude thrombin. Inert protein and a nonenzymatic inhibitor are removed from thrombin.

1. Procedure

a. Preparation of Stock Thrombin

1. Cellex-D and Cellex-P resins (Bio-Rad, Laboratories Calbiochem, Los Angeles, Calif.) are treated for the removal of fine particles. (Distilled water is deionized on ion exchange resin, passed through a millipore filter, HA grade, and stored in polyethylene containers.)
2. Cellex-D is packed tightly in a column (5 × 7 cm resin bed).
3. Cellex-P is handled similarly (2.5 × 7 cm).
4. Both columns are individually washed with acid and base, equilibrated with phosphate buffer at pH 7.0 and $\Gamma/2 = 0.1$, containing 5×10^{-4} M KCN to suppress growth of microorganisms.
5. The two columns are connected in series.
6. Parke-Davis Topical Thrombin (800 mg) is dissolved in 320 ml of equilibrating buffer in a polyethylene container.
7. The solution is applied to the Cellex-D column, followed by 400 ml of the same buffer (flow rate is 20 ml/min).
8. The Cellex-P column is disconnected and washed with 250 ml phosphate buffer at pH 7.0 and $\Gamma/2 = 0.15$. At this point, the inhibitor remains adsorbed on the Cellex-D resin and may be eluted with 1.0 M NaCl. The thrombin remains adsorbed on the Cellex-P resin.
9. Phosphate buffer at $\Gamma/2 = 1.0$, one-half due to NaCl at pH 6.75, is applied. Alternatively 0.15 M $CaCl_2$ may be applied to elute the thrombin.
10. The first 30 ml are discarded. The following 50 ml are collected. The entire procedure can be completed in 8 hours.

2. Analysis and Improvements

Over 91% of the original activity is obtained. At an ionic strength of 1.0, pH 7.0 at 4° C, this preparation loses activity to the maximum of 0.1% per week. At 23° C, in dilute solution, the loss averages 1.6% of its activity per day.

a. Concentration of Thrombin: Stock thrombin in 0.15 M $CaCl_2$ may be obtained by direct elution from Cellex-P or by appropriate dialysis of stock thrombin. The former procedure

requires an adjustment of pH to 7.0 before acetone addition.
1. At 0° C, cold acetone is added to a final concentration of 60 to 70 %.
2. The mixture is stirred gently for 15 min.
3. The precipitate is recovered by centrifugation, air dried, and dissolved in phosphate buffer $\Gamma/2 = 0.3$.

b. Gel Filtration: For analytical purposes, samples are applied to the column without concentration.
1. A column of Sephadex G-100 (140–400 mesh Pharmacia International), 0.95×100 cm is prepared, and washed with deareated column solution, for four days before use.
2. One ml of stock thrombin containing up to 5 absorbancy units is applied (1 absorbance unit is that amount/ml which for 1 cm path length has a unit corrected absorbance at pH 7.0 and $\lambda = 280$ mμ, corrected for scattering by subtracting 1.7 times the apparent adsorption at 320 mμ).
3. The column is developed with 1.0 M NaCl pH 7.0. The flow-rate is adjusted to 3–4 ml per hour.

3. Evaluation

Gel filtration of stock thrombin on Sephadex G-100 separates an average of 24 % of the absorbance of stock thrombin as an inactive protein and gives a single thrombin peak. From this study, a molecular weight of 36,000 is estimated.

G. Bovine Thrombin-Insoluble – Method of Hussain and Newcomb (1964)

Water insoluble thrombin is prepared by coupling soluble thrombin with a copolymer of p-amino-DL-phenylalanine and L-leucine. Alternatively prothrombin may be coupled to the copolymer and subsequently activated to yield water insoluble thrombin.

1. Procedure a

1. CG-50 type II resin is treated successively with acid and base and thereafter with 0.05 M sodium phosphate buffer pH 7.0, until the pH of the supernatant reaches 7.0.
2. A column 0.9×15 cm is prepared and equilibrated with the same buffer.
3. One hundred mg of bovine thrombin (Thrombin-Topical, Parke-Davis & Co.) dissolved in about 2 ml of the same buffer, are applied.
4. The inactive protein is washed off the column with 0.1 M sodium phosphate buffer pH 7.5.
5. The thrombin is subsequently eluted with 0.3 M sodium phosphate buffer, pH 8.0, containing 1.0 M NaCl.
6. The active effluent is concentrated by dialyzing against 10 % polyvinylpyrrolidone for 24 hours, at 4° C.
7. Dialysis is continued for an additional 4–6 hours against 0.154 M NaCl at 4° C. This concentrated thrombin has a specific activity of 665 NIH units/mg protein as compared to the starting material 57 NIH units/mg of protein.
8. The copolymer of p-amino-DL-phenylalanine and L-Leucine is prepared at the Weizman Institute of Science, Rehoboth, Israel, by the method of Bar-Eli and Katchalski (1963). This copolymer has a molar ratio of L-leucine and p-amino-DL-phenylalanine of 2:1:1.
9. Coupling of the thrombin to the copolymer is accomplished in a manner identical to that for preparation of insoluble papain (Cebra et al. 1961).
Diazotization of the copolymer results in an insoluble brownish-orange particle which is subsequently washed in phosphate buffer, pH 7.5.
Thrombin (5,000 NIH units in 5 ml of buffer) is mixed with the copolymer (100 mg weight before diazotization) and stirred at pH 7.5, 5° C for 24 hours.
10. The preparation is washed free of reaction products with sodium phosphate buffer, 0.1 M, pH 7.5. Siliconized glassware is used. Addition of 50 % glycerol to all solutions appear to improve the yield.

2. Procedure b

1. Normal oxalated beef plasma is adsorbed with $BaSO_4$ (100 mg/ml).
2. The $BaSO_4$ is eluted with 0.14 M pH 7.5 trisodium citrate.

3. The eluate is dialyzed against 0.05 M pH 7.0 phosphate buffer.
4. The dialysate is chromatographed on DEAE cellulose. The fraction containing prothrombin is eluted with 0.3 M sodium phosphate buffer and 1 M NaCl pH 8.0. This represents a 132 fold purification.
5. This material is concentrated and dialyzed as the thrombin was.
6. The prothrombin (41.25 mg protein in 12.5 ml) is coupled to the copolymer as above.
7. It is then washed in buffer and activated by a thromboplastin mixture containing Russel Viper Venom (Stypven® Burroughs Wellcome Co., Tuckahoe, N. Y.), factor V, and calcium.

The resulting insoluble thrombin is apparently identical to the insoluble thrombin prepared in the first procedure.

3. Evaluation

Water insoluble thrombin prepared as outlined has minimum clotting activity but excellent esterolytic activity. In this respect, it resembles acetylated thrombin (Landaburu and Seegers, 1959).

III. Discussion

A direct comparison of the specific activities of thrombin prepared by the above methods is not possible. The reason for this is because each laboratory throughout the years seems to have developed modifications of assay procedures, with concomitant individually fashioned conversion factors. This kind of individuality is to be admired, but with reservations, for it perpetuates a plethora of arguments which are totally unfounded.

In fact, as pointed out by Baughman and Waugh (1967), a careful examination of tyrosine content and clotting conversion factors as given by each laboratory, indicates that the average specific activity in terms of NIH units/mg of protein is approximately the same (about 2,200) for all products. With the exception of the latest developments in Seegers' laboratory, this generalization is true.

The physico-chemical parameters are all in general agreement. The variability in stability is apparently an effect of technologic maneuvers, in the last steps of purification, rather than the product isolated.

References

Aoki, N., Harmison, C. R., and Seegers, W. H. (1963). *Can. J. Biochem. Physiol. 41,* 2409.

Bar-Eli, A., and Katchalski, E. (1963). *J. Biol. Chem. 238,* 1690.

Baughman, D. J., and Waugh, D. F. (1967). *J. Biol. Chem. 242,* 5252.

Berg, W., Korsan-Bengsten, K., and Igge, J. (1966). *Thromb. Diath. Haemorrhag. 18,* 501.

Cebra, J. J., Givol, D., Silman, H. I., Katchalski, E. (1961). *J. Biol. Chem. 236,* 1720.

Flodin, P. (1962). A. B. Pharmacia, Uppsala, Sweden.

Hecht, E. R., Cho, M. H., and Seegers, W. H. (1958). *Am. J. Physiol. 193,* 584.

Hirs, C. H. W. (1955). In: "Methods in Enzymology" (S. P. Colowick and N. O. Kaplan, Eds.), p. 113, Academic Press, New York.

Hussain, Q. Z., and Newcomb, T. F. (1964). *Proc. Soc. Exptl. Biol. Med. 115,* 301.

Korsan-Bengsten, K., and Igge, J. (1961). *Scand. J. Clin. Lab. Invest. 13,* 591.

Landaburu, R. H., and Seegers, W. H. (1959). *Canad. J. Biochem. Physiol. 37,* 1361.

Magnusson, S. (1965). *Arkiv. Kemi 24,* 349.

Miller, K. D., and Copeland, W. H. (1962). *Proc. Soc. Exptl. Biol. Med. 111,* 512.

Miller, K. D., and Copeland, W. H. (1965). *Exptl. Mol. Pathol. 4,* 431.

Oncley, J. L., Melin, M., Richert, D. A., Cameron, J. W., and Gross, P. M., Jr. (1949). *J. Am. Chem. Soc. 71,* 541.

Owren, P. A. (1947). *Acta Med. Scand. 128,* Suppl. 194.

Rasmussen, P. S. (1955). *Biochim. Biophys. Acta. 16,* 157.

Schrier, E. E., Broomfield, C. A., and Scheraga, H. A. (1962). *Arch. Biochem. Suppl. 1,* 309.

Seegers, W. H. (1949). *Proc. Soc. Exptl. Biol. Med. 72,* 677.

Seegers, W. H. (1952). *Record Chem. Progress 13,* 143.

Seegers, W. H., McCoy, L., Kipfer, R. K., and Murano, G. (1968). *Arch. Biochem. Biophys. 128,* 194.

Seegers, W. H., Levine, G., Shephard, R. S. (1958). *Canad. J. Biochem. Physiol. 36,* 603.

Ware, A. G., and Seegers, W. H. (1949). *Am. J. Clin. Pathol. 19,* 471.

Purification of Ac-Globulin (Factor V)

Lowell E. McCoy

I. Introduction

While studying in vitro conversion of partially purified prothrombin to thrombin, Nolf (1908) hypothesized the existence of a "thrombogen" in plasma which was required for rapid thrombin generation. Quick (1943) reported that refractoriness of stored oxalated plasma to one-stage prothrombin reagents could be corrected by the addition of minute amounts of a "labile factor" present in fresh human plasma. Owren (1947) had applied the term factor V in describing the first Ac-globulin deficiency syndrome in man. Fahey et al. (1948) demonstrated that this activity could be preserved by citrate in lieu of oxalate as anticoagulant. Ware et al. (1947) and Ware and Seegers (1948) coined the term accelerator-globulin based on the finding that a concentrate obtained from plasma, accelerated the rate of zymogen activation and had an electrophoretic mobility of a β-globulin. They also found that thrombin treatment first increased the activity and subsequently destroyed it. That same year, Murphy and Seegers (1948) reported that Ac-globulin was destroyed during coagulation processes in man but not in the cow, cat, or rabbit. Sykes, Seegers, and Ware (1948) found that liver damage was associated with a reduction in plasma Ac-globulin concentration.

The first successful concentrate of Ac-globulin (Ware and Seegers, 1948) was prepared by ammonium sulfate and isoelectric fractionation of plasma. Aoki et al. (1963) reported a plasma fractionation method which gave products in improved yield and purity, and found the SH groups essential for activity.

Esnouf and Jobin (1967), employing chromatographic techniques were able to isolate a highly purified Ac-globulin. Barton and Hanahan (1967), by modifying the Esnouf and Jobin (1967) method were able to further refine Ac-globulin isolation to obtain even higher activity and demonstrate some effects of divalent metal ions on the activity and stability of the product. All procedures use bovine plasma as the source of Ac-globulin.

II. Method of Purification

A. Method of Aoki et al. (1963)

1. Materials

a. Plasma stored at –20° C in liter aliquots for not more than a week is obtained from nine volumes of fresh bovine blood anticoagulated with one volume of 1.85 % potassium oxalate with the formed elements being sedimented in the cold at 1,370 g for 20 min.

b. Barium carbonate.

c. 1 % (v/v) acetic acid.

d. Phosphate buffer, 0.05 M, pH 7.0 containing 2.69 gm $Na_2HPO_4 \cdot H_2O$ and 4.33 gm NaH_2PO_4 per liter of solution.

e. Phosphate buffer, 0.005 M, pH 7.0 obtained by diluting 1 volume of 0.05 M buffer with 9 volumes of distilled water.

f. 0.30 M phosphate (pH 8.0) containing 40.33 gm $Na_2HPO_4 \cdot H_2O$ and 2.19 gm NaH_2PO_4 per liter of solution.

g. Ammonium sulfate.

h. Saturated sodium carbonate solution.

i. IRC-50 (Bio Rex 70) cation exchange resin 200–400 mesh (Bio Rad Laboratories, Richmond, Calif.).

j. Imidazole buffer, 0.25 M (pH 6.8), containing 17.02 gm imidazole dissolved in distilled water adjusted to pH 6.8 using 1 M HCl, and diluted to 1 liter.

k. Phosphate buffered saline composed of 970 ml of 0.9 % (w/v) NaCl and 30 ml of 0.05 M phosphate buffer (pH 7.0).

2. Method (carried out at 5° to 0° C in an ice bath)

a. One liter of plasma is mixed with 40 gm of barium carbonate and stirred for 10 min.

b. The barium carbonate is sedimented and discarded by centrifugation in the cold at 1,370 g for 10 min.

c. Repeat steps *a* and *b* on the supernatant.

d. The supernatant from the second adsorption is diluted, with stirring, using 5 volumes of cold distilled water.

e. The solution is adjusted to pH 6.2 by addition of 1 % (v/v) acetic acid.

f. The precipitate which forms is sedimented in the cold at 1,370 g for 10 min.

g. Additional acetic acid is added to the stirred supernatant until the pH is 5.1.

h. The precipitate is collected by sedimentation at 4,000 g for 10 min.

i. The sides of the tubes are washed free of supernatant fluid using a stream of cold distilled water.

k. Using a glass rod, the precipitate is suspended in 1 liter of phosphate buffered saline.

l. The solution is cooled, with stirring, to –2° C and slowly brought to 45 % of saturation with solid ammonium sulfate (282 gm).

m. After all ammonium sulfate is dissolved the precipitate is collected by centrifugation at 2,500 g for 15 min.

n. Step *i* is repeated.

o. The precipitate is dissolved in a minimum volume of distilled water and dialyzed against neutralized distilled water (1 ml saturated Na_2CO_3/8 liters water) to a resistence of at least 1,000 ohms.

p. The dialyzed solution is adjusted to pH 6.3 by addition of 1 % (v/v) acetic acid.

q. The precipitate is sedimented at 1,370 g for 10 min and discarded.

r. Additional 1 % (v/v) acetic acid is employed to bring the supernatant pH to 5.2.

s. The sediment collected at 2,000 g for 10 min is triturated in phosphate buffered saline to dissolve.

3. Chromatography of the Ac-globulin concentrate (modified procedure of Landaburu and Seegers, 1961) conducted at 4° C

a. A 1.6 × 25 cm column of IRC-50 (sodium form) suspended in and equilibrated with 0.005 M phosphate buffer is poured, packed under gravity, and washed with 100 ml of the same buffer.

b. Two products of the Ac-globulin concentrate are pooled, applied to the column and allowed to enter the resin.

c. The sample is washed into the resin with two 5 ml aliquots of the equilibration buffer.

d. Phosphate buffer (0.005 M, pH 7.0) is used to elute non-adsorbed protein at a flow rate of 0.5 to 0.75 ml per minute while collecting 10 ml eluate fractions.

e. When all non-adsorbed protein has been eluted from the column (spectrophotometrically monitored) 0.05 M phosphate buffer (pH 7.0) is employed to further elute inactive protein.

f. When the eluted fractions become protein negative, 0.3 M phosphate buffer (pH 8.0) is used to elute the Ac-globulin.

g. The eluted Ac-globulin containing fractions are pooled, diluted with an equal volume of cold distilled water, brought to 38 % of saturation with solid ammonium sulfate, the precipitate sedimented for 10 min at 1,370 g and discarded.

h. Ammonium sulfate is used to bring the supernatant to 50 % of saturation.

i. The precipitate is collected at 2,500 g for 15 min and dissolved in imidazole buffer.

4. Comment

a. The Ac-globulin concentrate is stable for 8 hours at room temperature, 2 days at 4° C, 7 days at –20° C and in 50 % (v/v) glycerol for more then 3 weeks at –20° C.

b. The stability of the concentrate is also increased by addition of Ca^{++} ($CaCl_2$) to 0.08 M.

c. The chromatographed product although less stable at ambient or refrigerator temperatures has approximately the same stability as the non-chromatographed material when stored at –60° C in glycerol.

d. Ammonium sulfate can be removed from the chromatographed product by disc dialysis (Seegers, 1952) against carbonate neutralized 25 % (v/v) glycerol solution if the product is first diluted with an equal volume of glycerol.

e. The chromatographed product, after dialysis against water can be lypholized and stored for at least one month at –60° C.

B. Method of Esnouf and Jobin (1967)

1. Materials

a. Fresh bovine plasma is obtained from 9 volumes of blood anticoagulated with 1 volume of 1.34% (w/v) sodium oxalate and centrifuged at 4° C for 45 min at 1,000 g.

b. Barium sulfate.

c. M hydrochloric acid.

d. TEAE-cellulose (Serva Entwicklungs-Labor, Heidelberg, Germany).

e. Sodium phosphate buffers at pH 7.0 are made by addition of saturated sodium hydroxide to phosphoric acid to pH 7.0 and diluting aliquots of the solution to the molarities of phosphate as shown below.

(1) 0.01 M
(2) 0.03 M
(3) 0.10 M
(4) 0.15 M
(5) 0.30 M
(6) 0.40 M
(7) 0.50 M

f. Phosphorylated cellulose (Whatman P-70).

2. Method (carried out at ambient temperature)

a. One liter of fresh plasma is stirred for 20 min with 100 gm barium sulfate.

b. The supernatant is collected by centrifugation at 1,000 g for 30 min at 10° C and diluted with an equal volume of distilled water.

c. The solution is brought to pH 7.0 with M hydrochloric acid.

d. Dry TEAE-cellulose (15 gm) is added, and the mixture stirred for 20 min.

e. The TEAE-cellulose is collected by centrifugation at 1,000 g for 30 min at 10° C.

f. The cellulose is twice washed by stirring for 10 min in 1 liter of 0.03 M phosphate buffer.

g. The Ac-globulin is eluted by stirring the washed cellulose for 15 min with 200 ml ($^1/_5$ beginning plasma volume) of 0.40 M phosphate buffer.

h. After centrifugation at 1,000 g for 30 min to remove the cellulose, the eluate is dialyzed overnight at 4° C against distilled water to lower the phosphate concentration to 0.01 M.

i. The dialyzed eluate is centrifuged at 1,000 g for 30 min at 4° C to remove insoluble protein.

3. Chromatography of TEAE-cellulose Eluate (conducted at ambient temperatures)

a. A slurry of phosphorylated cellulose in 0.50 M phosphate buffer is poured into a 10 cm diameter column and allowed to settle to a height of 6 cm under gravity.

b. The packed cellulose is then washed with one liter of the suspending buffer and equilibrated with 0.01 M phosphate buffer.

c. The clarified dialyzed TEAE-cellulose eluate is applied to the column and washed into the resin with two 10 ml portions of the equilibration buffer.

d. A step elution of the column is accomplished using phosphate buffers at 0.01 M, 0.10 M, 0.15 M, 0.30 M, and 0.50 M in sequence at a flow rate of 1.9–2.0 ml/hr/cm² while collecting 45 ml fractions of eluate.

e. The eluates of a given buffer are monitored for protein content until the fractions are protein free, at which time the next buffer in the sequence is applied to the column.

f. The fraction eluted with 0.30 M buffer contains approximately 50% of the Ac-globulin activity and 3% of the protein.

g. Concentration of the pooled Ac-globulin fractions is accomplished by dilution of the fractions to 0.1 M phosphate and applying the solution at 8 ml/min to a 4 × 3 cm column of phosphorylated cellulose (prepared as in steps *a* and *b* above) and eluted at 1 ml/min with 0.30 M buffer.

h. Further concentration can be accomplished by ultrafiltration or with dry Sephadex G-200.

i. Dialysis overnight at 4° C followed by addition of an equal volume of glycerol and storage at –20° C gives a protein which retains its activity for months.

C. Method of Barton and Hanahan (1967)

1. Materials

a. Bovine plasma is obtained by centrifuging 9 volumes of fresh bovine blood anticoagulated with one volume of 0.1 M sodium oxalate for 20 min at 1,370 g and 4° C.

b. Veronal-acetate buffer pH 7.35 (Michaelis):

(1) 9.714 gm sodium acetate trihydrate
(2) 14.714 gm sodium diethylbarbiturate
(3) Dissolve in 500 ml distilled water

(4) Add sodium chloride to 4.25% (w/v) at 500 ml (21.25 gm)
(5) Add 434 ml 0.1 M hydrochloric acid
(6) Dilute to 2.7 liters with distilled water

c. Barium sulfate.

d. TEAE-cellulose (Cellex T, Bio Rad Laboratories, Richmond, Calif.): The resin (150 gm) is washed successively with 8 liter quantities of 0.1 M hydrochloric acid, 0.1 M sodium hydroxide, 0.1 M sodium chloride, distilled water, and finally equilibrated with 0.003 M sodium phosphate buffer at pH 7.0.

e. Phosphorylated cellulose (Whatman Chromedia P-11): The resin (500 gm) is washed with 10 liters M sodium phosphate buffer at pH 7.0, followed with 10 liters 0.4 M sodium phosphate, then three times with water, and finally equilibrated with 0.003 M sodium phosphate buffer at pH 0.7.

After use, regeneration is accomplished by successive washings with 0.4 M phosphate buffer, water, and 0.003 M phosphate buffer.

f. Sephadex G-200 (Pharmacia, Piscataway, N. J.).

2. Method (conducted at room temperature)

a. Ten liters of bovine plasma are stirred for 30 min with 1 kg barium sulfate and the adsorbed plasma clarified by centrifugation in the cold at 1,370 g for 10 min.

b. The adsorbed plasma is diluted with an equal volume of cold distilled water.

c. The pH of the solution is adjusted to 7.0 with M HCl.

d. A suspension of 140 gm of TEAE-cellulose in 2.2 liters of 3 mM phosphate buffer is added and the mixture stirred for 20 min.

e. After the resin has settled for 1 hour at 4° C all but 3 liters of supernatant fluid is siphoned off and discarded.

f. The settled resin and fluid are poured onto a Buchner funnel (12.5 cm) fitted with 2 pieces of Whatman No. 1 paper and the resin aspirated to a moist paste.

g. The residue on the filter is washed with successive 200 ml aliquots of 0.4 M phosphate buffer and the washes collected as separate fractions until a total volume of 2 liters has been collected.

h. Fractions 2–5 (200–1000 ml) usually contain most of the activity and are pooled.

i. The pooled fractions are dialyzed at 4° C against changes (at 90 min intervals) of 0.003 M phosphate buffer.

3. Phosphorylated Cellulose Chromatography

a. A column (1.0×9.4 cm) of phosphorylated cellulose in 0.003 M phosphate buffer (pH 7.0) is poured, and washed with 900 ml of the suspending buffer at a flow rate of 500–800 ml/hr.

b. The dialyzed TEAE-cellulose eluate is applied to the column and the column is washed with 0.1 M phosphate buffer (pH 7.0) until the eluate is protein free.

c. A second phosphate buffer (0.15 M, pH 7.0) is applied and with the aid of aspirator suction to maintain the above flow rate, chromatography is continued until the eluate is protein free.

d. Finally, 0.4 M phosphate buffer (pH 7.0) is applied to elute the Ac-globulin fraction. Elution is continued until the eluate is protein free.

e. The active fractions are pooled and dialyzed at 4° C against 20 liter portions of 0.003 M phosphate buffer for 12 hours with dialysate changes at 2 hour intervals.

f. The precipitate which forms during dialysis is removed by centrifugation for 10 min at 1,370 g.

g. The dialyzed eluate is applied to a second cellulose phosphate column (4.5 × 15 cm) equilibrated with 0.003 M buffer, and step eluted under N_2 pressure (2 lb/in^2) at a flow rate of 300 ml/hr employing 0.01 M, 0.1 M, 0.15 M, and finally 0.3 M phosphate buffer to elute the Ac-globulin.

h. Active fractions are pooled and dialyzed in the cold against 20 liter aliquots of veronal acetate buffer for 12 hrs with dialysate changes at 2 hour intervals.

i. The dialyzed eluate is concentrated in the dialysis tubing using dry G-200 Sephadex.

j. This concentrate can be further dialyzed for 12 hours at 4° C against veronal acetate buffer and stored in the freezer in glycerol.

4. Calcium Treatment of the Phosphorylated Cellulose Eluate

a. The concentrated phosphorylated cellulose eluate is brought to 8.5 mM Ca^{++} by addition of 0.4 M $CaCl_2$.

b. Upon warming for 2 min at 37° C, a precipitate is formed, which is collected by 10 min centrifugation at 4,000 g.
c. The supernatant is again mixed with the same volume of 0.4 M $CaCl_2$ as was used in step *a.*
d. The small amount of precipitate which forms is handled as in step *b.*
e. The precipitates from steps *b* and *d* are combined, washed with 8.5 mM $CaCl_2$, and dissolved in a minimum volume of veronal acetate buffer containing 2.5 mg EDTA/ml.
f. This sample is dialyzed for 6 hours, in the cold, against liter volumes of veronal acetate buffer with dialysate changes at hourly intervals.
g. The dialyzed sample can be mixed with an equal volume of glycerol and stored at –20° C.

III. Discussion

Although the above methods are designed to give the same end product, purified Ac-globulin, the individual methodologies have been selected to cover a range from precipitation (Aoki et al. 1963) to chromatography (Esnouf and Jobin, 1967) to a combination of both (Barton and Hanahan, 1967). Direct comparison of the final products derived from each method is impossible on a specific activity basis because of divergent assay methods. However, presentation of activity recoveries and degree of purification from plasma should permit the reader to evaluate the methods and select that which meets his requirements.

The method of Aoki et al. (1963) has given Ac-globulin activity recoveries of 15–20% having a purity level as measured by specific activity of 1150 times that of plasma. It must be pointed out that the isoelectric fractionation step at pH 5.1 must be rapidly and carefully conducted as the activity is less stable at this pH level.

Esnouf and Jobin (1967) reported an average activity recovery of 50% with the products having a 4,000 fold purification over plasma.

Barton and Hanahan (1967) have obtained 20–45% activity recoveries representing 3,500 to 8,500 fold purification over plasma. Calcium treatment of the above products nearly doubles the activity without causing appreciable loss of overall recovery. However, this shift in activity may be an ionic effect since the authors have demonstrated a molecular change using G-200 Sephadex.

All products, irregardless of method of purification, exhibit a lack of stability except when stored at freezer temperatures in stabilizing agents such as glycerine, sucrose, albumin, etc. Without such stabilizing agents the products will lose 50% or more activity when stored for 48 hours at refrigeration or higher temperatures. Freezing and thawing or drying of the unprotected samples caused irreversable activity losses as do certain chelating agents such as EDTA or citrate (Esnouf and Jobin, 1967).

Therefore, careful selection of the methodology is required since addition of stabilizing agents to the final products could present problems in further studies.

References

Aoki, N., Harmison, C. R., and Seegers, W. H. (1963). *Can. J. Biochem. Physiol. 41,* 2409.
Barton, P. J., and Hanahan, D. J. (1967). *Biochem. Biophys. Acta 133,* 506.
Esnouf, M. P., and Jobin, F. (1967). *Biochem. J. 102,* 660.
Fahey, J. L., Ware, A. G., and Seegers, W. H. (1948). *Am. J. Physiol. 154,* 122.
Landaburu, R. A., and Seegers, W. H. (1961). *Thromb. Diath. Haemorrhag. 6,* 435.
Murphy, R. C., and Seegers, W. H. (1948). *Am. J. Physiol. 154,* 134.
Nolf, P. (1908). *Arch. Int. Physiol. 6,* 1.
Owren, P. A. (1947). *Acta Med. Scand. Suppl. 1,* 194.
Quick, A. J. (1943). *Am. J. Physiol. 140,* 212.
Seegers, W. H. (1952). *Record Chem. Prog. 13,* 143.
Sykes, E. M., Jr., Seegers, W. H., and Ware, A. G. (1948). *Proc. Soc. Exptl. Biol. & Med. 67,* 506.
Ware, A. G., and Seegers, W. H. (1948). *J. Biol. Chem. 172,* 699.
Ware, A. G., Guest, M. M., and Seegers, W. H. (1947). *Science 106,* 41.

Purification of Factor VIII

Eberhard F. Mammen

I. Introduction

Factor VIII is a plasma protein which participates in the conversion of prothrombin to thrombin in the intrinsic pathway. It corrects the coagulation defect in the blood of patients with classical hemophilia (hemophilia A). This finding has generated great interest in its purification from plasma and most of the procedures were designed to obtain preparations which were clinically useful.

The iso-electric precipitation from plasma was one of the earliest techniques to obtain crude factor VIII concentrates (Addis, 1911; Bendien and van Creveld, 1936; Patek and Stetson, 1936; Patek and Taylor, 1937; Pohle and Taylor, 1937; Alexander and Landwehr, 1948). Salting-out procedures (Bidwell, 1955a, b; Brinkhous and Wagner, 1959; Janiak and Soulier, 1962; Schwick, 1967), fractionation with ethanol (Cohn et al. 1946; Blombäck, 1958; Niemetz et al. 1961; Achenbach et al. 1959; Baumgarten et al. 1963; Kalinke and Egli, 1967), precipitation with ether (Kekwick and Wolf, 1957; Holman and Wolf, 1963) and rivanol (Schwick, 1967) and finally cryoprecipitation (Pool et al. 1964; Pool and Shannon, 1965; Hershgold et al. 1966; Simson et al. 1966; Brown et al. 1967; Alexander and Odake, 1967) are a few of the more simple techniques to prepare crude Factor VIII concentrates from plasma. During the last few years the procedure of Pool et al. (1964) has found wide acceptance in the preparation of clinically useful concentrates. Factor VIII is usually 10–50 fold purified over plasma. Although these preparations are highly active and clinically useful, they are heavily contaminated with other plasma proteins, especially fibrinogen. Several groups of investigators have subsequently attempted to separate fibrinogen from factor VIII and a variety of different approaches was taken. For example, Lorand and Laki (1954) and Loeb (1959) employed kaolin to separate factor VIII from fibrinogen, Soulier (1959) used bentonite, and van Creveld et al. (1959a, b; 1961; 1966), Veder (1966) and Michael and Tunnah (1963, 1966) used various forms of column chromatography. All attempts to separate fibrinogen from factor VIII were marked by a considerable loss of factor VIII activity, and the extreme lability of factor VIII to various environmental changes has made its purification for physical-chemical characterization very difficult. This basic problem accounts for the fact that so little is known about the properties of factor VIII, as was pointed out in Chapter I.

Seegers and his associates, for example, have for many years attempted to characterize factor VIII from its physical-chemical point of view. The purification procedure was developed on the basis of the original work of Lorand and Laki (1954) (Seegers et al. 1957, 1959; Mammen, 1963). Although preparations could be obtained which sometimes approached homogeneity, the overall recovery of factor VIII was very low and the procedure lacked satisfactory reproducibility. This has made the procedure in the authors opinion impractical and highly discouraging to work with. In the following, several techniques are described which have been employed to obtain factor VIII preparations of fairly high yield and of fairly good quality.

II. Methods of purification

A. Procedure of M. Blombäck (1958)

1. Human blood is collected in trisodium citrate solution (3.2%) by adding 7 parts of blood to 1 part of trisodium citrate. The blood is immediately centrifuged for 30 min at 2,000 g at 4° C.

2. The supernatant plasma is separated and fractionated with ethanol as described by Cohn et al. (1946) (Cohn's fraction I). The plasma is cooled to 0° C and ethanol is added under

constant stirring to a final concentration of 0.027 M. The suspension is centrifuged for 25 min at 2,000 g at –3° C.

3. The precipitate is suspended in $^1/_4$ volume of the original plasma volume of a 0.055 M trisodium citrate solution, pH 6.8 ± 0.05, containing 6.5 % ethanol and 1 M glycine, chilled to –2° C to –3° C. The suspension is stirred for 60 min at –2° C to –3° C and centrifuged for 10–12 min at 2,000 g (Temp. –2° C).

4. The resulting precipitate is again suspended in cold trisodium citrate solution containing ethanol and glycine (see step 3) and after stirring for 60 min, centrifuged for 15 min at 2,000 g (Temp. –2° C).

5. The precipitate is dissolved in $^1/_{10}$ volume of 0.055 M citrate solution, pH 6.8 ± 0.05. The vessel containing the suspended precipitate is warmed to 37° C in order to dissolve the precipitate as rapidly as possible.

6. After a complete solution is obtained, it is shell-frozen and stored at –23° to –30° C. This fraction is called "Fraction I–0". It contains about 85 % fibrinogen and can be used clinically after further dilution with 0.05 M NaCl solution.

7. In order to remove most of the fibrinogen, Fraction I–0 is rapidly thawed and diluted with 0.055 M trisodium citrate solution, pH 6.8 ± 0.05, to a protein concentration of approximately 0.75 %. The solution is chilled to 0° C and a 10 % ethanol solution is added under constant stirring until a 0.5 % (v/v) concentration of ethanol is reached. The suspension is then stirred for 15 min at 0° C and centrifuged for 10 min at 2,000 g (0° C).

8. The precipitate is suspended to the original volume of Fraction I–0 in 0.055 M trisodium citrate solution and warmed to 30° C in a water bath for complete solution. The solution is shell-frozen and stored at –30° C. This fraction represents "Fraction I–1–A". It can be dried from frozen state.

B. Procedure of Simonetti et al. (1961, 1964)

1. Simonetti et al. (1961, 1964) start with Fraction I–0 of Blombäck (1958) (see steps 1–6 of above procedure), dilute Fraction I–0 to a protein concentration of approximately 2.5 % and add under continuous stirring a 1 % tannic acid-saline solution to a concentration of 0.08 ml tannic acid-saline/ml Fraction I–0. The suspension is centrifuged for 20 min at 2,000 g at 0° C.

2. The precipitate contains most of the fibrinogen and can be further processed to obtain highly purified fibrinogen.

3. The supernatant contains practically all of the factor VIII activity originally present in Fraction I–0. This fraction is called "Fraction I–0–Ta". The purification of factor VIII in Fraction I–0–Ta is stated as 200 times over plasma. Fraction I–0–Ta has been successfully used clinically.

C. Procedure of Hurt et al. (1966a)

The method to be described represents a modification of the procedure initially described by Wagner et al. (1964a, b). The authors used selected amino acids for the precipitation of factor VIII.

1. The blood is collected from normal subjects into acid citrate dextrose (ACD) solution (Formula A) at 0° C and the plasma immediately separated by centrifugation at 0° C.

2. Before further processing, a plasma sample is treated with a 10 % (w/v) Al $(OH)_3$ suspension (Moist Gel, British Drug House, Poole, England). That amount of Al $(OH)_3$ suspension is later on used which gives, after 30 min adsorption, a one-stage prothrombin time longer than 4 minutes and less than a 10 % decrease of factor VIII activity of the adsorbed plasma.

3. The main plasma batch (1,000 ml) is transfered to a plasma transfer set which contains the appropriate predetermined amount of 10 % Al $(OH)_3$ suspension and placed in an ice bath.

4. After 30 min of gentle agitation to keep the Al $(OH)_3$ in suspension, the plasma is centrifuged and the resulting precipitate discarded.

5. The supernatant plasma is mixed with an equal volume of 6 M beta alanine (Mann Research Laboratory, chromatographically pure beta alanine) at 0° C. The pH is adjusted to 6.8–6.9 by slowly adding 0.1 N acetic acid.

6. After constant stirring of the suspension at 0° C for 60 min it is centrifuged at 0° C and the supernatant discarded.

7. The precipitate is washed with 500 ml of a 6.5 % ethanol-water solution (v/v) at 0° C for 15 min and again centrifuged.

8. The washing with 500 ml 6.5 % ethanol-water is once repeated.

9. Next the precipitate is washed with 500 ml distilled water at 10° C for 10 min and once more precipitated by centrifugation.

10. The precipitate is dissolved in 100 ml citrate saline solution, pH 6.88 at 24° C (2 ml imidazole buffer, pH 6.88 plus 20 ml 3.2 % sodium citrate solution plus 80 ml 0.9 % saline solution) and quick frozen for storage at –30° C. This fraction is designated as "Fraction AA". It contains more than 75 % of the factor VIII activity originally found in plasma and is 60–80 fold purified over plasma.

Fraction AA can be further purified by three procedures, reprecipitation with beta alanine, adsorption on bentonite or adsorption on Florigel.

a. Reprecipitation with beta alanine

Hurt et al. (1966a) investigated several concentrations of beta alanine for the reprecipitation of fraction AA and two different time intervals for extraction. Optimal results were obtained with the use of 0.5 M beta alanine (final concentration) and 30 min extraction at 24° C.

1. Fraction AA is thawed and a 3 M beta alanine solution is added to give a final beta alanine concentration of 0.5 M. The suspension is stirred for 30 min at 24° C and centrifuged.

2. The resulting precipitate is dissolved in citrate saline solution, pH 6.88 and again quick frozen and stored at –30° C. Residual undissolved material becomes soluble after warming to 37° C. Analysis revealed a factor VIII recovery of 68–116 % with a 600–1,000 fold purification over plasma (Hurt et al. 1966b).

b. Adsorption on bentonite or Florigel

Hurt et al. (1966a, b) investigated various concentrations of bentonite and Florigel over various time intervals and concluded that best results were obtained with 20 mg bentonite or Florigel/ml of fraction AA.

1. Fifty grams of Wyoming Bentonite (Cenco) or Florigel (Fuller's earth, Floridin Company) are dissolved in 500 ml 0.9 % NaCl solution and stored at 4° C for 24 hours. Before use, the amount of adsorbent required is removed and centrifuged for 20 min at 1,850 g. The supernatant is aspirated and discarded.

2. Fraction AA (10 times concentrated) is rapidly thawed, brought to 24° C and added to the vial containing the appropriate amount of bentonite or Florigel (20 mg/ml fraction AA) and rapidly suspended with the adsorbent. After 16 min of incubation at 24° C under stirring, the suspension is centrifuged for 1 min at 4,300 g.

3. The supernatant is pipetted from the packed precipitate and again centrifuged for 2 min at 4,300 g to remove all traces of adsorbent.

4. The supernatant is quick frozen and stored at –30° C.

Analysis revealed a factor VIII recovery ranging from 30–70 % (fraction AA being 100 %) and a 4,000–5,000 times purification over plasma. By keeping all reagents sterile and pyrogen-free and by performing all purification steps under sterile conditions, the preparations have been used clinically.

D. Procedure of Johnson et al. (1967)

The procedure developed in the American Red Cross Research Laboratory in New York by A. J. Johnson and his associates (Johnson, 1967, 1968; Johnson et al. 1967) has only been published in principle, the technical details have not been reported. In view of the fact that high potency preparations are obtained, the procedure is outlined in principle.

In a first step, a 3 % ethanol supplemented cryoprecipitate is obtained from frozen plasma, utilizing the basic technique of Pool et al. (1964).

The cryoethanol precipitable protein is extracted with Tris-buffer and the precipitate, obtained by centrifugation, discarded. The supernatant is precipitated with 3 % polyethylene glycol and the obtained precipitate discarded.

In a next step, the supernatant is precipitated with 10 % polyethylene glycol and the resulting precipitate collected. The precipitate contains factor VIII 200–400 times purified over plasma.
By either using sucrose gradient centrifugation or agarose-gel chromatography, fibrinogen-free factor VIII preparations have been obtained that were 10,000 times purified over plasma.

E. Procedure of Brinkhous et al. (1968)

Recently, Brinkhous et al. (1968) described a procedure for the purification of factor VIII from human plasma in principle. The technical details are again not published. The procedure employes the cryoprecipitation technique of Pool et al. (1964), followed by precipitation with polyethylene glycol, presumably similar to the technique described by Johnson et al. (1967), followed by glycine precipitation according to Wagner et al. (1964a, b).
Cryoprecipitate from 200–500 units of citrated human plasma (4 % citrate) is pooled and precipitated with polyethylene glycol. Polyethylene glycol separates most of the fibrinogen from factor VIII. In a final step, the factor VIII is precipitated with glycine as described by Wagner et al. (1964). With this procedure more than 50 % of the factor VIII content of the original cryoprecipitate is recovered.
The preparation is lyophilized and commercially available from Hyland Laboratories as "Method Four". The factor VIII is purified 160–400 times over plasma.

III. Discussion

The factor VIII preparations obtained from human or animal plasma by employing any one of the above outlined techniques, vary considerably in their degree of purity. All human preparations have been clinically used in the treatment of hemophiliacs, but only the products prepared by Johnson et al. (1967) have been studied from the view-point of biochemical purity. In these products a 10,000 fold purification of factor VIII over plasma was achieved, but acrylamide-gel electrophoresis still revealed two components. This very likely indicates that these products are still contaminated with other plasma constituents which seems in this particular case not to be fibrinogen. It is remarkable that these fibrinogen-free factor VIII preparations are fairly stable upon storage. The chromatographic separation of fibrinogen from factor VIII described by other authors (Michael and Tunnah, 1963, 1966; van Creveld et al. 1959a, b, 1961; 1966) has usually resulted in a considerable loss of factor VIII activity which has been attributed to the fact that fibrinogen has a stabilizing effect on factor VIII. The extreme lability of the biological activity of factor VIII is unquestionably one of the greatest difficulties in its purification from plasma. The biological activity is not only destroyed by proteolytic enzymes, such as thrombin, plasmin and other esterases (Brinkhous and Wagner, 1959; Wagner et al. 1964a; Kekwick and Walton, 1962), but also by simple changes of the pH below 6.2 and above 6.9 (Surgenor, 1964; Weiss, 1965), by the addition of ammonium sulfate and by dialysis. The latter is apparently due to the removal of cations which leads to a rapid loss of factor VIII activity (Blombäck, 1964). These findings limit the availability of certain routine techniques for protein purification and make the task of purifying factor VIII extremely difficult.

The lack of adequate purification of factor VIII has not only limited physical-chemical studies on this coagulation factor, but also limited our understanding of its physiological function in the process of prothrombin activation.

References

Achenbach, W., Egli, H., Kesseler, K. H., and Overkamp, H. (1959). *Deut. Med. Wochschr. 84,* 675.

Addis, T. (1911). *J. Pathol. Bacteriol. 15,* 427.

Alexander, B., and Landwehr, G. (1948). *J. Clin. Invest. 27,* 98.

Alexander, B., and Odake, K. (1967). *Federation Proc. 26,* 478.

Baumgarten, W., Sanders, B. E., Belkin, B. D., Pagenkemper, F. E., Albers, W. G., and Ciminera, J. L. (1963). *Thromb. Diath. Haemorrhag. 9,* 354.

Bendien, W. M., and van Creveld, S. (1936). *Maandschr. Kindergeneesk. 5,* 179.

Bidwell, E. (1955a). *Brit. J. Haemat. 1,* 35.

Bidwell, E. (1955b). *Brit. J. Haemat. 1,* 386.

Blombäck, B. (1964). *In* "The Hemophilias" (K. M. Brinkhous, ed.), pp. 118—128. University of North Carolina Press, Chapel Hill, N. C.

Blombäck, M. (1958). *Arkiv Kemi 12,* 387.

Brinkhous, K. M., and Wagner, R. H. (1959). *Proc. 4th Intern. Congr. Biochem., Vienna 1958,* Vol. 10, pp. 1—12. Pergamon, New York.

Brinkhous, K. M., Shanbrom, E., Roberts, H. R., Webster, W. P., Fekete, L., and Wagner, R. H. (1968). *Am. Med. Assoc. J. 205,* 613.

Brown, D. L., Hardisty, R. M., Kosoy, M. H., and Bracken, C. (1967). *Brit. med. J. 1,* 79.

Cohn, E. J., Strong, L. E., Hughes, W. L., Mulford, D. J., Achworth, J. N., Melin, M., and Taylor, H. L. (1946). *J. Am. Chem. Soc. 68,* 459.

Hershgold, E. J., Pool, J. G., and Pappenhagen, A. R. (1966). *J. Lab. Clin. Med. 67,* 23.

Holman, S. A., and Wolf, P. (1963). *Lancet II,* 4.

Hurt, J. P., Wagner, R. H., and Brinkhous, K. M. (1966a). *Thromb. Diath. Haemorrhag. 15,* 327.

Hurt, J. P., Wagner, R. H., and Brinkhous, K. M. (1966b). *Federation Proc. 25,* 317.

Janiak, A., and Soulier, J. P. (1962). *Thromb. Diath. Haemorrhag. 8,* 406.

Johnson, A. J. (1967). *Blood 30,* 855.

Johnson, A. J. (1968). *Bibl. Haemat. 29,* 1109.

Johnson, A. J., Newman, J., Howell, M. B., and Puszkin, S. (1967). *Thromb. Diath. Haemorrhag. Suppl. 26,* 377.

Kalinke, H., and Egli, H. (1967). *Thromb. Diath. Haemorrhag. 18,* 389.

Kekwick, R. A., and Walton, P. L. (1962). *Nature 194,* 878.

Kekwick, R. A., and Wolf, P. (1957). *Lancet I,* 647.

Loeb, J. (1959). *Path. Biol. 7,* 2449.

Lorand, L., and Laki, K. (1954). *Biochim. Biophys. Acta 13,* 448.

Mammen, E. F. (1963). *Vox. Sang. 8,* 474.

Michael, S. E., and Tunnah, G. W. (1963). *Brit. J. Haemat. 9,* 236.

Michael, S. E., and Tunnah, G. W. (1966). *Brit. J. Haemat. 12,* 115.

Niemetz, J., Weilland, E., and Soulier, J. P. (1961). *Nouv. Rev. Franc. Hémat. 1,* 880.

Patek, A. J., and Stetson, R. P. (1936). *J. Clin. Invest. 15,* 531.

Patek, A. J., and Taylor, F. H. L. (1937). *J. Clin. Invest. 16,* 133.

Pohle, F. J., and Taylor, F. H. L. (1937). *J. Clin. Invest. 16,* 741.

Pool, J. G., and Shannon, A. E. (1965). *Federation Proc. 24,* 512.

Pool, J. G., Hershgold, E. J., and Pappenhagen, A. R. (1964). *Nature 203,* 312.

Schwick, H. G. (1967). *Blut 16,* 150.

Seegers, W. H., Landaburu, R. H., and Fenichel, R. L. (1957). *Am. J. Physiol. 190,* 1.

Seegers, W. H., Mammen, E. F., Lee, J. M., Landaburu, R. H., Cho, M. H., Baker, W. R., and Shepard, R. S. (1959). *In* "Hemophilia and other hemorrhagic states" (K. M. Brinkhous, ed.), pp. 38—46. University of North Carolina Press, Chapel Hill, N. C.

Simonetti, C., Casillas, G., and Pavlovsky, A. (1961). *Hémostase 1,* 57.

Simonetti, C., Casillas, G., and Pavlovsky, A. (1964). *In* "The Hemophilias" (K. M. Brinkhous, ed.), pp. 100—105. University of North Carolina Press, Chapel Hill, N. C.

Simson, L. R., Oberman, H. A., Penner, J. A., Lien, M. M., and Warner, E. L. (1966). *Am. J. Clin. Path. 45,* 373.

Soulier, J. P. (1959). *Path. Biol. 7,* 2451.

Surgenor, D. M. (1964). *In* "The Hemophilias" (K. M. Brinkhous, ed.), pp. 71—80. University of North Carolina Press, Chapel Hill, N. C.

van Creveld, S., Veder, H. A., Pascha, C. N., and Kroeze, W. H. (1959a). *Thromb. Diath. Haemorrhag. 3,* 572.

van Crefeld, S., Veder, H. A., and Pascha, C. N. (1959b) *Thromb. Diath. Haemorrhag. 4,* 211.

van Creveld, S., Pascha, C. N., and Veder, H. A. (1961). *Thromb. Diath. Haemorrhag. 6,* 282.

van Creveld, S., Mochtar, I. A., and Pascha, C. N. (1966). *Thromb. Diath. Haemorrhag. 15,* 338.

Veder, H. A. (1966). *Thromb. Diath. Haemorrhag. 16,* 738.

Wagner, R. H., McLester, W. D., Smith, M., and Brinkhous, K. M. (1964a). *Thromb. Diath. Haemorrhag. 11,* 64.

Wagner, R. H., Smith, M., and McLester, W. D. (1964b). *In* "The Hemophilias" (K. M. Brinkhous, ed.), pp. 81—86. University of North Carolina Press, Chapel Hill, N. C.

Weiss, H. J. (1965). *Thromb. Diath. Haemorrhag. 14,* 32.

Purification of Factor VII and Factor IX

GENESIO MURANO

I. Introduction

Several coagulation defects have been described in the literature. Factor VII and factor IX have been categorized as two proteins essential in the normal coagulation process. Apparently, in the event of a congenital aberration in the protein synthetic mechanism, two disease states known as "factor VII" and "factor IX deficiencies" respectively, are the result.

Factor VII was first described by Alexander et al. (1951), when it was noted that normal plasma corrected the abnormal coagulation tests of the plasma of a patient with a clotting defect which had not been recognized before. Similarly, after the observation by Pavlovski (1947) that the plasma of two patients with hemophilia clotted in a shorter time when mixed, as compared to each one separately, three groups of investigators in 1952 described a new type of hemophilia now known as hemophilia B, Christmas disease or PTC deficiency (Aggeler et al. 1952; Biggs et al. 1952; Schulman and Smith, 1952). The plasma was said to be lacking in a previously unrecognized coagulation factor, which was later named factor IX.

Several attempts at the purification of factor VII have been made to date (Williams and Norris, 1956; Soulier, 1962; Prydz, 1964, 1965; Osborn, 1965; Shaw et al. 1966; Deutsch et al. 1966; Tishkoff et al. 1968; Hogenauer et al. 1968).

Likewise, fractions containing factor IX activity have been prepared by Aggeler et al. (1954a, 1954b), Biggs et al. (1961), Yin and Duckert (1961), Bidwell (1962), Schiffman et al. (1963) and Bidwell et al. (1967).

It is to be noted that in all preparations of factor IX concentrates, significant amounts of prothrombin, factor VII and factor X are present.

Elaborate biophysical characterization of both factor VII and factor IX await further investigation.

II. Factor VII - Methods of Purification

A. Preparation of Factor VII – Method of Prydz (1964)

This procedure consists of adsorption of human serum on barium sulfate, elution with trisodium citrate, and chromatography on Sephadex and DEAE-Sephadex.

1. Procedure

a. Preparation of human serum:

1. Human serum is obtained from healthy, fasting donors, by letting the blood clot spontaneously for 4–5 hours at ambient temperature.

2. The clotted blood is centrifuged at 1,500 g for 30 min at 4° C.

3. The serum is suctioned off and stored at –22° C until ready for use.

b. Adsorption on barium sulfate:

1. To the serum are added the following: One-tenth volume of 0.1 M potassium oxalate and barium sulfate (100 mg/ml) at 2–3° C.

2. The mixture is stirred for 45 min and centrifuged for 30 min at 2,000 g.

3. The sediment is washed 3 times by resuspension with 0.15 M saline (0.2 volume).

c. Chromatography on Sephadex G-25:

1. Two or three grams of the washed barium sulfate-protein complex are mixed with 100 ml of Sephadex G-25 medium in 0.15 M saline. (This gel is suspended in 0.15 M saline the day before use).

2. The mixture is stirred until the barium sulfate-protein complex is homogeneously suspended.

3. The entire suspension is poured on top of a 3–4 cm bed of Sephadex G-25 in a column.

4. The barium sulfate-gel mixture is allowed to settle overnight at 2° C.

5. The column is washed with 0.15 M saline until no ultraviolet absorbing material is dedected.

6. A linear gradient of increasing trisodium citrate concentration is applied. The mixing bottle contains 500 ml of 0.15 M saline and the reservoir contains 500 ml of a 0.3 M sodium citrate solution, pH 7.5.

7. The eluent is collected in 4–6 ml fractions. The flow rate is adjusted at about 5 ml per hour.

The elution profile shows a major peak with a prolonged sloughing shoulder. The factor VII activity resides in this shoulder (citrate concentration level between 0.06 M and 0.13 M).

d. Dialysis:

The fractions containing peak activity are pooled and dialyzed against the appropriate buffer.

e. Chromatography on DEAE-Sephadex:

1. DEAE-Sephadex A-50 medium (capacity 3.9 meq/gram) is suspended in double glass-distilled water, washed successively with 0.5 N HCl, distilled water, 0.5 N NaOH, distilled water, 0.01 M NaH_2PO_4, and finally with 0.01 M sodium phosphate buffer at pH 8.0.

2. A column of this equilibrated adsorbant is prepared.

3. The dialyzed protein is applied to the column and allowed to adsorb.

4. The column is washed with 400 ml of 0.01 M sodium phosphate buffer at pH 8.0.

5. The protein is eluted by applying a linear gradient of increasing sodium chloride concentration. The mixing bottle contains 500 ml of 0.01 M sodium phosphate pH 8.0 buffer, and the reservoir, 500 ml of a 0.4 M sodium chloride solution in the same buffer.

6. The eluate is collected in 5–8 ml fractions at a flow rate of 15–30 ml per hour. The factor VII activity resides uniquely in fractions 85–100. Interestingly, factor IX, with traces of factor X and prothrombin activity, appear in fractions 100–120.

f. Concentration of the eluate:

1. The peak containing factor VII activity is dialyzed against a mixture of one volume of 0.1 M potassium oxalate and ten volumes of 0.15 M saline.

2. The eluate is treated with barium sulfate (10 mg/ml) to adsorb the protein.

3. The complex is washed 3 times with saline and the protein eluted in 0.1 volume of 0.5 M sodium citrate pH 7.5, at ambient temperature.

2. Evaluation

The product obtained from Sephadex G-25 represents a five fold purification over plasma, with a 95 % yield. The product obtained after chromatography on DEAE-Sephadex is found to be free of factor IX and factor X activity (Pryzd, 1963). The final recovery is about 50 % of the original serum factor VII activity. The specific activity ranges from 5,000 to 18,000 units/mg protein, representing a 500 to 1,300 fold purification over plasma.

B. Preparation of Factor VII-X Complex – Method of Shaw et al. (1966)

This procedure utilizes preparative electrophoresis with a polyvinyl chloride block to separate factor X from factor VII-X complex.

1. Procedure

a. Preparation of factor VII-X concentrate:

1. Fresh human serum (50 ml) is obtained from pooled blood of healthy donors. The blood is allowed to clot overnight at ambient temperature and the serum separated.
2. Barium sulfate powder (A. R.) is washed with water, to remove fine particles and dried at 120° C.
3. The VII-X complex is adsorbed from the serum by shaking 50 ml serum for 15 min with 5 gm of the washed barium sulfate, in a capped bottle.
4. The mixture is centrifuged for 10 min at 3,000 rpm. The supernatant is discarded.
5. The sediment is washed twice with 0.9 % saline.
6. The VII-X complex is eluted from the barium sulfate by shaking for 1 hour with 10 ml of 3.8 % trisodium citrate.
7. The suspension is centrifuged. The sediment is discarded.
8. The supernatant (containing VII-X complex) is concentrated to one tenth its volume by pressure dialysis in Visking tubing at 4° C against borate-phosphate buffer pH 8.5, ionic strength = 0.05, containing 2.34 gm $NaH_2PO_4 \cdot 2H_2O$ and 4.29 gm $Na_2B_4O_7 \cdot 10\,H_2O$/liter (Gedin and Porath, 1957).

b. Preparative electrophoresis:

1. Polyvinyl chloride powder (Stockholm Superfosfat Fabrik A. B. as Pevikon) is washed with 0.9 % saline and equilibrated to pH 8.5 with the borate-phosphate buffer.
2. A slurry of polyvinyl chloride (P. V. C) powder in buffer is poured into a Perspex former on glass to make a block 25×20×1 cm.
3. Electrical contact along each end of the block is made with layers of cellulose sponge (Wettex cloths). Each cellulose wick dips into a buffer reservoir which is connected to the electrode vessel with another cellulose wick.

The reservoir buffer is the same as that in the P. V. C. block.
4. The concentrated eluate from dialysis (1–2 ml) is applied as a line across the block, 3 cm from the cathode (bromophenyl blue may be used as a marker).
5. The block is covered with a sheet of parafilm, and electrophoresis carried out for 20 hours at 4° C (40–50 mA, 8 V/cm length).

c. Recovery of sample:
1. The block is cut transversely in 1 cm segments.
2. The P. V. C. is removed from each segment by vacuum filtration on a glass sinter.
3. The activity of factor VII-X complex and factor X alone are estimated in each segment.

2. Evaluation

A reasonably well defined separation of factor X from factor VII-X complex is obtained. Maximal factor VII activity is usually found in fractions 7, 8, and 9 about 12 cm from the origin. The recovery is about 50 %. The authors do not present any data on the full corrective activity of the VII-X complex.

C. Preparation of Factor VII – Method of Tishkoff et al. (1968)

Factor VII is isolated from "prothrombin complex", by two successive chromatographies on DEAE-Sephadex. Details concerning the technology up to the first chromatography can be obtained from the preparative procedure for prethrombin, "modified zymogen" (p. 120). Further purification of factor VII is obtained by a second chromatography on DEAE-Sephadex.

1. Procedure

a. Pooling of fractions:
1. Fractions D, E, and F, obtained from the first chromatography, constitute about 23 % of the total applied protein. They are pooled and concentrated by ultrafiltration as described under the preparation of "modified zymogen" (p. 120) (Tishkoff et al. 1968).
2. The concentrated material from three runs is diluted to a volume of about 8 ml in 0.05 M phosphate buffer, pH 5.92.

b. Rechromatography on DEAE-Sephadex:
1. About 18 mg of protein are applied to the column. Conditions for this second chromatography are exactly the same as for the first one described under "modified zymogen" (p. 120) (Tishkoff et al. 1968).
2. The protein profile indicates a discrete separation of factors VII and X. Activity measurements indicate that factor VII is eluted at about tube 160, while factor X is eluted at tube 190.
For physical analysis, the authors have combined only those fractions displaying peak activity.

2. Evaluation

This fraction is relatively free of factor X activity. It is inert in 25 % sodium citrate. It constitutes about 8 % of the total protein. In the ultracentrifuge, factor VII is homogeneous in the presence of dissociating agents.

III. Factor IX-Methods of Purification

A. Preparation of Factor IX – Method of Yin and Duckert (1961)

In this technique, principles of adsorption, heating, and salting out are employed for the preparation of factor IX.

1. Procedure

a. $BaSO_4$ adsorption:
1. Normal oxalated plasma or serum (1 part Na-oxalate, M/10, to 9 parts whole blood or serum) is allowed to age for at least 1 week at 1° C.
2. $BaSO_4$ (5 gm/200 ml) is added and the slurry is stirred at ambient temperature for 30 min.
3. The sediment is removed by centrifugation at 1,500 g for 15 min and discarded (prothrombin, factor VII, and factor X are adsorbed on the $BaSO_4$).
4. The supernatant is heated in a water bath at 56° C for 30 min.
5. After heating, the solution is rapidly cooled under tap water.

b. $(NH_4)_2SO_4$ precipitation:

1. To the cooled solution, $(NH_4)_2SO_4$ (saturated at room temperature pH 5.3–5.4) is added to 30 % saturation.
2. The slurry is allowed to stand at room temperature for 10 min, then it is centrifuged for 20 min at 1,500 g. The supernatant is discarded.
3. The precipitate is solubilized in one half the original plasma (or serum) volume of saline-buffer (3 volumes 0.9 % NaCl added to 1 volume of veronal-acetate buffer pH 7.35).
4. The solution is again treated with $(NH_4)_2SO_4$ to 40 % saturation.
5. The sediment is collected by centrifugation at 1,500 g for 25 min. The supernatant is discarded.
6. The precipitate is suspended in $^1/_3$ the original plasma (or serum) volume of the saline-veronal buffer described above.

c. Dialysis:

1. The solution is first dialyzed against running tap water for 4 hours, then against distilled water at 1° C for 48 hours.
2. A whitish precipitate (insoluble in water) is formed in the membrane.
3. The precipitate is collected by centrifugation at 1,200 g for 10 min, and dissolved in saline-veronal buffer ($^1/_5$ starting plasma or serum volume).
4. The solution is further dialyzed for 24 hours at 1° C against the same saline-veronal buffer.
5. At the end of dialysis, the solution is centrifuged at 1,000 g for 5 min. The supernatant is stored in glass tubes at –25° C.

This fraction constitutes the "clot promoting euglobulin" (CPE).

d. Celite adsorption:

1. The CPE solution is treated with Celite powder (Filter-Cel grade, Johns-Manville, Calif.) (50–75 mg/ml) at room temperature for 20 min, with continuous stirring.
2. The suspension is centrifuged for 3 min at 1,200 g.
3. The supernatant, containing factor IX is carefully pipetted into another test tube.
4. The centrifugation procedure is repeated 2 more times for 2 min at 1,200 g. This insures that all celite particles are removed.
5. The supernatant is examined under the microscope to insure complete removal of celite; it is then frozen at –25° C in siliconized tubes. It may be noted that Hageman factor activity may be eluted from the celite since this factor has a strong affinity for the reagent.

2. Evaluation

This fraction shortens the recalcification time of hemophilia B plasma to normal range. It does not effect the recalcification time or prothrombin consumption in normal plasma. The CPE fraction, prior to removal of Hageman factor with celite, retains its activity for over 1 year at –25° C. At 62° C, it is destroyed after 20 min. The authors provide no physical analysis for this protein.

B. Preparation of Factor IX – Method of Bidwell et al. (1967)

The purpose of this procedure is to obtain a concentrate of factor IX for therapeutic application. The concentrate contains considerable quantities of factors VII and X. One advantage of the technique is that from the same batch of plasma, both factor VIII and factor IX can be obtained.

1. Procedure

a. Preparation of fraction I–0 (Blombäck, 1958):

The preparation of this fraction is described in the factor VIII chapter (p. 140).

b. Preparation of "precipitate P":

1. The supernatant is brought to pH 5.85 ± 0.05, 19 % ethanol and –5° C.
2. Equilibration is carried out overnight at –5° C. To minimize handling losses, the precipitate is collected in plastic bags.
3. The sediment is collected by placing the plastic bags directly into metal buckets and centrifuged, at 1,800 g in a MSE Mistral 6L centrifuge. (This precipitate can be stored in the plastic bags at –40° C for several weeks and may be pooled if large scale purification is attempted).
4. The precipitate is washed with one half the original plasma volume of 20 % ethanol at –5° C.

5. The washed precipitate at this point is treated in a manner analogous to that used by Kekwick and MacKay (1954) for the precipitation of the globulins G_2. The precipitant, however, is ethanol instead of ether. The final conditions are as follows:

$$\mu = 0.01$$
$$\text{ethanol} = 10\text{–}12\,\%$$
$$\text{pH} = 5.2$$
$$\text{temperature} = -3^\circ\ \text{C}$$

6. The material is allowed to equilibrate overnight at –2.5° C.
7. The precipitate is collected by high speed centrifugation. The average yield is about 52 gm/liter of ACD plasma. This is "precipitate P".

c. Extraction of factor IX (Bidwell and Dike, 1966):

1. The "precipitate P" (or G_2 precipitate of Kekwick and MacKay, 1954) is suspended in one tenth the original plasma volume of ice cold saline. Stirring is facilitated by employing a Silverson Laboratory mixer.
2. The suspension is neutralized to pH 7.0–7.2 by dropwise addition of 10% w/v $NaHCO_3$.
3. The neutralized suspension is brought to ambient temperature (18–25° C).
4. Tricalcium phosphate (J. T. Baker, exclusively) is made into a thick slurry with water, and then added to the stirring suspension (5 gm/liter). Stirring is continued for 10 min. Factor IX adsorbs.
5. The adsorbent is recovered by centrifugation at 1,000 g for 1 min at 0° C.
6. The supernatant, together with the "sloppy" layer on top of the tricalcium phosphate is discarded.
7. The precipitate is washed (several times) with physiologic saline at 0° C (volume equal to original suspension) and again collected by centrifugation at 1,000 g for 1 min at 0° C.
8. The active fraction is eluted from the adsorbant by stirring the washed precipitate in one fifth the original suspension volume of 0.1 M trisodium citrate at ambient temperature.
9. The pH of the suspension at this point is about 8.0–8.3. The precipitate is removed by centrifugation (not less than 2,000 g for 20 min).
10. To the supernatant, heparin is added (1 unit/ml). This prevents the development of undesirable coagulant activity.

d. Removal of citrate and clarification:

1. The eluate is cooled to 0° C.
2. One third its volume of diethyl ether, cooled to –30° C is added.
3. With vigorous shaking, the mixture is frozen in a bath of acetone and solid CO_2.
4. The temperature of the frozen mass must fall to –30° C or lower. If required, this material may be stored at –40° C for several days.
5. Thawing is accomplished with running tap water, care being taken that the temperature not rise above 0° C.
6. Excess ether and denatured lipoproteins are removed by centrifugation at 0° C for 20 min at 1,000 g.
7. The organic phase (supernatant) is discarded. The aqueous subnatant is shaken again with one fifth its volume of cold ether but it is not frozen.
8. The organic phase (supernatant) is once again removed by centrifugation as in step 6.
9. The aqueous solution is dialyzed overnight at 2–4° C against 20 volumes of citrate-saline (0.38% w/v, trisodium citrate · $2H_2O$; 0.76% sodium chloride).
10. Nitrogen (O_2-free) is bubbled through the solution (1 liter/min) to facilitate stirring, and removal of excess ether.

e. Sterilization:

The solution is filtered successively through membranes, made by Millipore Filter Co., (Bedford, Mass., U.S.A.). In order of use, they are: Glass Pre-filter, R. A., H. A., and G. S. The pore size of the latter is $0.22 \pm 0.02\ \mu$. Alternatively, membranes manufactured by Membranfiltergesellschaft, Göttingen (Germany) and "Pasteur" type porcelain filter candles (Doulton Industrial Porcelain, Wilne Cote, Tamworth, Staffs., England) may be used. Seitz filtration is not used since the active fraction is adsorbed.

f. Preparation for clinical use:

1. The sterilized solution is sampled for sterility testing, assay, and general toxicity (Bidwell and Dike, 1966).

2. The solution is distributed in suitable amounts (50–150 ml) in blood bottles, shell frozen, and lyophilized.
To avoid denaturation, the temperature is kept at –30° C or below during the primary steps of lyophilization.
3. The dry material is stored in an atmosphere of dry nitrogen at 20° C.
4. For reconstitution, distilled water (sterile) is added. (Volume is equal to the volume from which the material was dried). The material dissolves immediately.

2. Evaluation

The lyophilized material (step *f*-3) is stable for at least two years. Routine preparations yield a product with a 200–300 fold purification. The authors present no physical data regarding the degree of heterogeneity in the preparation. Bidwell and Dike (1966) point out that factor II and factor X, when present in excessive quantities, may assay as factor IX activity.

IV. Discussion

Since the specific activity of all preparations of factors VII and IX are not reported by all authors, it is difficult to compare products. Both factors have rendered the task of their isolation a rather laborious and painstaking undertaking. The inability to obtain one factor free of another factor has perpetuated great frustration. It appears that when one deals with "factor VII", "factor X" tends to be isolated simultaneously and vice versa. When dealing with "factor IX", prothrombin tends to be isolated simultaneously and vice versa.
Of course, this ambivalence is not a rigid one, but it does occur and it must be logically explained.
Judging from the present data, the factor "VII-X complex" is probably analogous to the autoprothrombin III of Seegers et al. (1964) and Seegers and Marciniak (1965) ("factor X" section, p. 153).
Moreover, factor VII and factor X may be in reality one and the same protein – one being a structural variant of the other. In plasma, they exist in complex. As pointed out by Högenauer et al. (1968), the chemical similarities between "factor VII" and "factor X" are striking.
Similarly, factor IX may be a structural variant of prothrombin. In other words, "factor IX" deficiency may represent none other than a deadlock in one of the prothrombin activation pathways.
A detailed assessment of the aforementioned hypotheses is presently being made.

References

Aggeler, P. M., White, S. G., Glendening, M. B., Page, E. W., Leake, T. B., and Bates, G. (1952). *Proc. Soc. Exptl. Biol. Med. 79,* 692.
Aggeler, P. M., Spaet, T. H., and Emery, B. E. (1954a). *Science 119,* 806.
Aggeler, P. M., Spaet, T. H., White, S. G., Fowell, A. H., and Johnson, F. H. (1954b). *Rev. Hematol. 9,* 447.
Alexander, B., Goldstein, R., Landwehr, G., and Cook, C. D. (1951). *J. Clin. Invest. 30,* 596.
Bidwell, E. (1962). *Thromb. Diath. Haemorrhag. Suppl. 7,* 205.
Bidwell, E., and Dike, G. W. R. (1966). *In* "Treatment of Haemophilia and Other Coagulation Disorders" R. Biggs and R. G. MacFarlane, Eds.), pp. 43—69. Blackwell, Oxford.
Bidwell, W., Booth, J. M., Dike, G. W. R., and Denson, K. W. E. (1967). *Brit. J. Haematol. 13,* 568.
Biggs, R., Douglas, A. S., MacFarlane, R. G., Dacie, J. V., Pitney, W. R., Merskey, C., and O'Brien, J. R. (1952). *Brit. Med. J. 2,* 1378.
Biggs, R., Bidwell, E., Handley, D. A., MacFarlane, R. G., Trueta, J., Elliot-Smith, A., Dike, G. W. R. and Ash, B. J (1961). *Brit. J. Haematol. 7,* 349.
Blombäck, M. (1958). *Arkiv Kemi 12,* 387.
Deutsch, E., Lechner, K., and Schmer, G. (1966). *Thromb. Diath Haemorrhag. Suppl. 20,* 275.
Gedin, H. I., and Porath, J. (1957). *Biochem. Biophys. Acta 26,* 159.
Högenauer, E., Lechner, K., and Deutsch, E. (1968). *Thromb. Diath. Haemorrhag. 19,* 304.
Kekwick, R. A., and MacKay, M. E. (1954). *Medical Research Council Special Report Series,* No. 286. H. M. Stationary Office, London.
Osborn, E. C. (1965). *Clin. Chim. Acta 12,* 415.
Pavlovski, A. (1947). *Blood 2,* 185.
Prydz, H. (1963). *Scand. J. Clin. Lab. Invest. 15,* 450.
Prydz, H. (1964). *Scand. J. Clin. Lab. Invest. 16,* 101.
Prydz, H. (1965). *Scand. J. Clin. Lab. Invest. 17,* 78.
Schiffman, S., Rapoport, S. I., and Patch, M. J. (1963). *Blood 22,* 733.
Schulman, I., and Smith, C. H. (1952). *Blood 7,* 794.
Seegers, W. H., and Marciniak, E. (1965). *Life Sci. 4,* 1721.
Seegers, W. H., Cole, E. R., Aoki, N., and Harmison, C. R. (1964). *Can. J. Biochem. 42,* 229.
Shaw, S., Pegrum, G. D., Farthing, C. P., and Wolff, S. (1966) *Thromb. Diath. Haemorrhag. 15,* 294.
Soulier, J. P. (1962). *Nouv. Rev. franc. hematol. 2,* 27.
Tishkoff, G. H., Williams, L. C., and Brown, D. M. (1968). *J. Biol. Chem. 243,* 4151.
Williams, W. J., and Norris, D. G. (1956). *J. Biol. Chem. 241,* 1847.
Yin, E. T., and Duckert, F. (1961). *Thromb. Diath. Haemorrhag. 6,* 215.

Purification of Factor X (Autoprothrombin III-C)

Genesio Murano

I. Introduction

A plasma component necessary for the conversion of prothrombin to thrombin was first described by Hougie et al. (1957). It was designated as *factor X*. Milstone (1960a, b) described another potent procoagulant *thrombokinase* (Milstone, 1962; Milstone et al. 1963) and the term *autoprothrombin C* was introduced when it was noted that thrombin products differed in their ability to promote prothrombin consumption in hemophilic plasma (Kowarzyk and Marciniak, 1961; Marciniak, 1961).

Subsequently, several investigators (Ferguson et al. 1960; Pechet and Alexander, 1960; MacFarlane, 1961; Straub and Duckert, 1961; Esnouf and Williams, 1962) established that factor X can be activated by several physiologic and nonphysiologic agents prior to its participation in the prothrombin activation cycle. Once in the active form, it functions synergistically with factor V, lipids and calcium ions.

Seegers et al. (1962) postulated a precursor to autoprothrombin C and termed it *autoprothrombin* III. Fractions containing autoprothrombin III were obtained from bovine serum (Marciniak et al. 1962) and Seegers et al. (1964) were able to obtain autoprothrombin III from prothrombin preparations.

The activation characteristics of autoprothrombin III to autoprothrombin C as well as other modes of preparations have been described (Marciniak and Seegers, 1965; Seegers and Marciniak, 1965; Seegers et al. 1965).

This work, in conjunction with that of Seegers et al. (1963); Milstone (1964), Spaet (1964), Seegers et al. (1967), Seegers and Marciniak (1962), Marciniak and Seegers (1965), Kline (1965) and Lechner and Deutsch (1965) establishes with reasonable certainty, that activated factor X, thrombokinase and autoprothrombin C are analogous.

II. Methods of Preparation

A. Bovine Autoprothrombin C – Method of Seegers et al. (1966)

Purified prothrombin, prepared by the method of Seegers (1952), activated in strong salt solutions yields thrombin and autoprothrombin C. The activation is generated autocatalytically in ammonium sulfate. Autoprothrombin C is isolated from the activation mixture by salt and acetone fractionation, followed by chromatography on DEAE-cellulose.

1. Procedure

a. Prothrombin Activation: About 300,000 to 500,000 units of prothrombin (Seegers, 1952) with an average specific activity of 20,000 units/mg of tyrosine, are dissolved in 20–30 ml of 0.9 % saline buffered with imidazole at pH 7.1 to 7.2. The final prothrombin concentration should be 10,000 to 15,000 units/ml.

Crystalline ammonium sulfate is added rapidly with stirring. The final concentration is 300 mg/ml. (A slight precipitate may result and remain during the activation. This does not appear to influence the activation). As soon as all the salt is in solution, the pH is checked. It is usually necessary to readjust to 7.1 by adding a few drops of 1 M HCl.

The activation mixture is primed by adding purified thrombin (10 units/1000 units of prothrombin). The mixture is incubated at 28° C for 18–20 hours. At the end of this period, the mixture is assayed for thrombin and autoprothrombin C activity. Both activities develop simultaneously. The thrombin yield is about 75 to 100 % of the total thrombin potential. The autoprothrombin C yield is 15 to 20 units/100 units of prothrombin.

b. Ammonium Sulfate and Acetone Fractionation: The volume of the mixture is measured. The mixture is cooled to 0° C, in ice, and crystalline ammonium sulfate is added to a final concentration of 500 mg/ml. N.B.: It must be recalled that the mixture already contains $(NH_4)_2SO_4$ (300 mg/ml). The precipitate is collected by centrifugation in the cold at 3,800 g for 45 min. The supernatant is discarded. With the tube in an inverted position a gentle stream of cold distilled water is directed along the sides of the tube cautiously rinsing out the inner surface without touching the precipitate.

The precipitate is dissolved in 30 ml of cold (4° C) distilled water. An equal volume of dry cold acetone adjusted to pH 7.0 (–80° C) is added and stirred with a glass rod. The precipitate is recovered by centrifugation in the cold at 3,800 g for 5 min.

The supernatant is discarded. The precipitate is stirred with a glass rod and the remaining acetone is removed by hand warming the tube in front of an air flow. This process is continued until no acetone odor is detectable. The precipitate is next dissolved in a minimum volume of sodium phosphate buffer (0.05 M, pH 7.0). A clear solution is usually obtained.

c. Chromatography on DEAE-cellulose: Ten grams of DEAE-cellulose (Carl Schleicher and Schuell Co., Selectacel No. 70, Standard) are washed with 0.05 M pH 7.0 sodium phosphate buffer, using a mechanical stirrer. The process is continued until the cellulose is equilibrated at pH 7.0, allowed to settle and as much buffer as possible is decanted.

The activation mixture is added to the cellulose and stirred gently for 10 min. The protein-DEAE mixture is poured into a glass column, 2.5 cm in diameter, and allowed to settle. (Since thrombin does not adsorb under such conditions, it will appear immediately in the effluent. It may be saved in the cold and later fractionated with ammonium sulfate and acetone.) The column is packed with air pressure. Sodium phosphate buffer (0.05 M, pH 7.0) is applied and allowed to elute all the thrombin. When the thrombin titer in the eluate drops to less than 1 thrombin unit per ml, 0.1 M pH 7.88 sodium phosphate buffer is applied. The fraction eluted with this buffer is discarded.

Next, sodium phosphate buffer 0.4 M, pH 8.2 is applied. This buffer elutes autoprothrombin C.

d. Ammonium Sulfate and Acetone Fractionation: The peak tubes, as determined by tyrosine determination (Folin and Ciocalteau, 1927) are pooled, and cooled to 0° C. Phosphate crystals will appear. They may be removed by centrifugation. The volume of the sample is determined. Ammonium sulfate is added as rapidly as possible to a final concentration of 500 mg/ml. Vigorous stirring will aid in the solubilization of the ammonium sulfate. The precipitate is collected by centrifugation at 3,800 g for 45 min at 0° C.

The supernatant is discarded. With the tube in an inverted position, a gentle stream of cold distilled water serves to rinse the sides of the tubes, without disturbing the precipitate. The precipitate is dissolved in 20–30 ml of cold distilled water. An equal volume of dry acetone (–80° C) is added and a slight precipitate will be evident. The suspension is centrifuged at 3,800 g for 5 min. The supernatant is discarded. The remaining acetone is evaporated as previously described.

The precipitate is dissolved in 2–3 ml of 0.9 % NaCl solution buffered with imidazole at pH 7.0–7.2. An equal volume of glycerol is added for stability purposes, and the sample may be stored at –20° C.

The activity is determined by the method of Cole et al. (1962).

2. Evaluation

Physical analysis indicates that this fraction is relatively homogeneous. The average specific activity is 4,500 units per mg of protein or 67,000 units per mg of tyrosine. The average yield is near 1 mg per liter of plasma. It is difficult to appreciate the potency of this enzyme. In experiments performed by Seegers et al. (1966), it was established that one mg of autoprothrombin C can shorten the clotting time of about 30 liters of plasma from 150 seconds to 15 seconds under specified conditions.

B. Bovine Autoprothrombin III – Method of Seegers et al. (1964)

The zymogen autoprothrombin III, the immediate precursor of autoprothrombin C, may be isolated from prothrombin activation mixtures according to Seegers et al. (1964) or Seegers and Marciniak (1965). Various properties of this protein are described by Marciniak and Seegers (1965), and Seegers et al. (1965).

1. Procedure

About 200,000 units of prothrombin (Seegers, 1952) are diluted with imidazole-buffered saline, at pH 7.2, to a final concentration of 5,000 units/ml.
The following reagents are added:
$CaCl_2$ solution (0.025 M, final concentration), Ac-globulin (Aoki et al. 1963) (375 units/ml, final concentration),
Thrombin (Seegers et al. 1958) (100 units/ml, final concentration),
Crude Cephalin (2.1 mg/ml, final concentration).
The activation flask is incubated at 28° C. The activation is monitored by thrombin assays every 15–20 minutes. If the full titer of thrombin does not develop after two hours of incubation, additional Ac-globulin (80 units/ml of reaction mixture) will aid in the activation.
When the reaction is complete, the isolation procedure for autoprothrombin III is analogous to that of autoprothrombin C previously described (Seegers et al. 1966).

2. Evaluation

The physical properties of autoprothrombin III closely correspond to those of autoprothrombin C. In sodium citrate solution, the zymogen will not activate to the enzyme but it will readily do so with trypsin, Russell's Viper Venom, or tissue extracts and calcium ions. To assay for autoprothrombin III, it is necessary to first convert it to autoprothrombin C (Cole et al. 1962; Marciniak and Seegers, 1965; Reno and Seegers, 1967) and then test its activity either on purified prothrombin or plasma.

C. Bovine Autoprothrombin III – Method of Seegers and Marciniak (1965)

1. Procedure

a. Activation: About 250,000 units of purified prothrombin (Seegers, 1952) are diluted 1:2 in 0.025 M sodium phosphate buffer at pH 7.0. Purified thrombin is added to a final concentration of 45 units/1000 units of prothrombin and the mixture is incubated at 28° C for 90 min. The disappearance of prothrombin may be monitored by the two stage analytical procedure of Ware and Seegers (1949).

b. Chromatography: A column of DEAE-cellulose (40×1 cm) is equilibrated with 0.025 M phosphate buffer at pH 7.0. Slight pressure may be applied to aid in the packing of the cellulose. The effluent may be monitored either by tyrosine determination (Folin and Ciocalteau, 1927) or absorbancy at 280 mμ. The flow rate is adjusted to 2 ml/min.
The activation mixture is applied to the column and allowed to enter the cellulose bed. Sodium phosphate buffer (0.05 M, pH 7.0) is applied and a minor protein peak will be eluted.
Next, sodium phosphate buffer (0.075 M, pH 7.2) is applied. Another protein peak is eluted which contains prethrombin activity.
Further elution follows with sodium phosphate buffer (0.175 M, pH 7.4). The protein obtained contains an inhibitor of prothrombin activation (Marciniak et al. 1967).
Lastly, sodium phosphate buffer (0.40 M, pH 8.2) is applied and autoprothrombin III is eluted. This peak represents about 10 % of the total protein applied. The peak tubes are pooled and concentrated by ammonium sulfate and acetone precipitation as previously described (Seegers et al. 1966).

2. Evaluation

Like the fraction obtained by Seegers et al. (1964), this autoprothrombin III will not activate to autoprothrombin C in sodium citrate solutions. The active enzyme, however, is generated rapidly with the use of trypsin, or Russell's Viper Venom, or tissue extracts.

D. Human Factor X – Method of Kahn and Bourgain (1965)

A simplified procedure is described. Serum is subjected to isoelectric precipitation and preparative electrophoresis.

1. Procedure

a. Serum Preparation: Human blood is allowed to clot in a glass tube at room temperature for 24 hours. The clot is removed by centrifugation at 3,000 rpm for 20 min at 4° C.

b. Isoelectric Precipitation: A 24 ml aliquot of serum is diluted into 216 ml of distilled water at 0° C. While stirring the solution, 0.1 M acetic acid is added until a pH of 5.05 ± 0.05 is obtained. Stirring is continued for an additional 5 min. The opalescent solution is centrifuged at 3,500 rpm for 20 min at 0° C. The supernatant is discarded. The whitish precipitate is dissolved in 4 ml of veronal buffer (pH 8.6, ionic strength 0.05). The solution is kept for 20 min at 4° C.

c. Preparative Paper Electrophoresis: Four strips of Whatman 3 MM paper, 34/6 cm are superimposed. (In a Durrum Type cell, 4 sets of the 4 superimposed strips may be submitted to electrophoresis.) The strips are equilibrated for 1 hour, in the cold, with veronal buffer, pH 8.6, ionic strength 0.05. On each set of the four superimposed strips, one ml of the sample is applied transversally, in small portions in the middle. Electrophoresis follows with the following physical parameters: voltage = 190 volts, amperage = 40 m. a., time = 14 hours and temperature = 4° C.

Following electrophoresis, the paper strips are removed and cut transversally at one cm intervals at 3 cm distance on the negative side of the application area, and at 8 cm distance on the positive side. A total of 11 strips, 1 cm wide are obtained from each of the four sets of strips.

The corresponding 1 cm strips of each set are pooled and fixed with the aid of a rubber stopper, in the top of a glass tube. A total of 11 tubes are prepared. The tubes are centrifuged at 4° C at 2,000 rpm for 10 min. The paper strips, fixed at the top of the tube, are removed. About 1 to 1.5 ml solution is obtained in each tube.

A differential analysis by the tissue thromboplastin time and Stypven Time (Kahn and Bourgain, 1965) shows that the factor X activity resides in strip 2 and 3 on the positive side of the application area.

2. Evaluation

When this solution, representing factor X activity, is investigated for factor VII activity, only 1 to 5/100 parts of activity can be demonstrated. The solution does not correct factor IX deficient plasma. Further electrophoretic analysis of this solution demonstrates a homogeneous component migrating with the α_1-globulins. This material is stable for two weeks at 4° C.

E. Bovine Factor X – Method of Papahadjopoulos et al. (1964)

Factor X of bovine plasma is purified by combined $BaSO_4$ adsorption, elution with citrate and subsequent fractionation on DEAE-cellulose, and gel filtration on Sephadex.

1. Procedure

a. Preparation of the Plasma $BaSO_4$ Eluate: Bovine blood is obtained and mixed in plastic containers with 0.1 volume of 0.1 M sodium oxalate solution. The oxalated blood is centrifuged at 3,000 g for 40 min at 4° C. The plasma obtained, usually 2 liters per batch, is mixed with barium sulfate (U.S.P.) (75 mg/ml) and stirred for 30 min at room temperature. The mixture is centrifuged at 1,500 g for 30 min at 4° C. The clear supernatant is decanted and discarded. The solid cake of $BaSO_4$ is suspended in one volume of cold (0° C) 0.45 % NaCl. The suspension is centrifuged at 1,500 g for 30 min at 4° C. The supernatant wash is discarded. The NaCl washing procedure is repeated three times. Most of the yellow color is eliminated during these successive washes.

The $BaSO_4$ cake is next suspended in 0.1 volume of 5 % sodium citrate (pH 5.8). The mixture is stirred mechanically at 0° C for 1 hour. The suspension is centrifuged at 2,000 g for 30 min at 4° C. The supernatant, slightly yellow, is dialyzed for 24 hours against running tap water (10–12° C). The dialysate is centrifuged briefly to eliminate the small amount of white precipitate formed during dialysis and then stored at –20° C. A number of batches may be prepared up to this point and stored for further purification.

Once several batches are obtained, they are thawed, pooled and cleared of a small amount of white precipitate by centrifugation. The resulting clear solution is lyophilized and the white residue maintained in covered plastic containers at –20° C.

b. Chromatography on DEAE-cellulose: DEAE-cellulose (Brown Co. Lot 1272) is washed repeatedly with distilled water and finally with 0.15 M NaCl. The adsorbant is packed into a glass column with the aid of gentle air pressure, obtaining a bed of 2 × 20 cm. The column is equilibrated with distilled water at 4° C.
The lyophilized protein is dissolved in distilled water (100 mg/ml) and approximately 10 ml are applied to the column. A stepwise elution of the protein is accomplished with citrate buffers of increasing molarity from 0.04 to 0.08 M at pH 7.0. The flow rate is maintained near 10 ml per hour and the fraction volume is 10 ml.
Once the sample has entered the column, 0.04 M citrate buffer (pH 7.0) is applied. Prothrombin and factor VII, with trace amounts of factor V and thrombin activity can be assayed in this eluent (about 250 ml).
Next, 0.06 M citrate buffer (pH 7.0) is applied (about 300 ml). It serves to elute the remaining factor VII activity.
Further elution follows with 0.08 M citrate buffer (pH 7.0) and factor X is eluted.
The pooled fraction is frozen and lyophilized and reconstituted to a more concentrated solution in veronal buffer prepared according to Streuli (1959), and stored frozen in siliconized tubes at –20° C.
Under the conditions described, factor IX is not eluted. Duckert et al. (1960) have pointed out that this activity may be recovered at pH 5.8.
The column may be recycled by washing with 0.2 M citrate, and then with distilled water 4° C.

2. Evaluation

The recovery of factor X activity is 40–60 %. Approximately a 10,000 fold purification is achieved from a starting level of 3.6×10^{-3} units of factor X per mg of protein to a final value of 40 units of factor X per mg of protein. One unit is defined as the amount present in one ml of fresh, normal human plasma assayed according to Bachman et al. (1958).
The activity is stable for several months either in the lyophilized state or frozen at –25° C. Spontaneous activation of the frozen sample to active factor X is a common occurence. Filtration on Sephadex G-200 and G-100 results in a single peak. In electrophoresis, a single component is observed, migrating close to the α_1-globulin of whole human serum. Factor X prepared as outlined can be activated to the active form by: active factor X, trypsin, Russell's Viper Venom, 25 % sodium citrate + trypsin activated factor X, 25 % sodium citrate + purified prothrombin, and by 25 % sodium citrate + crude plasma $BaSO_4$ eluate.
In each instance, a change in molecular size and physico-chemical behavior is observed.

F. Bovine Factor X – Method of Lechner and Deutsch (1965)

Two procedures are described by these authors. One method consists of a slight modification of the procedure of Seegers and Landaburu (1960) in the preparation of DEAE chromatographed prothrombin (described in "purification of prothrombin", p. 101).
The second method is a modification of the Esnouf and Williams (1962) procedure.

1. Procedure a

Prothrombin is prepared according to Seegers (1952) and submitted to chromatography on DEAE-cellulose as described by Seegers and Landaburu (1960).
However, the chromatography is carried one step further. Sodium phosphate buffer (0.175 M, pH 7.45) containing 0.2 M NaCl is applied to the column. (Author's note: alternatively, 0.40 M phosphate buffer (pH 8.2) may be used (Marciniak and Seegers, 1965)). With this buffer, a small peak is eluted. The fraction is pooled and dialyzed against distilled water to remove the salt.
This fraction contains factor X activity with only traces of prothrombin activity. Assay according to Cole et al. (1962).

2. Procedure b

a. Preparation of $BaSO_4$ eluate: The methodology is the same as in the Esnouf and Williams (1962) procedure up to the elution of the barium sulfate complex with citrate (see following method).

To avoid activation of factor X in citrate, the latter is quickly removed by gel filtration on a column of Sephadex G-25 medium at 10° C.

The desalted eluate is adjusted to pH 6.0 with 0.1 N HCl and a variable amount of inactive protein precipitates. The precipitate is removed by centrifugation at 4° C at 3,000 rpm. The supernatant is recovered and adjusted to pH 4.8 at 4° C with 0.1 N HCl. The forming precipitate is collected by centrifugation and dissolved in 10 ml of 0.02 M phosphate buffer pH 7.0. The solution is dialyzed against the same buffer for 12 hours at 4° C. At the end of dialysis, the suspension is centrifuged to remove some insoluble protein.

b. Chromatography on DEAE Sephadex: DEAE Sephadex A-50 medium, 3.5 meq/gm 100–270 mesh (Pharmacia, Uppsala, Sweden), is pretreated with 0.5 N HCl and 0.5 N NaOH, and equilibrated with 0.02 M phosphate buffer pH 7.0.

A column 1.5 × 15 cm is prepared and the dialyzed material is applied to the column. After the eluate is washed into the column, an interrupted elution system is employed.

First, 0.02 M phosphate buffer (pH 7.0) containing 0.25 M NaCl is applied. Two unresolved protein peaks are eluted as monitored by 280 mμ absorbance.

Next, the same buffer containing 0.4 M NaCl is applied and a relatively homogeneous peak is eluted.

Finally, the same buffer containing 0.65 M NaCl is applied and a minor peak is apparent. This constitutes the factor X activity.

3. Evaluation

Factor X isolated by both procedures promotes the activation of DEAE-prothrombin, from the same chromatography, in 25 % sodium citrate. The same effect is evident when DEAE-prothrombin is activated with thromboplastin, Ac-globulin and calcium ions.

This factor X readily activates to the active form in 25 % sodium citrate, with thromboplastin and with Stypven.

The authors conclude that no basic differences exists between autoprothrombin III and factor X.

The properties are similar to those of the "unmodified" autoprothrombin III reported by Marciniak and Seegers (1965).

G. Bovine Factor X (Venom Substrate) - Method of Esnouf and Williams (1962)

1. Procedure

a. Preparation of Barium Sulfate Eluate: Blood is collected in plastic buckets containing 0.1 vol of 1.34 % (w/v) sodium oxalate. About 10 liters of blood are obtained from each of 4–5 animals immediately after slaughter.

The plasma (about 20 liters) is obtained by centrifugation at 1,000 g for 45 min at 4° C. The plasma is stirred for 15–20 minutes at room temperature with citrate washed barium sulfate (100 gm/liter) and the barium sulfate is recovered by centrifuging at 1,000 g for 45 min at 10° C.

The precipitate is washed twice with one quarter of the plasma volume of 0.15 M NaCl and once with water.

The barium sulfate is then stirred at room temperature for 10 min with one-tenth the original plasma volume of 0.2 M sodium citrate-citric acid buffer pH 6.8 and the suspension is centrifuged. The supernatant is dialyzed against 0.02 M sodium phosphate buffer, pH 7.2 at 4° C. The dialysis is carried out in Visking tubing for 24 hours against 4 changes of buffer, the volume of which is at least eight times that of the protein solution.

b. Preparation of DEAE-cellulose (Williams and Esnouf, 1962): 180 grams of DEAE-cellulose (Whatman DE-50) are washed with 2 M sodium chloride dissolved in 0.05 M sodium phosphate buffer pH 6.0. The slurry is packed in 5 equal portions into a glass column 9 × 28 cm. Each portion is packed under pressure from a nitrogen cylinder. The first portion is packed under a pressure of 50 mm Hg, and for each subsequent portion, the pressure is increased by 50 mm Hg.

The column is washed with 2 liters of the buffer used to prepare the slurry, and the cellulose is subsequently equilibrated with 0.02 M sodium phosphate pH 7.0.

c. Chromatography of Barium Sulfate Eluate: The dialyzed barium sulfate eluate (2 liters) is applied to the column and washed with 200 ml of 0.02 M sodium phosphate buffer pH 7.0. The flow rate is adjusted to 500 ml/hr. Sodium phosphate buffer (0.02 M, pH 7.0) containing 0.15 M sodium chloride is applied and 4.8 liters are run through the column.

Next, 0.02 M sodium phosphate buffer pH 7.0 containing 0.25 M sodium chloride is applied and 6 liters are run through the column. The effluent from these two buffers may be collected in bulk. It contains 96 % of the protein applied.

The columns are next treated with 0.02 M sodium phosphate buffer pH 7.0 containing 0.4 M sodium chloride. The flow rate is adjusted to 350 ml/hr and the effluent collected in 50 ml portions. After 1.3 liters of this buffer have passed through the column, a protein fraction representing 3 % of the protein applied to the column is eluted in the next one liter of effluent. This eluate contains the venom substrate.

d. Concentration of Venom Substrate: The effluent containing the venom substrate is diluted with an equal volume of distilled water. Barium sulfate (50 gm/liter) is added to the diluted effluent and stirred at room temperature for 15 min. The venom substrate readily adsorbs to the barium sulfate. The barium sulfate is collected by centrifugation.

The precipitate is stirred at room temperature for 7 min with 0.2 M sodium citrate buffer pH 6.8 (one twentieth the volume of the diluted effluent) and the suspension is centrifuged to remove the barium sulfate. The supernatant contains 68 % of the adsorbed protein. The elution of the barium sulfate is repeated with sodium citrate (one fortieth of the original volume of column effluent) and the suspension is centrifuged. The supernatant contains 25 % of the adsorbed protein.

The two sodium citrate eluates are pooled and dialyzed at 4° C for 15 hrs against two changes of 30 vol of 0.15 M sodium chloride. The dialysed material is lyophilized. The residue is dissolved in 6 ml of water and dialyzed at 4° C for 14 hrs against 400 vol of 0.1 M sodium chloride buffered with 0.01 M Tris-hydrochloric acid, pH 7.3.

2. Analysis and Improvements

The yield of venom substrate is about 150 mg from 20 liters of plasma. Electrophoretically, at pH 6.5 and 7.3, this material is homogeneous. In the ultracentrifuge, two components are resolved. The specific activity, estimated from the clotting time of recalcified normal citrated plasma, is 5.1 units/μg of protein. This represents a 3,640 fold purification.

Preparative Ultracentrifugation: Two ml of the protein solution, dissolved in 0.1 M sodium chloride buffered with 0.01 M tris-hydrochloric acid pH 7.3, are layered on 2.5 ml of a buffered salt solution containing 10 % (w/v) sucrose in a centrifuge tube.

The tube is centrifuged at 40,000 rpm for 6 hrs at 2° C in a S.W. 39 L rotor (Spinco Model L Ultracentrifuge). The rotor is allowed to come to rest without breaking.

The contents of the tube are fractionated by piercing the bottom of the tube with a pin and collecting five 0.9 ml fractions. 25 μl of each of the fractions are added to 2.5 ml of 0.9 % sodium chloride and E_{280} is measured to locate the light component (venom substrate). The heavy component is packed to the bottom of the tube. About 70 % of the light component is found in the third sample at the interface of the two layers. This fraction is dialyzed against 0.1 M sodium chloride buffered with 0.01 M tris-hydrochloric acid pH 7.3. This removes the glucose.

3. Evaluation

In the ultracentrifuge, this material is homogeneous. The specific activity is 5.6 units/μg. This represents a 4,000 fold purification. Coagulant as well as esterolytic activity is displayed by this protein. It is readily transformed into its active form by Russell's viper venom.

H. Bovine Factor X – Method of Jackson et al. (1968)

With this procedure, 100 liters of bovine plasma may be processed in a period of 2–3 days. Factor X is adsorbed onto barium sulfate, eluted by concentrated citrate solution, selectively adsorbed on DEAE cellulose, and finally chromatographed on Sephadex G-100.

1. Procedure

a. Collection of blood: Immediately after being stunned, the animals are hung by the hind legs, and the great vessels are cut directly above the heart. A polyethylene bucket is held into the incision and 8–16 liters of blood are collected from each animal within a period of 1–3 min.

The blood is transferred to a 25 gal plastic barrel, and one volume of 0.1 M sodium oxalate is added for each nine volumes of blood. Vigorous stirring with a spatula usually prevents any clotting. If small clots appear, they may be skimmed off and discarded.

b. Plasma preparation: The blood is centrifuged in a continuous flow, disk-type separator (De Laval PBRX 207) with a bowl speed of 6,000 rpm. Separation and recovery are optimum when a 86 mm specific gravity disk is used and the flow rate is 2–3 gal/min. The blood is pumped to the centrifuge by a variable speed peristaltic pump (Vanton "Flex-i-liner", Model XB-T60A) constructed of Teflon and Viton. Foaming of the plasma is minimized by maintaining a back pressure of 60 psi with the separator exit port valve. The entire procedure is carried out at 30 to 40° C. The plasma is collected in 1 gal polyethylene jars and immediately frozen at –28° C.

Approximately 24 hrs prior to commencement of the next step in the procedure, the plasma is thawed at 28° C. As some of the plasma proteins fail to dissolve at this temperature, the plasma is filtered by gravity through a Buchner funnel, fitted with a pad of glass wool.

c. Barium sulfate ($BaSO_4$) adsorption

1. With vigorous stirring, at ambient temperature, barium sulfate (suitable for X-Ray diagnosis, Merk) is added (10 gm/liter of plasma).
2. The suspension is stirred for at least 30 min.
3. The $BaSO_4$ is separated from the plasma either by centrifugation using the BRPX-207 separator as previously described, or allowed to settle in the barrel overnight (Jackson and Hanahan (1968) recommend the centrifugation procedure).
4. The $BaSO_4$ sediment is transferred (with saline) to 1 liter centrifuge cups, and centrifuged at ambient temperature at 1,300 g (International PR-2, or Lourdes, 30-R Centrifuge).
5. The small amount of saline is decanted and discarded.
6. The $BaSO_4$ cake is transferred into a high speed homogenizer (Waring, CB-5), and dispersed at high speed.
7. The blendor speed is reduced and 2 liters of wash solution are added (0.40 %, w/v, in NaCl, and 0.001 M in trisodium citrate, pH 7.5).
8. The finely divided $BaSO_4$ is rapidly stirred for 2–3 min (n-octyl alcohol is used to control the foaming).
9. The $BaSO_4$ is collected by centrifugation at 1,300 g.
10. Steps 7–9 are repeated five to seven times.

d. Elution of factor X from $BaSO_4$

1. The $BaSO_4$ cake obtained from the last wash (step *c*-10) is finely divided in the homogenizer.
2. Five liters of 0.06 M trisodium citrate, adjusted to pH 5.8 with concentrated HCl, are added to the $BaSO_4$ which is kept in suspension for 30 min.
3. The barium sulfate is collected by centrifugation of 1,300 g. The supernatant is saved.
4. Steps 1–3 are repeated.
5. To reduce the possibility of degradation of factor X, 1 M DFP, in anhydrous isopropyl alcohol, is added to the $BaSO_4$ eluate (final concentration 5×10^{-4} M DFP).

e. DEAE-cellulose adsorption: Prior to use, DEAE-cellulose (Selectacel, Type 20, 1.0 meq/gm, lot 1544, Schleicher and Schuell, N. Y.) is washed in 1 N NaOH, distilled water, 1 N HCl, distilled water until neutral, then with 95 % ethanol, and finally with absolute ethanol. The ethanol is removed in vacuo using a water aspirator for 24–48 hours.

1. Dry DEAE-cellulose is added to the $BaSO_4$ eluate, 2 mg/unit of factor X activity (Bachman et al. 1958).

2. The pH of the suspension is adjusted to 7.1 with 1 M NaOH, and stirring is continued for 15 min.

3. The adsorbent is rapidly removed from the solution by filtration on a Buchner funnel, fitted with a piece of 400 mesh nylon net.

4. The filter cake with its adsorbed proteins is transferred to 600 ml centrifuge cups for batchwise washings. This removes a large portion of the loosely bound protein.

5. The cellulose is stirred with 0.06 M sodium citrate in 0.05 M Tris-HCl, pH 6.7 (one tenth the $BaSO_4$ eluate volume).

6. The suspension is centrifuged at 1,370 g, 20° C, the supernatant discarded, and the washing repeated with the same buffer at pH 8.0. The supernatant is discarded.

7. The cake is transferred to a 2 liter filter flask with 1 liter of 0.08 M sodium citrate in 0.05 M Tris-HCl (pH 8.0).

8. The slurry is deareated using a water aspirator.

9. The deareated DEAE-cellulose with its adsorbed protein is immediately packed into a Lucite chromatographic column (4.5×40 cm) into which a 3.5 cm high clean DEAE bed has been previously packed.

10. The packed column is washed with 0.08 M sodium citrate in 0.05 M Tris-HCl (pH 8.0) until the absorbance (at 280 mμ) of the effluent is less than 0.1. About 1 liter of buffer is required.

11. Next, about 100 ml of the same buffer containing 0.01 M DFP, is passed through the column.

f. Elution of factor X from DEAE-cellulose

1. A linear gradient in sodium chloride, 0 to 0.5 M (in a buffer mixture containing 0.1 M sodium citrate and 0.05 M Tris, adjusted to pH 8.0 with 12 N HCl) is applied to the column.

Each of the reservoirs contain a volume of buffer, two to three times the volume of the packed cellulose.

2. The flow rate is adjusted to 30–50 ml/(cm^2hr). Fractions of about 20 ml are collected.

3. Factor X activity is eluted as a single peak skewed toward the trailing edge. The active fractions are pooled immediately after elution, and DFP is added to 10^{-3} M final concentration. All operations are performed at ambient temperature.

4. The solution (about 400 ml) is concentrated to a final volume of 10–20 ml using a "Diaflo" ultrafiltration cell (Amicon Co., Modell 400). The ultrafiltrator and membranes are rinsed with 100 ml of distilled water containing 0.001 M DFP, prior to the application of the sample.

g. Sephadex gel filtration: The chromatography is carried out in an upward direction with the aid of flow adaptors (Pharmacia).

1. The concentrated material is warmed and applied immediately to a column of Sephadex G-100 (Pharmacia) (2.5×95 cm) packed in 0.01 M Tris-HCl (pH 7.5) and 0.5 M NaCl.

2. The flow rate is adjusted to 7–10 ml/(cm^2 hr) and 2.2 ml fractions are collected. A typical elution profile displays a single peak with a slight trailing shoulder.

2. Evaluation

The specific activities (clotting and esterolytic-TAMe) are essentially constant across the peak. In the ultracentrifuge, this preparation displays a homogeneous Schlieren pattern. The final product represents a 16,000 fold purification. The average yield is approximately 1 mg/liter of plasma – the same as that reported by Seegers et al. 1966.

III. Discussion

The physical properties of the very powerful procoagulants herein discussed vary considerably from one preparation to another and are discussed in the biochemistry section. There appears to be little doubt however, that inactive factor X and autoprothrombin III are one and the same protein. The same holds true for activated factor X, thrombokinase and autoprothrombin C. Qualitatively, on an activity basis, it is impossible to differentiate between these proteins.

An accurate assessment of the optimal specific activity of the products isolated by the various procedures described is impossible. This is, of course, due to the variance in method of assay in different laboratories. One characteristic common to all preparations is the strikingly powerful procoagulant activity.

References

Aoki, N., Harmison, C. R., and Seegers, W. H. (1963). *Can. J. Biochem. Physiol. 41,* 2409.
Bachman, F., Duckert, F., and Koller, F. (1958). *Thromb. Diath. Haemorrhag. 2,* 24.
Cole, E. R., Marciniak, E., and Seegers, W. H. (1962). *Thromb. Diath. Haemorrhag. 8,* 434.
Duckert, F., Yin, E. T., and Straub, W. (1960). *8th Collog. Prot. Biol. Fluids.* Brugge, Belgium, Amsterdam, Elsevier, 410.
Esnouf, M. P., and Williams, W. J. (1962). *Biochem. J. 84,* 62.
Ferguson, J. H., Wilson, E. G., Iatridis, S. G., Rierson, H. A.. and Johnston, B. R. (1960). *J. Clin. Invest. 39,* 1942.
Folin, O., and Ciocalteau, U. (1927). *J. Biol. Chem. 73,* 627.
Hougie, C., Barrow, E. M., and Graham, J. B. (1957). *J. Clin. Invest. 36,* 485.
Jackson, C. M., Johnson, T. F., Hanahan, D. J. (1968). *Biochemistry* 7, 4492.
Jackson, C. M., Hanahan, D. J. (1968). *Biochemistry 7,* 4506.
Kahn, M. J. P., and Bourgain, R. H. (1965). *Hemostase 5,* 413
Kline, D. L. (1965). *Ann. Rev. Physiol. 27,* 285.
Kowarzyk, H., and Marciniak, E. (1961). *Polski Tygod. Lekar 16,* 1641.
Lechner, K., and Deutsch, E. (1965). *Thromb. Diath. Haemorrhag. 13,* 314.
MacFarlane, R. G. (1961). *Brit. J. Haematol. 7,* 496.
Marciniak, E. (1961). *Bull. Acad. Polon. Sci. Ser. Sci. Biol. 9,* 381.
Marciniak, E., and Seegers, W. H. (1965). *New Istanbul Contrib. Clin. Sci. 8,* 117.
Marciniak, E., Cole, E. R., and Seegers, W. H. (1962). *Thromb Diath. Haemorrhag. 8,* 425.
Marciniak, E., Murano, G., and Seegers, W. H.'(1967). *Thromb. Diath. Haemorrhag. 18,* 161.
Milstone, J. H. (1960a). *Nature 187,* 1127.
Milstone, J. H. (1960b). *Proc. Soc. Exptl. Biol. Med. 103,* 361.
Milstone, J. H. (1962). *J. Gen. Physiol.* 45, No. 4 pt. 2 (Suppl.), 103.
Milstone, J. H. (1964). *Federation Proc. 23,* 742.
Milstone, J. H., Oulianoff, N., and Milstone, V. K. (1965). *J. Gen. Physiol. 47,* 315.
Papahadjopoulos, D., Yin, E. T., and Hanahan, D. J. (1964). *Biochemistry 3,* 1931.
Pechet, L., and Alexander, B. (1960). *Federation Proc. 19,* 64.
Reno, R. S., and Seegers, W. H. (1967). *Thromb. Diath. Haemorrhag. 18,* 198.
Seegers, W. H. (1952). *Record. Chem. Progress 13,* 143.
Seegers, W. H., and Landaburu, R. H. (1960). *Can. J. Biochem. Physiol. 38,* 1405.
Seegers, W. H., and Marciniak, E. (1962). *Thromb. Diath. Haemorrhag. 8,* 1.
Seegers, W. H., and Marciniak, E. (1965). *Life Sci. 4,* 1721.
Seegers, W. H., Levine, W. H., and Shepard, R. S. (1958). *Can. J. Biochem. Physiol. 36,* 603.
Seegers, W. H., Aoki, N., and Marciniak, E. (1962). *New Istanbul Contrib. Clin. Sci. 5,* 170.
Seegers, W. H., Cole, E. R., Harmison, C. R., and Marciniak, E. (1963). *Can. J. Biochem. Physiol. 41,* 1047.
Seegers, W. H., Cole, E. R., Aoki, N., and Harmison, C. R. (1964). *Can. J. Biochem. 42,* 229.
Seegers, W. H., Marciniak, E., and Heene, D. (1965). *Texas Rept. Biol. Med. 52,* 449.
Seegers, W. H., Heene, D., and Marciniak, E. (1966). *Thromb. Diath. Haemorrhag. 15,* 1.
Seegers, W. H., Marciniak, E., Kipfer, R., and Yasunaga, K. (1967). *Arch. Biochem. Biophysics 121,* 372.
Spaet, T. H. (1964). *Federation Proc. 23,* 757.
Straub, W., and Duckert, F. (1961). *Thromb. Diath. Haemorrhag. 5,* 402.
Streuli, F. (1959). *Thromb. Diath. Haemorrhag. 3,* 194.
Ware, A. G., and Seegers, W. H. (1949). *Am. J. Clin. Pathol. 19,* 471.
Williams, W. J., and Esnouf, M. P. (1962) *Biochem. J. 84,* 52.

Purification of Hageman Factor (factor XII)

Gary L. Grammens and Eberhard F. Mammen

I. Introduction

Since the discovery of Hageman Factor (HF) several attempts have been undertaken to concentrate or purify this coagulation component from both plasma and serum of various species. A basic premise utilized in almost all techniques is the property of Hageman factor to be easily adsorbed on various surfaces from which HF can be subsequently eluted. Glass powder, glass wool, CM-cellulose, celite, diatomaceous earth and kaolin have been used as adsorbing agents. The agent of choice by various investigators has been largely based on technical feasability and not so much on superior adsorbing qualities. It is pertinent here to interject the warning that this principle of adsorption can be a detriment as well as a useful purification tool. It is for this reason that it is advisable to scrupulously avoid unsiliconized glassware during purification or storage. The use of siliconized glassware or plastic equipment will result in considerably higher yields. In the process of adsorption, Hageman factor becomes activated so that the end product is always "activated Hageman factor".

The techniques described here are those which have produced good preparations with worthwhile yields.

II. Methods of Purification

A. Procedure of Schoenmakers et al. (1963, 1965)

Day 1: Nine volumes of bovine blood are added to one volume of 3.8 % trisodium citrate solution. The mixture is centrifuged in polystyrene bottles at 3,500 g for 60 minutes at 4° C. The platelet poor plasma is separated and incubated for 10 minutes at 37° C with $^1/_{10}$ volume of an $Al(OH)_3$-gel suspension. The alumina-suspension is prepared by stirring 10 gm of moist gel in 40 ml of distilled water for 10 minutes prior to use.

Day 2: After storing the plasma-alumina-gel suspension overnight at 4° C it is centrifuged at 6,000 g for 15 minutes at 3° C, and the precipitate is discarded. Two liters of the supernatant plasma are percolated over chromatographic columns (diameter 7 cm, length 90 cm) packed with glass powder (Pyrex, 100–350 mesh; or P-3, Pulles and Hanique, Eindhoven, Netherlands). Prior to use the glass powder was stirred with 4 N HCl, the acid discarded and the glass powder washed with water until neutral. Next, the glass powder was stirred with 2 N NaOH, the alkaline discarded and the glass powder washed with distilled water until a pH of 6.0 was reached.

After percolation the column is washed with 0.15 M NaCl solution until the U.V. absorption of the eluate at 280 mμ is less than 0.04. These washings are discarded.

Next, glycine-saline buffer pH 9.6 (50 gm NaCl in 1.0 liter of 0.1 M glycinate buffer, pH 9.6) is employed to elute Hageman factor from the glass powder columns. The use of a fraction collector is advisable, the elution of the protein can be followed by U. V. absorption. The elution flow-rate should not exceed 2.5 ml/minute.

The Hageman factor active eluates are combined and immediately cooled to 0° C. Alcohol fractionation follows. The eluate is further cooled at –6° C and pre-cooled ethanol (96 %) is slowly added with gentle stirring until a final concentration of 25 % (v/v) is obtained. Next, the pH of the mixture is adjusted to 6.9 with 1 M acetic acid and the suspension is stored overnight at –6° C.

Day 3: The precipitate formed overnight is removed by centrifugation at 9,000 g for 10 minutes at –6° C and discarded.

Zinc acetate 0.25 M (pH 5.5) in 25 % ethanol is added to the remaining supernatant to produce a final concentration of 20 mM of Zn^{++}. After adjustment of the pH to 5.8 the suspension is stored at –6° C overnight.

Day 4: The Zn-protein precipitate is collected by centrifugation at 9,000 g for 10 minutes at –6° C. The supernatant is discarded and the precipitate is redissolved in 10 ml of 0.1 M EDTA.

In order to remove the Zn-EDTA and excess of EDTA, the preparation is filtered on a 2.5 cm × 35 cm Sephadex G-25 column, previously equilibrated in 0.15 M acetate buffer (pH 5.2). Elution follows with the same buffer at a flow-rate of 60 ml/hr.

The protein is collected as a single fraction and lyophilized. The yield of protein should be at this stage about 50 % of the protein from the glass eluates.

Day 5: Two such samples are pooled and redissolved in water to their original volume and dialyzed against 0.15 M acetate buffer (pH 5.2). Four hours of dialysis with two buffer changes are usually sufficient.

The dialyzed solution is next chromatographed on a 2 cm × 30 cm column of CM-Sephadex (C-50, medium, 4.7 meq/gm) previously equilibrated with 0.15 M sodium acetate buffer (pH 5.2). After application of the protein, the first elution is performed with 0.15 M acetate buffer (pH 5.2) until no more protein is detectable at 254 mμ. A 300 ml linear gradient progressing to 1 M sodium chloride in 0.15 M acetate buffer (pH 5.2) is now utilized to elute the Hageman protein from the column. The tubes containing peak Hageman factor activity are collected and dialyzed against 0.15 M acetate buffer (pH 5.2) as before.

The dialysate can be frozen and kept at –20° C overnight.

Day 6: The dialysate is thawed and rechromatographed on a similar column of CM-Sephadex, pre-equilibrated with 0.15 M acetate buffer (pH 5.2). After application of the protein to the column the elution follows with 0.15 M acetate buffer (pH 5.2) until no more protein is removed. A second linear gradient of 0.30 to 1.0 M sodium chloride in 0.15 M acetate buffer (pH 5.2) is now used to elute Hageman factor from the column. The active fractions are again dialyzed, this time for at least 15 hours against distilled water. The dialysate is lyophilized and stored at 4° C over P_2O_5 in a vacuum.

Day 7: Two CM-Sephadex batches are now dissolved in 20 ml of 0.05 M Tris-chloride buffer (pH 7.5) and dialyzed against 1 liter of buffer for approximately 2 hours.

The dialysate is applied to a 2 cm × 25 cm column of DEAE-Sephadex (A-50, medium, 3.0 meq/gm previously equilibrated with 0.05 M Tris-chloride buffer (pH 7.5). First elution follows with 0.05 M Tris-chloride buffer (pH 7.5) until no more protein is detected. The Hageman protein is next eluted using a 300 ml linear gradient rising to 0.4 M sodium chloride in 0.05 M Tris-chloride buffer (pH 7.5). The active fractions are now combined and dialyzed for at least 15 hours against distilled water. The dialysate is next lyophilized and stored at 4° C over P_2O_5 under vacuum.

This procedure yields approximately 16 mg of purified Hageman protein from about 20 liters of bovine plasma. The product thus recovered is homogeneous by means of the analytical ultracentrifuge, shows a single boundary on disc electrophoresis and exhibits esterase activity towards substituted arginine esters, such as N-benzoyl-L-arginine ethyl ester (BAEE) and p-tosyl-L-arginine methyl ester (TAMe).

B. Procedure of Speer et al. (1965)

Day 1: Three hundred grams of Hyflo-Super-Cel (Johns Manville Celite) is slurried in distilled water and filtered on filter cloth in a large Buchner funnel. Next, the celite is washed with 2 liters of 0.007 N ammonium hydroxide and then with distilled water to a pH of 7.0. This pretreated celite is added to 2 liters of outdated (30 days old) ACD human plasma and the mixture is stirred for 10 minutes at room temperature.

The mixture is again filtered in a large Buchner funnel and the celite is washed with distilled water until the U.V. absorption of the eluate at 280 mμ is less than 0.05.

In order to remove the Hageman protein from the celite, the celite is stirred with 1 liter of 0.007 N ammonium hydroxide for about 10 minutes and then filtered.

The elution with 1 liter of 0.007 N ammonium hydroxide is repeated once more.

The two ammonium hydroxide filtrates combined as crude Hageman factor preparations are stable at 4° C for at least one month.

Day 2: The pH of the ammonium hydroxide filtrates is adjusted to pH 7.0 by the addition of 25 % acetic acid with stirring. The mixture is now chilled overnight at 4° C.

Day 3: The suspension is centrifuged at 9,000 g for 10 minutes at 4° C and the obtained precipitate is discarded. The pH of the supernatant is again adjusted to 5.2 by adding 25 % acetic acid under stirring. The suspension is once more chilled overnight at 4° C.

Day 4: The suspension is centrifuged once more at 9,000 g for 10 minutes at 4° C and the precipitate is collected. The supernatant is discarded. The precipitate is dissolved in approximately 30 ml of dilute ammonium hydroxide and if necessary, this ammonium solution can be stored at –20° C for several months.

Next saturated ammonium sulfate (pH 9.0) is added until a 40 % (v/v) concentration is reached. This mixture is stored overnight at 4° C.

Day 5: The precipitate formed overnight is removed by centrifugation at 9,000 g for 10 minutes at 4° C and discarded. To the supernatant further saturated ammonium sulfate solution (pH 9.0) is added until a 50 % (v/v) concentration is achieved. This mixture is again stored overnight at 4° C.

Day 6: The precipitate is again removed by centrifugation at 9,000 g for 10 minutes at 4° C and discarded. To the supernatant saturated ammonium sulfate solution (pH 9.0) is added to raise the concentration to 67% (v/v). Again this mixture is stored overnight at 4° C.

Day 7: The suspension is once more centrifuged at 9,000 g for 10 minutes at 4° C and the precipitate is recovered. The supernatant is discarded. The precipitate is dissolved in 5 ml of distilled water. If necessary, this product can again be stored at –20° C for several months without losing Hageman factor activity.

The ammonium sulfate precipitated Hageman preparation is next dialyzed thoroughly against distilled water and finally against 0.1 M ammonium acetate buffer (pH 7.0).

CM-Sephadex (C-50, medium, Pharmacia) is allowed to swell overnight in an excess of distilled water. It is next filtered and soaked for 10 minutes in 0.5 N HCl. After filtration, the Sephadex is washed with distilled water until a neutral pH is reached. Next, the Sephadex is soaked for 10 minutes in 0.5 N NaOH, again filtered and once more washed with distilled water until neutral.

The Sephadex gel is then equilibrated overnight at room temperature with 500 ml of 0.1 M ammonium acetate buffer (pH 7.0). The gel is filtered, resuspended in fresh 0.1 M ammonium acetate buffer (pH 7.0) and loaded into a chromatographic column as a slurry, forming a filtration bed of 45 cm × 3.5 cm. The column is allowed to cool to 4° C while settling.

Day 8: The dialyzed Hageman preparation is applied to the column and chromatography is started with 75 ml of 0.1 M ammonium acetate buffer (pH 7.0). Subsequently, by means of a two reservoir system, gradient elution is accomplished, wherein there is a simultaneous increase in ionic strength and in pH through gradual mixing of 75 ml of starting buffer in the lower reservoir and dropwise addition of 200 ml of 0.2 M ammonium acetate buffer (pH 7.0) from the upper reservoir.

When 100 ml of this mixture remains in the lower reservoir, 1 liter of 0.2 M ammonium acetate buffer (pH 9.7) is introduced into the upper reservoir and the gradient elution is continued until all protein has been completely eluted.

The initial flow rate of 1 to 2 ml per minute decreases with the progressive increase in pH and ionic strength to a final flow-rate of 0.5 ml/minute. The active Hageman protein is the last protein to be eluted, emerging from the column as the pH rises above 9.2 (approximately 950 ml) and requires 400 to 500 ml for its complete elution.

All column fractions are collected in siliconized glass tubes, and when the pH of the effluent reaches 9.0, each tube receives 3 ml of 0.05 M sodium pyrophosphate. Thus a 20 ml column fraction is collected directly in dilute sodium pyrophosphate in order to stabilize the purified factor XII activity.

Even under these circumstances, the factor XII activity is not completely stable and therefore it is best to freeze these fractions immediately at –20° C or below.

For analysis, the fractions are at least 5 times diluted prior to assay in order to avoid interference of the assay due to pyrophosphate and ammonium acetate.

Day 9: The contaminating salts are removed from the Hageman factor preparations by gel filtration on a Sephadex G-50 column with ammonium hydroxide as eluent at 4° C. The active fractions are frozen and stored at –20° C. At this time, the preparations are lyophilized and stored at –20° C.

Rechromatography of the purified Hageman preparations on cellulose phosphate (Whatman) utilizing gradient elution revealed only one peak which emerged with an 0.1 M ammonium acetate buffer (pH 9.8).

According to Speer et al. (1965) the overall recovery of the Hageman factor was 25% with a purification of 10^6 fold over plasma. The preparations were homogeneous in the analytical ultracentrifuge, upon rechromatography, and in the Tiselius moving-boundary electrophoresis. In contrast to the preparations manufactured by the procedure of Schoenmakers et al. (1963, 1965) these preparations do not exhibit esterolytic activity towards p-tosyl-L-arginine methyl ester (TAMe).

C. Procedure of Mammen and Grammens (1967)

Day 1: Nine volumes of fresh bovine blood are collected in one volume of 3.2 % trisodium citrate in plastic containers. The blood is centrifuged either in polystyrene bottles at 3,500 g for 60 minutes at 4° C, or by means of a Sharples centrifuge. The plasma may be used fresh or it may be stored in plastic bottles in lots of 3 to 4 liters at –20° C. Even after six months of storage excellent Hageman preparations were obtained from the plasma.

Three liters of plasma are exposed to glass wool (Corning No. 3950) in the following manner: Three gauze pouches containing glass wool are used. Approximately 20 gm of glass wool are placed in the center of an appropriately sized double layer of gauze. The four corner edges are pulled together and a piece of twine is used as a purse string.

One of these glass wool pouches is immersed into the plasma and periodically removed and reimmersed to insure uniform exposure. The exposure time found to be most effective in terms of yield and time is about 3 minutes. After exposure to the plasma, the glass wool pouch is rerinsed for about 3 minutes under running cold tap water and excess water is squeezed out. Next, the glass wool pouch is rinsed in 1.5 liters of 10 % sodium chloride solution (pH 8.0) for approximately 3 minutes in order to elute the proteins which have been adsorbed onto the glass wool. The glass wool pouch is rinsed under running cold tap water, the excess water is squeezed out and the pouch is again exposed to the original plasma. Using 3 pouches, considerable time can be saved for while one is being exposed to the plasma, the second is being washed under the running cold tap water and the third is undergoing the exposure to the same 10 % sodium chloride solution. Repeated exposure of the plasma to the glass wool pouches is carried out for about 3 hours.

The 10 % sodium chloride solution containing the eluted protein is now chilled to 2° C and ammonium sulfate salt is added until a 25 % (w/v) concentration is reached. The ammonium sulfate salt is added under stirring of the solution. After the salt has been added, the mixture is stirred for about 15 minutes at room temperature, and the pH is adjusted to 7.0 by adding 0.1 N NaOH solution. The mixture is now allowed to remain for approximately 60 minutes in the refrigerator at 4° C.

The precipitate formed is removed by centrifugation of the mixture in plastic centrifuge tubes at 3,000 g for 15 minutes at 0° C. The precipitate is discarded.

The supernatant solution is again chilled to 2° C and ammonium sulfate salts are added under stirring until a 55 % (w/v) concentration is obtained. After stirring this mixture for 15 minutes at room temperature, the pH is again adjusted to 7.0 by adding 0.1 N NaOH. After storage in the refrigerator at 4° C for about 60 minutes the suspension is once more centrifuged in plastic centrifuge tubes at 3,000 g for 15 minutes at 0° C. The supernatant is now discarded, but the precipitate is resuspended in approximately 20 ml of distilled water and the pH is adjusted to 7.0 by adding either 1 % acetic acid or 0.1 N NaOH, depending upon the initial pH.

Some insoluble material can be removed by centrifugation at 3,000 g for 15 minutes at 0° C.

The supernatant solution is dialyzed against distilled water at 4° C to an electrical resistance greater than 3,000 Ohms. The dialysis may be started in the late afternoon and may be continued overnight.

Day 2: After dialysis the pH of the dialysate is adjusted to 6.0 by adding 0.01 N NaOH. Any precipitate formed may be removed by centrifugation at 3,000 g for 15 minutes at 0° C.

Next the supernatant solution is cooled in an ice salt water bath to 4° C and pre-cooled (–50° C) ethanol (96 %) is added to reach a concentration of 40 % (v/v). After stirring the suspension for about 15 minutes it is centrifuged for 15 minutes at 3,000 g at 0° C.

The supernatant is discarded but the precipitate is resuspended in approximately 10 ml of 0.05 M phosphate buffer (pH 7.9). This resuspended precipitate contains most of the original Hageman factor activity. If necessary, this resuspended precipitate can be stored at –20° C.

Next the preparation is chromatographed on DEAE-cellulose. Previously several grams of DEAE-cellulose had been suspended in 0.05 M phosphate buffer pH 7.9, adequately stirred and stored overnight. The supernatant solution is decanted to remove fine particles and new buffer is added. The procedure is repeated until the pH of the supernatant is 7.9. The buffer cellulose suspension is now poured into a siliconized chromatography column (actual DEAE-cellulose column 2.5 cm × 30 cm, hold up volume 60–70 ml) and packed under slight air pressure. The packed column is washed with 0.05 M phosphate buffer pH 7.9 until the pH of the effluent is 7.9.

The ethanol precipitate, dissolved in 0.05 M phosphate buffer, pH 7.9, is now applied to the column and elution is started with an 0.05 M phosphate buffer pH 7.9. Under these conditions the Hageman factor protein is not adsorbed onto the column and emerges behind the hold up volume in a sharp peak. The fractions are collected in siliconized glass tubes in volumes of approximately 15 ml. The emerging protein peak contains about 90 % of the initial Hageman factor activity placed onto the column and contains at this point approximately 5–10 % impurities.

The tubes containing highest protein concentration are combined and dialyzed against distilled water for about 3 hours. The electrical resistance should be greater than 3,000 Ohms. The dialysate is next lyophilized overnight in a siliconized container.

Day 3: The lyophilized protein is dissolved in approximately 10 ml of distilled water and chromatographed on a siliconized Sephadex G-150 column (2.5 cm × 50 cm) using distilled water as the eluant. The Hageman factor protein emerges in a sharp peak and again the fractions are collected in siliconized glass tubes in volumes of approximately 15 ml.

The tubes containing the highest protein concentration are combined and again lyophilized in a siliconized container. The lyophilized products can be stored in a dessicator over P_2O_5 at room temperature.

This procedure yields approximately 15 to 25 mg of purified protein from 1 liter of bovine plasma. The protein is homogeneous by means of ultracentrifugation, immunoelectrophoresis, cellulose acetate electrophoresis, and polyacrylamide electrophoresis. Also these preparations have no esterolytic activity when p-tosyl-L-arginine methyl ester (TAMe) is used as the substrate.

D. Procedure of Ratnoff and Davie (1962)

Day 1: Approximately 1,200 ml of pooled citrated normal human plasma are mixed with $^1/_{10}$ volume of aqueous aluminum hydroxide gel, stirred for 5 minutes at room temperature and then centrifuged for 10 minutes at 1,000 g. The aluminum hydroxide gel (Cutter Laboratories, Berkley, Calif. (0.6 % aluminum oxide)) was diluted to 0.55 % by the addition of water.

The precipitate is discarded and the supernatant plasma is mixed with 7.5 mg of diatomaceous earth per ml of plasma, stirred for 10 minutes and recentrifuged. The precipitate is discarded. The supernatant is incubated in a silicone coated flask at 37° C overnight and a few drops of toluol are added as a preservative.

Day 2: The preparation is diluted with an equal volume of 0.15 M sodium acetate buffer (pH 5.2), and the pH is adjusted to 5.2 by adding 1 M acetic acid. Next, an equal volume of distilled water is added. Eighteen mg of carboxymethylcellulose (prepared by the procedure by Ellis and Simpson (1956)) are added per ml of acidified diluted plasma. The suspension is stirred for 10 minutes at room temperature and then centrifuged to remove the carboxymethylcellulose. The Hageman factor is adsorbed onto the CM-cellulose. Next, the carboxymethylcellulose is washed repeatedly with 0.075 M sodium acetate buffer (pH 5.2) containing 10^{-4} M versene. The washings are repeated until material can no longer be precipitated from the supernatant by adding an equal volume of 10 % trichloracetic acid. Six washings are usually sufficient. Each time the acetate buffer is removed by centrifugation.

The washed carboxymethylcellulose is now eluted repeatedly with 0.6 M sodium acetate buffer (pH 5.2) until the eluting fluid contains only traces of material precipitated by trichloracetic acid. Each elution is performed with a volume of buffer equivalent to $^1/_3$ the volume of the original plasma. The various eluates are combined and recentrifuged to remove traces of carboxymethylcellulose.

The Hageman factor protein is now precipitated from the eluate by means of ammonium sulfate fractionation. Solid ammonium sulfate is added to give a 60% (w/v) saturation. After addition of the ammonium sulfate the suspension is stored overnight at 4° C.

Day 3: The precipitated protein is collected by centrifugation at 37,000 g and dissolved in approximately 60 ml of 0.025 M phosphate buffer (pH 6.8) containing 1×10^{-4} M versene. The dissolved precipitate is dialyzed against 2 liters of the same buffer for 4 hours. Dialysis is then continued for an additional 4 hours against 2 liters of 0.025 M barbital buffer (pH 7.45) containing 1×10^{-4} M versene. The dialysate is centrifuged for 10 minutes at 10,000 g and the precipitate is discarded.

The supernatant is divided in half and each portion is placed on a 2 cm × 22 cm DEAE-cellulose column, previously equilibrated with 0.025 M barbital buffer (pH 7.45). Elution from the column is performed by a buffer gradient established by placing 175 ml of 0.025 M barbital buffer (pH 7.45) in the mixing chamber and 175 ml of a mixture of 0.025 M barbital buffer (pH 7.45) in 0.25 M NaCl in the upper reservoir. The fractions are collected in 10 ml samples in plastic tubes. The flowrate is about 25 ml per hour. After chromatography the tubes containing Hageman factor activity of both columns are combined and dialyzed overnight against 4 liters of 1×10^{-4} M versene.

Day 4: The dialysate is lyophilized.

Day 5: The lyophilized protein is dissolved in 30 ml of 0.025 M sodium acetate buffer (pH 5.2) and again chromatographed on a 2 cm × 22 cm CM-cellulose column previously equilibrated 0.025 M sodium acetate buffer (pH 5.2). Elution from the column follows by a buffer gradient established by placing 150 ml of 0.025 M sodium acetate buffer (pH 5.2) in the mixing chamber and 150 ml of 0.6 M sodium acetate buffer (pH 5.2) in the upper reservoir. Elution is continued with the 0.6 M sodium acetate buffer (pH 5.2) until the Hageman protein is completely eluted. The fractions are collected in 10 ml aliquots in plastic tubes at a flow-rate of 25 ml per hour. The fractions containing most of the Hageman factor activity are combined and dialyzed overnight against 4 liters of 1×10^{-4} M versene.

Day 6: The preparations are lyophilized.

This purification procedure yields between 10 and 50% of original plasma Hageman factor activity with an overall 3,000 to 5,000-fold purification. The Hageman factor preparations are free of most of the known coagulation constituents but the homogeneity of the preparations by means of physical-chemical measurements has apparently not been studied.

References

Ellis, S., and Simpson, M. E. (1956). *J. Biol. Chem. 220,* 939.

Mammen, E. F., and Grammens, G. L. (1967). *Thromb. Diath. Haemorrhag. 18,* 306.

Ratnoff, O. D., and Davie, E. W. (1962). *Biochemistry 1,* 967.

Schoenmakers, J. G. G., Kurstjens, R. M., Haanen, C., and Zilliken, F. (1963). *Thromb. Diath. Haemorrhag. 9,* 546.

Schoenmakers, J. G. G., Matze, R., Haanen, C., and Zilliken, F. (1965). *Biochim. Biophys. Acta 101,* 166.

Speer, R. J., Ridgway, H., and Hill, J. M. (1965). *Thromb Diath. Haemorrhag. 14,* 1.

Purification of Plasma Thromboplastin Antecedent (PTA, factor XI)

EBERHARD F. MAMMEN and GARY L. GRAMMENS

I. Introduction

Plasma thromboplastin antecedent (PTA) deficiency or factor XI deficiency was in 1953 described by Rosenthal et al. (1953). Studies on various properties of plasma thromboplastin antecedent (Rosenthal, 1955) revealed that the activity is present in normal plasma and serum and that it migrates electrophoretically in the region of the β_2-globulins (Rosenthal, 1955; Lewis et al. 1958). The activity could be precipitated from plasma at 25 to 33 % ammonium sulfate saturation and Cohn fractions IV-1 and III also contained PTA activity. Like Hageman factor, only small amounts of PTA are adsorbed from plasma and serum on barium sulfate (Rosenthal, 1955). Partial separation from Hageman factor has been achieved by adsorbing plasma with low concentrations of Celite (10–15 mg/ml), whereas higher concentrations of Celite (30 mg/ml) will adsorb both PTA and Hageman factor (Soulier and Prou-Wartelle, 1960).

Schiffman et al. (1960) separated PTA and Hageman factor from normal human plasma employing chromatography on DEAE-cellulose. Elution was performed by continuously increasing the sodium chloride concentration from 0.05 M to 0.3 M in the presence of 0.02 M sodium diethyl barbiturate buffer. The pH was kept constant at 7.12. Lucite columns with ash free filter paper support were used. The fractions were collected in polyethylene tubes in a cold room. PTA activity was eluted before Hageman factor activity and assays of both fractions for factors II, V, VII, VIII, IX and X activities revealed less than 1 % of their normal plasma activity.

II. Methods of Purification

A. Preparation from Hageman Deficient Plasma

In 1961 Ratnoff et al. (1961) described a technique for the preparation of Hageman factor from PTA deficient plasma und PTA from Hageman deficient plasma. The latter procedure will be described here.

Blood was drawn from patients with Hageman deficiency using No. 18 gauge needles coated with Arquad-2C (Monocote-E, Armour) and glass syringes coated with silicone (G.E. Dri-Film, SC-87). The blood was mixed with one-ninth volume of 0.13 M trisodium citrate and centrifuged in silicone-coated Lusteroid tubes for 15 min at 2,700 g. The plasma was re-centrifuged twice for 10 and 30 min, respectively at 27,000 g. The platelet poor plasma was stored in silicone-coated Lusteroid tubes and either used within a few hours or stored at –25° C until used.

The plasma was next adsorbed with dilute aluminum hydroxide gel to remove factors II, VII, IX and X. One part of commercial aluminum hydroxide (Cutter Laboratories, Berkely, Calif.) was diluted with 3 parts of water. Ten parts of plasma were mixed with 1 part of dilute aluminum hydroxide gel for 3 min at 37° C in silicone-coated Lusteroid tubes. The mixture was centrifuged for 5 min at 2,700 g to remove the aluminum hydroxide gel. The adsorbed plasma was either processed immediately or stored at –25° C until used.

In order to remove fibrinogen and to decrease the levels of factors V and VIII, the adsorbed plasma was heated for 30 min at 56° C.

The adsorbed, heated plasma was next diluted to twice its volume with 0.15 M sodium acetate (pH 5.2). The pH of the mixture was adjusted to 5.2 by adding 1 M acetic acid. The acidified plasma was further diluted with an equal volume of water and 75 mg of carboxymethyl cellulose for each original ml of plasma were added. The mixture was stirred for 10 min at room temperature and centrifuged for 5 min at 2,700 g.

The carboxymethyl cellulose was washed twice with $^1/_2$ of the original plasma volume of 0.075 M sodium acetate buffer (pH 5.2). Elution of PTA from the carboxymethyl cellulose followed by twice washing the cellulose for 5 min with $^1/_2$ of the original plasma volume of 0.067 M sodium phosphate buffer (pH 6.8) and 1 M sodium chloride in equal amounts. The two eluates were combined and recentrifuged in order to remove traces of the carboxymethyl cellulose.

Dialysis of the eluate for 16 to 24 hours against 0.067 M sodium phosphate buffer (pH 6.8) completed the purification procedure. The preparations were stored at –25° C.

B. Preparation from Normal Human Serum

The partial purification of activated PTA from normal human serum was described by Ratnoff and Davie (1962). The preparations were further purified by Kingdon et al. (1964). Venous blood was drawn using No. 18 gauge needles coated with Arquad 2-C (Monocote-E, Armour) and glass syringes coated with silicone (G. E. Dri-Film, SC-87) and allowed to clot in glass tubes. The serum was separated by centrifugation.

In order to remove factors VII, IX, X and traces of II, one liter of serum was mixed for 10 min at room temperature with barium sulfate (Baker) (100 mg/ml serum). The barium sulfate was removed by centrifugation.

Next the serum was heated for 30 min at 56° C in order to remove traces of factor V and VIII activity.

The serum was acidified by adding an equal volume of 0.15 M sodium acetate buffer (pH 5.2). The pH was adjusted to 5.2 by the addition of 1 M acetic acid.

The adsorbed, heated, and acidified serum was placed on a 6.5 × 12 cm carboxymethyl cellulose column at room temperature, previously washed with 0.15 M sodium acetate buffer (pH 5.2). Occasionally the serum had to be pressed into the columns by positive air pressure.

Next, the column was washed with a volume of 0.05 M sodium acetate buffer (pH 5.2) equal to $^1/_2$ of the original serum volume. Elution followed with $^1/_4$ volume of equal parts of 0.067 M sodium phosphate buffer (pH 6.8) and 1 M sodium chloride.

The eluate was fractionated with solid ammonium sulfate and the precipitate obtained between 35–50 % saturation was collected by centrifugation. The precipitate was dissolved in $^1/_5$ volume of 0.067 M sodium phosphate buffer and dialyzed against four liters of the same buffer. The dialysate was dried from the frozen state.

Approximately 400 mg of material, $^2/_5$ of it protein, was obtained from one liter of serum. At this point, the PTA was purified about 50–60 fold compared with the original serum. The total yield was around 15 %.

Two of these products (each from 1 liter of serum) were dissolved in about 10 ml of distilled water and dialyzed overnight against one liter of acetate buffer (0.15 M acetic acid-sodium acetate, pH 5.2) and rechromatographed on carboxymethyl cellulose.

Two CM-cellulose columns (1.6 × 50 cm) were prepared from 15 gm CM cellulose each. The cellulose had been washed three times with the acetate buffer prior to packing the columns.

Approximately 76 mg of protein were placed on each of the two columns and after complete application, the column was layered with 5 ml acetate buffer. Elution followed by establishing the following gradient: 200 ml acetate buffer were placed in the mixing chamber and 200 ml phosphate-saline buffer (0.05 M sodium phosphate in 0.35 M NaCl, pH 6.3) in the reservoir. The eluting solution was pumped through each column at a constant rate of 50 ml/hr. Five ml fractions were collected every 6 min. The optical density of each fraction at 280 mμ was recorded and each tube was assayed for activity. Those fractions containing more than 10 % of the total activity were combined.

The protein was precipitated by adding solid ammonium sulfate to 70 % saturation. After stirring the suspension for 15 min, the precipitate was recovered by centrifugation (20 min, 35,000 g). The supernatant was discarded and the precipitate either frozen at –20° C without loss of activity, even when stored for several months, or the precipitate was dissolved in acetate buffer and dialyzed overnight against 1 liter of acetate buffer.

In a concentration of 1–3 mg protein/ml solution, the biological activity was stable at 4° C for a period of up to 4 weeks. However, the stability was decreased in lower protein concentrations or in pH ranges from 7–8 at concentrations of below 0.5 mg/ml.

The rechromatography on CM-cellulose resulted in an additional purification of 2 to 4 fold with a yield of 60–80 %.

III. Discussion

The purification of PTA from Hageman deficient plasma is obviously dependent upon the availability of such a deficiency plasma. This fact is limiting the usefulness of the above described procedure. The advantage of the procedure is that the crude PTA preparations are not only free of other coagulation factors, but also free of Hageman factor. The latter seems to be present at least in traces in the preparations obtained from serum (Kingdon et al. 1964; Davie and Ratnoff, 1965).

The preparations from Hageman deficient plasma seem to be purified 10–20 fold over the original plasma but the loss of activity is great. Adsorption on diluted aluminum hydroxide gel and heating of the adsorbed plasma are responsible for the loss of activity (Ratnoff et al. 1961).

The preparations from normal human serum are purified more then 150-fold, but still are impure (Kingdon et al. 1964). Apparently, further purification can be obtained by column chromatography on hydroxyl apatite (Kingdon et al. 1964) but no further experimental details seem to be available. The overall recovery is also low with this procedure and only 10–12 % of the original PTA activity seems to be recovered. Physical-chemical data on PTA are not as yet available.

References

Davie, E. W., and Ratnoff, O. D. (1965). *In:* "The Proteins" (H. Neurath, ed.), Vol. III, pp. 359—443. Academic Press, New York.

Kingdon, H. S., Davie, E. W., and Ratnoff, O. D. (1964). *Biochemistry 3,* 166.

Lewis, J. H., Walters, D., Didisheim, P., and Merchant, W. R. (1958). *J. Clin. Invest. 37,* 1323.

Ratnoff, O. D., and Davie, E. W. (1962). *Biochemistry 1,* 677.

Ratnoff, O. D., Davie, E. W., and Mallett, D. L. (1961). *J. Clin. Invest. 40,* 803.

Rosenthal, R. L. (1955). *J. Lab. Clin. Med. 45,* 123.

Rosenthal, R. L., Dreskin, O. H., and Rosenthal, N. (1953). *Proc. Soc. Exptl. Biol. Med. 82,* 171.

Schiffman, S., Rapaport, S. I., Ware, A. G., and Mehl, J. W. (1960). *Proc. Soc. Exptl. Biol. Med. 105,* 453.

Soulier, J. P., and Prou-Wartelle, O. (1960). *Brit. J. Haematol. 6,* 88.

Purification of Tissue Thromboplastin

Eberhard F. Mammen

I. Introduction

Tissue extracts from almost all mammalian organs contain a powerful clot promoting activity. This activity has been designated as "tissue thromboplastin" or "tissue thrombokinase". In the laboratory, extracts of tissues play a key role in the determination of several coagulation factors for clinical and research purposes. Extracts from brain, lung, placenta, testes, thymus and other organs have been used in the past, but brain and lung thromboplastins have found widest acceptance for clinical studies and research purposes in blood coagulation.

The most commonly used thromboplastins are, in principle, crude extracts of various tissues, obtained by extracting the tissues with saline or buffer solutions. The crude preparations cannot be considered as a chemical entity. Besides clot promoting activity, they frequently contain clot delaying substances and material which does not affect the coagulation of blood or plasma. For research purposes, the crude tissue extracts have been further purified to yield material which has been chemically characterized as either lipoprotein or predominantly lipid. Details on the chemical composition of these thromboplastins were outlined in Chapter I.

In order to characterize the type of thromboplastin prepared or used, Hecht et al. (1958) recommended a nomenclature which is adopted in this contribution. According to this nomenclature, "lung extract thromboplastin (bovine)" indicates a preparation from lung, obtained by extraction of fresh lung tissue with physiological saline or buffer solutions. The word "extract" implies the heterogeneous composition. In addition, the term designates the type of tissue and the species from which it was derived. Such lung extract thromboplastin (bovine) can be further purified to yield "lung thromboplastin (bovine)". This material is essentially a lipoprotein.

By the same token, "brain extract thromboplastin (bovine)" represents a crude extract of bovine brain tissue which is heterogeneous in its composition. Upon further purification, "brain thromboplastin (bovine)" is obtained which is chemically a complex lipid, as outlined in Chapter I.

Since thromboplastins from lung and brain tissue are most commonly used today, only methods for the preparation of lung extract thromboplastin, lung thromboplastin, brain extract thromboplastin and brain thromboplastin are described in the following. The methods for preparation can, in principle, be applied to other types of tissue as well.

II. Methods of Preparation

Tissue material for the preparation of tissue thromboplastin should be carefully separated from blood, in order to avoid contamination with blood constituents, especially platelet phospholipids, erythrocyte stroma and plasmatic coagulation factors.

A. Lung Extract Thromboplastin (Bovine)

The outlined method was in principle described by Cohen and Chargaff (1941) and Chargaff et al. (1944).

1. A bovine lung, freshly obtained from the slaughter house, is dissected free of the trachea, major bronchi and major blood vessels, and carefully washed under running tap water.
2. The washed lung is ground through a domestic meat grinder and the ground material mixed with an equal volume of 0.9 % sodium chloride solution.
3. To insure complete mixing, the entire material is reground once again.
4. The resulting suspension is placed in a refrigerator at 4° C and stored for about 24 hours under frequent stirring.
5. The suspension is pressed out through a canvas bag or gauze and the filtrate centrifuged for 10 min at about 800 g (4° C).
6. The precipitate is discarded. The supernatant can serve as a crude lung extract thromboplastin, and can be stored for months at –20° C. For use, it is thawed and rehomogenized. As a preservative, phenol is added to a final concentration of 0.5 % to prevent bacterial growth. When stored with phenol at 4° C, the activity will be stable for at least one month.

B. Lung Thromboplastin (Bovine)

Lung extract thromboplastin can be further purified, and in the following the procedure of Chargaff et al. (1942) is described.

1. The procedure for the preparation of lung extract thromboplastin (bovine) is followed as described above (Steps 1–4), with the exception that 1 kg of ground lung tissue is extracted

with 600 ml cold 0.9% sodium chloride solution.

2. The suspension is pressed out through a canvas bag or gauze, and the filtrate subjected to three centrifugations at 45 min at 2,700 g (4° C).

3. The turbid, reddish supernatant is centrifuged for 25 min in an ultracentrifuge at 30,000 g (4° C).

4. The supernatant is discarded and the precipitate dissolved in about $^1/_3$ of the original volume of borate buffer, pH 8.6 (ionic strength 0.15) and again sedimented at around 30,000 g for 25 min (4° C).

5. The supernatant is discarded and the precipitate dissolved in the same amount of borate buffer as before.

6. In order to remove undissolved particles, the material is centrifuged for 20 min at 5,000 g (4° C).

7. The supernatant is once again centrifuged in the ultracentrifuge at around 30,000 g for 25 min.

8. The precipitate is once more dissolved in the same amount of borate buffer as before and again cleared from undissolved particles by centrifuging at 5,000 g for 20 min.

9. The alternate high and low speed centrifugation is repeated 2–4 times more until the supernatant becomes clear and colorless.

10. The final precipitate can be dissolved in borate buffer, pH 8.6 (ionic strength 0.15) and used for assay, or it can be dissolved in water, dialyzed for 48 hours against running tap water and for 48 hours against frequent changes of ice cold distilled water and dried from frozen state.

This procedure yields 65 mg of lung thromboplastin (bovine) from 100 gm of starting tissue.

This method was used with minor modifications by Williams (1964) to obtain the starting material for the purification of lung microsomes.

C. Brain Extract Thromboplastin

Brain extract thromboplastins usually represent acetone dried extracts from brain. The original preparation of such extracts was described by Quick (1938, 1942) and later procedures, such as for example described by Owren (1949), Thies (1957), Gollub et al. (1962), Deutsch et al. (1964), Hecht (1965) and many other authors represent minor modifications of this original procedure. The preparation of acetone dried rabbit and human brain is described in this volume by Rizza and Walker and for details the reader is referred to Chapter III, p. 93. The described procedures can be applied to brain of any animal species. The dried brain powder preparations, stored in the dark and under refrigeration, are stable over an almost indefinite period of time (Deutsch et al. 1964; Hecht, 1965). However, when stored at 4° C in watery suspensions, they gradually lose their activity despite the addition of bactericides (Powell, 1957).

Long contact of the brain tissue with acetone will impair the activity of the resulting preparations (Hecht, 1955). For this reason, the acetone must be carefully removed during the preparation.

D. Brain Thromboplastin

Hecht et al. (1958) used brain extract thromboplastin (rabbit) as starting material for a further purification which resulted in brain thromboplastin (rabbit). This procedure was used by Deutsch et al. (1964) for the further purification of human brain extract thromboplastin.

1. About 40 gm of dried brain extract thromboplastin powder are suspended in 700 ml distilled water and continuously stirred for approximately 5 min.

2. The suspension is centrifuged for 10 min at 3,000 g and the supernatant discarded.

3. The precipitate is again suspended in 700 ml distilled water and continuously stirred with the aid of a stirring apparatus for 30 min in a 37° C waterbath.

4. The suspension is once more centrifuged for 10 min at 3,000 g.

5. The milky supernatant is temporarily stored at 4° C until further use.

6. The precipitate is again suspended in 350 ml distilled water and stirred for an additional 30 min at 37° C.

7. The suspension is centrifuged for 10 min at 3,000 g and the precipitate discarded.

8. The supernatant is combined with the first supernatant (Step 5) and centrifuged in an ultracentrifuge for 60 min at 100,000 g.
9. The resulting supernatant is discarded, while the precipitate is resuspended in the original volume of 0.85 % sodium chloride solution.
10. The suspension is again centrifuged for 60 min at 100,000 g and the supernatant is discarded.
11. At this time, the precipitate usually appears in form of two layers. The bottom layer has a gray color, while the top layer has a more transparent and yellow color. With the aid of a spatula, the top layer is carefully separated from the gray bottom layer and resuspended in 0.85 % saline solution. The gray bottom layer is discarded.
12. The resuspended top layer is centrifuged for 60 min at 100,000 g, the supernatant discarded and the top layer again separated from the gray bottom layer.
13. The top layer is again resuspended in 0.85 % saline solution and the procedure repeated until no gray bottom layer can be identified anymore. Usually 4–6 washings are sufficient to remove the gray material.
14. The finally resulting transparent, slightly yellow precipitate can be emulsified in a desired quantity of saline solution, or may be dried from frozen state. Storage in both forms should be at –20° C. Deutsch et al. (1964) recommended storage in dried form at –20° C under nitrogen. The activity was stable for an almost indefinite period of time.

The chemical nature of brain thromboplastin is discussed in Chapter I.

E. Partial Thromboplastin Preparations

With the description of the partial thromboplastin time technique by Langdell et al. (1953), the need for the preparation of suitable "partial thromboplastin" became apparent. Such material can be obtained from platelets, erythrocyte stroma, vegetable phospholipids, and from tissue thromboplastin. Most preparations use brain extract thromboplastin as starting material and usually acetone dried brain powder is extracted with ether. The "partial thromboplastin" is ether soluble and can be obtained by evaporating the ether. The exact procedure for the preparation of partial thromboplastin is described by Langdell and the interested reader is referred to Chapter III, p. 16.

The description of the chemical nature of partial thromboplastin, its effect on coagulation and its difference to "full" thromboplastin is outlined in Chapter I.

References

Chargaff, E., Moore, D. H., and Bendich, A. (1942). *J. Biol. Chem. 145,* 593.
Chargaff, E., Bendich, A., and Cohen, S. S. (1944). *J. Biol. Chem. 156,* 161.
Cohen, S. S., and Chargaff, E. (1941). *J. Biol. Chem. 140,* 689.
Deutsch, E., Irsigler, K., and Lomoschitz, H. (1964). *Thromb. Diath. Haemorrhag. 12,* 12.
Gollub, S., Ottolenghi, A. C., Lisbinsky, L., and Ulin, A. W. (1962). *Thromb. Diath. Haemorrhag. 7,* 95.
Hecht, E. (1955). *Biochem. Z. 326,* 325.
Hecht, E. (1965). "Lipids in Blood Clotting". Thomas, Springfield, Ill.
Hecht, E., Cho, M. H., and Seegers, W. H. (1958). *Am. J. Physiol. 193,* 584.
Langdell, R. D., Wagner, R. H., and Brinkhous, K. M. (1953). *J. Lab. Clin. Med. 41,* 637.
Owren, P. A. (1949). *Scand. J. Clin. Lab. Invest. 1,* 131.
Powell, D. E. B. (1957). *J. Clin. Pathol. 10,* 262.
Quick, A. J. (1938). *J. Am. Med. Ass. 110,* 1658.
Quick, A. J. (1942). "The Hemorrhagic Diseases and the Physiology of Hemostasis". Thomas, Springfield, Ill.
Thies, H. A. (1957). "Menschliche und tierische Gewebsthrombokinasen. Ihre Eigenschaften und ihre Bedeutung für die Anwendung von Antikoagulantien". Thieme, Stuttgart.
Williams, W. J. (1964). *J. Biol. Chem. 239,* 933.

Purification of Platelet Factor 3

Genesio Murano

I. Introduction

Ever since Denys, in 1887, proved the clinical correlation between thrombocytopenia and severe hemorrhages, several chemical entities associated with thrombocytes have been described. These have been named "factors" 1 through 10. Johnson (1967) has assessed the properties of these "factors".

In platelets, the properties of heparin neutralization (Conley et al. 1948) and the interaction of platelet material with one or more plasma components (van Creveld and Paulssen, 1952; Jürgens, 1954, and Johnson et al. 1952) have been attributed to platelet factor 4 and factor 3 respectively. Johnson et al. (1952) demonstrated that platelet factor 3 interacts with antihemophilic globulin (factor VIII) in promoting the intrinsic activation of prothrombin to thrombin. Bergsagel and Hougie (1956), showed that platelets form complexes with autoprothrombin C (factor X) in the presence of calcium ions. It was later demonstrated that platelet factor 3, specifically, is involved in this reaction (see Introductory Chapter).

Several degrees of purification of platelet factor 3 have been reported (Garret and Klein, 1957; Vandendriessche, 1959; Deutsch et al. 1957; van Creveld and Paulssen, 1952; Deutsch, 1954; Alkjaersig et al. 1955). Most of the methods result in the isolation of the lipid moiety alone. The method of Alkjaersig et al. (1955) will be described, since it is the only one that isolates platelet factor 3 in toto.

II. Method of Purification (Alkjaersig et al. 1955)

The purification of platelet factor 3 is based on the removal of impurities by adsorption after the platelets have been disrupted by ultrasonication.

1. Procedure

a. Preparation of platelets (modification of Seegers et al (1954))

1. Four liters of oxalated bovine blood (1:9) are brought to the laboratory about 1 hour after collection.
2. The blood is centrifuged in a Sharpless centrifuge at 1,800 rpm.
3. The platelet rich plasma (p.r.p.) is collected in a plastic beaker (2 liters or more).
4. The p.r.p. is centrifuged at 4,000 g for 10 min in the cold using 100 ml siliconized tubes.
5. The precipitate is suspended in a minimum amount of oxalated saline.
6. The suspension is centrifuged for 50 min in two 40 ml conical tubes at 250 g at ambient temperature.
7. Three layers are clearly distinguishable. The two top layers (containing platelets) are cautiously collected, and resuspended in a minimum amount of oxalated saline.
8. The suspension is centrifuged at ambient temperature for 20 min at 250 g.
9. The top layer is collected and resuspended in physiologic saline (0.9 %).
10. The suspension is placed in specially designed plastic tubes (Fig. 1) and centrifuged at 1,000 g for 20 min at ambient temperature. Alternatively, regular conical plastic centrifuge tubes may be used.
11. The supernatant is discarded. The platelet layer is carefully dislodged from the walls utilizing a wooden swab. A few ml of saline will facilitate this operation.
12. The platelet suspension is transferred into 12 ml siliconized, graduated, heavy duty, centrifuge tubes. A siliconized syringe and needle *must* be employed.
13. The suspension is centrifuged at 4,000 g in the cold for 15 min. The supernatant is discarded.
14. The volume of the packed platelets is recorded and diluted $\times$ 5 with 0.9 % saline.

15. The suspension is decanted into a storage vessel and may be stored at –20° C.

b. Extraction of platelet factor 3

1. A 20 ml suspension of packed platelets is thawed and diluted to 200 ml with 0.9 % saline.
2. The suspension is emulsified with a mechanical homogenizer, and subsequently subjected to ultrasonication at 800 Kc for 4 min.
3. To the suspension are added 3 ml of purified thrombin (100 U/ml). The mixture is allowed to stand at ambient temperature for 30 min. This procedure removes the "clottable factor" (Ware et al. 1948).
4. The mixture is agitated to break up the clot and centrifuged for 10 min at 3,000 g. The precipitate is discarded.
5. To the platelet preparation are added 8.5 grams of kaolin, and the mixture is agitated mechanically in a centrifuge tube for 20 min at ambient temperature. The kaolin adsorbs various impurities, including platelet factors 1 and 4, but not platelet factor 3.
6. The kaolin with adsorbed impurities is removed by centrifugation at 3,000 g for 10 min in the cold.
7. The opalescent supernatant, containing platelet factor 3 activity, is centrifuged for 2.5 hours at 106,000 g in a Spinco Ultracentrifuge.
8. The supernatant is discarded. The sediment (platelet factor 3) is suspended in 10–20 ml of 0.9 % saline or distilled water and stored at –80° C.

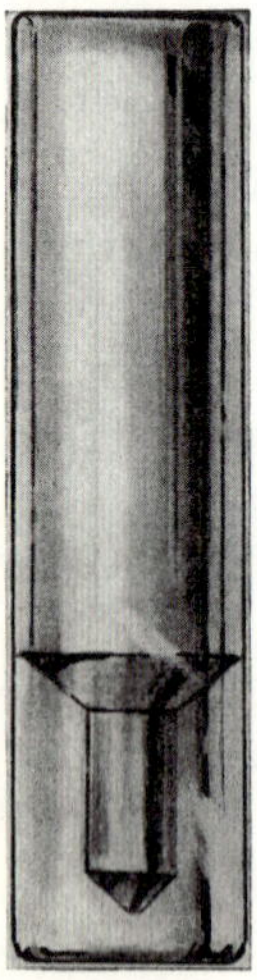

Fig. 1. Special centrifuge tube with recessed bottom.

2. Evaluation

The total activity recovered represents a 65 % yield. About 96 % of the nitrogen, tyrosine, and carbohydrate and 85 % of the phosphorous is removed by the procedure. All other coagulation factors are removed. The platelet factor 3 is easily suspended in saline solution; it can be preserved in a deep freeze, and it is stable at 56° C for at least 30 minutes.

III. Discussion

Platelet factor 3 prepared as outlined above possesses *no* platelet factor 1, 2, 4, antifibrinolysin, serotonin, clottable factor, and clot retracting activity. Its ability to retain over 30 % of the activity after heating at 100° C for 30 min, indicates a nonproteineous substance. The N/P ratio is 8.4 to 1. All indications are that it is a lipoprotein whose activity lies in the lipid moiety. Its precise mechanism of action still represents a web of chimerical conjecture. There is little doubt that platelet factor 3 functions in the intrinsic pathway of thrombin formation: Intrinsically, it mediates the complex formation of plasma factor VIII and factor IX. In addition, it mediates the complex formation of plasma factor V and active factor X. In other words, the lipid appears to function as a stage, upon which the protagonists (clotting factors) can perform.

References

Alkjaersig, N., Abe, T., and Seegers, W. H. (1955). *Am. J. Physiol. 181,* 304.
Bergsagel, D. E., and Hougie, C. (1956). *Brit. J. Haemat. 2,* 113.
Conley, C. L., Hartman, R. C., and Lalley, J. S. (1948). *Proc. Soc. Exptl. Biol. Med. 69,* 284.
Denys, J. (1887). *La Cellule 3,* 445.
Deutsch, E. (1954). *Rev. Hémat. 9,* 483.
Deutsch, E., Wawersich, E., and Franke, G. (1957). *Tromb. Diath. Haemorrhag. 1,* 397.
Garrett, J. U., and Klein, E. (1957). *Proc. Soc. Exptl. Biol. Med. 96,* 824.
Johnson, S. A., Smathers, W. M., and Schneider, C. L. (1952). *Am. J. Physiol. 170,* 631.
Johnson, S. A. (1967). *In:* "Blood Clotting Enzymology" (W. H. Seegers, ed.), pp. 379—420, Academic Press, New York.
Jürgens, R. (1954). *Arch. Exptl. Path. u. Pharmakol. 222,* 107.
Seegers, W. H., Johnson, S. A., Felin, C., and Alkjaersig, N. (1954). *Am. J. Physiol. 178,* 1.
van Creveld, S., and Paulssen, M. M. (1952). *Lancet 262,* 23.
Vandendriessche, R. (1959). *Acta Med. Scand. 165,* 217.
Ware, A. G., Fahey, J. L., and Seegers, W. H. (1948). *Am J. Physiol. 154,* 140.

CHAPTER 5

Assay for Prothrombin

HEINZ SCHRÖER

I. Introduction

The quantitative determination of prothrombin in plasma, serum or purified systems plays an important role in the investigations of the blood coagulation mechanism. Prothrombin is the mother molecule of the enzymes thrombin and autoprothrombin C and has a central position in the coagulation process.

Since there is no chemical method for the assay of prothrombin it is not possible to determine its concentration accurately. Therefore one has to depend on the amount of thrombin formed during the activation of prothrombin. However, thrombin cannot be determined chemically either*, but is instead measured by its clotting effect on fibrinogen. Therefore, it has to be assured that all prothrombin is converted to thrombin, and that the latter is present in full activity during the assay procedure. "Two-stage methods" for the determination of prothrombin as first described by Warner et al. (1936) are based on this basic principle.

"One-stage assays" for prothrombin do not comply with this presupposition. However, there is an approximate proportionality between the clotting time and the prothrombin concentration of a one-stage test system provided the system is standardized and contains all procoagulant components in excess with the exception of prothrombin. This offers the possibility to determine the relative prothrombin content of a substrate by comparing the clotting times measured with the values obtained by assaying different dilutions of a normal plasma. The one-stage prothrombin time methods require only little expenditure of time, energy and money, but they are not very specific. Their accuracy, however, has been found sufficient for many clinical purposes. Their inaccuracy becomes especially evident when prothrombin-rich plasma – for instance the plasma of certain animals is assayed. For determining the activity of purified prothrombin one-stage methods are not suitable.

The thrombin concentration of a solution is usually determined by the velocity with which fibrinogen is converted to fibrin. Under standardized conditions a certain clotting time corresponds to a certain thrombin activity. It is up to the individual investigator to express the activity as the reciprocal value of the clotting time, or in percent of the thrombin potential of a normal plasma, or to assign a unit to a certain clotting time and convert clotting times into units of thrombin. For biochemical purposes the activity in thrombin units is preferred because this allows an accurate standardization as well as the creation of quantitative relationships between thrombin units and units of other clotting components of a test system.

Since the thrombin potential of plasma is directly dependent upon the prothrombin concentration, the activities of prothrombin and thrombin can be expressed by one and the same unit of measure. According to the specific conditions established by Seegers and Smith (1942) a prothrombin unit is defined as the amount of prothrombin which, after complete conversion to thrombin, converts 1 ml of a standardized fibrinogen solution into fibrin at 28° C in 15 seconds (Iowa unit). A second thrombin (prothrombin) unit frequently used

---

* An indirect chemical determination of thrombin activity is based on the quantitative determination of N-terminal glycine which appears during the thrombin-induced conversion of purified fibrinogen to fibrin (Jorpes et al. 1958; Magnuson, 1958, 1960).

is the National Institutes of Health (NIH) unit; it is defined as the amount of thrombin which coagulates 1 ml of a standardized 1 % human fraction I (Cohn) at 25° C in 45 seconds. 1 NIH unit is equivalent to 1.25 Iowa units. Other assigned units (Bayerle and Marx, 1949; Gerendás, 1948; Owren, 1947) are no longer in use.

II. Original Two-Stage Procedure

The "classical" two-stage method of Warner et al. (1936), modified by Ware and Seegers (1949), is the basic procedure for all two-stage methods later on developed. In those laboratories where this procedure is performed several times a day it has given an excellent account of itself, and is among the most reliable methods for the quantitative determination of prothrombin concentrations. In the following this two-stage method is described taking into account some technical improvements introduced by Seegers (1962).

A. Principle

In a diluted sample containing prothrombin a complete conversion to thrombin is obtained by the addition of tissue thromboplastin, Ac-globulin (factor V) and calcium ions in optimal concentration and at standard pH. At regular time-intervals small amounts of the activation mixture are added to a standard solution of fibrinogen and the clotting times measured. After a few minutes of activation shortest clotting times will be reached indicating a maximum thrombin concentration in the mixture. From these clotting times the prothrombin concentration is calculated in units/ml taking into account the dilutions of plasma.

If prothrombin is determined in plasma, the plasma has to be defibrinated first by the addition of a small amount of thrombin because the plasma fibrinogen would otherwise interfere with the test results. After addition of thrombin the formed clot is removed, and the defibrinated plasma is allowed to stand for a few minutes in order for the antithrombin to neutralize the excess traces of thrombin.

The sample to be assayed is so diluted that clotting takes place within a range of 15 seconds. In this range the relationship between clotting time and thrombin concentration is optimal (a change of 1 second means approximately a 10 % change in thrombin concentration). Normal human plasma usually has to be diluted 250 times because it contains about 250 ± 50 Iowa units/ml.

B. Reagents

1. Tissue Thromboplastin

Extracts of brain or lung tissue are used. The commercial thromboplastin preparations from rabbit or monkey brain are prepared according to the recommendations of the manufacturer. In the original two-stage prothrombin assay lung extract was used as thromboplastin.

To obtain lung extract thromboplastin, a bovine lung is dissected free of trachea, bronchi and major blood vessels and is ground through a domestic meat grinder. The ground material is mixed with an equal amount of physiological saline solution. This mixture is reground to insure complete mixing. The resulting suspension is placed in the refrigerator, and an extract is allowed to form during the next 24 hours. Occasional stirring is necessary. The first extract is strained through gauze and the filtrate is discarded. The remaining crude homogenate is mixed with another equal volume of saline, extracted for 48 hours at 4° C and filtered. The filtrate is homogenized, and at this stage can be used for analyses. As a preservative, phenol is added to a final concentration of 0.5 % to prevent bacterial growth. If the lung thromboplastin is to be saved for a longer time it can be frozen before mixing with phenol. Stability and purity of this reagent can be improved by repeated sedimentation at high speed centrifugation and resuspension in physiological saline (Chargaff et al. 1942), see also Chapter IV, p. 170.

2. Acacia

Fine ground acacia is dissolved in physiological saline solution to a concentration of 15 %. This procedure is slow, and continuous mechanical stirring is necessary to obtain suspension of the material. Unsoluble debris is removed by light centrifugation. As the commercial acacia contains calcium in various amounts the calcium content must be determined for each new supply. Little variations in the calcium content can be neglected; it is only important that the calcium concentration of the prothrombin converting incubation mixture is within the optimal range (0.0025–0.01).

3. Calcium Chloride

0.7–0.8 % (the definite concentration depends on the calcium content of the acacia batch used) in physiological saline solution is used.

4. Imidazole

1.75 gm imidazole is dissolved in 90 ml 0.1 N hydrochloric acid and diluted to 100 ml volume with distilled water. If the pH is not 7.2–7.4 which is the optimal range for the determinations, it can be adjusted with a few drops of strong hydrochloric acid or sodium hydroxide.

5. Thrombin for Defibrination

By dissolving commercial thrombin preparations in distilled water a solution is prepared which should have an activity of 200 units/ml. This solution is mixed with an equal volume of glycerol to stabilize thrombin activity (Milstone, 1942; Seegers, 1944). When stored at 4° C the thrombin retains sufficient activity for months.

6. $BaCO_3$ Adsorbed Bovine Serum (source of Ac-globulin)

Bovine blood is collected and allowed to clot. After 1–2 hours centrifuge for 20 minutes at 600 g and remove serum. In order to remove the remaining prothrombin, 200 mg barium carbonate are mixed with 5 ml serum. Agitate for about 10 minutes at room temperature, and remove the barium carbonate by centrifugation. The prothrombin free bovine serum retains its Ac-globulin activity at room temperature for about 18 hours; at 5° C for about 2—3 weeks, at –10 to –20° C for at least a year. When diluted 600 times it furnishes sufficient Ac-globulin in the two-stage procedure to provide for maximum conversion of prothrombin to thrombin. The adsorbed serum should be stored in small portions (about 1 ml) in the deep freezer.

7. Fibrinogen

Purified bovine fibrinogen prepared by any method is used in 1 % solution (concentration data on the basis of clottable protein). A mixture of 9 parts physiological saline solution and 1 part imidazole buffer serves as solvent. Each new solution is tested for its reactivity by using the solution as the clotting substrate in the two-stage assay of a standard bovine plasma. If the result corresponds to the normal prothrombin content of this bovine plasma standard (262 U/ml) the reactivity of the fibinogen is considered to be normal; its "correction factor" (see below) is 1.0. If the result is greater than 262, the correction factor is less than 1.0. Conversely, if the result is lower than 262, the correction factor is greater than 1.0. The correction factor for a given fibrinogen is always used in the two-stage prothrombin assay.

8. Standard Bovine Plasma

Equal volumes of plasma from five cows are mixed. The prothrombin content of this "standard plasma" can be considered as constant (Ware and Seegers, 1949; Seegers, 1962); it is 262 units/ml by definition. In the frozen state (stored in 1 ml portions at –10 to –20° C) it remains stabile for more than 2 years.

C. Preparation of mixtures

Shortely before the assay is performed the following solutions are prepared:

1. Thromboplastin-calcium-mixture

1 ml tissue thromboplastin is suspended in 4 ml physiological saline solution. To this suspension 10 ml of the following mixture are added:

15 % Acacia, dissolved in physiol. saline	2 parts
$CaCl_2$ (0.7–0.8 %**), dissolved in physiol. saline	2 parts
Imidazole buffer, pH 7.2	1 part
Physiol. saline	1 part

** The concentration used depends on the calcium content of the acacia solution.

The latter mixture may be prepared ahead of time and stored in the refrigerator since it is also used for the determination of thrombin activity.

2. Diluted Adsorbed Bovine Serum (1:75)

A 14.8 ml volume of physiological saline solution is thoroughly mixed with 0.2 ml of the barium carbonate-treated bovine serum. To prevent an untimely inactivation of the Ac-globulin, the test tube with the diluted serum is stored in ice water.

D. Performance of the Two-Stage Assay

1. Defibrination of the Plasma

A mixture is prepared of 0.4 ml 0.9% NaCl solution +0.1 ml thrombin solution (100 units/ml) +0.5 ml plasma in a small glass tube (10 × 75 mm). Within 15–20 seconds fibrin forms which is wound out as it forms with an applicator stick. The defibrinated plasma is allowed to stand for 10 minutes at room temperature.

2. Dilution and Addition of Ac-globulin

To 2.4 ml of the diluted bovine serum (1:75) 0.1 ml of the defibrinated plasma is added. Mix well.

3. Preparation of the Reaction Mixture (Prothrombin-Thrombin Conversion)

A 1.0 ml sample of the diluted defibrinated plasma is mixed thoroughly with 3.0 ml of the thromboplastin-calcium mixture. Time the beginning of this reaction by a stop-watch. The test tube containing the reaction mixture is placed into a water bath of 28° C.

4. Clotting of Fibrinogen to Measure Thrombin Formation

At 1–2 minutes intervals, 0.4 ml of the incubation mixture is pipetted into a test tube (10 × 75 mm) containing 0.1 ml of the 1% fibrinogen solution. The clotting times are measured by a second stop-watch. Usually, the shortest clotting times are obtained after 4–6 minutes. At this time the thrombin formation in the reaction mixture has reached its maximum. The clotting times should be around 15 seconds, corresponding to a thrombin activity of 1 unit/ml in the test system.

E. Calculation of Activity in Units/ml

1. Plasma dilution with defibrination	1:2
2. Dilution with saline-Ac-globulin diulent	1:25
3. Dilution with the reaction mixture	1:4
4. Dilution with the fibrinogen	1:1.25
Total dilution	1:250

Thus, the prothrombin activity of the plasma assayed is 250 units/ml, provided the clotting time was exactly 15.0 seconds, and the reactivity of the fibrinogen used was normal.

If the clotting time diverges from the 15 second value, the unit number has to be multiplied with a factor resulting from the relation between clotting time and thrombin concentration (Table 1). However, the calculation offers reliable values only if the shortest clotting times are within the range of 13 to 17 seconds. At higher deviations the test has to be repeated with the use of another total dilution whereby the variation of the dilution should be placed in step D-2 by changing the relationship (1:25) between the defibrinated plasma and the diluted bovine serum. A fairly correct dilution range can be predicted as follows: 10 seconds clotting – dilute twice as much; 22 seconds clotting – dilute half as much.

Example for calculation: The shortest clotting time was 13.0 seconds. The corresponding unit conversion factor is 1.2. If the dilution was 250 times, the prothrombin activity of the plasma assayed was 250 × 1.2 = 300 units/ml. This value can also be related to the prothrombin activity of a normal plasma and expressed in percent of normal.

F. Use of Correction Factor

In order to eliminate variations in reagents, especially fibrinogen, a "fibrinogen correction factor" may be helpful. The two-stage procedure is performed on a standard bovine plasma with the use of the listed reagents and fibrinogen. The quotient of the activity of the stan-

Table 1: Concentration of Thrombin Related to Clotting Time

Seconds	Units	Seconds	Units	Seconds	Units	Seconds	Units
11.0	1.50	15.0	1.00	19.0	0.75	23.0	0.65
.2	1.47	.2	0.97	.2	0.74	.2	0.64
.4	1.44	.4	0.96	.4	0.73	.4	0.64
.6	1.41	.6	0.95	.6	0.73	.6	0.64
.8	1.38	.8	0.94	.8	0.72	.8	0.64
12.0	1.34	16.0	0.92	20.0	0.72	24.0	0.64
.2	1.31	.2	0.91	.2	0.72	.2	0.63
.4	1.28	.4	0.89	.4	0.71	.4	0.63
.6	1.25	.6	0.88	.6	0.71	.6	0.63
.8	1.23	.8	0.86	.8	0.70	.8	0.61
13.0	1.20	17.0	0.85	21.0	0.70	25.0	0.60
.2	1.17	.2	0.84	.2	0.69	26.0	0.49
.4	1.16	.4	0.83	.4	0.68	27.0	0.47
.6	1.13	.6	0.82	.6	0.68	28.0	0.44
.8	1.12	.8	0.81	.8	0.68	29.0	0.43
14.0	1.10	18.0	0.80	22.0	0.67	30.0	0.40
.2	1.07	.2	0.79	.2	0.66	31.0	0.38
.4	1.05	.4	0.77	.4	0.66	33.0	0.34
.6	1.03	.6	0.76	.6	0.65	35.0	0.31
.8	1.02	.8	0.76	.8	0.65	37.0	0.28

dard plasma (262 units/ml) and the activity really measured using the given reagents is the correction factor.

Example: The prothrombin activity determined on a standard plasma was 250 units/ml. Thus, the fibrinogen correction factor is 262/250 = 1.05.

Using such a "correction factor" it is possible to compare the assay results not only of different investigators but also of different laboratories with each other. The accuracy becomes still greater when each analyst determines his own correction factor.

Table 2:
1. Determination of the Fibrinogen Correction Factor

Material	Incubation time (min)	Clotting time (sec)	Dilution and Calculations
Standard	2	38.0	Total dilution: 1:250
bovine	4	17.2	
plasma,	5	15.2	15.0 sec = 1.00 unit
262 U/ml	6	15.0*	1.00** × 250 = 250 U/ml
(by	7	15.2	Fibrinogen correction
definition)			factor: 262/250 = *1.05*
	8	15.8	

* Shortest clotting time
** Unit conversion factor (see table 1)

G. Example for Recording Data and Calculations

The results and calculations of the two-stage procedure are best recorded in tabular form (Seegers, 1962) (Tables 2 and 3).

H. Remarks

The increase of the clotting time after it had reached its shortest value during the incubation of the reaction mixture is due to anti-

Table 3:
2. Prothrombin Assay on the Unknown Plasma

Material	Incubation time (min)	Clotting time (sec)	Dilution and Calculation
Human	2	30.9	Dilution steps:
plasma			1:2; 1:25; 1:4; 1:1.25
XY	3	19.6	
	4	16.8	
	5	15.2	Total dilution: 1:250
	5.5	14.4	14.2 sec = 1.07 units
	6	14.2*	1.07** × 250 = 267 U/ml
	6.5	14.3	
	7	15.0	1.05*** × 267 = 280 U/ml
	8	15.6	

* Shortest clotting time
** Unit conversion factor (see table 1)
*** Fibrinogen correction factor

thrombin which is still slightly active, although the plasma has been diluted several hundred times. With low plasma dilutions antithrombin becomes more of a consideration. This has to be taken into account when a plasma with a very low prothrombin content is to be assayed because such a plasma cannot be tested using considerable dilutions. In those cases the clotting times should be measured in about half-minute intervals.

If the prothrombin assay is performed on an unknown plasma sample a correction should be made for the dilution introduced by the anticoagulant. This involves the hematocrit value. For instance, if the hematocrit is 40% for blood which had been mixed with an anticoagulant in the usual way (9 parts of blood and 1 part of anticoagulant), each 10 ml of blood will contain 4 ml cells and 6 ml diluted plasma. Of this diluted plasma 1 ml is anticoagulant, so the actual prothrombin value of the unknown plasma is multiplied by $^6/_5$. This correction is not necessary in routine work unless the unknown has a very abnormal hematocrit value.

When the two-stage method is used to determine the prothrombin content in purified prothrombin solutions, the initial defibrination procedure is omitted. Instead, the purified prothrombin solution is diluted with physiological saline solution corresponding to the prothrombin concentration to be expected. However, the dilution in the second step (mixing with diluted serum) should always be kept constant at 1:10 instead of 1:25.

III. Other Two-Stage Assays

In attempts to reduce the expenditure of the two-stage method, and if possible, to increase its accuracy, different modifications of the original procedure have been introduced (Marbet and Winterstein, 1954; Rieben, 1947b, 1951; Schwick and Störiko, 1966). The simplifications suggested consist essentially in the possible use of commercially available reagents, and in renouncing certain methodical details which do not necessarily influence the reliability of the results. The initial plasma defibrination or the use of thrombin respectively may be omitted, and instead, the unknown plasma can be directly diluted (1:30 or 1:50) with physiological saline solution. As a relatively high dilution of plasma is reached the fibrin formation in the mixture is insignificant; the loss of thrombin activity due to adsorption on fibrin does not or not considerably effect the result. The addition of acacia to the reaction mixture is not necessary either, but it aids in the determination of the clotting time because, in the presence of acacia, the change from the fluid to the gelatinous state occurs very rapidly, thus facilitating a better reading of the end-point of the clotting time. No advantage can be seen in the use of partially purified preparations of factor V instead of the $BaCO_3$-adsorbed bovine serum, all the more as it is generally known that the activity of those purified preparations undergoes considerable changes. In the original two-stage method socalled "factor VII" is not considered because this "cofactor of tissue thromboplastin" (Koller et al. 1951, 1952) is only a prothrombin conversion accelerator, but does not increase the thrombin yield.

A procedure frequently used is the two-stage method of Schultze and Schwick (1953) or Schwick and Störiko (1966). This method first developed by Rieben (1946a, 1947b, 1951), later modified by Schultze (1949, 1950) has the practical advantage that all reagents are commercially available (Behringwerke, Marburg, Germany). The initial defibrination of the unknown plasma as well as the use of reagents to enhance the sensitivity of fibrinogen are omitted. Instead of imidazole buffer different barbiturate-acetate buffers (pH 7.6 and pH 6.7) are used. Figure 1 illustrates the assay. Corresponding to the original two-stage method the thrombin activity is tested on a solution of purified bovine fibrinogen (0.6%) by measuring the shortest clotting time during the incubation of the reaction mixture. The prothrombin activity is not expressed in units/ml, but in percent of normal and can be calculated from a standard curve (Fig. 2).

A number of attempts have been made to eliminate the disturbing influence of antithrombin on the prothrombin assay (Rieben, 1946a, 1946b, 1947a; Sternberger, 1947; Marbet and Winterstein, 1954, 1955; Jürgens and Beller,

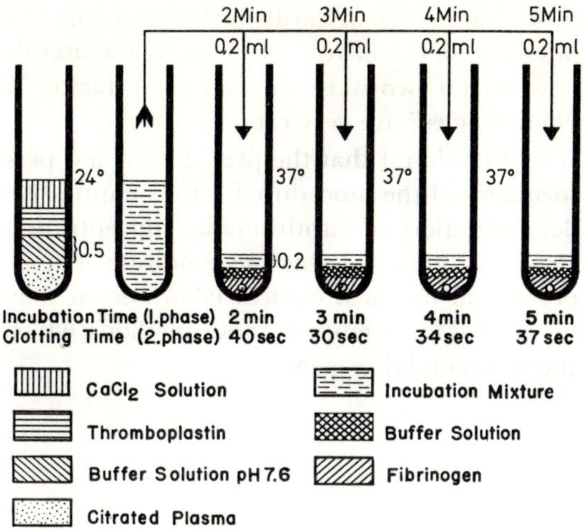

Fig. 1. Two-stage prothrombin assay of Schultze and Schwick (1953). The activation mixture (first tube from the left side) contains all components in equal amounts. The citrated plasma (1 part of 3.8% sodium citrate solution + 9 parts of blood) is previously diluted 1:30 or 1:50 with physiological saline solution. The details are described by Schwick and Störiko (1966).

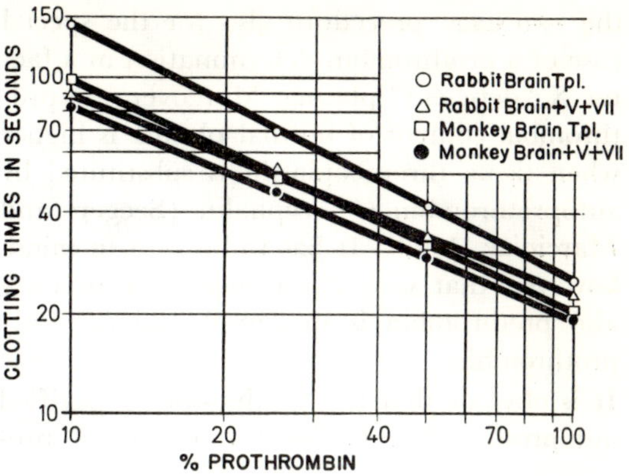

Fig. 2. Standard curves for the two-stage prothrombin assay of Schultze and Schwick (1953). The plasma was diluted 1:30 (according to Schwick and Störiko [1966]).

1959; Biggs and MacFarlane, 1962), but its actual value is uncertain.

In the original two-stage method, modified by Ware and Seegers (1949) the effect of antithrombin is reduced by a sum of different factors:

1. Dilution of plasma
2. The use of a relatively low reaction-temperature (28° C)
3. Indirectly, by the presence of acacia in the reaction mixture; the acacia increases the sensitivity of the fibrinogen to thrombin, thus allowing a greater dilution of the plasma.

IV. Role of Autoprothrombin C in the Assays

Autoprothrombin C (Marciniak and Seegers, 1962) is the most powerful catalyst of prothrombin activation. It is probably identical with active factor X (Esnouf and Williams, 1962; Lechner and Deutsch, 1965). Its presence in the activation mixture of the two-stage procedure has to be regarded as being essential because no thrombin can be generated from prothrombin without autoprothrombin C (Mammen, 1968). During the two-stage analysis of prothrombin, autoprothrombin C is generated from either prothrombin or from autoprothrombin III according to the following equation (Marciniak and Seegers, 1965):

$$\text{Autoprothrombin III} \xrightarrow[\text{Thromboplastin}]{Ca^{++}} \text{Autoprothrombin C}$$

Therefore, under normal circumstances, it is not necessary to add autoprothrombin C to the reaction mixture.

On the other hand, Hougie et al. (1957) observed that in a factor X "deficient" plasma the conversion of prothrombin to thrombin by tissue thromboplastin and calcium was incomplete; normal serum which is supposed to be a potential source for autoprothrombin C (Seegers, 1962), could correct this "deficiency". This finding is in accordance with an observation of Seegers and Marciniak (1962) who found that in the two-stage analysis of a factor X "deficient" plasma, the thrombin yield as well as the rate of thrombin formation could be fully normalized by the use of autoprothrombin C + cephalin instead of tissue thromboplastin. Therefore, it would be ideal to generally add autoprothrombin C to the reaction mixture in order to guarantee the reliability of the two-stage procedure also for the special case of a prothrombin determination in a factor X "deficient" plasma. Moreover, the prothrombin content of normal plasma is higher when tissue thromboplastin is substituted by autoprothrombin C + cephalin (Seegers and Marciniak, 1962). It has to be kept in mind, however, that with this change in procedure also prethrombin is measured and not only prothrombin.

It is obvious that the routine-use of purified autoprothrombin C for the two-stage prothrombin assay can hardly be realized, but this of course does not restrict seriously the usefulness of the two-stage method since factor X "deficiencies" are very rare.

It is of no doubt that the preparation and performance of the procedure for the quantitative determination of prothrombin concentration requires a relatively high expenditure. For its occasional use in a clinical laboratory it may be advisable to employ those methods which use commercial reagents.

References

Bayerle, H., and Marx, R. (1949). *Hoppe-Seylers Z. Physiol. Chem. 283,* 248.

Biggs, R., and MacFarlane, R. G. (1962). "Human Blood Coagulation and its Disorders". 3rd edition, Blackwell, Oxford.

Chargaff, E., Moore, D. H., and Bendich, A. (1942). *J. Biol. Chem. 145,* 593.

Esnouf, M. P., and Williams, W. U. (1962). *Biochem. J. 84,* 62.

Gerendás, M. (1948). *Acta Physiol. Hung. 1,* 4.

Hougie, C., Barrow, E. M. and Graham, J. B. (1957). *J. Clin. Invest. 36,* 485.

Jorpes, E., Vrethammer, T., Ohmann, B., and Blombäck, B. (1958). *J. Pharm. Pharmacol. 10,* 561.

Jürgens, J., and Beller, F. K. (1959). "Klinische Methoden der Blutgerinnungsanalyse". Thieme, Stuttgart.

Koller, F., Loeliger, A., and Duckert, F. (1951). *Acta Haematol. 6,* 1.

Koller, F., Loeliger, A., and Duckert, F. (1952). *Rev. Hematol. 7,* 156.

Lechner, K., and Deutsch, E. (1965). *Thromb. Diath. Haemorrhag. 13,* 314.

Magnusson, S. (1958). *Acta Chem. Scand. 12,* 355.

Magnusson, S. (1960). *Thromb. Diath. Haemorrhag. 4,* 167.

Mammen, E. F. (1968). *Thromb. Diath. Haemorrhag. Suppl. 25,* 15.

Marbet, R., and Winterstein, A. (1954). "Prothrombin" Hoffmann-LaRoche, Basel.

Marbet, A., and Winterstein, A. (1955). *Medizinische 1,* 1.

Marciniak, E., and Seegers, W. H. (1962). *Can. J. Biochem. Physiol. 40,* 597.

Marciniak, E., and Seegers, W. H. (1965). *New Istanbul Contrib. Clin. Sci. 8,* 117.

Milstone, H. (1942). *J. Gen. Physiol. 25,* 679.

Owren, P. A. (1947). "The Coagulation of Blood". Gundersen, Oslo.

Quivy, D., and Breynaert, R. (1952). *Rev. Hematol. 7,* 122.

Rieben, W. K. (1946a). *Helv. Med. Acta 13,* 295.

Rieben, W. K. (1946b). *Schweiz. Med. Wochschr. 76,* 725.

Rieben, W. K. (1947a). "Beiträge zur Kenntnis der Blutgerinnung". Schwabe, Basel.

Rieben, W. K. (1947b). *Bull. Soc. Chim. Biol. 29,* 111

Rieben, W. K. (1951). *Wien. Med. Wochschr. 38,* 670.

Schultze, H. E. (1949). *Naunyn-Schmiedebergs Arch. Exptl. Pathol. Pharmakol. 207,* 173.

Schultze, H. E. (1950). *Deutsch. Med. Wochschr. 75,* 607.

Schultze, H. E., and Schwick, G. (1953). *Medizinische 1354,* 1386.

Schwick, H. G., and Störiko, K. (1966). Beiträge zur Diagnostik von Gerinnungsstörungen". Laboratoriumsblätter für die Medizinische Diagnostik, Behringwerke, Marburg.

Seegers, W. H. (1944). *Arch. Biochem. 3,* 363.

Seegers, W. H. (1962). "Prothrombin". Harvard Univ. Press, Cambridge.

Seegers, W. H., and Marciniak, E. (1962). *Thromb. Diath. Haemorrhag. 8,* 1.

Seegers, W. H., and Smith, H. P. (1942). *Am. J. Physiol. 137,* 348.

Sternberger, L. A. (1947). *Brit. J. Exp. Pathol. 28,* 168.

Ware, A. G. and Seegers, W. H. (1949). *Am. J. Clin. Pathol. 19,* 471.

Warner, E. D., Brinkhous, K. M., and Smith, H. P. (1936). *Am. J. Physiol. 114,* 667.

Thrombin Clotting Assays

Zbigniew S. Latallo

I. Introduction

Thrombin clotting assays reflect the unique ability of this enzyme to convert fibrinogen into fibrin. This conversion involves a number of reactions which are conventionally divided into three steps (Scheraga and Laskowski, 1957).

Step 1. Proteolysis $F \overset{T}{\rightleftharpoons} f + P$ (1)
Step 2. Polymerization $nf \rightleftharpoons f_n$ (2)
Step 3. Clotting $mf_n \rightleftharpoons \text{fibrin}$ (3)
(F = fibrinogen, T = thrombin, f = fibrin monomer, P = fibrinopeptides, n and m variable numbers).

Thrombin is required only for the proteolytic step. Proteolysis of fibrinogen by this enzyme is highly specific and very limited. It consists in liberating about 3% of the total Nitrogen present in the substrate in the form of fibrinopeptides A and B. Two moles of each fibrinopeptide are released from one mole of fibrinogen. The proteolytic reactions may be written as follows:

$$F \rightleftharpoons f_B + P_A \quad (5)$$
$$f_B \rightleftharpoons f + P_B \quad (4)$$
$$F \rightleftharpoons f_A + P_B \quad (6)$$
$$f_A \rightleftharpoons f + P_A \quad (7)$$

(P_A and P_B = fibrinopeptides, f_B = fibrinogen deprived of P_A only, f_A = fibrinogen deprived of P_B only).

The sequence of these reactions is not exactly known except that at the very initial stage (4) the liberation of P_A occurs much faster than that of P_B (Bettelheim, 1956, Blombäck and Yamashina, 1957).

Even greater diversity of reactions occurs in steps 2 and 3. Not only the final fibrin monomer f but also its intermediate f_B is capable of polymerization and spontaneous clotting (Blombäck et al. 1957). On the other hand both f and f_B may copolymerize with F and under certain conditions will not form a clot (Shainoff and Page, 1962; Lipinski et al. 1967).

II. Methods

Three types of assays may be employed for measurement of the clotting activity of thrombin: Determination of the rate of fibrinogen to fibrin monomer conversion; measurement of fibrin gel formation e. g. the sum total of steps 1, 2 and 3; and the titration of the enzyme with a suitable stoichiometric inhibitor.

A. Determination of the Rate of Fibrinogen to Fibrin Monomer Conversion

Two approaches for the measurement of the rate of step 1 reaction have been proposed. Either the rate of release of nonprotein (i. e. fibrinopeptide) nitrogen can be determined (Lorand, 1951; Laskowski et al. 1956), or the rate of appearance of N-terminal glycine in fibrin monomer can be registered (Blombäck and Yamashina, 1957; Blombäck, 1958; Ehrenpreis et al. 1958).

Although these two approaches have proven valuable in providing information about the kinetics of the initial phases of the fibrinogen-fibrin conversion, the methods are too cumbersome for routine purposes.

B. Determination by Fibrin Gel Formation

This type of assay has been traditionally employed for measuring thrombin activity and is still widely used. An aliquot of unknown thrombin solution is mixed with a standard solution of fibrinogen, and the time elapsed before visible gel formation is recorded. Although the first fibrin is visible long before completion of gelation, experience has shown that the use of this endpoint results in a sensitive method for thrombin activity.

The observation by Ferry and Morrison (1947) that tensile strength or rigidity in a fibrinogen-thrombin coagulation mixture changes predictably during clotting, as well as the observation by Nygaard (1941) indicating that reproducible changes in optical density occur under similar conditions, have led to the introduction of various instrumental procedures for the assay of thrombin activity (Nygaard, 1941; Burstein and Guinand, 1955). However, simple visual registration of the moment of clot formation in a test tube seems to be a method of equal accuracy although somewhat more prone to human error. Early thrombin assays employed either oxalated (Mellanby, 1933; Astrup and Darling, 1941) or citrated plasma (Lenggenhager, 1940) as the source of fibrinogen. Antithrombins and prothrombin greatly influence the clotting times and limit application of plasma as a substrate for thrombin. Great species variations in the amount of thrombin required to clot 1 ml of plasma in 15 seconds have been observed (Seegers and Smith, 1942).

1. Procedure of Seegers and Smith (1942)

Warner et al. (1936) and Smith et al. (1937) first proposed a thrombin assay based on a fixed clotting time of a standardized fibrinogen preparation. Seegers and Smith (1942) subsequently defined the conditions which formed the basis for many current assays. The units of thrombin are either expressed in Iowa or N.I.H. units. An Iowa unit is that amount of thrombin which will clot 1.0 ml of a standardized fibrinogen solution in 15 seconds at 28° C. An N.I.H. unit is the amount of thrombin which converts 1 ml of fibrinogen (Cohn Fraction I) at 25° C to fibrin in 45 sec. One N.I.H. unit is equal to 1.25 Iowa units (Seegers, 1962).

a. Reagents: Fibrinogen can be prepared from oxalated prothrombin free bovine plasma by ammonium sulphate precipitation (Seegers and Smith, 1942), or by any other procedure (see Chapter VI, p. 229).

Acacia: Calcium is removed from a 5 % solution of commercial acacia by precipitation with potassium oxalate. Upon centrifugation, the excess of oxalate is removed by dialysis and the acacia precipitated and dried with ethanol.

Imidazole Buffer: 1.75 gm of imidazole is dissolved in 90 ml of 0.1 N HCl and diluted to 100 ml with water. The pH should be 7.25.

Reaction Mixture:

15 % acacia in 0.9 % NaCl	2 parts
1 % $CaCl_2$ in 0.9 % NaCl	1 part
Imidazole buffer	1 part
0.9 % NaCl	1 part

Before use 5 ml of the reaction mixture are diluted with 10 ml of 0.9 % saline.

b. Performance of the test and calculation: Place 0.3 ml of the diluted reaction mixture in a 12 × 75 mm clean test tube containing 0.1 ml of the fibrinogen substrate and add 0.1 ml thrombin solution (the dilution of the thrombin will vary and must be made in 0.9 % NaCl). Start the stop watch as the thrombin is blown into the tube. The first appearance of fibrin is the end point. When a 15 second clotting time is obtained on repeated tests at 28° C, the thrombin concentration in the final clotting mixture is one unit. If the clotting is not exactly 15 sec, but in the range of 13 to 17 sec, the conversion table (Chapter V, p. 179) may be used to convert clotting times into thrombin units; if, on the other hand the clotting times are less than 13 sec or greater than 17 sec appropriate dilutions of the sample to be tested must be made. These dilutions have to be taken into account when calculating the thrombin activity of the unknown sample.

c. Comments

Fibrinogen preparations employed in this procedure may vary in terms of purity and therefore clottability. These variations make it necessary to restandardize every new batch of fibrinogen to be used. Samples of a standard thrombin preparation are made available by the N.I.H. The potencies of these standards as designated on the label are stated to be accurate within a standard error of ±4.5 %.

2. Author's Procedure

The following procedure employs the use of highly purified fibrinogen. Bovine fibrinogen must contain at least 97 % clottable protein. Fibrinogen prepared according to Kekwick et al. (1955) or Blombäck and Blombäck

(1956) are equally suitable. A stock solution of 1.8 % fibrinogen in 0.3 M NaCl is kept frozen at –20° C. When stored under these conditions no appreciable deterioration is observed over a period of several months. Prior to testing the stock solution is thawed at 37° C for 30 min and subsequently diluted with 3 volumes of 0.05 M Tris-HCl buffer containing 0.1 M NaCl, pH 7.4 and 1 volume of distilled water. Aliquots of 0.5 ml are pipetted into clean glass test tubes of 8 mm internal diameter and placed in a water bath at 37° C.
Serial dilutions of thrombin (range 2–30 units/ml) are made with the Tris-HCl buffer in siliconized or paraffinized tubes, prewarmed and 0.1 ml aliquots of each dilution added to the fibrinogen solution. A stop watch is simultaneously started, the content of the tube mixed thoroughly and the time of the appearance of the clot recorded. Tris buffer may be substituted by imidazole buffer of the same molarity. In order to convert clotting times into thrombin units, serial dilutions of reference thrombin are utilized to plot a standard calibration curve. A double logarithmic plot of clotting times in seconds versus thrombin units will give a straight line for clotting time values between 10 and 100 sec. Thrombin activity of an unknown sample can be read directly off the standard calibration curve.

3. General Comments

The thrombin-fibrinogen interaction is for one influenced by factors which influence enzyme reactions in general and is also determined by specific conditions which influence the nonenzymatic polymerization phase. The temperature optimum for the overall reaction lies by 40° C. The optimal ionic strength for the proteolytic action of thrombin is 0.1 (Blombäck, 1958). Increasing the ionic strength delays clotting, an effect which may be due to inhibition of polymerization (Latallo et al. 1962). Although calcium ions are not required for thrombin action, they enhance the rate of polymerization of fibrin monomer. Conversely phosphate and citrate ions decrease polymerization rates (Latallo, 1966). Optimum pH for thrombin proteolysis is between 8.5 and 9.0 (Blombäck, 1958), the optimum pH for polymerization is around 6.0 (Latallo et al. 1962). The apparent pH optimum for the clotting process is pH 6.5 to 7.5, depending on ionic strength and fibrinogen concentration.
The optimum fibrinogen concentration in the final mixture lies between 0.1 and 0.4 %. An increase of the fibrinogen concentration results in a prolongation of the clotting times.

C. Titration with Hirudin

1. Principle

A new approach to the determination of thrombin clotting potency was proposed by Markwardt (1957a, 1963). It is based on titration of the enzyme with its specific inhibitor hirudin. Hirudin has been obtained in a highly purified state (Markwardt, 1957b, 1963) and has been shown to form a stoichiometric complex with thrombin. For practical purposes, the complex does not dissociate at pH 7.4 and 20° C.
Thrombin affinity to hirudin is higher than its affinity to fibrinogen. The formation of the hirudin-thrombin complex therefore occurs even in the presence of fibrinogen. Hirudin is a protein of molecular weight of 16,000 ± 1,000. It is soluble in distilled water. One mg of hirudin neutralizes 8,500 units of thrombin. Its potency is expressed in antithrombin (AT) units: 1 AT unit neutralizes 1 NIH unit of thrombin.

2. Procedure

A sample of 0.1 ml of hirudin solution containing 100 AT units/ml is mixed with 0.2 ml of 0.5 % fibrinogen in Tris buffer, pH 7.4. Aliquots of 0.005 ml of the thrombin solution to be tested are added to the mixture at 1 min intervals until a clot is formed. This end point indicates that a total of 10 units of thrombin has been exceeded. For high accuracy, thrombin should be so diluted to make a total volume added of no less than 0.1 ml. The method as described obviates many difficulties inherent in the classical clotting time assays. Plasma may be used as a source of fibrinogen as well.

References

Astrup, T., and Darling, S. (1941). *Acta Physiol. Scand.* *2*, 22.

Bettelheim, F. R. (1956). *Biochim. Biophys. Acta 19*, 121.

Blombäck, B. (1958). *Arkiv Kemi 12*, 321.

Blombäck, B., and Blombäck, M. (1956). *Arkiv Kemi 10*, 415.

Blombäck, B., and Yamashina, I. (1957). *Acta Chem. Scand. 11*, 194.

Blombäck, B., Blombäck, M., and Nilsson, I. M. (1957). *Thromb. Diath. Haemorrhag. 1*, 76.

Burstein, M., and Guinand, A. (1955). *Rev. Hematol. 10*, 571.

Ehrenpreis, S., Laskowski, M. Jr., Donelly, T. H., and Scheraga, H. A. (1958). *J. Am. Chem. Soc. 80*, 4255.

Ferry, J. D., and Morrison, P. R. (1947). *J. Am. Chem. Soc. 69*, 388.

Kekwick, R. A., Mackay, M. E., Nance, M. H., and Record, B. R. (1955). *Biochem. J. 60*, 671.

Laskowski, M. Jr., Donelly, T. H., Van Tijn, B. A., and Scheraga, H. A. (1956). *J. Biol. Chem. 222*, 815.

Latallo, Z. S. (1966). *Postepy Higieny i Medycyny Doswiadczalnej 20*, 657.

Latallo, Z. S., Fletcher, A. P., Alkjaersig, N., and Sherry, S. (1962). *Am. J. Physiol. 202*, 675.

Lenggenhager, K. (1940). *Helv. Med. Acta 7*, 262.

Lipiński, B., Wegrzynowicz, Z., Budzyński, A. Z., Kopeć, M., Latallo, Z. S., and Kowalski, E. (1967). *Thromb. Diath. Haemorrhag. 17*, 65.

Lorand, L. (1951). *Nature 167*, 992.

Markwardt, F. (1957a). *Arch. Pharmaz. Ber. dtsch. pharmaz. Ges. 290*, 280.

Markwardt, F. (1957b). *Hoppe-Seyler's Z. Physiol. Chem. 308*, 147.

Markwardt, F. (1963). Blutgerinnungshemmende Wirkstoffe aus blutsaugenden Tieren. G. Fischer, Jena.

Mellanby, J. (1933). *Proc. Roy. Soc. Lond. B, 113*, 93.

Nygaard, K. K. (1941). Haemorrhagic Diseases. Henry Kimpton, London.

Scheraga, H. A., and Laskowski, M. Jr. (1957). *Advances in Protein Chemistry 12*, 1.

Seegers, W. H. (1962). Prothrombin. Harvard Univ. Press, Cambridge, Mass.

Seegers, W. H., and Smith, H. P. (1942). *Am. J. Physiol. 137*, 348.

Shainoff, J. R., and Page, I. H. (1962). *J. Exptl. Med. 116*, 687.

Smith, H. P., Warner, E. D., and Brinkhous, K. M. (1937). *J. Exptl. Med. 66*, 801.

Warner, E. D., Brinkhous, K. M., and Smith, H. P. (1936). *Am. J. Physiol. 114*, 667.

Assays of Factor V

Herbert I. Horowitz

I. Introduction

The existence of a heat and storage labile plasma factor distinct from prothrombin and necessary for normal prothrombin conversion was discovered by Quick in 1943 and confirmed by Ware and Seegers (1948) and by Stefanini and Crosby (1950). Meanwhile, Owren (1947) had studied a young woman with a prolonged clotting time and prothrombin time. Her congenital coagulation defect was corrected by plasmas from which prothrombin had been removed by adsorption. The coagulant lacking in this patient's plasma was named factor V by Owren; it has subsequently been found to be identical to Quick's labile factor and Seegers' Ac-globulin.

II. Methods of Assay

Methods for measurement of factor V have employed substrates naturally or artificially depleted of the factor. When patients with severe deficiency are available then their platelet-poor plasma provides a convenient and useful reagent. In view of the rarity of congenital factor V deficiency methods involving artificially depleted substrates are in general use. One-stage and two-stage procedures have been described. For the most part clotting is accelerated by tissue thromboplastin but an assay using Stypven both to deplete the substrate of factor V and as the thromboplastic agent has also been advocated.

A. Two-stage method

1. Method of Ware and Seegers (1948)

a. Principle of the Method

The thrombin generation test, used to such good advantage by Seegers and his associates (1954), has been adapted to the assay of factor V (Ware and Seegers, 1948). Partially purified reagents are used to generate thrombin; these include prothrombin prepared from beef plasma and tissue thromboplastin extracted from lung. In setting up this assay highly dilute (1:800) bovine serum serves as a reference source for factor V. Results are expressed in units of Ac-globulin, the unit being defined as that amount of plasma which when diluted 1,000 times will convert a standard solution of prothrombin to thrombin at a minimal rate. The interested reader is referred to the original article (Ware and Seegers, 1948) or to subsequent summaries (Seegers, 1962; Johnson and Seegers, 1964) for full details of this method.

b. Evaluation

Except for those laboratories using similar techniques routinely, preparation of reagents and standardization of results will be difficult. It gives reproducible and reliable results and has been advocated as a research procedure.

B. One-stage methods

Basically, two methods have been proposed. The most commonly employed method relies on the storage lability of factor V. A new method is based on the ability of Russell's viper venom to activate factor V, thereby markedly enhancing its storage lability.

1. Method of Spaet

The following means of preparing factor V deficient substrate is based on Spaet's (unpublished) modification of earlier procedures.

a. Preparation of Deficient Substrate

1. Collect approximately 60 ml of blood into $^1/_{10}$ volume of 0.1 M sodium oxalate.
2. Separate platelet-poor plasma by centrifuging for 15 minutes at 5,000 RPM.
3. Incubate plasma at 37° C until the prothrombin time using 0.1 ml of plasma and 0.2 ml of commercial thromboplastin reagent (Simplastin, Warner-Chilcott, Morris Plains, New Jersey) prolongs to 60 to 80 seconds. This requires approximately 5 days.
4. Dialyze the resultant plasma for 24 hours at 4° C against large volumes (5 liters) of a solution prepared by diluting one volume of 3.8 % sodium citrate with nine volumes of normal saline.
5. The plasma is now alloted in 1 ml aliquots to glass or nalgene tubes and stored at –20° C.

b. Preparation of Dilution Curves

1. A dilution curve should be established every time a new artificially deficient reagent is prepared and whenever a new lot of Simplastin is used.
2. Pool citrated platelet-poor plasma from at least 5 normal individuals.
3. Dilute 1:10, 1:20, 1:40, 1:80 in distilled water.
4. Perform test as directed below using these dilutions.
5. Plot on log-log paper. A straight line should be obtained.

c. Assay Procedure

1. Dilute test plasma 1:10 in distilled water.
2. Prewarm factor V deficient substrate and test plasma at 37° C for five minutes.
3. Add 0.1 ml diluted test plasma to 0.1 ml factor V deficient substrate.
4. After 30 seconds add 0.2 ml of Simplastin and time clot formation.
5. Estimate factor V content from dilution curve.

d. Evaluation of Method

Factor V and other procoagulants are much more stable in citrate than in oxalate. The method employs these differences; factor V is allowed to inactivate relatively rapidly in oxalate. When the reagent has been prepared it is stabilized for storage by substituting citrate for the oxalate. Though other commercial or home-made tissue extracts can be substituted, Simplastin has proven to be a reliable reagent. Our results with the method have correlated well with those obtained from naturally deficient substrate assays. The method is sufficiently sensitive to even accurately detect mild factor V deficiency in heterozygotes (levels of up to 60 % of normal). The reagent may be used as a factor V deficient plasma in other tests as for example in correcting the prothrombin consumption abnormality of a suspected factor V deficiency.

2. Method of Borchgrevinck et al. (1960)

An alternate means of preparing factor V deficient plasma and assaying for this factor was described by Borchgrevinck et al. (1960).

a. Principle of Method

Stypven is used to activate factor V in citrated plasma. Activated factor V is rapidly inactivated at 37° C. The residual Stypven in the plasma (with added phospholipid) serves as the thromboplastic coagulation accelerator in the final clotting test.

b. Preparation of reagent

1. Cephalin (Rapaport et al. 1959) is diluted to optimal concentration for the particular preparation in veronal buffer, pH 7.3 (Hjort et al. 1955).
2. Stypven is dissolved in the cephalin suspension to a concentration of 1:100,000 (10 μg per ml).
3. Mix equal parts of the Stypven-cephalin suspension and normal platelet-poor plasma; adjust pH to 8.5 ± 0.1 with 1 NaOH.
4. Place 10 ml quantities in scrupulously clean 15 ml test tubes; stopper and incubate at 37° C.
5. Test incubation mixture until "blank time" reaches 60–70 seconds. This requires about 4 hours.
6. Pool all tubes and readjust pH to 7.3 with 1 N HCl. The reagent may be stored in small aliquots at –20° C.

c. Establishing a Calibration Curve

1. Ten percent, 5 %, 2 %, 1 % and 1/2 percent dilutions of normal plasma are made in veronal buffer.
2. Four tenths ml of reagent is preincubated at 37° C for 3 to 10 minutes in a 10 × 70 mm test tube. Two tenths ml of diluted test plasma is added. Exactly 2 minutes later the mixture is recalcified with 0.2 ml of 0.035 M calcium chloride and the clotting time recorded.
3. The concentration of diluted plasma and the clotting time when plotted on log-log paper should describe a straight line.

d. Assay of Factor V

The unknown plasma is diluted 1 to 10 in veronal buffer and tested as above. Concentration of factor V may then be read off the calibration curve.

e. Evaluation

This procedure permits preparation of a reagent suitable for accurate assays in one work day. Materials for the procedure should be readily available to most coagulation laboratories (though "off concentrations" such as 0.035 M $CaCl_2$ are used). Since Stypven remains in the reagent it cannot be used in other types of studies.

3. Method of Schultze and Schwick (1953)

A commercial reagent for assay of factor V is available from Behringwerke, A.G., Marburg, Germany, and is said to contain prothrombin, factors VII and X, fibrinogen and thromboplastin. We have had limited experience with this reagent. In a one-stage test system similar to that described for the artificially depleted factor V reagent it gave a dilution curve parallel to the artificially depleted reagent and to the naturally deficient plasma. Assays of normal and deficient plasma were in good agreement with other methods. However, using the naturally deficient substrate small amounts of factor V activity could be detected. From this brief experience the reagent can be recommended for clinical evaluation of factor V deficiency.

References

Borchgrevinck, C. F., Pool, J. C., and Stormorken, H. (1960). *J. Lab. Clin. Med. 55,* 625.

Hjort, P. F., Rapaport, S. I., and Owren, P. A. (1955). *J. Lab. Clin. Med. 46,* 89.

Johnson, J. F., and Seegers, W. H. (1964). In "Blood Coagulation, Hemorrhage and Thrombosis" (L. M. Tocantins and L. A. Kazal, eds.), pp. 197—210, Grune & Stratton, New York.

Owren, P. A. (1947). *Acta Med. Scand. Supp. 194.*

Quick, A. J. (1943). *Am. J. Physiol. 140,* 172.

Rapaport, S. I., Aas, K., and Owren, P. A. (1954). *Blood 9,* 1185.

Schultze, H. E., and Schwick, G. (1953). Laboratoriumsblätter, Behringwerke No. 3.

Seegers, W. H. (1962). "Prothrombin". Harvard Press. Cambridge.

Seegers, W. H., Johnson, J. F., and Fell, C. (1954). *Am. J. Physiol. 176,* 97.

Spaet, Th., unpublished.

Stefanini, M., and Crosby, W. H. (1950). *Proc. Soc. Exptl. Biol. Med. 74,* 370.

Ware, A. G., and Seegers, W. H. (1948). *Am. J. Physiol. 152,* 567.

Assays for Antihemophilic Factor (Factor VIII)*

George D. Penick, Harold R. Roberts and Campbell W. McMillan

I. Introduction

Most specific methods of assaying factor VIII utilize hemophilic blood or plasma as a test substrate, although a number of artificial media have been devised. Over the years different investigators have used a variety of end points to measure the amount of factor VIII present in test samples added to the substrate, e. g., whole blood clotting time (Patek and Taylor, 1937; Alexander and Landwehr, 1948); amount of prothrombin utilized (Graham et al. 1951, 1955); partial thromboplastin time (Langdell et al. 1953; Stapp, 1961a; Fischer, 1964); amount of thromboplastin generated (Biggs et al. 1955); etc. We have found the last two of these indices to be reliable and reproducible and have consequently accumulated most of our experience with these two methods. They will be described in detail.

II. Partial Thromboplastin Method (Langdell et al. 1953)

A. Principle

The assay is based upon the observations that the partial thromboplastin time (PTT) of hemophilic plasma is prolonged, and that the degree of correction of this prolonged time is proportional to the concentration of factor VIII added as test material. When various dilutions of normal plasma are added to hemophilic plasma, the resulting PTT's are linearly related to the logarithms of the plasma concentrations. By similarly determining and plotting the PTT's of mixtures of an unknown sample and hemophilic substrate plasma, the factor VIII concentration of the unknown material can be expressed in per cent of the normal control.

* Supported by USPHS Grants HE-06350, HE-5652, FR-46 and HE-08498

B. Materials and Reagents

1. Hemophilic Plasma (Substrate)

Blood is drawn from a patient with severe classic hemophilia into 3.2% trisodium citrate (1 part citrate to 8 parts blood). It is centrifuged for 30 min at 2,000 rpm in a refrigerated centrifuge; the plasma is carefully aspirated and stored in 6 ml aliquots in clean glass tubes at –20° C.

2. Control Plasma

Blood is drawn from ten normal individuals into 3.2% trisodium citrate (1:8). Plasma is prepared as described above, pooled, and stored in 6 ml aliquots at –20° C.

3. Cephalin

Thrombofax (Ortho Pharmaceutical, Raritan, N.J.), diluted 1:10 in normal saline, is used as the partial thromboplastin.

4. Citrated Saline, Buffered

Stock solution is made by mixing 1 part 0.9% saline, 1 part imidazole buffer (pH 7.2) and 0.4 parts 3.2% trisodium citrate. It is stored at 5° C.

5. Calcium-Imidazole-Saline

Add 1.4 parts of 1.2% $CaCl_2$ in 0.9% saline to 1.2 parts imidazole buffer (pH 7.2).

6. Kaolin

Kaolin (Fisher Scientific Co., Fair Lawn, N.J.), is used for activation of plasma samples.

C. Procedure

Serial dilutions of the control and test plasmas are made accurately and rapidly with careful mixing as follows:

10% sample: 0.1 ml plasma + 0.9 ml citrated saline

5% sample: 0.5 ml 10% sample + 0.5 ml citrated saline

2.5 % sample: 0.5 ml 5 % sample + 0.5 ml citrated saline
1.25 % sample: 0.5 ml 2.5 % sample + 0.5 ml citrated saline; discard 0.5 ml of the 1.25 % sample.
A blank control tube contains 0.5 ml citrated saline.
To 6 ml hemophilic plasma add 30 mg kaolin, mix well and then add 0.5 ml of the mixture to each of the diluted plasma samples.
Cap tubes with parafilm and incubate for 15 min at 28° C, tilting frequently to keep the kaolin suspended.
Prepare a calcium-cephalin mixture by adding 5 ml of the cephalin reagent to 5 ml of calcium-imidazole-saline, mix thoroughly, and warm to 37° C.
After 15 min incubation period, place the plasma mixtures into the ice bath.
Determine partial thromboplastin times on the plasma samples as follows, beginning with that containing the 10 % dilution of control plasma:
Place 0.2 ml plasma mixture into a 10×75 mm test tube at 37° C for 60 sec;
Add 0.2 ml cephalin-calcium mixture; simultaneously start a stopwatch;
Tilt the tubes until the first evidence of fibrin formation appears; stop the stopwatch and record the clotting time;
Repeat the same procedure on another 0.2 ml aliquot of the 10 % sample;
In a like manner, determine duplicate PTT values on the 10 % test sample mixture, and then proceed to each other paired dilution.

D. Calculations

Average the duplicate PTT's for each diluted sample.

Using semilogarithmic paper, plot the plasma concentrations on the logarithmic scale against the PTT's on the arithmetic scale and connect points with the best fitting (visually) straight line (see Fig. 1).

For any common clotting time, compare concentrations of the test and control samples. (In the illustration, the clotting time of the 10 % sample of the test plasma is comparable to that of a 2.6 % concentration of the control plasma.)

Calculate factor VIII activity of the test materials as follows:

$$\frac{\text{Concentration of Normal Control}}{\text{Concentration of Test Sample}} \times 100 = \%\text{ of factor VIII activity} \qquad (1)$$

Example:

$$\frac{2.6}{10} \times 100 = 26\,\%\text{ of factor VIII activity} \qquad (2)$$

Note: The blank control sample (hemophilic plasma) should have a PTT value of >200 sec.

III. Thromboplastin Generation Method

A. Principle

The amount of "intrinsic thromboplastin" generated when serum, calcium, phospholipid and adsorbed plasma are incubated is directly proportional to the amount of factor VIII in the plasma sample. Generated thromboplastin is measured by its shortening effect on hemophilic substrate plasma. By selecting a standard period of incubation, the thromboplastin generated when a test plasma sample is used can be compared with that formed when a normal plasma sample is used. An expression of factor VIII in terms of per cent activity of the control can then be calculated.

B. Materials and Reagents

1. Glass and Plastic Ware

Test tubes and pipettes are soaked overnight in a soap solution, rinsed, soaked in 0.1 N HCl, rinsed and oven-dried. Plastic lusteroid tubes are air-dried.

2. 0.025 M $CaCl_2$

Prepare with anhydrous $CaCl_2$ and distilled-demineralized water. Store at 5° C.

3. Imidazole Buffer

Add 3.4 gm imidazole to 1,000 ml distilled-demineralized water. Neutralize to pH 7.3

by slow addition of HCl acid reagent (36.5-38.0 %) with stirring (usually requires about 1.6 ml). Store at 5° C in 30 ml quantities.

4. 0.9 % NaCl

Add 9.0 gm of NaCl (J. T. Baker Chemical Co., Phillipsburg, N. J.) to 1,000 ml distilled-demineralized water with stirring. Store in 30 ml quantities at 5° C.

5. 3.2 % Trisodium Citrate

Add 8.0 gm trisodium citrate (J. T. Baker Chemical Co., Phillipsburg, N. J.) to 250 ml distilled-demineralized water. Store at 5° C.

6. $Al(OH)_3$ Gel

Add 50 ml aluminum hydroxide gel (Amphogel, Wyeth Labs., Inc., Philadelphia, Pa.) to 50 ml distilled-demineralized water. Store in dark at room temperature.

7. Inosithin, 3.8 %

Add 3.8 gm inosithin (Associated Concentrates, Inc., Long Island, N. Y.) to 100 ml 0.9 % NaCl and dissolve at 37° C with periodic mixing (usually requires 4–6 hrs). Store in 5.0 ml and 0.2 ml quantities at –20° C.

8. Adsorbed Normal and Hemophilic Plasmas

Select a normal donor and a donor with severe classic hemophilia. From each, draw 9.0 ml blood and add in each case to 1.0 ml 3.2 % trisodium citrate in a glass centrifuge tube. Centrifuge at 2,500 rpm for 15 min at 5° C. Add to each decanted plasma $^1/_{10}$ volume $Al(OH)_3$ gel. Invert carefully 4 times and place in 37° C waterbath for 3 min. Recentrifuge as above. Immediately decant adsorbed plasmas and store in carefully measured 0.2 ml quantities at –20° C.

9. Normal Serum

Draw 30 ml blood from a normal donor and place in 5 ml quantities into each of six glass tubes. Incubate at 37° C for exactly 6 hrs. Centrifuge at 5° C for 15 min at 2,500 rpm. Carefully decant serum into glass tubes and store at 5° C for exactly 12 hrs. Pool samples and store at –20° C in 0.2 ml aliquots.

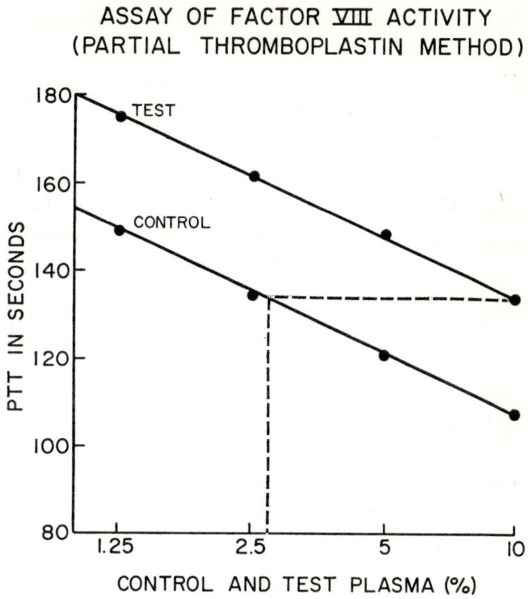

Fig. 1. Assay of factor VIII activity by means of the partial thromboplastin method (Langdell et al. 1953).

10. Substrate Plasma

Draw 180 ml blood from a normal donor and add with gentle mixing to 20 ml of 3.2 % trisodium citrate. Centrifuge for 30 min at room temperature and 3,000 rpm. Aspirate plasma (avoid red cell contamination) and store in 3 ml aliquots at –20° C.

C. Procedure

Thaw tube containing 0.2 ml normal serum at 37° C. Dilute 1:20 with imidazole buffer. Incubate at room temperature for exactly 2 hrs. Transfer to plastic tube in melting ice bath. (Do not allow pipette to rest in the serum.) Prepare test sample to be assayed by same procedure described above for adsorbed normal plasma.

Thaw adsorbed normal and hemophilic plasmas at 37° C. Dilute normal sample 1:5 with imidazole buffer and place in ice bath with 0.1 ml pipette inserted. Dilute hemophilic sample 1:20 with imidazole buffer and place in ice bath with 1.0 ml pipette inserted.

Thaw 0.2 ml tube of Inosithin at 37° C and dilute 1:35 with 6.8 ml 0.9 % NaCl. Further dilute to 1:140 by mixing 1.0 ml of the 1:35 Inosithin with 3.0 ml 0.9 % NaCl.

Thaw substrate plasma at 37° C and insert 1.0 ml pipette.
Warm $CaCl_2$ solution to 37° C in about 3 ml quantities in each of two tubes into which 1.0 ml pipettes have been inserted.
Label 9 glass tubes as follows: 10, 20, 40, 80, 160, 320, 640, 1280, control. Add exactly 0.1 ml imidazole buffer to each. Add 0.1 ml adsorbed normal plasma (1:5 dilution) to the first tube and mix thoroughly; transfer 0.1 ml to the next and repeat to the 1280 dilution tube (0.1 ml of this last dilution is discarded; do not add plasma to the blank control tube). Discard tubes 10, 20, and 40 and transfer the others to the melting ice bath.
Add to each tube, beginning with the control tube and working backwards, the following:
0.1 ml 1:140 dilution of Inosithin
0.1 ml 1:20 adsorbed hemophilic plasma (source of factor V)
0.1 ml 1:20 normal serum.
Recalcify tube "80" by placing in 37° C water bath and forcibly adding 0.1 ml $CaCl_2$. Start stopwatch. Similarly recalcify each of the remaining tubes at 1 min intervals. Insert 0.1 ml pipettes into each of these incubating tubes.
Place 0.1 ml $CaCl_2$ into each of a series of tubes in front of incubating tubes.
After about 5 min 45 sec incubation, add 0.1 ml incubating mixture to the corresponding tube containing $CaCl_2$. At exactly 6 min incubation, add 0.1 ml substrate plasma and start a second stopwatch. Record clotting time. (Control tube should clot in 30–40 sec range.)
Repeat this procedure for each of the incubating mixtures.
Follow the same way with the test sample.

D. Calculations

Plot clotting times vs. plasma dilutions on log-log paper. (Resulting curves for normal and test plasmas should be parallel straight lines at 15° angle with abscissa.)
Compare any two points on test and control curves for any selected clotting time.

Express factor VIII activity as follows:

$$\frac{\text{Reciprocal of Test Plasma Dilution}}{\text{Reciprocal of Normal Dilution}} \times 100 = \%\ \text{factor VIII activity} \qquad (3)$$

Procedure may be adapted to *micro-method* by following modifications:
Obtain capillary blood sample by applying tourniquet to forearm, making hemolet stab wound, discarding first drop of blood, and collecting 0.1 ml blood in a 0.2 ml pipette.
Wipe pipette tip and add blood to 0.45 ml citrated saline (1 part 3.2 % trisodium citrate to 41 parts 0.9 % NaCl). Rinse pipette gently 3–5 times.
Fill 2 heparinized microhematocrit tubes and determine hematocrit in duplicate.
Dilute $Al(OH)_3$ gel by adding 0.05 ml stock reagent to 5.0 ml 0.9 % saline; add 0.5 ml of this diluted gel to the citrated blood sample.
Mix and incubate at 37° C for exactly 3 min.
Centrifuge at 2,500 rpm for 15 min at 5° C.
Decant supernatant and assay as above, assuming initial dilution to be 1:20.
Correct for hematocrit values as follows:

$$\frac{\text{Assay value of factor VIII in }\% \times 50}{100 - \text{hematocrit value}} = \text{corrected factor VIII activity in }\% \qquad (4)$$

E. Interpretation

The factor VIII activity of normal individuals varies from 75 to 150 %; severe classic hemophiliacs generally have less than 1 % activity. Moderate to mild hemophiliacs have plasma levels ranging between 3 to 30 %.

References

Alexander, B., and Landwehr, G. (1948). *J. Clin. Invest.* *27,* 98.
Biggs, R., Eveling, J., and Richards, G. (1955). *Brit. J. Haematol.* *1,* 20.
Graham. J. B., Collins, D. L., Jr., Godwin, I. D., and Brinkhous, K. M. (1951). *Proc. Soc. Exptl. Biol. Med.* *77,* 294.
Graham, J. B., Penick, G. D., and Brinkhous, K. M. (1955). In: "The Coagulation of Blood. Methods of Study" (L. M. Tocantins, ed.) pp. 77—80, Grune & Stratton, New York.
Langdell, R. D., Wagner, R. H., and Brinkhous, K. M. (1953). *J. Lab. Clin. Med.* *41,* 637.
Patek, A. J., Jr., and Taylor, F. H. L. (1937). *J. Clin. Invest.* *16,* 113.

Addendum

Prepared by E. Deutsch and K. Lechner

Partial Thromboplastin Method with Artificial Factor VIII-free Reagents (Stapp, 1961a)

A. Principle

A thrombin defibrinated, dialysed, normal human plasma is used as a source of prothrombin, and a stored, dialysed bovine serum as a source of factor V. Both reagents contain factors VII, IX, X, XI and XII. Tachostyptan (Hormon-Chemie, Munich, Germany) replaces platelets. This system contains all the factors necessary for the endogenous system, except factor VIII. Therefore, the clotting time depends on the concentration of factor VIII in the test sample.

B. Materials and Reagents

1. Water bath (37° C);
2. Two stopwatches;
3. Siliconized glass tubes;
4. Non-siliconized glass tubes
(19 mm diameter) already used several times and well-cleaned, with a nonrepellent surface are recommended. (If not available boil new tubes with chrome sulphuric acid, rinse with tap water, incubate several hours with 10% potassium hydroxide, rinse first with tap water and then with distilled water);
5. Buffer solutions:
a. 0.2 M imidazole stock solution: 17.2 gm imidazole to be dissolved in 1,000 ml distilled water;
b. 0.1 N HCl;
c. Imidazole buffered saline (pH 7.35):
250 ml imidazole stock solution
180 ml 0.1 N HCl
570 ml distilled water
Mix and dilute ten times with distilled water. Add 8.5 gm sodium chloride per liter;
d. Imidazole buffer (pH 7.08):
250 ml imidazole stock solution
250 ml 0.1 N HCl
500 ml distilled water
Mix and dilute ten times with distilled water;
e. Imidazole buffered saline (pH 7.08):
Add to imidazole buffer 8.5 gm sodium chloride per liter;
f. Buffered citrate-saline solution (pH 7.32):
Add to 500 ml buffered saline (e) 100 ml 3.8% sodium citrate;
6. 3.8% citrate solution:
Dissolve 38 gm trisodium citrate in 1,000 ml distilled water;
7. Glycerol;
8. 0.03 M calcium chloride solution:
Dissolve 3.33 gm anhydrous calcium chloride in 1,000 ml distilled water;
9. Thrombin solution (1,000 U/ml):
Dissolve 1 ampule "Topostasin-Roche" with 3,000 U in 1.5 ml saline and add 1.5 ml glycerol. Store at –20° C;
10. 1% Merthiolate;
11. Tachostyptan:
Dilute the contents of an original ampule 10 times with imidazole buffered saline pH 7.08; mix, wait 5 min and dilute 50 times with the same buffer, which results in a final dilution of 1:500. This solution should be freshly prepared every day; it may stay at room temperature for the day only. The ampules are stable at 4° C for at least 1 year (Fischer, 1964);
12. Thrombin defibrinated, dialysed normal human plasma (TD-Plasma):
Citrated whole blood (1 part trisodium citrate and 9 parts blood) are centrifuged twice in siliconized tubes at room temperature for 30 min at 4,500 rpm. The platelet-free plasmas of several donors with at least 80% prothrombin may be pooled, and at least 200 ml plasma should be used for one batch.
To each 10 ml portion of the pooled platelet-poor plasma in glass tubes in a water bath of 37° C, 0.2 ml thrombin solution (1,000 U/ml) is added; mix by inverting the tube quickly and remove the fibrin by winding it onto a wooden or glass applicator stick. Repeat the same pro-

cedure after 15 min with another 0.2 ml portion of thrombin. Incubate for 3 to 5 hrs at 37° C; centrifuge at 4,500 rpm 30 min; mix the portions and dialyse against 20 to 30 volumes of imidazole buffered saline pH 7.08 for 2 days at 4° C. Change dialyzing fluid several times. Small parts of the TD-Plasma are quick-frozen and stored at –20° C. Thawed samples should not be refrozen;

13. Stored dialyzed bovine serum:
Blood which is withdrawn by canulating the jugular vein of healthy cattle is collected in cylindrical glass containers and defibrinated by stirring with glass rods for 30 min. It is then centrifuged twice for 60 min at 4,500 rpm, 4° C. Transfer the cell-free serum into an Erlenmeyer flask; 1 part 1 % Merthiolate is added to 100 parts of serum; stored at 37° C for several days until factor VIII activity has ceased and only 100 to 250 % factor V remains. Both factors should be determined every day during incubation, from the third day on twice daily. The factor VIII-free serum is dialyzed as described under 12.

C. Test Plasma

After a clean venipuncture with a wide bore needle the first ml of blood is discarded and 9 ml whole blood is mixed with 1 ml 3.8 % trisodium citrate in a siliconized tube, then mixed by inverting three times, and at once centrifuged at 3,500 rpm for 30 min. The platelet-poor plasma is transferred to another siliconized tube with a siliconized pipette and factor VIII is determined at once, or the sample may be quick-frozen and stored at –20° C for several days.

D. Performance of the Test

Pipette the following reagents into a glass tube at 37° C in the following order:

0.2 ml platelet-poor test plasma
0.1 ml thrombin defibrinated dialyzed normal human plasma
0.1 ml stored dialyzed bovine serum
0.1 ml buffered saline
0.2 ml imidazole buffer pH 7.08
0.1 ml diluted Tachostyptan (1:500)

Start stopwatch, shake tube vigorously for 10 sec and incubate 50 sec at 37° C and add 0.2 ml of 0.03 M $CaCl_2$; start a second stopwatch, shake vigorously for 10 sec, incubate for 50 sec at 37° C and then tilt the tube every 10 sec until a solid clot appears. The test is performed in triplicate, and at least in two dilutions with citrated saline pH 7.32. A dilution of 1:5 is best suited for normals and carriers of hemophilia.

E. Standardization

Pool ten normal plasmas. Test the pooled plasma undiluted (100 %), diluted 1:2 (50 %), 1:4 (25 %), 1:5 (20 %) and 1:8 (12.5 %). Plot clotting times vs plasma dilutions on log-log paper, and extrapolate the straight line for further dilutions (Further dilutions cannot be made because the reagents do not contain enough fibrinogen, and fibrinogen becomes the limiting factor). A straight line up to a dilution of 1:100 is obtained, if plasma of a severe hemophiliac A or factor VIII-free bovine fibrinogen (Stapp, 1961b) for further dilution is used.

F. Comments

In addition to the advantages held in common with other one-stage methods with respect to simplicity and accuracy, this method has the advantage that no hemophilic substrate plasma is necessary. The disadvantages are the rather complicated method of preparation of the reagents, and the fact that plasma cannot be diluted by more than 1:8. Fibrinogen becomes the limiting factor in higher dilutions. The preparation of factor VIII-free fibrinogen is too complicated to be used as a routine reagent (Stapp, 1961b).

References

Stapp, W. (1961a). *Proc. VIIIth European Congr. Hematol. Vienna, Vol. II. No. 424.*
Stapp, W. (1961b). *Thromb. Diathes. Hemorrhag. 6,* 287.

Assays for Factors VII and X

M. P. Esnouf and Karl Lechner

I. Introduction

The function of factor X in the clotting process has been most thoroughly investigated. It has been shown that it is activated by tissue thromboplastin-factor VII (extrinsic system: Nemerson and Spaet [1964], Lechner and Deutsch [1965], Williams and Norris [1966]), by a mixture of factor VIII and IX_a (intrinsic system: Macfarlane and Ash [1962]), and by the action of Russell's viper venom (Esnouf and Williams [1962]). A new enzyme is produced, activated F X (F X_a), plasma thrombokinase or autoprothrombin C. It converts prothrombin to thrombin in the presence of phospholipid, calcium and factor V (Esnouf and Jobin [1967]).

Factor X can be assayed either by its clot promoting activity in certain test systems (biological assay) or by measuring the esterase activity after activation (biochemical assay).

II. Assay for Factor X

A. Biological Assay

1. Principle

Factor X is activated to factor X_a by Russell's viper venom and calcium. In a one-stage procedure factor X_a activates prothrombin, in the presence of factor V and phospholipids, to thrombin which converts indicator fibrinogen to fibrin. The clotting time is measured. The necessary factors II, V and fibrinogen are supplied by a substrate free of factor X. This is a rate assay, that is the clotting time of the indicator fibrinogen is influenced by the rate of activation of factor X which, other things being equal, is a function of the concentration of factor X in the sample.

2. Reagents

a. Substrate plasma: The substrate plasma should be essentially free of factor X, but should contain prothrombin, factor V and fibrinogen. The best reagent for this purpose would be the plasma of a patient with a severe isolated deficiency of factor X. These patients are rare and their plasma is available only in limited amounts. Therefore, most laboratories use plasma from which the factor X has been removed. Several methods for the preparation of a substrate plasma for the factor X assay have been described. The main problem in the techniques described below is to find a simple method of separating factor X from prothrombin.

b. Seitz-filtered bovine plasma (Bachmann et al. 1958): Two 14 cm diameter asbestos filter pads, for pressure filtration, are placed in a 2 liter original Seitz filter. The lower pad is of 30 % asbestos and the upper of 20 % asbestos (Filtrox, St. Gallen, Switzerland). About 1,500 ml bovine oxalated plasma (1 part sodium oxalate + 9 parts bovine blood, centrifugation 30 min, 2,500 rpm) are filtered at room temperature at a rate of one drop per second. The first 200 ml are discarded, and the rest of the filtrate is collected in 50 ml portions. In each portion prothrombin times and the stypven times (0.1 ml filtrate, 0.1 ml buffer, 0.1 ml stypven-lipid reagent – see below – and 0.1 ml 0.025 M $CaCl_2$) are determined. The fractions with a prothrombin activity of more than 25 % of normal plasma and a stypven time of more than 80 sec can be used as reagents. Small aliquots of these fractions are stored deep frozen at –20° C.

c. Charcoal-filtered bovine plasma (Denson, 1961): A pyrex tube of 3.2 cm internal diameter is stoppered at one end with glass wool. 7.5–15 gm (usually 10 gm) powdered wood charcoal (Griffin and George Ltd, Alperton, Middlesex) or beechwood charcoal (Thomas Hill Jones, London, E 3; code No. G. L. 90) are introduced into this column and covered with a layer of glass wool. After washing with 25 ml physiological saline solution, 50 ml bovine oxalated plasma are applied to the column. The rest of the washing fluid which emerges first from the column is discarded, and the filtered plasma is collected and tested in the same way as described for Seitz-filtered plasma.

d. Bentonite absorbed human plasma (Hougie, 1962): Normal citrated, platelet poor human plasma is stirred with 17 mg/ml bentonite (Prolabo, 12, Rue Pelee, Paris) for 10 min at room temperature with a glass rod. After centrifugation (3,000 rpm, 20 min) the supernatant is checked for prothrombin and factor X activity as described above and frozen at –20° C. Because bentonite also adsorbs factor V and fibrinogen, these factors must be replaced by the addition of an equal amount of $Al(OH)_3$ (0.5 ml Alumina gel/10 ml plasma) adsorbed citrated human plasma or barium sulfate (100 mg/ml) adsorbed oxalated bovine plasma. This mixture should have a prothrombin concentration of more than 25% and a stypven time (see 2b) of more than 60 sec.

e. Remarks: With all three methods suitable substrate plasmas for the determination of factor X can be obtained. Each method, however, has its specific advantages and disadvantages.
The simplest method is the bentonite adsorption according to Hougie (1962). It seems, however, that good results are obtained only if bentonite PROLABO is used. Bentonite tends to clump and must be carefully dispersed in the plasma with glass rods. The concentration of adsorbent necessary for the separation of prothrombin and factor X is critical and may vary from plasma to plasma. A pilot adsorption with different concentrations of bentonite (17 mg/ml, 20 mg/ml and 23 mg/ml) is recommended to determine the optimal concentration.
Some experience is needed to get good results with Seitz filtration. The procedure is time consuming and with some batches of bovine plasma no suitable fractions may be obtained. Exact control of the filtration rate is essential for the best results. A further problem is that fibrinogen often precipitates and impedes the flow through the filter.
Substrate plasma for the determination of factor X may be obtained commercially from Thame Diagnostic Reagents, Ltd, Thame, Oxford, England (charcoal filtered bovine plasma according to Denson), and from Hoffman La Roche, Grenzach, Germany.

f. Russell's viper venom-cephalin reagent: Russell's viper venom (Burroughs Wellcome, Tuckahoe, N. Y.) is dissolved in 0.9% saline to give a concentration of 50 μg/ml. This stock solution is usually kept frozen in small portions (for one day's use) at –20° C, but it may be kept at +4° C for weeks.
The Russell's viper venom-cephalin reagent is prepared by mixing 1 part of the Russell's viper venom stock solution with 9 parts of a phospholipid suspension. The phospholipid preparations and their concentrations are the same as for the partial thromboplastin times (Chapter III, p. 76). The Russell's viper venom-cephalin reagent must be freshly prepared each day. A preparation of Russell's viper venom already mixed with phospholipid can be obtained from Thame Diagnostic Reagents.

g. Plasma to be tested: Platelet poor citrated plasma is prepared. This plasma is diluted 1:10 in veronal-buffer pH 7.3 (Owren, 1947) before testing.

h. 0.025 M $CaCl_2$.

3. Performance of the Test

To an aliquot of 0.1 ml substrate plasma, 0.1 ml Russell's viper venom-cephalin reagent and 0.1 ml diluted patient plasma are pipetted in this order in a glass test tube and warmed to 37° C. Then 0.1 ml prewarmed 0.025 M $CaCl_2$ is added and the clotting time is recorded at 37° C. A calibration curve is obtained by testing different dilutions (1:10, 1:20, 1:50, 1:100) of pooled plasma from five normal donors. The 1:10 dilution is arbitrarily defined as 100%. A linear relationship exists between the log of the clotting time and the log of the concentration (fig. 1).

B. Biochemical Assay

1. Principle

If the preparations of Factor X to be assayed are reasonably pure, a more accurate form of assay can be used. Esnouf and Williams (1962) demonstrated that factor X_a has esterase activity and synthetic amino acid esters are split. However, 50–100 μg factor X are needed for this assay. Recently, Leveson and Esnouf (1967) have found that considerably lower concentrations of factor X_a can be assayed using carbobenzoxyphenylalanine p-nitrophenyl ester and measuring the rate of release of p-nitrophenol.

2. Materials and Reagents

These assays are conveniently carried out using a recording spectrophotometer with a cell compartment which can be maintained at 37° C. The following reagents are needed:
Factor X in 0.01 M tris hydrochloric acid buffer pH 7.5.
Coagulant protein of Russell's viper venom.
0.01 M Tris hydrochloric acid buffer pH 7.5.
0.3 mM carbobenzoxy-phenylalanine p-nitrophenyl ester in acetone.
0.05 M Tris hydrochloric acid buffer pH 8.0.
0.1 M calcium chloride in 0.01 M Tris hydrochloric acid pH 7.5.

3. Procedure

To each of two cuvettes the following reagents are added: 0.1 ml of the coagulant protein containing 1 μg of protein, to one cuvette is added a sample of factor X. 0.01 M Tris hydrochloric acid buffer is added to both cuvettes to bring the volume to 0.9 ml. When the cells are equilibrated at 37° C, 0.1 ml of the calcium chloride solution is added, and the mixtures are incubated for at least 10 min. Then 1.0 ml of pH 8.0 buffer at 37° C and 0.1 ml of the substrate are added. The rate of appearance of p-nitrophenol is measured at 400 mμ.

4. Calculations

The rate of hydrolysis of the substrate by factor X_a is the difference between the rates of hydrolysis found in the two cuvettes.

With this procedure one observes hydrolysis rates of the order of 0.5 mM/min/mg of factor X_a. Since p-nitrophenol has a molar extinction coefficient of 15×10^3, it can be seen that a rate of change of optical density of 0.0075 units per min can be obtained with factor X_a at a concentration of 1 μg/ml.

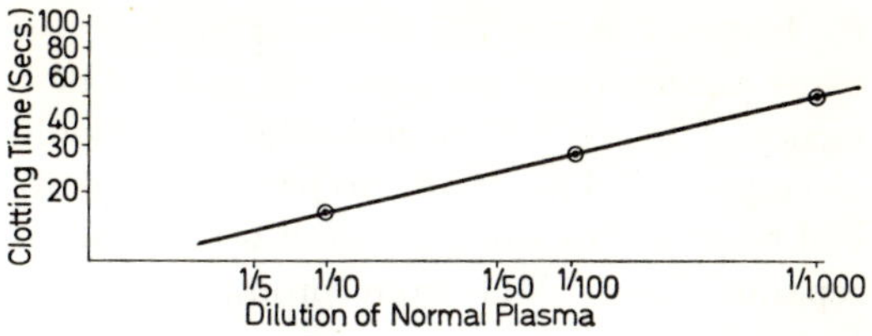

Fig. 1. Calibration curve for the estimation of factor X activity.

III. Assays of Factor VII

A. Specific Assay of Factor VII

1. Principle

In a one-stage test system containing fibrinogen, prothrombin, factor V, factor X, tissue thromboplastin and calcium ions, but no factor VII, the clotting time is prolonged. It is shortened by the addition of small amounts of factor VII, the clotting times ranging with the amount of factor VII added. This is a rate assay in which the rate of activation of factor VII determines the rate of formation of fibrin from the indicator fibrinogen.

2. Reagents

Substrate plasma for the assay of factor VII must contain fibrinogen, prothrombin, factor X and factor V in amounts which should be at least 50 % of their normal plasma concentration. The activity of factor VII should be below 1 % of the activity of normal plasma.

a. Congenital factor VII-deficient plasma: The best substrate plasma is platelet poor citrated plasma from a patient with an isolated severe deficiency of factor VII (F. VII less than 1 %). Because factor VII and factor X deficiency are often combined, it is essential to determine that substrate plasma contains normal amounts of factor X.

The substrate plasma may either be kept at –20° C for up to 2 months or may be lyophilized. If, after prolonged storage, the activity of factor V falls below 50 %, the addition of an equal amount of barium sulfate (100 mg/ml) adsorbed bovine plasma is advisable.

b. Artificial factor VII-deficient plasma: Because plasma from patients with isolated deficiency of factor VII is generally unavailable, attempts have been made, to prepare an artificial reagent. For this purpose it is necessary to separate factor VII from prothrombin and factor X.

Method of Lechner and Deutsch (1967):

1. Barium sulfate (100 mg/ml) adsorbed oxalated bovine plasma (1 part 1.33 % sodium oxalate and 9 parts bovine blood are centrifuged in the cold to remove the blood cells and platelets).

2. Human factor II–X concentrate. This is prepared by chromatography of human plasma on DEAE-cellulose in the following way:

45 ml blood from a donor with a normal prothrombin time, are mixed with 5 ml 3.8 % trisodium citrate in siliconized centrifuge tubes, and platelet poor plasma is obtained by centrifugation at 3,000 rpm for 30 min at 4° C. The platelet poor plasma is removed and diluted with 0.15 M saline to the original blood volume of 50 ml. One gm DEAE-cellulose (Serva, Heidelberg) is suspended in citrated saline (1 part 3.8 % trisodium citrate + 9 parts 0.15 M saline) and introduced into a small chromatographic column (1.0 to 1.5 cm diameter). After equilibration of the column with citrated saline for at least 2 hrs the diluted plasma is applied to the column and the flow rate adjusted to 30 ml/hr. When the plasma has entered the column, it is washed with citrate-saline solution (1 part 3.8 % trisodium citrate and 19 parts 0.15 M saline) until the optical density of the effluent at 280 mμ is below 0.05. The column is then eluted with 0.02 M phosphate buffer, pH 7.0, containing 1.0 M NaCl. The fractions eluted contain factor II and factor X (and factor IX) but only very small amounts of factor VII. Factor VII had passed the column without being adsorbed. The fractions containing factor II and factor X are combined and dialysed overnight against a mixture of 1 part 3.8 % citrate and 4 parts 0.15 M NaCl. After dialysis the solution is adjusted to a factor II and X concentration of approximately 100 %.

3. Equal parts of the barium sulfate adsorbed plasma and the factor II and factor X concentrate are mixed, divided into small portions and stored quick-frozen at –20° C.

A similar reagent can be obtained by the addition of purified factor X to Seitz-filtered or charcoal-filtered bovine plasma. Methods of purifying factor X for such purposes have been described by Denson (1961) (paper electrophoresis of the citrate eluate prepared from barium sulphate after i.v. has been slined with bovine plasma) and Shaw et al. (1966) (polyvinylblock-electrophoresis of a human serum eluate).

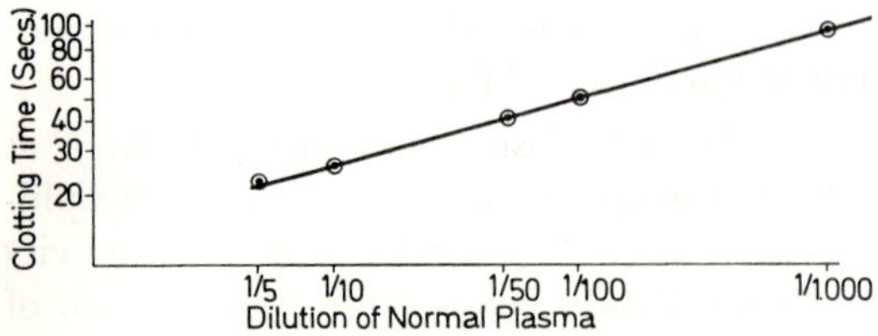

Fig. 2. Calibration curve for the estimation of factor VII activity.

c. Plasma to be tested: Platelet poor citrated or oxalated plasma of the patient is obtained. The plasma is diluted (usually 1:10) with veronal buffer, pH 7.3, for the assay.

d. Tissue thromboplastin: Preferably a tissue thromboplastin preparation from human brain should be used (for details of preparation see Chapter IV, p. 170). Lung thromboplastin is not sensitive to factor VII. Tissue thromboplastin preparations from bovine sources are not suitable because the reaction between tissue thromboplastin and factor VII and X is species specific.

e. 0.05 M $CaCl_2$.

3. Performance of the Test

0.1 ml of factor VII deficient plasma (either natural or artificial) and 0.1 ml tissue thromboplastin suspension are pipetted in this order into a glass test tube and warmed to 37° C. Then 0.1 ml 0.05 M $CaCl_2$ is added and the clotting time is recorded at 37° C.

4. Calibration Curve

This curve is obtained by testing different dilutions (1:10, 1:20, 1:50, 1:100) of pooled normal plasma (Fig. 2).

5. Comments

The artificial factor VII deficient plasma still contains small amounts of factor VII. Therefore, the test gives too high an estimate of the values for plasma samples with factor VII activity below 10 %. In such a case plasma from a patient with a severe factor VII deficiency is needed for the exact determination of factor VII.

B. Assay of Factor VII and X

1. Principle

In a system containing fibrinogen, factor V and prothrombin, the thromboplastin time depends on the amounts of both factor VII and factor X in the plasma.

2. Reagents

a. Substrate plasma: Seitz-filtered or charcoal filtered bovine plasma (as used for the determination of factor X) is used. This plasma contains prothrombin, factor V and fibrinogen, but not factors VII and X.

b. Plasma to be tested: The platelet poor plasma of the patient is diluted with veronal buffer (usually 1:10).

c. Human brain thromboplastin (as in A).

d. 0.05 M $CaCl_2$.

3. Performance of the Test

Aliquots of 0.1 ml substrate plasma, 0.1 ml patient's plasma in an appropriate dilution and 0.1 ml human thromboplastin are pipetted in a glass test tube and warmed to 37° C. Then 0.1 ml 0.05 M $CaCl_2$ is added and the clotting time determined at 37° C.

4. Calibration Curve

This is obtained by testing different dilutions of normal pooled plasma (see A).

5. Comments

Although this test is often used as "factor VII-test", it does not measure specifically factor VII, but the combined activities of both factors VII + X.

If the activity of the patient's plasma is found to be reduced, this may be caused by a reduced activity of factor VII, of factor X or of both. If factor X is found to be normal with a specific factor X test (see p. 195), it can be assumed that the reduced activity of the plasma in this test is due to a decreased activity of factor VII. In this case, however, the reading obtained from the calibration curve is higher than the actual factor VII activity.

If factor X is lacking or greatly reduced in the patient's plasma, the test is not practicable. Thus, this assay is very limited in its application.

References

Bachmann, F., Duckert, F., and Koller, F. (1958). *Thromb. Diath. Haemorrhag. 1,* 169.

Denson, K. W. E. (1961). *Acta Haematol. 25,* 105.

Esnouf, M. P., and Jobin, F. (1967). *Biochem. J. 102,* 666.

Esnouf, M. P., and Williams, W. J. (1962). *Biochem. J. 84,* 62.

Hougie, C. (1962). *Proc. Soc. Exptl. Biol. Med. 109,* 754.

Lechner, K., and Deutsch, E. (1964). *Thromb. Diath. Haemorrhag. 13,* 314.

Lechner, K., and Deutsch, E. (1967). *Thromb. Diath. Haemorrhag. 18,* 252.

Leveson, J. E., and Esnouf, M. P. (1967). Unpublished observations.

Macfarlane, R. G., and Ash, B. J. (1962). *Brit. J. Haematol. 10,* 217.

Nemerson, Y., and Spaet, T. (1964). *Blood 23,* 657.

Owren, P. A. (1947). "The Coagulation of Blood". Gundersen, Oslo.

Shaw, S., Pegrum, G. D., Farthing, C. P., and Wolff, S. (1966). *Thromb. Diath. Haemorrhag. 15,* 294.

Williams, W. J., and Norris, D. G. (1966). *J. Biol. Chem. 241,* 1847.

Assays for Factor IX

(Christmas Factor, Plasma Thromboplastin Component [PTC], Platelet Cofactor II, Antihemophilic Globulin B [AHF B])

H. G. Schwick

I. Introduction

Today almost two decades after the discovery of factor IX and the first description of hemophilia B by Biggs et al. (1952), assay techniques for this procoagulant still fall short of absolute and exact quantitation. The assays described in the following, although not as accurate and reproducible as for instance the prothrombin assay, have proven adequate for clinical purposes i. e., the diagnosis and treatment of hemophilia B, the diagnosis of the von Willebrand-Jürgens syndrome with factor IX deficiency, the diagnosis of hemorrhagic states in the newborn and in hemorrhagic complications during anticoagulant therapy.

factor IX can be assayed in three principally different assay systems: (1) the thromboplastin generation test (2) the prothrombin consumption test and (3) the partial thromboplastin time test. As of this time, most workers in the field would agree that the quantitation of factor IX, irrespective of the assay system employed, requires plasma or serum from patients suffering from hemophilia B. Although artificial substrates have been proposed, their accuracy and reliability in factor IX assays remain doubtful.

One assay technique representing each of the three procedures will be described in detail in the following; suggested modifications for each of these three outlined techniques will be covered only through references to the literature.

II. Assay for Factor IX by the Thromboplastin Generation Test (Biggs and Douglas, 1953) (modified by Schwick, 1954; and Schwick and Störiko, 1966)

A. Principle

In this two-stage assay, formation of active "plasma thromboplastin" takes place under the participation of factors XII, XI, VIII, IX, X and V in addition to platelet factor 3 and calcium ions. In the second stage of the test the activity of formed "plasma thromboplastin" is measured using as a substrate platelet-poor plasma containing constant quantities of prothrombin and fibrinogen. The rate of thromboplastin formation and especially the maximal recorded activity of plasma thromboplastin depends on the concentration of participating factors. On the basis of these established correlations factor IX can be quantitated indirectly.

B. Reagents

1. Aluminum hydroxide suspension, 1 percent

2. Plasma adsorbed to aluminum hydroxide

Human venous blood is withdrawn and collected in a siliconized test tube containing 1 ml of a 0.1 mol/L sodium citrate solution for 9 ml of blood. Plasma is obtained by centrifuging for 15 minutes at 3000 g in siliconized centrifuge tubes. A 0.1 ml aliquot of 1 percent aluminum hydroxide suspension is added to 1 ml of this citrated plasma. The mixture is kept at 37° C for 3 minutes with gentle agitation and subsequently centrifuged for 5 minutes at 3000 g. The supernatant plasma is essentially free of factors II, VII, IX and X, all adsorbed by the treatment with aluminum hydroxide. The plasma must be diluted 1:5 with saline for the test.

3. Normal serum and hemophilia B serum

One ml of citrated plasma from a healthy donor and one ml from a patient suffering from hemophilia B are pipetted into each of two test tubes, mixed with 0.1 ml of a 1:10 dilution of any potent commercial tissue thromboplastin solution and caused to coagulate by addition of 1 ml of a 0.025 M $CaCl_2$ solution. The serum is incubated for 30 minutes at 37° C, then centrifuged for 15 minutes at 3000 rpm. In order to inactivate the free thrombin, the serum is re-incubated for 30 minutes at 37° C.

4. Platelets

Blood is obtained as described under section II, B, 2 with sodium citrate and is centrifuged for 10 minutes at 1500 rpm in siliconized centrifuge tubes in order to remove the erythrocytes.

The supernatant plasma containing platelets is centrifuged in a siliconized tube for 15 minutes at 3000 rpm. The plasma is poured off, the platelets are washed three times with saline, and are then resuspended in saline amounting to one-third the original plasma volume.

5. Substrate plasma

Platelet-poor plasma remaining after preparing the platelet suspension (section II, B, 4) can be used as substrate plasma in the second stage of the test.

C. Test Procedure

Immediately prior to the start of the test, 0.1 ml of substrate plasma and 0.1 ml of diethylbarbiturate-acetate buffer pH 6.7 are pipetted into each of 5–6 test tubes kept in a water bath at 37° C; into one additional test tube also kept in the water bath at 37° C is mixed: 0.3 ml of a 1:5 dilution of aluminum hydroxide adsorbed plasma, 0.3 ml of a 1:10 dilution of serum and 0.3 ml of platelet suspension. The mixture is shaken and 0.3 ml of a $CaCl_2$ solution 0.025 moles/L is added; a stopwatch is started at that point. At one minute intervals a 0.1 ml aliquot is removed from the incubation mixture and pipetted into one tube containing substrate plasma together with 0.1 ml of $^1/_{40}$ M $CaCl_2$ solution. The coagulation time for each tube at each one minute interval is recorded. If the plasma and serum described under sections II, B, 2 and 3 come from a healthy donor, activation times will be from 2 to 4 minutes, and coagulation times from 10 to 13 seconds.

For quantitative determination of factor IX, the measured plasma thromboplastin activity is plotted against concentrations of factor IX. One part (by volume) of a 1:10 dilution of normal serum is mixed with e.g., 8, 32 and 128 parts (by volume) of a 1:10 dilution of serum deficient in factor IX (taken from a donor known to have severe hemophilia B); these mixtures are added to the standard incubation mixtures in 0.1 ml aliquots and tested in the manner described above. When the shortest coagulation times obtained are plotted on a logarithmic scale against the dilutions on an arithmetic scale, a straight line graph results. For quantitation of factor IX activity in an unknown sample, the serum to be tested is diluted with known hemophilia B serum instead of with normal serum. This method ensures that in the various dilution stages all the coagulation factors involved, except factor IX, remain unchanged in concentration i. e., plasma thromboplastin activity is influenced only by the concentration of factor IX.

Further modifications of the plasma thromboplastin generation test which have been proposed especially for determining factor IX include the method suggested by Egli et al. (1957). According to this modification, maximum surface activation is accomplished through contact of the test serum with glass wool. Another modification proposed by Cattan (1965) and by Didisheim et al. (1958, 1962) is claimed by its authors to provide improved reliability in studies of hemophilia B carriers.

D. Comments

For the plasma thromboplastin generation test in the modifications described here, standardized reagents are available: aluminum hydroxide suspension, standardized substrate plasma and normal serum, as well as dry platelets can be obtained from Behringwerke, Marburg/Lahn, Germany.

III. Assay for Factor IX by the Prothrombin Consumption Test

A. Principle (Quick, 1947, 1966)

When normal blood clots in a glass test tube at 37° C, prothrombin is converted to thrombin and a linear decline in the prothrombin level ensues. After clotting has been allowed to proceed for one hour, approximately 5 percent of the original prothrombin levels are demonstrable in the serum. If any coagulation factor necessary for intrinsic prothrombin activation is lower than normal or absent, the rate of prothrombin to thrombin conversion is reduced and higher levels of prothrombin are demonstrable in the serum at any given time interval. The prothrombin consumption test, therefore, reflects the combined activities of factors responsible for intrinsic prothrombin activation i. e., factors XII, XI, IX, VIII, X and V; and this is accomplished by determination of serum prothrombin under specified standard conditions.

The following assay system devised by Quick (1966) permits the specific demonstration of factor IX deficiency.

B. Reagents

1. Hemolysate

Erythrocytes contain phospholipids which when released possess a coagulant activity similar to platelet factor 3.

10 ml of oxalated blood is centrifuged for 5 minutes at 1000 rpm; the erythrocytes are washed four times with saline and re-centrifuged for 20 minutes at 2000 rpm. The washed erythrocytes are brought up to the original blood volume by addition of saline, and frozen for 12 hours at –20° C. The thawed solution of completely hemolyzed erythrocytes is used as a hemolysate; if stored in small aliquots at –20° C, it can be used for a period of about six weeks.

2. Aged normal serum

Fresh blood from healthy donors is allowed to clot in a glass test tube; 15 minutes after coagulation it is centrifuged at 3000 rpm; and the supernatant serum is then incubated for 45 minutes at 37° C. The serum is aged for 48 hours at 4° C. Serum aged in this manner can be kept for several weeks if stored at –20° C. It is practically free of Factors II, V and VIII.

3. Tissue Thromboplastin

4. Oxalated rabbit plasma adsorbed to $Ca_3(PO_4)_2$

Fresh oxalated rabbit plasma is mixed with $Ca_3(PO_4)_2$ (20 mg/ml plasma) and kept at 37° C for 5 minutes under gentle agitation. After centrifugation the clear plasma is kept frozen at –20° C until used for the test.

C. Test Procedure

The blood to be tested for factor IX is withdrawn with siliconized syringes and needles and transferred into glass tubes. 1 ml of the blood is placed in each of three test tubes, the first of which (tube 1) contains 0.1 ml of hemolysate, the second (tube 2) 0.1 ml of hemolysate and 0.03 ml of aged human serum, and the third (tube 3) no additional substances. The test mixtures are kept at 37° C; 15 minutes after clotting the mixtures are centrifuged at 3000 rpm, and the supernatant serum is incubated for 45 minutes at 37° C to insure complete inactivation of free thrombin.

The prothrombin content of the serum samples in tubes 1, 2, and 3 can be determined either by a one-stage or two-stage test. For the qualitative demonstration of factor IX deficiency the one-stage modification (Quick et al. 1963) is well suited. Serum prothrombin in the one-stage test is assayed by mixing 0.1 ml of the serum samples with 0.1 ml of thromboplastin, 0.1 ml of a 0.02 moles/L $CaCl_2$ solution and 0.1 ml of $Ca_3(PO_4)_2$ adsorbed oxalated rabbit plasma (providing a source of factor V and I). The clotting time of this mixture is determined.

Normal values by this technique lie between 16 and 35 seconds. In case of factor IX deficiency, the serum from tube 1 shows a shortened coagulation time of about 8–11 seconds, whereas the coagulation time in serum tube 2 where factor IX was replaced by aged serum is normal.

The procedure is well suited for qualitative demonstration of factor IX deficiency in cases of hemophilia B. The prothrombin consumption test described by Graham et al. (1955) for quantitative demonstration of factor VIII could conceivably with suitable modifications be used for the quantitation of factor IX as well.

IV. Assay for Factor IX by the Partial Thromboplastin Time

A. Principle

The differentiation between hemophilia A and B as well as other coagulopathies can be accomplished through the combined use of the partial thromboplastin time (PTT) and the complete thromboplastin time (Quick test), (Langdell et al. 1953). In the PTT test, platelet factor 3 or suspensions of certain phospholipids are added to the plasma in addition to calcium ions. The PTT test reflects the levels of the following factors of the intrinsic pathway; XII, XI, IX, VIII, X, V, II and I. In this test system, factor IX activity can be determined by the shortening of the partial thromboplastin time of plasma known to be deficient in factor IX.

MacPherson and Hardisty (1961), Proctor and Rapaport (1961) and Aggeler et al. (1964) have introduced surface activation of the plasma by means of kaolin or celite as a means of standardizing the PTT test.

B. Reagents

1. Normal plasma and hemophilia B plasma

Nine parts (by volume) of venous blood are mixed during withdrawal with one part (by volume) of a 3.8 percent sodium citrate solution; the plasma is obtained by centrifugation of the blood for 15 minutes at 3000 rpm.

2. Plasma adsorbed to $BaSO_4$

One-hundred mg of $BaSO_4$ are added per ml of oxalated plasma and the mixture is gently shaken for 30 minutes at 5° C. It is then centrifuged for 10 minutes at 3000 rpm, and the supernatant plasma is used.

3. Platelet factor 3 or phospholipid suspension

According to Bell and Alton (1954) and Rodman et al. (1958), phospholipids with platelet factor 3 activity can be obtained from acetone-dried chloroform-extracted brain homogenates. Such preparations are available commercially as reagents for the PTT test: Cephaloplastin (Dade Reagents, Miami, Florida, USA); Hyland Partial Thromboplastin Time Test (Hyland, Los Angeles, California, USA); Platelin (Warner-Chilcott, Morris Plains, New Jersey, USA); PTT-Reagenz (Behringwerke Marburg/Lahn, Germany); Tachostyp-Test (Hormonchemie, Munich, Germany); Thrombofax (Ortho Research Foundation, Raritan, New Jersey, USA).

C. Test Procedure

A 0.2 ml aliquot of citrated plasma is pipetted into a test tube placed in a water bath followed by 0.2 ml of PTT reagent (phospholipid with platelet factor 3 activity). If the reagent contains kaolin or a similar substance suitable for surface activation, the mixture is allowed to stand for 2 to 3 minutes at 37° C. At time zero 0.2 ml of a 0.02 M $CaCl_2$ solution prewarmed to 37° C is added and the coagulation time recorded.

Coagulation times for normal plasma lie between 70 and 90 seconds, depending on the platelet factor 3 activity of the phospholipid preparation used. If the preparation contains a surface-activation additive, the times fall between 35 and 50 seconds. In severe cases of factor VIII or factor IX deficiency values will be around 200 seconds or longer. For differentiating between hemophilia B and other coagulopathies, e.g., hemophilia A, the plasma to be tested is mixed with an equal volume of known hemophilia B plasma. This mixture is then tested as described above.

In hemophilia B, coagulation time is greatly prolonged; if a known hemophilia B plasma is used, factors V and VIII must be present at normal concentrations.

For quantitative determination of factor IX, plasma from a patient with severe hemophilia B is used as a substrate. Serial dilutions of the plasma to be tested are added, and the coagulation times of the mixtures are determined, observing the testing volumes given for the PTT test (Barrow et al. 1960).

V. Assays for Factor IX using Artificial Substrates

Methods have been proposed for determining factor IX without using hemophilia B plasma. The author has no experience with such methods and, thus confines himself here to describing their principle.

Stapp (1965) obtained human plasma free of factor IX by treatment with bentonite. This plasma is said to be suitable as a substitute for hemophilia B plasma in a modified PTT test for determining factor IX.

Egli and Schneider (1962) have proposed a modification based on the assumption that plasma which has not been surface-activated contains no factor IX. According to them, this absence of factor IX activity in normal plasma obtained with certain precautions makes it possible to use such normal plasma instead of hemophilia B plasma as factor IX deficient plasma in a one-stage test based on the principle of the PTT test.

References

Aggeler, P. M., Hoag, M. S., Kropatkin, M. L., and Kaplan, S. S. (1964). *In* "The Hemophilias" (K. M. Brinkhous, Ed.), pp. 131—147. University of North Carolina Press, Chapel Hill, N. C.

Barrow, E. M., Bullock, W. R., and Graham, J. B. (1960). *J. Lab. Clin. Med. 55,* 936.

Bell, W. N., and Alten, H. G. (1954). *Nature 174,* 880.

Biggs, R., Douglas, A. S., MacFarlane, R. G., Dacie, J. V., Pitney, W. R., Merskey, C., and O'Brien, J. R. (1952). *Brit. Med. J. 2,* 1378.

Biggs, R., and Douglas, A. S. (1953). *J. Clin. Pathol. 6,* 23.

Cattan, A. (1965). *Rev. Franc. Etudes Clin. Biol. 10,* 225.

Didisheim, P., Ferguson, J. H., and Lewis, J. H. (1958). *Arch. Intern. Med. 101,* 347.

Didisheim, P., and Vandervoort, R. L. E. (1962). *Blood 20,* 150.

Egli, H., Kesseler, K., and Klesper, R. (1957). *Acta Haematol. 17,* 338.

Egli, H., and Schneider, W. (1962). *Thromb. Diath. Haemorrhag. 7,* 523.

Graham, J. B., Penick, G. D., and Brinkhous, K. M. (1955). *In* "Blood Coagulation, Hemorrhage and Thrombosis" (L. M. Tocantins and L. A. Kazal, eds.), p. 112. Grune and Stratten, New York-London.

Langdell, R. D., Wagner, R. H., and Brinkhous, K. M. (1953). *J. Lab. Clin. Med. 41,* 637.

MacPherson, J. C., and Hardisty, R. M. (1961). *Thromb. Diath. Haemorrhag. 6,* 492.

Proctor, R. R., and Rapaport, S. J. (1961). *Am. J. Clin. Pathol. 36,* 212.

Quick, A. J. (1947). *Am. J. Med. Sci. 214,* 272.

Quick, A. J., Hussey, C. V., and Geppert, M. (1963). *Am. J. Med. Sci. 246,* 517.

Quick, A. J. (1966). *J. Am. Med. Assoc. 197,* 138.

Rodman, N. F., Barrow, E. M., and Graham, J. B. (1958). *Am. J. Clin. Pathol. 29,* 525.

Schwick, G. (1954). *Klin. Wochschr. 32,* 171.

Schwick, H. G., and Störiko, K. (1966). *In* „Beiträge für Diagnostik von Blutgerinnungsstörungen", Laboratoriums-Blätter, Frankfurt/Main.

Stapp, W. F. (1965). *Scand. J. Clin. Invest. 17* (Suppl. 84), 109.

Assays for Autoprothrombin I, II, III, C, and Prethrombin

HEINZ SCHRÖER

I. Introduction

The assay methods described in this chapter are mainly employed in biochemistry to clarify the prothrombin complex and its activation. Obviously, there are several similarities between the functions and properties of the procoagulant prothrombin derivatives on one hand, and certain plasma clotting factors designated by Roman Numerals on the other hand. Autoprothrombin I seems to be related to factor VII, autoprothrombin II to factor IX, autoprothrombin III to inactive factor X, and autoprothrombin C may be the same as active factor X. But, as long as the possible identities have not been proven on a molecular basis they can hardly be of any consequence for the practical performance of the quantitative determinations concerned. Therefore, no speculative attempt is made in the following to correlate the methods described to those procedures being in use to assay for the plasma „factors" which may correspond to prothrombin derivatives.

The conditions for the generation and functions of the different split products of prothrombin are described in the introductory chapter.

The principle of all methods for the determination of procoagulant activity of a certain prothrombin derivative is always the same. The test system has to be composed in such a way that the speed of thrombin formation and/or the terminal thrombin yield is representative of the activity of the components concerned. Special attention has to be focused on attaining maximal specifity and sensitivity of the different test systems by creating optimal conditions for the reaction in which the unknown component is involved. To arrange those conditions it is important to find the most suitable reaction-constituents as well as their optimal concentrations in the test system.

II. Assay for Autoprothrombin I_p

From purified, not chromatographed prothrombin, in the presence of calcium ions and platelet factor 3, a derivative is obtained (Seegers, 1952b) which acts as an accelerator in clotting systems containing tissue extract (Seegers et al. 1955). Since platelets are needed for its generation from prothrombin, it has been called autoprothrombin I_p. This procoagulant corrects the clotting defect of a factor VII deficient plasma (Seegers and Alkjaersig, 1955), and its activity is destroyed by antithrombin (Seegers et al. 1964c). Purification methods have not been devised, but it has been possible to enrich its activity (Mammen et al. 1960a).

A. Procedure

The main requirement for the determination of autoprothrombin I_p is the presence of tissue extracts (tissue thromboplastin) as a basic component of the reaction mixture (Mammen et al. 1960a; Seegers et al. 1955; Seegers and Kagami, 1964). This is used in such a low concentration that in the absence of autoprothrombin I_p, only a small percentage of the prothrombin present in the mixture is converted to thrombin. The most accurate results are obtained when purified prothrombin is used as the substrate. The requirements mentioned are considered in the assay method of Seegers et al. (1955). According to this method the composition of the test system – and that of the control – is the following:

Reagents	Test System (ml)	Control System (ml)
Purified prothrombin (3,000 U/ml)	1.0	1.0
Diluted thromboplastin (1:25)	0.5	0.5
Bovine adsorbed serum (1:50)	0.5	0.5
$CaCl_2$ (0.16 M in imidazole buffer)	0.5	0.5
Physiological saline	0.0	0.5
Autoprothrombin I_p	0.5	0.0

The thrombin yield as well as the rate of thrombin formation increases after addition of autoprothrombin I_p depending on the concentration of the latter. By comparing the final thrombin activities obtained by using different concentrations of autoprothrombin I_p in the system described above (standard curves*), the activity of the unknown preparation can be quantitated. Approximately 1 unit of autoprothrombin I_p is needed to accelerate 1 unit of substrate thrombin (1 unit of autoprothrombin I_p is equivalent to the activity derived from 1 unit of prothrombin) (Seegers et al. 1955).

* Standard curves are prepared by standard autoprothrombin I_p samples generated from purified prothrombin in the presence of platelet factor 3 and calcium ions.

III. Assay for Autoprothrombin I_c

Seegers et al. (1962) found that a prothrombin derivative with the accelerator properties of autoprothrombin I is obtained from purified bovine prothrombin when autoprothrombin C is added to the solution at alkaline pH. To indicate that this protein is generated by the action of autoprothrombin C it has been called autoprothrombin I_c. On the basis of solubility, pH-stability and heat resistance it was distinguished from autoprothrombin I_p (Seegers et al. 1962). By precipitation with 50% ammonium sulfate from the activation mixture and following chromatography and gel filtration, purified preparations of autoprothrombin I_c were obtained with a specific activity between 32,000 and 34,000 units/mg tyrosine or 1,550 units/mg dry weight. The molecular weight of these preparations was determined to about 34,300. The amino acid composition was found to be quite similar to that of autoprothrombin C (Harmison et al. 1965).

Autoprothrombin I_c accelerates the thrombin formation from prothrombin by thromboplastin, Ac-globulin and calcium ions. It is more effective in correcting the prothrombin time of Stuart plasma than that of factor VII deficient plasma. The autoprothrombin I_c, when added to prothrombin, does not reduce the prothrombin activity („two-stage refractoriness" is not produced), and this distinguishes it from autoprothrombin C.

A. Procedure

The most reliable method for the quantitative determination of the autoprothrombin I_c concentration is that described by Seegers and Kagami (1964) which is a modification of the partial thromboplastin time test of Langdell et al. (1953). In this procedure use is made of the observation that plasma from dogs treated with Dicumarol shows a prolonged partial thromboplastin time. This becomes shortened when autoprothrombin I_c is added to the test system. The shortening effect is dependent on the concentration of autoprothrombin I_c. By using cephalin instead of tissue thromboplastin the sensitivity of the test is increased. The presence of Ac-globulin in the Dicumarol plasma is essential.

1. Reagents

a. Dicumarol dog plasma: This is citrated plasma obtained from a 20 kg dog given a single dose of 50 mg Dicumarol 3 days before the blood sample was taken. The prothrombin concentration usually ranges from 15 to 20 units/ml plasma. If the plasma is stored in a deep freezer it remains suitable over a period of at least 3 months.

b. Crude "cephalin" suspension: This material is prepared in the usual manner by ether extraction of the acetone-dried gray substance of calf brain (Cole et al. 1962). A freshly obtained calf brain is dissected free of the meninges, rinsed in water, the gray matter collected, and ground in acetone with a mortar and pestle. About three changes of acetone are required to dry the brain. The acetone is removed and the material is allowed to air dry. It is then finely ground and extracted with 300–400 ml ether for 2–3 days in the dark. The flask is shaken occasionally. The extract is filtered and placed in a large evaporating dish, and the ether is evaporated. The crude lipid is washed 2 times with acetone, and the acetone is decanted and discarded. After air drying, the lipid is weighed and suspended in saline to a 5% concentration. The lipid suspension is homogenized and stored in a deep freezer until needed. Before use, it is thawed and diluted with saline to get the desired concentration.

c. Calcium chloride solution, 0.05 M in imidazole buffer, pH 7.2.

2. Performance of the Assay

The test system should be composed as follows:

Dicumarol dog plasma	0.1 ml
0.2% Cephalin suspension	0.1 ml
0.05 M $CaCl_2$, pH 7.2	0.05 ml
Unknown test material	0.05 ml

The Dicumarol plasma and the cephalin suspension are placed in a test tube and the latter is kept at 37° C. The calcium chloride solution (0.1 ml) and the unknown substrate (0.1 ml) are warmed separately to 37° C and then mixed. Immediately after complete mixing, 0.1 ml of this solution is added to the plasma-cephalin mixture and the clotting time is measured. The end point of the clotting time can be determined very exactly because of the extremely rapid gelatination of the system.

The curve in figure 1 shows the relations between clotting time and concentration of purified autoprothrombin I_c. It may be used as a standard curve for the calculation of the activity. By definition, the test system contains 1 unit autoprothrombin I if the clotting time is 20 seconds. In this case the activity of the unknown solution is 1 unit/0.05 ml or 20 units/ml. The clotting time should be within the range of 18 to 22 seconds. Otherwise the assay has to be repeated by using different dilutions.

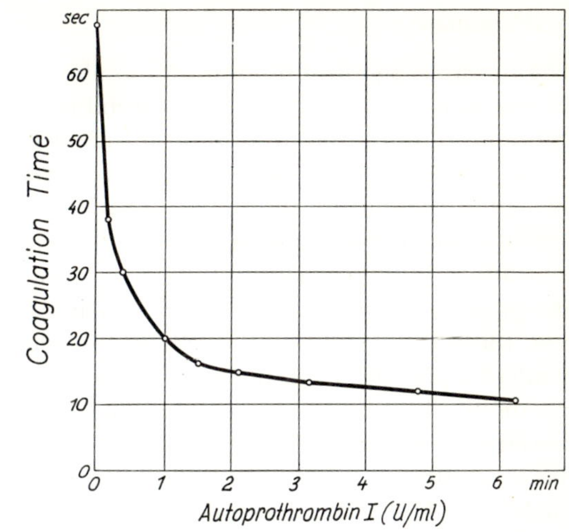

Fig. 1. Standard curve for the autoprothrombon I_c assay according to Seegers and Kagami (1964). The prothrombin content of the Dicumarol plasma was 17 units/ml.

3. Remarks

The prothrombin content of the Dicumarol plasma is within certain limits, of no influence on the clotting times. When blood samples were taken daily from a dog treated with Dicumarol there was practically no autoprothrombin I activity in the plasma before or during the time the prothrombin concentration decreased and returned to normal. From this finding it became obvious that normal dog plasma does not contain significant amounts of autoprothrombin I.

IV. Assay for Autoprothrombin II

This activity was first found in serum (Johnson et al. 1954), it is closely related to the plasma deficiency of patients with hemophilia B (Johnson and Seegers, 1954). The serum of those patients, in contrast to normal serum, contains autoprothrombin II in low concentration (Johnson et al. 1955). During treatment with Dicumarol its concentration in serum is also diminished (Johnson and Seegers, 1956; Johnson et al. 1957).

Autoprothrombin II is activated from purified, not chromatographed bovine prothrombin at pH 8.1–8.2 in the absence of calcium ions with thrombin added to the prothrombin solution. Surfaces play an important role in this reaction (Schröer et al. 1965). By precipitation at half saturated ammonium sulfate followed by chromatography on IRC-50 at pH 7.0 autoprothrombin II can be isolated from the activation mixture (Mammen et al. 1960a). A similar procedure was used for its isolation from activated human prothrombin. The molecular weight, calculated on the basis of the physical-chemical data of autoprothrombin II and its amino acid composition, is about 49,900 (Harmison and Seegers, 1962). When blood clots after thrombin has been added an increase in autoprothrombin II concentration of the serum is observed. However, practically no autoprothrombin II in serum is found after addition of autoprothrombin C instead of thrombin. This is due to the fact that autoprothrombin C in suitable concentration causes a rapid and almost complete conversion of prothrombin to thrombin. In the "thromboplastin generation test" autoprothrombin II substituted for normal serum (factor IX) (Ulutin et al. 1961a, 1961b). Its activity was found in serum when purified prothrombin was added to blood from dogs that were treated with Dicumarol. In tests with hemophilia B plasma as substrate, the serum concentration of autoprothrombin II was proportional to the amount of prothrombin added to Dicumarol plasma before clotting (Schröer et al. 1965).

A. Procedure

The accelerating effect of autoprothrombin II on the activation of purified prothrombin to thrombin in the presence of platelet factor 3, Ac-globulin (factor V) and calcium ions can be used as an indicator for the quantitative determination of the autoprothrombin II concentration. If all participants of the reaction, except autoprothrombin II, are present in excess, the resulting thrombin yield is only dependent upon the concentration of autoprothrombin II. This procedure was first employed by Seegers et al. (1957) to determine the concentration of platelet cofactor I (factor VIII). The assay procedure was modified by Mammen et al. (1960b). The high Ac-globulin concentration required for the reaction mixture is reached by adding $BaCO_3$-adsorbed bovine serum (Murphy et al. 1947). Originally, instead of this reagent, a prothrombin preparation was used which was not purified from Ac-globulin. However, the large differences in Ac-globulin content of those preparations was found to be a source of error.

1. Reagents

Purified prothrombin (Seegers, 1952a), platelet factor 3 (Alkjaersig et al. 1955), $CaCl_2$ solution (0.15 M in imidazole buffer), $BaCO_3$-adsorbed bovine serum (1:25) (see chapter „Assay for Prothrombin").

2. Performance of the Assay

The reaction mixture is composed as follows:

Purified prothrombin (3,000 U/ml)	1.0 ml
Platelet factor 3 (80 U/ml)	0.5 ml
$CaCl_2$ (0.15 M in imidazole buffer)	0.5 ml
Bovine adsorbed serum (1:25)	0.5 ml
Unknown in saline	0.5 ml
Total	3.0 ml

This mixture is incubated at 28° C. At regular time intervals samples are taken from the mixture and added to a fibrinogen solution for determining the thrombin activity (Seegers and Smith, 1942). The maximum of thrombin activity which is reached after 1 hour of incubation serves as a relative measure for the autoprothrombin II content. This can be expressed in units/ml corresponding to the thrombin activity found. Actual concentration data can be formulated by relating the thrombin activity measured to the thrombin activity obtained by testing different amounts of an autoprothrombin II preparation (Table 1).

Table 1: Thrombin Yields after One-hour Incubation of the Reaction Mixture (see text) in Dependence of the Autoprothrombin II Concentration. (According to Seegers, 1962.)

Autoprothrombin II (γ/ml)	Thrombin (U/ml)
0	127
132.8	131
265.6	358
398.4	450
531.2	550
664.0	691
796.8	742
929.6	873
1062.4	995

When all of the prothrombin substrate is converted to thrombin, the concentration of the latter is 1,000 units/ml. Sometimes the autoprothrombin II concentrates have to be diluted before being placed in the reaction mixture. If the unknown is plasma or adsorbed plasma, it is first defibrinated (technical advise, see chapter "Assay for Prothrombin") and thereby becomes diluted 1:2; consequently its dilution in the activation mixture is 1:2.

The method described can be adapted by suitable modifications to any requirements which may result from the scientific questions concerned (Harmison and Mammen, 1967; Mammen et al. 1960b; Seegers, 1962).

V. Assay for Autoprothrombin III

This precursor of autoprothrombin C (Marciniak and Seegers, 1965) is derived from purified prothrombin under those conditions which favor the generation of a considerable thrombin activity, but not the generation of much autoprothrombin C (Marciniak and Seegers, 1962). In a prothrombin solution (pH 7.2) containing calcium ions, Ac-globulin and crude cephalin, besides thrombin, autoprothrombin

III is produced (Seegers et al. 1964a). This can be purified from the activation mixture by precipitation with acetone followed by chromatography (Seegers et al. 1964a). Autoprothrombin III can likewise be prepared from purified prothrombin by first digesting the prothrombin with thrombin at neutral pH. The prothrombin derivatives, prethrombin, autoprothrombin III and inhibitor, appearing under these conditions, can be separated by fractionation on DEAE-cellulose (Seegers and Marciniak, 1965). The physical-chemical properties of both autoprothrombin III preparations are very similar and almost equal to those of autoprothrombin C. Its molecular weight is only a little higher than that of the active enzyme. Autoprothrombin III can be activated in different ways. Under biological conditions, the activation by tissue thromboplastin is considered to be the most effective way. Experimentally, the fastest activation is reached by Russel's Viper Venom (Stypven) (Mammen, 1968). With tissue thromboplastin, Ac-globulin and calcium ions, the yield is only 50 % of that by using the snake venom. To a lesser extend, the activation occurs when purified platelet cofactor I (factor VIII) is present (Marciniak and Seegers, 1965). Autoprothrombin III can also be converted to autoprothrombin C by trypsin or in a 25 % sodium citrate solution (Seegers et al. 1965).

A. Procedure

To determine the concentration of autoprothrombin III, a two-stage principle is applied (Cole et al. 1962). In a first step a maximal conversion of autoprothrombin III to autoprothrombin C is achieved by adding Russel's Viper Venom. Details of the procedure were described by Reno and Seegers (1967).

1. Reagents

Russel's Viper Venom (Stypven), Burroughs-Wellcome Co. (0.1 mg/ml).
Imidazole buffered saline (dilution 1:9)
$CaCl_2$ (0.25 M)
Crude cephalin suspension (0.1 % in NaCl)
Buffered bovine plasma (1 part oxalated platelet-poor plasma plus 1 part imidazole buffered NaCl).

2. Performance of the Assay

Add in order, mix and place at 37° C the following activation mixture:

Buffered NaCl	1.65 ml
Stypven	0.05 ml
$CaCl_2$	0.20 ml
Diluted autoprothrombin III	0.10 ml
Total	2.00 ml

A timer is started when the autoprothrombin III is added.
At 2 min and at each 30 sec intervals thereafter, 0.1 ml of the activation mixture is pipetted into a test tube (10 × 75 mm) containing 0.2 ml buffered bovine plasma and 0.2 ml cephalin suspension at 37° C.
The clotting times of the test medium are noted.
The shortest clotting times are usually attained between 3 and 5 min of incubation.
The shortest clotting times must fall between 13 and 16 sec. If not, another autoprothrombin III dilution must be prepared.
From the shortest clotting times the units of autoprothrombin III per ml of activation mixture can be determined. One unit of autoprothrombin III equals one unit of autoprothrombin C. Table 2 can be used for the conversion of clotting times to thrombin units.
The total unitage of autoprothrombin III per ml of sample can be calculated by multiplying the units read in Table 2 times the dilution of

Table 2: Conversion of Clotting Times to Thrombin Units. (Autoprothrombin III Assay.)

Times Clotting sec	Thrombin Units	Clotting Times sec	Thrombin Units
12.0	0.272	15.0	0.146
12.2	0.263	15.2	0.140
12.4	0.247	15.4	0.135
12.6	0.236	15.6	0.131
12.8	0.225	15.8	0.126
13.0	0.217	16.0	0.122
13.2	0.210	16.2	0.118
13.4	0.200	16.4	0.113
13.6	0.190	16.6	0.110
13.8	0.182	16.8	0.105
14.0	0.177	17.0	0.102
14.2	0.170	17.2	0.100
14.4	0.163	17.4	0.097
14.6	0.155	17.6	0.094
14.8	0.150	17.8	0.090
		18.0	0.087

the sample in the activation mixture (usually 20 ×). The dilution of the sample in the clotting mixture (1:5) is taken into account in Table 2.

As a control of the test system, 0.1 ml of 0.025 M $CaCl_2$ solution is added to the buffered bovine plasma-cephalin mixture. Clotting times greater than 35 sec should be obtained.

All assays should be performed in triplicate and averaged to minimize errors of dilution and timing.

VI. Assay for Autoprothrombin C

Autoprothrombin C is most likely identical (Seegers, 1966) with active factor X of various authors (Esnouf and Williams, 1962; Lechner and Deutsch, 1965; Milstone et al. 1963; Spaet and Cintron, 1963; Tishkoff et al. 1960). In plasma of patients with hemorrhagic diseases, except parahemophilia, it normalizes the partial thromboplastin times as well as the prothrombin consumption (Seegers and Marcininak, 1962). Autoprothrombin C is inactivated by antithrombin (Seegers et al. 1964) but not by hirudin (Markwardt et al. 1964), it is not found in serum in appreciable concentrations (Seegers et al. 1967a). When purified prothrombin is brought into a salt solution of high concentration it activates spontaneously to thrombin and autoprothrombin C (Fig. 2). Both enzymes are end-products of prothrombin activation. They appear with the same speed, and the time-course of their release is typical for an autocatalytic process.

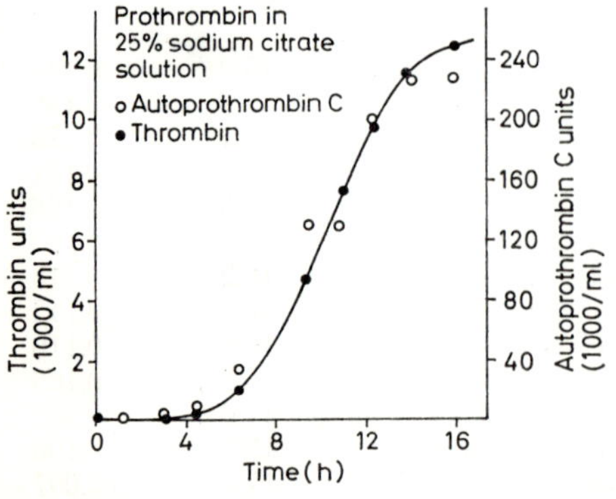

Fig. 2. Activation of purified prothrombin in 25 per cent sodium citrate solution. (According to Seegers, 1966.)

After the activation in strong salt solutions is complete, the autoprothrombin C can be separated from the mixture by precipitation with acetone, followed by chromatography on DEAE-cellulose (Seegers et al. 1966). In another purification procedure (Seegers et al. 1963) purified prothrombin is first activated to thrombin and autoprothrombin C by tissue thromboplastin, Ac-globulin and calcium ions. The protein of the mixture is precipitated with acetone, and the autoprothrombin C is then isolated by chromatography on DEAE-cellulose and Amberlite IRC-50. Its physical-chemical and immunological properties differ considerably from those of thrombin (Harmison et al. 1961; Seegers et al. 1963; Seegers ct al. 1958; Barnhart, 1967). The molecular weight is about 24,000. When tissue extract is present, the prothrombin activation always leads to the generation of thrombin and autoprothrombin C (Marciniak and Seegers, 1962; Seegers, 1964). This effect of tissue extract may be partially due to its content of cathepsin (Purcell and Barnhart, 1963).

Two quantitative procedures for autoprothrombin C have been described by Cole et al. (1962). In one of these (A), purified prothrombin is used as a substrate. In this procedure, a reaction mixture is used in which the thrombin titer developing in 20 min is proportional to the amount of autoprothrombin C in the reaction mixture. In the other method (B) a standard bovine plasma is recalcified and the clotting times are noted. Autoprothrombin C shortens the clotting time, and the extend of this is a quantitative measure for autoprothrombin C activity, provided the unknown does not contain thrombin which would interfere with the result.

A. Procedure Using Purified Prothrombin

1. Reagents

Purified prothrombin, isolated from bovine plasma according to Seegers (1952a).

Cephalin suspension (0.4% in physiological saline) (preparation see "Assay for Autoprothrombin I_c").

$BaCO_3$ – adsorbed bovine serum (as source for Ac-globulin) diluted 1:50 with physiological saline. (Adsorbing procedure see "Assay for Prothrombin".)
$CaCl_2$ (0.32 M, pH 7.2 in imidazole buffer).

2. Performance of the Assay

The following activation mixture is prepared in silicone coated test tubes to prevent the adsorption of prothrombin and thrombin on glass; temperature 28° C:

Purified prothrombin (4,500 U/ml)	0.4 ml
0.4% suspension crude "cephalin"	0.2 ml
Serum Ac-globulin	0.3 ml
$CaCl_2$ (0.32 M in pH 7.2 imidazole buffer)	0.1 ml
Autoprothrombin C in 0.9% saline	0.2 ml
Total	1.2 ml

Prothrombin is the last component to be added, and the generation of thrombin is followed by removing a sample of the mixture at various time intervals in order to assay for thrombin (Seegers and Smith, 1942). For this purpose 0.1 ml of the reaction mixture is added to 0.4 ml of a mixture containing 0.1 ml of a 1% fibrinogen solution and 0.3 ml acacia-calcium mixture (see chapter "Assay for Prothrombin"). The clotting times are measured at 28° C. In almost all cases activation of prothrombin to thrombin is complete within 12 min. The amount of thrombin generated is expressed as thrombin units per ml of reaction mixture. The activity generated depends on the quantity of autoprothrombin C in the reaction mixture (Fig. 3). The amount of prothrombin added should be such that about 300–700 units of thrombin are produced. This is considered the most accurate range. The autoprothrombin C units are determined from a set of standard curves such as shown in Fig. 3. The appropriate dilution and correction factors are applied in order to express the autoprothrombin C concentration of the solution being assayed.

3. Example of Calculations

An autoprothrombin C sample of unknown concentration was diluted in saline 40 times. The dilution in the activation mixture was 1:6. The generation of thrombin followed a curve like that obtained with 4 units of standard autoprothrombin C in Fig. 3.

The activity of autoprothrombin C in the sample was $40 \times 6 \times 4 = 960$ units/ml.

If the unknown sample contains thrombin, the amount of thrombin should be determined by a thrombin assay (Seegers and Smith, 1942), and the thrombin units per ml of activation mixture contributed by the autoprothrombin C sample can then be calculated and subtracted from the total thrombin titer in the activation mixture.

4. Comments

One unit of autoprothrombin C, under standard conditions, catalyzes the generation of 70 units of thrombin. Under the same standard conditions, 4 units of autoprothrombin C generate about 460 units of thrombin (instead of $4 \times 70 = 280$ units), 16 units of autoprothrombin C, however, generate about 810 units of thrombin (instead of $16 \times 70 = 1120$ units). Thus, there is an optimum for the procoagulant effect of autoprothrombin C depending on the specified conditions of temperature, pH and ionic strength. These findings support an observation made by Mertz et al. (1939) that an appreciable amount of thrombin generates easily with small amounts of a procoagulant.

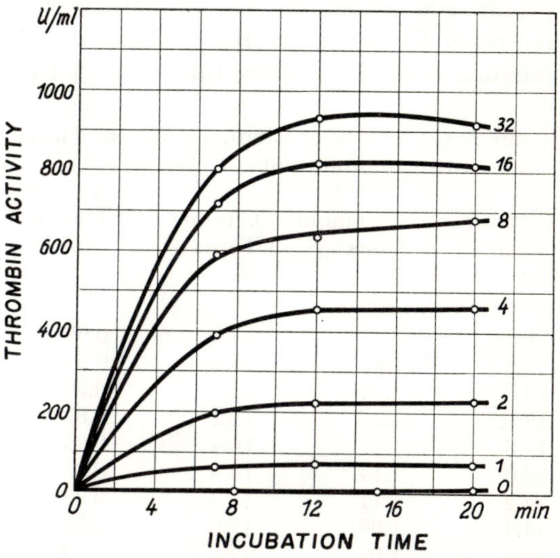

Fig. 3. Quantitative relationship between thrombin and autoprothrombin C. The numbers on each curve represent units of autoprothrombin C in the reaction mixture. (According to Cole et al. 1962.)

As prothrombin approaches complete activation, a relatively large amount of procoagulant is needed to convert the last remaining traces of prothrombin to thrombin. With anticoagulants just the opposite holds (Hecht et al. 1957). The accuracy of the method described above is only sufficient within a certain range of final thrombin concentration (300–700 U/ml).

B. Procedure Using Standard Bovine Plasma

This method is easier to perform but can only be used if the unknown autoprothrombin C sample is free of thrombin.

1. Reagents

Bovine oxalated platelet-poor plasma (diluted immediately before use with an equal volume of imidazole buffered saline)
Crude "cephalin" suspension (0.1 % in 0.9 % NaCl)
$CaCl_2$ (0.025 M)

2. Performance of the Assay

Mix 0.2 ml of diluted plasma with 0.2 ml crude cephalin suspension and warm to 37° C. Autoprothrombin C sample is diluted to desired concentration with 0.025 M $CaCl_2$. Immediately add 0.2 ml of the diluted autoprothrombin C sample to the plasma-cephalin mixture. Note the clotting time. The clotting times should be in the range of 13 to 18 sec. If not, autoprothrombin C has to be diluted differently.

Table 3: Conversion of Clotting Times to Thrombin Units. (Autoprothrombin C Assay.)

Clotting Times sec	Thrombin Units	Clotting Times sec	Thrombin Units
13.0	1.32	15.6	0.93
13.2	1.27	15.8	0.91
13.4	1.24	16.0	0.89
13.6	1.20	16.2	0.87
13.8	1.17	16.4	0.85
14.0	1.14	16.6	0.83
14.2	1.11	16.8	0.82
14.4	1.08	17.0	0.80
14.6	1.05	17.2	0.79
14.8	1.03	17.4	0.77
15.0	1.00	17.6	0.76
15.2	0.98	17.8	0.75
15.4	0.95	18.0	0.73

3. Calculation

The clotting times in sec are converted to thrombin units using Table 3. Since in this test 1 unit of autoprothrombin C generates 40 units of thrombin, the units of autoprothrombin C per ml sample are equal to the thrombin units (Table 3) times the dilution with $CaCl_2$ times 3 (dilution in assay mixture) divided by 40.
As a control, 0.2 ml $CaCl_2$ substitutes for the autoprothrombin C sample. The clotting times should be greater than 35 sec.

VII. Assay for Prethrombin

The fact that the dissociation of prothrombin occuring during the first minutes of its activation in a strong salt solution does not coincide with the appearance of thrombin and autoprothrombin C activity suggests the existance of a subunit of prothrombin which contains the thrombin molecule in an inactive state. This prothrombin derivative was discovered and isolated by Seegers and Marciniak (1965). It was called prethrombin.
A conversion of this proenzyme into active thrombin does not occur under the classical conditions for prothrombin activation (thromboplastin, Ac-globulin, calcium ions); it only happens when autoprothrombin C is present. This reaction is accelerated by lipids, Ac-globulin and calcium ions. Thrombin is not able to activate prethrombin, but trypsin is.
The easiest way to obtain prethrombin from purified prothrombin is to add thrombin to the prothrombin solution at pH 7.0. The dissociation products arising, prethrombin, autoprothrombin III and an inhibitor, can be separated by chromatography. Further purification of the prethrombin is achieved by ammonium sulfate precipitation, and gel filtration on Sephadex.
The specific activity of prethrombin is about 45,000 U/mg tyrosine, its molecular weight is near 36,000 (Seegers et al. 1967b). The amino acid analysis for prethrombin is much like that of thrombin. Evidently prethrombin is a sub-

unit closely related to thrombin, and most likely a peptide bond is broken when thrombin activity appears (Seegers, 1966).

A. Procedure

Prethrombin is determined quantitatively by using a two-stage procedure. The method developed for this purpose by Marciniak and Seegers (1965) corresponds to the two-stage procedure of Ware and Seegers (1949). However, since prethrombin, in contrast to prothrombin, has no source of autoprothrombin C needed for its activation the latter has to be added together with cephalin, thus replacing tissue thromboplastin in the assay for prothrombin. This proceeding is in accord with the modified two-stage assay of Seegers and Marciniak (1962). The cephalin suspension (Cole et al. 1962) is prepared as described in the chapter on "Assay for Autoprothrombin I_c". To obtain the high Ac-globulin concentration required for the reaction, purified Ac-globulin (Aoki et al. 1963) has to be used instead of bovine serum treated with $BaCO_3$. The other reagents required are the same as the ones used for the two-stage prothrombin assay (Chapter V, p. 175).

Composition of the Reaction Mixture:

Acacia-calcium buffer reagent	1.9 ml
Crude cephalin (0.1 % in saline)	0.9 ml
Autoprothrombin C (10–20 U/ml)	0.1 ml
Ac-globulin preparation (200 U/ml)	0.1 ml
Diluted prethrombin	1.0 ml

In this mixture ("first stage") prethrombin activates to thrombin. The measurements of thrombin activity and the calculations are carried through as in the two-stage assay of Ware and Seegers (1949).

References

Alkjaersig, N., Abe, T., and Seegers, W. H. (1955). *Am. J. Physiol. 181,* 304.

Aoki, N., Harmison, C. R., and Seegers, W. H. (1963). *Can. J. Biochem. Physiol. 41,* 2409.

Barnhart, M. I. (1967). *In:* "Blood Clotting Enzymology" (W. H. Seegers, Ed.), p. 218. Academic Press, New York.

Cole, E. R., Marciniak, E., and Seegers, W. H. (1962). *Thromb. Diath. Haemorrhag. 8,* 434.

Esnouf, M. P., and Williams, W. J. (1962). *Biochem. J. 84,* 62.

Harmison, C. R., and Mammen, E. F. (1967). *In:* "Blood Clotting Enzymology" (W. H. Seegers, Ed.), p. 23. Academic Press, New York.

Harmison, C. R., and Seegers, W. H. (1962). *J. Biol. Chem. 237,* 3074.

Harmison, C. R., Landaburu, R. H., and Seegers, W. H. (1961). *J. Biol. Chem. 236,* 1693.

Harmison, C. R., Schröer, H., and Seegers, W. H. (1965). *Thromb. Diath. Haemorrhag. 13,* 587.

Hecht, E., Landaburu, R. H., and Seegers, W. H. (1957). *Am. J. Physiol. 189,* 203.

Johnson, S. A., and Seegers, W. H. (1954). *J. Appl. Physiol. 6,* 429.

Johnson, S. A., and Seegers, W. H. (1956). *Circulation Res. 4,* 182.

Johnson, S. A., Rutsky, J., Schneider, C. L., and Seegers, W. H. (1954). *Proc. 4th Intern. Congr. Hematol.* Grune & Stratton, New York, 1954.

Johnson, S. A., McClaughry, R. J., and Seegers, W. H. (1955). *J. Michigan State Med. Soc. 54,* 797.

Johnson, S. A., Seegers, W. H., Koppel, J. L., and Olwin, J. H. (1957). *Thromb. Diath. Haemorrhag. 1,* 2.

Langdell, R. D., Wagner, R. H., and Brinkhous, K. M. (1953). *J. Lab. Clin. Med. 41,* 637.

Lechner, K., and Deutsch, E. (1965). *Thromb. Diath. Haemorrhag. 13,* 314.

Mammen, E. F. (1968). *Thromb. Diath. Haemorrhag. Suppl. 25,* 15.

Mammen, E. F., Thomas, W. R., and Seegers, W. H. (1960a). *Thromb. Diath. Haemorrhag. 5,* 218.

Mammen, E. F., Yoshinari, M., and Seegers, W. H. (1960b). *Thromb. Diath. Haemorrhag. 5,* 38.

Marciniak, E., and Seegers, W. H. (1962). *Can. J. Biochem. Physiol. 40,* 597.

Marciniak, E., and Seegers, W. H. (1965). *New Istanbul. Contrib. Clin. Sci. 8,* 117.

Markwardt, F., Hoffmann, A., and Landmann, H. (1964). *Thromb. Diath. Haemorrhag. 11,* 230.

Mertz, E. T., Seegers, W. H., and Smith, H. P. (1939). *Proc. Soc. Exptl. Biol. Med. 41,* 657.

Milstone, J. H., Oulianoff, N., and Milstone, V. K. (1963). *J. Gen. Physiol. 47,* 315.

Murphy, R. C., Ware, A. G., and Seegers, W. H. (1947). *Am. J. Physiol. 151,* 338.

Purcell, G. M., and Barnhart, M. I. (1963). *Biochim. Biophys. Acta 78,* 800.

Reno, R. S., and Seegers, W. H. (1967). *Thromb. Diath. Haemorrhag. 18,* 198.

Schröer, H., Heene, D. L., and Seegers, W. H. (1965). *Thromb. Diath. Haemorrhag. 13,* 187.

Seegers, W. H. (1952a). *Record Chem. Progr. (Kresge-Hooker Sci. Lib.) 13,* 143.

Seegers, W. H. (1952b). *Harvey Lectures 47,* 180.

Seegers, W. H. (1962). "Prothrombin". Harvard Univ. Press. Cambridge, Mass.

Seegers, W. H. (1964). *Federation Proc. 23,* 749.

Seegers, W. H. (1966). "Prothrombin in Enzymology, Thrombosis and Hemophilia". Charles C. Thomas, Springfield, Ill.

Seegers, W. H., and Alkjaersig, N. (1955). *Circulation Res. 3,* 514.

Seegers, W. H., and Kagami, M. (1964). *Can. J. Biochem. 42,* 1249.

Seegers, W. H., and Marciniak, E. (1962). *Thromb. Diath. Haemorrhag. 8,* 1.

Seegers, W. H., and Marciniak, E. (1965). *Life Sci. 4,* 1721.

Seegers, W. H., and Smith, H. P. (1942). *Am. J. Physiol. 137,* 348.

Seegers, W. H., Alkjaersig, N., and Johnson, S. A. (1955). *Am. J. Physiol. 181,* 589.

Seegers, W. H., Landaburu, R. H., and Fenichel, R. L. (1957). *Am. J. Physiol. 190,* 1.
Seegers, W. H., Lenine, W. G., and Shepard, R. S. (1958). *Can. J. Biochem. Physiol. 36,* 603.
Seegers, W. H., Cole, E. R., and Marciniak, E. (1962). *Thromb. Diath. Haemorrhag. 7,* 239.
Seegers, W. H., Cole, E. R., Harmison, C. R., and Marciniak, E. (1963). *Can. J. Biochem. Physiol. 41,* 1047.
Seegers, W. H., Cole, E. R., Aoki, N., and Harmison, C. R. (1964a). *Can. J. Biochem. 42,* 229.
Seegers, W. H., Cole, E. R., Harmison, C. R., and Monkhouse, F. C. (1964b). *Can. J. Biochem. 42,* 359.
Seegers, W. H., Schröer, H., and Kagami, M. (1964c). *Can. J. Biochem. 42,* 1425.
Seegers, W. H., Marciniak, E., and Heene, D. L. (1965). *Texas Rept. Biol. Med. 23,* 675.
Seegers, W. H., Heene, D. L., and Marciniak, E. (1966). *Thromb. Diath. Haemorrhag. 15,* 1.
Seegers, W. H., Schröer, H., and Marciniak, E. (1967a). *In:* "Blood Clotting Enzymology" (W. H. Seegers, Ed.), p. 103, Academic Press, New York.
Seegers, W. H., Kipfer, R. K., and Yasunaga, K. (1967b). *Arch. Biochem. 121,* 372.
Spaet, T. H., and Cintron, J. (1963). *Blood 21,* 745.
Tishkoff, G. H., Pechet, L., and Alexander, B. (1960). *Blood 15,* 778.
Ulutin, O. N., Johnson, J. F., and Seegers, W. H. (1961a). *Am. J. Physiol. 201,* 660.
Ulutin, O. N., Mammen, E. F., and Seegers, W. H. (1961b). *Thromb. Diath. Haemorrhag. 5,* 456.
Ware, A. G., and Seegers, W. H. (1949). *Am. J. Clin. Pathol. 19,* 471.

Assays for Hageman Factor (factor XII) and Plasma Thromboplastin Antecedent (factor XI)*

OSCAR D. RATNOFF

I. Introduction

Hageman factor (Factor XII) and plasma thromboplastin antecedent (PTA, Factor XI) are agents which participate in the early stages of the coagulation of cell-poor plasma in glass tubes. Both were originally identified through the discovery of individuals whose plasmas appeared to be deficient in these agents (Ratnoff, 1954; Rosenthal et al. 1953). Those deficient in Hageman factor, said to have Hageman trait, have been essentially asymptomatic, while those with PTA deficiency have usually had a mild hemorrhagic diathesis, although some are asymptomatic. Both Hageman trait and PTA deficiency are inherited as autosomal recessive traits. Heterozygous carriers are asymptomatic, but a partial deficiency of Hageman factor or PTA can often be found in the laboratory. In addition to its hereditary deficiency, an acquired deficiency of PTA has been noted in hepatic disease.

* That portion of this chapter which reflects studies carried out in the laboratories of Case Western Reserve University was supported by Grant No. HE 01661 from the National Heart Institute, United States Public Health Service, and by a Grant from the American Heart Association.

Assays for Hageman factor and PTA are based upon their role in the initiation of clotting through the so-called intrinsic pathway for the formation of thrombin. Both factors appear to be inactive in freshly shed blood. When plasma comes in contact with glass or a number of other insoluble substances such as kaolin, diatomaceous earth, barium carbonate or asbestos, Hageman factor is changed to an activated form. Hageman factor can also be activated by *solutions* of ellagic acid (4,4',5,5',6,6'-hexahydroxydiphenic acid 2,6,2',6'-dilactone), a derivative of tannic acid, and, to a minor extent, by precipitation of the euglobulin fraction of plasma. The nature of the activation process is not known, but purified human Hageman factor is altered, during activation, from a substance with a sedimentation coefficient of 4.5-5.5, as determined by sucrose gradient ultracentrifugation, to one which sediments rapidly to the bottom of the gradient tube. Moreover, activated human Hageman factor, unlike its precursor, is excluded from columns of Sephadex G-200 and from polyacrylamide gel.

Once activated, Hageman factor changes PTA from an inert to an activated form, an alteration which is apparently enzymatic. Activation does not require the presence of calcium ions and can therefore take place in citrated plasma. Activated PTA – often misnamed contact factor – next converts Christmas factor (plasma thromboplastin component, Factor IX) into an activated form. In this step, activated PTA behaves enzymatically. It can also hydrolyze p-toluenesulfonyl-L-arginine methyl ester (TAME) and is inhibited by diisopropylphosphofluoridate (DFP) which is bound to a serine residue. The activation of Christmas factor requires the presence of calcium ions and is inhibited by small amounts of heparin. Once activated, Christmas factor can initiate a chain of reactions leading to the formation of thrombin.

Plasma also possesses inhibitory activity directed against activated PTA and probably against activated Hageman factor as well. Assays designed to estimate the concentration of either Hageman factor or PTA must take into account this inhibitory property.

Activated Hageman factor, besides acting in the clotting process, participates in the induction of certain experimental inflammatory states. It increases vascular permeability in guinea pig skin and promotes leukocytic infiltration in the rabbit ear chamber. Incubated with human plasma, activated Hageman factor brings about the elaboration of the permeability-increasing factor known variously as PF/Dil or simply PF. Either directly or through its activation of PF/Dil, it activates one of the plasma kallikreinogens, leading to the formation of biologically active polypeptide kinins which increase vascular permeability, dilate blood vessels, lower blood pressure, contract smooth muscle and induce pain. Activated Hageman factor has also been implicated in the activation of plasminogen to plasmin, but this effect is probably indirect.

The assays for Hageman factor and PTA which have proved most successful are those based upon Margolis' (1958) technique of activating these agents by exposing plasma to kaolin. This property was adapted by Rapaport et al. (1961a) to the measurement of PTA, and by Davie and Ratnoff and Davie (1962) to the assay of Hageman factor, Christmas factor and antihemophilic factor (Factor VIII). The literature concerning the nature and function of Hageman factor and PTA has been the subject of a recent review (Ratnoff, 1966).

II. Assay for Hageman Factor (Adapted from Ratnoff, 1964)

A. Principle

The technique for the assay of Hageman factor is derived from an assay for PTA first described by Rapaport et al. (1961a). The preparation to be tested is incubated with kaolin to bring about maximal activation of Hageman factor. The mixture is then incubated with plasma deficient in Hageman factor, obtained from a patient with Hageman trait. In this step, any Hageman factor in the preparation to be assayed presumably activates PTA contained in the Hageman factor-deficient plasma. After a suitable interval, the mixture is recalcified and its clotting time is measured. The addition of calcium ions allows the reactions which lead to the formation of fibrin to proceed beyond the step at which PTA is activated. The clotting time of the mixture appears to be a function of the concentration of Hageman factor in the preparation tested. Small amounts of phospholipid are included in the kaolin mixture to accelerate the formation of thrombin.

B. Reagents

1. Preparation to be tested

Plasma is prepared from blood to which one-ninth volume of 0.13 M trisodium citrate buffer (pH 5.0) has been added. The assay can also be performed upon serum or upon fractions of plasma or serum, dissolved or diluted in barbital-saline buffer.

2. Barbital-saline buffer

A solution containing 7.30 gm of sodium chloride, 2.76 gm of barbital and 2.06 gm of sodium barbital is diluted to a volume of 1 liter with distilled water; the pH is approximately 7.5.

3. Kaolin

Acid-washed, American standard (Fisher Scientific Company, Fair Lawn, New Jersey).

4. Soybean phosphatides

Gliddex "P", a crude preparation of soybean phosphatides (Chemurgy Division, Glidden Paint Company, Chicago) is suspended at a concentration of 0.1 % in 0.15 M sodium chloride solution, using a mechanical homogenizer, divided into 5 ml lots and stored at –25° C until needed.

5. Plasma substrate

Hageman factor-deficient plasma. Platelet-deficient citrated plasma is prepared in silicone-coated tubes from the blood of a patient with Hageman trait and stored at –25° C in polystyrene containers previously rinsed with silicone fluid SF 96 (200) (General Electric Company, Waterford, New York), after quick freezing in an ethanol-dry ice mixture. The citrated plasma is obtained from venous blood to which one-ninth volume of 0.13 M trisodium citrate buffer (pH 5.0) has been added.

6. Calcium chloride solution, 0.025 M.

C. Performance of the test

1. On the day of the test, a tube containing 5 ml of 0.1 % Gliddex "P" is thawed, and to it is added 50 mg of kaolin. The kaolin and Gliddex "P" are suspended with the aid of a mechanical homogenizer. One-tenth ml of the suspension is pipetted into each of a suitable number of disposable glass tubes (internal diameter 8 mm). These tubes are kept in a melting ice bath until needed.

2. The plasma or serum to be tested is diluted 20-fold in a silicone-coated polypropylene tube by the addition of barbital-saline buffer, just before use. The diluted plasma is kept in a melting ice bath during the few moments until it is needed. Further dilutions are made separately, and not as serial dilutions of those already tested. Duplicate determinations are made on separately prepared dilutions to obviate errors in dilution.

3. One-tenth ml of diluted plasma or serum is added with a silicone-coated 0.2 ml pipette to 0.1 ml of the kaolin-Gliddex mixture. The tube is tapped gently to mix its contents and incubated at 37° C for 2 minutes. Then, 0.1 ml of Hageman factor-deficient plasma is added with a silicone-coated 0.2 ml pipette. The tube is once again tapped and incubated at 37° C for 8 more minutes. Finally, 0.1 ml of 0.025 M calcium chloride solution, pre-warmed at 37° C, is added and a stop watch started. After 30 seconds, the tube is tilted continuously until a clot forms. The end point is sharp and usually unmistakable.

Two determinations can be carried out simultaneously, but duplicate determinations are never performed at the same time. With skill, successive determinations can be overlapped, speeding the assay procedure.

4. Fractions of plasma or serum are tested in a similar manner, diluting the preparations in silicone-coated polypropylene tubes with barbital-saline buffer, or, better still, barbital-saline buffer to which one percent bovine albumin has been added. The preliminary incubation period of 2 minutes is omitted when purified Hageman factor preparations are assayed, unless they are stabilized by the bovine albumin solution. The fraction to be tested must be added to the kaolin-Gliddex mixture before the addition of Hageman factor-deficient plasma, or a falsely low value will be obtained. The greatest accuracy is obtained if fractions of plasma or serum are tested as soon after dilution as is feasible, since these are often unstable.

D. Calculations and unitage

1. No absolute standard for the concentration of Hageman factor in plasma is as yet available. Arbitrarily, the activity in 1 ml of the average normal human plasma has been assigned a value of 1 unit (Ratnoff and Davie, 1962). An approximation of this unit has been made by assaying the Hageman factor activity of a fresh pool of plasma obtained from 20 normal subjects whose age ranged from 21 to 30 years. A secondary standard of lyophilized plasma prepared from a large pool of human plasmas has proved useful.

2. The relative concentrations of Hageman factor in different samples of plasma or serum or in fractions of plasma or serum can be estimated in the following way. The most active

sample – that is, the one which accelerates the clotting of Hageman factor-deficient plasma the most – is diluted by two-fold steps in barbital-saline buffer; each dilution is freshly prepared and is not a serial dilution of a previously tested sample. Successive dilutions are tested until a concentration is found such that the clotting time exceeds that of the weakest sample under study. A calibration curve is constructed on doubly logarithmic paper; over a wide range, the logarithm of the concentration of Hageman factor is an inverse linear function of the logarithm of the clotting time. The activity of each unknown sample can then be calculated by interpolation into the calibration curve. The values obtained can be translated into arbitrary units of activity by constructing the calibration curve from determinations of the activity of a lyophilized plasma sample which has previously been compared with a pool of 20 normal plasmas.

E. Precautions and sources of error

Meticulous care in pipetting and attention to the order and timing of additions of the various reagents are necessary to insure accuracy. Serial dilutions are to be avoided to minimize error. Duplicate determinations are never made from the same dilution, lest this be in error. Similarly, duplicate determinations are never assayed simultaneously, lest an error in technique lead to false results, even though the duplicate determinations may be in good agreement.

In the technique described, the sample to be tested is incubated with kaolin for two minutes before the addition of Hageman factor-deficient plasma. This interval is needed to insure full activation of Hageman factor in plasma. Hageman factor-deficient plasma has the property of inhibiting the clot-promoting property of kaolin, glass and other agents. Were the sample to be tested added directly to Hageman factor-deficient plasma, full activation of Hageman factor would not occur. When purified preparations of Hageman factor are tested, the preliminary incubation period of two minutes must be eliminated because significant deterioration occurs during this time (Haanen and Schoenmakers, 1963). This deterioration can be obviated to a large degree by suspension of the fraction in a solution of one per cent bovine albumin in barbital-saline buffer.

Activation of Hageman factor, in the method outlined, is brought about by exposure to kaolin. Attemps to substitute solutions of ellagic acid for kaolin have been unsuccessful, apparently because this agent does not bring about complete activation of Hageman factor. An accurate assay for Hageman factor cannot be carried out in the presence of other *activated* clotting factors, since these will accelerate clotting and lead to falsely high values.

F. Interpretation of results

Using the technique described, the concentration of Hageman factor in normal plasma ranged from 0.36 to 1.52 units per ml, with a coefficient of variation of the individual values in two series of 8.6 and 9.6 per cent**. Similarly, Iatridis and Ferguson (1962) found values ranging from 0.42 to 2.05 units per ml and Veltkamp et al. (1965), from 0.65 to 1.75 units per ml, transposing these investigators' units to our own. No significant difference has been found in the titer of Hageman factor in normal individuals of different race or sex. During the first week of life, its concentration is less than 25 % of that in adults, arising to adult levels after about two weeks (Kurkcuoglu and McElfresh, 1960). In Hageman trait, the deficiency of Hageman factor is probably incomplete, traces of an activity resembling this substance being found in plasma. In one case, the concentration of Hageman factor was 0.036 units per ml, that is, 3.6 % of normal, unlike the usual finding in Hageman trait (Bok et al. 1965). Heterozygous carriers usually have a partial deficiency of Hageman factor, detected only by specific assay. In some carriers, the concentration of Hageman factor is approximately half of normal, while in others its concentration is much lower, suggesting the possibility that at least two normally occurring alleles are involved in the production of Hageman factor (Ratnoff, 1965; Veltkamp et al. 1965). No variations in the concentration of Hageman factor have been recognized in the

** This was stated incorrectly in a recent publication (Ratnoff, 1966).

plasma of individuals with disease states other than Hageman trait.

G. Other assays for Hageman factor

Haanen and Schoenmakers (1963) have published a modification of the assay technique described above in which the initial period of incubation of the test sample and kaolin is omitted. In our experience, this modification leads to an underestimation of the Hageman factor content of purified samples of Hageman factor which tend to be unstable in aqueous solution.

A minor modification of the method outlined in this chapter has been described by Iatridis and Ferguson (1962). An adaptation of the thromboplastin generation test for the assay of Hageman factor has been published by Colman and Alexander (1965).

No quantitative assays have been devised taking advantage of the participation of Hageman factor in experimental inflammatory reactions. A crude estimate of the Hageman factor present in human plasma can be made immunologically, using the technique of passive hemagglutination inhibition (Smink et al. 1967).

III. Assay for PTA (Adapted from Rapaport et al. 1961a)

A. Principle

The preparation to be tested is incubated with kaolin and plasma believed to be deficient in PTA. During this incubation, the kaolin activates Hageman factor present in the PTA-deficient plasma, and this, in turn, activates any PTA in the preparation under study. After an appropriate time, the mixture is recalcified and its clotting time measured. Upon recalcification, the activated PTA in the mixture brings about the activation of Christmas factor and, ultimately, the formation of a fibrin clot. The clotting time of the mixture is a function of the concentration of PTA in the preparation tested. Small amounts of phospholipid are included in the kaolin mixture to accelerate the formation of thrombin.

B. Reagents

The reagents used are the same as those for the determination of Hageman factor activity, except for the substrate plasma deficient in PTA. This is prepared in the same manner as Hageman factor-deficient plasma, from blood obtained from a patient with hereditary PTA deficiency. Alternatively, artificial PTA-deficient plasma may be prepared either from normal human plasma, as suggested by Soulier and Prou-Wartelle (1960), or from horse plasma, which is often partially deficient in PTA (Wartelle, 1958). The end point of the assay is not as sharp when horse plasma is used as a substrate. Platelet-deficient human or equine plasma is prepared in silicone-coated containers, from blood to which one-ninth volume of 0.13 M trisodium citrate buffer (pH 5.0) has been added. The plasma is mixed in a silicone-coated beaker with 15 mg of diatomaceous earth (Filter-Cel Celite, Johns Mansville Co.) per ml of plasma, and stirred with a magnetic stirrer at room temperature for 5 minutes. The plasma is then centrifuged twice at 2° C for 15 minutes at 3500 rpm in an International PR-2 centrifuge. The supernatant plasma is then incubated at 37° C for 5 hours in silicone-coated polypropylene tubes, divided into 2 ml lots, quick-frozen in ethanol-dry ice and stored at –25° C.

C. Performance of the test

1. On the day of the test, a mixture of Gliddex "P" and kaolin is prepared as in the technique for measuring Hageman factor, and a series of tubes filled with 0.1 ml of the suspension. The tubes are kept in a melting ice bath until needed.

2. The plasma to be tested is diluted 20-fold in a silicone-coated polypropylene tube by the addition of barbital-saline buffer, just before use, and is kept in a melting ice bath during the few moments until used. Further dilutions are made freshly, and not as serial dilutions of those already tested. Duplicate determinations are made on separately prepared dilutions to obviate errors in dilution.

3. One-tenth ml of diluted plasma or serum and 0.1 ml of PTA-deficient plasma are added

with silicone-coated 0.2 ml pipettes to 0.1 ml of the kaolin-Gliddex mixture. The tube is tapped gently to mix its contents and incubated at 37° C for 8 minutes. Then, 0.1 ml of 0.025 M calcium chloride solution, pre-warmed at 37° C, is added and a stop watch started. After 30 seconds, the tube is tilted continuously until a clot forms. The end point is sharp and usually unmistakable.

Two determinations can be made simultaneously, but duplicate determinations are never performed at the same time.

4. Fractions of plasma or serum are tested in the same way, diluting the preparations in silicone-coated polypropylene tubes with barbital-saline buffer. The 8 minute period of incubation must be omitted, since the activated PTA deteriorates rapidly. Thus, results obtained by this technique are not comparable to those obtained with diluted plasma or serum.

D. Calculations and unitage

1. No absolute standard for the concentration of PTA in plasma is a yet available. Arbitrarily, the activity in 1 ml of the average normal human plasma has been assigned a value of 1 unit. An approximation of this unit has been made by assaying the PTA activity of a fresh pool of plasma obtained from 20 normal subjects whose age ranged from 21 to 30 years. A secondary standard of lyophilized plasma obtained from a large pool of human plasma has proved useful.

2. The relative concentrations of PTA in different samples of plasma or serum or in fractions of plasma or serum are estimated using the same technique used for the assay of Hageman factor. As in the case of Hageman factor, over a wide range the logarithm of the concentration of PTA is an inverse linear function of the logarithm of the clotting time. The activity of each unknown sample is calculated by interpolation into a calibration curve. The values obtained can be translated into arbitrary units of activity by constructing the calibration curve from determinations of the activity of a lyophilized plasma sample which has previously been compared with a pool of normal plasma.

E. Precautions and sources of error

The same problems described in the assay of Hageman factor are met in the assay of PTA. The preliminary incubation period of two minutes, needed in the assay for Hageman factor, is not required. The assay is vitiated by the presence of *activated* clotting factors which participate in clotting at a later stage than PTA, since these will accelerate clotting. For reasons already mentioned a direct comparison of the activity of plasma or serum and that of purified PTA fractions cannot be made.

Much has been made in the literature of the spontaneous correction of the defect in PTA-deficient plasma upon storage in the frozen state. I have not observed this phenomenon in carefully prepared platelet-deficient plasma handled in such a way that it never comes in contact with glass.

F. Interpretation of results

In normal human plasma, the concentration of PTA in four different series has varied from 0.75 to 1.37 units per ml (Egeberg, 1961), 0.63 to 1.36 units per ml (Rapaport et al. 1961b), 0.80 to 1.08 units per ml (Leiba et al. 1965) and 0.55 to 1.85 units per ml (Ratnoff et al. 1964), the last representing our experience with the method described. In our own experience (Ratnoff et al. 1964), the coefficient of variation of individual values was 4.2 %. No sex or racial difference has been noted. During pregnancy, the titer of PTA slowly falls, reaching on the average 0.62 units per ml at term (Hilgartner and Smith, 1965). For the first ten days of life, the titer is low, in one series averaging 0.41 units per ml. It then gradually rises, but even at a year, the average concentration in infants is still below that of the adult.

The titer of PTA in patients with hereditary PTA deficiency who are homozygous for the abnormal allele is 20 % of normal or less, that is, 0.20 units per ml or less (Rapaport et al. 1961b; Nossel et al. 1966). Heterozygous individuals have titers between 0.30 and 0.60 units per ml. It is doubtful that any patients yet observed have had an absolute deficiency of PTA. Titers of 0.03 to 0.20 units per ml are the rule (Rapaport et al. 1961b; Leiba et al. 1965; Nossel et al. 1966).

Acquired deficiencies of PTA have been noted in hepatic disorders (Naeye, 1957; Rapaport, 1961; Horowitz et al. 1963) and in congenital heart disease (Hilgartner et al. 1965). These deficiencies have been partial and not as severe as in hereditary PTA deficiency. A marginally low titer of PTA has also been reported in two of three patients with paroxysmal nocturnal hemoglobinuria (Egeberg, 1962).

G. Other Assays for PTA

A clever technique for the assay of PTA has been devised by Nossel and his associates (1966), making use of the ready absorption of this substance to celite. The virtue of this assay is in its use of normal platelet deficient plasma as a substrate. I have had no experience with this method.

Nossel (1964, 1966) prepares an eluate of celite which has been treated with the plasma to be tested, adapting a method of Waaler (1959). The plasma is adjusted to pH 7.8–8.0 with 0.1 N hydrochloric acid and added to a silicone-treated tube containing 20 mg of celite 512 (Johns Manville Company) for each ml of plasma. The mixture is incubated at 37° C for 10 minutes, mixing by inversion over parafilm every 2 minutes. The celite is then separated by centrifugation and the supernatant plasma discarded. The celite is washed five times in normal saline solution or distilled water. The celite is then eluted by the addition of a volume of 10 % sodium chloride solution equal to the volume of plasma originally used, again incubating the mixture at 37° C for 10 minutes, inverting the tube over parafilm every 2 minutes. The celite is again separated from the supernatant fluid by centrifugation, the eluate is removed with a silicone-coated pipette and dialyzed for a minimum of an hour against 0.15 M sodium chloride solution. The clot-promoting activity of the eluate is then tested by incubating a mixture of 0.1 ml suitably diluted eluate, 0.2 ml of platelet-poor normal plasma which has not been in contact with glass, 0.1 ml of crude brain phospholipids and 0.1 ml 0.02 M calcium chloride. The clotting time is a measure of the concentration of PTA in the plasma to be tested.

The results of Nossel's test correlate fairly well with that obtained by an assay using as substrate plasma from a patient with PTA deficiency. The variations reported are, however, disturbing. For example, the celite eluate technique is said to have given a value of 40 to 50 per cent of normal for samples containing 110 to 120 per cent of normal activity by Rapaport's method. Greater accuracy is achieved when the concentration of PTA is less than 20 per cent of normal (Nossel et al. 1966). Like other assays, its results are vitiated by the presence of activated clotting factors participating subsequent to PTA in the clotting process. Moreover, since the formation of an active clot-promoting eluate depends upon the presence of Hageman factor, one cannot distinguish Hageman trait from PTA deficiency by this method.

A number of other minor modifications of Rapaport's technique have been published (Leiba, 1965; Nossel, 1966), the most notable of which, the use of artificially PTA-deficient plasma as a substrate, has been emphasized by Horowitz (1963).

References

Bok, J., Veltkamp, J. J., and Loeliger, E. A. (1965). *Thromb. Diath. Haemorrhag. 13,* 8.

Colman, R., and Alexander, B. (1965). *Thromb. Diath. Haemorrhag. 13,* 176.

Egeberg, O. (1961). *Scand. J. Clin. Lab. Invest. 13,* 140.

Egeberg, O. (1962). *Scand. J. Clin. Lab. Invest. 14,* 217.

Haanen, C., and Schoenmakers, J. G. G. (1963). *Thromb. Diath. Haemorrhag. 9,* 557.

Hilgartner, M. W., and Smith, C. H. (1965). *J. Pediat. 66,* 747.

Horowitz, H. I., Wilcox, W. P., and Fujimoto, M. M. (1963). *Blood 22,* 35.

Iatridis, S. G., and Ferguson, J. H. (1962). *Thromb. Diath. Haemorrhag. 8,* 46.

Kurkcuoglu, M., and McElfresh, A. E. (1960). *J. Pediat. 57,* 61.

Leiba, H., Ramot, B., and Many, A. (1965). *Brit. J. Haematol. 11,* 654.

Margolis, J. (1958). *J. Clin. Pathol. 11,* 406.

Naeye, R. L. (1957). *Proc. Soc. Exptl. Biol. Med. 94,* 623.

Nossel, H. L. (1964). "The Contact Phase of Blood Coagulation". Blackwell Scientific Publications, Oxford.

Nossel, H. L., Niemetz, J., Mibashan, R. S., and Schulze, W. G. (1966). *Brit. J. Haematol. 12,* 133.

Rapaport, S. I. (1961). *Proc. Soc. Exptl. Biol. Med. 108,* 115.

Rapaport, S. I., Schiffman, S., Patch, M. J., and Ware, A. G. (1961a). *J. Lab. Clin. Med. 57,* 771.

Rapaport, S. I., Proctor, R. R., Patch, M. J., and Yettra, M. (1961b). *Blood 18,* 149.

Ratnoff, O. D. (1954). *J. Lab. Clin. Med. 44,* 915.

Ratnoff, O. D. (1964). *In:* "Blood Coagulation, Hemorrhage and Thrombosis" (L. M. Tocantins and L. A. Kazal, eds.), p. 141. Grune and Stratton, New York.

Ratnoff, O. D. (1965). Selected papers from the 10th Congress of the International Society of Haematology, Suppl. *Scand. J. Haematol., Series Haematologica 7,* 29.

Ratnoff, O. D. (1966). *In:* "Progress in Hematology" (E. B. Brown and C. V. Moore, eds.), Vol. 5, p. 204. Grune and Stratton, New York.

Ratnoff, O. D., and Davie, E. W. (1962). *Biochem. 1,* 967.

Ratnoff, O. D., Botti, R. E., Breckenridge, R. T., and Littell, A. S. (1964). Unpublished observations.

Rosenthal, R. L., Dreskin, O. H., and Rosenthal, N. (1953). *Proc. Soc. Exptl. Biol. Med. 82,* 171.

Smink, M. McL., Daniel, T. M., Ratnoff, O. D., and Stavitsky, A. B. (1967). *J. Lab. Clin. Med. 69,* 819.

Soulier, J.-P., and Prou-Wartelle, O. (1960). *Brit. J. Haematol. 6,* 88.

Veltkamp, J. J., Hemker, H. C., and Loeliger, E. A. (1965). *Thromb. Diath. Haemorrhag. Suppl. 17,* 181.

Waaler, B. A. (1959). *Scand. J. Clin. Lab. Invest. 11, Suppl. 37,* 1.

Wartelle, O. (1958). Thesis, University of Paris.

CHAPTER VI

Fibrinogen

ROLF M. HUSEBY and NILS U. BANG

I. Introduction

Blood coagulation ultimately depends on the thrombin-catalyzed conversion of fibrinogen to fibrin. Fibrinogen occur in blood plasma in concentration of about 2–4 g per liter and constitutes about 5 percent of the total protein (Oncley et al. 1947; Cohn et al. 1950). The purpose of this review is twofold; first, we shall briefly survey current knowledge on the biochemical and biophysical characteristics of fibrinogen and the sequential changes occuring during fibrinogen-fibrin conversion and secondly, we shall consider in some detail the major published procedures for purification and quantitative assays for fibrinogen.

II. Biophysical and Chemical Properties of Fibrinogen

A. Chemical Composition

Fibrinogen may be considered a globulin-type protein containing about 3 percent carbohydrate. The earliest reports of the amino acid composition of both human and bovine fibrinogen were based on paper chromatography (Bailey, 1944; Brand and Edsall, 1947; and Tristam, 1949). More recently, automated analysis has been used to determine the amino acid composition of bovine and human fibrinogen (Mihalyi et al. 1963; Henschen and Blombäck, 1964; Murray and Huseby, 1965; and Huseby and Murray, 1967a). The composition of bovine fibrinogen is given in Table 1. All species of fibrinogens studied to date show similar composition.

The carbohydrate composition has been investigated by a number of workers (Consden, 1953; Blombäck, 1958a; Laki and Mester, 1962; and Brown, 1964). The carbohydrate content has been estimated to be between 1 and 5 percent. A carbohydrate analysis on bovine fibrinogen is shown in Table 2 (Brown, 1964).

Table 1: Amino Acid Composition of Bovine Fibrinogen (moles per 100,000 gm).

Amino Acid	Mihalyi	Murray and Huseby	Henschen and Blombäck	Average
Aspartic acid	103.4	107.0	102.0	104.1
Serine	58.0	59.0	66.8	61.3
Threonine	55.0	54.5	58.7	56.0
Glutamic acid	95.3	95.7	92.1	94.4
Proline	45.0	40.5	38.3	41.3
Glycine	83.3	76.4	83.3	81.0
Alanine	36.0	34.5	41.8	37.5
Cystine (half)	20.6	27.6	17.8	22.0
Valine	42.5	42.5	38.7	41.2
Methionine	15.6	16.2	14.8	15.5
Isoleucine	36.5	31.4	35.2	34.4
Leucine	51.0	40.4	49.7	47.0
Tyrosine	27.7	22.7	32.5	29.63
Phenylalanine	25.8	23.2	24.8	24.6
Lysine	64.5	63.6	58.4	62.16
Hisitidine	17.1	16.8	15.3	16.4
Arginine	46.4	43.8	44.5	44.9
Tryptophan	20.3	–	21.6	20.9
Ammonia	110.1	–	64.2	87.1

Table 2: Carbohydrate Composition of Bovine Fibrinogen*.

Carbohydrates	Moles per 340,000 gm
N-Acetylneuraminic acid (sialic acid)	10
Glucosamine	9
Galactose } Mannose }	29

* Brown, 1964

B. Biophysical Characteristics

1. Molecular Weight

The molecular weight of fibrinogen has been estimated by a number of methods. On the basis of diffusion and sedimentation data, the molecular weight of bovine fibrinogen is between 320,000 and 340,000 (Shulman, 1953; Caspary and Kekwick, 1957; and Scheraga and Laskowski, 1957). The molecular weight of human fibrinogen is also of this magnitude (Caspary and Kekwick, 1957). The S°_{20w} is between 7.7 and 7.9 Svedberg units. Using sedimentation equilibrium methods the molecular weight of bovine fibrinogen was estimated to be 400,000 (Johnson and Mihalyi, 1965) with an S°_{20w} value of 8.14 Svedberg units.

The molecular weight of fibrinogen has also been determined by light scattering techniques (Steiner and Laki, 1951a, b; Hocking et al. 1952; and Edsall, 1953) and osmotic pressure measurements (Nanninga, 1946, and Oncley et al. 1947). However, values usually found by these techniques are not in agreement with the accepted value for the molecular weight of fibrinogen.

2. Titration Behavior

The titration behavior of highly purified fibrinogen and fibrin solutions has not yet been completely elucidated. The pioneer work in this area was done by Mihalyi (Mihalyi, 1954a, b) who found that, based on differential titration, 3.6 new alpha-amino groups are released with clotting. This, of course, is well recognized today as the proteolytic action of thrombin on fibrinogen. Other titrations giving different values have been reported (Chaudhuri, 1948, and Shulman and Ferry, 1950). Their work, however, is open to question since high extrapolations were made in the carboxylic acid regions of the titration curves.

3. Conformation Data

Only a small amount of conformation work has been done on fibrinogen (Cohen and Szent-Györgyi, 1957; Yang and Doty, 1957; Kay and Marsh, 1961; Mihalyi, 1965; and Huseby and Murray, 1967a, b). In the three earliest works the optical rotation was measured into the visible, and only one value was presented. However, Mihalyi (1965) and Huseby and Murray (1967b) made observations on the optical rotary dispersion. Mihalyi reported that fibrinogen contained some 34–35 percent helix which decreases upon denaturation to values ranging from 22 to 0 percent helix depending on the mode of denaturation (see Table 3).

Table 3: Helical Content (percent) of Fibrinogen in Various Solvents Calculated from the Optical Rotation Data*.

	λc	$[\alpha]$	b^0
Native	34	37	34
Dioxane 20 percent	31	39	28
Acid-denatured	22	22	23
Alkali-denatured	18	20	18
Urea, native	24	29	25
Urea, denatured	19	15	21
Guanidine HCl, denatured	5	0	6
Guanidine HCl, reduced	7	3	5
Guanidine HCl, sulfite-treated	8	2	6

* from Mihalyi (1965)

Native and denatured fibrinogen was similarly studied in the far ultraviolet (Huseby and Murray, 1967a) with the theoretical absorption values first employed by Rosenheck and Doty (1961). This technique gave helical contents for fibrinogen ranging from 43 to 30 percent as seen in Fig. 1. Recently, the far ultraviolet optical rotary dispersion and circular dichroism of fibrinogen was reported (Huseby and Murray, 1967b), and these preliminary experiments indicated that fibrinogen is a helical protein. These results are in substantial agreement with low-angle x-ray diffraction studies of Stryer et al. (1963) in which a value of 30 percent helix was found for fibrinogen.

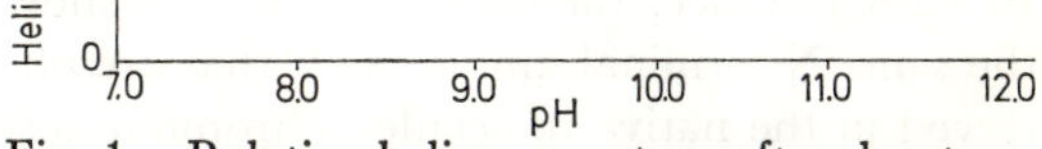

Fig. 1. Relative helix percentage after denaturation of fibrinogen at various pHs (Huseby and Murray, 1967a).

4. Other Biophysical Characteristics

The partial specific volume v, has been determined for both human and bovine fibrinogen (Armstrong et al. 1947; Koenig, 1950; and Laskowski, 1957). A slightly higher value has been reported for human fibrinogen (0.725) than for bovine fibrinogen (0.705–0.718). The intrinsic viscosity $[\eta]$ = ATA is about the same for both species of fibrinogen with averages between 0.23 to 0.25 (Nanninga, 1946; Hocking et al. 1952; Shulman, 1953; Scheraga et al. 1957). Fibrinogen has been studied by electron microscopy (Hall, 1949, 1963; Seigel et al. 1953; Hall and Slayter, 1959; and Bang, 1964a). According to the work of Hall, the molecule is a triglobular one interconnected with a strand-type structure. The outer globular spheres are about 60 Å in diameter while the middle sphere is about 50 Å in diameter. The interconecting strands are 15 Å in width and about 140 to 165 Å in length. The overall length of the molecule was estimated to be between 450–500 Å at pH 9.5. At pH values approaching the iso-electric point the molecule shortens, probably because of charge effects.

5. Fibrinogen Structure

Fibrinogen is thought to exist as a dimer, based on the observations that fibrinogen can be split into two identical sets of three different peptide chains (Clegg and Bailey, 1962, and Henschen, 1964a). Recently (Capet-Antonini and Guinand, 1967) the dimer structure of fibrinogen was shown to disassociate into subunits of a molecular weight of 180,000 ($S^{\circ}_{20,w} = 6.5$) at a temperature of 37° C. A number of investigators have shown that fibrinogen contains less than one detectable free sulfhydryl group per molecule (Bagdy et al. 1948; Carter and Warner, 1954; Loewy et al. 1961a; and Henschen, 1964a). The total number of disulfide linkages in fibrinogen is 28 or 29 (Henschen, 1964b). After oxidation of the fibrinogen molecule, the individual peptide chains have been isolated (Clegg, 1962; Henschen, 1964b). In each instance, the individual chains show the same N-terminal amino acids that are observed in the native molecule. Thrombin acts on two of the three chains to release the fibrinopeptides A and B, each chain having a molecular weight of 50–65,000 (Henschen, 1963; and Johnson and Mihalyi, 1965). However, recent preliminary reports (Gerbeck et al. 1967) do not support such a simple 6-chain structure for fibrinogen. The possibility of heterogeneous fibrinogens as shown by Mosesson (Mosesson and Finlayson, 1963) may account for Gerbeck's findings.

III. Fibrinogen-Fibrin Conversion

A. Thrombin Action on Fibrinogen

During the course of events leading to coagulation a complex series of conversions occurs culminating in the generation of thrombin from its precursor prothrombin. Thrombin has a proteolytic action on fibrinogen that is highly specific for only four peptide bonds in the fibrinogen molecule. Thrombin has also been reported to cause proteolytic activation of plasminogen, chymotrypsinogen-A, trypsinogen, and other zymogens. Fibrinogen may be acted upon by a variety of enzymes to form gels, including staphylococcal coagulase (Murray and Gohdes, 1959), papain (Eagle and Harris, 1937), vasculokinase (Murray, 1961), and reptilase (Blombäck and Yamashima, 1958). Thrombin has esterolytic action on a number of synthetic amino acid esters and shows a specificity closely resembling trypsin but of a more restricted nature. The enzyme also acts on cold insoluble globulins (Murray and Huseby, 1967; Lipinski et al. 1964), chymotrypsinogen-A (Engel and Alexander, 1966a), trypsinogen and plasminogen (Engel et al. 1966), other portions of the fibrinogen molecule (Blombäck et al. 1967), and several synthetic esters (Lorand et al. 1962).

The first indication that thrombin might act proteolytically on fibrinogen came from end-group analysis (Bailey et al. 1951) and the release of non-protein nitrogen observed by Lorand during fibrin formation (Lorand, 1951, 1952). It is now well established that thrombin acts on fibrinogen in the initial phases of clotting to release the fibrinopeptides A and B (see below). Thrombin interaction with fibrinogen from several species results in similar changes in the N-terminal amino acids (Blombäck and Yamashima, 1958; von Korff et al. 1963; and Blombäck et al. 1966a) as is illustrated in Fig. 2 taken from the paper of Blombäck and Yamashima (1958).

Recently, Blombäck reported that both alanine and aspartic acids appear to be present as terminal amino acids in human fibrin; however, the aspartic acid arises from the removal of N-terminal alanine from the A-chain in fibrinogen (Blombäck et al. 1963a).

B. Fibrinopeptides

Fibrinopeptides are released during coagulation, and the identification of peptide material in clot supernatant solutions confirmed the proteolytic action of thrombin (Bettelheim and Bailey, 1952; Lorand, 1952).

Since this finding a great number of fibrinopeptides derived from fibrinogen from several species have been isolated, and their amino acid sequences have been deduced by conventional techniques (Fig. 3A and B). The amino acid sequence for bovine fibrinopeptide A was reported from three different laboratories (Blombäck et al. 1959; Folk et al. 1959; and Sjöquist et al. 1960), and their results are in agreement. The amino acid sequence of bovine fibrinopeptide B has also been published by three groups of investigators although there is some disagreement in their results (Folk and Gladner, 1960; Sjöquist et al. 1960; and Blombäck and Doolittle, 1963).

Additional peptides that are analogs or degraded portions of the A and B peptides have been isolated, including phosphorylated A peptides from man and dog (Blombäck et al., 1962; and Osbahr et al. 1964). The phosphorylated residue in human and canine peptides is the serine in position three from the N-terminal end of fibrinopeptide A. The tyrosine residue

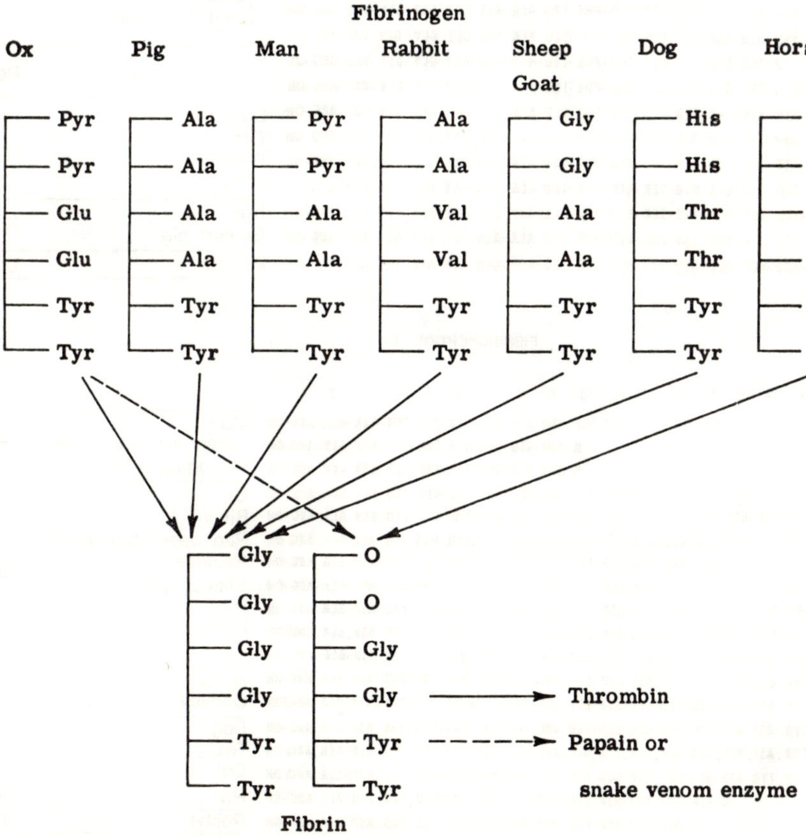

Fig. 2. Pattern changes in N-terminal amino acids of various fibrinogens after thrombin action (Blombäck and Yamashima, 1958).

in the fibrinopeptides from several species is sulfated. Although the amino acid sequence of the fibrinopeptides has been elucidated, their secondary and tertiary structures have not been investigated.

The partial amino acid sequences of the three individual chains in the fibrinogen molecule have been reported (Blombäck et al. 1967; Iwanaga et al. 1967; Pirkle and Henschen, 1968) and, are listed in Figure 4. In addition, fibrinogen from a congenital dysfibrinogenaemia has been isolated and a specific amino acid substitution in the A chain of fibrinogen has been shown to partially explain the abnormal coagulation characteristics of this fibrinogen (Blombäck et al. 1968b). The specific substitution occurs in residue 19 of the alpha (A) chain of fibrinogen from the N-terminal

FIBRINOPEPTIDE A

19 18 17 16 15 14 13 12 11 10 9 8 7 6 5 4 3 2 1

Sequence	Species	Order
H-ALA-ASP-SER-GLY-GLU-GLY-ASP-PHE-LEU-ALA-GLU-GLY-GLY-GLY-VAL-ARG-OH	Man	Primates
H-ALA-ASP-THR-GLY-GLU-GLY-ASP-PHE-LEU-ALA-GLU-GLY-GLY-GLY-VAL-ARG-OH	Green monkey (C. aeth.)	
H-ALA-ASP-THR-GLY-GLU-GLY-ASP-PHE-LEU-ALA-GLU-GLY-GLY-GLY-VAL-ARG-OH	Macaques (Rh. Cyn.)	
H-GLU-ASP-GLY-SER-ASP-PRO-PRO-SER-GLY-ASP-PHE-LEU-THR-GLU-GLY-GLY-GLY-VAL-ARG-OH	Ox	Artiodactyls
H-GLU-ASP-GLY-SER-ASP-PRO-ALA-SER-GLY-ASP-PHE-LEU-ALA-GLU-GLY-GLY-GLY-VAL-ARG-OH	Bison	
H-ALA-ASP-GLY-SER-ASP-PRO-ALA-SER-SER-ASP-PHE-LEU-ALA-GLU-GLY-GLY-GLY-VAL-ARG-OH	Red deer (C. elaphus	
H-ALA-ASP-GLY (SER, ASP, PRO, ALA, SER, SER, GLU, PHE, LEU, ALA, GLU, GLY, GLY, GLY, VAL, ARG)-OH	Sika deer	
H-ALA-ASP-GLY-SER-ASP-PRO-ALA-GLY-GLY-GLU-PHE-LEU-ALA-GLU-GLY-GLY-GLY-VAL-ARG-OH	Reindeer	
H-ALA-ASP-ASP-SER-ASP-PRO-VAL-GLY-GLY-GLU-PHE-LEU-ALA-GLU-GLY-GLY-GLY-VAL-ARG-OH	Sheep, goat	
H-ALA-GLU-VAL-GLN-ASP-LYS-GLY-GLU-PHE-LEU-ALA-GLU-GLY-GLY-GLY-VAL-ARG-OH	Pig	
H-THR-ASP-PRO-ASP-ALA-ASP-LYS-GLY-GLU-PHE-LEU-ALA-GLU-GLY-GLY-GLY-VAL-ARG-OH	Llama	
H-THR-ASP-PRO-ASP-ALA-ASP-GLU-GLY-GLU-PHE (LEU, ALA, GLU, GLY, GLY, GLY, VAL, ARG)-OH	Camel (C. drom.)	
H-THR-GLU-GLU-GLY-GLU-PHE-LEU-HIS-GLU-GLY-GLY-GLY-VAL-ARG-OH	Horse	Perissodactyls
H-THR-LYS-THR-GLU-GLU-GLY-GLU-PHE-ILU-SER-GLU-GLY-GLY-GLY-VAL-ARG-OH	Donkey, Mule	
H-THR-ASN-SER-LYS-GLU-GLY-GLU-PHE-ILU-ALA-GLU-GLY-GLY-GLY-VAL-ARG-OH	Dog, fox	Carnivores
H-GLY-ASP-VAL-GLN-GLU-GLY-GLU-PHE-ILU-ALA-GLU-GLY-GLY-GLY-VAL-ARG-OH	Cat	
H-THR-ASP-VAL-LYS-GLU-SER-GLU-PHE-ILU-ALA-GLU-GLY-ALA-VAL(-GLY-ARG)-OH	Badger	
H-THR-ASN-VAL-LYS-GLU-SER-GLU-PHE-ILU-ALA-GLU-GLY-ALA(-ALA-GLY-ARG)-OH	Mink	
H-ALA-ASP-THR-GLY-THR-THR-SER-GLU-PHE-ILU(-ASP, GLU, GLY, ALA, GLY, ILU, ARG)-OH	Rat	Rodents
H-THR-ASP-THR-GLU-PHE-GLU-ALA-ALA-GLY-GLY-GLY-VAL-ARG-OH	Guinea pig	
H-VAL-ASP-PRO-GLY-GLU-SER-THR-PHE-ILU-ASP-GLU-GLY-ALA-THR-GLY-ARG-OH	Rabbit	Lagomorphs

FIBRINOPEPTIDE B

21 20 19 18 17 16 15 14 13 12 11 10 9 8 7 6 5 4 3 2 1

Sequence	Species	Order
ᶜGLU-GLY-VAL-ASN-ASP-ASN-GLU-GLU-GLY-PHE-PHE-SER-ALA-ARG-OH	Man	Primates
H-ASN-GLU-GLU-GLY-LEU-PHE-GLY-GLY-ARG-OH	Green monkey (C. aeth.)	
H-ASN-GLU-GLU-SER-PRO-PHE-SER-GLY-ARG-OH	Macaques (Rh., Cy.)	
ᶜGLU-PHE-PRO-THR-ASP-TYR-ASP-GLU-GLY-GLN-ASP-ASP-ARG-PRO-LYS-VAL-GLY-LEU-GLY-ALA-ARG-OH	Ox	Artiodactyls
(GLU, PHE, PRO, THR, ASP, TYR, ASP, GLU, GLY, GLU, ASP, ASP, ARG, PRO, LYS)-VAL-GLY-LEU-GLY-ALA-ARG-OH	Bison	
(GLU, SER, HIS, THR, ASP, TYR, ASP, GLU, GLU, GLU, GLU, ASP, ARG)(ALA-LYS)(LEU, HIS, LEU, ASP, ALA, ARG)-OH	Red deer (C. elaphus)	
HIS-GLU-LEU-ALA-ASP-TYR-ASP-GLU-VAL-GLU-ASP-ASP-ARG-ALA-LYS-LEU-HIS-LEU-ASP-ALA-ARG-OH	Reindeer	
H-GLY-TYR-LEU-ASP-TYR-ASP-GLU-VAL-ASP-ASP-ASN-ARG-ALA-LYS-LEU-PRO-LEU-ASP-ALA-ARG-OH	Sheep, goat	
H-ALA-ILU-ASP-TYR-ASP-GLU-ASP-GLU-ASP-GLY-ARG-PRO-LYS-VAL-HIS-VAL-ASP-ALA-ARG-OH	Pig	
H-ALA-THR-ASP-TYR-ASP-GLU-GLU-GLU-ASP-ASP-ARG-VAL(-LYS, VAL, ARG, LEU, ASP, ALA, ARG)-OH	Llama	
H-ALA-THR-ASP-TYR-ASP-GLU-GLU-GLU-ASP-ASP-ARG-VAL-LYS-VAL-ARG-LEU-ASP-ALA-ARG-OH	Camel (C. drom.)	
H-LEU-ASP-TYR-ASP-HIS-GLU-GLU-GLU-ASP-GLY-ARG-THR-LYS-VAL-THR-PHE-ASP-ALA-ARG-OH	Horse	Perissodactyls
H-LEU-ASP-TYR-ASP-HIS-GLU-GLU-GLU-ASP-GLY-ARG(THR-LYS)(VAL, THR, PHE (ASP, ALA, ARG))OH	Donkey	
H-HIS-TYR-TYR-ASP-ASP-THR-ASP-GLU-GLU-GLU-ARG-ILU-VAL-SER-THR-VAL-ASP-ALA-ARG-OH	Dog	Carnivores
(GLU, TYR, TYR, ASP, ASP, THR, ASP, GLU, GLU, GLU, ARG, ILU, VAL, SER, THR, VAL, ASP, ALA, ARG)-OH	Fox	
H-ILU-ILU-ASP-TYR-TYR-ASP-GLU-GLY-GLU-GLU-ASP-ARG-ASP-VAL-GLY-VAL-VAL-ASP(-ALA, ARG)-OH	Cat	
H-ALA-THR-THR-ASP-SER-ASP-LYS-VAL-ASP(ILU, SER, LEU, ALA, ARG)-OH	Rat	Rodents
H-ALA-ASP-ASP-TYR-ASP-ASP-GLU-VAL-LEU-PRO-ASP-ALA-ARG-OH	Rabbit	Lagomorphs

Fig. 3. Amino acid sequences of fibrinopeptides A and B according to Blombäck et al. (1966b).

end. The arginine at this position has been replaced by a serine residue. This change could be achieved by a single base substitution in one of the RNA codons for arginine.

The nature of the N-terminal portions of the fibrinogen molecule has been shown to exist in a compact "disulfide knot" (Blombäck et al. 1968a). This "disulfide knot" contains the N-terminal portions of all three chains in the fibrinogen molecule. In this portion of the molecule, comprising only 15 percent by weight of the fibrinogen; are found 36 percent of the total half-cystine in fibrinogen. The possible unique conformation in this region of the molecule, imposed by disulfide linkages, may form the polymerization site of fibrinogen.

Blombäck has shown that the presence of phosphorus in human fibrinogen is not necessary for clotting (Blombäck et al. 1963b). The phosphorylated serine in fibrinopeptide A is in the same amino acid sequence that is found in several proteolytic enzyme active sites (Trypsin, chymotrypsin and thrombin). Laki (1951a) and Gladner et al. (1963) have made the interesting observation that bovine fibrinopeptide B has vasoactive properties. Thus, the possibility arises that the fibrinogen-fibrin conversion plays an additional role in physiological hemostasis, and, therefore, fibrinogen probably should be included among the biologically important kininogens.

ALPHA (A) CHAIN (HUMAN)

Ala-Asp-Ser-Gly-Glu-Gly-Asp-Phe-Leu-Ala-Glu-
Gly-Gly-Gly-Val-Arg-Gly-Pro-Arg-Val-Val-Glu-Arg-
His-Glm-Ser-Ala-Cys-Lys-Asp-Ser-Asp-Trp-Pro-Phe-(
Asp-Asp-Cys-Glu-Trp-Tyr-Ser)-Lys-Cys-Pro-
Ser-Gly-Cys-Arg-Met

BETA (B) CHAIN (HUMAN)

Glu-Gly-Val-Asn-Asp-Asn-Glu-Glu-Gly-Phe-Phe-Ser-Ala-
Arg-Gly-His-Arg-Pro-Leu-Asp

GAMMA (C) CHAIN (BOVINE)

Try-Val-Ala-Thr-Arg-Asp-Asn

Fig. 4. Partial amino acid sequences of the individual chains of human fibrinogen (chain A and B) and bovine fibrinogen (chain C). (Blombäck et al. 1967; Iwanaga et al. 1967; and Pirkle and Henschen, 1967).

C. Formation of Fibrin

We stated earlier in this discussion that the fibrinopeptides are released during the initial phases of fibrinogen activation. The scheme at present may be summarized as follows:

Fibrinogen	$\xrightarrow{\text{Thrombin}}$	Fibrin Monomer and Peptide A and Peptide B
Fibrin Monomer	$\rightleftharpoons$	Aggregates
Fibrin Aggregates	$\rightleftharpoons$	Fibrin_S
Fibrin_S	$\xrightarrow{\text{FSF (F XIII)}}$	Fibrin_I

1. Phase I - Release of Fibrinopeptides and Formation of Fibrin Monomer

During the release of peptide material the dipole moment of the fibrinogen molecule undergoes marked changes (Haschemeyer and Tinoco, 1962, and Haschemeyer, 1963). These data indicate that the two A peptide fragments are released from the same side of the fibrinogen molecule, whereas the B peptides are located symmetrically in the molecule. By all other parameters, however, fibrinogen and fibrin monomers appear to be the same. The events leading to fibrin monomer polymerization after the release of the fibrinopeptides still elude explanation.

2. Phase II - Aggregation

The initial phases of fibrin polymerization have been studied by a number of investigators. Ferry and Shulman (1949) found that hexamethylene glycol inhibited the formation of fibrin gels, although the formation of intermediate polymers was observed in ultracentrifuge experiments. Similar observations were made in urea (Ehrlich et al. 1952) and 1 M sodium bromide pH 5.6 (Donnelly et al. 1955). The studies in hexamethylene glycol systems show that initial polymers are formed that have a molecular weight of about 4.95×10^6 and a length of 4000 Å possessing twice the molecular width of the original fibrinogen. These observations led to the hypothesis of intermediate fibrin polymer formation through staggered overlapping. This concept was later confirmed through electron microscopical observations of sequential changes during fibrin polymerization (Bang, 1964a).

Kinetic studies on the formation of fibrin are in no way complete. The difficulties in such a study are obvious since one is dealing with a series of complex equilibrium constants in the overall reaction (Sturtevant et al. 1955; Ehrenpreis et al. 1958; Laskowski et al. 1960; and Endus et al. 1966). For the present the knowledge of the release of the fibrinopeptides is limited to the fact that the release rate of fibrinopeptide A exceeds that of the B peptide (Blombäck and Vestermark, 1958). A first order relationship has been found between fibrinogen and fibrin monomer formation (Ehrenpreis et al. 1958). In a series of papers Waugh and co-workers (Waugh and Livingstone 1951a, b, and Waugh, 1954) have shown that the reaction of thrombin with fibrinogen is first order with respect to the enzyme, but not first order with respect to fibrinogen. A detailed kinetic analysis for each individual reaction sequence in the formation of fibrin has yet to be accomplished.

The mode of aggregation of fibrin polymers is still unknown. In a series of papers by Scheraga's group (Sturtevant et al. 1955; and Scheraga, 1958) the original association was thought to be of a hydrogen bonding type calculated from observable thermodynamic relationships and to occur between tyrosine or lysine as donor and histidine as acceptor. Recently this same group (Endus et al. 1966) brought evidence that the original estimation of hydrogen bond energy formation of –6 kcal/mole was too large, and a revision to –1.5 kcal/mole was used in a recalculation of the association. From these data a co-ordinate covalent bond formation between ionizable groups was postulated. It was originally found by Belister (Belister and Kotbova, 1960) that photooxidation of the histidine residues in fibrin monomers prevents coagulation. Some controversy exists regarding the exact mechanism of polymerization, and a definite picture is not available, since most studies have centered only on the initial and final states of fibrin polymerization. Individual pathways are largely unknown because means of reliable experimental analysis are still lacking.

3. Role of Carbohydrate in Fibrin Formation

The carbohydrate content of fibrinogen and fibrin has been studied by a number of investigators. Recent experiments seem to indicate that carbohydrate is not released during the initial phases of clotting. Tyler (1966) did not observe the release of carbohydrate upon clotting. Some workers noted a small difference in hexose content of fibrinogen and fibrin (Laki, 1951b; Szara and Bagdy, 1953; Bagdy and Szara, 1955; and Blombäck, 1958b). In addition, carbohydrate containing peptides have been isolated (Haschemcyer et al. 1966) supporting the structural theories first proposed by Laki and Gladner (1964) which indicate that the carbohydrate in fibrinogen is connected through glucosamine in peptide linkage with aspartic acid. Some intriguing observations have been made concerning the role of the fibrinogen carbohydrate moiety in coagulation. Selective periodate oxidation of the carbohydrate moiety renders fibrinogen unclottable (Laki and Mester, 1962) but when sialidase is allowed to react with fibrinogen, thus removing terminal sialic acid from the carbohydrate chains, fibrinogen becomes more susceptible to clotting (Chandrasekar et al. 1962). As mentioned earlier, the exact amount of carbohydrate in fibrinogen is debatable; however, the latest values reported are those by Brown (1964) listed in section II, A of this chapter. The postulate has been made (Laki and Gladner, 1964) that if carbohydrate is released from fibrinogen during clotting, this release may occur in the second enzymatic phase during the action of fibrin stabilizing enzyme (F XIII) on fibrin. In general, it can be said that at the present time reliable information on the role of carbohydrate in fibrinogen is still not available.

4. Fibrin Crosslinking and Fibrin Stabilizing Enzyme (F XIII)

The final stage of coagulation is the formulation of a relatively insoluble polymer. The resultant insoluble fibrin is the product of the action of an enzyme that is akin to the transamidases. This enzyme was first isolated and partly purified by Lorand and Jacobsen (1958). Further work (Loewy et al. 1961a) has led to the isolation of the enzyme (Factor XIII, Fibrinase, Laki-Lorand Factor) in an 8000-fold purification over plasma. It has a molecular weight of 350,000 with subunits of about 111,000 (Loewy, 1961b), and is found in several tissues (Tyler and Loek, 1964). The postulate that this enzyme requires ionized calcium for its activation (Lorand, 1965) is now disputed (Kisselback and Wagoner, 1966). At the present time the enzyme is believed to transpeptidize specific epsilon amino groups of lysine with specific asparagine and glutamine residues in the fibrin molecule with the release of ammonia (Lorand et al. 1962; Loewy et al. 1964; and Lorand and Jacobsen, 1964).

The carbohydrate moiety in fibrinogen (see previous section) has been postulated as the possible site of action, but arguments both for and against this mechanism now exist (Laki and Chandrasekar, 1963; Chandrasekar and Laki, 1964; Chandrasekar et al. 1964; Rosenberg and Carmen, 1964; and Tyler, 1966).

IV. Isolation and Assay of Fibrinogen

A. Assay of Fibrinogen

The assay of fibrinogen has been the subject of numerous reports in the last twenty-five years. However, in the final analysis they are all variations of only a few methods. These include turbidimetric estimation of fibrinogen after salting out procedures; estimation of fibrinogen by zone electrophoresis; spectrophotometric assays of the purified protein; assays of fibrinogen as fibrin after coagulation; gravimetric and heat precipitation methods. Limitations are found in all the assays listed.

1. Estimation of Plasma Fibrinogen using Sodium Sulfite Fractionation

This method has been explored by a large number of investigators, but the method below is essentially that employed by Goodwin (1961, 1965). The assay is based on the precipitation of the fibrinogen by a salt followed by quantitation of the protein using the biuret reaction.

a. Reagents: Sodium sulfite solution, 13 percent. Dissolve 130 gm of sodium sulfite in 500 ml of water. After the material has dissolved dilute to 1 liter.

Five percent sodium phosphate. Dissolve 5 gm of $Na_3PO_4 \cdot 12H_2O$ in 100 ml of water.

Cupric sulfate, 4 percent. Dissolve 4 gm of $CuSO_4 \cdot 5H_2O$ to give 100 ml solution.

Protein standard solution (Albumin). Dissolve any high purity salt-poor human serum albumin to give a final concentration of 1 gm per 100 ml in 0.85 percent sodium chloride. The concentration should be determined by Kjeldahl analysis.

Diluted standard solutions. Standards are made from the stock albumin by diluting from 9:1 to 1:9 in 10 ml volumetric flasks with 0.85 percent sodium chloride.

Blood collection. Blood should be collected in 7 ml amounts using 20 mg of solid potassium oxalate as the anticoagulant; mix well.

b. Procedure: The blood is collected and centrifuged. Into a clean 15 × 120 mm Pyrex screw-cap tube, calibrated at the 8 or 10 ml mark, one ml of the plasma is introduced. Next, 9.0 ml of the 13 percent sodium sulfite solution is mixed with the plasma, and the tube is allowed to stand at 37° C for 10 minutes. The tube is centrifuged at 3000 rpm for 10 minutes in a small clinical centrifuge. Pour off the supernatant fluid, and allow the tube to drain for one minute; wipe the lip clean. Add 5 ml of sodium sulfite, and break up the precipitate. Cap the tube and shake. Remove the cap, and add 3 ml of sulfite solution being careful not to leave the precipitate on the side of the tube. Recentrifuge and drain as before. Add 8 or 10 ml of the sodium phosphate reagent to the precipitate, and place the tubes in boiling water until the protein dissolves. Cool the tube, and replace the evaporated solution with sodium phosphate solution to the original mark. To each tube add 0.2 ml of the copper sulfate reagent, cap and shake. Remove the cap and centrifuge for 10 minutes at 3000 rpm. Decant the supernatant solution and record the optical density at 560 mμ using a blank with all reagents and employing water in place of plasma or standard albumin. The standard curve is constructed using the diluted standards 1 ml, sodium phosphate 8 ml, and copper sulfate solution 0.2 ml as in the determination of the unknown.

2. Determination of Fibrinogen by zone Electrophoresis

Early attempts at quantitation of fibrinogen by zone electrophoresis (Hirsch and Cattaneo, 1956) were not encouraging. The difficulties encountered can be assumed to have been caused by the choice of filter paper as a supporting medium. Fibrinogen significantly interacts with the paper support and under the standard conditions of paper electrophoresis (barbital buffers, pH 8.6–8.9 and ionic strength, 0.05 to 0.1). Fibrinogen as well as other unidentified plasma proteins remain at the point of application and spuriously high values for fibrinogen are obtained (Bang, unpublished observations). These difficulties were largely eliminated with the introduction of cellulose acetate electrophoresis (Bang and Almy, 1965). Minimal or no protein is absorbed onto the cellulose acetate support. No detectable interaction between fibrinogen and cellulose acetate occurs with this procedure.

The electrophoretic separation of plasma proteins takes place in a thin layer of buffer along the upper surface of the strip. Within certain limits of pH and ionic strength this method bears close resemblance to moving boundary electrophoresis. Plasma fibrinogen and purified human fibrinogen (Blombäck, Fraction I_4) are found to exhibit identical electrophoretic mobilities in a pH range of 8.4 to 9.2 and at ionic strengths of 0.05 and 0.1. The electrophoretic mobilities of either purified human fibrinogen or human plasma fibrinogen are in close agreement with reported data for mobilities in free electrophoresis (Applying the Durrum correction factor for increased migration paths). The details of the experimental procedure which has become routine in our laboratories is given below:

a. Reagents and Materials:

2.5 × 18 cm Cellulose Acetate Membrane Strips (Oxo Co. Ltd, London, England)

Procion Brilliant Blue

Tris (Hydroxymethyl Amino Methane)

Ethylene Diamine tetraacetic Acid (EDTA)

Sodium Barbital (Sodium Diethyl Barbituric Acid)

Ethylene Dichloride, Diethylene Glycol, Propylene Glycol

Electrophoresis Apparatus (Gelman Instrument Co., Ann Arbor, Mich.)

Electrophoresis Buffer: Tris 12.11 gm; sodium Veronal 5 gm; EDTA (acid form) 2.15 gm; distilled water to 1000 ml; pH 8.8; and ionic strength 0.025.

Fixative Stain: The combined fixative-stain is a modification of that reported by Fazekas de St. Groth et al. (1963). The fixative-stain is made up as follows: Procion Blue, 5 gm; Picric Acid, 50 gm; HCl concentrated, 20 ml; Absolute Methanol to 1000 ml Rinsing: Absolute Methanol.

b. Procedure: Each strip is soaked in Tris-EDTA-Barbital buffer prepared as outlined above, taking care to place the strips on the surface of the buffer with their shiny side facing upwards. The buffer is allowed to soak into the strips from below for two to five minutes, and the strips are then immersed completely in the buffer for an additional fifteen to thirty minutes.

A 500–600 ml volume of buffer with diethylene glycol or propylene glycol admixed to the buffer to 3 percent v/v is added to each electrophoresis chamber making sure that the levels of buffer in each of the chamber sections are identical. Each of 6–8 cellulose acetate strips are now tensioned between the designated supports by magnetic bars as for example outlined in the procedures manual of the Gelman Electrophoresis Chambers.

Exactly 3 microliters of platelet-poor plasma or serum or purified fibrinogen are applied as an even streak close to the cathodal end of the cellulose acetate membrane strip using an applicator. With any of a number of commercially available power supplies it is possible to handle six electrophoresis chambers loaded with 6–8 strips each; for optimum separation a 180-minute run at a constant voltage of 200 V is recommended. Under these conditions the observed increase in amperage is in the order of 0.01 to 0.015 m amp/cellulose acetate strip, and only a fraction of a degree rise in the buffer temperature is encountered. The total length of the separated pattern is 8 to 9 cm.

At the completion of the 180-minute electrophoresis, individual strips are rapidly removed from the electrophoresis chambers and are transferred without drying, their shiny side facing downwards onto the surface of the fixative-stain mixture. Fixation is complete instantaneously with no blurring or "running" of individual zones. After two to five minutes of immersion in the fixative-stain, maximum color intensity of the separated bands is achieved. The strips are ready for transfer into the rinsing bath of absolute methanol. Rinsing for one to two minutes in each of three rinses of clean absolute methanol is sufficient to completely destain the background of the strips.

The rinsed cellulose acetate strips are dried under pressure between blotters of filter paper. Drying is complete after five to ten minutes.

The stained bands of the electrophoretically separated plasma proteins are cut out, and each band is dissolved in one ml of a mixture of ethylene-dichloride: absolute ethanol (9:1). The resultant fluids are colored, non-turbid and show an O.D. maximum of approximately 600 mμ. Readings are made in a 1 cm light path cuvette. The blank cuvettes contain the same solvent mixture and the same quantity of dissolved cellulose acetate from an unstained electrophoresis strip.

Conversion from optical density into fibrinogen expressed in mg/ml is made with the aid of a reference calibration curve. The reference calibration curve is made following an electrophoretic run of serial dilutions of a highly purified human fibrinogen preparation. Fibrinogen standards can be prepared routinely with the method of Blombäck and Blombäck (1956). The standard reference purified fibrinogen is 97–99 percent clottable. Most lots of a commercial preparation of human fibrinogen obtainable from KABI Pharmaceuticals, Stockholm 35, Sweden, are better than 95 percent clottable, and quite suitable for use in establishing a refence calibration curve. Individual stained bands are cut out, dissolved, and spectrophotometric readings are made exactly as outlined above. Reference calibration curves for fibrinogen are highly reproducible, and Lambert-Beer's law is valid over a range of 4 to 30 micrograms of fibrinogen, the higher value corresponding to 10 mg/ml of fibrinogen dilution.

The final value of plasma fibrinogen, as determined from the fibrinogen standard curve, must be corrected by subtracting from it a blank band in the fibrinogen area of a serum sample from the same patient.

c. Comments

The low conductivity of the buffer system prevents extensive changes in temperature and evaporation from the strips during the electrophoresis run. It was found advisable to add either diethylene or propylene glycol to the buffer system to insure only minimal changes in temperature. The addition of urea at a concentration of 3 M (w/v) to the plasma sample significantly increases the separation between the fibrinogen, gamma, and beta globulins. The electrophoretic mobility for fibrinogen as well as other plasma proteins differs significantly from that obtained in free electrophoresis. In the outlined procedure, the clear separation of fibrinogen from neighboring proteins is the determinant factor. Though fibrinogen is heat labile and also precipitates at approximately 4 to 5° C, particularly at low ionic strength, it remains readily soluble and undergoes no detectable denaturation in the electrical field during the time period and at temperatures of 23 to 25° C.

Lambert-Beer's law is obeyed over a wide range of concentrations not only for fibrinogen, but also for highly purified human serum albumin, purified 7 S gamma globulin, and human plasma or serum applied to the strip, fixed, stained, and dissolved without electrophoretic separation. Moreover, all four proteins or mixtures diluted to protein concentrations comparable to those used in the standard reference fibrinogen curve, give slopes identical to that obtained for fibrinogen in concentration versus O.D. curves or graphs. Because of this, spectrophotometric scanning techniques and calculation of fibrinogen concentration by planimetry or automated integration are considered acceptable. The values for fibrinogen contents determined by the colorimetric and by the photometric scanning and integration techniques are in good agreement.

The technique is reproducible for plasmas from the same individuals or from plasma pools whether the anticoagulant is citrate, oxalate, or EDTA. Electrophoretic mobilities and staining intensities for fibrinogen in plasma collected in these three anticoagulants agree excellently. For one citrate plasma pool the following values for fibrinogen were obtained using different techniques; fibrinogen as fibrin 430 mg percent (technique outlined in section IV, A, 3, c); fibrinogen as fibrinogen (determined from a standard curve in the manner outlined above) 322 mg percent; and planimetry 368 mg percent.

Values for fibrinogen measured as fibrinogen by zone electrophoresis are found to be consistently 10 to 25 percent lower than fibrinogen measured as fibrin. Thus, it is possible that the contribution of occluded plasma proteins in the fibrin clot in the conventional assays of fibrinogen as fibrin is somewhat larger than previously suspected by other authors. The relative merits of the different methods of fibrinogen measurement are discussed more completely in section IV, C.

3. Spectrophotometric Assay for Clottability of Fibrinogen in Purified Systems

When working with purified fibrinogen systems, the assay for the protein may be carried out quite readily by spectrophotometry. Many variations of this technique exist. The methods developed by Laki (1951c) and Blombäck (1956) have been used in the authors' laboratory with minor modifications and are quite suitable.

a. Determination of Total Clottable Protein

According to Laki (1951c) this method is simple in design and is based on the ultraviolet absorption of fibrinogen. The method is based on measuring the amount of tyrosine and tryptophane absorption at 278 mμ before and after coagulation. As given below, it is a modification of the original Laki procedure (1951c). The purified fibrinogen solution concentration is diluted with 0.1 M KCl so that the absorption at 278 mμ is 1.0 in a one cm cell, although any readible optical density may be used. With appropriate instrumentation, such as the Cary spectrophotometer, optical densities of up to 2.5 may be accurately measured. However, it is recommended that with ordinary spectrophotometers the optical density should not exceed 1.0 because of the error inherent in the detector systems. A blank may be prepared using 0.1 M KCl. After the O.D. has been checked three solutions are prepared as follows:

	Tube 1	*Tube 2*	*Tube 3*
Fibrinogen Solution	1.0 ml	1.0 ml	
0.5 M Phosphate Buffer (pH 7.0)	0.1 ml	0.2 ml	0.2 ml
0.1 M KCl	2.5 ml	2.5 ml	3.5 ml
Thrombin (250 NIH u/ml)	0.1 ml		

All three tubes are allowed to stand for one hour at 37° C. Tube 1 forms a clot. The other two tubes should remain clear. At the end of one hour the clot in Tube 1 is removed carefully and compressed so that the supernatant solution is collected. The optical density of Tube 1 supernatant solution is now measured at 278 mμ and 325 mμ, Tube 3 being used as a blank. This process is repeated with Tube 2, again using Tube 3 as the blank. The optical density recorded for Tubes 1 and 2 are calculated in a 1 cm cell by subtracting the O.D. at 325 from the O.D. at 278 in a 1 cm cell. This subtraction of optical density at 325 mμ in nonabsorbing regions of the spectrum will help correct for light scattering. Two optical densities are now available for the calculation of percent clottable protein (the optical density of the fibrinogen remaining in Tube 1 after coagulation and the optical density of the fibrinogen in Tube 2 before coagulation). The percent clottable protein may now be calculated from the following formula:

$$\%\ \text{clottable protein} = \frac{(A_{\text{fibrinogen}}) - (A_{\text{supernatant}})}{(A_{\text{fibrinogen}})} \times 100$$

b. Assay for Clottable Protein in Purified Systems or Plasma, Method of Blombäck and Blombäck (1956)

Although the foregoing method is simple and rapid, it is sometimes advantageous to know the amount of coagulable protein existing as fibrinogen in a system. The following method, based with minor modifications on the original method of Blombäck and Blombäck (1956) has that advantage.

Standard fibrinogen solutions: It is suggested that standard fibrinogen solutions be prepared from the protein by the method of Seegers (1947) as described in section IV, B, 5. Two methods are available for the calculation of fibrinogen concentration in the samples. The fibrinogen is dissolved in a phosphate buffer solution of pH 6.35 and ionic strength 0.15. The buffer is 0.05 M in phosphate and 0.07 M in NaCl. The protein concentration is adjusted to give between 0.15 and 0.3 percent fibrinogen. This may be done quite readily by checking the optical density of the solution at 278 mμ where a 0.3 percent solution will have an optical density of about 4.5. (The solution should, of course, be diluted below an optical density of 1.0 to check this value.) At this point the standards are treated in the same manner as the unknowns. Serial dilutions are now made of the standard fibrinogen as desired.

The standard solutions and the unknowns in 1 ml aliquots are next pipetted into small beakers and mixed with 2.0 ml of the pH 6.35 buffer (ionic strength 0.15) and 0.15 ml of standard (100 NIH u/ml) thrombin. The clotting mixture is allowed to stand for two hours. The clots are then carefully poured on silk cloth over filter paper, allowed to synerese, then washed three times with 0.15 M NaCl, and transferred carefully to a test tube with a glass stopper. Ten ml of 40 percent urea in 0.2 N NaOH are added, and the clot is dissolved. One ml of 0.3 M NaCl is then added, and the contents are mixed. A blank is prepared from 40 percent urea in 0.2 N NaOH and 0.3 M NaCl. The O.D. values are determined at 278 and 325 mμ. The values A_{278}–A_{325} of the samples will give the true optical density.

The standard fibrinogen solution before dilution is also clotted in a second experiment to determine the nitrogen content. It is, therefore, best to use a relatively large sample and coagulate it in the same manner as the serial dilutions and the unknown. The fibrin sample is not dissolved in urea but is dialyzed exhaustively and dried. The total nitrogen is determined by the micro Kjeldahl method. The method of Lang (1958) has been used by this laboratory and is quite satisfactory.

The nitrogen to protein conversion factor for fibrin is 6.02. From the absolute nitrogen content of the standard solutions, the concentration of fibrinogen in the serial dilutions are plotted against the optical densities, and the unknown in mg of fibrin may be found.

An alternative method is to measure the optical density of the unknown in 40 percent urea, 0.2 N NaOH and then using the extinction coefficient of fibrin in alkali as 16.17 ($E^{1\%}_{1\,cm}$), to calculate the concentration of fibrin. The concentration is calculated with the following equations:

$$\%\ \text{fibrin} = \frac{A_{278}\text{–}A_{325}}{16.17 \times \text{cm (usually 1 cm)}}$$

$$\text{mg fibrin/ml} = \% \times 10\,\text{mg}$$

c. Modified Ratnoff and Menzie Method (1951)

The following technique, which is a modification of that published by Ratnoff and Menzie (1951), has been standard in the authors' laboratory for a number of years. The technique lends itself equally well to fibrinogen determinations in human plasma and to fibrinogen quantitation of partly or highly purified fibrinogen.

Principle: Fibrinogen is converted into fibrin by the addition of thrombin and calcium chloride. Glass beads are utilized in the clotting mixture since thrombin adsorbs onto glass, and the dense fibrin polymer which forms around the glass beads effectively expels solvent and nonclottable proteins. Epsilon-aminocaproic acid is added to the clotting mixture to prevent fibrinolytic degradation of fibrinogen or fibrin during clot formation.

Quantitation is obtained by hydrolysis of the fibrin, and determination of fibrin tyrosine using the Folin-Ciocalteau reagent.

Reagents:
Epsilon-aminocaproic acid (EACA) chromatographically pure
Glass Beads (Super Brite® type No. 140-5005)
Folin-Ciocalteau phenol reagent
Topical bovine thrombin (Parke-Davis)
Plastic test tubes
Epsilon aminocaproic acid saline mixture:

1.32 gm EACA dissolved in 100 ml of 0.14 M NaCl (10^{-1} M EACA)

Glycine buffer: 12.2 gm glycine (0.163 M glycine) per liter of 0.25 N sodium hydroxide

Procedure: The following mixture of fibrinogen-thrombin coagulation diluent may be prepared in advance and stored at 4° C in stoppered plastic tubes.

6.0 ml EACA saline, 0.2 ml glass beads, 0.2 ml of 0.2 M calcium chloride.

To each tube of diluent add in rapid succession 0.2 ml plasma or fibrinogen solution, and 0.2 ml thrombin (100 NIH u/ml). Immediately stopper the tube with pliofilm, and mix its contents by repeated inversion; continue inverting until the fibrin clot formed around the glass beads falls freely to the bottom of the tube.

Allow the tubes to stand for 20 minutes at room temperature.

If additional fibrin has formed repeat the inversion of the tube several times; add more glass beads if necessary.

Place the tube at 4° C for 3 hours or overnight.

Centrifuge 1000 × G for 5 minutes.

Decant, add 6 ml of saline and mix well.

Repeat the centrifugation and saline washes twice as outlined above.

Decant well, and wipe the last drop from lip of the tube.

Pour 0.4 ml of 2.5 N NaOH over the clot.

Transfer the tubes to a boiling water bath for 1–2 minutes, and let stand at room temperature for an additional 5–10 minutes.

Add to each tube 4.6 ml of glycine buffer, 0.8 ml distilled water and 1.5 ml 5 percent trichloroacetic acid, and mix well.

Add 1.5 ml of Folin-Ciocalteau reagent diluted 1:3 with distilled water. Mix immediately and well by inversion or by use of a Vortex mixer. Allow at least 10 minutes and no more than 30 minutes for maximum color development.

Read the optical density in a spectrophotometer at 650 mμ in a cuvette of 10 mm light path against a reagent blank.

Preparation of reagent blank: Substitute the patient's serum for patient's plasma and subject this to the entire procedure outlined above.

The optical density is converted into fibrinogen in mg/100 ml using a standard calibration curve.

A washed, dried preparation of bovine fibrin available commercially from many different supply houses in the United States and western Europe is suitable for the construction of a standard calibration curve.

A stock solution is prepared by dissolving 10 mg/ml washed dried bovine fibrin in 2.5 normal sodium hydroxide. Serial dilutions are made from the stock solution utilizing 2.5 normal sodium hydroxide as the diluent. For each dilution admix 0.4 ml of fibrin solution, 4.6 ml glycine buffer, 1.5 ml 5 percent trichloroacetic acid, and 1 ml distilled water. Mix well; then add 1.5 ml Folin reagent diluted 1:3. Color development and spectrophotometric readings are made exactly as above.

A reagent blank is prepared by substituting 0.4 ml water for the fibrin solution.

4. Gravimetric Determinations of Fibrinogen

The simplest method for the determination of fibrinogen is the gravimetric procedure. Several reported procedures may be used but the following methods are based upon the observations of Ingram (1952), Wycoff (1956), Bang (1957), and Persson (1963).

a. Macro Method

The blood is collected in a graduated centrifuge tube containing 10 mg of oxalate. The tube is filled to the 5 ml mark. The oxalate is a mixture of 60 percent ammonium oxalate and 40 percent potassium oxalate and may be prepared by dissolving 1.2 gm of the ammonium salt and 0.8 gm of the potassium salt in 100 ml of water. To each collection tube, 0.5 ml of the anticoagulant is added and dried. The tube is inverted after the addition of blood.

The tube is centrifuged for 2–3 minutes at 3000 rpm, and 1 ml of the plasma is added with mixing to a test tube containing 5 ml of 0.9 percent sodium chloride. A 0.2 ml volume of thrombin (100 NIH/ml) is then added, and the tube is rapidly shaken. Gelation is complete within a few minutes, but it is best to allow the clot to stand for 30 minutes. The clot is now loosened from the tube and poured on several layers of fine filter paper, and the water is removed from the clot by pressure with additional filter papers.

The clot is rinsed in 0.9 percent saline for a short time, then in 99 percent ethanol for 5 minutes, and finally in ether for 5 minutes. The clot is now dried at 37° C for 2 hours and is weighed. The calculation of fibrinogen content per 100 ml of blood plasma is as follows:

$$\text{weight of clot} \times 100 = \text{mg fibrinogen/100 ml plasma}$$

b. Micro Method

Equipment and Reagents:

Microbalance

Ten percent alcoholic saline: Mix 100 ml of 95 percent ethanol with 900 ml of 0.85 percent sodium chloride solution.

Thrombin: 10 mg of Parke-Davis Topical Thrombin is dissolved in 100 ml of the above saline solution (final concentration of thrombin is about 2.5 u/ml).

Reagent grade sulfuric acid.

Thirty percent H_2O_2

Ammonium sulfate standard solution: Dissolve 0.472 gm of dry ammonium sulfate in 1 liter of water. This solution contains 0.10 mg of nitrogen per ml.

Nessler's Reagent: Prepared according to Koch and McMeekin (1924).

Procedure: The citrated or oxalated blood is centrifuged for 10 minutes at 2000 rpm, and 0.1 ml of plasma is pipetted into small (195 × 85 mm) test tubes. Two ml of the thrombin solution are added and mixed. The clot is allowed to form for one hour. The fibrin is then collected on small glass needles of about 3 inches in length made by drawing a 3 mm Pyrex glass rod to a diameter of 0.3 to 0.5 mm and leaving 3 inches of the rod intact above the needle for a handle. The fibrin is collected by rotating the rod. The collected fibrin is washed by placing the needle into distilled water for a short time, and then into ethanol. The needle and fibrin are dried at 80° C for 30 minutes and are weighed on a microbalance to constant weight. Calculation:

mg/fibrin 100 mls plasma = weight fibrin in mg × 100.

If a microbalance is not available, the fibrin may be estimated by digestion and colorimetric determination. After the fibrin has been washed with water and ethanol, the needles are inserted in 18 × 155 mm Pyrex tubes containing 0.15 ml of concentrated sulfuric acid. The tubes are then placed in a sand bath on a hot plate so that the acid refluxes. When the tubes have been heated for five minutes, each is removed from the sand bath and agitated so that the fibrin comes in contact with the acid. The tubes are returned to the sand bath and a drop of the peroxide is added. This procedure is repeated, and the tubes are then heated for 10 minutes to complete the reaction. The tubes are cooled, and 6.0 ml of water are added and mixed with the contents of each tube. Then 4.0 ml of Nessler's reagent are added and mixed. The samples are read in a spectrophotometer at 500 $m\mu$ using the appropriate blank with no fibrin. A standard curve of ammonium sulfate standards are plotted to obtain the mg of nitrogen in the fibrin sample. In the original method of Wycoff (1956), the conversion value of 6.25 was used to determine the mg of protein in 0.1 ml of plasma.

5. Plasma Fibrinogen Titer (Method of Bowman, 1957)

This assay for fibrinogen is rapid and may be used as a semiquantitative evaluation of fibrinogen content.

a. Reagents

Test plasma: Five ml of freshly drawn venous blood are placed into a collection tube containing 0.1 ml of a 10 percent sodium citrate solution. The specimen is centrifuged at 1500 × G for 200 minutes to obtain the supernatant platelet-poor plasma. Other anticoagulants may be used, but lower titration values may be obtained. EDTA plasma is less desirable, according to the authors.

Thrombin: 1000 units of bovine "topical" thrombin are reconstituted with 5 ml of distilled water and are added to a vial containing 5 ml of CP (chromatographically pure) glycerol. The bovine thrombin-glycerol solution when stored at 4° C may be used for repeated assays over a one-month period.
Normal saline: 0.85 percent sterile solution.

b. Procedure: Arrange a series of seven test tubes (13 × 100 mm). Pipette no saline into the first tube, 4.5 ml saline into the second tube, 0.5 ml saline into the third tube, 2.0 ml saline into the fourth tube, and 1.0 ml saline into the fifth, sixth, and seventh tubes.
Place 0.5 ml of the test plasma into the first tube, and another 0.5 ml of the test plasma into the second. With a fresh pipette, mix the contents of the second tube by drawing up and discharging six times with the pipette.
With a fresh pipette, transfer 0.5 ml of the plasma mixture from tube No. 2 to tube No. 3. Also, transfer an additional 0.5 ml of the plasma mixture from tube No. 2 to tube No. 4. Mix the contents of tube No. 3 well.
With a fresh pipette, mix the contents of tube No. 4 well, then transfer 1.0 ml of its plasma mixture to tube No. 5. Mix well by drawing up and discharging six times with the pipette, and in a similar way transfer 1.0 ml of the plasma dilution in tube No. 5 to tube No. 6 and 1.0 ml of the plasma dilution of tube No. 6 to tube No. 7.
Discard the final 1.0 ml residual from tube No. 7. Avoid air bubbles in preparing dilutions.

At room temperature, add 0.1 ml of thrombin solution to each tube. Shake each tube lightly to mix. Let the tubes stand for a minimum of 90 seconds.
Examine each tube by tilting gently in a horizontal position against a good light source. In tube No. 1 a firm fibrin clot and in tube No. 2 a gelatinous fibrin clot will normally form. These adhere to the tubes when the tubes are inverted. A transparent white pellicle forms in the remaining tubes. When the end point is reached in tube No. 6 or No. 7, the fibrin clot is small, filmy, and often attached to the meniscus of the plasma-saline mixture. The highest dilution in which a visible single coagulum of fibrin is seen is the fibrinogen or "thrombin" titer. Reciprocals of the plasma dilutions are: Tube No. 1: 1; Tube No. 2: 10; Tube No. 3: 20; Tube No. 4: 50; Tube No. 5: 100; Tube No. 6: 200; Tube No. 7: 400. The normal range is 100–400.

6. Heat Precipitate Determination of Fibrinogen (Goodwin, 1965)

a. Reagents:
Alkaline potassium tartrate-copper sulfite. 20 gm Na_2CO_3 and 0.5 gm potassium tartrate in 1 liter of 0.1 N NaOH. To 45 ml of this solution add 5 ml of $CuSO_4$ solution made by dissolving 1.0 gm of $CuSO_4 \cdot 5H_2O$ in 1 liter of distilled water.
Lowry Reagent (commercial)
Benedict's Qualitative Solution (commercial) or according to Prunty et al. (1959).

b. Procedure: Place from 0.5 to 1.0 ml of plasma in a Pyrex tube. Incubate the mixture at 60° C for 10 minutes. Centrifuge the tube and drain. To the precipitate add 0.5 ml of saline and mix with a suitable mechanical mixer. Add an additional one ml of saline, mix, centrifuge and drain.
Repeat this step two times. To the precipitate add 5 ml of 2.5 percent NaOH and dissolve the fibrin. The fibrin content of the plasma may be determined by either biuret or Lowry methods with the use of human albumin as a standard.

a. Method I. Modified Biuret Method:
Add 1.0 ml of Benedict's Qualitative Solution to the dissolved fibrin, and dilute to 7 ml with water. Allow to stand 20 minutes and measure the O.D. at 555 mμ. The blank is prepared in a similar manner substituting 5 ml of 2.5 percent NaOH for the protein.

b. Method II. Lowry Method:
Add 0.4 ml of dissolved fibrin to 10 ml of alkaline potassium tartrate-copper sulfate and allow to stand for 10 minutes. Prepare the blanks in the same manner using 0.4 ml of 2.5 percent NaOH. Next, add 1.0 ml of Lowry phenol biuret reagent to both the unknowns and the standards. Mix and allow to stand for 30 minutes and read at 700 mμ.
The standards for either method are made from human albumin in water and treated the same as the fibrin unknowns.

B. Isolation of Fibrinogen

1. Method of Blombäck and Blombäck (1956)

The method devised by Blombäck and Blombäck is based on ionic strength and alcohol precipitation techniques. The method is applicable to either human or bovine material. The convenience of the procedure makes it adaptable to isolation on a large scale. It is convenient to have at hand large quantities of stock citrate buffers for the procedures. The composition of the standard citrate buffers is given below.

Citrate solution for blood collection: 4 percent solution trisodium citrate, $Na_3C_6H_5O_7 \cdot 2H_2O$ dissolved in water.

Citrate buffer pH 6.0, 0.055 M, ionic strength 0.30: For each liter of buffer, 16.18 gm of trisodium citrate $Na_3C_6H_5O_7 \cdot 2H_2O$ are dissolved in 900 ml of water. The pH is adjusted to 6.0 with concentrated HCl, and the solution is diluted to 1 liter.

Citrate buffer pH 6.35, 0.055 M, ionic strength 0.30: For each liter of buffer, 16.18 gm of trisodium citrate $Na_3C_6H_5O_7 \cdot 2H_2O$ are dissolved in 900 ml of water. The pH is adjusted to 6.35 with concentrated HCl, and the solution is diluted to 1 liter.

Citrate buffer, pH 7.0, 0.055 M, ionic strength 0.30: For each liter of buffer, 16.18 gm of trisodium citrate $Na_3C_6H_5O_7 \cdot 2H_2O$ are dissolved in 900 ml of water. The pH is adjusted to 7.0 with concentrated HCl, and the solution is diluted to 1 liter.

Precipitation of Cohn Fraction I: The blood to be collected is diluted with 4 percent citrate solution to a final volume ratio of 9 parts blood and 1 part anticoagulant. The material is stirred gently to insure against coagulation. The blood is separated from the plasma by either centrifugation or by the use of a laboratory separator such as the DeLaval separator. Careful handling is necessary to prevent hemolysis. The plasma is stirred gently and cooled as quickly as possible to 0° C without permitting the formation of ice. The pH of the plasma is adjusted to 7.2 with a stock 0.8 M acetate buffer-ethanol solution. The 0.8 M acetate buffer is prepared from sodium acetate buffered to 4.0 with acetic acid. This buffer has a mole ratio of sodium acetate to acetic acid of 0.2 and is conveniently prepared by taking 200 ml of 4 M sodium acetate, 400 ml of 10 M acetic and sufficient water to make 1 liter. When diluted 80 times with water, it should have a pH of 4.0 ± 0.02 when measured with a glass electrode at 25° C. The plasma at 0° C is stirred while, for each liter of plasma, a mixture of 177 ml of a 53.3 percent ethanol-water solution and 1 ml of the acetate buffer is added over a period of one and one-half hours. The ethanol-water-acetate buffer may be added through capillary jets. After this addition, the mixture is allowed to stand for one additional hour at –3° C with gentle stirring.

The precipitate is now centrifuged at a temperature of between –2° C and –3° C. The weight of the precipitate is recorded, and the supernatant solution may be kept for further fractionation, if desired. The precipitate, which is largely fibrinogen, is labelled Cohn Fraction I. The material may be stored at –20° C or used immediately in the next step of the Blombäck procedure.

Extraction I. The first step involves the extraction of the Cohn Fraction I material with a citrate-glycine-ethanol buffer, pH 6.0. For each 100 gm of the wet paste labelled Cohn Fraction I, 1000 ml of this buffer is needed. The buffer is prepared by dissolving 75 gm (1 mole/liter) of glycine and 65 ml of absolute ethanol in 900 ml of the stock citrate buffer pH 6.0. The pH is checked and adjusted, if necessary, to 6.0. The solution is then diluted to 1000 ml with additional stock citrate buffer pH 6.0.

The precipitate from Cohn Fraction I is mixed with a small known amount of the citrate-glycine-ethanol buffer, pH 6.0 until a homogeneous paste is formed. The rest of the buffer is added and the temperature is brought to –3° C with stirring. After one hour, the mixture is centrifuged. The supernatant solution is discarded and the weight of the precipitate is recorded.

Extraction II (bovine): A second extraction with a citrate-glycine-ethanol buffer, pH 7.0 is now made. For each 100 gm weight of the material from Extraction I, 1000 ml of this buffer is needed. The buffer is prepared by dissolving 75 gm (1.0 mole) of glycine and 65 ml of absolute ethanol in 900 ml of the stock citrate buffer, pH 7.0. The pH is checked and adjusted, if necessary, to 7.0. The solution is then diluted to 1000 ml with additional stock citrate buffer pH 7.0. The precipitate from Extraction I is mixed with a small amount of the citrate-ethanol-glycine buffer, pH 7.0 until a homogeneous paste is formed. The rest of the buffer to be used is added and the temperature of the suspension is brought to –3° C and stirred for one hour. The suspension is centrifuged, and the supernatant solution is discarded. The weight of the precipitate is recorded and denoted Fraction I–0.

Extraction II (human): If human material is used, Extraction I is repeated for Extraction II.

Further purification of fibrinogen I–0: The precipitate denoted I–0 is dissolved at 30° C in the stock citrate buffer, pH 6.35 to a protein concentration of 1.5 percent. The solution is filtered if cloudy. The solution is then diluted to 0.67 percent protein with a citrate-glycine buffer, pH 6.35. This buffer is prepared by dissolving 75 gm (1 mole) glycine in 900 ml of stock citrate buffer, pH 6.35. The pH is adjusted if necessary and the solution is diluted to 1 liter with stock citrate buffer, pH 6.35. For every 100 gm of wet paste denoted I–0 the final volume will be about 1300 ml (or 650 ml of stock citrate buffer, pH 6.35 plus 650 ml of glycine-citrate buffer, pH 6.35).

Precipitation of I–1 (Cold Insoluble Globulins): To every 1000 ml of dissolved fraction I–0 chilled to 0° C, a mixture of 23.6 ml of absolute ethanol, 21.7 ml of 1 M glycine in citrate buffer, pH 6.35, and 135.7 ml citrate buffer, pH 6.35 (total 181 ml) is added over a period of 45 minutes. The temperature is kept at 0° C with gentle stirring and then centrifuged. The precipitate should be weighed and labelled "cold insoluble globulins, I–1"; the supernatant solution is preserved for Step I–2.

Precipitation of I–2: For each 1000 ml of the supernatant of I–1, 305 ml of cold citrate buffer, pH 6.35, and 69.4 ml of absolute ethanol (total 374.4 ml) are added over a period of one hour, and the temperature is lowered to –4° C. The suspension is stirred for another half hour of complete precipitation and then is centrifuged. The precipitate is labelled "I–2" and weighed.

For additional purification of I–2, different procedures are employed for material of human or bovine origin.

Further purification of I–2 (bovine material): The precipitate I–2 is dissolved in 0.3 M sodium chloride (17.55 gm NaCl/100 ml) to a protein concentration of 1.8 percent. Then for each 100 ml of this solution, add dropwise a mixture of 145 ml of 2 M glycine (prepared by dissolving 150 gm of glycine in 1000 ml water for each liter needed), 55 ml of demineralized water, and 280 ml of a 0.04 M phosphate buffer, pH 7.3 to 7.5. The phosphate buffer may be prepared from stock solutions of 0.2 M KH_2PO_4 (27.22 gm/1000 ml) and 0.2 M K_2HPO_4 (34.84 gm/1000 ml). The pH 7.0 buffer is then prepared by mixing 45 ml of the 0.2 M KH_2PO_4 and 155 ml of the 0.2 M K_2HPO_4 and diluting to 1000 ml. The pH of the solution should be checked. After the addition of the above solutions, the temperature of the protein solution is lowered to 0° C.

Fraction I–3 (bovine): To each 1000 ml of the diluted solution from the above step cooled to 0° C, 100 ml of 0.5 M glycine-ethanol solution is added. This solution is prepared from 37.5 gm of glycine, 82.5 ml of absolute ethanol, and sufficient demineralized water to yield a final volume of 1000 ml.

After the addition of this solution, the protein solution is allowed to stand for at least two hours at 0° C with gentle stirring. The solution is centrifuged, and the precipitate is weighed and labelled "cold insoluble protein". The supernatant solution must be clear for Step I–4.

Fraction I–4 (bovine-purified fibrinogen): To each 1000 ml of the supernatant solution from the above step (I–3), 123 ml of 53.3 percent ethanol-water (volume percent) are added. The temperature is lowered to –4° C and the solution is stirred for thirty minutes. The material is centrifuged, and the precipitate is labelled "Fraction I–4 Purified Fibrinogen". The material can be stored for long periods at –20° C without loss of clotting ability.

Further purification of I–2 (Human): The precipitate of I–2 human is dissolved in the stock 0.055 M trisodium citrate buffer, pH 6.35 to give a protein concentration of 0.7 percent.

The volume is measured, and twice the volume of 0.75 M glycine (56.25 gm glycine/1000 ml) is added dropwise with gentle stirring. The solution is then cooled to 0° C. If a small precipitate is formed, it is not removed until the end of Step I–3.

Fraction I–3 (human): The diluted fraction from the preceding step is cooled to 0° C. To each 1000 ml of this solution, 100 ml of 0.5 M glycine-ethanol solution is added. This solution is prepared from 37.5 gm of glycine, 82.5 ml of absolute ethanol, and enough demineralized water to give a final volume of 1000 ml. The mixture is allowed to stand for two hours at 0° C with gentle stirring, and is then centrifuged. The precipitate is weighed and represents insoluble protein, Fraction I–3. The supernatant solution is preserved for the final I–4 step.

Fraction I–4 (human-purified fibrinogen): To each 1000 ml of the supernatant solution from I–3, 123 ml of 53.3 percent ethanol-water are added dropwise with gentle stirring. The temperature is brought to –4° C and the solution is stirred for an additional 30 minutes. The material is centrifuged, and the precipitate is labelled "Human Fraction I–4". The material may be preserved for long periods at –20° C.

2. Method of Laki (1951c)

The preparation is based on the further purification of Cohn Fraction I. Although this method is applicable to large scale fractionation, the following small scale preparation may be used as an example.

Two grams of dry lyophilyzed Cohn Fraction I (Armour Bovine Fibrinogen 60–70 percent clottable protein) are dissolved in 100 ml of 0.1 M buffer, pH 6.64. The solution is diluted with 100 ml of water; the pH is now 6.52. The solution is left standing overnight at 0 to 4° C. The precipitate is removed by centrifugation and discarded. The remainder of the supernatant solution containing the fibrinogen is subjected to further purification. The volume of the supernatant solution is measured. A volume of a saturated ammonium sulfate solution equal to one-third of the supernatant solution volume is added at room temperature with stirring. The flocculent precipitate is collected by centrifugation and dissolved in 60 ml of 0.3 M KCl at room temperature. The pH of the solution is adjusted to 7.4 with ammonium hydroxide.

The material is dialyzed against several changes of 0.3 M KCl for 72 hours. The material contains about 95 percent fibrinogen.

3. Preparation by a double salt complex — Method of Brown (1967)

Recently Brown has developed a method based on the specific precipitation of fibrinogen from plasma using a heavy metal complex. The method is simple and yields a product of high purity free of contaminants.

Preparation of double salt: Thirty grams (0.0875 moles) of mercuric nitrate ($Hg[NO_3]_2 \cdot H_2O$) are dissolved in approximately 200 ml of distilled water with the aid of approximately 40 drops of 6 N HNO_3. Then sufficient 3.5 M potassium thiocyanate solution (usually about 40 ml) is added slowly until the visual precipitation of the mercuric thiocyanate occurs. The mercuric thiocyanate ($Hg[SCN]_2$) is allowed to settle and then is thoroughly washed by decantation with distilled water. The moist mercury thiocyanate paste contains approximately 43 percent water after vaccum filtration through a Buchner funnel.

Approximately 34 ml of a 3.5 M KSCN solution (or a sufficient volume to just dissolve the $Hg[SCN]_2$) are added to the freshly prepared mercuric thiocyanate paste. The white needles of potassium trithiocyanate ($KHg[SCN]_3$) are allowed to form overnight at 4° C. These crystals are collected on a Buchner funnel, washed with cold absolute alcohol, and dried in a desiccator. The over-all yield of the ($KHg[SCN]_3$) crystals is usually between 20–25 percent of the theoretical yield.

The potassium tetrathiocyanate crystalline reagent is prepared by dissolving 10 gm of fresh moist mercury thiocyanate ($Hg[SCN]_2$) paste prepared as described above, and 30 gm (0.031 moles) of potassium thiocyanate crystals in 20 ml of distilled water. To this solution is added 25 gm (0.060 moles) of potassium mercury trithiocyanate ($KHg[SCN]_3$). After constituents have dissolved the potassium mercuric tetrathiocyanate monoclinic prisms are allowed to form at room temperature during the next 24 hours. The tabular crystals are washed in cold alcohol and air dried. The over-all yield of the $K_2Hg[SCN]_4$ crystals is approximately 80 percent of the theoretical.

Preparation of Fibrinogen: Fresh plasma (200 ml) is separated from whole blood collected on Dowex 50 W × 8 (sodium form). This may be accomplished by a Cohn fractionator or by centrifugation. The plasma is collected in a plastic container containing 10 gm of wet barium sulfate. Epsilon aminocaproic acid is added to give a final concentration of EACA of 0.1 moles/liter of plasma. The material is gently stirred for one hour at room temperature or several hours at 2° C. The solution is centrifuged and the supernatant plasma is treated with 5 gm of wet TEAE cellulose for each 50 ml of plasma. (The triethylaminoethyl cellulose should be treated with 0.5 M NaOH, washed to neutrality, and filtered before use.) After the addition of the TEAE cellulose, the suspension is stirred for 10 minutes at room temperature and then is centrifuged for 15 minutes at 8000 × G. The plasma is decanted and kept, while the cellulose precipitate is washed with a volume of 0.15 M NaCl and 0.1 M epsilon amino caproic acid, pH 7.2, equal to the plasma volume. This wash is combined with the plasma to yield a volume of about twice the original plasma volume. This diluted plasma is adjusted to pH 7.2 with 0.1 M sodium acetate buffer pH 4.0. The solution is cooled to 0° C and is now made 4 mM in $K_2Hg[SCN]_4$ by the addition of an appropriate volume of a 50 mM solution. The suspension is allowed to stand at 0° C for one hour with occasional stirring. The material is centrifuged for 15 minutes at 8000 × G. The fibrinogen-containing precipitate is washed twice with 50 ml of cold buffer (0.15 M sodium acetate, 0.1 M epsilon aminocaproic acid, pH 6.5). The washed precipitate is now dissolved at room temperature in 25 ml of a solution containing 0.3 M NaCl and 0.1 M epsilon aminocaproic acid, pH 7.2. The material is passed through a column of Sephadex G-25 with a solution of 0.3 M NaCl, pH 7.2, as the eluting phase. The elution is monitored at 254 mμ. Two peaks appear: the first is the fibrinogen; the second is the co-ordination complex. The protein solution is treated with Chelex 100 (Calbiochem) 4 gm/100 ml to remove mercuric ions. The solution is centrifuged and the solution containing the fibrinogen has a final purity of 94 to 99 percent as determined by coagulable protein.

4. Isolation of Heterogeneous Fibrinogens (Method of Mosesson and Sherry (1966). Subfractions of Fibrinogen)

Most methods that are employed for the isolation of fibrinogen take little cognizance of the fact that these preparations contain fibrinogen fractions of various solubilities and coagulability. In a series of articles on this subject (Finlayson and Mosesson, 1962; and Mosesson and Finlayson, 1963), definitive chromatography was used to separate these fractions. More recently (Mosesson and Sherry, 1966) a fractionation of these materials by precipitation methods has been employed. The purification yields several fibrinogen-like proteins, all clottable by thrombin.

Human outdated plasma is made 2.1 M in glycine by the addition of 165.0 gm of glycine per liter of plasma. The temperature of the mixture is brought to 5° C and the solution is allowed to stand with gentle stirring. The precipitate is collected by centrifugation.

The precipitate is now dissolved in a volume of 0.15 M NaCl, 0.01 M sodium phosphate, pH 6.4 buffer ($\Gamma/2 = 0.16$) equal to one-third of the original plasma volume. Again the solution is made 2.1 M in glycine (vide supra) and brought to 5° C. The precipitate is again collected by centrifugation. This fraction is designated I–G_2.

The fraction (I–G_2) is dissolved and brought to one-tenth of the original plasma volume with 0.10 M sodium phosphate pH 6.4. The I–1 Fraction (Laki, 1951c) is removed by diluting this solution with an equal volume of water and allowing the mixture to stand at 2° C overnight. The cold insoluble material (I–1) is removed by centrifugation. The volume of the supernatant solution is now increased to twice its original volume with the addition of 0.3 M NaCl. The solution is cooled to –2° C to –3° C while 95 percent ethanol is added with stirring to yield a final concentration of ethanol of 8 percent (91.9 ml of 95 percent ethanol/liter of solution). The precipitate I–2 is removed by centrifugation at –3° C. This material may be further purified by the method of Blombäck and Blombäck (1956) for fractions I–3 and I–4.

The supernatant solution from Fraction I–2 is then quantitatively precipitated by raising the ethanol concentration to 16 percent and lowering the temperature to –4° C. (This step will require the addition of 10.1 ml of 95 percent ethanol for each 100 ml of the above solution that is already 8 percent in ethanol.) The resulting fraction (I–5) is collected by centrifugation at –4° C. The I–5 fraction is next dissolved in 0.27 M NaCl, 0.1 M sodium phosphate pH 6.4 and brought to a concentration of 0.1 to 0.15 percent in total protein. The solution is now made 8 percent in ethanol by the addition of 95 percent ethanol (9.27 ml/100 ml of the protein solution) while the temperature is lowered to –2 to –3° C. The precipitate (I–6) is collected by centrifugation at a –3° C. The supernatant solution from the above step is brought to 16 percent in ethanol (1.01 ml 95 percent ethanol for 10 ml of supernatant solution), and the temperature is lowered to a –4° C. The resultant precipitate (I–7) is collected by centrifugation at –4° C.

The final fraction (I–8) is collected by redissolving fraction I–7 in 0.1 M NaCl and 0.01 M sodium phosphate pH 6.4. The solution is made 2.1 M in glycine by the addition of solid glycine. The precipitate, fraction I–8, is collected by centrifugation and is about 98.7 percent clottable.

5. Cryoprecipitation — Method of Ware, Guest, and Seegers (1947)

Twenty liters of blood are mixed with one liter of oxalate anticoagulant (1.85 percent $K_2C_2O_4 \cdot 2H_2O$ and 0.5 percent $H_2C_2O_4 \cdot 2H_2O$). The oxalated blood is centrifuged. A one gallon stainless steel or plastic container is then filled with the plasma and frozen solid at –30° C. This is then placed in an ordinary refrigerator at 5° C. After the frozen plasma has thawed part of the cold plasma is poured into two clean cups that have been previously cooled in an ice bath, and centrifuged at room temperature (2.500 rpm for 1 minute). After decanting the supernatant solution the centrifugation step is repeated until the fibrinogen has been collected. The centrifuge cups are again placed in an ice bath. A total of 110 ml of *ice cold* saline (0.9 percent NaCl) is now poured over the fibrinogen. Thorough but gentle mixing is achieved by using a single glass rod fitted on one end with a No. 7 rubber stopper. The mixture is then centrifuged at room temperature for 1 minute at 2,500 rpm and, after decantation, the cups are returned to the ice bath. One hundred and ten ml of iced saline are again added and mixed with the fibrinogen, and this mixture is centrifuged for one minute at 2,500 rpm. The washing is repeated five more times with 100, 90, 80, 70 and 50 ml portions of ice cold saline. To remove the last 50 ml of saline, three minutes are allowed for centrifugation. The fibrinogen is then suspended in 200 ml of saline and set in a water bath at 35° C. The special stirrer is used to keep the mixture in constant motion until temperature is 33° C. The fibrinogen solution is centrifuged for two hours at room temperature at 2,500 rpm. The clear fibrinogen is then decanted.

The solution may either be frozen at –20° C or lyophilized and stored at –20° C.

6. Preparation of Fibrinogen Free from Plasminogen Activity — Method of Bergström and Wallén (1961)

Fraction I–4, prepared as discubed by Blombäck and Blombäck (see section IV, B, 1) is used as starting material for the further purification of bovine fibrinogen. This highly purified preparation is free from plasmin activity. However, plasmin activity can be detected after activation with urokinase. In the final step of this preparation, fibrinogen is precipitated under the following conditions: ethanol 6.5 percent (v/v), glycine 0.45 M, protein concentration about 0.15 percent, pH about 7.0, and ionic strength about 0.08. Concentrated solutions of this fraction in 0.3 M NaCl were stored frozen at –15° C until used (Section IV, B, 1).

The purification of fibrinogen-free plasmin is performed by reprecipitation of fraction I–4 with ethanol in the presence of lysine monohydrochloride and glycine. The following procedure is used.

To every 100 ml of diluted fibrinogen solution are added with stirring 480 ml of a mixture consisting of 72.5 ml of 2 M glycine, 72.5 ml of 2 M lysine HCl, 55 ml of distilled water, and 280 ml of a phosphate buffer, pH 7.3–7.5, ionic strength 0.1. This buffer may be prepared from 45 ml of 0.2 M KH_2PO_4, 155 ml of 0.2 M K_2HPO_4 and distilled water to give a total volume of 1000 ml. After cooling to 0° C in a low-temperature thermostat heater, 137 ml of 53.3 percent ethanol are added. During this addition, the temperature is lowered to –4° C. After standing for 15 minutes the mixture is centrifuged for 5–10 minutes at 2000 × G. The precipitate is dissolved in 100 ml of 0.3 M NaCl, and the above procedure is repeated twice.

After the third precipitation, the fibrinogen is dissolved in 0.3 M NaCl to yield a protein concentration of approximately 2.5 percent. The solution is dialyzed for about 48 hours against several changes of 0.3 M NaCl at 0° C. To provide a suitable sample of the starting material for comparative analyses, lysine is added to the solution in low concentration (about 1 mM of lysine/gm of protein), whereupon the solution is dialyzed as stated above. The dialyzed solution is stored frozen at –15° C to –20° C.

7. Preparation of Fibrin Monomer

The following method for the preparation of fibrin monomer is that described by Donnelly et al. (1955) as modified by Lorand (1966).

Fibrin is prepared from a 3 percent solution of fibrinogen in 1 M NaBr. The fibrinogen solution is made 1 mM in iodoacetic acid to inactivate Factor XIII. To this solution nineteen volumes of buffered thrombin are added. The final concentrations of the clotting mixture are: 0.15 percent fibrinogen, 0.2 u/ml thrombin, 0.09 M KCl, 0.05 M NaBr, 0.015 M Na_2HPO_4, 0.03 M KH_2PO_4. The pH of the solution is 6.2 to 6.4. The fibrin clot is removed as it is formed by using a rotating glass rod. The removed fibrin is immediately redissolved at room temperature in sufficient NaBr to make the final concentration 1 M in NaBr at pH 5.3 (0.05 M acetate buffer). The solution of the fibrin is facilitated by the use of a magnetic stirrer. The solution is again diluted twenty-fold as before but without thrombin. The fibrin clot is again collected, and the process of redissolution and dilution is repeated a total of three times. The final solution of fibrin is dissolved as before in 1 M NaBr at pH 5.2 to 5.3, and then is dialyzed against this solution. The solution may be stored at –20° C for long periods.

C. Factors Influencing Analytical Results in Fibrinogen Assays:

Although the various analytical procedures enumerated in this chapter have been well established as useful laboratory tools in both the clinical and the biochemical laboratory, a number of uncontrollable and partly unknown variables can be assumed to cause significant errors and are discussed below.

The determination of fibrinogen as fibrin in native plasma and in partly or highly purified fibrinogen preparations, has won the widest acceptance. However, in all modifications of this procedure, important sources of errors must be recognized.

The simple expedient of measuring the dry weight of the washed synerized clot may produce high values unless correction is made for the salt content of the dried fibrin.

Different values for clottable fibrinogen may be obtained, depending on the protein assay utilized. Since the fibrinogen-fibrin conversion is accompanied by the release of 3 percent peptide material, the most highly purified fibrinogen preparation can be no more than 97 percent clottable. This figure is readily confirmed within the limits of experimental error if the calculations are based on micro Kjehdahl nitrogen determinations. However, if protein and peptide determinations are based on adsorption at 280 mμ, a highly purified fibrinogen preparation will appear to be 100 percent clottable. This experimental error is introduced by the extremely low absorption of the fibrinopeptides at 280 mμ.

Ferry and Morrison (1947a, b) noted that the physical properties of the fibrin clot depend on the pH and ionic strength of the fibrinogen-thrombin clotting mixture. Two extreme types of fibrin clots were observed. One was transparent, gelatinous, very friable, and almost perfectly elastic within the range in which it was deformed without rupture, and would not readily synerize. The other was opaque, nonfriable, and plastic; it compacted readily under expulsion of solvent. The first clot type which was observed under conditions of alkaline pH and relatively high ionic strength, was termed fine. The second clot type formed at lower pH (approaching the isoelectric point for fibrin monomer) and at a lower ionic strength, was termed coarse. The clot type most suitable for fibrinogen quantitation is the coarse variety, since adequate syneresis is necessary for the effective removal of all contaminating nonclottable protein material. Clotting at relatively low ionic strengths and in a pH range of 6 to 6.5 usually provides a fibrin gel with only minor contamination of occluded proteins. However, the thrombin concentration in the system must be relatively high to insure complete conversion of fibrinogen to fibrin monomer, because the pH is far from the pH optimum of 8 for the thrombin catalyzed phase of the fibrinogen-fibrin conversion. In practice we recommend that any suggested procedure for fibrinogen quantitation should take place at a pH of 8 or lower, since the quantity of occluded nonclottable plasma proteins rapidly increases above this pH value.

Little attention has been given to factors that may give rise to spuriously low or spuriously high fibrinogen values under clinical pathological conditions.

The clarification of the coagulation defect occurring in clinical states associated with hyperplasminemia, which is discussed by Triantaphyllopoulos and Triantaphyllopoulos in Chapter VIII, provided important information concerning the limitations on the widely used assay procedures for plasma-fibrinogen levels. The recognition of the antithrombin properties as well as the polymerization inhibitors among proteolytic molecular fragments of fibrinogen occurring in hyperplasminemic states, led to important changes in recommended assay procedures. The need for addition of epsilon-aminocaproic acid and longer incubation periods to insure complete coagulation in plasmas obtained from patients during fibrinolytic episodes soon became apparent. However, gross errors in fibrinogen quantitation may be made under these clinical circumstances. The major problems encountered can be explained through the recognized physical and ultrastructural changes of the fibrin polymer observed in fibrinolytic states, i. e., the observation that some large molecular fragments of fibrinogen may be incorporated in the fibrin clot resulting in "defective fibrin polymerization". The incorporation of fibrinogen-like molecular fragments may give high values. The extremely friable, low tensile strength physical properties of the defective fibrin clot allow fragments to be washed away during the washing procedures, thus yielding low values for the fibrinogen content.

Techniques other than the estimation of fibrinogen as fibrin in fibrinolytic states can be equally misleading. As pointed out in Chapter VIII by Triantaphyllopoulos and Triantaphyllopoulos, these problems can all be attributed to the difficulties inherent in separating some of the early large molecular products of fibrinogen degeneration from the parent fibrinogen molecule. These "early fibrinogen breakdown products" are largely thermolabile and are, therefore, counted as fibrinogen when a heat precipitation technique is utilized. Similarly, the salting out properties of these large degradation products closely resemble those of fibrinogen. They are largely precipitable by ammonium sulfate at 25 percent saturation, and they show the same electrophoretic mobility as intact fibrinogen. Hence, no procedure which depends on either salt fractionation or electrophoretic quantitation of plasma fibrinogen can be utilized.

Finally, immunochemical techniques have several limitations in that large molecular degradation products of fibrinogen possess antigen determinants almost identical to those of the parent fibrinogen molecule. The large molecular fibrinogen derivatives readily react with fibrinogen antibody, and in routine immunological quantitation that utilize immunoprecipitin systems no distinction can be made between the parent fibrinogen molecule and its proteolytic degradation products.

The determination of "fibrinogen and fibrinogen-like molecules" in plasma and in serum as discussed by Barnhart, and Triantaphyllopoulos and Triantaphyllopoulos, although not ideal, provides the only practical solution to the problem today. However, none of these techniques offers more than a semiquantitative measure of the ratio of fibrinogen to degradation products since some of the "early products" may be incorporated in the clot. Residual fibrinogen may remain in serum if the coagulation defect is severe enough. However, for all practical clinical purposes the combination of fibrinogen determinations in plasma and the assay for fibrinogen breakdown products in serum has proven its value in following a patient in a clinical situation of fibrinolytic purpura.

Uncertainty in fibrinogen assays may arise in clinical situations such as multiple myeloma and macroglobulinemia. Considerable controversy has arisen in the literature concerning fibrinogen levels in these disease states, probably because of unrecognized problems in fibrinogen assays. The presence of specific antithrombin ("antithrombin V") has been postulated by several authors (Loeliger and Hers, 1957; Benda et al. 1958; Larrieu et al. 1958), and this thrombin inhibitor may account for some of these experiences (Bang, 1967). Fibrinogen measured as fibrin is usually normal or elevated if clotting is allowed to continue for 12 hours or longer and if thrombin is added in sufficiently high concentration. However, usually fibrinogen measured as fibrinogen through plasma electrophoresis on cellulose acetate is lower than normal in some patients with myeloma or macroglobulinemia.

Immunoelectrophoresis against human fibrinogen antibody results in two complete precipitin arcs formed in the fibrinogen and paraprotein regions, indicating immunological similarity of the two antigens. Sera from these patients give a weakly positive precipitation arc in the region corresponding to the fibrinogen band in plasma and a strongly positive precipitin arc corresponding to the paraprotein band. From these preliminary data, it has been concluded that paraprotein from some patients readily conjugates with fibrinogen, producing a complex that reacts abnormally slowly with thrombin. These findings, may in part, explain the conflicting reports on fibrinogen levels in paraproteinemic states.

Recently, Bang (1964b) noted the striking similarity in published reports in the literature enumerating diseases associated with high fibrinogen levels and diseases associated with high levels of acidic glycoproteins (Winzler, 1955). Because of this observation, a study was undertaken to determine the effect of acidic mucoproteins on the physical properties of fibrinogen formed in coagulation mixtures of purified fibrinogen and thrombin. The acidic mucoproteins in these experiments were reprecipitated bovine or human Cohn Fraction VI. The gelation rates for fibrinogen-thrombin mixtures and fibrinogen-thrombin-mucoprotein mixtures were followed by continuous spectrophotometric recording of changes at a wavelength of 340 mμ. Striking enhancement in gelation rates was found in the presence of Fraction VI. In both systems, (1) fibrinogen-thrombin and (2) fibrinogen-mucoprotein-thrombin, electrophoretically homogeneous plasma proteins including the alpha, beta, and gamma globulins, and albumin were each tested for a possible effect on the gelation rates. The presence of these plasma proteins did not change gelation rates in either system. However, each individual protein could be recovered almost quantitatively from the washes of the clots when *no* mucoprotein was present; in the presence of mucoproteins the recovery of individual plasma proteins from the clot liquor was nil.

These observations suggest that mucoproteins may change the properties of the fibrin gel so that it retains plasma proteins in quantity. Fibrinogen with increasing purification shows a tendency toward conjugation with other proteins and phospholipoproteins in addition to glycoproteins. An experimental system has not yet been devised that would clearly establish whether high concentrations of mucoproteins in pathological plasma may enhance the tendency of fibrin to occlude plasma proteins but this possibility should be kept in mind in interpreting high fibrinogen values in many chronic disease states.

The major preparative techniques covered in the foregoing all possess specific advantages making them of special usefulness for specific research purposes.

The one fibrinogen preparation which is used the most widely in coagulation laboratories is

Cohn Fraction I. This is quite an impure preparation containing only 40–60 percent fibrinogen. All other plasma protein components are present, although the degree of contamination contributed by individual plasma proteins may vary somewhat from preparation to preparation. Moreover, most preparations of fraction I contain small but significant quantities of all other procoagulants as attested to by the fact that most fraction I fibrinogen preparations will coagulate when ionized calcium is added in optimal quantities.

All preparations of fraction I contain sizable quantities of plasminogen, a property which makes this kind of preparation suitable for substrate preparations in assays for plasminogen activators (see section 373). Occasional batches of fraction I may contain trace quantities of plasmin a property which seriously reduces the stability of the product and such batches of fraction I fibrinogen in general should be discarded and not used for coagulation assays of any kind.

The preparation techniques of Laki (1951c) and Blombäck and Blombäck (1956) uniformly produces a highly purified fibrinogen preparation suited for physical-chemical studies since these materials by most physical-chemical and immunochemical criteria seem to consist of only one component. Fraction I–0 of Blombäck and Blombäck has a special clinical interest since this fraction by itself or following further purification for an excellent source of antihemophilic globulin (Factor VIII). Although both fraction I–4 of the Blombäck and Laki's highly purified fibrinogen behave as single proteins by physical-chemical analysis they possess multiple biologic activities. Fraction I–4 was originally claimed to be free of plasminogen but most batches of this fraction will lyse when exposed to plasminogen activators such as urokinase. Similarly, fibrinogen purified according to Laki contains small but significant quantities of plasminogen. Both preparations contain significant quantities of factors V and VIII and occasional batches will contain sufficient prothrombin and other procoagulants to clot upon addition of ionized calcium. Both preparations contain significant quantities of fibrin stabilizing factor and both preparations readily yield fibrin I. The method of Brown as outlined in this section appears to represent a significant advancement in that Brown has arrived at a fibrinogen preparation free of factor II, V, VII, X and XIII. Its freedom of demonstrable factor XIII is of particular importance since this unique feature will make this preparation useful in specific and quantitative assays for fibrin stabilizing factor as described on page 262. Whether treatment of fibrinogen with the mercuric double salt complex as advocated by Brown alters the molecular structure of fibrinogen is another question which awaits clarification.

The preparation devised by Bergström and Wallén (1961) reproducibly yields a fibrinogen which is free of plasminogen and such preparations are now being employed widely for fibrinolytic assays i. e., plasminogen or plasminogen activator assays. The preparation of Brown (1967) apparently is free of plasminogen contamination.

The method of preparing fibrinogen by cryoprecipitation has won wide and well-deserved acceptance in coagulation laboratories since this technique is simple, requires little apparatus and reproducibly yields a fibrinogen preparation of high stability. The cryoprecipitation technique is best applied to isolation of fibrinogen from bovine plasma since the yield of cryoprecipitated fibrinogen from bovine plasma is considerably higher and more constant than for human plasma. The preparation was originally claimed to be free of fibrinolytic enzymes and procoagulants. However, a number of batches of cryoprecipitated fibrinogen prepared in the author's laboratory contained trace quantities of procoagulants as well as plasminogen.

One of the more exciting advances in fibrinogen fractionation is the discovery of fibrinogens with various solubilities (Mosesson and Finlayson, 1963). The exact physiological role of high and low soluble fibrinogens has not yet been elucidated. The isolation of highly soluble fibrinogen and its structure similarity to a fragment arising from plasmin proteolysis may indicate that this fibrinogen is a breakdown product of circulating fibrinogen (Fletcher et al. 1966, see also p. 248 and 406). It remains to be seen what significance these various fractions of fibrinogen of varying solubility play in hemostasis. Although the chromatography of fibrinogen has not been discussed in this chapter, even the most homogeneous preparations of fibrinogen contain two or more components separable on DEAE cellulose. The details of these studies have been published (Finlayson, 1968). As pointed out, fibrinogens from almost all sources are heterogeneous under chromatography conditions.

References

Armstrong, S. H., Jr., Budka, M. J. E., Morrison, K. C., and Hasson, M. (1947). *J. Am. Chem. Soc. 69,* 1747.

Bagdy, D., and Szara, I. (1955). *Acta Physiol. Acad. Sci. Hung. 7,* 179.

Bagdy, D., Guba, F., Lorand, L., and Mihalyi, E. (1948). *Hung. Acta Physiol. 1,* 197.

Bailey, K. (1944). *Advances in Protein Chem. 1,* 310.

Bailey, K., and Sanger, F. (1951). *Ann. Rev. Biochem. 20,* 118.

Bailey, K., Bettelheim, F. R., Lorand, L., and Middlebrook, W. R. (1951). *Nature 167,* 233.

Bang, H. O. (1957). *Scandinav. J. Clin. Lab. Invest. 9,* 205.

Bang, N. U. (1964a). *Thromb. Diath. Haemorrhag. Suppl. 13,* 73, 131.

Bang, N. U. (1964b). *Federation Proc. 23,* 577.

Bang, N. U. (1967). *In* "Blood Clotting Enzymology" (W. H. Seegers, ed.), pp. 487—549. Academic Press, New York.

Bang, N. U., and Almy, T. P. (1965). *Federation Proc. 25,* 386.

Bang, N. U., Fletcher, A. P., Alkzaersig, N., and Sherry, S. (1962). *J. Clin. Invest. 41,* 935.

Belister, V. A., and Kotbova, K. I. (1960). *Ukrain Biokhim. Zhur. 32,* 3.

Benda, L., Deutsch, E., and Mammen, E. (1958). *Wien. Klin. Wochschr. 50,* 559.

Bergström, K., and Wallén, P. (1961). *Arkiv Kemi 17,* 505.

Bettelheim, F. R., and Bailey, K. (1952). *Biochim. Biophys. Acta 9,* 578.

Blombäck, B. (1958). *Arkiv Kemi 12,* 99.

Blombäck, B., and Blombäck, M. (1956). *Arkiv Kemi 10,* 415.

Blombäck, B., and Doolittle, R. F. (1963). *Acta Chem. Scand. 17,* 1816.

Blombäck, B., and Vestermark, A. (1958). *Arkiv Kemi 12,* 173.

Blombäck, B., and Yamashina, I. (1958). *Arkiv Kemi 12,* 299.

Blombäck, B., Sjöquist, J., and Wallén, P. (1959). *Acta Chem. Scand. 13,* 819.

Blombäck, B., Blombäck, M., Edman, P., and Hessel, B. (1962). *Nature 193,* 883.

Blombäck, B., Blombäck, M., Doolittle, R. F., Hessel, P., and Edman, P. (1963a). *Biochim. Biophys. Acta 78,* 563.

Blombäck, B., Blombäck, M., and Searle, J. (1963b). *Biochim. Biophys. Acta 74,* 148.

Blombäck, B., Blombäck, M., Edman, P., and Hessel, P. (1966a). *Biochim. Biophys. Acta 115,* 371.

Blombäck, B., Blombäck, M., Hessel, B., and Iwanaga, S. (1967). *Nature 215,* 1445.

Blombäck, B., Blombäck, M., Hessel, B., and Iwanaga, S. (1967). *Nature 215,* 1445.

Blombäck, B., Blombäck, M., Henschen, A., Hessel, B., Iwanaga, S., and Woods, R. (1968a). *Nature 218,* 130.

Blombäck, B., Blombäck, M., Mammen, E., and Prasad, S. (1968b). *Nature 218,* 134.

Bowman, H. S., and Yelito, M. (1957). *Am. J. Obstet. Gynecol. 74,* 670.

Brand, E., and Edsall, J. T. (1947). *Ann. Rev. Biochem. 16,* 223.

Brown, M. (1964). Ph. D. Dissertation, Boston College.

Brown, M. (1967a). *Science 157,* 1017.

Brown, M. (1967b). Private Communication.

Carter, J. R., and Warner, E. D. (1954). *Am. J. Physiol. 179,* 549.

Capet-Antonini, F., and Gunand, S. (1967). *C. R. Acad. Sci., Paris 265,* 2093.

Caspary, E. A., and Kekwick, R. A. (1957). *Biochem. J. 67,* 41.

Chandrasekhar, N., and Laki, K. (1964). *Biochim. Biophys. Acta 93,* 392.

Chandrasekhar, N., Warren, L., Osbahr, A., and Laki, K. (1962). *Biochim. Biophys. Acta 63,* 337.

Chandrasekhar, N., Osbahr, A. J., and Laki, K. (1964). *Biochim. Biophys. Res. Commun. 15,* 182.

Chaudhuri, D. R. (1948). *Hung. Acta Physiol. 1,* 238.

Clegg, J. B., and Bailey, K. (1962). *Biochim. Biophys. Acta 63,* 525.

Cohen, C., and Szent-Györgyi, A. (1957). *J. Am. Chem. Soc. 79,* 248.

Cohn, E. J., Gurd, F. R. N., Surgenor, D. M., Barnes, B. A., Brown, R. K., Derouaux, G., Gillespie, J. M., Kahnt, F. W., Lever, W. F., Liu, C. H., Mittelman, D., Mouton, R. F., Schmid, K., and Uroma, E. (1950). *J. Am. Chem. Soc. 72,* 465.

Consdin, R. (1953). Discussion, Faraday, Inc. *13,* 282.

Donnelly, T. H., Laskowski, M., Jr., Notley, N., and Scheraga. H. A. (1955). *Arch. Biochem. Biophys. 56,* 369.

Eagle, H., and Harris, T. N. (1937). *J. Gen. Physiol. 20,* 543.

Edsall, J. T. (1953). *In* "Blood Cells and Plasma Proteins" (J. L. Tullis, ed.), p. 121. Academic Press, New York.

Ehrenpreis, S., Laskowski, M., Jr., Donnelly, T. H., and Scheraga, H. A. (1958). *J. Am. Chem. Soc. 80,* 4255.

Ehrlich, P., Shulman, S., and Ferry, J. D. (1952). *J. Am. Chem. Soc. 74,* 2258.

Engel, A., and Alexander, B. (1966). *Biochemistry 5,* 3590.

Engel, A., Alexander, B., and Pechet, L. (1966). *Biochemistry 5,* 1543.

Endus, G. F., Ehrenpreis, S., and Scheraga, H. A. (1966). *Biochemistry 5,* 1561.

Fazekas de St. Groth, S., Webster, R. G., and Datyner, A. (1963). *Biochim. Biophys. Acta 71,* 377.

Ferry, J. D., and Morrison, P. R. (1947a). *J. Am. Chem. Soc. 69,* 388.

Ferry, J. D., and Morrison, P. R. (1947b). *J. Am. Chem. Soc. 69,* 400.

Ferry, J. D., and Shulman, S. (1949). *J. Am. Chem. Soc. 71,* 3198.

Finlayson, J. S. (1968). *In* "Fibrinogen" (K. Laki, ed.), Chapter III, p. 39. Dekker, Inc., New York.

Finlayson, J. S., and Mosesson, M. W. (1963). *Biochemistry 2,* 42.

Fletcher, A. P., Alkjaersig, N., Fischer, S., and Sherry, S. (1966). *J. Lab. Clin. Med. 68,* 78.

Folk, J. E., and Gladner, J. A. (1960). *Biochim. Biophys. Acta 44,* 383.

Folk, J. E., Gladner, J. A., and Levin, Y. (1959). *J. Biol. Chem. 234,* 2317.

Gerbeck, C. M., Yoshikawa, T., and Montgomery, R. (1967). *Federation Proc. 26,* 1537.

Gladner, J. A., Murtasign, P. A., Folk, J. E., and Laki, K. (1963). *Ann. N. Y. Acad. Sci. 104,* 47.

Goodwin, J. (1961). *Am. J. Clin. Pathol. 35,* 227.

Goodwin, J. (1965). *Clin. Chem. 11,* 63.

Hall, C. E. (1949). *J. Biol. Chem. 179,* 857.

Hall, C. E. (1963). *Lab. Invest. 12,* 998.

Hall, C. E., and Slayter, H. S. (1959). *J. Biophys. Biochem. Cytol. 5,* 11.

Haschemeyer, A. E. V. (1963). *Biochemistry 2,* 851.

Haschemeyer, A. E. V., and Tinoco, I. (1962). *Biochemistry 1,* 996.

Haschemeyer, R. H., Cynkin, M. A., Han, L. C., and Trindle, M. (1966). *Biochemistry 5,* 3443.

Henschen, A. (1963). *Arkiv Kemi 22,* 1.

Henschen, A. (1964a). *Arkiv Kemi 22,* 355.

Henschen, A. (1964b). *Arkiv Kemi 22,* 375.

Henschen, A., and Blombäck, B. (1964). *Arkiv Kemi 23,* 347.

Hirsch, A., and Cattaneo, C. (1956). *Hoppe-Seylens Z. Physiol Chem. 304*, 53.
Hocking, C. S., Laskowski, M., Jr., and Scheraga, H. A. (1952). *J. Am. Chem. Soc. 74*, 775.
Huseby, R. M., and Murray, M. (1967a). *Biochim. Biophys. Acta 133*, 243.
Huseby, R. M., and Murray, M. (1967b). *Federation Proc. Abstracts 26*, 537.
Ingram, G. I. C. (1952). *Biochem. J. 51*, 583.
Iwanaga, S., Wallén, P., Grondahl, N., Henschen, A., and Blombäck, B. (1967). *Biochim. Biophys. Acta 147*, 609.
Johnson, P., and Mihalyi, E. (1965). *Biochim. Biophys. Acta 102*, 467.
Kay, C., and Marsh, M. (1961). *Nature 189*, 307.
Kiesselback, T., and Wagner, R. (1966). *Am. J. Physiol. 211*, 1472.
Koch, F. C., and McMeekin, T. L. (1924). *J. Am. Chem. Soc. 46*, 2066.
Koenig, V. L. (1950). *Arch. Biochem. 25*, 241.
Laki, K. (1951a). *Science 114*, 435.
Laki, K. (1951b). *Trans. 4th Josiah Macy Jr. Conf. on Blood Clotting and Allied Problems*, p. 217.
Laki, K. (1951c). *Arch. Biochem. Biophys. 32*, 317.
Laki, K., and Chandrasekhar, N. (1963). *Nature 197*, 1267.
Laki, K., and Gladner, J. A. (1964). *Physiol. Reviews 44*, 127.
Laki, K., and Mester, L. (1962). *Biochim. Biophys. Acta 57*, 152.
Lang, C. A. (1958). *Anal. Chem. 30*, 1692.
Larrieu, M. J., Beaumont, J. L., Caen, J., Seligman, M., and Bernard, J. (1958). *Rev. Franc. Etudes Clin. Biol. 3*, 617.
Laskowski, M. Jr., Ehrenpreis, S., Donnelly, T. H., and Scheraga, H. A. (1960). *J. Am. Chem. Soc. 82*, 1340.
Lipinski, B., Budzynski, A., Latallo, Z., and Kowalski, E. (1964). *Acta Biochim. Pol. 11*, 527.
Loeliger, A., and Hers, J. F. (1957). *Thromb. Diath. Haemorrhag. 1*, 499.
Loewy, A. G., Dunathan, K., Kriel, R., and Wolfinger, H. L., Jr. (1961a). *J. Biol. Chem. 236*, 2625.
Loewy, A. G., Dahlburg, A., Dunathan, K., Kriel, R., and Wolfinger, H. L., Jr. (1961b). *J. Biol. Chem. 236*, 2634.
Loewy, A. G., Dahlburg, J. E., Dorwart, W. V., Jr., Weber, M. J., and Eisele, J. (1964). *Biochem. Biophys. Res. Commun. 15*, 177.
Lorand, L. (1951). *Nature 167*, 992.
Lorand, L. (1952). *Biochem. J. 52*, 200.
Lorand, L. (1965). *Federation Proc. 24*, 784.
Lorand, L., and Jacobsen, A. (1958). *J. Biol. Chem. 230*, 421.
Lorand, L., and Jacobsen, A. (1964). *Biochemistry 3*, 1939.
Lorand, L., Konishi, K., and Jacobsen, A. (1962). *Nature 194*, 1148.
Lorand, L., and Ong, H. H. (1966). *Biochem. 5*, 1747.
Mihalyi, E. (1954a). *J. Biol. Chem. 209*, 723.
Mihalyi, E. (1954b). *J. Biol. Chem. 209*, 733.
Mihalyi, E. (1963). *Biochim. Biophys. Acta 67*, 73.
Mihalyi, E. (1965). *Biochim. Biophys. Acta 102*, 487.
Mosesson, M. W., and Finlayson, J. S. (1963). *J. Clin. Invest. 42*, 747.
Mosesson, M. W., and Sherry, S. (1966). *Biochemistry 5*, 2829.
Murray, M. (1961). *Am. J. Clin. Pathol. 36*, 500.
Murray, M., and Gohdes, P. J. (1959). *J. Bacteriol. 78*, 450.
Murray, M., and Huseby, R. M. (1965). Technicon Symp. 713.
Murray, M., and Huseby, R. M. (1967). *Biochem. Med. 1*, 15.
Nanninga, L. B. (1946). *Arch. Neerl. Physiol. 28*, 241.
Oncley, J. L., Scatchard, G., and Brown, A. (1947). *J. Phys. and Colloid Chem. 51*, 184.
Osbahr, A. J., Jr., Colman, R. W., Laki, K., and Gladner, J. A. (1964). *Biochem. Biophys. Res. Commun. 14*, 555.
Persson, J. (1963). *J. Lab. Clin. Invest. 15*, 353.
Pirkle, H., and Henschen, A. (1968). *Biochemistry 7*, 1362.
Prunty, F. T. G., McSweeney, R. R., and Hawkins, J. R. (1959). A Laboratory Manual of Chemical Pathology. Pergamon, New York.
Ratnoff, O. D., and Menzie, C. (1951). *J. Lab. Clin. Med. 37*, 316.
Rosenberg, A., and Carman, R. H. (1964). *Nature 204*, 994.
Rosenheck, K., and Doty, P. (1961). *Proc. Natl. Acad. Sci. 47*, 1775.
Scheraga, H. A. (1958). *Ann. N. Y. Acad. Sci. 75*, 189.
Scheraga, H. A., and Laskowski, M. (1957). *Advances in Protein Chem. 12*, 2.
Seegers, W. H., Nieft, M. L., and Vandenbelt, J. M. (1947). *Arch. Biochem. 7*, 15.
Seigel, B. M., Mernan, J. P., and Scheraga, H. A. (1953). *Biochim. Biophys. Acta 11*, 329.
Shulman, S. (1953). *J. Am. Chem. Soc. 75*, 5846.
Shulman, S., and Ferry, J. D. (1950). *J. Phys. and Colloid Chem. 54*, 66.
Sjöquist, J., Blombäck, B., and Wallén, P. (1960). *Arkiv Kemi 16*, 405.
Steiner, R. F., and Laki, K. (1951a). *J. Am. Chem. Soc. 73*, 882.
Steiner, R. F., and Laki, K. (1951b). *Arch. Biochem. Biophys. 34*, 24.
Stryer, L., Cohen, C., and Langridge, R. (1963). *Nature 197*, 793.
Sturtevant, J. M., Laskowski, M., Jr., Donnelly, T. H., and Scheraga, H. A. (1955). *J. Am. Chem. Soc. 77*, 6168.
Szara, S. T., and Bagdy, D. (1953). *Acta Physiol. Acad. Sci. Hung. 4*, 229.
Tristam, G. R. (1949). *Advances in Protein Chem. 5*, 83.
Tyler, H. M. (1966). *Nature 210*, 1045.
Tyler, H. M., and Lack, C. H. (1964). *Nature 202*, 1114.
von Korff, R. W., Pollara, B., Cayne, R., Runquist, J., and Kapoor, R. (1963). *Biochim. Biophys. Acta 24*, 698.
Ware, A. G., Guest, M. M., and Seegers, W. H. (1947). *Arch. Biochem. 13*, 231.
Waugh, D. F. (1954). *Advances in Protein Chem. 9*, 325.
Waugh, D. F., and Livingstone, B. J. (1951a). *Science 113*, 121.
Waugh, D. F., and Livingstone, B. J. (1951b). *J. Phys. and Colloid Chem. 55*, 1206.
Winzler, R. J. (1955). *In:* "Methods of Biochemical Analysis" (D. Glick, ed.), Vol. II, pp. 279—312. Wiley (Interscience), New York.
Wycoff, H. D. (1956). *J. Lab. Clin. Med. 47*, 645.
Yang, J. T., and Doty, P. (1957). *J. Am. Chem. Soc. 79*, 761.

Fibrinogen and Fibrin Derivatives

D. C. Triantaphyllopoulos and E. Triantaphyllopoulos

I. Introduction

The first study concerning fibrinogen and fibrin derivatives was published in 1945 (Seegers et al. 1945). The biological significance of these products, however, was appreciated only in the last decade, after it was reported independently by two different laboratories that fibrinogen digests have anticoagulant properties (Triantaphyllopoulos, 1958; Niewiarowski and Kowalski, 1958). The ability of these derivatives to inhibit the clotting of fibrinogen by thrombin varies greatly with the degree of fibrinogenolysis. The most active inhibitors are obtained, when the parent fibrinogen becomes completely uncoagulable (Triantaphyllopoulos, 1958; Triantaphylopoulos and Triantaphyllopoulos, 1965a, b, 1967a).

The development of quantitative assays for fibrinogen and fibrin derivatives has encountered several difficulties.

1. The fibrinogen derivatives are largely heterogeneous. Experimental evidence indicates that fibrinolysin breaks down fibrinogen in a long series of reactions with the liberation of several peptides and free amino acids (Triantaphyllopoulos and Triantaphyllopoulos, 1967c, 1968a, b) while the remainder of the molecule is split into macromolecular fragments of various sizes (Kowalski et al. 1960; Triantaphyllopoulos, 1961; Nussenzweig et al. 1961a; Triantaphyllopoulos and Triantaphyllopoulos, 1965a, b, 1967b; Fletcher et al. 1966). A whole spectrum of derivatives with weights ranging from about 300,000 to less than a thousand is successively produced. The fragments which have anticoagulant activity vary in size from about 300,000 to 30,000.

2. The degradation products do not possess any specific property, which could be used as a means of isolation or characterization. Unlike fibrinogen, which has the unique ability among the other plasma proteins to be clotted by thrombin and thus be easily isolated from plasma, the derivatives are largely unclottable.

3. Initial derivatives cannot be easily distinguished from fibrinogen. They can be clotted by thrombin, they can be precipitated by ammonium sulfate at 25% saturation, by ether and heating at 56° C and show the same electrophoretic mobility as intact fibrinogen (Triantaphyllopoulos and Triantaphyllopoulos, 1962, 1965a, b, 1967a).

4. Limitations in the application of immunological procedures. Fibrinogen reacts with the same antisera and must be removed before the determinations. Clottable derivatives will be clotted along with fibrinogen and will not be measured. Nonclottable derivatives may also be incorporated into the clot (Alkjaersig et al. 1962). In the presence of large amounts of very potent derivatives, the blood can remain unclottable even at normal fibrinogen concentrations (Triantaphyllopoulos, 1958). Unless the plasma is diluted with distilled water and thrombin is added, all or part of the fibrinogen will remain in the "serum" and will be determined together with the fragments. Although the immunological procedures determine only the fragments which have been shown to possess anticoagulant properties, they cannot provide information about the degree of the coagulation abnormality. Detection of a large amount of these fragments in the serum does not necessarily mean a significant coagulation abnormality. There is a great variation in specific activity among derivatives.

Only one isolation procedure has been described so far (Triantaphyllopoulos and Triantaphyllopoulos, 1964). The method is well suited for investigative purposes. The anticoagulant derivatives are obtained from plasma semiquantitatively and their activity can be determined. The isolated fractions can further be purified by electrophoretic or chromatographic techniques (section II).

The immunological procedure of Merskey et al. (1966) is based on the inhibition of the immune agglutination of sheep erythrocytes coated with fibrinogen, by the fibrinogen and fibrin derivatives (see p. 407). The highest dilution of test serum which will prevent this agglutination permits the calculation of the concentration of these derivatives in the test serum. This method has been claimed to be accurate and sensitive. It has, however, the disadvantage that it is a multiple step procedure and requires attention to detail in order to give reproducible results.

The immune flocculation method of Ferreira et al. (1964) depends on a rapid semiquantitative precipitin test. The immune serum is prepared by immunizing rabbits against a fine suspension of fibrin isolated by recalcification of ACD-plasma and exhibits a heavier cross reaction with gamma globulins than antifibrinogen sera. Adsorption of the immune serum with normal serum abolishes the ability of the immune serum to detect physiological concentrations of fibrinogen-fibrin derivatives.

The nephelometric method of Schultze and Schwick (1959) is based on measurements of the turbidity, which is produced when fibrinogen derivates combine with the antibodies of specific antisera. It is simple, fast and reasonably accurate (Section III).

When specific antisera are not available, a quick presumptive diagnosis of the presence of fibrinogen derivatives in the plasma can be obtained by:

1. Demonstration of increased fibrinolytic activity (see also Chapter IV).
2. Determination of clottable fibrinogen after dilution of the plasma with saline and after dilution with water. When thrombin is added to normal plasma in the absence of calcium chloride, a larger clot is obtained, if the plasma is diluted with distilled water than if it is diluted with saline. The opposite is observed with lysed plasma (Section IV) (Triantaphyllopoulos et al. 1962).

II. Chemical Procedures

A. Isolation From Plasma

Principle

Prothrombin and its derivatives are removed from plasma by adsorption on tricalcium phosphate. The fibrinogen and fibrin derivatives are precipitated by saturation of the lysed plasma with ammonium sulfate to 25 % and 50 %. In cases of normal or partially lysed plasma, ammonium sulfate saturation is preceded by addition of ether to 11 % by volume in order to precipitate intact fibrinogen and clottable derivatives.

Materials

1. *Protease inhibitor.* a) Trasylol, a preparation containing 5000 kallikrein inhibitor units (KIU)/ml, can be purchased either from FBA Pharmaceuticals, New York or from Bayer A. G. Leverkusen, Germany. b) Iniprol, pancreatic trypsin inhibitor is manufactured by Choay Laboratories, Paris, France. This preparation contains 200,000 anti-Schwert-Takenaka (1400 anti-caseinolytic) units per ml (Soulier, 1961).

2. *Thrombin.* The preparation Thrombin Topical of Parke, Davis and Company is adequate. The contents of a vial of 10,000 NIH units are dissolved in 5 ml saline. An equal volume of glycerol is added to prevent freezing during storage at –20° C. This stock solution (1000 NIH units/ml) is stable for months.

3. *Ether.* Only ether of high purity, same as used for anesthesia, should be employed. The cans should be kept sealed or tightly stoppered in the deep-freezer. They should be opened only shortly before use in order to avoid formation of peroxides.

4. *Tricalcium phosphate.* The powder can be purchased from Merck and Co., Inc. Rahway, N. J.

5. *Calcium chloride* in stock molar solution.

6. *Sodium oxalate* 0.1 M.

7. *Ammonium sulfate.* Water is saturated with the salt at room temperature under continous stirring. The solution is allowed to equilibrate for at least one day before it is filtered and used.

Procedure

About 50 ml of blood obtained by venipuncture are mixed, 9 volumes to 1, with 0.1 M sodium oxalate. A protease inhibitor, (Iniprol to a concentration of 14 anticaseinolytic (2000 anti-Schwert-Takenaka) units, or Trasylol to a concentration of 50 KIU per ml), is added immediately, and the blood is centrifuged to obtain the plasma. The latter is adsorbed on tricalcium phosphate (final suspension 0.01 M) in order to remove the prothrombin complex. The adsorbed plasma is then checked for the presence of clottable protein. One ml is mixed with 5 ml distilled water containing 0.01 M calcium chloride and 10 NIH units of thrombin per ml. The mixture is allowed to stand at room temperature for 10 minutes and is then inspected for the presence of fibrin. Care must be taken not to confuse a precipitate of euglobulins for a true fibrin network. If there is fibrin formation, the clottable protein must be removed first by ether precipitation. If there is no clot formation, the step with ether is omitted and the plasma is treated with ammonium sulfate directly after adsorption.

Ether precipitation. The adsorbed plasma is cooled in an ice-bath to 0° C. Ether of the same temperature is then added to the plasma to a concentration of 11% by volume. The erlenmeyer flask containing the mixture is tightly stoppered and kept at 0° C for 16 hours. After completion of the precipitation the plasma-ether mixture is centrifuged at about 12,000 × G for 10 minutes in a refrigerated centrifuge kept at 0° C. The precipitate is dissolved in a small volume of saline containing about 2.1 anticaseinolytic units of pancreatic trypsin inhibitor (or 7 KIU of Trasylol) per ml and stored at –20° C.

Ammonium sulfate precipitation. The supernatant is freed o ether under reduced pressure and then saturated with ammonium sulfate to 25% (3 volumes of plasma: 1 volume of saturated salt solution). The mixture is allowed to stand at room temperature for at least 10 minutes and then centrifuged at about 27,000 × G for 10 minutes (longer, if lower speeds are used). The supernatant is saturated further to 50% by addition of the saturated ammonium sulfate solution at a ratio of 1 to 2 volumes of supernatant. The suspension is again allowed to stand for at least 10 minutes and then centrifuged as before. Both precipitates are dissolved in as small a volume of saline as possible. They are then dialysed against saline at 4° C under continuous stirring, until they are free of sulfate anions (addition of a few drops of barium chloride to the dialysates does not produce turbidity). The solutions are clarified by centrifugation, the volumes are recorded and the protein contents are determined by the biuret method of Kingsley for total protein (see Hawk et al. 1954) or any other suitable method. Pancreatic trypsin inhibitor at 2.1 anticaseinolytic units or Trasylol at 7 KIU per ml is added and the fractions are stored at –20° C, if they are not used immediately for further purification or determination of their antithrombic activity (Section II, B, C).

Comments

The ether precipitation must be carried out at 0° C throughout. If the temperature is allowed to rise, some or all of the precipitate will redissolve.

By this fractionation procedure the fibrinogen and fibrin derivatives, which have antithrombic activity, are obtained mainly in one fraction. High inhibitory activity (80–90% inhibition of the control value) is always exhibited by the 0–25% fraction from both partially and completely lysed plasmas. An ether precipitate is obtained only from normal or partially lysed plasmas. The precipitate from normal plasmas represents intact fibrinogen; it shows no inhibitory effect. The precipitate from partially lysed plasmas contains mostly or exclusively initial derivatives. These can be distinguished from fibrinogen by the fact that their thrombin time is longer and the clot which is formed is cloudy, loose and smaller. Addition of these derivatives to solutions of intact fibrinogen prolongs the thrombin time of the latter (Triantaphyllopoulos and Triantaphyllopoulos, 1967a), while addition of fibrinogen at the same concentration has the opposite or no effect. The later the stage these fragments are isolated, the greater are the differences from fibrinogen. Very early derivatives can be distinguished only by the difficulty with which they can be dissolved in saline or 0.3 M potassium chloride, since they show very slight or no detectable clotting abnormalities. The 25–50% fraction exhibits a slight inhibitory effect (about 9%) occasionally.

These findings are at variance with results obtained when fractionation is applied to pure fibrinogen solutions lysed in vitro. The 25–50% ammonium sulfate saturation fraction from these solutions always shows the highest antithrombic activity (Triantaphyllopoulos and Triantaphyllopoulos, 1965a, 1967a) regardless of the degree of fibrinogenolysis. If such a fraction is added to normal plasma, the activity of the new fraction, which can be isolated at the same degree of saturation (25–50%) from the mixture, shows only 38% of the specific activity of the added anticoagulant. The greatest inhibitory activity is detected in the 0–25% fraction of the mixture (80%) and the ether precipitate exhibits 26% of the specific activity of the added anticoagulant. (Ether precipitate from normal human plasma shows no inhibitory effect). It is interesting to note, however, that the 0–25% fraction from normal plasma can exert an approximately 20% inhibition on control values (Triantaphyllopoulos and Triantaphyllopoulos, 1964).

B. Determination of Antithrombic Activity

Principle

The thrombin clotting time of a solution of intact fibrinogen is determined in the presence and in the absence of fibrinogen-fibrin derivatives. The values are translated into units of thrombin activity by means of a thrombin calibration curve. The percent difference between the two values is the measure of the antithrombic activity of the preparation.

Materials

1. *Saline,* 0.85 % sodium chloride (w/v).

2. *Antiprotease,* section II, A, 1.

3. *Imidazole buffer 0.25 M, pH 7.25.* The buffer is prepared as described by Mertz et al. (1939). Imidazole, 1.72 g. (Eastman Organic Chemicals, Rochester 3, N. Y) is dissolved in 90 ml 0.1 N hydrochloric acid. The pH is adjusted to 7.25 and the solution diluted to 100 ml with demineralized water. The buffer is kept at 4° C.

4. *Fibrinogen.* a) A stock solution can be prepared by any of the known methods, which give a protein of high clottability. We have used the method of Laki (1951) with minor modifications, extensively. Two grams of bovine fibrinogen (fraction I of Cohn, Armour Pharmaceutical, Kankakee, Ill.) are dissolved in 100 ml 0.1 M phosphate buffer, pH 6.4 with the help of a magnetic stirrer. An equal volume of deionized water is added and the solution is kept overnight at 4° C. The cold precipitated protein is removed by filtration and the clear filtrate is allowed to warm up to room temperature. Ammonium sulfate is added to 25 % saturation (1 volume of the saturated solution [Section II, A] to 3 volumes of filtrate). The mixture is allowed to stand at room temperature for 1–2 hours until the precipitate aggregates on the top. Most of the fluid can be siphoned off through narrow tubing and the remaining mixture is then centrifuged at 4° C. The precipitate is transferred into a beaker, cut into small pieces with two spatulas and dissolved in a small volume of 0.3 M sodium or potassium chloride with the help of a magnetic stirrer. The solution is dialyzed against 0.3 M sodium or potassium chloride until it is free of sulphate ions (the dialysate does not form a precipitate with barium chloride). Sodium citrate 0.2 M is added in a volume equal to $^1/_{10}$ the volume of the dialysed solution and the protein concentration is determined by the biuret (Hawk et al. 1954) or any other method. The solution is then distributed into small tubes (about 1 ml per tube), stoppered tightly and stored at –25° C. The clottability of this product, if properly prepared, is 95 % and over. b) Working solution. One tube is taken from storage and the solution is melted in a water bath at 37° C immediately before use. The required amount is added to a mixture of saline, imidazole buffer and the protease inhibitor, all calculated to give a solution containing 2 mg fibrinogen, 2.1 anticaseinolytic (300 anti-Schwert-Takenaka) units of Iniprol or 7 kallikrein inhibitor units of Trasylol per ml and 0.04 M imidazole.

5. *Thrombin.* Working solution. The stock thrombin solution (1000 NIH units/ml) described in section II, A, 2, is diluted 1:100 with water immediately before use. This solution contains 10 NIH units/ml and should be kept in a siliconized container, since thrombin is adsorbed on glass.

6. *Test solution.* The solution containing the fibrinogen and/or fibrin derivatives is diluted to 4 mg per ml with saline immediately before determination.

Procedure

Fibrinogen and saline, 0.1 ml each, are pipetted into a 10 × 100 mm test tube and mixed. One tenth ml dilute thrombin solution is forcibly blown in and a stop watch started. The contents of the tube are well mixed and the solution is carefully inspected for clot formation. Clot detection is facilitated by gently shaking the tube over a magnifying mirror and looking at the reflection. At the appearance of a clot the watch is stopped and the time recorded. This represents the control value. The antithrombic effect of a test solution is determined by adding 0.1 ml of the freshly prepared dilution (4 mg/ml) instead of saline. The test is performed for at least 3 times with both the control and the test solutions and the values are averaged.

Thrombin calibration curve. Calculation of antithrombic activity.

The relationship between clotting time and thrombic activity is established by adding 0.1 ml of varying dilutions of a standard thrombin solution to mixtures of fibrinogen (0.1 ml) and saline (0.1 ml). The standard thrombin solution should be diluted to concentrations which will give clotting times between 6 and 30 seconds. This is the most sensitive range of the reaction. Over and below these values, the experimental error is high. The clotting times in seconds are plotted versus the reciprocal of the corresponding thrombin concentrations. From the intercept (I) and the slope (S) of the straight line, which is obtained, the constants of the appropriate equation are determined.

$$C = \frac{S}{tt - I} \qquad (1)$$

S = slope
C = thrombin concentration in NIH or any other units.
tt = thrombin time in seconds
I = intercept

Applying this equation the units of thrombin activity in the presence and in the absence (saline control) of the fibrinogen-fibrin derivatives can be calculated. The difference between these two values represents the number of thrombin units, which were neutralized by each anticoagulant. This difference in percent $\left(\frac{C-A}{C} \times 100\right.$, where C are the NIH units of the control, A the NIH units in the presence of the anticoagulant) is the measure of the antithrombic activity of each preparation. Since the concentration of all anticoagulant preparations is adjusted to a constant level (4 mg protein/ml), these values can be considered as representing specific activities.

Comments

The test is performed at room temperature in order to have a uniform temperature throughout the experiment. If the determination is started in the water bath, the tube will have to be removed from the water for inspection of clotting and this will bring down the temperature of the solution. Since the clotting time of the control and anticoagulant solution can vazywidely, the temperature in each case will be lowered to a different degree and errors due to these differences will be introduced. All manipulations, especially the shaking of the tubes during observation, should be standardized, otherwise considerable difference in the triplicate values may result. In the presence of fibrinogen-fibrin derivatives the clot is usually loose or scattered and the solution remains fluid during the initial stages of clotting.

For comparative purposes, it is essential to adjust the concentration of all anticoagulant preparations to the same protein concentration (4 mg/ml). When such a concentration cannot be obtained, the concentration of fibrinogen should be reduced so that it is always equal to half the concentration of the anticoagulant being tested.

C. Fractionation

1. Column Electrophoresis

Column or continuous flow paper (curtain) electrophoresis has been used extensively by us for the fractionation of preparations isolated by 0–25 % and 25–50 % ammonium sulfate saturation from lysed fibrinogen solutions or lysed plasmas. These methods have the advantage over other types of electrophoresis that the separated zones can be easily eluted and collected in fractions with a fraction collector. Unlike ordinary column chromatography in the column electrophoretic procedure a new column needs not to be packed every time. The same column can be used over and over again for many separations. The technique can be mastered easily and does not require much of the operators time. Fractions in quantities sufficient for several studies (60–100 mg of large peak, 10–20 mg of small peak) can be separated within 36 hrs. For a description of curtain electrophoresis see Triantaphyllopoulos and Triantaphyllopoulos (1962).

Reagents

1. *Veronal buffer* 0.02 M, pH 8.6. Sodium diethylbarbiturate, 30.8 g and barbituric acid, 5.55 g are dissolved in 5 liters demineralized water. The pH is adjusted carefully to 8.6 by

addition of the acid or the salt and the volume is brought to 7.5 liters.

2. *Munktell's cellulose* powder especially developed for zone electrophoresis can be purchased from Grycksbo Paperback A. B. Sweden.

3. *Bromphenolblue*

4. *Saline* (0.85 % sodium chloride w/v).

Procedure

A column electrophoresis apparatus of the Porath type can be obtained from the LKB Company of Stockholm, Sweden (No. 3340). The column is filled to $^1/_3$ with the veronal buffer and a filter paper is allowed to settle over the perforated disk at the bottom of the column. The cellulose powder suspended in the veronal buffer is poured in, through an extension tube attached to a funnel and another filter paper is allowed to settle on the top after packing. The packing is usually done at room temperature, all operations from then on, however, must be carried out at 4° C. The sample, 3–5 ml, at a concentration of 40–70 mg protein/ml, is stained by the addition of a very small amount of bromphenolblue, so that the migration of the proteins through the column can be observed. The stained sample is dialysed against veronal buffer under continuous stirring in order to a) equilibrate the sample with the electrophoretic buffer and b) eliminate the excess of the dye, which is not bound to protein. The buffer is changed at hourly intervals, 3–4 times. The sample is centrifuged and the clear supernatant is transferred on the column with the special applicator supplied with the instrument. Current is applied at 17 mamp and ≃ 560 V until the first blue colored band reaches the bottom of the column (15–18 h). The power is switched off and elution is started at a flow rate of one drop/10 seconds. Fractions are collected at 20 min intervals and the absorbancy at 280 mμ is determined. Three to five components are usually eluted by this method (Fig. 1), depending on the degree of fibrinogenolysis, the origin and the method of preparation of the parent fibrinogen solution (Triantaphyllopoulos and Triantaphyllopoulos, 1965a). Three of the components appear at low concentrations insufficient for coagulation or other studies and sometimes do not show at all. Of the two others (main anticoagulants) the smaller peak (β-derivative of Seegers et al. 1945 or component E of Nussenzweig et al, 1961a) is more electronegative and is eluted before the larger. The central fractions belonging to each main peak, designated as the large and the small peak fractions for easy identification, are pooled together, dialyzed against demineralized water 2–3 times and concentrated by freeze-drying. The dry powders are dissolved in and dialyzed against saline until the dialysate is free of veronal (no absorption at 240 mμ). The protein concentration in each fraction is determined either spectrophotometrically at 280 mμ or by the method of Lowry et al. (1951). The fractions are stored at –20° C, if they are not used immediately. It is not advisable to freeze and melt a preparation more than once. If several tests are planned, the sample should be distributed into several tubes so that a different aliquot can be melted each time.

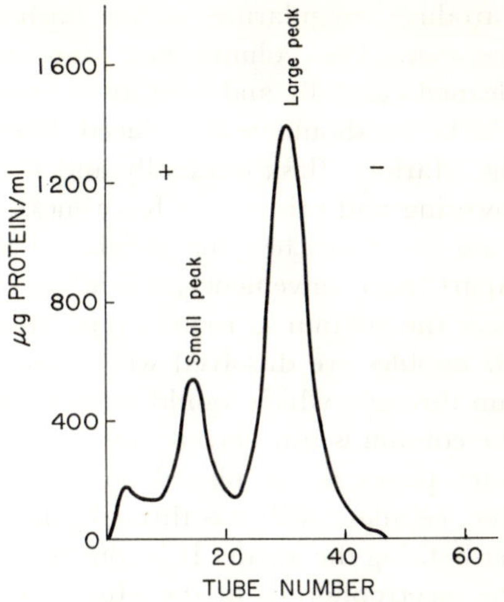

Fig. 1. Column electrophoresis in 0.02 M veronal buffer, pH 8.6 of a fraction isolated by 25–50 % ammonium sulfate saturation from a solution of human fibrinogen during relatively advanced stages of spontaneous fibrinogenolysis. Current was applied at 17 mamp and 560 V. The plus and minus signs indicate the anode and cathode respectively.

Comments

Care should be taken to avoid trapping air bubbles within the perforated disc. This will increase the resistance of the system and will introduce irregularities in the buffer flow at the exit. The column and disc should be cleaned carefully and kept away from grease. The buffer should be introduced slowly, raising the Mariotte flask gradually and if necessary lowering and raising it a few times, when the fluid level reaches the height of the disc. Apart from convenience, it is advantageous to pack the column at room temperature. Small air bubbles are dissolved when cold buffer is run through, which should be done as soon as the column is transferred to the cold room. If filter paper is not placed on the perforated disc, cellulose will pass through, into the buffer bathing the anode. It is convenient to start the electrophoresis in the afternoon, half an hour before leaving the laboratory. By next morning the first colored band will be close to the bottom of the column and elution can be started.

Irregularities of the colored band, which is formed on the top of the column after the application of the sample indicate either poor packing or channeling of the upper layer by impurities introduced with the sample. The filter paper and the top cellulose layer (in case of channeling) should be removed and the upper 2–3 cm of cellulose should be stirred and then allowed to settle and a new filter paper applied. If this does not improve separation, a new column should be packed.

The large and small peak fractions correspond to the alpha and beta derivatives of Seegers et al. (1945) or components D and E of Nussenzweig et al. (1961a). The large peak can be detected from the beginning of fibrinogenolysis and shows initially the same electrophoretic mobility as intact fibrinogen. The small peak appears at about the time when the parent solution can no longer be clotted by thrombin and is more electronegative than the large. The concentration of the former fraction increases gradually with fibrinogenolysis and may reach 30% of the total protein. The mobility of both of these fractions increases with increasing proteolysis and may reach the mobility of the alpha globulins (large peak) or the albumin (small peak). The small peak (component E) has been shown to be a single component by further electrophoresis, thermostability (Nussenzweig et al. 1961a; Triantaphyllopoulos and Triantaphyllopoulos, 1965a, b) and ultracentrifugal studies. The large peak seems to be heterogeneous (Triantaphyllopoulos and Triantaphyllopoulos, 1963, 1965a, b).

2. Column Chromatography on DEAE Cellulose (Method of Nussenzweig et al. 1961a)

The final products of fibrinogenolysis are separated by column chromatography on DEAE cellulose into four fractions containing 5 components: A, B + C, D and E. Components D and E correspond to the large and small peak fractions which are obtained by column or continuous flow paper electrophoresis (Triantaphyllopoulos and Triantaphyllopoulos, 1965a, 1966) or to the alpha and beta derivatives of Seegers et al. (1945).

Materials

1. Sodium carbonate buffer 0.01 M, pH 8.9.
2. Same carbonate buffer containing 0.1 M sodium chloride.
3. Same carbonate buffer as (1) containing 0.2 M sodium chloride.
4. Diethyl-amino-ethyl (DEAE) cellulose, standard type.

Procedure

The cellulose is activated with 1 M sodium hydroxide and then washed with distilled water until the effluent becomes neutral. The washing is continued with the plain 0.01 M sodium carbonate, pH 8.9, buffer until the effluent acquires the pH of the buffer. The resin is poured into the column and allowed to settle by sedimentation to a height of about 40 cm and a pressure of 40 cm of water is applied. The preparation of the fibrinogen derivatives, 5–6 ml at 6–7 mg protein per ml, is dialyzed at 4° C against the plain carbonate buffer and then applied on the column. Elution is started with the same buffer at a flow rate of about 90 ml per hour until the first component is eluted (about 200 ml). Gradient elution is then applied by increasing the ionic strength with the No. 2 buffer. The concentrated solution flows into a one liter mixing flask, which has been filled with the initial buffer and the mixture is continuously agitated with a magnetic stirrer to secure proper mixing. The pro-

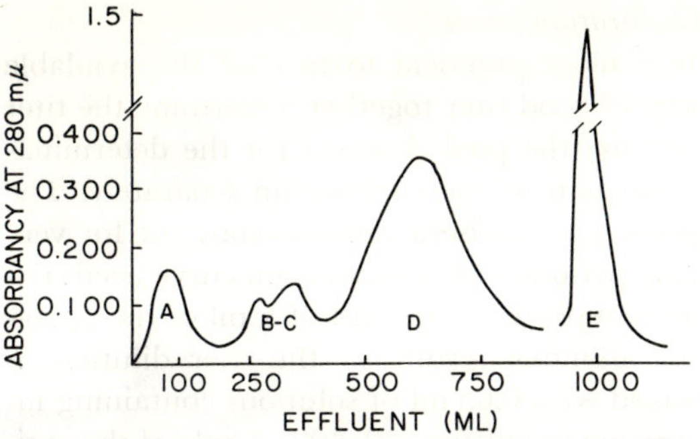

Fig. 2. Column chromatography of final products of fibrinogenolysis on DEAE cellulose according to Nussenzweig et al. (1961a), without previous fractionation.

tein content of the eluate is determined by measuring the absorbancy at 280 mμ. The last buffer which contains 0.2 M sodium chloride is started after the fourth component (D) is eluted (after about 900 ml of effluent) and is applied directly on the column. Four fractions in all, containing 5 components, A, B + C, D and E, are obtained (Fig. 2). The aliquots belonging to each fraction are pooled and dialyzed against demineralized water. They are then concentrated by freeze-drying and dialyzed against physiological saline to remove excess salt. The protein concentration is determined by a micromethod (Lowry et al. 1951 or adsorption at 280 mμ) and the fractions are stored in the deep freezer, if they are not used immediately.

III. Immunological Determination (Based on the Method of Schultze and Schwick, 1959)

Principle

The test serum is mixed under standard conditions with an antiserum prepared against fibrinogen or fibrinogen derivatives. The turbidity which is produced is proportional to the concentration of the derivatives in serum. Fibrinogen has at least four antigenic determinants. Its main fibrinolytic derivatives, the large and small peak or component D and E of Nussenzweig et al. (Section II, C, 1 and 2) react with antifibrinogen sera but each has different antigenic determinants, which combine with antibodies of different specificities. At least one of the fibrinogen determinants is lost during the degradation (Nussenzweig et al. 1961b). One antigenic determinant is similarly lost during clotting (Salmon, 1959).

Materials

1. *Antiprotease.* See section II, A, 1.
2. *Buffered saline (pH 7.5).* Monosodium (NaH_2PO_4) and dipotassium phosphate (K_2HPO_4) are dissolved in saline (0.85 % sodium chloride), each separately, to give M/15 solutions. The working buffer is prepared by mixing 14.8 ml of the monobasic with 85.2 ml of the dibasic solution.
3. *Preparation of Antigen.* a) Human Fibrinogen. This protein can be isolated from outdated Red Cross blood or any other normal human blood by any procedure, which gives a product of high clottability. b) *Fibrinogen* or fibrin *derivatives* can be used as antigens for special purposes. Most preparations of human fibrinogen even, when they show a clottability of 97 %, contain traces of profibrinolysin, which becomes spontaneously activated and lyses the fibrinogen in a matter of days or weeks. Human fibrinogen dissolved in buffered citrated saline (imidazole, 0.025 M, pH 7.3, sodium citrate 0.02 M, sodium chloride 0.85 %) at 10 mg/ml is sterilized by Seitz filtration and then incubated at 37° C under sterile conditions. Every day an aliquot (about 1 ml) is removed with a sterile technique and tested for coagulability by adding 5 ml of a solution of thrombin in distilled water (20 NIH units/ml). The mixture is allowed to stand at room temperature for 10 minutes and then is examined for the presence of fibrin strands. The incubation may be stopped as soon as the stage of uncoagulability is reached (the products isolated at this stage have the highest antithrombic effect. (Triantaphyllopoulos, 1958; Triantaphyllopoulos and Triantaphyllopoulos, 1965a) or allowed to continue for longer periods. Final products are obtained when the incubation is allowed to continue for about 4–5 times longer than the clottable period (initial period of incubation when the solution is still clottable by thrombin). The solution may be fractionated by column chromatography (section II, C, 2) or column electro-

phoresis (section II, C, 1) or used as unfractionated digest after dialysis against saline for the preparation of the antigen.

4. *Preparation of immune antiserum.* We have followed the procedure recommended by Kabat and Meyer (1961). A saline solution of fibrinogen derivatives containing 1.5 mg protein per ml is sterilized by Seitz filtration. To a hundred ml of the sterilized antigen 5 ml of a 1% sterile alum solution are added. Sodium hydroxide N/10, is carefully pipetted to the mixture until a strongly turbid suspension is obtained or a precipitate is formed. The suspension is then poured into small sterilized bottles, which are tightly covered and stored in the deep-freezer. Injections are given to rabbits four times a week according to the following pattern:

3 injections of 1 ml
3 injections of 1.5 ml
4 of 2 ml
3 of 5 ml

The antigen is introduced intravenously except for the first injection of each week which is given intraperitoneally.

The animal is bled one week after the last injection by heart puncture. If it is not intended to be used again for further production of antibodies, it is bled by inserting a catheter into the heart through the right external jugular vein following ether or Nembutal (27 mg/kg b. w. intravenously) anesthesia. The blood is allowed to clot, the cells are removed completely by two centrifugations and the serum is stored in the deep freezer after addition of a 1% merthiolate solution at 1 ml/100 ml of serum. Immune sera can be kept for years without loss of potency.

Determination of titer

The immune serum is diluted serially with buffered saline and 0.5 ml of each dilution is mixed into small spectrophotometric cuvettes with 0.05 ml of a solution of antigen containing 200–250 μg protein/ml. Similar aliquots are mixed with 0.05 ml buffered saline and serve as blanks. The mixtures are incubated at 37° C for one half hour. The highest dilution which shows a good turbidity (absorbancy, at 418 mμ, 0.2–0.4) is considered as the titer of the antiserum.

Calibration curve

It is more practical to mix all the available sera of good titer together, determine the titer and use the pooled serum for the determinations than to use each serum separately. The potency of antisera remains constant for very long periods, and a calibration curve needs not to be repeated. One half of a ml of the (pooled) immune serum, at the titer dilution, is mixed with 0.05 ml of solutions containing increasing quantities (50–400 μg/ml) of the antigen dissolved in buffered saline. A mixture of 0.05 ml buffered saline plus 0.5 ml of the diluted immune serum serves as a blank. The mixtures are placed in an incubator at 37° C for half an hour and the resulting turbidity is determined in a spectrophotometer at 418 mμ (the samples should be mixed carefully before reading). The amount of antigen used in each determination is plotted against the corresponding absorbancy (optical density) and a straight line is obtained for most of the concentrations of antigen used.

1. Determination of the Concentration of Fibrinogen and Fibrin Derivatives in the Serum

The blood is mixed with a potent antiprotease immediately after it is obtained from the vein of the subject in order to inhibit the in vitro breakdown of fibrinogen (50 KIU of Trasylol or 14 anticaseinolytic units of Iniprol per ml of blood). The serum is centrifuged at least twice until it is completely free of blood cells and clear. It is then diluted at different ratios with buffered saline and 0.05 ml of each dilution (antigen) is mixed with 0.5 ml of the diluted immune serum (antibody). Similar 0.05 ml aliquots are mixed with 0.50 ml of buffered saline in order to measure the nonspecific absorbancy of the serum at each dilution. The mixtures are left at 37° C for half an hour and the turbidity is again measured at 418 mμ. The nonspecific absorbancy (mixtures with buffered saline) is substracted from the absorbancy of the respective mixtures with the immune serum. The amount of derivatives corresponding to the difference of these values is read from the calibration curve. The amount of protein found (in μg) is multiplied by the original dilution of the serum of the subject and by the further dilution of this serum in the test mixture (0.05 + 0.50) i.e. μg from curve x dilution of serum x 11. (If the antigen values in the calibration curve are plotted as μg/ml, the dilution in the test mixture is taken care of and the result does not need to be multiplied by 11.)

Comments

Results obtained by this method show that the serum of healthy persons contains 20–50 mg of derivatives per 100 ml. It should be mentioned in this connection that fractions obtained by 25 % ammonium sulfate saturation from normal plasmas, after removal of fibrinogen with ether (section II, A), show inhibitory activity (up to 20 % of the control value).

Normal gamma globulins react with antifibrinogen sera. This may be due to: a) contamination of the antigen with the globulins, b) contamination of the globulin preparations with fibrinogen derivatives. c) It may also indicate that some of the gamma globulins are fibrinogen derivatives. Electrophoresis of fractions obtained from lysed fibrinogen solutions has shown the presence of components with the mobility of gamma globulins (Triantaphyllopoulos, 1961; Triantaphyllopoulos and Triantaphyllopoulos, 1965a). Additional procedures for the immunologic determination of fibrinogen and fibrin related molecules are rescribed in Chapter X, p. 457.

IV. Presumptive Tests

A. Thrombin Clotting Time of Plasma

Principle: The test is based on the ability of fibrinogen derivatives to prolong the thrombin clotting time of solutions of intact fibrinogen. A prolongation of the thrombin clotting time of plasma is suggestive of the presence of these anticoagulant derivatives.

Materials: Thrombin: One tenth ml of the stock solution (see Section II, A, 2) is diluted to 10 ml with saline in a siliconized or plastic tube.

Procedure: Two tenths ml oxalated (0.01 M) or citrated (0.01 M) plasma are pipetted into a 10 × 100 mm test tube. One tenth ml of the diluted thrombin solution is added and a stop watch started. The contents of the tube are mixed at room temperature and the exact time of the formation of a clot is recorded. Clot detection is facilitated by gently shaking the tube over a magnifying mirror and looking at the reflection. A control determination with normal plasma must always be performed. Normal values should be between 10 and 12 seconds.

Comments: The test must be performed immediately after the collection of the blood. If the plasma is stored in an unstoppered tube at room temperature, CO_2 escapes and the pH of the plasma becomes more alkaline. This results in an appreciable non-specific prolongation of the thrombin clotting time. The diluted thrombin solution should always be freshly prepared since the activity of the enzyme in dilute solutions rapidly deteriorates.

An increase in thrombin clotting time is only a presumptive indication for the presence of fibrinogen derivatives. Similar prolongation can also be caused by hypo- and dysfibrinogenemia, heparin, heparinoids and antithrombin V.

Differentiation between heparin and fibrinogen derivatives can be made by the addition of 10 μg protamine sulfate per ml plasma. This small concentration of protamine while it will neutralize the anticoagulant effect of heparin, it will shorten the thrombin clotting time of plasma containing fibrinogen derivatives only by a few seconds. Another way of differentiating between the two anticoagulants is based on the ease with which heparin is adsorbed on tricalcium phosphate. The fibrinogen derivatives, like fibrinogen itself are not adsorbed on this salt. If shaking the suspected plasma with a 0.01 M suspension of tricalcium phosphate (see II, A, 4) does not restore the thrombin clotting time to normal, it can be concluded that the anticoagulant involved is not heparin.

B. Reversal of Clottability of Plasma Fibrinogen

Principle: When normal plasma is clotted by thrombin in the absence of calcium chloride, a larger clot (about 14 %) is obtained if the plasma is diluted with distilled water rather than with saline. When fibrinogenolysis is initiated the difference becomes gradually smaller and a point is reached when the clot formed in saline is larger than the clot formed in distilled water (Triantaphyllopoulos et al. 1962). Clottability in distilled water disappears earlier than clottability in saline.

Materials: Thrombin: See Section II, A, 2.
Saline: 0.85 % sodium chloride (w/v).

Procedure: One ml aliquots of plasma are diluted with a) 25 ml distilled water containing 0.2 ml of the stock thrombin solution (8 NIH units/ml final solution), b) 25 ml saline containing the same amount of thrombin. The resulting clot is collected and its protein content can be determined by one of the methods described in the special chapter for fibrinogen on p. 222 ff.

Note: It is important to avoid addition of calcium chloride to the diluents. In the presence of calcium the clot which is formed in the distilled water is always larger, regardless if the plasma is normal or partially lysed (Triantaphyllopoulos et al. 1962).

References

Alkjaersig, N., Fletcher, A. P., and Sherry, S. (1962). *J. Clin. Invest. 41,* 917.

Ferreira, H. C., Murat, L. G., and Ferri, R. G. (1964). *Transfusion 2,* 21.

Fletcher, A. P., Alkjaersig, N., Fisher, S., and Sherry, S. (1966). *J. Lab. Clin. Med. 68,* 780.

Hawk, P. B., Oser, B. L., and Summerson, W. H. (1954). "Practical Physiological Chemistry." 13th Edition, McGraw-Hill, New York.

Kabat, E. A., and Mayer, M. M. (1961). "Experimental Immunochemistry." 2nd Edition, Charles C. Thomas, Springfield, Illinois.

Kowalski, E., Budzynski, A., Kopec, M., and Murawski, K. (1960). *Blood 15,* 164.

Laki, K. (1951). *Arch. Biochem. 32,* 317.

Lowry, O. H., Rosebrough, N. J., Farr, A. L., and Randall, R. J. (1951). *J. Biol. Chem. 193,* 265.

Merskey, C., Kleiner, G. J., and Johnson, A. J. (1966). *Blood 28,* 1.

Mertz, E. T., Seegers, W. H., and Smith, H. P. (1939). *Proc. Soc. Exptl. Biol. Med. 41,* 657.

Niewiarowski, S. E., and Kowalski, E. (1958). *Rev. Hematol. 13,* 320.

Nussenzweig, V., Seligmann, M., Pelmont, J., and Grabar, P. (1961a). *Ann. Inst. Pasteur 100,* 377.

Nussenzweig, V., Seligmann, M., and Grabar, P. (1961b). *Ann. Inst. Pasteur 100,* 490.

Salmon, J. (1959). *Clin. Chim. Acta 4,* 767.

Schultze, H. E., and Schwick, H. G. (1959). *Clin. Chim. Acta 4,* 15.

Seegers, W. H., Nieft, M. L., and Vandenbelt, J. M. (1945). *Arch. Biochem. 7,* 15.

Soulier, J. P. (1961). *In* "International Symposium: Anticoagulants and Fibrinolysins" (R. L. MacMillan and J. F. Mustard, eds.), pp. 403—412. Lea and Febiger, Philadelphia.

Triantaphyllopoulos, D. C. (1958). *Can. J. Biochem. Physiol. 36,* 249.

Triantaphyllopoulos, D. C. (1960). *Can. J. Biochem. Physiol. 38,* 909.

Triantaphyllopoulos, D. C. (1961). *Thromb. Diath. Haemorrhag.* 7 (Suppl. 1), 79.

Triantaphyllopoulos, D. C., Greene, T. L., and Triantaphyllopoulos, E. (1962). *Thromb. Diath. Haemorrhag. 7,* 421.

Triantaphyllopoulos, D. C., and Triantaphyllopoulos, E. (1964). *Can. J. Physiol. Pharmacol. 42,* 169.

Triantaphyllopoulos, E., and Triantaphyllopoulos, D. C. (1962). *Am. J. Physiol. 203,* 595.

Triantaphyllopoulos, E., and Triantaphyllopoulos, D. C. (1963). *Federation Proc. 22,* 620.

Triantaphyllopoulos, E., and Triantaphyllopoulos. D. C. (1965a) *Am. J. Physiol. 208,* 521.

Triantaphyllopoulos, E., and Triantaphyllopoulos. D. C. (1965b). *Brit. J. Haematol. 11,* 331.

Triantaphyllopoulos, E., and Triantaphyllopoulos, D. C. (1966). *Nature 209,* 265.

Triantaphyllopoulos, E., and Triantaphyllopoulos. D. C. (1967a). *Brit. J. Haematol. 13,* 28.

Triantaphyllopoulos, E., and Triantaphyllopoulos. D. C. (1967b). *Biochem. J. 105,* 393.

Triantaphyllopoulos, E., and Triantaphyllopoulos. D. C. (1967c). *Thromb. Diath. Haemorrhag. 18,* 300.

Triantaphyllopoulos, E., and Triantaphyllopoulos. D. C. (1968a). *Life Sci. 7,* 431.

Triantaphyllopoulos, E., and Triantaphyllopoulos. D. C. (1968b). *Brit. J. Haemat. 15,* 337.

Isolation and Purification of Fibrin Stabilizing Enzyme (F XIII, FSF, Laki-Lorand Factor, Fibrinase)

Rolf M. Huseby

I. Introduction

In the final stage of blood coagulation fibrin becomes insoluble. This insolubility is the direct result of crosslinking in the fibrin polymer by the action of a transpeptidating enzyme. This enzyme was first isolated by Lorand and Jacobsen (1958). The initial experiments with the enzyme illustrating its possible role in the fibrinogen-fibrin transformation were demonstrated by Laki and Lorand (Laki and Lorand, 1948; Lorand, 1948, 1950). As a result the enzyme was termed the Laki-Lorand Factor. In a separate series of papers (Loewy et al. 1961a, 1961b, 1961c, and 1961d) the enzyme was isolated and purified 8000-fold over plasma. Loewy termed the enzyme fibrinase. The enzyme for clarity here will be referred to as the Fibrin Stabilizing Enzyme (F XIII). The enzyme is found to occur in tissue (Tyler and Lack, 1964) and also in platelets (Kesselback and Wagner, 1966). In a series of investigations, the action of the enzyme on fibrin was elucidated. It was first thought that the enzyme might act as a transamidase utilizing the free-N-terminal residues of fibrin as donor groups (Lorand et al. 1962; Loewy et al. 1964; and Loewy et al. 1966). Evidence has now accumulated to show that this crosslinking of fibrin occurs through a transpeptidation reaction between the epsilon amino group of lysine and the beta or gamma carbonyl groups of asparagine or glutamine (Lorand et al. 1962, 1963; Lorand and Jacobsen, 1958; Loewy et al. 1964; and Lorand and Jacobsen, 1964). In more recent articles the role of lysine as the donor in these reactions has been clearly demonstrated (Lorand et al. 1966; Fuller and Doolittle, 1966) and the acceptor has been shown to be either glutamic or aspartic residues, possibly in their amide forms (Lorand and Ong, 1966).

The mechanism for this transpeptidation is at the present time not known. The release of ammonia from the reaction may indicate that the enzyme is dependent on asparagine or glutamine for action coupled with a specific sequence of amino acids at the site of action. A number of inhibitors of this enzyme are known and compete with the donors and acceptors in fibrin crosslinking. These include alpha-N-p-toluenesulfonyl-L-lysine methyl ester (Lorand, 1965), glycine methyl ester and carbobenzoxy-L-asparagine (Lorand and Jacobsen, 1964) and dansyl cadaverine (N-1,5-aminopentyl-5-dimethylamino-1-naphthalene sulfonamide).

II. Isolation of FSF (F XIII)

A. Preparation of Crude Fibrin Stabilizing Enzyme from Plasma – Method of Loewy et al. (1961a)

Outdated plasma is used as the source of material in the first step of the procedure as outlined by Loewy et al. (1961a) for the isolation of fibrin stabilizing enzyme (F XIII). It is convenient to start with six to twelve liters of plasma.

Fraction 1. For each of the steps of the fractionation, a solution of saturated ammonium sulfate is required and Dixon's nomogram (1953) is utilized for calculation of percent $(NH_4)_2SO_4$ saturation.

Ammonium sulfate, saturated at room temperature (760 to 770 grams $(NH_4)_2SO_4$ for each liter of water) is adjusted to pH 7.0 with ammonium hydroxide and is added to the plasma to give a final concentration of 20 percent saturation (1 part ammonium sulfate solution to 4 parts plasma). A precipitate will form and the mixture is allowed to stand for at least 2–3 hours at 4° C. The mixture is centrifuged, and the supernatant solution is discarded. The resulting precipitate is dissolved in one-tenth the original plasma volume in 0.15 M KCl.

Fraction 2. The solution of Fraction 1 in 0.15 M KCl is adjusted to pH 5.4 with 1 N HCl. The stock solution of saturated ammonium sulfate is adjusted to pH 5.4 and added to the fraction 1 solution to a final concentration of 16 percent (1 part of the ammonium sulfate solution to 5.25 parts of the fraction 1 in 0.15 M KCl, pH 5.4). The mixture is stirred for one hour at 4° C and centrifuged. The supernatant solution is discarded, and the precipitate is dissolved in one-twentieth of the original plasma volume of 0.5 M KCl.

Fraction 3. The solution of Fraction 2 in 0.5 M KCl is adjusted to pH 7.0, and saturated ammonium sulfate, pH 7.0 is added to a final concentration of 16 percent (1 part ammonium sulfate solution to 5.25 parts of the Fraction 2 in 0.5 M KCl). The mixture is allowed to stand at 4° C for 1 hour and then is centrifuged. The supernatant solution (Loewy Fraction 6) can be used for the preparation of fibrin stabilizing enzyme (F XIII) free fibrinogen in low yields (Loewy et al. 1961a). The precipitate that has been collected is Fraction 3 and is the crude starting material for further purification of the enzyme.

B. Purification of FSF by DEAE-Cellulose Chromatography – Method of Loewy et al. (1961a)

The Fraction 3 precipitate containing the crude fibrin stabilizing enzyme is used for the final purification of the enzyme. It is next dissolved in one-fiftieth the original plasma volume of 0.15 M KCl.

The desired amount of Fraction 3 is heat treated at 56° C for 3 minutes. A circulating water bath operated at 80 to 85° C is used, and the crude fibrin stabilizing enzyme in an Erlenmeyer flask of several volume excess over the volume of Fraction 3 is immersed into the bath. The temperature of the flask is measured with a thermometer placed into the center of the solution. The temperature of the flask is allowed to rise rapidly to 56° C and is held at this point for 3 minutes. Copious amounts of fibrinogen are precipitated, and care must be taken to keep the bulb of the thermometer from this precipitate. The temperature is kept at 56° C by periodic immersions of the flask. After 3 minutes the flask is transferred to an ice bath at 4° C and rapidly cooled. The supernatant solution is filtered through gauze and then is centrifuged. A saturated solution of ammonium sulfate, pH 7.0 is added to a final concentration of 36 percent (1 part saturated ammonium sulfate to 1.78 parts of the heat treated Fraction 3). The resulting mixture is stirred at 4° C for one hour and then is centrifuged. The collected precipitate is dissolved in $^1/_{1000}$ of the original plasma volume in 0.1 M phosphate buffer, pH 7.0 and is dialyzed against 100 volumes of this buffer for 18–24 hours. The dialyzed solution is centrifuged, and the supernatant solution is stored at 4° C or frozen. This fraction (Loewy Fraction 5) contains semipurified fibrin stabilizing enzyme purified

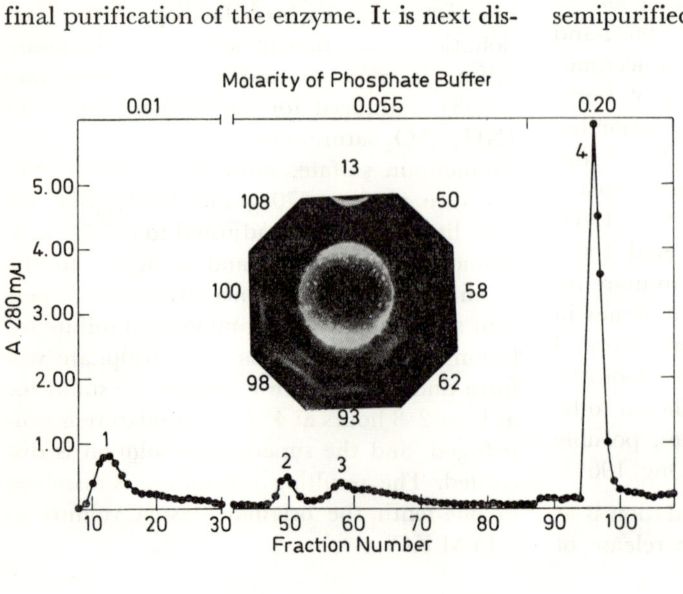

Fig. 1. DEAE-Cellulose chromatograph of Loewy Fraction V with batch elution schedule and Ouchterlony experiment. From Loewy et al. 1961a.

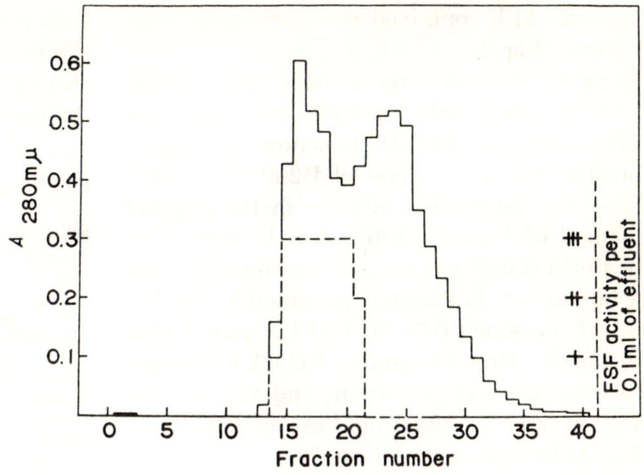

Fig. 2. Chromatograph of stabilizing enzyme on Bio-Gel P 200. Right-hand ordinate indicates absorbance of fraction at 280 mμ (broken line).
Left-hand ordinate indicates fibrin stabilizing enzyme activity (solid line), (Konishi and Lorand, 1966).

6200-fold over plasma according to Loewy (1961a).

Following dialysis against 0.01 M phosphate buffer, pH 7.0 the Fraction 5 solution (15 to 60 mg total) is applied to a DEAE-cellulose column (40 × 1 cm or 90 × 2 cm) equilibrated with the same buffer. A gradient elution is used (Fig. 1). In the original experiments of Loewy, 120 ml of 0.01 M phosphate buffer, pH 7.0 was washed over the column followed by 200 ml of 0.055 M phosphate, pH 7.0. Three minor peaks were eluted containing no activity. Finally, the purified FSF (F XIII) is eluted in a single peak with 0.20 M phosphate buffer, pH 7.0. The material was purified some 8000 times over plasma. In the author's laboratory, the elution of small inactive peaks has not always been observed; however, the fibrin stabilizing enzyme is eluted with the 0.2 M phosphate buffer, pH 7.0.

C. Purification of Fibrin Stabilizing Enzyme – On Bio-Gel P200 – Method of Lorand (1966)

The method described in detail by Lorand and Konishi (1965) uses Loewy Fraction 3 as starting material, and the preparation and purification of the enzyme is carried out on Bio-Gel (California Biochemical Corporation) P 200 columns.

The Fraction 3 of Loewy et al. (1961a) is heat treated as indicated in Section II, A, and is precipitated, dialyzed, and applied to a column, and eluted with Tris buffer, pH 7.0. In the original work, two peaks were seen, the

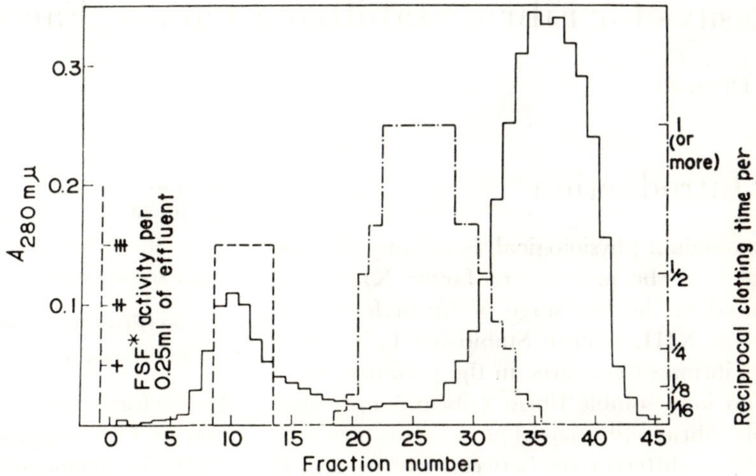

Fig. 3. Separation of fibrin stabilizing enzyme from thrombin after activation on Bio-Gel P 200 columns.
Absorbance of fractions at 280 mμ (solid line).
Activated fibrin stabilizing enzyme activities (broken line).
Right-hand ordinate thrombin activities (dots and dashes), (Konishi and Lorand, 1966).

first of which contained the fibrin stabilizing enzyme (Fig. 2).

In the same manner, the activated fibrin stabilizing enzyme may be separated from thrombin after activation (Fig. 3). This procedure again involves the use of Bio-Gel P 200 for separation. The incubation mixture in the original method of Lorand (1966) for the activation of fibrin stabilizing enzyme was formed from a mixture of Tris buffer, presumably pH 7.0, 0.1 M cysteine, 0.01 M $CaCl_2$, and 100 u/ thrombin. After 10 minutes, EDTA was added to terminate the activation, and the mixture was chromatographed on Bio-Gel P 200 (see Fig. 3) to separate the thrombin.

D. Assay of Chromatographic Fractions from the Activated Purification of Fibrin Stabilizing Enzyme (F XIII)

Bovine topical thrombin is purified by the chromatographic procedure of Rasmussen (1955). In the work of Lorand (1966), 0.25 ml aliquots of the eluted fractions are mixed with 1.85 ml of Tris buffer and 0.1 ml of 0.1 M $CaCl_2$. To this is added 0.3 ml of 1.5 percent fibrin solution prepared by the method of Donnelly et al. (1955) with the modification that one mM iodoacetate was added to the fibrinogen 0.5 hours before clotting. The mixture is allowed to incubate for 30 minutes and then is dissolved in 2.5 ml of 2 percent monochloroacetic acid. The fractions containing the enzyme produce larger insoluble clot cores than inactive fractions.

References

Dixon, M. (1953). *Biochem. J. 54,* 457.
Donnelly, T. H., Laskowski, M. Jr., Notley, N., and Scheraga, H. A. (1955). *Arch. Biochem. Biophys. 56,* 369.
Fuller, G. M., and Doolittle, R. F. (1966). *Biochim. Biophys. Res. Comm. 25,* 694.
Kesselback, T. A., and Wagner, R. H. (1966). *Am. J. Physiol. 211,* 1472.
Laki, K., and Lorand, L. (1948). *Science 108,* 280.
Lorand, L. (1948). *Acta Physiol. Acad. Sci. Hung. 1,* 192.
Lorand, L. (1950). *Nature 166,* 694.
Lorand, L. (1965). *Federation Proc. 24,* 784.
Lorand, L., and Jacobsen, A. (1958). *J. Biol. Chem. 230,* 421.
Lorand, L., and Jacobsen, A. (1964). *Biochemistry 3,* 1939.
Lorand, L., and Konishi, K. (1966). *Biochim. Biophys. Acta 121,* 177.
Lorand, L., and Ong, H. H. (1966). *Biochim. Biophys. Res. Comm. 23,* 188.
Lorand, L., Konishi, K., and Jacobsen, A. (1962). *Nature 194,* 1148.
Lorand, L., Ong, H. H., Lipinski, B., Rule. N. G., Downey, J., and Jacobsen, A. (1966). *Biochim. Biophys. Res. Comm. 25,* 629.
Lorand, L., Doolittle, R. F., Konishi, K., and Riggs, S. K. (1963). *Arch. Biochem. Biophys. 102,* 171.
Loewy, A. G., Dunathan, K., Kriel, R., and Wolfinger, H. L., Jr. (1961a). *J. Biol. Chem. 236,* 2625.
Loewy, A. G., Dahlburg, A., Dunathan, K., Kriel, R., and Wolfinger, H. L., (1961b). *J. Biol. Chem. 236,* 2634.
Loewy, A. G., Dunathan, K., Gallant, J. A., and Gardner, B. (1961c). *J. Biol. Chem. 236,* 2644.
Loewy, A. G., Gallant, J. A., and Dunathan, K. (1961d). *J. Biol. Chem. 236,* 2648.
Loewy, A. G., Dahlburg, J. E., Dorwart, W. M., Jr., Weber, M. J., and Eisele, J. (1964). *Biochim. Biophys. Res. Comm. 15,* 177.
Loewy, A. G., Matacic, S., and Darnell, J. A. (1966). *Arch. Biochem. Biophys. 113,* 435.
Rasmussen, P. S. (1955). *Biochem. Biophys. Acta 16.* 157.
Tyler, H. M., and Lack, C. H. (1964). *Nature 202,* 1114.

Assays for Fibrin Stabilizing Factor (Factor XIII)

F. Duckert

I. Introduction

To obtain a physiological, hemostatically normal clot, the presence of factor XIII is required in the last stage of fibrin formation. Factor XIII, (Fibrin Stabilizing Factor, FSF or Fibrinase) converts, in the presence of calcium ions, soluble fibrin ($fibrin_S$) into insoluble fibrin ($fibrin_I$). The solvents generally used to differentiate between $fibrin_S$ and $fibrin_I$ are 5 M urea or 1 or 2 % acetic acid. The ability of very small quantities of FSF to produce insoluble fibrin makes its quantitative assay somewhat difficult.

Three different types of test systems have been devised based on:

1. The formation of insoluble fibrin after addition of FSF containing solutions to a Factor XIII free fibrinogen substrate.

2. The variable stability of plasma clots sensitized to the dissolving action of urea by an inhibitor of Factor XIII, the monoiodoacetic acid.
3. Immunologic assay using a specific FSF neutralizing antibody.

II. Substrates for the FSF Assay

Various sources of FSF free fibrinogen have been proposed.

A. Patient's Plasma

The plasma of patients with a total congenital deficiency of Factor XIII activity is, if available, the best substrate. The fibrinogen is unaltered and free of inhibitors (Duckert et al. 1960).

B. FSF Free Fibrinogen

Fibrinogen free of Factor XIII has been prepared according to various methods.
1. Isolation by precipitation and chromatography (Loewy et al. 1961).
2. Preparation by absorption of fibrinogen with a mercuric double salt complex (Brown et al. 1967).
3. By inhibition with SH blocking agents, for example, p-chloromercuribenzoic acid (Swigert et al. 1963).

C. Test for Absence of FSF from Fibrinogen Substrate

According to specifications defined by Loewy et al. (1961) and Lorand (1964), fibrinogen preparations are considered free of FSF if clots obtained by the addition of thrombin in the presence of cysteine and calcium ions incubated for at least 18 hours at 37° C remain soluble in an suitable solvent like monochloracetic acid or urea solution. In order to prove the absence of FSF, the purified fibrinogen solution after being adjusted to a concentration of 5 mg/ml is assayed in the following test system (Heene, 1968):
0.2 ml purified fibrinogen solution (5 mg/ml in imidazole-buffered saline (IBS), pH 7.8).
0.4 ml IBS, pH 7.8
0.2 ml 0.05 M cysteine
0.2 ml thrombin calcium chloride (10 NIH u/ml in 0.025 M $CaCl_2$).
The fibrin clot is covered with a thin layer of mineral oil and incubated for 18 to 20 hours at 37° C. At the end of the incubation time the clot is gently removed and placed in 2.0 ml of solvent, either 0.05 M urea oxalate or 0.2 M monochloracetic acid. A stopwatch is started. The test tube is continuously agitated and the time of dissolution of the clot recorded in seconds. Fibrin clots free of FSF are readily dissolved in less than 60 seconds, usually 15 to 20 seconds. Lysis times in excess of 60 seconds indicate that the substrate is unsuitable for FSF measurements.

III. Assay Using FSF Free Fibrinogen (Loewy et al. 1961)

The assay consists of incubating the FSF free substrate with a dilution series of the unknown FSF before adding the solvent.

A. Performance of the Test

The test system is as follows:
0.1 ml FSF free fibrinogen (2 mg/ml) in 0.15 M ammonium acetate buffer, pH 7.0;
0.1 ml of FSF unknown made up in serial dilutions in 0.15 M KCl, pH 7.0;
0.1 ml thrombin (50 u/ml) in a mixture of 0.15 M KCl and 0.1 M $CaCl_2$.
After incubation for 1 hour, 2 ml 2% acetic acid is added, the clot gently detached from the test tube and left for 18 hours in the solvent. The endpoint is very sharp. A clot is either totally soluble or insoluble. When a $^1/_{200}$ dilution gives an insoluble clot while a $^1/_{400}$ dilution does not, the undiluted solution contains by definition 200 units/ml.

IV. Assay Using Plasma from Patients with FSF Deficiency

A. Principle

The FSF activity is partially blocked by addition of monoiodoacetic acid which enhances the solubility of plasma clots. The effect of monoiodoacetic acid is directly proportional to the concentration of FSF present in the tested plasma (Sigg, 1966; Sigg and Duckert, 1963).

B. Reagents

Oxalated plasma (1 part 0.1 M sodium oxalate plus nine parts of blood);
Na-monoiodoacetate (MIA) serially diluted to 0.035, 0.025, 0.015 and 0.005 M;
$CaCl_2$ solution (0.05 M);
5 M urea, pH 7.0.

C. Procedure

Aliquots of 0.1 ml of MIA in serial dilutions (0.035, 0.025, 0.015, and 0.005 M) are added into test tubes each containing 0.2 ml aliquots of the oxalated test plasma, and 0.1 ml $CaCl_2$ (0.05 M) is subsequently added to each tube. After coagulation has occured, the four tubes are incubated for 30 minutes at 37° C. Three ml 5 M urea are then added to each tube. The clots are carefully separated from the wall of the test tube using a glass rod, so that the clots float in the urea solution. Incubation at 37° C is continued. At 30, 45, 60 and 90 minutes after the addition of urea, each tube is shortly but vigorously shaken. Each time the condition of the clot is observed and graded according to the following scale (Fig. 1):

Clot intact, solution clear	4 points
Clot broken up in large fragments, solution clear	3 points
Clot in smaller fragments, solution slightly turbid	2 points
Clot in very small fragments, solution turbid	1 point
Clot completely dissolved, solution turbid	0 point

D. Calculation of FSF Activity

A sum of points for the four tubes read at different incubation times is made up. An example is given in Table 1. The values for normal

Table 1: Example of Point Tabulation in FSF Assay

Incubation Time in min.	30	45	60	90
MIA 0.035	3	0	0	0
0.025	4	2	0	0
0.015	4	4	4	3
0.005	4	4	4	4

Total: 40 points

plasma were found to vary between 36 and 48 points. A calibration curve may be obtained by diluting normal plasma with FSF free plasma (Fig. 2). This plasma can be replaced by purified fibrinogen devoid of Factor XIII. In this case a standard thrombin solution (33 NIH units/ml) in 0.05 M $CaCl_2$ should be used instead of $CaCl_2$ alone. The fibrinogen must give 0 points when used alone in the test. For factor XIII concentrations below 10% of the normal value, the MIA concentration is reduced to 0.005, 0.002, 0.001 and 0.0005 M respectively.

V. Immuno Assay (Bohn and Haupt, 1968)

A. Principle

Serial dilutions of specific anti-FSF antiserum are incubated with the plasma sample and clotted with Ca-Thrombin. The clots are exposed to a 1% monochloracetic acid solution for 90 min. The highest dilution of antiserum which inhibits factor XIII in plasma determines the FSF level of the unknown by comparison to a standard reference plasma.

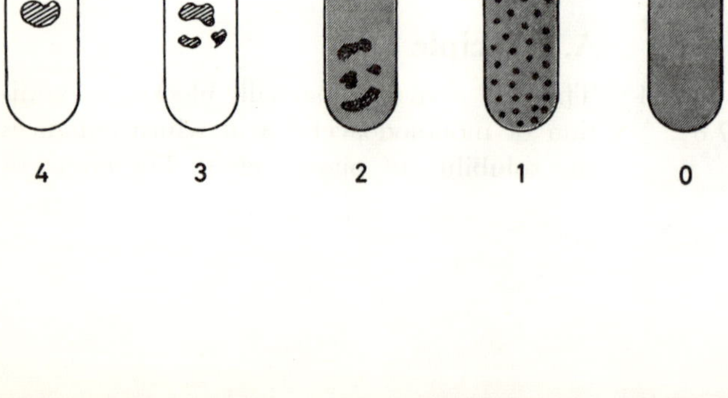

Fig. 1. Graphic illustration of point tabulation system for the MIA Tolerance Test.

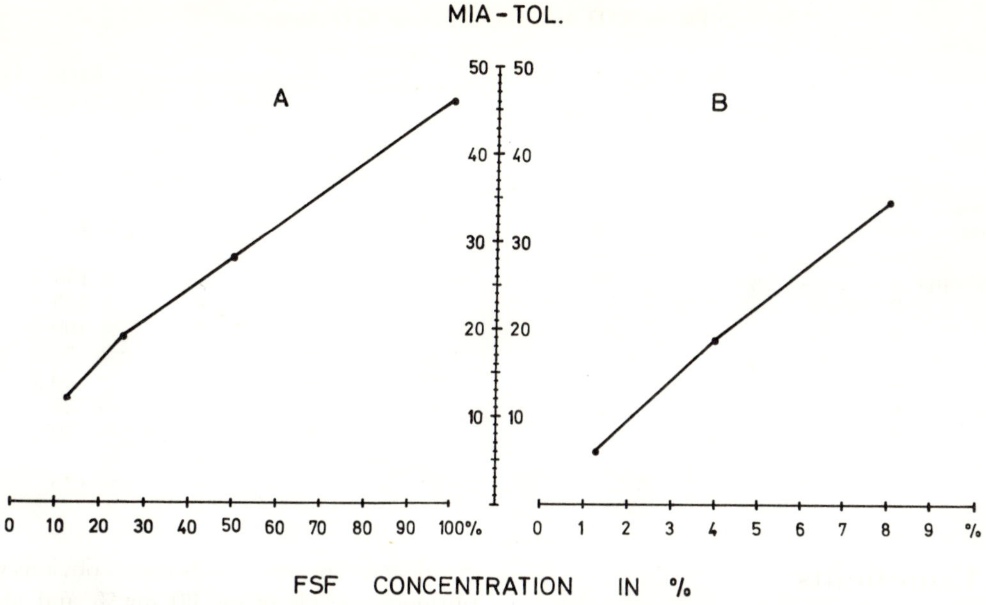

Fig. 2. Calibration curve for MIA Tolerance Test. A. Range between 10 and 100 % FSF activity. B. Range between 0 and 10 % FSF activity. Values on the ordinate represent test score in arbitrary point units. For explanation see text.

B. Reagents

Commercially available antihuman factor XIII rabbit antiserum (Behring Werke, Marburg, Germany; Certified Blood Donor Service, Inc. Woodbury, N. Y.).

Ca-thrombin solution: 60 NIH units of thrombin dissolved in 3.5 ml of 0.05 M $CaCl_2$ solution.

Monochloracetic acid (1 % in water).

A pool of platelet poor citrated normal plasma (obtained from at least 10 donors.

C. Procedure

Aliquots of 0.2 ml patient's plasma are incubated at 20° C with 0.1 ml aliquots of serially diluted antiserum. After 30 minutes, 0.1 ml of the Ca-thrombin solution is added. After 1 hour at 20° C the clots are transferred into 3 ml of a 1 % monochloracetic acid solution and the tubes shaken at 10–15 min intervals. The tubes are inspected for clot lysis after 90 minutes of incubation at room temperature. In a parallel series of test tubes, 0.2 ml aliquots of the normal pooled reference plasma are tested in an identical manner.

D. Calculation of Results

The reciprocal of the highest dilution of antiserum which prevents stabilization of fibrin, i. e. permits total lysis in monochloracetic acid, is determined for the reference plasma and test plasma. If the FSF content of the reference plasma is arbitrarily set at 100 %, the FSF content of the test plasma in percent can be calculated from the following equation:

$$\frac{\text{Reciprocal Antiserum Dilution Reference Plasma}}{\text{Reciprocal Antiserum Dilution Test Plasma}} \times 100 = \text{FSF content in } \% \qquad (1)$$

The application of this calculation for a series of test plasma is illustrated in Table 2.

Table 2: Factor XIII Assay using Factor XIII Antiserum.

	Dilution of Antiserum (0.1 ml) 1:6	1:7,2	1:9	1:12	1:18	1:36	1:90	1:180	Control without antiserum (0.1 ml NaCl)	Factor XIII Activity in % of normal
Reference Plasma	—	—	—	+	+	+	+	+	+	= 100
Testplasma 1	—	+	+	+	+	+	+	+	+	= 150
2	—	—	+	+	+	+	+	+	+	= 125
3	—	—	—	+	+	+	+	+	+	= 100
4	—	—	—	—	+	+	+	+	+	= 75
5	—	—	—	—	—	+	+	+	+	= 50
6	—	—	—	—	—	—	+	+	+	= 25
7	—	—	—	—	—	—	—	+	+	= 10
8	—	—	—	—	—	—	—	—	+	= 5
9	—	—	—	—	—	—	—	—	—	= <5

VI. Comments

Assay systems using a factor XIII free fibrinogen give reproducible results. The performance of the test is simple. Unfortunately the preparation of an adequate substrate is difficult. The possible denaturation of Factor XIII introduces certain problems: a) The fibrinogen may be altered during purification. b) If one uses inhibitors of Factor XIII the inhibition is partly reversible and traces of the inhibitor can remain in the preparation. These preparations tested by means of the MIA tolerance always show a residual activity of about 10%. Moreover, they do not behave like a factor XIII deficient plasma in the simple urea solubility test. More FSF is required in order to render the substrate clot insoluble in urea.

The separation of fibrinogen and Factor XIII gives by far the best substrate, but as mentioned this preparation is complicated. All these tests are less reliable in the presence of large quantities of fibrinogen and/or low Factor XIII activity.

Different problems arise with the use of monoiodoacetic acid and whole plasma test system and errors are higher than when FSF free fibrinogen is used. This is largely due to variation in interpretation of the degree of clot dissolution (see criteria). Moreover, the test system is sensitive to varying plasma fibrinogen levels. Therefore this test is not an absolute measure for Factor XIII. The influence of the fibrinogen concentration becomes obvious with fibrinogen levels below 80 mg% and above 800 mg%.

The fibrin monomers can also be used in a 2-stage assay system (Buluk et al. 1961; Lorand, 1964). This allows a distinction between the precursor form and the active form of factor XIII. The first stage is the activation of factor XIII by thrombin in presence of calcium ions, the second one the formation of a clot by addition of the fibrin monomers with subsequent cross linking of the fibrin network by the activated factor XIII.

The introduction of specific FSF neutralizing antisera may represent a significant advancement in FSF quantitation. However, the practical experiences with this test are still limited. The purity and specificity of commercial antisera remain potential problems precluding complete evaluation at this time.

The factor XIII antiserum cannot however differentiate between active or potentially active factor XIII and inactive or denatured one. For the detection of the abnormal protein the antiserum is a valuable tool as demonstrated recently (Duckert, 1969) but it cannot be used for the exact determination of factor XIII activity when both the normal and the abnormal proteins are present in the tested system.

Finally this short review would remain incomplete if no quotation is made of the determination of factor XIII transamidase activity.

It has been shown that factor XIII can incorporate small molecules into casein. Loewy (1968) and Lorand et al. (1969) made use of the incorporation of ^{14}C-glycine ethyl ester and fluorescent dansylcadaverine respectively. These test systems are quite attractive if it can be demonstrated that the factor XIII reaction with the artificial reagents parallels exactly the cross linking of fibrin under variable conditions.

References

Bohn, H., and Haupt, H. (1968). *Thromb.Diath. Haemorrhag. 19,* 309.
Buluk, K., Januszko, T., and Olbromski, J. (1961). *Nature, 191,* 1093.
Brown, M., and Rothstein, F. (1967). *Science 155,* 1017.
Duckert, F. (1969). *Thromb. Diath. Haemorrhag. Suppl. 34,* 11.
Duckert, F., Jung, E., and Shmerling, D. H. (1960). *Thromb. Diath. Haemorrhag. 5,* 179.
Heene, D. L. (1968). *Thromb. Diath. Haemorrhag. Suppl. 28,* 33.
Loewy, A. G. (1968). *Thromb. Diath. Haemorrhag. Suppl. 28,* 41.
Loewy, A. G., Dunathan, K., Kriel, R., and Wolfinger, H. L. (1961). *J. Biol. Chem. 236,* 2625.
Lorand, L. (1964). *In:* "Blood Coagulation, Hemorrhage and Thrombosis". (L. M. Tocantins and L. A. Kazal, eds. pp. 239—245. Grune and Stratton, New York.
Lorand, L., Urayama, T., de Kiewiet, J. W. C., and Nossel, H. L. (1969). *J. Clin. Invest. 48,* 1054.
Sigg, P. (1966). *Thromb. Diath. Haemorrhag. 15,* 238.
Sigg, P., and Duckert, F. (1963). *Schweiz. Med. Wochschr. 93,* 1455.
Swigert, S., Koppel, J. L., and Olwin, J. H. (1963). *Nature 198,* 797.

Chapter VII

Determination of Antithrombin

Eberhard F. Mammen

I. Introduction

One of the physiological functions of antithrombin is the inactivation of thrombin activity. Since Morawitz (1905) introduced the term antithrombin for the ability of plasma or serum to neutralize thrombin, several apparently different forms of antithrombin activities have been described. Astrup and Darling (1943) differentiated between an activity which inactivated thrombin progressively and an activity which functioned together with heparin immediately in the neutralization of thrombin. In 1945, Seegers et al. (1945c) described the adsorption of thrombin on fibrin, and in 1952, Seegers noted a fourth antithrombin effect during the activation of prothrombin in ether-treated defibrinated plasma.

In an attempt to easier describe the various mechanisms of thrombin inactivation, Seegers et al. (1954) proposed a number system for the various antithrombin activities which is widely adopted today. Antithrombin I was defined as the ability of fibrin to adsorbe thrombin; the term antithrombin II was used to describe the plasma cofactor of heparin; antithrombin III was recommended to designate the substance in plasma or serum which neutralizes thrombin activity; and antithrombin IV was used to describe the material in ether-treated plasma which would act in relationship to prothrombin activation.

In 1957, Loeliger and Hers described an antithrombin activity, subsequently termed antithrombin V, in a patient with rheumatoid arthritis and hypergammaglobulinemia. Similar activities had been demonstrated in patients with gamma myeloma (Craddock et al. 1953; Frick, 1955; Gehmacher et al. 1954; Lüscher and Labhart, 1949, Lüscher et al. 1949; Ratnoff, 1953; Uehlinger, 1949; Benda et al. 1958; and Verstraete and Vermylen, 1959).

In 1958, Niewiarowski and Kowalski introduced the term antithrombin VI to describe the anticoagulant activity which develops when fibrinogen is digested by fibrinolysin (plasmin). This anticoagulant activity was first documented by Triantaphyllopoulos (1957), and independently described by Niewiarowski and Kowalski (1957), and by Stormorken (1957).

Not covered by the number system are substances which interfere with thrombin activity in vitro, like antibodies against thrombin, diisopropylfluorophosphate (DFP), or other enzyme inhibitors. Theoretically, these also are antithrombins in the strict sense of the terminology.

Practically, however, the word antithrombin is restricted to the native power of plasma or serum to neutralize thrombin activity. In defining the term antithrombin, a distinction must be made between antithrombin activity due to a specific substance in plasma, and a number of nonspecific antithrombin reactions. Such a differentiation is important for the discussion of the various methods of antithrombin determination. Antithrombin I, or the ability of fibrin to adsorbe thrombin, is a nonspecific antithrombin reaction. This phenomenon has so far only been demonstrated in vitro, and its physiological importance in vivo is not fully recognized. Nevertheless, antithrombin determinations in vitro have to take this phenomenon into account. By the same token, the ability of glass to adsorbe and neutralize thrombin activity (Seegers et al. 1952) has to be taken into consideration.

The use of the terms antithrombin II and III might indicate that these activities are associated with two different plasma constituents, although one has to encounter the possibility that they are expressions of one and the same substance. The work of Lyttleton (1954), Burstein (1955), Burstein and Loeb (1956), Monkhouse et al. (1955), Monkhouse and Clarke (1957), and Monkhouse (1967) make it seem possible that heparin-cofactor activity and the progressive enzymatic antithrombin activity of plasma or serum are functions of one substance only. In other words, antithrombin II and antithrombin III activities are likely associated with an identical substance (Verstraete, 1966).

With respect to the possible identity of antithrombin III and IV it should be recalled that Seegers et al. (1954) stated in their original publication: "It is our belief that these two antithrombins are not the same substances, but it is hardly possible to come to a definite conclusion on the basis of our experiments". Subsequently, the identity between these two activities was established (Sokal, 1955; Seegers et al. 1964a; Monkhouse and Milojevic, 1965; Seegers, 1962), and antithrombin IV is a kinetic effect rather than a substance different from antithrombin III.

Antithrombin V was detected in association with hypergammaglobulinemia or gamma myeloma. The activity is apparently not occuring in plasma or serum under physiological conditions. Most likely the antithrombin V effect is due to elevated levels of gamma globulin or paraproteins interfering with the polymerization of fibrin monomers (Vermylen and Verstraete, 1960), rather than due to the neutralization of the enzymatic activity of thrombin. Therefore, antithrombin V is possibly a nonspecific antithrombin effect.

The physiological function of fibrinogen derivatives (split products) as antithrombin VI may be of certain relevance, since small amounts of these derivatives can be detected in normal plasma and serum. But there is at present no conclusive evidence as to the role that these split products play in the neutralization of thrombin activity under physiological conditions. Their antithrombin effect in states of hyperfibrinolysis is well documented. Apparently, the fibrinogen derivatives compete with native fibrinogen molecules for thrombin molecules and thereby make less thrombin available for the conversion of fibrinogen. The mechanism of inhibition is of competitive nature (Triantaphyllopoulos, 1959; Triantaphyllopoulos and Triantaphyllopoulos, 1966).

These considerations leave antithrombin III as the only plasma or serum constituent which blocks thrombin activity, and Monkhouse (1967) regards this type of thrombin neutralization as the only true antithrombin activity.

This antithrombin (antithrombin III) has been concentrated from plasma and serum (Monkhouse et al. 1955; Shinowara and Buckley, 1959; Monkhouse and Milojevic, 1963; Hensen and Loeliger, 1963b), and it apparently is a protein which is associated with the alpha-globulin fraction (Monkhouse and Clarke, 1957). Certain physical-chemical properties of this compound have recently been described (Seegers et al. 1964b).

II. Methods of Measurement

A. General Considerations

For the determination of antithrombin activities in plasma or serum it is of importance to consider the difference between nonspecific and specific antithrombin reactions. If possible, the nonspecific reactions should be eliminated in order to obtain more accurate results. Since thrombin is readily adsorbed on glass surfaces, all determinations should be performed in siliconized or paraffinized glassware, or in plastic containers. Since thrombin is furthermore adsorbed on fibrinogen or fibrin, plasma should be defibrinated before the actual antithrombin determination. For defibrination, heating of the plasma samples to 56° C for 3–5 minutes is advisable. Heating of the plasma up to this temperature does not interfere with the antithrombin activity (Seegers et al. 1952). However, higher temperatures will begin to inactivate antithrombin. Heating of the plasma will not only remove fibrinogen, and thereby the antithrombin I effect, but will also remove the fibrinogen derivative which has the highest antithrombin activity. This derivative corresponds to the alpha-derivative of Seegers et al. (1945b) and components D and D–E of Nussenzweig et al. (1961). With the removal of these split products of fibrinogen, most of the antithrombin VI effect is eliminated. Not precipitated is the beta-derivative or component E, but the antithrombin effect of this derivative is negligible (Triantaphyllopoulos, 1965).

The actual temperature at which antithrombin determinations are performed is of further importance. With increasing temperatures the rate of thrombin inactivation, and the amount of thrombin neutralized will become greater (Seegers et al. 1952). Therefore, it is recommended to adopt a certain standard temperature for all antithrombin determinations. This standard temperature may range between 28° C and 37° C, and subsequently all determinations should be performed at the selected temperature in order to obtain reproducable and comparable data.

The stability of antithrombin activity in whole blood, plasma or serum is remarkable, and up to 4 weeks of storage at +4° C no loss of activity was noted (Seegers et al. 1952). Therefore, no special precautions with regard to the time between withdrawal of blood and actual assay of antithrombin have to be observed.

Due to the enzymatic nature of antithrombin, the concentration of thrombin in plasma will only decrease progressively. Therefore, ideally, methods of antithrombin determination should consist of a series of measurements at different time intervals. The rate of neutralization varies with the concentration of both thrombin and antithrombin. When the concentration of thrombin is high relative to the antithrombin concentration, the neutralization is facilitated slowly, and some thrombin will always remain in an active state. Actually, the initial inactivation proceeds rapidly, but after about 30 minutes of incubation, the inactivation process begins to slow down considerably, and only after about two hours an equilibrium condition is reached (Klein and Seegers, 1950). When the concentration of thrombin is small relative to the antithrombin concentration, a large amount of thrombin will be neutralized rather rapidly. But even under these conditions small traces of thrombin will remain in active form (Klein and Seegers, 1950). Even in the presence of a considerable excess of antithrombin, small traces of thrombin remain in active form (Seegers, 1962). Therefore, methods that utilize large amounts of thrombin relative to the concentration of antithrombin are of greater accuracy. Generally, the amount of thrombin which remains after a fixed quantity of antithrombin has been allowed to react with the thrombin, depends on the quantity of thrombin available.

Of further importance is the purity of thrombin preparations used for the determination of antithrombin. It has been demonstrated that autoprothrombin C activity (activated factor X, plasma thrombokinase) is readily neutralized in plasma (Seegers and Marciniak, 1962). When plasma was first incubated with thrombin, the subsequent capacity for inactivation of autoprothrombin C was reduced. When plasma was first incubated with autothrombin C, the subsequent capacity for inactivation of thrombin was reduced. Experiments with purified antithrombin III revealed that antithrombin had the capability to neutralize both thrombin and autoprothrombin C activities (Seegers et al. 1964b). Since commercial thrombin preparations may be contaminated with autoprothrombin C (Cole et al. 1964; Kerwin and Milstone, 1967), erroneous antithrombin results may be obtained because part of the antithrombin activity is utilized in the inactivation of autoprothrombin C, rather than in the neutralization of thrombin. Therefore, higher levels of remaining thrombin activity will be measured, leading to the interpretation of decreased levels of antithrombin. It is, therefore, advisable to purify the commercial thrombin preparations further in order to remove autoprothrombin C. The further purification can be achieved by column chromatography on either cation exchange resin IRC-50 (XE-64) (Seegers et al. 1958), on phosphate cellulose (Cellex-P) (Seegers and Landaburu, 1960), or by combined barium sulfate adsorption and chromatography on DEAE-cellulose (Kerwin and Milstone, 1967).

In reviewing the present literature, a considerable number of procedures for the determination of antithrombin have been described.

It will be impossible to review them all, and, therefore, only a few methods will be considered in detail which chiefly measure the specific enzymatic antithrombin activity in either plasma or serum. An attempt will be made, however, to list the principle of other procedures as well. Basically, the methods for the antithrombin determination can be divided into two groups: those which utilize an excess amount of thrombin relative to the antithrombin concentration, and those which use small amounts of thrombin.

B. Procedures Using Excess Amounts of Thrombin

1. Method of Seegers et al. (1952)

In 1952, Seegers et al. described a procedure for the determination of antithrombin activity in plasma or serum. In this method excess amounts of thrombin are added to plasma or serum. The amount of thrombin added is sufficient so that always some thrombin activity remains. This thrombin activity is measured by clotting fibrinogen at various intervals of incubation, or after 2 hours of incubation, when an equilibrium between thrombin and antithrombin concentrations is established.

Materials and Reagents: Thrombin: The purest available thrombin is added as a substrate. It may be prepared from purified prothrombin as described by Hecht et al. (1958), Seegers et al. (1958), or Seegers and Landaburu (1960). Also commercial thrombin preparations may be used, but if these are contaminated with autoprothrombin C, they should be further purified as suggested above. A constant check of the thrombin activity is necessary, since thrombin may change its activity during storage. Loss of thrombin activity during storage can be minimized in a 50 % glycerol solution. In 50 % glycerol thrombin activity is fairly stable for months when stored in a deep freeze at –20° C. Thrombin in weaker solutions of glycerol is also stable, but will freeze at deep freeze temperatures. The thawing process may then reduce the activity. For the antithrombin determination, thrombin is made up to a strength of 1,200 units/ml. It is buffered with 5 % imidazol buffer at pH 7.2 to 7.4 in a concentration of 12.5 % by volume of solution.

Plasma: Plasma is obtained from blood collected in either 1.85 % potassium oxalate solution or 3.2 % trisodium citrate solution in a proportion of one part anticoagulant plus nine parts of blood. The cellular elements of the blood are removed by centrifugation at approximately 2,000 g for about 10 to 15 minutes. The supernatant plasma is separated. It is not necessary to perform the antithrombin determination immediately since, as outlined above, the antithrombin activity is extremely stable from the storage point of view (Seegers et al. 1952). Before analysis of antithrombin activity, the plasma must be defibrinated in order to remove the antithrombin I and antithrombin VI effect. About 1 ml of plasma is heated in a water bath to 56° C for 3 to 5 minutes. The heat coagulated fibrinogen is removed by centrifuging the sample for 10 minutes at about 2,000 g. The supernatant defibrinated plasma can be decanted or pipetted off. Plasma may also be defibrinated by the addition of small amounts of thrombin. For this purpose 0.5 ml of plasma are mixed with 0.4 ml of 0.9 % saline, and 0.1 ml of a thrombin solution containing 100 units/ml is added. The clot is removed as it forms with a glass rod or a wooden applicator stick. The plasma is allowed to stand for 10 minutes at room temperature. The addition of these small amounts of thrombin apparently does not materially affect the antithrombin concentration. Comparative analysis after both defibrination procedures revealed the same results (Johnson and Seegers, 1964).

Serum: Blood is withdrawn and transferred to a clean glass tube and allowed to clot at 37° C. After two hours incubation at 37° C the tube is centrifuged for 10 minutes at 2,000 g and the supernatant serum is pipetted off. The serum can be stored at room temperature or refrigerator temperature for several hours, or may be frozen at –20° C in a deep freeze. It is not necessary to defibrinate the serum before analysis, unless the serum is from patients with states of hyperfibrinolysis. Under these circumstances the heat precipitable fibrinogen derivatives should be removed.

Glassware: Because thrombin is readily adsorbed on glass surfaces, all glassware must be coated with either silicone or paraffin. If any commercial products are applied for coating, the manufacturer's directions are suitable for this procedure. Instead of siliconized or paraffinized glass ware, polyethylene tubes may be used. It is not advisable to re-use siliconized or paraffinized glassware for repeated determinations. The author uses paraffinized test tubes. We use tubes that have broken rims and are to be discarded, paraffinize them and discard them after the antithrombin determination.

Actual Procedure: In brief, the method consists of allowing plasma or serum to react with a known amount of thrombin for a given period of time. The remaining thrombin activity is measured on fibrinogen. In detail, 0.5 ml of defibrinated plasma or serum are placed in a siliconized or paraffinized glass tube or plastic tube and 0.5 ml of thrombin (preferably 1,200 units/ml in 50 % glycerol) are added. The mixture is incubated at 28° C or 37° C, whatever temperature the individual investigator prefers. After two hours of incubation the mixture is placed in an ice bath to slow the reaction and the remaining thrombin activity is promptly measured by means of a routine thrombin determination procedure, such as, for example, described by Seegers and Smith (1942). In principle, this analysis consists of the dilution of the mixture until a 1 % fibrinogen solution is clotted at 15 seconds by the thrombin contained therein. A clotting time of 15 seconds represents under these conditions one Iowa unit of thrombin. The unitage represented by clotting times slightly deviating from 15 seconds may be obtained from a correction table published by Ware and Seegers (1949) (see Chapter V, p. 179). If instead of Iowa units, National Institute of Health (NIH) units should be preferred, one NIH unit of thrombin is equivalent to 1.25 Iowa units of thrombin (Seegers, 1962). The thrombin assay need not be performed in coated glassware of plastic tubes.

Computation of Results: The results of this antithrombin determination procedure can be expressed by calculating the percentage of thrombin destroyed per ml of plasma or serum according to Eq. 1.

$$\frac{(T-2t) \times 100}{T} \qquad (1)$$

"T" is the standard concentration of thrombin used, and "t" the thrombin concentration in the incubation mixture after 2 hours of incubation. In actual figures, when 0.5 ml of thrombin, containing 1,200 units/ml (T) were added to 0.5 ml of defibrinated plasma, and 300 units/ml of thrombin were measured in the incubation mixture (t), 50 % of the thrombin was destroyed by antithrombin in this particular ml of plasma or serum. It is advisable to run at least three determinations of thrombin at the endpoint of incubation. These should check within a fraction of a second of each other. Only the triple determination assures that an equilibrium between antithrombin and thrombin has been established, and that the dilution utilized in the thrombin analysis was correct. It is further advisable to run a control sample along with the analytical specimens. In the control sample 0.5 ml of 0.9 % saline is used instead of 0.5 ml of defibrinated plasma or serum. No destruction of thrombin should be found in the control. The control sample, furthermore, governs the activity of the reagents.

Normal Values: A survey of the antithrombin activities in plasma of 306 human subjects conducted by Seegers et al. (1952) gave values ranging between 30 % and 50 %. These figures are in agreement with the ones the author routinely obtains from normal human plasma. The antithrombin activity in serum is generally lower than in defibrinated plasma (Seegers et al. 1952; Blombäck et al. 1963).

Comments: The procedure is specific for the determination of the enzymatic antithrombin activity, and practically all the nonspecific antithrombin effects are eliminated. The method gives accurate and reproducable results, and can be routinely applied. A disadvantage of this procedure is the fairly large quantities of thrombin needed. Furthermore, in the presence of heparin the results become inaccurate due to its interference with the thrombin determination.

2. Method of Monkhouse et al. (1955)

In principle, this procedure is similar to the method of Seegers et al. (1952), but thrombin activity is measured by its capability to hydrolyze p-toluenesulfonyl-arginine-methyl ester (TAMe).

Materials and Reagents: Thrombin: The same specifications as outlined above apply for the thrombin used in this procedure, only the stock solution is made up of 2,000 units/ml in 50% glycerol solution. This stock solution of thrombin is kept at –20° C in a deep freeze, and before analysis the activity should be checked to assure accurate conditions.

Plasma: The plasma is obtained and defibrinated as outlined above.

Tris-buffer: 15.8 gm of trimethylol amino methane are dissolved in 1,500 ml of distilled water and the pH adjusted to 8.5 by the addition of 1 N HCl. The volume is made up to exactly 2,000 ml.

TAMe: P-toluenesulfonyl-arginine-methyl ester (TAMe) is freshly prepared daily in a 0.4 M solution.

Glassware: Siliconized glassware or polyethylene containers should be used during incubation of thrombin with antithrombin.

Actual Procedure: Basically, a constant amount of thrombin is added to various amounts of defibrinated plasma or serum. After incubation for one hour at 28° C the remaining thrombin activity is measured on TAMe as substrate.

In detail, 200 units of thrombin (0.1 ml of the stock solution containing 2,000 units/ml) are placed in each of a number of siliconized test tubes. Varying amounts of defibrinated plasma, from 0.1 ml to 0.8 ml are added, and the volume adjusted to 1 ml with tris-buffer. The tubes are incubated for one hour at 28° C. After this time interval, the tubes are placed in an ice bath and the remaining thrombin activity is measured against TAMe. A procedure for the determination of the esterolytic activity is described in detail in Chapter VIII, p. 365.

Computation of Results: The total amount of thrombin destroyed is calculated for each test tube. A curve is constructed plotting volume of plasma or serum added per tube against the units of thrombin utilized. To estimate the potency of antithrombin in this particular plasma or serum sample, the point on the curve which represents 100 units of thrombin destroyed (50% destruction) is located and a perpendicular dropped to the abscissa. This gives the volume of plasma or serum having destroyed 100 units of thrombin. By defining 1 unit of antithrombin as the amount which will neutralize one unit of thrombin in one hour at 28° C, the units of antithrombin can be obtained. By simple multiplication, the potency of antithrombin, in terms of units per ml of plasma, can be calculated. Defibrinated normal plasma samples contain around 250 units/ml of antithrombin.

Comments: The method is specific for the enzymatic antithrombin activity and has the advantage that the antithrombin activity can be measured more accurately in the presence of heparin.

3. Method of Hallén (1962)

The procedure described by Hallén (1962) is also utilizing large excesses of thrombin relative to antithrombin concentration.

Materials and Reagents: Buffer: Tris-buffer is used for the dilution of plasma, thrombin, and fibrinogen. The ionic strength of the buffer is 0.15 and the pH 7.4.

Plasma: Blood is collected in trisodium citrate (3.8%) under siliconized conditions, the plasma is separated as described above and defibrinated by heat as outlined before. The plasma is diluted in a proportion of 1:5 with tris-buffer.

Thrombin: Thrombin from commercial sources is diluted to 200 NIH units/ml and kept in ice water in a siliconized test tube.

Fibrinogen: Hallén used fibrinogen prepared by the method of Blombäck and Blombäck (1956) and diluted to a final concentration of 0.8% with Tris-buffer.

Actual Procedure: In principle, thrombin is added to defibrinated plasma and after incubation, the remaining thrombin is measured on fibrinogen as a substrate. In detail, 1 ml of defibrinated, 1:5 diluted plasma is placed in each of two siliconized glass tubes and warmed for 3 minutes at 37° C. One ml of thrombin (200 NIH units/ml) is added to each tube, and the mixture is incubated for 60 minutes at 37° C. After incubation 0.5 ml of the mixture of each tube is placed in different siliconized tubes and immediately diluted with 3 ml of cold Tris-buffer. The tubes are placed in an ice bath and the residual thrombin is measured within an hour.

Thrombin is determined by diluting the contents of one of the tubes with Tris-buffer to such an extent that 0.2 ml of this dilution clots 0.6 ml of 0.8 % fibrinogen in 35 to 45 seconds. Usually the dilution has to be 1:18 or 1:20. This dilution is now directly applied to the second incubation tube, and 0.2 ml of this diluted mixture is added to 0.6 ml of 0.8 % fibrinogen. The coagulation time is recorded. Three determinations are made and the mean of the three values is calculated.

The clotting times are converted to units of thrombin by means of a standard curve. The standard curve is prepared by diluting the standard thrombin solution (200 NIH units/ml) to four units/ml, two units/ml, and one unit/ml. 0.2 ml of each dilution are added to 0.6 ml of the 0.8 % fibrinogen solution and the clotting times are noted. At least four determinations of each dilution are made and the mean values calculated. The above obtained clotting times of 35 to 45 seconds should correspond to 2–2.5 units of thrombin. By plotting clotting times in seconds against the strength of each thrombin dilution in units per ml on double logarithmic paper, a straight line should be obtained.

Computation of Results: The results are expressed in units of antithrombin, whereby one unit of antithrombin is defined as the amount of antithrombin which neutralizes one unit of thrombin under the experimental conditions. Equation (2) is used for calculation.

$$AT = (100 - a \times b) \times 10 \qquad (2)$$

"AT" is the number of antithrombin units per ml of plasma, "a" is the residual thrombin in units per ml of mixture used for the analysis, and "b" is the ratio between the volume of added tris-buffer plus reaction mixture.

Normal Values: Hallén found in the plasma of 42 healthy persons a mean of 554 antithrombin units per ml of plasma with a standard deviation of 59.92 units.

Comments: This procedure determines the enzymatic antithrombin activity in plasma, and should also be applicable to serum. The reason for preparing plasma in siliconized tubes is not quite clear to the author, and the assumption is made that it is not absolutely necessary. The dilution of thrombin with Tris-buffer without the addition of glycerol necessitates quick handling, because thrombin in diluted form readily loses its activity, even at low temperatures. Hallén stresses the importance of the 0.8 % fibrinogen solution, because apparently lower concentrations of fibrinogen are sometimes labile. With a drop in fibrinogen concentration, erroneous results are obtained. According to Hallén, it is also important to dilute the sample to be tested to clotting times around 35 to 45 seconds. When the thrombin concentration is high there is apparently the tendency for the antithrombin values to be high and vice versa. This difficulty can be avoided by diluting the sample appropriately.

C. Procedures Using Small Amounts of Thrombin

1. Modified Method of Gerendas (1946)

A simple and useful procedure for the determination of antithrombin was introduced by Gerendas (1946; 1946–48) and subsequently modified by Mihályi (1954) and by Monkhouse (1963). The method is based on the principle that when small amounts of thrombin react with large concentrations of antithrombin, the rate of disappearance of thrombin activity follows a first order reaction. Monkhouse (1963) used the procedure for the determination of antithrombin in plasma and antithrombin fractions, while Mihályi determined antithrombin activity in serum.

a. Modification of Monkhouse (1963)

Materials and Reagents: Thrombin: Commercial thrombin preparations can be used and diluted to 10 NIH units per ml with 0.9 % saline containing 0.006 M Tris-buffer. The same Tris-buffer is used as described in Section II B 2.

Fibrinogen: Monkhouse (1963) used fibrinogen prepared by the method of Jaques (1943).

Phosphate Buffer: 0.05 M phosphate buffer pH 7.8 was used.

Plasma: The preparation and defibrination of plasma is the same as described above.

Glassware: Siliconized glassware or polyethylene tubes should be used.

Actual Procedure: An 0.3 ml aliquot of defibrinated plasma is diluted with 0.2 ml of

0.05 M phosphate buffer pH 7.8 in a siliconized glass tube or polyethylene tube, and 0.3 ml of the thrombin solution (10 NIH units/ml) are added. After 30 seconds and minute intervals thereafter, 0.1 ml of the reaction mixture is added to 0.2 ml fibrinogen solution, and the clotting times are recorded.

Computation of Results: By plotting log clotting times against incubation times, a straight line should be obtained, the slope of which is the rate K. The slope of this line varies directly with the antithrombin concentration as demonstrated in Fig. 1. Such a plasma dilution curve can be best obtained from a normal plasma, or even better, from a pool of three to five normal plasmas, in order to reduce possible individual variations. In using such a set of standard dilution curves it is important to use not only always the same concentration of thrombin, but also the same concentration of fibrinogen.

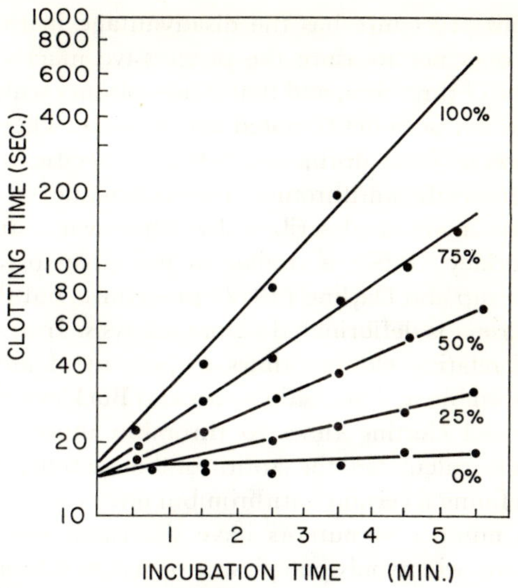

Fig. 1. Relation between plasma dilution and rate of thrombin inactivation.

b. Modification of Mihályi (1954)

Materials and Reagents: Thrombin: Thrombin was prepared from prothrombin purified by the procedure of Seegers et al. (1945a). Prothrombin was activated to thrombin according to Seegers et al. (1950).

Fibrinogen: Commercial fibrinogen, bovine fraction I from Armour Laboratories was used in the original work.

Phosphate Buffer: 0.5 M phosphate buffer pH 7.23 was used in this procedure.

Serum: Human blood was collected and allowed to clot. The clot was gently pressed with a glass rod and centrifuged. After centrifugation, the serum was allowed to stand at room temperature for one hour. Mihályi used serum not older than 24 hours.

Actual Procedure: An 0.8 ml sample of serum was mixed with 0.2 ml of 0.5 M phosphate buffer pH 7.23 and sufficient saline solution to give a total volume of 1.5 ml after the addition of thrombin. The tube was incubated at 24° C and after reaching temperature equilibrium, thrombin was added. The amount of thrombin added varied between 30 and 40 units in the final 1.5 ml of reaction mixture. At different time intervals 0.2 ml of the reaction mixture were added to a fibrinogen solution and the clotting times recorded. The incubation was followed for six minutes.

Computation of Results: The clotting times were plotted against incubation time as described above and a straight line resulted. The values are calculated as described in Section II C 1 a.

2. Other Methods

A method devised by Astrup and Darling (1942) has been extensively used in various modified forms. In principle, 1 ml of standardized thrombin solution with known activity is added to various dilutions of plasma or serum, and after incubation of the mixture for thirty minutes, the remaining thrombin is measured on fibrinogen. The modification of this procedure introduced by Biggs and Macfarlane (1953) consists of shortening the incubation time to 15 minutes (see also Biggs and Macfarlane, 1962). The coagulation times of the fibrinogen solution are dependent upon the amount of thrombin remaining in the various plasma and serum dilutions. By plotting the various remaining concentrations of thrombin against dilutions, a straight line is obtained which is used to correct for any given value. The amount of antithrombin is arrived at by subtracting the thrombin activity remaining from the original amount of thrombin added.

This procedure has the disadvantage in that it does not measure the progressive inactivation of thrombin, and that it uses plasma which has not been defibrinated before assay. Therefore, no clear distinction between specific and nonspecific antithrombin effects is made.

The method described by Shinowara and Buckley (1960) is similar in principle to the Astrup and Darling (1942) procedure, but the plasma is defibrinated before analysis. Instead of relating clotting times to percent of antithrombin activity, Shinowara and Buckley converted clotting times to thrombin units and then calculated the antithrombin activity by defining a certain antithrombin unit.

A number of authors have described procedures where only one plasma or serum dilution is added to a standard amount of thrombin (Herbert, 1940; Quick, 1951; Schultze and Schwick, 1953; Witte and Dirnberger, 1953; Sokal, 1955; Jürgens, 1956; Hensen and Loeliger, 1963a). After a certain incubation time, which varies from one author to the other, the remaining thrombin activity is determined by clotting fibrinogen or barium sulfate adsorbed normal human plasma. The clotting times are either directly converted to percent of antithrombin activity by using a standard curve obtained by diluting a normal serum or plasma, or the clotting times are converted to thrombin units by means of a standard thrombin dilution curve. In the latter instances the remaining thrombin units are subtracted from the original thrombin units added to plasma or serum and then expressed in percent of antithrombin activity or units of antithrombin, whereby arbitrary antithrombin units are designed.

All of these procedures are technically easy to perform and probably useful for routine clinical antithrombin determinations. However, they do not take into consideration the progressive destruction of thrombin by antithrombin. Furthermore, most authors advocate an incubation time of 30 minutes or less, whereas a true equilibrium between thrombin and antithrombin is reached at the earliest after 60 minutes of incubation, better even after two hours. Since in all of the methods small amounts of thrombin are used relative to the antithrombin concentration, both substances may continuously change in concentration, which is due to the fact that both inactivate each other. This may lead to erroneous results, especially when thrombin determinations are made only after *one* particular time of incubation.

References

Astrup, T., and Darling, S. (1942). *Acta Physiol. Scand. 4,* 293.

Astrup, T., and Darling, S. (1943). *Acta Physiol. Scand. 5,* 13.

Benda, L., Deutsch, E., and Mammen, E. F. (1958). *Wien. Klin. Wochschr. 70,* 559.

Biggs, R., and Macfarlane, R. G. (1953). "Human Blood Coagulation and its Disorders". Blackwell Scientific Publications, Oxford.

Biggs, R., and Macfarlane, R. G. (1962). "Human Blood Coagulation and its Disorders". Third Edition, Davis, Philadelphia.

Blombäck, B., and Blombäck, M. (1956). *Arkiv Kemi 10,* 415.

Blombäck, B., Blombäck, M., and Olsson, P. (1963). *Thromb. Diath. Haemorrhag. 9,* 368.

Burstein, M. (1955). *Arch. Intern. Pharmacodynam. 101,* 285.

Burstein, M., and Loeb, J. (1956). *Rev. franc. études clin. biol. 1,* 752.

Cole, E. R., Koppel, J. L., and Olwin, J. H. (1964). *Nature 202,* 301.

Craddock, Ch. G., Adams, W. S., and Figueroa, W. G. (1953). *J. Lab. Clin. Med. 42,* 847.

Frick, P. G. (1955). *Am. J. Clin. Pathol. 25,* 1263.

Gehmacher, K., Herold, G., and Reimer, E. E. (1954). *Wien. Z. Inn. Med. 35,* 245.

Gerendas, M. (1946). *Nature 157,* 837.

Gerendas, M. (1946—48). *Hung. Acta Physiol. 1,* 97.

Hallén, A. (1962). *Thromb. Diath. Haemorrhag. 8,* 56.

Hecht, E. R., Cho, M. H., and Seegers, W. H. (1958). *Am. J. Physiol. 193,* 584.

Hensen, A., and Loeliger, E. A. (1963a). *Thromb. Diath. Haemorrhag. Suppl. 10,* 18.

Hensen, A., and Loeliger, E. A. (1963b). *Thromb. Diath. Haemorrhag. Suppl. 10,* 46.

Herbert, F. K. (1940). *Biochem. J. 34,* 1554.

Jaques, L. B. (1943), *Biochem. J. 37,* 344.

Johnson, J. F., and Seegers, W. H. (1964). *In:* "Blood Coagulation, Hemorrhage and Thrombosis" (L. M. Tocantins and L. A. Kazal, eds.), pp. 329—333. Grune and Stratton, New York.

Jürgens, J. (1956). *Materia Medica Nordmark 8,* 10.

Kerwin, D. M., and Milstone, J. H. (1967). *Thromb. Diath. Haemorrhag. 17,* 247.

Klein, P. D., and Seegers, W. H. (1950). *Blood 5,* 742.

Loeliger, A., and Hers, J. F. Ph. (1957). *Thromb. Diath. Haemorrhag. 1,* 499.

Lüscher, E., and Labhart, A. (1949). *Schweiz. Med. Wochschr. 79,* 598.

Lüscher, E., Labhart, A., and Uehlinger, E. (1949). *Helv. Med. Acta 16,* 283.

Lyttleton, J. W. (1954). *Biochem. J. 58,* 8.

Mihályi, E. (1954). *J. Gen. Physiol. 37,* 139.

Monkhouse, F. C. (1963). *Thromb. Diath. Haemorrhag. 9,* 387.

Monkhouse, F. C. (1967). *In:* "Blood Clotting Enzymology" (W. H. Seegers, ed.), pp. 323—344. Academic Press, New York.

Monkhouse, F. C., and Clarke, D. W. (1957). *Can. J. Biochem. Physiol. 35,* 374.

Monkhouse, F. C., and Milojevic, S. (1963). *Thromb. Diath. Haemorrhag. 9,* 221.
Monkhouse, F. C., and Milojevic, S. (1965). *Can. J. Physiol. Pharmacol. 43,* 819.
Monkhouse, F. C., France, E. S., and Seegers, W. H. (1955). *Circulation Res. 3,* 397.
Morawitz, P. (1905). *Ergeb. Physiol. 4,* 307.
Niewiarowski, S., and Kowalski, E. (1957). *Bull. Acad. Polon. Sci. Classe II, 5,* 169.
Niewiarowski, S., and Kowalski, E. (1958). *Rev. Hématol. 13,* 320.
Nussenzweig, V., Seligmann, M., Pelmont, J., and Grabar, P. (1961). *Ann. Inst. Pasteur 100,* 377.
Quick, A. J. (1951). "The Physiology and Pathology of Hemostasis". Kimton, London.
Ratnoff, O. D. (1953). *J. Clin. Invest. 32,* 596.
Schultze, H. E., and Schwick, G. (1953). "Laboratoriumsblätter", Behring-Werke, Nr. 2.
Seegers, W. H. (1952). *Arch. Biochem. Biophys. 36,* 484.
Seegers, W. H. (1962). "Prothrombin". Harvard University Press, Cambridge, Mass.
Seegers, W. H., and Landaburu, R. H. (1960). *Can. J. Biochem. Physiol. 38,* 1405.
Seegers, W. H., and Marciniak, E. (1962). *Nature 193,* 1188.
Seegers, W. H., and Smith, H. P. (1942). *Am. J. Physiol. 137,* 348.
Seegers, W. H., Loomis, E. C., and Vandenbelt, J. M. (1945a). *Arch. Biochem. 6,* 85.
Seegers, W. H., Nieft, M. L., and Vandenbelt, J. M. (1945b). *Arch. Biochem. 7,* 45.
Seegers, W. H., Nieft, M. L., and Loomis, E. C. (1945c). *Science 101,* 520.
Seegers, W. H., McClaughry, R. I., and Fahey, J. L. (1950). *Blood 5,* 421.
Seegers, W. H., Miller, K. D., Andrews, E. B., and Murphy, R. C. (1952). *Am. J. Physiol. 169,* 700.
Seegers, W. H., Johnson, J. F., and Fell, C. (1954). *Am. J. Physiol. 176,* 97.
Seegers, W. H., Levine, W. G., and Shepard, R. S. (1958). *Can. J. Biochem. Physiol. 36,* 603.
Seegers, W. H., Schröer, H., and Kagami, M. (1964a). *Can. J. Biochem. 42,* 1425.
Seegers, W. H., Cole, E. R., Harmison, Ch. R., and Monkhouse, F. C. (1964b). *Can. J. Biochem. 42,* 359.
Shinowara, G. Y., and Buckley, D. J. (1959). *Thromb. Diath. Haemorrhag. 4,* 17.
Sokal, G. (1955). *Acta Haematol. 14,* 34.
Stormorken, H. (1957). *Brit. J. Haematol. 3,* 229.
Triantaphyllopoulos, D. C. (1957). *Proc. Western Group Div. Med. Res. Natl. Council Can. 11,* 21.
Triantaphyllopoulos, D. C. (1959). *Am. J. Physiol. 197,* 575.
Triantaphyllopoulos, D. C. (1965). *Federation Proc. 24,* 800.
Triantaphyllopoulos, D. C., and Triantaphyllopoulos, E. (1966). *Brit. J. Haematol. 12,* 145.
Uehlinger, E. (1949). *Helv. Med. Acta 16,* 508.
Vermylen, C., and Verstraete, M. (1960). *Thromb. Diath. Haemorrhag. 5,* 267.
Verstraete, M. (1966). *Thromb. Diath. Haemorrhag. Suppl. 20,* 385.
Verstraete, M., and Vermylen, C. (1959). *Acta Haematol. 22,* 240.
Ware, A. G., and Seegers, W. H. (1949). *Am. J. Clin. Pathol. 19,* 471.
Witte, S., and Dirnberger, P. (1953). *Klin. Wochschr. 31,* 598.

Heparin Assays in Blood

J. Erik Jorpes

I. Introduction

Physiologically there is very little, if any, heparin in the blood. Even with techniques sensitive enough for recovery of minute amounts of heparin added to plasma, no heparin can be found in the circulating plasma (Masure, 1960; Jaques et al. 1949; Monkhouse et al. 1949; Monkhouse and Jaques, 1950; Gibson et al. 1952). With the octylamine method of Monkhouse et al. (1949), in which the heparin, after further precipitation with brucine, was assayed colorimetrically with the Azur-A stain, 0.02–0.36 mg of heparin added to 10 ml of citrated blood could be recovered with 90 percent yields. If added to plasma the yield was 100 percent (Jaques, 1949). Normal human blood was considered by the authors to contain no more than possibly 0.009 mg of heparin per 100 ml. Zöllner et al. (1962) and Zöllner and Lorenz (1963) precipitated heparin with 5-amino-acridine, removed the base with sodium hydroxide and determined the heparin either with the meta-chromatic stain Azur 17 or by the ribonuclease inhibition technique of Lorenz et al. (1960). Since such small quantities as 0.15–0.40 μg of heparin per ml could be recovered from human plasma, endogenous plasma heparin in excess of 0.15 μg/ml could be excluded. The lowest concentration exerting an anticoagulant effect was found to be 1 μg/ml, one tenth of this concentration still having a lipemia clearing effect (König et al. 1959).

However, with the extensive use of heparin in the treatment of thrombo-embolic conditions, in hemodialysis and in extracorporeal circulation methods for checking the heparin content of the circulating blood became essential.

II. Assays for Anticoagulant Activity of Heparin

Assays for potency of a heparin sample or determining the heparin concentration in a biological medium rely on the use of biological systems in which heparin due to its strong electric charge interferes with one or several enzyme reactions. The conventional medium used for this purpose is blood, but single enzyme reactions may prove as useful (Zöllner and Lorenz, 1963). Heparin samples derived from different sources and almost identical in chemical composition, except possibly for variations in molecular weight and size, vary considerably in strength. Chemical methods are, therefore, less specific. The same applies to methods based on metachromatic color reactions. A substantial number of techniques depending on the anticoagulant properties of heparin have appeared in the literature.

In the following this literature will be briefly reviewed, emphasizing only the principle features of different types of suggested assays. Towards the end of this presentation a few selected assay procedures will be described in detail.

Fresh whole blood was the first medium used and it is still the most reliable one. Fresh blood taken directly from the blood vessel was filled into series of small test tubes containing increasing amounts of heparin and the coagulation time measured (Howell, 1924; Charles and Scott, 1933; Jorpes, 1935). These techniques (Jaques and Bell, 1959; Jorpes, 1946) are suited for the assay of samples in preparative work and for that purpose they are superior to other techniques. Jaques et al. stated in 1955 that "the biological activity of heparin in terms of its action on freshly drawn whole blood alone gives relative values corresponding to what is found when materials are injected intravenously. In addition, we have never found other types of assay to have the reproducibility of the whole blood method."

The main advantage of the fresh whole blood methods is that the technique ensures the presence of the heparin co-factor and all the labile factors entering into the coagulation system without any admixture of additional salts or thromboplastin. In fact, the whole blood in vitro method as elaborated for bovine blood by Jalling et al. (1946) gave the same values for the strength of a series of heparin preparations as found by an in vivo technique. In view of the difficulties in obtaining uniform results by the use of the in vitro methods using citrated or oxalated plasma, Jorpes et al. (1954) devised an in vivo method in which heparin in suitable increments was injected intravenously in unanesthetised sheep and the coagulation times measured 4 minutes after injection. The increments in clotting time closely paralleled the increasing doses of heparin. This method has no practical applicability.

Whole blood preserved with sodium sulfate, as suggested by Hewson (1771), (50 ml of a 7 percent solution to 250 ml of fresh bovine blood) has proved to be a very suitable medium. It can be stored below 4° C for several weeks. The coagulation time is reduced to a few minutes by the addition of bovine brain thromboplastin. The blood is diluted with one volume of a dilute heparin solution containing one-fifth volume of a thromboplastin solution. Three different concentrations of heparin, both of the unknown and of the standard, differing in strength by 20 percent, are used. The method as described by Adams and Smith (1950) was accepted as the official method of the British Pharmacopoeia of 1953. It has proven very useful.

The use of *oxalated or citrated blood or plasma,* which can be stored, is much more convenient than the use of fresh whole blood, and promised to simplify laboratory routine. Reinert and Winterstein (1939) measured the influence of different amounts of heparin on the coagulation time of *recalcified citrated sheep plasma,* a technique later applied by Foster (1942) and by Kuizenga et al. (1943), and finally accepted as the official method of U.S.P., XIV, 1950.

The method has its drawbacks and has met with criticism (Studer and Winterstein, 1951; Blombäck et al. 1953; Winterstein, 1957). The citrated plasma undergoes changes through disruption of platelets with formation of partial thromboplastin and the addition of ionized calcium is a delicate step. Suitably modified, however, the method can give values in conformity with the thrombin and whole blood methods (Pritchard, 1956).

The weaknesses of the earlier methods for the assay of the anticoagulant activity of a heparin preparation were discussed by Winterstein (1957). For one and the same heparin sample the U.S.P. XIV, 1950 method gave in different laboratories values varying between 15.6 and 25.8 units per mg and the B.P. 1953 method values between 18 and 68 units per mg.

Walton et al. (1966) compared the two methods in assaying the strength of heparin samples from different animal species and different organs, lungs, intestinal mucosa etc. against standard samples of the lung heparin and the mucosal heparin. There were wide variations in the results. Belks and Warren (1958), however, found the recalcification technique useful and time-saving for the routine control of heparinemia, the values differing only slightly from those of the whole blood coagulation time.

Likewise, McGoon (1950) found the use of recalcified citrated blood and specially constructed "hour glass" tubes very simple. The error of the technique was considered to be below 5 percent.

The inconveniences of recalcification can be avoided by *inducing coagulation with thrombin,* which shortens the coagulation time in proportion to the amount added to a range between 10 and 120 seconds, and furthermore, makes the end-point sharper. Because of the specific antithrombic action of heparin, thrombin is the appropriate reagent to neutralize the action of heparin. Thrombin methods as introduced by Jaques and Charles (1941) for oxalated whole blood and further elaborated by Kjems and Wagner (1948) for oxalated bovine plasma and by Studer and Winterstein (1951) for citrated plasma soon became the most commonly used techniques. Kjems and Wagner (1948) stated that "it is possible by this procedure to determine the potency of an unknown heparin sample with great accuracy and more rapidly than by existing methods". If properly applied the thrombin methods give good results (Jaques and Bell, 1959; Blombäck et al. 1953, 1955).

The details of the method of Studer and Winterstein were discussed by Winterstein (1957) and by Mercier (1959). Because of the sensitivity of the coagulation system to even small changes in the pH of the medium the thrombin is dissolved in a buffer solution, pH 7.3. Besides the advantages of rapid performance, easy reproducibility and insignificant cost, the relative standard deviation of the method is claimed to be only $\pm$ 2 percent.

Instead of using plasma as the substrate, the test can be performed with fibrinogen, thrombin and a plasma fraction containing the heparin co-factor (Winterstein, 1957).

Equipment suitable for bedside determination of the coagulation time, the prothrombin and the antithrombin time of blood and plasma has been described by Marbet and Winterstein (1953).

In using the thrombin methods precautions must be taken to ensure that enough heparin co-factor is present in the system, allowing the heparin, if present in higher concentrations, to exert its full action (Burstein, 1954). Since human plasma can be deficient in this respect, Blombäck et al. (1955) added an equal volume of citrated bovine plasma to the human plasma to be analyzed.

III. Control of Heparinemia

The techniques applied in routine determination of the heparin content of blood are based on the determination of the coagulation time of either unaltered or citrated whole blood or of blood or plasma after adding a heparin neutralizing agent.

The most elaborate technique of measuring the coagulation time was introduced by Hartert (1955) with the *thrombelastograph* (Chapter III, p. 70).

In the techniques using fresh whole blood every detail, such as venipuncture technique, glassware, whether siliconized or not, possible exclusion of air, temperature and moisture in the coagulation chamber must be carefully considered (Olwin et al. 1958). Jaques and

Bell (1959) modified the Lee and White clotting time technique utilizing protamine sulfate for the in vitro titration of heparin. A modification of the moving watchglass method of Bergquist (1945) is described by Jorpes et al. (1954). In other techniques use is made of glass capillaries or nonsiliconized small test tubes containing moving glass beads (Hedenius, 1936).

According to Struver et al. (1962) a cephalin (partial thromboplastin) time method gives greater precision and reproducibility than the Lee-White technique and also allows serial determinations to be made within the operating room.

Since heparin interferes with thromboplastin formation in the intrinsic system, the thromboplastin generation test (Biggs et al. 1953; MacMillan and Brown, 1954) can be used for its assay. However, the mechanism of this reaction is complicated and the analytical technique time-consuming.

With a well controlled thromboplastin preparation added before recalcification, straight line curves for the coagulation times can be obtained over a much wider range of heparin concentration than with the thrombin technique, in which the thrombin concentration must be carefully adjusted according to the heparin content of the plasma (Hiepler, 1959).

For in vitro titration of the heparin content of blood the thrombin and heparin precipitating agents *protamine* or *polybrene* are the most frequently used reagents. A rapid nonspecific turbidometric method based on the use of streptomycin was described by Altescu (1963). Marbet and Winterstein (1951a) also elaborated a nephelometric technique for the determination of heparin in urine.

The possibility of neutralizing heparin with protamine, as first described by Chargaff and Olson (1938) was utilized by Jaques and Waters (1941) for the in vitro titration of the heparin content of the blood. For references see LeRoy et al. (1950) and Refn and Vestergaard (1954). The latter authors improved the method by titrating with thrombin the small amounts of heparin still present in excess close to the neutralization point. The method was worked out for 5–10 ml of citrated blood with 10–20 μg heparin per ml plasma.

In 1939 Jorpes et al. found that pyrogen-free protamine preparations could be given intravenously in man for the in vivo neutralization of heparin, and in 1953 Preston and Parker introduced Polybrene, Hexadimethrine bromide (Abbott), a quaternary ammonium salt, a polymer of N_1 N_1 N_1' N_1' tetramethylhexamethylene and trimethylene bromide, molecular weight 5000–10,000 as a heparin neutralizer.

The heparin equivalent of protamine was determined by Jaques (1943) by measuring the coagulation time after adding 0.5 ml of whole blood to a series of test tubes containing protamine in different amounts, ranging from 0.5 to 0.005 mg per 0.5 ml. Birkinshaw and Smith (1962) quantitated the excess of heparin or protamine in mixtures by staining a spot of the solution on Whatman No. 1 filter paper with bromocresol green, and found that 1 mg of protamine sulfate neutralizes 100 units of heparin, with small variations depending on the samples of heparin and protamine used.

Perkins et al. (1956) titrated out the minimal amount of protamine which restores normal clotting times at the end of surgical procedures by adding 1 ml of whole blood to a series of test tubes, containing from 0 to 50 μg of protamine in 5 μg increments. Even if the amount of heparin neutralized by a definite amount of protamine sulfate varies somewhat with the degree of purity of the two components (Godal, 1960), the amount of circulating heparin can be determined by in vitro titration either with protamine or with polybrene.

Applying the technique of Perkins et al. (1956) of protamine titration in 27 cases of cardiopulmonary bypass, Hawksley (1966) found that over half of the cases required half or less than half the standard dose of protamine generally recommended. A rigid standard dose of protamine, based solely on previous heparin given could lead to considerable and possibly dangerous overdosage.

The thrombin time of heparinized plasma is influenced by a number of factors, the content of heparin co-factor, calcium, ionic strength and pH. However, according to Godal (1961) none of these factors affect the heparin-antiheparin ratio as determined by titration with polybrene. Godal found this synthetic antiheparin more reliable than protamine for the titration of heparin in plasma. Increasing amounts of polybrene were added to the plasma until the thrombin time was shortened no further. He calculated that 0.9 mg of polybrene is equivalent to 1 mg of heparin.

For restoration of normal coagulability at the end of surgery Keats et al. (1959) found protamine and polybrene effective in equivalent doses. None of a series of 40 patients required additional amounts of the antiheparin agents in the postoperative period. The subjective effects produced by both drugs at twice the heparin neutralizing dose were mild and transient. Heparin, 1.5 mg/kg, had been administered just before cardiopulmonary bypass and the neutralizing agent, 2.5–3 mg/kg, intravenously upon removal of the catheters.

In spite of adequate neutralization of the circulating heparin with protamine a state of hypocoagulability accompanied by a bleeding tendency may develop within a few hours, a situation referred to as "heparin rebound" by Hyun et al. (1962). The hypocoagulability can be corrected by injecting additional protamine, the dose of which is determined by special titration techniques as described by Frick and Brögli (1966) and Bollub (1967).

Andersen et al. (1959) found protamine administered in doses exceeding the heparin dosage by 100–200 percent to be sufficient. They considered the "heparin rebound" phenomenon to be caused by protamine excess rather than release of bound heparin.

Raby and Servelle (1962) found dosages of protamine or polybrene exceeding the heparin dosage by 1.5 to 2 times to be sufficient for restoration of normal clotting in most cases. However, they recommended a determination of the actual heparinemia 5–10 minutes after the last protamine or polybrene injection. In some cases the dose 1.5 mg of hexadimethrine per mg of heparin administered proved to be too low. The thotal dose necessary for exact neutralization corresponded to about three times the amount of residual heparin measured at the end of bypass. The same applies to protamine (Raby and Fernand-Laurent, 1962).

Lately the general use of polybrene has been seriously questioned. In 1962 Kimura et al. showed that there is a definite trend for the toxicity of hexadimethrine to increase in parallel with the increase in the average polymer size. Both the intravenous toxicity and the disrupting effects on the mast cells are interrelated through the average molecular size of the samples. In the same year Haller et al. (1962) observed lethal toxic symptoms in a number of patients due to severe renal tubular lesions after dosages of 5 mg polybrene/kg or higher. The symptoms were consistently reproducible in dogs. Likewise, Karlson and Lerner (1962) found in dogs that a polybrene excess of 1 mg/kg upset the coagulation mechanism prolonging the coagulation time, causing a poor clot retraction and reducing the platelet count, and the fibrinogen content. A polybrene excess of 5 mg/kg caused severe clotting changes. Evidently, the old story about the unreliability of synthetic compounds, foreign to the animal body, as compared to biological products, protamine in this case, has once more been repeated. If during preparation due attention is paid to freedom from pyrogens protamine can be made atoxic.

In order to avoid the threat of bleeding in the use of the artificial kidney hemodialysis Gordon et al. (1956) introduced a technique of *regional heparinization in the dialyzer circuit*. This procedure consisted of the infusion of heparin into the blood leaving the patient and of protamine into the blood re-entering the patient. The excess of heparin is in both situations to be determined by in vitro titration.

Darby et al. (1960), who applied the principle in 35 six-hour dialyses reduced the volume of blood necessary for a heparin analysis to 1 ml by performing the test with 0.2 ml plasma and 0.1 ml thrombin solution of a suitable strength.

According to Beall (1963), the renal hemodynamic effects of protamine sulfate and hexadimethrine bromide are similar.

Because of the imminent risk of osteoporosis in administering heparin in daily doses above 10,000 IU or 100 mg heparin (Griffith et al.

1965; Jaffee and Willis, 1965) to patients undergoing periodic extracorporeal dialysis, Thurnherr et al. (1967) supervised the patients by Ca-balanced studies and X-ray examinations. They reduced the heparin to the minimum necessary for anticoagulation without risk of clotting in the dialysis apparatus. A micromodification of the thrombin method elaborated by Blombäck et al. (1955, 1959) proved efficient.

In addition to sources of error already discussed in connection with the determination of heparin content of the blood there is one which always is to be kept in mind, namely hypofibrinogenemia. In extracorporeal circulation and hemodialysis a more or less pronounced fibrinogenolysis may take place, and in septic conditions a multiple peripheral fibrin deposition may lead to hypo- or afibrinogenemic conditions simulating hyperheparinemia. Routine analyses for fibrinogen are, therefore, recommended.

IV. Technical Procedures

A. Determination of Strength of Heparin Preparations According to Howell as Modified by Jaques and Charles (1941)

Principle: 0.1, 0.2, 0.3 ml of the standard heparin solution (2.5 u/ml) and of four dilutions of the unknown heparin varying by 10 percent in concentration are placed in calibrated test tubes. Fresh arterial blood is added to the 1 ml mark. After 2 hours, the degree of clotting in the tubes of unknown solution is matched with that of the standard tubes. The method was adopted officially in the *British Pharmacopoeia,* 1948.

Procedure: Wash Pyrex culture tubes (8 mm i.d., marked at 1.0 ml) thoroughly, using cleaning solution, and boil in distilled water. Select fifteen tubes of uniform bore for each assay. Prepare a standard heparin solution containing 2.5 International units per ml. All solutions are made up in 0.85 percent saline containing 0.3 percent tricresol. Dilute the unknown solution to approximately the same strength as the standard, as indicated by preliminary assay, and prepare four such dilutions differing by 10 percent. Measure 0.1, 0.2, 0.3 ml of each solution (standard and four dilutions of the unknown) into the tubes, and add saline to 0.3 ml.

Anesthetize a cat by intraperitoneal injection of sodium amytal (80 mg/kg). Expose one carotid artery and insert a clean glass cannula. Fill the tubes to the 1 ml mark with blood, the 0.1 ml tubes first, then 0.2 ml tubes in the reverse order, and finally the 0.3 ml tubes. As each tube is filled, the contents are mixed by inverting twice in such a manner that the blood covers the inside area of the tube. Three such racks may be filled at the same time placed in a water bath at 25° C, and covered. It is advisable to inspect the tubes at intervals. After 2 hours read the tubes by tipping each tube and judging the degree of clotting. A complete clot which does not break upon tipping is recorded as plus, completely fluid blood as minus. Intermediate stages may be designated by D^+, D, dd, d. At least four intermediate stages can be distinguished, and, with practice, eight. After completing the reading, the data are examined. For acceptance, the readings for the tubes containing the standard must match either those for one middle dilution of unknown solution or lie between the readings for the two mid-dilutions. The potency of the unknown is calculated from the matching dilution which contains 2.5 u/ml. Instead of cats, dogs can be used equally well.

B. Determination of Heparin as an Antithrombin According to Studer and Winterstein (1951)

Principle: Increasing amounts of heparin are added to beef plasma and this is clotted with thrombin. A curvilinear relation is found between heparin (0.1–0.3 mg of standard) and clotting time (30–70 seconds). The amount of heparin in the unknown is determined by comparison with the standard in this range.

Procedure: Collect ox blood in citrate, centrifuge, and, after standing for 24 hours at 0° C, store the plasma in wide-mouthed flasks at –10° C. Before use, liquefy by warming with warm water, filter, and keep during the day in the refrigerator. Prepare 0.1 percent solution of standard heparin (100–130 u/mg). Adjust the pH of all heparin solutions to 6–8. With a 0.1 percent thrombin solution (0.60 NIH units/ml), determine the amount of thrombin to give a time difference of 5 seconds between the clotting times without heparin and with 0.1 mg, and about 10 seconds difference between the values for 0.1 and 0.2 mg. With 0.3 mg of heparin, the clotting time should be about 60 seconds. Optimal conditions must be determined for each plasma. For this, place 1 ml of plasma in a 10 cm test tube in a water bath at 37° C. In another test tube, put 0.5 ml of distilled water or heparin solution (0.1, 0.2, or 0.3 ml standard and water to 0.5 ml). Add 5 ml of thrombin. Dilute the mixture accurately 1:20, add 1.0 ml to the plasma, and start a stop watch. With a platinum loop make a series of movements from below upward (two per second). The first fibrin strand remains on the loop, and at this moment stop the watch and read the clotting time. Having established the thrombin concentration required, make three to five determinations for each of 0, 0.10, 0.20. 0,25, and 0.30 mg of heparin. Single values should not fluctuate by more than 1 second.

To determine the potency of heparin preparations of unknown activity, follow the same procedure as in the establishment of the standard curve to find the concentrations of the unknown preparation which give clotting times of 30–75 seconds. Then take five dilutions of standard and five dilutions of unknown, giving clotting times in quintuplicate. Calculate the potency of the unknown in International units from the potency of the standard either graphically or by least squares, testing for linearity and parallelism.

C. Determination of Heparin in Blood from Coagulation Times (Jaques and Ricker, 1948; and Jaques and Bell, 1959)

To determine the amount of heparin in a blood sample from the clotting time, it is necessary to know whether the same clotting times are obtained when heparin and blood are mixed in vitro and in vivo. Careful analysis has shown that, after injection of heparin, the peak clotting time obtained is higher than when the same concentration of heparin is added to the blood from the same subject in vitro. When blood is removed by using silicone-treated syringes, mixed with heparin in a silicone-treated tube, and after 5 minutes transferred to a glass tube, the clotting time is the same as in vivo. This procedure (ex vivo) must then be followed when determining clotting times for the estimation of heparin levels in blood.

Procedure: For silicone-treated syringes and glassware, the dry glassware is rinsed with General Electric Dri-Film No. 9987-petroleum ether (1:4). The excess is drained off and the articles rinsed thoroughly with distilled water (*Warning:* HCl is set free!). The treatment is repeated twice and the articles are wrapped to keep them dust-free. They can be sterilized by boiling in distilled water but should be recoated after each use. The silicone can be removed by soaking overnight in 7.5 percent NaOH in acetone or by boiling in an Alconox solution. Twenty-gauge needles are boiled for 2 minutes in 1 percent Arquad (Armour and Co., Chicago), rinsed, and allowed to dry.

To collect blood in silicone, the vein is distended by exercise, shut off with a tourniquet or cuff set below arterial pressure, and the treated needle passed directly through the skin into the vein. Blood is drawn into the silicone-treated syringe at the same rate of flow as it enters the vein, care being taken to avoid eddies in the syringe or collapsing or distending the vein. When sufficient blood is obtained, withdraw the needle quickly, detach, discard about 10 percent of the blood, and use 80 percent, leaving a further 10 percent (first blood into syringe) for discard. It must be remembered that the silicone technique is like sterile technique-one break in technique by contact with damaged tissue or uncoated glass nullifies it.

To determine coagulation times by the Lee and White method, wash 8 × 75 mm Pyrex test tubes thoroughly, treat with chromate-sulfuric acid cleaning solution, rinse, and finally boil in distilled water three times. Place 1 ml of blood in a tube in a water bath and tilt gently at 15 or 30 second intervals until clotting occurs (the tube can be turned upside down). Time with a stop watch.

To establish the relation between heparin concentration and coagulation time, place suitable amounts of heparin (e.g., 0.1, 0.2, 0.3, 0.5, 1.0 units) in silicone-treated 5 ml beakers. Take blood from the subject by using the silicone-treated syringe and Arquad needle, and add 1.0 ml to the heparin solutions and mix. After 5 minutes, determine the clotting times on these mixtures by drawing the sample into a plain glass syringe, transferring it to an 8 mm test tube, and timing the coagulation as described above. This gives the ex vivo curve.

To measure circulating heparin after injection or liberation of endogenous heparin, draw 3 ml of blood with a 5 ml plain syringe, observing the precautions described for collecting blood in silicone. Discard 1 ml and transfer the second ml to an 8 mm test tube in the water bath, and determine the clotting time. The concentration of heparin equivalent to this is read from the ex vivo test.

D. Protamine Titration of Heparin in Blood According of Refn and Vestergaard (1954)

In the original description of this test by Jaques (1943) protamine was added directly to heparinized blood resulting in a reduction of clotting times to normal values when the equivalent amount of protamine was used. The exact amount of protamine required to give a concentration of protamine in the blood which completely depresses dissociation of the heparin-protamine compound is proportional to the concentration of heparin present and thus can be used for estimating the amount of heparin. In the modification by Refn and Vestergaard to be described below thrombin is added to assure that the titration is not effected by a larger or smaller amount of thromboplastin in the plasma samples. The antithrombin effect of heparin is utilized for determining the equivalence point, as a small excess of heparin in proportion to protamine has a marked effect on the coagulation time.

Procedure:

Reagents: 0.9 percent NaCl solution
40 percent trisodium citrate solution and the following stock solutions prepared in 0.9 percent NaCl solution:
heparin 400 γ/ml
protamine sulphate 1 mg/ml
Thrombin (Hoffmann la Roche) 1 mg/ml.

By venipuncture withdraw 10 ml of blood and transfer it directly from the syringe into a centrifuge tube containing 0.1 ml 40 percent trisodium citrate solution. Mix the sample and centrifuge, then remove the plasma with a Pasteur pipette. Transfer 0.5 ml plasma to a test tube with an inside diameter of 7 mm and a length of 70 mm. Add 0.3–0.7 ml of a diluted protamine sulphate solution and then 0.2 ml diluted thrombin solution. Immediately after addition of the thrombin start a stopwatch, close the tube with a paraffined cork and tilt it continuously until coagulation occurs. Excess of protamine will produce a short clotting time independent of the excess amount. If there is a protamine deficit – i.e. excess of heparin – the effect will be a prolonged clotting time, due to the antithrombin effect of heparin, even very small differences in the quantity of free heparin involving great variations in the clotting time. Utilizing 5 to 7 plasma samples, 0.5 ml each, and varying amounts of protamine, the equivalence is determined, corresponding to the smallest amount of protamine that gives a short clotting time.

The equivalence ratio between protamine and heparin:

$$= \frac{\gamma \text{ protamine sulphate}}{\gamma \text{ heparin}}$$

is about 1.3 but varies with the protamine sulphate employed. In order to avoid marked variations in the volume of the reaction mixture, the concentration of the protamine sulphate solution is varied according to the expected heparin content. With a heparin content of 10 γ/ml plasma, a protamine sulphate solution of about 15 γ/ml will be suitable.

As a guide in the choice of a suitable dilution of thrombin for the assay it may be stated that 0.2 ml solution should give a clotting time lying between 10 and 20 seconds with 0.5 ml normal plasma.

The equivalence ratio is determined from the difference observed when titrating normal plasma samples after addition of known quantities of heparin, e. g. 10 and 20 γ hep./ml plasma.

If it is found that a plasma sample of which the heparin content is to be determined contains less than 5 γ/ml, it is of advantage to add a known amount of heparin in vitro.

In a series of dog experiments the titres were determined on two samples taken one immediately after the other by venipuncture. In these titrations the standard deviation of a single determination was 15 percent.

It is essential that all glass surfaces are thoroughly cleaned and that the test tubes employed have equal diameters. It has been found that the addition of NaCl solution to compensate for variations in volume of protamine solution is unnecessary. The analyses can be made at room temperature, though stock solutions should be kept cold.

The earlier methods of titration give increasing clotting times when excess of protamine is increased and therefore a minimum in clotting time at equivalence is obtained. In the method described here excess of protamine does not alter the clotting time. According to Chargaff (1938) the explanation is that the anticoagulant effect of protamine is not an antithrombin effect. This constancy of the clotting time with excess of protamine makes the equivalence point less well defined, theoretically, but in practice it is an advantage, because a prolonged coagulation time unequivocally shows that more protamine must be added, and therefore the equivalence point is found more quickly and with the use of a smaller quantity of plasma.

The method has been applied in control of sublingual heparin dosage (Refn and Raaschou, 1952) and subcutaneous application of heparin (Raaschou, Refn and Vestergaard, 1954).

References

Adams, S. S., and Smith, K. L. (1950). *J. Pharm. Pharmacol. 2,* 836.

Altescu, E. J. (1963). *J. Pharm. Pharmacol. 15,* 488.

Andersen, M. N., Mendelow, M., and Alfano, G. A. (1959). *Surgery 46,* 1060.

Beall, A., Jr. (1963). *Cardiovasc. Res. Center Bull. Bylor Univ. Coll. Med. 1,* 76.

Belko, J. S., and Warren, R. (1958). *Arch. Surgery 76,* 210.

Bergquist, E. (1945). *Acta Chir. Scand. 92,* Suppl. 101.

Biggs, R., Douglas, A. S., and Macfarlane, K. G. (1953). *J. Physiol. 122,* 554.

Birkinshaw, V. J., and Smith, K. L. (1962). *J. Pharm. Pharmacol. 14,* Suppl. 95.

Blombäck, B., Blombäck, M., Corneliusson, E. V., and Jorpes, J. E. (1953). *J. Pharm. Pharmacol. 5,* 1031.

Blombäck, B., Blombäck, M., and Wallén, P. (1955). *Rev. Hématol. 10,* 45.

Blombäck, B., Blombäck, M., Olsson, P., William-Olsson, G., and Senning, A. (1959). *Acta Chir. Scand.,* Suppl. *245,* 259.

British Pharmacopoeia (1953). pp. 257, 833.

Burstein, M. (1954). *Semaine d'Hôpit. 30,* 1.

Chargaff, E. (1938). *J. Biol. Chem. 125,* 671.

Chargaff, G., and Olson, K. B. (1938). *J. Biol. Chem. 122,* 1953.

Charles, A. F., and Scott, D. A. (1933). *J. Biol. Chem. 102,* 425, 437.

Darby, J. P., Sorensen, R. J., O'Brien, Th. F., and Teschan, P. E. (1960). *New England J. Med. 262,* 654.

Foster, R. H. K. (1942). *J. Lab. Clin. Med. 27,* 820.

Frick, P. G., and Brögli, H. (1966). *Surgery 59,* 721.

Gibson, R. B., Carr, T. L., Green, S., and Fowler, W. M. (1952). *Proc. Soc. Exptl. Biol. Med. 79,* 577.

Godal, H. C. (1960). *Scand. J. Clin. Lab. Invest. 12,* 446.

Godal, H. C. (1961). *Scand. J. Clin. Lab. Invest. 13,* 153.

Gollub, S. (1967). *Surg. Gynecol. Obstet. 124,* 337.

Gordon, L. A., Simon, E. R., Rukes, J. M., Richards, V., and Perkins, H. A. (1956). *New England J. Med. 255,* 1063.

Griffith, G. C., Nichols, D., Jr., Asher, J. D., and Flanagan, B. (1965). *J. Am. Med. Assoc. 193,* 85.

Haller, J. A., Jr., Ransdell, H. T., Stovens, D., and Rubel W. F. (1962). *J. Thorac. Cardiovasc. Surg. 44,* 486.

Hartert, H. (1955). *Z. Klin. Med. 153,* 432.

Hawskley, M. (1966). *Lancet 1,* 563.

Hedenius, P. (1936). *Acta Med. Scand. 88,* 5.

Hiepler, E. (1959). *Arzneimittelforschung 9,* 763.

Howell, W. H. (1924). *Am. J. Physiol. 71,* 553.

Hyun, B. H., Pence, R. E., Davila, J. C., Butcher, J., and Custer, R. P. (1962). *Surg. Gynecol. Obstet. 115,* 191.

Jaffe, M. D., and Willis, P. W. (1965). *J. Am. Med. Assoc. 193,* 152.

Jalling, O., Jorpes, J. E., and Linden, G. (1946). *Quart. J. Pharm. Pharmacol. 19,* 96.

Jaques, L. B. (1943). *Biochem. J. 37,* 1898.

Jaques, L. B. (1949). *Acta Haematol. 2,* 188.

Jaques, L. B., and Bell, H. J. (1959). *Methods of Biochem. Analysis 7,* 253.

Jacques, L. B., and Charles, A. F. (1941). *Quart. J. Pharm. Pharmacol. 14,* 1.

Jaques, L. B., and Ricker, A. G. (1948). *Blood 3,* 1197.

Jaques, L. B., and Waters, E. T. (1941). *J. Physiol. 99,* 454.

Jacques, L. B., Monkhouse, F. C., and Stewart, M. (1949). *J. Physiol. 109,* 41.

Jaques, L. B., Bell, H. J., and Cho, M. H. (1955). *Proc. International Conf. on Thrombosis and Embolism,* Basle 1954, p. 281.

Jorpes, J. E. (1935). *Biochem. J. 29,* 1817.

Jorpes, J. E. (1946). "Heparin". Oxford University Press.

Jorpes, J. E., Edman, P., and Thaning, T. (1939). *Lancet 237,* 975.

Jorpes, J. E., Blombäck, M., and Blombäck, B. (1954). *J. Pharm. Pharmacol. 6,* 694.
Karlson, K. E., and Lerner, B. (1962). *Ann. Surg. 156,* 875.
Keats, A. S., Denton, A. C., and Telford, J. (1959). *J. Thorac. Cardiovasc. Surg. 38,* 362.
Kimura, T., Young, P. R., and Barlow, G. H. (1962). *Proc. Soc. Exptl. Biol. Med. 111,* 37.
Kjems, H., and Wagner, H. (1948). *Acta Pharmacol. Toxicol. 4,* 155.
König, E., Seitz, W., and Zöllner, N. (1959). *Zeitschr. Physiol. Chem. 314,* 177.
Kuizenga, M. H., Nelson, J. W., and Cartland, G. F. (1943). *Am. J. Physiol. 139,* 612.
LeRoy, G. V., Halpern, B., and Dolkart, R. E. (1950). *J. Lab. Clin. Med. 35,* 446.
Lorenz, B., Lorenz, R., and Zollner, N. (1960). *Z. Ges. Exptl. Med. 133,* 144.
Mac-Millan, R. L., and Brown, K. G. W. (1954). *J. Lab. Clin. Med. 44,* 378.
Marbet, R., and Winterstein, A. (1951a). *Helv. Physiol. Acta 9,* 17.
Marbet, R., and Winterstein, A. (1951b). *Helv. Physiol. Acta 9,* 24.
Marbet, R., and Winterstein, A. (1953). *Praxis 42,* 61.
Masure, R. (1960). "Les Inhibiteurs Normaux et Pathologiques de la Coagulation Sanguine." Mason, Paris.
Mercier, J. (1959). *Bull. Soc. Chim. Biol. 41,* 1101.
McGoon, D. C. (1950). *J. Lab. Clin. Med. 35,* 111.
Monkhouse, F. C., and Jaques, L. B. (1950). *J. Lab. Clin. Med. 36,* 782.
Monkhouse, F. C., Stewart, M., and Jaques, L. B. (1949). *Am. J. Physiol. 8,* 112.
Olwin, J. H., Arscott, P. M., and Koppel, J. L. (1958). *Geriatrics 13,* 773.
Perkins, H. A., Osborn, J., Hurt, R., and Gerbode, F. (1956). *J. Lab. Clin. Med. 48,* 223.
Preston, F. W., and Parker, R. P. (1953). *Arch. Surg. 66,* 545.
Pritchard, J. (1956). *J. Pharm. Pharmacol. 8,* 523.
Raby, C., and Fernand-Laurent, J. (1962). *Hemostase 2,* 329.
Raby, C., and Servelle, M. (1962). *Hemostase 2,* 325.
Raaschou, R., Refn, I., and Vestergaard, L. (1954). *Ugeskr. f. Laeger 116,* 281.
Refn, I., and Raaschou, F. (1952). *Nord. Med. 47,* 1952.
Refn, I., and Vestergaard, L. (1954). *Scand. J. Clin. Lab. Invest. 6,* 284.
Reinert, M., and Winterstein, A. (1939). *Arch. Int. Pharmacodyn. 62,* 47.
Struver, G. P., Bitner, D. L., and Wall, A. (1962). *Surg. Forum 13,* 127.
Studer, A., and Winterstein, A. (1951). *Helv. Physiol. Pharmacol. Acta 9,* 6.
Thurnherr, N., Tholen, H., and Duckert, F. (1967). *Helv. Med. Acta 33,* 334.
Walton, P. L., Ricketts, C. R., and Bangham, D. R. (1966). *Brit. J. Haematol. 12,* 310.
Winterstein, A. (1957). *Pharmaceut. Weekblad 92,* 982.
Zöllner, N., Lorenz, B. (1963). *In:* "Methods of Enzymatic Analysis" (N. U. Bergmeyer, ed.), pp. 79—86. Academic Press, New York.
Zöllner, N., Burger, Chr., and Braun, R. (1962). *Zeitschr. Physiol. Chem. 329,* 76.

Circulating Anticoagulants

E. Deutsch and K. Lechner

I. Introduction

Circulating anticoagulants have been observed in patients with already existing plasmatic bleeding disorders; in these instances, the inhibitors usually developed after treatment with plasma or plasma fractions. These inhibitors and those which also develop in rare cases post partum are isoantibodies. Circulating anticoagulants may develop also in the course of several diseases, such as collagen diseases (especially disseminated lupus erythematosus and rheumatoid arthritis), dermatological diseases (Pemphigus vulgaris, Dermatitis herpetiformis Duhring Brocq), liver disorders, diseases of the reticuloendothelial and lymphatic systems, and in the course of drug allergies. Occasionally, circulating anticoagulants were detected in patients without an associated disease state (Deutsch, 1961). These inhibitors belong to the autoantibodies.

Inhibitors can develop against any one of the known coagulation factors; most frequently, however, they seem to be directed against factor VIII.

According to their mode of action, the circulating anticoagulants can be categorized into two groups. One group of inhibitors apparently inactivates individual coagulant factors in a progressive and time-consuming reaction. The other group of circulating anticoagulants inhibits the reaction between coagulation factors in an almost immediate type of reaction. They probably interfere with the activation of the coagulation factor without actually destroying the factor. In this type of inhibition, the coagulation factor can be recovered when the inhibitor is separated.

The presence of circulating anticoagulants should be considered:

a. When patients with a known hemorrhagic diathesis suddenly become refractory against therapy.

b. When a coagulopathy suddenly develops in a previously healthy person.

c. When certain coagulation tests give contradictory results which are no longer in agreement with the pattern known for the typical plasmatic hemorrhagic diseases. Especially discrepancies between test systems using undiluted plasma, such as highly abnormal whole blood coagulation times, plasma recalcification times, prothrombin times, partial thromboplastin times and thrombelastogram on one hand, and normal individual coagulation factor activities (usually tested on diluted plasma), on the other hand, are indicative of the presence of certain types of circulating anticoagulants.

The search for anticoagulants can be followed in three steps. First, the demonstration of the presence of an inhibitor by means of test methods which measure the overall coagulability of blood or plasma (these tests will be discussed later). Obviously only those test systems should be used which give clearly abnormal results with the patient's plasma. In view of the possible presence of two different types of inhibitors, it is important to perform the tests immediately and upon incubation over a certain period of time. Second, the localization of the exact site of action of the inhibitor, and third, the purification and biochemical characterization of the inhibitor.

II. Demonstration of Inhibitors by Means of Test Systems Measuring the Overall Coagulability of Plasma

A. Recalcification Times of Mixtures of Plasma

1. Reagents

a. Platelet poor patient's plasma. Nine ml of blood are added to 1 ml of a 3.8% trisodium citrate solution in a siliconized container and after thorough mixing the blood is centrifuged at 4,000 g for 30 minutes at 4° C. The plasma is pipetted off using siliconized pipettes and placed in siliconized test tubes.

b. Platelet poor normal plasma. The plasma is obtained from the blood of a control person in the same way as outlined for patient's plasma.

c. 0.025 M calcium chloride solution.

2. Test Mixture

A 0.2 ml aliquot of calcium chloride solution is added into a test tube containing 0.2 ml of normal plasma, patient plasma, or mixtures of both. The contents are well mixed and placed in a water bath at 37° C. The coagulation times are determined.

3. Procedure

a. Before analysis, the patient's plasma and the normal plasma are stored in icewater. If possible, the test should be performed within an hour after withdrawal of the blood.

b. The two plasma samples are mixed in plastic containers as outlined in Table 1. At zero time 1 ml of the patient's plasma is pipetted into a plastic tube, and two 0.2 ml aliquots of plasma are removed and pipetted into two glass tubes. The plastic tube is stoppered and placed in a water bath at 37° C and a stop watch is started. The plasma samples in the two glass tubes are recalcified (see above) and the clotting times are recorded. After 10 minutes, the second mixture of the two plasmas is made (see Table 1) and two aliquots of 0.2 ml of this plasma mixture are removed for the determination of the recalcification times. The plastic tube is again stoppered and incubated in a water bath at 37° C. Further plasma mixtures are made at the specified time intervals as outlined in Table 1. After 60 minutes of incubation, again two times 0.2 ml are removed from mixture 1 and the recalcification times are once more determined. The remaining plasma mixtures are then processed at the designated time intervals in an identical manner.

4. Computation of the Results

The results are best expressed graphically, plotting coagulation times in seconds against plasma mixtures in percent (Fig. 1).

Table 1:

Mixture	1	2	3	4	5	6	7
Patient Plasma ml	1.0	0.9	0.8	0.5	0.2	0.1	0
Normal Plasma ml	0	0.1	0.2	0.5	0.8	0.9	1.0
Time of Mixture and First Assay	0'	10'	20'	30'	40'	45'	50'
Time of Second Assay	60'	70'	80'	90'	100'	105'	110'

5. Evaluation of the Results

a. The presence of an inhibitor is likely when the addition of 50 % normal plasma to the patient's plasma (mixture 4) does not completely normalize the recalcification times in one of the two sets of tests. If the addition of 10 to 20 % of patient's plasma to normal plasma (mixture 5 or 6) results in a considerable prolongation of the recalcification times of the normal plasma with or without incubation, the presence of an inhibitor is almost certain (Fig. 1, part 2).

b. The presence of an inhibitor must also be suspected when the shape of the tracing obtained after incubation differs significantly from the tracing prior to incubation.

c. When inhibition increases or becomes apparent only after incubation, an anticoagulant with a progressive mode of action may be suspected (Fig. 1, part 3). When inhibition is observed prior to incubation and does not increase during incubation, an anticoagulant with an immediate mode of action can be postulated (Fig. 1, part 2).

d. The amount of patient's plasma needed to inhibit the clotting times of normal plasma may be taken as a rough quantitative estimate of inhibitor level.

B. Miscellaneous Procedures

The basic principle of the test procedure outlined above also applies to any test system in which the overall coagulability of blood or plasma is measured. But the special conditions of each individual test procedure have to be considered. No further details will be dis-

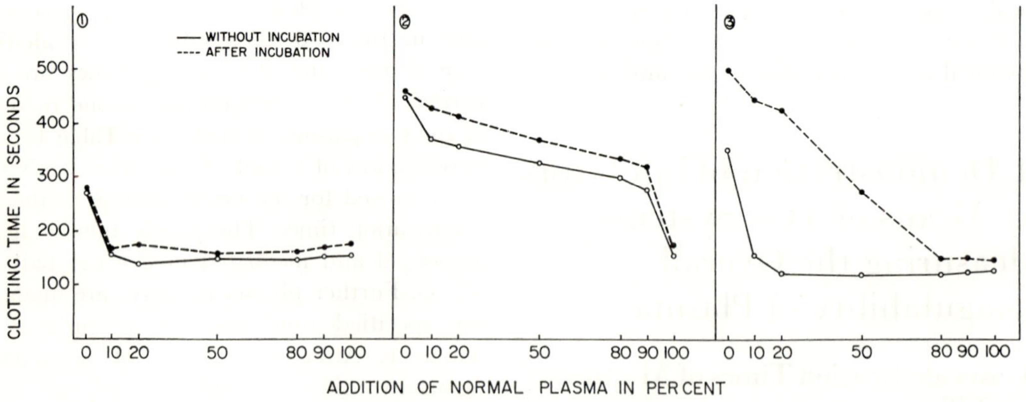

Fig. 1: Recalcification Times of Mixtures of Plasma.

O——O Coagulation times without incubation.

O - - - O Coagulation times after 60 minutes of incubation.

Part 1: Hemophilia A plasma without an inhibitor. Normalization of the prolonged clotting times is achieved by the addition of 10 % of normal plasma.

Part 2: Inhibitor with an immediate mode of action in a patient with L. E. No significant differences in the coagulation times with or without incubation. Already 10 % of the patient's plasma inhibits the coagulation times of normal plasma considerably.

Part 3: Inhibitor with a progressive mode of action in a patient with severe hemophilia A after several transfusions. Without incubation the coagulation defect is normalized by the addition of 20 % normal plasma. This is normal and under these circumstances an inhibitor would easily be missed. After incubation 50 % patient's plasma inhibits the coagulation of normal plasma considerably.

cussed; however, the usefulness of mixtures of whole blood for the determination of inhibitors of the contact phase might be emphasized at this point. This test system is especially useful when the clotting times are determined in both, glass and siliconized tubes. A further advantage of this procedure is that the blood is not diluted.

In principle, 20 ml of patient's blood and 20 ml of normal blood with an identical blood group are collected in siliconized tubes. Using siliconized pipettes, mixtures of the two blood samples are immediately made in glass tubes and siliconized tubes and the coagulation times are determined in each sample. The following scheme can be followed:

Normal Blood:	2.0	1.8	1.6	1.0	0.4	0.2	0.0 ml
Patient Blood:	0.0	0.2	0.4	1.0	1.6	1.8	2.0 ml

The tests can be performed at room temperature.

The results are evaluated as described above for recalcified plasma. Due to the long coagulation times of the blood in siliconized tubes both immediate inhibitors and those with a progressive mode of action are registered.

III. Determination of the Site of Action of an Inhibitor

The site of action of an inhibitor may be estimated by the simultaneous determination of the prothrombin times, partial thromboplastin times, and thrombin times, as outlined in Table 2.

However, the positive confirmation requires more elaborate techniques, which will be outlined below.

A. Inhibitors with a Progressive Mode of Action

In the presence of an inhibitor with a progressive mode of action low values for one of the coagulation factors can be expected. The presence of an inhibitor is then determined in this particular test system.

In principle, normal plasma or the purified coagulation factor and aluminum hydroxide adsorbed patient plasma or the purified inhibitor are incubated together at 37° C, and after varying time intervals the remaining activity of the coagulation factor in question is determined.

As an example, the procedure for the detection of an inhibitor against factor VIII is outlined:

1. The Determination of a Factor VIII — Inhibitor with a Progressive Mode of Action

A 0.2 ml sample of normal citrated plasma (source of factor VIII) and 0.2 ml of aluminum hydroxide adsorbed patient plasma are mixed and incubated in a plastic tube at 37° C. Immediately and as frequently as possible within the first 20 minutes of incubation a sample is removed, and after appropriate dilution, the factor VIII activity is measured either by means of a one-stage method using hemophilia A plasma as a substrate (Chapter V, p. 189), or by means of the thromboplastin generation test (Chapter III, p. 82). A parallel determination with a sample of aluminum hydroxide adsorbed hemophilia A plasma instead of the patient plasma is performed as a control. According to Shapiro (1967) one inhibitor unit is the amount of inhibitor which inactivates 30 %, of a 50 u/ml solution of factor VIII in 15 minutes at 37° C.

2. Determination of Factor VIII-Inhibitors According to Biggs and Bidwell (1959)

a. Reagents:

a. Bovine AHG (Maws Pharmacy Supplies Ltd. Ethical Division, Aldusgate House, Barnet, England): A solution is prepared with an activity of 1,000–2,000 % (approximately 10 mg dry substance/ml).

b. Aluminum hydroxide adsorbed patient plasma.

c. Aluminum hydroxide adsorbed plasma of a patient with hemophilia A without inhibitor.

d. Reagents for the thromboplastin generation test according to Biggs et al. (1955).

b. Technique:

a. Incubation: 0.1 ml bovine AHG is incubated with 0.9 ml of the adsorbed patient plasma for one hour at 37° C. At the same

Table 2:

Site of Action	Prothrombin Times	Partial Thromboplastin Times	Thrombin Times
Factor VIII, IX, XI, XII	Normal	Abnormal	Normal
Factor VII, Tissue Thromboplastin	Abnormal	Normal	Normal
Factor II, V, X	Abnormal	Abnormal	Normal
II. Stage	Normal (Abnormal)	Normal (Abnormal)	Abnormal

time bovine AHG is incubated with the adsorbed hemophilia A plasma. The concentration of the inhibitor should be selected in such a way that approximately 70–90% of the added factor VIII will be destroyed.

b. Determination of the remaining AHG: After one hour of incubation the control specimen is diluted with cold citrated saline solution in a proportion to 1:32 and 1:128. The sample containing the inhibitor is diluted to 1:16 and 1:64. The factor VIII activity is determined in 0.1 ml of these dilutions according to Biggs et al. (1955).

The inhibitor concentration is proportional to the logarithm of the residual factor VIII activity.

One inhibitor unit is defined as the amount of inhibitor which inactivates 75% of the added factor VIII after one hour of incubation.

c. Critical evaluation of the Procedure:

The disadvantage of this procedure is the elaborate technique and the use of reagents of different species (bovine AHG) in a human test system.

B. Inhibitors with an Immediate Mode of Action

These inhibitors commonly block the activation of a coagulation factor or the effect of an intermediate product. The effect of these inhibitors upon the test system can be reduced or eliminated by dilution. For the determination of the exact site of action multistage test systems of the intrinsic and extrinsic coagulation systems are best used which have to be composed ad hoc (see for example Breckenridge and Ratnoff [1963] and Yin and Gaston [1965]). The following sequence of steps of study may help to select an appropriate multistage system:

1. The inhibitor prolongs the prothrombin time and partial thromboplastin time, but not the thrombin time: Probable site of action: Factor X, V or Prothrombin.

2. The inhibitor interferes only with the prothrombin time: Probable site of action: Factor VII or tissue thromboplastin. It should be tested for species specifity in the latter case.

3. The inhibitor interferes only with partial thromboplastin time: Probable site of action: Factor XII, XI, IX or VIII.

4. The inhibitor prolongs the thrombin time: It interferes either with the effect of thrombin on fibrinogen or with the formation of fibrin itself. For the determination of such an inhibitor, the thrombin time test (Chapter V, p. 89) has to be modified by selecting a thrombin solution which clots a normal plasma in 20–25 seconds. Then mixtures of plasma are prepared as outlined above (II, A, 3, b). To 0.2 ml of each of the plasma mixtures, 0.2 ml of the thrombin solution are added and the coagulation times are determined.

If the thrombin times are prolonged, the presence of either heparin, a heparin-like substance, an antithrombin, abnormal proteins, or fibrin (-ogen) split products can be suspected. For further differentiation, the reader is referred to the appropriate chapters in this book.

In case of a dysproteinemia or paraproteinemia with prolongation of the thrombin times, individual plasma fractions should be prepared from the patient's plasma and individually tested in order to clearly demonstrate that the abnormal protein is responsible for the inhibition of clotting.

IV. Methods for the Biochemical Characterization of Inhibitors

Almost all of the circulating anticoagulants are gamma globulins in nature. For their characterization, the use of appropriate procedures of protein chemistry are recommended, such as ammonium sulfate precipitation, gel filtration on Sephadex G-200, chromatography on DEAE-cellulose, starchblock electrophoresis, immuno-electrophoresis, and immunoprecipitation techniques. Especially the loss of inhibitor activity after treatment with the specific antiserum and the isolation of the inhibitor by immunadsorption, etc. is recommended. For details of these individual techniques the reader is referred to special text books such as, for example, Heremans and Schultze (1966).

References

Biggs, R., and Bidwell, E. (1959). *Brit. J. Haematol. 5,* 379.

Biggs, R., Eveling, J., and Richards, G. (1955). *Brit. J. Haematol. 1,* 20.

Breckenridge, R. T., and Ratnoff, O. D. (1963). *Am. J. Med. 35,* 813.

Deutsch, E. (1961). *In:* "The Coagulation Balance" (I. S. Wright and F. Koller, eds.) p. 112. Schattauer Verlag, Stuttgart.

Heremans, J. F., and Schultze, H. E. (1966). Molecular Biology of Human Proteins. Vol I. Elsevier, Amsterdam-London-New York.

Shapiro, S. S. (1967). *J. Clin. Invest. 46,* 147.

Yin, E. T., and Gaston, L. W. (1965). *Thromb. Diath. Haemorrhag. 14,* 88.

Chapter VIII

Physiology and Biochemistry of Fibrinolysis

Nils U. Bang, M. D.

I. Introduction

The continuous rise in the number of publications dealing with fibrinolysis appearing in the literature over the last two to three decades attests to the intensive interest in the subject shared by workers in many fields of biological sciences. Indeed, the total literature on fibrinolysis has now expanded to the point where it can no longer be covered by any single review.

Several factors have contributed to this remarkable upsurge in interest in the fibrinolytic enzyme system in man and experimental animals. From the teleological standpoint an enzyme system capable of hydrolyzing fibrin and removing fibrin deposits intravascularly or extravascularly would seem to be desirable as a fundamental physiological defense mechanism. The importance of fibrin formation is not limited to its role in intravascular thrombotic occlusion but the deposition of fibrin is an integral part of tissue inflammatory response to any injury; be it traumatic, thermal, microbial or immunological. Indeed, it can be fairly stated that the deposition of fibrin, the rate at which it is deposited, the physical, chemical and morphological characteristics of deposited fibrin play a fundamental role in determining the natural history of a wide variety of pathological processes in man. Conversely, fibrinolysis may be considered a fundamental mechanism of repair of tissue injury.

The introduction of immunofluorescent techniques in experimental pathology has recently provided the means of confirming what had previously been suspected, that fibrin in tissues under suitable pathological circumstances may acquire tinctorial and morphological characteristics making it difficult or impossible to identify by standard histological techniques.

The use of special fibrin stains and of fluorescine-labelled fibrinogen or fibrin antibodies established the presence of fibrin in a wide variety of pathological lesions, e. g. the hyaline material accumulating in the arterioles in benign essential hypertension, in fibrinoid, as seen in collagen diseases, in the generalized Schwartzman reaction, in toxemias of pregnancy and as a component of at least some cases of amyloid deposits (Lendrum, 1961; Gitlin and Craig, 1957; Gitlin et al. 1953; Gitlin et al. 1957; Crawford and Wolf, 1960; Duguid, 1959; and Horowitz et al. 1965) (see also Morris et al. 1964). These recent examples serve to illustrate the omnipresence of fibrin in human pathology.

The demonstration of unusually rapid turnover rates of many clotting factors has lead several authors to the belief that blood coagulation and fibrin deposition is a continuous ongoing process. If this is true, it provides the fibrinolytic enzyme system with a logical purpose of maintaining the proper hemostatic balance by continuously removing deposited fibrin and, thus, maintaining patency of blood vessels and fluidity of circulating blood. As more fundamental knowledge on the biochemistry and physiology of the fibrinolytic enzyme system is gathered, the concept of a dynamic equilibrium between clotting and lysis is winning more supporters since such a hypothesis would seem to fit many recent experimental observations (Duguid, 1946; Astrup, 1959). A critical review of these concepts was furnished recently by Hjort and Hasselback (1961).

The development of pharmacological agents and enzyme preparations suitable for clinical trials in the treatment of thromboembolic diseases has further stimulated interest in fibrinolytic phenomena and has lead to a better, more concise formulation of the biochemistry of fibrinolysis and a better characterization of individual components of the system as well as the elucidation of the major pathways of activation of fibrinolysis. Assay systems have been developed for clinical trials which have proven adequate for the exact quantitation of fibrinolytic enzyme activity in the blood of patients receiving these agents providing useful guidelines for effective and safe therapy.

Experience gained in the area of therapeutic fibrinolysis has undoubtedly aided in elucidating many obscure aspects of the fibrinolytic enzyme system and its role in normal physiology and pathology and have lead to the formulation of important new concepts. Most importantly, the intensive studies in many laboratories focusing on the exact mechanism of the coagulation defect developing in the course of fibrinolytic enzyme therapy have substantially altered current thinking concerning the mechanisms of physiological and pathological fibrinolysis. The demonstration of the anticoagulant properties of products of fibrinogen proteolysis arising as a consequence of an active fibrinolytic state suggests another potential role for the fibrinolytic enzyme system in maintaining the appropriate dynamic equilibrium of fibrin formation and resolution. It is speculated that the release of fibrinogen products with anticoagulant properties may be as important a hemostatic regulatory mechanism as the removal of already deposited fibrin (section III).

It should be emphasized, however, that current hypotheses regarding the role of fibrinolysis in health and disease although extremely attractive remain hypothetical. The one major requirement for continued progress in this entire field is the development of more sensitive and specific assay systems than heretofore available. It is a serious shortcoming in this area currently that no methods are available which predictably and accurately register subtle variations in fibrinolytic activity under varying physiological circumstances in whole undiluted blood or blood plasma. Although Sawyer et al. (1960a), using a sensitive ^{131}I-labelled fibrin substrate, was able to demonstrate fibrinolytic activity in normal freshly drawn plasma from non-stressed subjects wide variations was demonstrated within this group of normal plasmas requiring a large number of samples and statistical analysis to confirm the presence of significant levels of fibrinolytic activity under normal circumstances. Increased sensitivity in assays for fibrinolytic activity can be accomplished through a variety of techniques depending on dilution and/or acidification of the test plasma by which normal inhibitors are separated from the activators and enzymes of the system. Although a multitude of observations on fluctuations in fibrinolytic activity under physiological or pathological circumstances have been made utilizing such assay systems and although the results in many instances showed differences which turned out to be significant on statistical analysis in support of some of these most interesting hypotheses; it would be wise, in the author's view, to treat all these postulates with some reservation until we learn to understand the relevance and true significance of the information obtained through assay systems separating activators and inhibitors.

Another area of intensive interest in recent years has been the delineation of the exact role played by the fibrinolytic enzyme system in a wide variety of disease states associated with generalized bleeding tendencies. The description of severe hemorrhagic state associated with low plasma fibrinogen levels and rapid lysis of blood clots by in vitro testing was first described in the obstetrical literature which is not suprising since the most severe and extreme cases of bleeding associated with enhanced fibrinolysis are seen in obstetrical cases. However, since the first descriptions of pathological fibrinolysis in cases of abruptio placentae and other obstetrical emergencies by De Lee at the turn of the century (De Lee, 1901), it has become apparent that pathologically-enhanced levels of fibrinolytic activity in plasma may account for bleeding tendency in a wide variety of diseases such as traumatic injuries (Scott et al. 1954), major surgery

(Meyers et al. 1957; von Kaulla and Swan, 1958; von Kaulla et al. 1960; Marchal et al. 1961; Soulier et al. 1952a, b), cirrhosis of the liver (Goodpasture, 1914), lymphomas (Schulz and Knoblock, 1954; Cooperberg and Neiman, 1955; Baker et al. 1964) and severe progressive strokes (Bang, 1965). With improved assay techniques and improved understanding of basic mechanisms involved, it has also become apparent that fibrinolysis may contribute not only to serious bleeding problems but also may account for a mild generalized hemorrhagic diathesis in many clinical situations.

The diagnosis of fibrinolysis as the major etiological factor in cases of clinical bleeding represents a problem which is no longer of merely academical interest. Since the introduction of specific pharmacological agents capable of inhibiting fibrinolysis such as epsilon aminocaproic acid (EACA, Amicar®, Lederle), 1-aminomethyl) cyclohexane-4-carboxylic acid (AMCHA), (Okamoto and Okamoto, 1962) and p-aminomethyl benzoic acid (PAMBA), (Lohmann et al. 1964) as well as the introduction of broad-spectrum protease inhibitors (Trasylol®, Bayer), the problem of accurately differentiating between pathological fibrinolysis on one hand and the so-called defibrination syndrome (see section by Maki and Beller) on the other hand presents a major challenge with theoretical, biochemical as well as practical therapeutical implications.

The foregoing introductory remarks have served to outline the scope and diversification of ongoing research in fibrinolysis. The remainder of this review will deal with specific aspects of the overall problems as outlined. However, an exhaustive review at this time would follow too closely a number of excellent and detailed surveys of fibrinolysis appearing within the last few years and would, therefore, be unduly repetitious. Moreover, individual contributors of specific subsections in this book have all provided an adequate and detailed coverage of their specific subjects. The following, therefore, can be considered a brief summary of recent reviews in the literature and the appropriate sections in this book.

The reader who is interested in going beyond this book in studying the problems of fibrinolysis at greater depths is urged to consult other recent reviews by Astrup (1958), Sherry et al. (1959a), Albrechtsen (1959), von Kaulla (1963), Bang et al. (1964), Pechet (1965), Fearnley (1965) and Sherry (1965). In addition, the following recent symposia all devoted to this subject are warmly recommended to the interested reader: Thrombolytic Activity and Related Phenomena (1961), Fibrinolysis (1964), and The Fibrinolysin System (1966).

II. General Scheme and Nomenclature

Physiological and therapeutical activation of the fibrinolytic enzyme system depends on the presence in mammalian plasma and other body fluids of a proteolytic enzyme precursor in large quantities. This protease zymogen is termed plasminogen or profibrinolysin; the activated protease is termed plasmin or fibrinolysin. Plasminogen can be converted into plasmin under the influence of a number of physiological or pharmacological plasminogen activators such as tissue kinases, blood kinase, urokinase, streptokinase and staphylokinase. Plasmin is a broad-spectrum proteolytic enzyme, an endopeptidase similar but not identical to trypsin.

Some controversy has emerged in recent literature concerning the proper terminology for the proenzyme and activated protease. The proponents adhering to the older nomenclature plasminogen-plasmin correctly claim that this enzyme possesses a substrate specificity which is far from limited to fibrin in as would be implied in the term fibrinolysin. Plasmin, like trypsin, aside from fibrin digests several biologically important proteins and peptides. Fibrinogen and the fibrinogen related coagulation moieties, Ac globulin (Factor V) and antihemophilic globulin (Factor VIII) are all avidly hydrolyzed and irreversibly inactivated by plasmin. In addition, plasmin digests ACTH, somatotropin and glucagon (Mirsky et al. 1959a, 1959b). Plasmin has also been credited with hydrolyzing certain of the components of complement (Lepow et al. 1953; Pillemer et al. 1952; and Alagille and Soulier,

1956) although these latter claims currently are being re-examined in several laboratories.

Although the author favors the old nomenclature of plasminogen-plasmin over the more recent term profibrinolysin-fibrinolysin for the above mentioned reasons, he sees nothing wrong with this latter terminology which is utilized by several of the contributors in this book as long as it is implicitly understood that the name fibrinolysin refers *only* to one of the major biological functions of this enzyme and does not in any way imply substrate specificity for fibrin. One important property of plasminogen is its great affinity for fibrinogen-fibrin. When a fibrin clot forms somewhere between 20 and 30 percent of the plasminogen content in plasma is trapped in the clot and all fibrin formed in vivo is, therefore, heavily contaminated with plasminogen. Plasminogen activators, therefore, have two points of attack. These activators will activate plasminogen into plasmin and nonspecific proteolytic activity will arise in spite of the presence of plasmin inhibitors in plasma. At the same time activators will also absorb onto or diffuse into fibrin thrombi and activate intrinsic plasminogen in the strategic position as an integral part of the fibrin polymer.

The affinity between fibrinogen-fibrin and plasminogen is readily demonstrable in vivo since plasminogen levels closely correlate with fibrinogen levels in a variety of body fluids; it is also readily observed in pathological states associated with the defibrination syndrome where the rate and severity of diffuse intravascular fibrin deposition correlate well with the decrease in circulating plasminogen levels. According to the prevalent opinion as formulated by Sherry and co-workers (Sherry et al. 1959a) this breakdown of the fibrin clot from within through activation of its large plasminogen impurities is the most important thrombolytic mechanism in vivo. It is evident that the activated nonspecific protease plasmin in plasma will contribute somewhat to lysis of in vivo fibrin deposits. However, the relative contribution of this latter mechanism remains a question of some controversy. In vitro experiments in Sherry's laboratory (Alkjaersig et al. 1959a) demonstrate convincingly that the rate of lysis of a preformed fibrin clot increases in parallel with both the quantity of plasminogen entrapped in the clot and the concentration of plasminogen activator in the surrounding medium. It is apparent from some of these experiments that only very high concentrations of auto-activated plasmin devoid of plasminogen activator will dissolve a preformed standardized fibrin clot while an identical standard clot will dissolve readily and completely under the influence of low concentrations of plasminogen activator in the surrounding medium. However, these views are not universally accepted. A second hypothesis proposed by Ambrus and Markus (1960) and further elaborated on by Ambrus in this book (p. 39) proposes that a reversible plasmin-plasmin-inhibitor complex is of crucial importance for in vivo fibrinolysis. This assumption is based on experiments which suggest that activated plasmin circulates as an inactive complex with a plasmin inhibitor but that plasmin is dissociated from its inhibitor when the complex is brought into contact with fibrin. In these authors' view plasmin possesses a greater affinity for fibrin than for the specific inhibitor. Nanninga and Guest (1964) have published evidence in support of this hypothesis but other work in Sherry's laboratory failed to confirm this concept (Fletcher, 1960).

Under the physiological circumstances, plasmin evolved from plasminogen circulating in the blood will be inactivated by antiplasmins. Although large quantities of plasmin inhibitors are readily demonstrable in the blood the conversion of even a small percentage of the total plasma-plasminogen will always result in a state of temporary hyperplasminemia. This is difficult to reconcile with published laboratory data (Fletcher, 1960; Fletcher et al. 1961; and Norman, 1958) indicating that the total capacity of plasmin inhibitors in the blood of a given individual is potent enough to inhibit several fold as much plasmin as could ever be formed; in other words, if all plasmin circulating in the blood stream was instantaneously converted into plasmin there would still be a great excess of inhibitors, more than sufficient to inhibit all active free plasmin. On the other hand, there is unassailable clinical evidence to indicate that plasmin or nonspecific protease activity is present in the circulation in severe fibrinolytic states. The further work in Norman's laboratory (Norman and Hill, 1958) has helped to clarify these discrepancies. This work demonstrated that at least two plasmin inhibitors are normally present in plasma; these two inhibitors react with plasmin to form inactivate complexes. However, the rate of complex formation is markedly, different for the two inhibitors. One of the inhibitors, an $alpha_1$ globulin, partially inhibits plasmin immediately upon contact in a temperature independent reaction. The other, an $alpha_2$ globulin, inhibits plasmin at a certain rather slow but constant rate to form an inactive complex. Hence, some of the plasmin formed at any given time will be inhibited immediately but the remainder will stay in the circulation for varying periods of time. According to the concentration of plasminogen activators present in the blood stream at a given time and the levels of circulating plasminogen (i. e., the rate of conversion of plasminogen into plasmin) hyperplasminemia of all degrees of severity and of varying duration will arise. But even at low concentrations of plasminogen activators in the blood a state of temporary hyperplasminemia will ensue. Although free plasmin activity is demonstrable in vitro only in extremely severe fibrinolytic states the effects of even mild temporary hyperplasminemia can readily be recognized by a decrease in plasma fibrinogen (Factor I) accelerator globulin (Factor V) and antihemophilic globulin (Factor VIII).

The sequence of events in enhanced plasma fibrinolysis are illustrated in Figure 1. (1) a rise in plasminogen activators in plasma will (2) result in conversion of plasminogen into plasmin and (3) the complexing of plasmin with plasmin inhibitors to form proteins which possess neither enzyme nor enzyme inhibitor activity. As can be noticed from Figure 1, the end result of a fibrinolytic episode at the time when all circulating plasmin has been inhibited will be a fall in plasminogen as well as plasmin inhibitor levels in plasma. As previously noted, circulating plasminogen activator will also attack plasminogen in any preformed fibrin deposit causing thrombolysis from within. Plasmin while free and circulating in the bloodstream aside from breaking down a number of proteins necessary for normal hemostasis (Factors I, V and VIII) will also result in the release of large molecular fibrinogen fragments with anticoagulant properties as described later in section IV. Mechanisms responsible for the generation of activator activity in the circulation as well as the exact

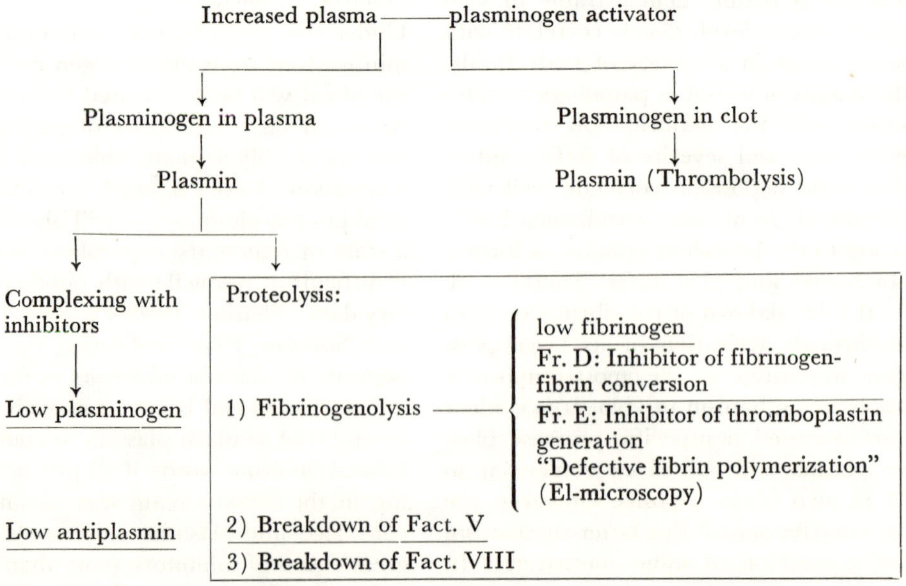

Fig. 1. Scheme of activation of the fibrinolytic enzyme system and the development of the fibrinolytic coagulation defect.

mechanisms involved in plasminogen-plasmin conversion although intensely studied in many laboratories are still matters of controversy.

Although low levels of a blood activator plasminogen have been consistently demonstrated in plasmas from normal healthy humans (Sawyer et al. 1960a); it is as yet unresolved whether it represents tissue kinases entering the bloodstream in different quantities under a variety of physiologic and pathologic conditions. Experiments have been presented by Iatridis and Ferguson (1962) which might support the concept of a fibrinolytic activator existing normally as an inactive precursor. These authors provide evidence that plasminogen activator activity is generated in increasing amounts upon glass activation of whole blood concomitantly with activation of Hageman factor (Factor XII). It is indeed possible from these experiments that at the time when intravascular fibrin formation occurs the compensatory mechanism, that of fibrinolysis in situ, is also initiated. The increasing realization of an association between clotting, fibrinolysis and the release of bradykinin and possibly other vasoactive peptides with a central role of Hageman factor (Eisen, 1964) lend support to the concept that significant quantities of plasminogen activator may be produced locally and may be of major importance in the physiologic control of hemostasis.

Regarding the origin of tissue activators entering the bloodstream attention has focused on the release of plasminogen activator from vascular endothelium. Evidence in support of this line of reasoning has been supplied through techniques developed by Todd (1959) who demonstrated zones of lysis around small vessels when he incubated tissue slices in contact with thin fibrin films and subsequently fixed and stained the preparation. Evidence has been presented by Kwaan et al. (1957a) and Chakarbarti et al. (1963) to support the idea that normal capillaries and venous endothelium is a reservoir for plasminogen activator. The actual trigger required to release activator from the endothelial layer is unknown although vascular injury and/or ischemia is presumed to be a major factor as discussed further in Section V.

The major source of confusion in the understanding of the mechanism of plasminogen activation arose from studies of the activation of plasminogen by streptokinase, an extracellular bacterial protein which is synthesized by several strains of actively growing streptococci. It was observed originally (Müllertz, 1957) that streptokinase is incapable of activating bovine plasminogen and plasminogen from other animal species; however, the admixing of streptokinase with small quantities of human plasma, serum or euglobulin would produce a plasminogen activator capable of activating plasminogen of all mammalian species studied. Because of these results Müllertz invoked the existence of a separate and specific protein in human blood termed proactivator which when incubated with streptokinase would form a "universal activator complex". The existence of such a distinct and separate entity has later been disputed for a number of reasons. Several different authors have confirmed that "activator complex activity" can be generated from plasminogen preparations at all stages of purification and no one has accomplished to produce a purified preparation of proactivator devoid of plasminogen. Sherry et al. (1959a) noted that Tillett (1935, 1938) many years earlier had found that hemolytic streptococci isolated from different animals sources produce a principle which incites fibrinolysis in animal species different from that observed with the streptokinase produced by human strains. It is, therefore, possible that the experiments which led to the postulate of the proactivator apply to strain differences in streptococci rather than mammalian species differences. Current evidence would favor the concept that streptokinase combines with either human plasminogen or plasmin; this complex, in turn, becomes the universal activator capable of converting all mammalian species plasminogen into plasmin (De Renzo et al. 1965; Kline and Fishman, 1961; and Alkjaersig, 1964).

The existence of inhibitors against physiological kinases both urokinase and tissue kinase have been firmly established in normal plasmas (Johnson and McCarty, 1960b) and partly characterized as an alpha$_2$ globulin in human plasma. Streptokinase is inhibited by two types of inhibitors; it is neutralized by streptokinase neutralizing antibodies found in titers varying considerably from individual to individual and in the same individual at different times. Recent streptococcal infections and previous infusions of streptokinase can produce a very sizable increase in streptokinase neutralizing antibodies (Fletcher et al. 1958). In addition, streptokinase is inhibited by a physiological kinase inhibitor which may or may not be identical to the inhibitor described for urokinase and tissue kinases (Johnson and McCarty, 1960a). The properties and functions of activators as well as plasmin inhibitors will be further discussed in section II, B and C and section VI.

III. Individual Components

A. Plasminogen and Plasmin

The physical-chemical properties of a variety of plasminogen preparations will be enumerated in the section by Heberlein and Barnhart (p. 336) which will cover those aspects of the biochemistry of plasminogen which pertain to its purification. In the following, we shall cover only some of the broader aspects of the physiology and physiological chemistry of this enzyme system.

Plasminogen is widely distributed in tissues, body fluids and circulating blood where it is normally found in concentrations varying from 3.5–4.5 Remmert and Cohen (1949) caseinolytic units per ml plasma. An important characteristic of plasminogen as well as plasmin is its high affinity for fibrinogen and fibrin; until very recently all attempts to prepare fibrinogen free of plasminogen were unsuccessful and numerous observers have agreed that all fibrin formed from plasma in vivo or in vitro contains large impurities of plasminogen entrapped in its meshwork unless special procedures for its removal or destruction are employed such as continuous washing for 48–72 hours or heat treatment (Sherry et al. 1959a; and Lassen, 1958).

The precise tissue site of plasminogen synthesis has not been elucidated. Although Barnhart and Riddle (1963) using immunofluorescent techniques have provide convincing evidence indicating that eosinophilic leukocytes play a role in the synthesis and/or transport of plasminogen, the fact that this proenzyme has been identified in many tissues through chemical means makes it uncertain whether eosinophils serve as the sole source of plasminogen production as suggested by Barnhart and Riddle. The turnover rate of this protein has not been established. Indirect evidence from clinical trials involving the infusion of large quantities of streptokinase would indicate that the rate of synthesis of plasminogen is quite rapid. Following the cessation of the I.V. administration of high doses of streptokinase at which time the levels of circulating plasminogen were zero, normal plasminogen levels were restored within 12–18 hours (Fletcher et al. 1959a; and Balstrup et al. 1962). Several authors have confirmed the existence of plasminogen isoenzymes as discussed by Heberlein and Barnhart (page 336).

Of particular interest is Bergström's demonstration of genetically different forms of bovine plasminogen (Bergström, 1963). When plasminogen was prepared separately from 10 individual animals and analyzed by starch gel electrophoresis at pH 8.0, it was found that two of the preparations contained a single component whereas the rest of them separated into two fractions both containing plasminogen activity. Slotta and Gonzalez (1964) suggested that highly purified plasminogen may exist in two different molecular forms; the native plasminogen, an unstable carbohydrate containing euglobulin and a pseudoglobulin derived from the native plasminogen by acid treatment. These preparations have identical specific caseinolytic activity; however, when fibrin is used as the substrate the activity of euglobulin plasminogen is 50 percent higher than the pseudoglobulin plasminogen. The native plasminogen was found to contain about 92 percent protein, 5 percent hexose, 2.8 percent hexoseamine and 0.6 percent sialic acid. Although hexose and hexoseamine were found to be essential for activity, sialic acid was not. When submitted to starch gel electrophoresis both forms of plasminogen separated into several bands. It was concluded that plasminogen exists as aggregates or complexes of subunits with proenzyme activity. In this connection it is noteworthy that carboxypeptidase and alpha chymotrypsin split insoluble plasminogen into soluble products preserving the activity of the original preparation (Fishman and Kline, 1963).

Alkjaersig (1964) in her exhaustive treatise of the subject observed numerous differences in physical-chemical behavior between a euglobulin native-type plasminogen prepared by column chromatography and the acid extracted pseudoglobulin type plasminogen. Plasminogen prepared by these two different methods exhibited significant differences in sedimentation behavior. Whereas the $S^{\circ}_{20,w}$ value for the acid purified material was 4.3 and showed clear interdependence of S value with protein concentration, the comparable S value for column plasminogen was 4.9 and this value was virtually independent of protein concentration. However, column plasminogen preparations could easily be converted by brief treatment at acid pH into products with physical-chemical characteristics indistinguishable from those prepared by acid purification procedures.

Furthermore, substances like lysine and epsilon aminocaproic acid which have been extensively used for the solubilizing effect in several reported purification procedures were also found to induce molecular changes. Alkjaersig (1964) was lead to hypothesize from these observations that the plasminogen molecule possesses a high degree of plasticity in its secondary and tertiary structure not unlike that described for many other proteins and that the differences observed among the various preparations can most readily be attributed to structural changes during different purification procedures. Such a view if confirmed can clarify a most confusing situation.

Recently Robbins and co-workers (1967) have further elucidated the molecular structure of native plasminogen and the probable events at the molecular level in the course of plasminogen to plasmin conversion. Human plasminogen appeared to be a single polypeptide chain molecule (monomer) which following activation by urokinase is transformed into a two polypeptide chain plasmin molecule (monomer) connected by a single interchain disulfide bond. Although plasminogen and plasmin contain approximately 22 disulfide bonds the apparent cleavage of a single disulfide bond at pH 9.0 by reduction with 2-mercaptoethanol in 8 M urea resulted in complete loss in enzymatic activity with formation of the two chains.

At pH 3.0 different disulfide bonds appeared to be cleaved since the reduction of approximately five disulfide bonds at this pH resulted only in 50 percent loss in activity. The cleavage of the single interchain disulfide bond of plasmin at pH 9.0 resulted in the formation of two major chains (alpha and beta).

The amino-terminal amino acid residue of plasminogen and one plasmin chain was found to be lysine in the amino-terminal of the second plasmin chain was found to be valine. The carboxy terminal amino acid sequence of plasminogen and one plasmin chain was found to be Leu-Asn-COOH and the carboxyterminal of the second plasmin chain was found to Lys-Arg-COOH. From this data the authors concluded that the activation of human plasminogen monomer to plasmin monomer by urokinase is due to the cleavage of a single arginyl valine bond which results in a two chain molecule held together by a single disulfide bond.

Human plasminogen and plasmin according to these investigations would have the same molecular weights, namely, $89{,}000 \pm 1500$ and similar amino acid compositions. It should be emphasized, however, that these more recent data await further confirmation and that some of the findings of Robbins and co-workers (1967) conflict with previous published data. The data on disulfide bond cleavage of plasminogen and plasmin were not in agreement with the data of Taylor and Staprans (1966) whose reduction experiments were carried out under somewhat different conditions. The recent findings of no molecular weight change during plasminogen-plasmin conversion conflicts with earlier reports indicating that the activation of plasminogen to plasmin is accompanied by the release of substantial quantities of trichloroacetic acid soluble fragments and a reduction of molecular weight of the parent molecule varying somewhat depending on the mode of activation (Alkjaersig et al. 1958; Rife and Shulman, 1963; and Ablondi and Hagan, 1960).

The kinetics of plasminogen activation by urokinase, streptokinase or trypsin are first-order in nature (Alkjaersig et al. 1958). Plasmin is an endopeptidase with many but not all characteristics in common with trypsin. The active centers of the two enzymes seem to be functionally identical (Ronwin, 1962). The substrate spectra of the two enzymes show many similarities although differences exist in terms of their specificities for hydrolysis of a number of synthetic amino acid esters (Ronwin, 1962). In contrast to trypsin, plasmin does not activate trypsinogen or chymotrypsin. Plasmin like trypsin attacks lysyl-lysine or lysyl-arginine bonds in fibrinogen and fibrin; however, plasmin exerts greater specificity than trypsin in that the total number of susceptible peptide bonds cleaved by plasmin is less than the number cleaved by trypsin.

As mentioned, plasmin, aside from fibrinogen and fibrin, will readily hydrolyze and destroy the fibrinogen-like procoagulants antihemophilic globulin (Factor VIII) and accelerator globulin (Factor V). Protein substrates for plasmin which have been utilized for its quantitative assay in the laboratory include casein (Remmert and Cohen, 1949), gelatin (Kaplan, 1944) and Protamine-Heparin complexes (Kjeldgaard and Ploug, 1957). Markus and Ambrus (1960) have provided some evidence to support the contention that plasmin may exist in different functionally active forms. Depending on the amount of streptokinase added to purified plasminogen for its activation, plasmins with different amino acid ester substrate specificity and different caseinolytic rate characteristics would evolve; these authors suggested the nomenclature alpha and beta plasmin for these different entities. It should be noted, however, that this work was done utilizing less pure plasminogen preparation than those available today and it would therefore, seem wise to reserve final judgement as to the existence of functionally different molecular species of plasmin until Markus and Ambrus's observations have been repeated in more highly purified systems.

B. Plasmin Inhibitors

An extensive review of this subject will be presented by Ambrus (p. 336). In this space we shall consider only some of the broader aspects of the problem of plasmin inhibitors. Plasma and serum as well as most animal tissues studied possess a substantial inhibitory capacity against plasmin. It was suspected for many years that several protein fractions in human plasma were capable of inhibiting plasmin. Grob (1949) utilizing alcohol fractionation in the cold noted plasmin inhibitors to be present in both Cohn fractions IV and VI; Norman and Hill (1958) also using the Cohn scheme of fractionation noted different plasmin inhibitors in fraction IV_1 and IV_4. The total antiplasmin capacity of normal plasma is still a matter of some dispute.

While Norman (1958) estimated the antiplasmin content of plasma to exceed the total plasmin potential by approximately 30-fold, Fletcher et al. (1959a, b) observed an average antiplasmin content in plasma of 5.9 caseinolytic units per ml as compared to an average plasminogen content of 3.8 caseinolytic units per ml. The normal range of antiplasmin activity in our laboratory is 12–20 caseinolytic units (Bang, unpublished).

Reference has been made previously to the results of Norman and Hill (1958) indicating the presence of two functionally distinct and separate plasmin inhibitors in plasma. One is a heat stabile, rapidly acting $alpha_2$ globulin combining with plasmin at a rate which shows no temperature dependence, the other inhibitor is a heat labile slowly acting $alpha_1$ globulin combining with plasmin at rates which depend on temperature as well as the concentration of both plasmin and inhibitor. A dramatic improvement in our understanding of the exact nature and characterization of antiplasmin was recently provided by Schwick et al. (1967).

These authors successfully isolated and purified five protease inhibitors from human plasma and characterized them in terms of their individual inhibitory spectra and, therefore, elucidated some controversial aspects regarding the exact identity of plasmin, trypsin and thrombin inhibitors. The purified inhibitors were designated $alpha_1$ antitrypsin, $alpha_1$ chymotrypsin, inter-alpha-trypsin inhibitor, antithrombin III, and $alpha_2$ antiplasmin ($alpha_2$ macroglobulin). The $alpha_1$ antitrypsin does not only combine with trypsin but also with chymotrypsin, with elastase and with plasmin. Based on the findings that this inhibitor represents 90 percent of the antiprotease activity of plasma as well as kinetic data, it was established that $alpha_1$ antitrypsin is identical with a slow acting $alpha_1$ antiplasmin described by Norman and Hill (1958). The $alpha_2$ antiplasmin was demonstrated to be identical with the $alpha_2$ immediate inhibitor of Norman and Hill (1958); this latter inhibitor was found to be broad spectrum protease inhibitor reacting with all proteases tested including thrombin. Antithrombin III was found to inactivate thrombin in a progressive reaction catalyzed by heparin; this antithrombin also reacted with trypsin and with plasmin. The inter-alpha-trypsin inhibitor was found to inhibit plasmin as well; among the five inhibitors tested only the $alpha_1$ chymotrypsin inhibitor was found to be specific for one enzyme.

The concentrations of all five inhibitors in human plasma were determined by quantitative precipitation with specific antisera. For 100 ml of plasma the following values were found: $alpha_1$ antitrypsin 210–500 mg, $alpha_1$ antichymotrypsin 14–35 mg, inter-alpha-trypsin inhibitor 10–30 mg, antithrombin III approximately 40 mg and $alpha_2$ antiplasmin 220–380 mg.

C. Plasminogen Activators

1. Urokinase

Normal urine contains a plasminogen activator capable of activating plasminogen of several animal species. As early as 1913 Johansson suggested that urine and fibrin might contain interacting enzymatic substances, a proenzyme and an activator yielding an active fibrinolytic enzyme. Even earlier Hedin (1903) had noted that an enzyme present in an isolated serum globulin fraction and urine each showed a weak proteolytic effect on casein whereas the combination of the two enzymes resulted in a caseinolytic activity which was much higher than the sum of their individual activities. Almost four decades after Johansson's publication three groups (Williams, 1951; Astrup and Sterndorff, 1952; and Sobel et al. 1952) independently arrived at the conclusion that the fibrinolytic activity of urine is due to the presence of a plasminogen activator for which the name urokinase was suggested by Sobel and co-workers (1952).

Partial purification of urokinase was first reported by von Kaulla (1954) through absorption and elution from human urine on barium sulfate. A thromboplastic substance in urine was noted in these early preparations and although von Kaulla (1956) later described methods the separation of urokinase from thromboplastic substances and obtained a partial purification of the thromboplastic material; the presence of uroplastin as a minor contaminent even in high purification urokinase preparations has remained a significant problem until recently (Alkjaersig et al. 1965).

Celander et al. (1955) published their method which lends itself to large scale production of urokinase. They discovered that urokinase following the simple expedient of foaming large volumes of urine would be concentrated 10–20 fold in the foam fraction. Ploug and Kjeldgaard (1956-7) first published techniques suitable for the preparation of urokinase of high specific activity. Their method involved the adsorption of urokinase onto silica gel, elution with ammonia and chromatography on Amberlite IRC50. Moving boundry electrophoresis of the purified material exhibited three peaks; the one peak corresponding to urokinase was estimated to account for 37 percent of the total protein in the preparation.

Most recently, Lesuk et al. (1965) and White and co-workers (1966) independently reported on urokinase preparations which can be considered pure and homogeneous by all physical-chemical criteria. Lesuk et al. (1965) starting with aqueous solutions of highly purified human urokinase succeeded in obtaining urokinase in crystalline form. Crystallization was induced at pH 5.0–5.3 and at a temperature of 4° C by the addition of sodium chloride; urokinase crystals appeared to be colorless thin plates "of unusual fragility and brittleness". Specific activity reached a maximum plateau after two to three recrystallizations. Maximum specific activity attained was 104,000 ± 4800 CTA units* per mg of estimated protein.

Solutions of crystalline urokinase when subjected to polyacrylamide gel disc electrophoresis produced a single band; the preparation also appeared homogeneous on moving boundry electrophoresis. When examined for homogeneity in the analytical ultracentrifuge a single symmetrical peak was observed exhibiting some boundry spreading at a pH of 6.8 and at that pH the weight-average molecular weight of the crystalline enzyme showed marked concentration dependence indicating reversible aggregation. The calculated molecular weight for urokinase at zero protein concentration was 54,000 ± 900 assuming a partial specific volume of 0.735 ml per gm at 10° C.

White et al. (1966) provided a detailed protocol for a purification procedure which eventually resulted in two distinct and separate types of highly purified urokinase. Briefly, the successive steps in their purification scheme are: (1) foaming and ammonium sulfate precipitation (2) adsorption on and elution from Amberlite IRC50 (3) gel filtration on Sephadex G100 (4) refiltration on Sephadex G100 (5) chromatography on hydroxyl apatite (6) separate refiltration of each type of urokinase on Sephadex G100.

The two highly purified types designated S_1 and S_2 were analyzed by physical-chemical and immunochemical techniques. Type S_1 urokinase exhibited a specific activator activity of 218,000 CTA units/mg protein and a molecular weight of 31,500 by either sedimentation-diffusion or sedimentation-equilibrium techniques. Type S_2 urokinase, a larger molecule showed a specific activity of 93,500 CTA units/mg and a molecular weight of 54,700 as calculated by the sedimentation-equilibrium technique.

Unlike the S_1 type, type S_2 showed an equilibrium plot deviating from linearity although the S_2 type like the S_1 type was homogeneous by all other criteria. The S_2 type can be considered closely related to or perhaps identical to Lesuk's crystalline preparation.

White and co-workers (1966) postulated that the S_1 type urokinase represents the purest form of urokinase so far accomplished whereas the S_2 type in these authors' opinion represented a conjugate between urokinase and inert protein. This theory was convincingly reputed by Lesuk et al. (1967), who were able to show that the S_1 type urokinase represents a breakdown product of urokinase containing the active center and arising as a consequence of the purification procedures as reported by White et al. (1966).

Fraction C_1 prepared as described by White et al. (1966) was found by Lesuk et al. (1967) to undergo gradual degradation from an initial molecular weight of 54,000 to active fragments in the region of 36,000 molecular weight upon simple maintenance of fraction C_1 under the conditions of temperature, buffer composition and urokinase concentration observed by White et al. during their purification procedure. Moreover, Lesuk and coworkers (1967) observed that crystalline urokinase can be cleaved by trypsin to yield an active fragment of molecular weight 36,000 in stoichiometric amounts.

Urokinase must be characterized as a proteolytic enzyme, for in high concentrations it hydrolyzes casein (Alkjaersig et al. 1958) it splits a heparin protamine complex (Kjeldgaard and Ploug, 1957) and hydrolyzes a number of amino acid esters: tosylarginine methyl ester (TAMe) and lysine ethyl ester (LEe) (Sherry and Alkjaersig, 1957). Recently a series of synthetic substrates with considerably higher sensitivity for urokinase than TAMe and LEe have been described: alpha-N-acetyl-L-lysine methyl ester (ALMe) (Sherry et al. 1964), carbobenzoxy-L-tyrosine-p-nitrophenyl ester (CTNe) (Lorand and Mozen, 1964) and alpha-N-acetylglycyl-L-lysine methyl ester (AGLMe) (Walton, 1967).

* The CTA unit reference to the standard unit of urokinase activity adopted by the Committee on Thrombolytic Agents, National Heart Institute (Sherry et al. 1964).

For a more detailed description of urokinase esterolytic activity see Troll (p. 365).

As mentioned, urokinase probably activates plasminogen by splitting lysyl-lysine, lysyl-arginine or lysyl-valine bonds (Shulman et al. 1958; Robbins et al. 1967) but the special biochemical properties which provide urokinase with the specificity as an activator for plasminogen are obscure.

Urokinase as a plasminogen activator possesses characteristics which theoretically would make it a most effective thrombolytic agent. Sawyer and co-workers (1960b) convincingly demonstrated in in vitro experiments that the fibrinolytic to fibrinogenolytic ratio for urokinase in a plasma-plasma fibrin clot system is considerably higher than that observed with another plasminogen activator, streptokinase or activated plasmin. From these experiments it could be predicted and was indeed later confirmed in clinical trials with prolonged I.V. administration of urokinase that substantial elevations of circulating thrombolytic activity can be maintained throughout the infusion at the expense of only a moderate decline in circulating plasminogen levels and only a slight reduction in circulating fibrinogen levels (Johnson et al. 1964b; Fletcher et al. 1965).

It has been postulated that urokinase serves a physiological role in maintaining the patency of the urinary tract during pathological circumstances leading to hemorrhage and intraluminal clot formation. Urinary urokinase has been demonstrated to substantially contribute to the frequent complication of post-operative bleeding following prostatic surgery (McNicol et al. 1961a); and this realization in turn led to the formulation of rational and highly successful therapy with the synthetic plasminogen activation inhibitor epsilon aminocaproic acid (McNicol et al. 1961b and Andersson and Nilsson, 1961). Postoperative bleeding following prostatectomy was demonstrated to be perpeturated by constant contact between the surgical wound and urokinase and prevented by the high concentration of epsilon aminocaproic acid which is readily achieved in urine because of the substantial clearance rate of this compound (McNicol et al. 1962).

The question of the cellular site of synthesis of urokinase has not been completely clarified and it is a matter of dispute whether urokinase largely represents excreted blood and tissue kinases or whether it is locally produced in the urinary tract. Smyrniotis et al. (1959) observed significant alterations in urinary urokinase excretions in certain disease states; the tendency toward greater or less urokinase excretions parallels the levels of plasma thrombolytic activity similarly studied by Sawyer et al. (1960a) in a variety of diseases. Colgan and co-workers (1952) observed a striking increase in fibrinolytic activity of the urine 4–5 days prior to the occurrence of fatal pulmonary hemorrhage following total body irradiation in dogs. Guest and Celander (1960) noticed higher urokinase values in urine samples obtained after exercise; physical exercise has been documented by many observers to be accompanied by significant enhancement of plasma-plasminogen activator.

Von Kaulla and Swan (1958) noticed a close correlation between the development of systemically enhanced fibrinolytic activity in a series of patients observed during and after cardiac surgery; the enhanced urokinase excretion returned to normal as the intensity of the fibrinolytic state of these patients declined. On the other hand, Kucinski and Fletcher (1966a, b) found that a specific antiserum against human urokinase does not react with the plasminogen activator released from blood vessels into plasma in vivo while it neutralizes the activity of urokinase. Bernik and Kwaan (1967) similarly demonstrated that a plasminogen activator immunologically identical to urokinase is present in the media of a number of primary human kidney cultures.

The earlier findings by Kwaan and Fisher (1965) and Kwaan and Astrup (1967) indicated that plasminogen activator activity as demonstrated by a histochemical technique resides largely in the capillaries vasa rectae and the collecting tubules of the renal medulla, whereas glomerular capillaries contain very low levels of activator activity. Such a distribution of plasminogen activator activity would speak in favor of the local production of urokinase in the renal medulla and would not support the contention that urokinase represents merely excreted blood and tissue kinases.

2. Tissue kinases

The presence of plasminogen activators was first demonstrated in different animal tissues by Astrup and Permin (1947), Permin (1949) and Astrup and Sterndorff (1956). In human tissues Albrechtsen (1957a, b and 1959) has reported that large amounts of tissue activator are present in the uterus, adrenal lymph nodes, prostate, lungs and ovary whereas moderate or small amounts are present in the pituitary, kidney, striated muscle, myocardium, testicles and spleen with no demonstrable activator present in the liver.

It should be noted that the term tissue kinase or fibrokinase as it was formulated by Astrup's group refers to any substance possessing plasminogen activator activity which is extractable from tissues with 1 M KSCN.

In these earlier experiments it proved impossible to purify and reliably characterize tissue activators from different tissues and even at this state when improved purification procedures yielding high specific activity highly-purified preparations of tissue activators from certain tissues such as pig heart (Bachmann et al. 1964), no firm proof is as yet available to indicate that tissue activators extract from different tissues and organs are identical enzymes.

Conversely, the possibility has not been excluded that a number of cathepsins and lysosomal proteases may function as plasminogen activators. Ali and Lack (1965) obtained on subcellular fractionation of rabbit kidney by differential and density-gradient centrifugation a high proportion of plasminogen activator which was particulate and displayed sedimentation properties similar to the lysosome-rich fraction as judged by the acid phosphate activity. Plasminogen activator activity was found to be closely associated with a latent protease the activity of which was enhanced by detergents such as Triton X-100 or sodium desoxycholate. The tissue activator purification scheme reported by Bachmann and coworkers (1964) does not involve the initial extraction of tissue with KSCN but rather acetate buffers and the final product following purification by chromatography and gel filtration is 1700-fold purified over the starting tissue extract. The material is somewhat unstable and quite insoluble at normal pH but it is relatively homogeneous displaying only minor impurities by physical-chemical analysis.

Subsequently, Ali (1967) reported on the purification of a tissue activator from rabbit kidney yielding a final product with an increase in specific activity 2200-fold over the initial tissue extract. This enzyme fraction was soluble and stable at neutral pH and appeared to be biophysically homogeneous.

An improved variety of the purification procedure utilizing thiocyanate extracts of a pregnant hog ovary as the starting material has recently been published (Astrup and Kok, 1965) and is further described on page 332.

It has been proposed repeatedly that local activation and release of tissue activator is a major mechanism for the resolution of inflammatory or traumatic exsudates (Astrup, 1956a, b).

Astrup (1956b) has further proposed that the local release of tissue activator in high concentrations may be responsible for local hemorrhage and a large number of authors have postulated that the release of tissue activator into the general circulation may be one mechanism for the hemorrhagic diathesis with laboratory evidence of enhanced proteolysis as seen in a wide variety of disease states (see section VI). There is as yet no clue as to the exact mechanism controlling the release of the tissue activator into the general circulation. The finding by Moltke (1958) would indicate that the leptomeninges of the brain are a particularly rich source of tissue activator and this observation may provide a possible explanation for the later findings by Schneck and von Kaulla (1961). These authors demonstrated a marked increase in systemic fibrinolytic activity following procedures such a pneumoencephalography, ventriculography, cerebral angiography, diagnostic manipulations which could all be expected to cause a transient increase in intracranial pressure and/or transient ischemia of the cerebral circulation; ischemia in particular has been noted to cause release of tissue activator into the general circulation (Tagnon, 1942).

The release of tissue activator from miningeal tissues could similarly explain the striking enhancement in circulating fibrinolytic activity following electric shock (Fantl and Simon, 1948), the shock seen following rapid intravenous injection of cardiazol (Meneghini, 1950) and circulatory collapse for a variety of other reasons (Fischer et al. 1956). We shall return to a further discussion concerning the physiologic role and hemostatic regulations of tissue activator of plasminogen in section V.

3. Tissue Culture Kinases

It is an old observation in tissue culture work that clot lysis can be produced by a variety of tissue cultures grown in plasma clots (Fisher, 1946, and Goldhaber et al. 1947). There have been scattered reports in the literature in recent years indicating that the tissue cultures of kidneys of mammalian species are capable of synthesizing and excreting into the culture medium a urokinase-like plasminogen activator. Barnett and Baron (1959) reported the presence of plasminogen activator in the supernatant medium from serum-free monkey kidney cultures. The plasminogen activator described by Barnett and Baron (1959) was not proteolytic in the absence of serum and like tissue activator (see page 332); it was readily dissolved by KSCN. The activator appeared to be the product of a metabolic process and not the result of a cell breakdown since only a small fraction of the activity found in the supernatant could be extracted from the cells.

Painter and Charles (1962) using primary cultures of monkey kidney cells and an established line of dog kidney cells confirmed these observations and achieved a substantial purification of plasminogen activator from both sources. The purification procedures closely resemble methods previously utilized for the purification of urokinase such as foaming and calcium phosphate gel absorption and elution.

In parallel experiments, Painter and Charles (1962) obtained partially purified preparations of urokinase from human and monkey urine utilizing purification procedures identical to those employed with the tissue culture media as a starting material. The urokinases and tissue culture kinases fractionated very similarly and starch gel electrophoresis at pH 3.6 in 8 M urea produced sharply defined bands containing plasminogen activator activity in almost identical positions in the starch gel slab.

These experiments, therefore, provided strong evidence to support the contention that the plasminogen activator content in urine and tissue culture media from growing kidney cell lines are closely related if not identical substances.

Bernik and Kwaan (1967) examined primary cultures from human kidneys and noticed again the release of a plasminogen activator in such cultures. By means of histochemical slide techniques the fibrinolytic activity was accurately localized to the active cells. The sole site of plasminogen activator release in these experiments appeared to be cells which emerged from small vessels and no significant fibrinolytic activity was exhibited by tubular cells, fibroblasts, macrophages or lymphocytes in the outgrowth.

The concentration of plasminogen activator in the culture media increased with the age of the culture during the exponential growth phase; the titre of activity changed after repeated changes of fluid and as the interval between refeedings was lengthened. Preliminary immunologic characterization of the plasminogen activator in the tissue culture media shows that this plasminogen activator is identical to urokinase. In a later communication, Bernik and Kwaan (1968) have recently reported that the human kidney tissue culture activator exhibits partial immunologic identity with a plasminogen activator derived from a lung tissue culture but no identity with plasminogen activator produced from other cell lines.

The continued development of work aimed at the characterization of tissue culture plasminogen activators must be viewed with considerable interest. With further refinement of immunologic techniques such as those utilized by Bernik and Kwaan (1967), a final answer to the problem of the exact cellular origin and properties of urokinase and other tissue kinases should be within reach. Furthermore, it is a distinct possibility that tissue cultures may come to be a useful and convenient source of urokinase-like plasminogen activator for clinical trials.

4. Blood activator

The existence of a physiological blood activator has been known for a long time but information concerning the origin and characterization is still in short supply and it has never been sufficiently isolated or purified to determine its properties as an enzyme protein. It is largely the striking lability of the blood activator in freshly-drawn blood (Astrup and Sterndorff, 1956, and Mullertz, 1957) which has hindered progress in further characterization of this substance. Although the lability of blood activator would seem to set it apart from tissue activators and urokinase which are very stable substances their partial or complete identity cannot be excluded on this basis; the presence of inhibitors or enzymes in the blood capable of irreversibly degrading plasminogen activator could account for these differences. The blood activator is partially absorbed onto fibrin during coagulation and a major but unfortunately variable portion of this activator is precipitated in the plasma euglobulin fraction (Mullertz, 1957; and Sherry et al. 1959a).

Although the levels of blood activator can be reproducibly quantitated in the euglobulin fraction (Mullertz, 1953) and through techniques involving high dilutions of the plasma sample (Fearnley and Lackner, 1955; and Fearnley et al. 1957) the physiologic significance of activator measurements performed by such techniques are questionable since in both instances the pre-requisite for detection and quantitation of activity is the removal from the activator of normally occurring inhibitors. Utilizing a highly sensitive ^{131}I labelled fibrin substrate, Sawyer et al. (1960a) finally provided the unequivocal evidence for the presence of significant levels of plasminogen activator activity in normal fresh plasma but it required the collection of a substantial number of cases before statistically valid figures emerged.

The recent finding of the stabilizing effect of inorganic polyphosphates such as hexa-metaphosphate (Brakman and Astrup, 1964) may provide the means for further characterization and urgently needed additional information concerning the exact nature of the blood activator. Currently the lack of an assay system sufficiently sensitive and specific to accurately record the subtle variations in plasminogen activator activity in whole undiluted plasma under normal physiologic circumstances is one serious impediment to progress in understanding of the exact physiologic role of the fibrinolytic enzyme system.

5. Trypsin

Trypsin has long been recognized as a plasminogen activator (Lewis and Ferguson, 1952; Kocholaty et al. 1952; Jacobsson, 1953; Jackson and Mertz, 1954). The mechanism of plasminogen-plasmin conversion by trypsin is principally different from that caused by specific activators such as urokinase as evidenced by a substantially slower rate and the splitting off of greater amounts of trichloroacetic acid soluble peptide-material during activation (Alkjaersig et al. 1958).

In addition, epsilon aminocaproic acid was found to be a competitive inhibitor of plasminogen-plasmin conversion by urokinase whereas it functioned as a noncompetitive inhibitor for plasminogen-plasmin conversion by trypsin (Alkjaersig et al. 1959b). The physiologic or pathologic significance of plasminogen activation by trypsin in such disease states as acute hemorrhagic pancreatic necrosis has not been elucidated.

6. Streptokinase

Streptokinase is a protein of bacterial origin which can be harvested and purified utilizing the broth of actively growing hemolytic streptococci as the starting material. Streptokinase has been produced commercially for quite some time and according to available information most streptokinase is produced by a Lancefield group C organism (Sherry et al. 1959a). Some physical-chemical parameters of streptokinase have been reported and a molecular weight of 47,000 estimated from ultracentrifugal analysis (Davies et al. 1964) and 51,000 according to gel filtration analysis (Doleschel and Auerswald, 1967). Streptokinase is highly soluble over a wide pH range but its activity is rapidly and irreversibly destroyed at pH values above 9 and at pH 2 in the presence of 1 M NaCl under which conditions plasmin is precipitated from solution (Troll and Sherry, 1955). This latter effect has been effectively utilized in studies of the enzyme kinetics of the plasminogen to plasmin conversion by streptokinase (Alkjaersig et al. 1958).

Extensive efforts have been made in many laboratories in attempts to define synthetic amino ester or protein substrates other than plasminogen for streptokinase but no success has as yet been encountered. It would appear, therefore, that the enzymatic action of streptokinase on human plasminogen is nonproteolytic in nature confirming the previously mentioned observations by Robbins and co-workers (1967) which led these authors to postulate that plasminogen to plasmin conversion involves no reduction in molecular weight and no splitting off of detectable quantities of peptide material. The activation of human plasminogen by streptokinase was long felt to take place in a two-step reaction. During the first phase streptokinase was felt to react immediately and stoichiometrically with a serum factor termed proactivator by Astrup's group (Astrup, 1956a). The complex formed between activator and plasminogen was then supposed to mediate plasminogen to plasmin conversion enzymatically in a first-order reaction (Alkjaersig et al. 1958). As mentioned, the original basis for the idea of the necessity for a distinct and separate protein, proactivator, in streptokinase catalyzed plasminogen activation was the observation that streptokinase readily activates plasminogen in human serum whereas it was found to be almost completely inactive in bovine and porcine plasma (Cliffton and Downie, 1950). On the other hand, it was observed that the addition of small amounts of human serum or plasma or human euglobulin fraction to streptokinase produces a "universal activator" capable of readily activating plasminogen of all animal species (Geiger, 1952; Müllertz, 1955; and Müllertz and Lassen, 1953).

In spite of extensive work in many laboratories the existence of a separate proactivator protein remains unproven since all attempts to separate this hypothetical entity from plasminogen have met with failure. The extensive work by DeRenzo and co-workers (1963, 1965 and 1967; Davies et al. 1964; Barg et al. 1965; and Hummel et al. 1966), convincingly revealed the true identity of the "universal activator" as being either a streptokinase-plasminogen or streptokinase-plasmin conjugate. They demonstrated the appearance of a new discreet component as a result of plasminogen-streptokinase interaction by starch electrophoresis, analytical ultracentrifugation and gel filtration. Plasminogen and streptokinase seem to undergo complexing in an equimolar ratio. The exact nature of the mechanism of streptokinase-plasminogen conjugation and conformational changes which the two participating proteins undergo in the formation of the "universal activator complex" awaits further clarification.

The specific problems arising from the antigenic properties of streptokinase as it pertains to the therapeutic use of this plasminogen activator will be discussed later in section VII.

7. Others

Staphylokinase – – staphylococcal culture filtrates have been observed by many authors to possess the properties of plasminogen activator (Lack, 1948; Gerheim et al. 1948; Lewis and Ferguson, 1951; Hayashi and Mackawa, 1954; Celander and Guest, 1959; and Davidson, 1960). Staphylokinase differs from streptokinase in that this activator activates a wider range of animal plasminogens (Davidson, 1960); all animal species plasminogens with the exception of ox plasminogen were readily activated by staphylokinase. The addition of human euglobulin or plasminogen did not affect the spectrum of staphylokinase as a plasminogen activator. Staphylokinase in contrast to streptokinase has definite caseinolytic properties (Davidson, 1960) and plasminogen to plasmin conversion by staphylokinase is probably enzymatic in nature analogous to urokinase activation (Lewis and Ferguson, 1951). The physical-chemical properties of staphylokinase have not been adequately studied and the potential usefulness of this plasminogen activator for therapeutic purposes is not known.

Organic Solvents -- when a mixture of chloroform and serum is gently agitated activation of plasminogen eventually occurs (Christensen, 1946; Loomis et al. 1947; and Baumgarten et al. 1957) and the first plasmin preparations intended for therapeutic uses were chloroform activated human plasminogen. Christensen's studies (1946) as well as the later work by Baumgarten and co-workers (1957) convincingly demonstrated that the activation of plasminogen which occurs upon addition of chloroform to human plasma or plasma fractions is due to the immediate inactivation of inhibitors followed by a slow probably autocatalytic conversion of plasminogen to plasmin.

The usefulness of this procedure for activating plasminogen is limited and the results of activation experiments unpredictable because chloroform and other organic solvents denatures plasminogen to a variable degree in different experiments.

Peptone -- Ungar and Mist, 1949, reported that euglobulin precipitated from guinea pig serum in the presence of peptone showed an increase in fibrinolytic activity. He also reported the production in guinea pig euglobulin following antigen-antibody reactions and formulated a concept of inflammatory response based on the release of a blood protease (Ungar, 1952). Olesen (1957) and Astrup and Olesen (1957) obtained partial purification of a component in peptone capable of activating plasminogen in several animal species including man. It has recently been postulated by Astrup's group (Brakman and Astrup, 1964) that peptone induced activation of fibrinolysis involves dissociation between activators and inhibitors in the system and that this system may reflect the state of inhibitor-activator equilibrium in plasma (Brakman and Astrup, 1964). The significance of these observations for human physiology and pathology remains to be established.

D. Activator Inhibitors

1. Physiologic Inhibitors

Inhibitors of physiologic activators have been found in the blood circulation (Schmitz, 1937). Müllertz (1955) observed that a crude preparation of bovine globulin inhibited the activation of bovine plasminogen by human streptokinase activated globulin. He also showed that the inhibitory effect of bovine globulin on the activation process was markedly reduced in the presencee of fibrin and he tentatively concluded that fibrin serves an important role in protecting the active components of the fibrinolytic enzyme system from their respective inhibitors. Von Kaulla and Schneck (1963) during their studies of pharmacologic induction of fibrinolysis in man observed that the shortening of the fibrinolysis euglobulin time after the intravenous injection of the triggering compound was occasionally preceded by a marked prolongation of the euglobulin lysis time. However, the prolongation alone was frequently observed when the drug failed to induce increase in the fibrinolytic activity. These authors tentatively explained this phenomenon on the basis that an anti-activator is released and precipitated with the euglobulin fraction together with any activator normally present. Nilsson et al. (1961) extensively studied an activator inhibitor demonstrated in a patient with a serious clinical problem of recurrent thrombo embolism. This patient exhibited, besides high levels of plasmin inhibitors, very strikingly enhanced inhibition of plasminogen activation by both streptokinase and urokinase. Streptokinase inhibition was 10–20 times enhanced over normal values and urokinase inhibition was 5–10 fold enhanced over normal levels. The activation inhibitor was present in both plasma and serum. It was destroyed by heating at 56° C for 30 minutes and was found to be concentrated largely in Cohn fraction IV-1. Cohn fractions II + III which contain essentially all plasma gamma globulin inhibited activation by streptokinase by virtue of its content of immunologic streptokinase neutralizing antibodies but did not inhibit activation by urokinase. Electrophoretic analysis revealed the activator inhibitor to be distributed in the alpha$_1$, alpha$_2$ and beta$_1$ globulins with a peak of activity concentrated in the alpha$_2$ globulin fraction. Johnson and McCarty (1960a) similarly provided evidence for the existence of an antiactivator predominantly concentrated in the alpha$_2$ globulin fraction which appeared to be distinct and separate from the immunologic streptokinase neutralizing inhibitor. The role of streptokinase neutralizing antibody is further discussed in section VII.

2. Synthetic Inhibitors

Lysine and arginine amino acid esters (see Troll (p. 365) being substrates for urokinase and tissue kinase inhibit activation of plasminogen competitively (Alkjaersig et al. 1958). An additional inhibitor, epsilon aminocaproic acid, a close analog of lysine, was originally discovered as an antifibrinolytic agent by Okamoto and co-workers (1957). These authors considered the main effect of epsilon aminocaproic acid in the fibrinolytic system to be plasmin inhibition. It was subsequently shown by Alkjaersig et al. (1959b) and Ablondi et al. (1959) that the main action of epsilon aminocaproic acid is a competitive inhibition of plasminogen activation. Competitive inhibition of activation of human and bovine plasminogen by streptokinase, urokinase and tissue activators can be detected at epsilon aminocaproic acid concentrations as low as 10^{-4} M. EACA also functions as a noncompetitive inhibitor of plasmin at concentrations above 5×10^{-2} M. It was shown by Alkjaersig et al. (1959b) that EACA in concentrations around 10^{-5} M enhances the proteolytic activity of plasmin in analogy with the findings previously reported for certain quarternary amines (Astrup and Alkjaersig, 1952).

Sjoerdsma and Nilsson (1960) investigated a number of aliphatic amino acids in an attempt to elucidate the structure-activity relationship for plasminogen activation inhibition. Maximum activity was in the 6-carbon compound EACA with about 50 percent of the activity of EACA demonstrable in delta-amino valeric acid and 33 percent of the activity in delta-amino laevulinic acid. The terminal position of the amino group is critical since alpha aminocaproic acid (norleucine) is without activity. The structure around the carboxyl end is of significance since the addition of one amino group in the alpha position of EACA producing alpha epsilon aminocaproic acid (or lysine) results in an almost total loss of activity.

Bickford et al. (1964) conducted an even more extensive investigation on the structure-activity relationship of the omega amino carboxylic acids and alkylamines. Glycine, beta-alanine, gamma-amino-butyric acid, glutaric acid, valeric acid, cadaverine and lysine did not inhibit with concentrations less than 10 mM ($K_i > 10$ mM). Competitive inhibition was found with delta-aminovaleric acid ($K_i = 4.7$ mM), EACA ($K_i = 2.8$ mM), ω-aminocaprylic acid ($K_i = 1.0$ mM), propylamine ($K_i = 3.3$ mM), butylamine ($K_i = 3.0$ mM) and amylamine ($K_i = 1.0$ mM). The authors concluded that inhibition around the active center probably occurs because of both electrostatic and hydrophobic bonding of the inhibitor to the enzyme because inhibition is competitive and because inhibition is dependent on the positive charge and increases with increasing chain lengths of either the omega amino carboxylic acid or the alkyalmine series.

Similarly, Skoza et al. (1968) systematically investigated the effect of aliphatic or cyclic amino acids and derivatives on fibrinolytic inhibition. In agreement with Sjoerdsma and Nilsoon (1960) these authors found the terminal amino group to be quite specific since substitution with guanidino, trimethyl amino, or quartenary amino ions resulted in a 100-fold loss of activity. Skoza et al. (1968) also established the degree of ionization of the terminal amino group to be important for optimal activity. The negatively-charged carboxyl group provides an important but less specific effect on inhibitory potential since replacement of the carboxyl group by sulphonic or phosphonic groups could be accomplished without significant loss of inhibitory potential, leading Skoza to suggest that the terminal carboxyl group helps to control orientation of the inhibitor molecule. The best inhibitors to fibrinolysis are found among structures the most closely related to EACA; in each instance of inhibitors of optimal efficacy the terminal amino and carboxyl groups are separated by a distance approximately equal to the length of six co-valently bonded carbon atoms. In the case of the cyclic amino acids, 4-(aminomethyl)-cyclohexane-1-carboxylic acid and 4-(aminomethyl)benzoic acid (see below) and analogs thereof. Skoza et al. (1968) established that optimum activity is achieved when the amino group is distanced 3 Å from the ring, e.g. separated from the ring structure by one-methylene group.

Two amino acids incorporating the cyclohexane or the benzene ring were subsequently found to be very potent inhibitors of plasminogen activation: 1-(aminomethyl)cyclohexane-4-carboxylic acid (AMCHA) (Okamoto and Okamoto, 1962) and *p*-aminomethylbenzoic acid (PAMBA) (Lohman et al. 1964).

According to Okamoto and Okamoto (1962) the activity of AMCHA is 10–20 times higher than EACA; upon isolation of the cis- and trans-stereoisomers they found all activity to reside in the trans-form of the molecule. PAMBA may be somewhat more potent than AMCHA but appears to be considerably more toxic (Lohman et al. 1964; Maki and Beller, 1966).

An extensive clinical experience with EACA as an antifibrinolytic agent has accumulated and the pharmacology of this compound has been the subject of a careful and extensive study by McNicol et al. (1962) utilizing an assay technique of ion exchange resin loaded paper chromatography for quantitation of EACA. EACA was found to be rapidly and predictably absorbed from the gastrointestinal tract with peak plasma levels being achieved in about two hours. A very high clearance rate of this compound was demonstrated corresponding to approximately 75 percent of endogeneous creatinine clearance; if sufficient EACA has been administered to produce plasma levels in the therapeutic range of 10^{-3} M the greater part of this dosage can be found in the urine after 12 hours. Sustained plasma and urine levels of EACA can be maintained readily by repeated oral doses or by continuous intravenous infusion. When the compound is given at a rate of one gram per hour plasma levels sufficient to produce a fibrin inhibition of plasminogen activator activity in plasma is achieved. With a priming dose of 4–6 grams therapeutic levels in plasma can be attained rapidly within 1–2 hours. Since EACA is cleared by the kidneys at a high rate therapeutically effective urinary levels can be achieved with dosages which do not produce excessive plasma levels. EACA readily diffuses across the cellular membrane and equilibrium within or compartments of the total water space is readily achieved as evidenced by the observations that the excretion of EACA following a 12-hour intravenous injection is prolonged occurring over a 72-hour period. In the intact isolated rat diaphragm preparation McNicol (1962) reported that EACA competes effectively with essential amino acids for transmembrane transport and that EACA in this preparation substantially inhibits the incorporation of lysine into trichloroacetic acid precipitable protein.

Sherry et al. (1959c) first reported on the use of EACA in man; they found that the intravenous infusion of EACA inhibited the fibrinolytic activity induced by systemic administration of streptokinase, nicotinic acid and bacterial pyrogen. Nilsson et al. (1960b) showed that oral or intravenous administration of EACA inhibited pathological fibrinolytic activity in a patient with cirrhosis of the liver and in another with acute leukemia. Other investigators have reported that EACA is effective in the control of the hemorrhagic states, probably due to hyperplasminemia, in carcinoma of the prostate (Andersson and Nilsson, 1961); surgical operations (Andersson, 1962; McNicol, 1962); heart surgery with the extracorporeal circulation (Gans and Krivit, 1962); and aplastic anemia and leukemia (Mikata et al. 1959). Grossi et al. (1961) found EACA to be of doubtful value in the treatment of the hemorrhagic state associated with cirrhosis of the liver.

The potential hazards of EACA in defibrination syndromes will be discussed later by Beller in Chapter II. The high plasma and tissue levels which have to be achieved with EACA for therapeutic efficacy makes this agent potentially hazardous in chronic liver disease where depressed protein synthesis is present. EACA competing effectively with essential amino acids for transmembrane transport could be expected to further limit the capacity for protein synthesis of the diseased hepatic parenchyma and in our laboratory we have observed hepatic coma developed in two patients to whom EACA was given in an attempt to control hemorrhage secondary to pathologic fibrinolysis (unpublished). It is our policy to withhold EACA when bleeding diathesis develops in the cirrhotic but it should be emphasized that no extensive clinical evaluation of this situation has as yet been reported. Because of the excessively high clearance rate of EACA chronic renal disease with significant depression of renal function can be expected to produce excessively high levels of plasma and tissue levels of EACA and in our laboratory chronic renal disease is considered a contraindication to the use of EACA.

The demonstration in animal experiments of substantial hyperkalemia associated with EACA administration (Carroll and Tice, 1966) would further emphasize the potential hazards of EACA administration in the presence of depressed renal function.

Although the clinical use of AMCHA and PAMBA has not as yet been fully established in large-scale clinical trials, agents such as AMCHA which produces effective inhibition of plasminogen activation at lower plasma levels than EACA should offer a very significant advantage in therapeutic fibrinolytic bleeding states. The excellent and exhaustive studies of the pharmacology of AMCHA in man by Andersson et al. (1968) further emphasizes the potential value of this drug. Comparing the activity of AMCHA to EACA these authors found that the 24-hour urinary recovery after a single dose of AMCHA of 10 mg/kg was 90 percent after I.V. injection and 38.5 percent after oral administration as opposed to 71 and 64 percent respectively of EACA following a single I.V. or oral dose of 100 mg/kg. The relatively low recovery of AMCHA after oral administration was first attributed to incomplete absorption from the GI tract but was later documented to be the result of the long, sustained retention of AMCHA in tissues. These sustained tissue levels of AMCHA were demonstrated to effectively inhibit local tissue activator as documented by assays for tissue activator activity in surgical tissue specimens.

Andersson et al. (1968) found that AMCHA when used in doses of 20 mg/kg by mouth as premedication before surgery would maintain adequate antifibrinolytic activity in serum for 7–8 hours, in tissues for up to 17 hours and in urine for up to 48 hours. In contrast, EACA in oral doses of 100 mg/kg was found to produce adequate serum levels for only 3 hours, tissue levels for about 6 hours and urine levels for up to 24 hours.

In agreement with earlier investigations, Andersson et al. (1968) found AMCHA to be eight times more potent than EACA as an inhibitor of urokinase but 10 times more potent than EACA as an inhibitor of tissue activators.

In a preliminary survey of 53 patients, side effects were found to be milder and less frequent after AMCHA than after EACA.

Trasylol® (Bayer Compound A 128) is a polypeptide of bovine origin the structure of which including its amino acid sequence has been completely elucidated (Anderer, 1965). This polypeptide, broad-spectrum protease inhibitor has been demonstrated to be identical to the Kunitz-Northrup trypsin pancreatic inhibitor since the two substances have been demonstrated to be of identical amino acid sequence (Kassell et al. 1965). A protease inhibitor of pancreatic origin has been market in France under the trade name Iniprol®. Both preparations have been found to inhibit plasmin as well as plasminogen activation (Steichele and Herschlein, 1961; Beck et al. 1963; Soulier et al. 1964). Although a massive number of reports on the clinical usefulness of Trasylol® in particular has accumulated in the German literature, we must await large scale fully controlled clinical trials before the clinical efficacy of these preparations can be completely assessed. Such information in our view is urgently needed since Trasylol appears to possess some obvious advantages over EACA. It is suprisingly nontoxic and can be infused in very large quantities without untoward effects (Beck et al. 1963). Moreover, in vitro experiments as well as in vivo experiments (Amris, 1964; Amris, 1965; Amris and Hilden, 1968;

Nordström et al. 1968) have suggested that Trasylol in high doses functions as an inhibitor of thromboplastic activity. If this effect can be substantiated in the clinical situation, we may have a very useful drug in Trasylol which could be administered in a clinical situation where the clear differentiation between diffuse intravascular coagulation and fibrinolysis is impossible to make.

IV. Fibrinogenolysis

Triantaphyllopoulos and Triantaphyllopoulos on p. 247 will provide an extensive discussion on the biophysics and biochemistry of the molecular fragments of plasminogen arising upon incubation with plasmin and Maki and Beller on p. 404 will enumerate available techniques for their quantitation in plasma. In this section we shall confine our remarks to those aspects of the problem which have relevance to the clinical situation and to the understanding of the role of fibrinogen breakdown products in the development of the coagulation defect encountered in pathologic fibrinolytic states and in patients receiving fibrinolytic enzyme preparations for therapeutic purposes.

Fletcher et al. (1959b) and Fletcher (1960) observed that the crucial parameter in the coagulation defect was the raised thrombin clotting time; the severity of the defect correlated with the prolongation of the thrombin clotting time. It was, therefore, assumed that the biochemical defect involved either an inhibition of thrombin action or a defect in steps II and III, the polymerization-gelation reaction of fibrin formation. Niewiarowski and Kowalski (1957, 1958) had previously shown that the products of proteolytic degradation of fibrinogen possessed a marked "antithrombic activity"; they obtained a partially purified fibrinogen derivative that prolonged the thrombin clotting time when added to plasma or to purified fibrinogen solutions. Niewiarowski and Kowalski assumed that fibrinogen breakdown products exerted a specific inhibitory effect on thrombin and consequently named the abnormal fibrinogen derivative "antithrombin VI". Triantaphyllopoulos (1958) arrived at essentially the same conclusion.

Fletcher (1960) later revised this concept. Using methods modified from Ehrenpreis et al. (1958), they demonstrated that the proteolytic action of thrombin on fibrinogen at either pH 5.3 or pH 7.6 was not in any way inhibited by the presence of fibrinogen breakdown products, and therefore concluded that the defect must reside in the polymerization-gelation phase (Fletcher, 1960). Consequently the coagulation anomaly was designated "defective fibrin polymerization" by Fletcher et al. (1962). Latallo et al. (1962b) corroborated this hypothesis by recording the rate of gelation in a system of purified fibrin monomer with and without the fibrinogen degradation products added. Polymerization rates were recorded spectrophotometrically at 3500 Å. Optical density changes at this wavelength represent changes in light scattering properties of the coagulation mixture. Since thrombin was absent in this system it was possible to record the specific changes in phases II and III caused by the fibrinogen breakdown products. These studies demonstrated unequivocally that fibrinogen breakdown products (FBP) would alter the rate of fibrin polymerization. Initially the rate was slowed down in defective fibrin polymerization. However, the opacities of the normal fibrin clot and of the "defective" fibrin clot were usually identical after several hours of incubation below a certain concentration of FBP in the coagulation mixture. Optical density values for the final defective fibrin clot were sometimes higher than for the normal fibrin clot. The influence of FBP on the polymerization rate seemed to be pH-dependent. When the same amount of FBP was added to coagulation mixtures at different pH, the decrease in polymerization rates was more marked at higher pH values with a pH range of 6.5–8.5.

Further investigation by Alkjaersig et al. (1962) was aimed at a biophysical characterization of the polymerization inhibitor.

The proteolytic breakdown products of fibrinogen had previously been investigated in several laboratories. Holmberg (1944), who studied the breakdown of fibrinogen incubated with streptokinase, suggested that fibrin was split into two large fragments as a result of proteolysis. Seegers et al. (1945) confirmed this observation in electrophoretic studies of fibrinogen degraded by allowing the solution to stand at room temperature until none of it could be clotted by thrombin. These authors isolated and partly purified two fibrinogen derivatives through ammonium sulfate precipitation. The degradation product, which was termed alpha-fibrinogen derivate, exhibited an electrophoretic mobility only slightly higher than that of fibrinogen, while the other, termed beta-fibrinogen derivate migrated at a somewhat higher rate. More recently the existence of at least four proteolytic degradation products of fibrinogen were demonstrated in the ultracentrifugation and electrophoresis studies by Shulman (1952) and through two-dimensional paper chromatography by Sherry and Alkjaersig (1957). Sherry and Alkjaersig (1957), Kaplan (1955) and Kowalski et al. (1960) established that the majority of the fibrinogen breakdown products were relatively large protein molecules, since approximately 50 percent of the fibrinogen digest could be precipitated by trichloroacetic acid, even after prolonged incubation with plasmin. With the exception of Kaplan (1955), all these authors agree that the fibrinogen degradation products exhibit physical properties different from those of fibrinogen. An important development began when the various components in the fibrinogen digest became adequately separated and characterized (Nussenzweig and Seligman, 1960; Nussenzweig et al. 1961a; Latallo et al. 1962a; Alkjaersig et al. 1962). Nussenzweig et al. (1961a) obtained four distinct fractions through column chromatography on DEAE-cellulose of fibrinogen totally degraded by plasmin. All these fractions showed homogeneity on biophysical analysis. The first two protein peaks in the eluated, termed fractions A and B-C, were small molecular thermostable peptides. The third protein peak, termed fraction D, was a high molecular thermolabile protein exhibiting a sedimentation constant ($S^{\circ}_{20,w}$) of 5 and a diffusion constant of 5.3×10^{-7} cm²sec⁻¹. A molecular weight of 83,000 was calculated for fraction D on the basis of these data. The final fraction to be eluted was termed fraction E; it was a thermostabile protein with a sedimentation constant ($S^{\circ}_{20,w}$) of 3, a diffusion constant of 7.5×10^{-7} cm^2sec^{-1}, and an estimated molecular weight of 35,000.

Approximately 50 percent of the total protein of the digest was fraction D. Fraction E represented 15–20 percent of the total protein. The thermolability of fraction D, the thermostability of fraction E, and the electrophoretic mobilities of these two fractions made it plausible that fraction D was identical with Seegers' alpha-fibrinogen derivative and fraction E with the beta-derivative. Subsequent immunochemical analyses of the fibrinogen digest (Nussenzweig et al. 1961b) revealed that both the large molecular degradation products, fractions D and E, could be precipitated with antisera against fibrinogen. Distinctly different bands of precipitation with antifibrinogen sera were demonstrated by immunoelectrophoresis for each of the purified fractions D and E. The lower molecular fractions (A and B-C) showed no precipitate with antifibrinogen sera.

Latallo et al. (1962a) obtained partial purification of the larger molecular fibrinogen degradation products through alcohol fractionation in the cold. The studies by Alkjaersig et al. (1962) provided strong evidence that the fibrin polymerization inhibitor resided among the larger molecular fragments of fibrinogen proteolysis. The purified fraction obtained through gel filtration consisted mainly of a protein with a sedimentation constant ($S^{\circ}_{20,w}$) of 5.25. However, significant amounts of another protein exhibiting a sedimentation constant ($S^{\circ}_{20,w}$) of 3 were also present in the purified fractions utilized in the experiments. The fibrinogen derivatives studied must, therefore, have been mixtures of the fractions D and E of Nussenzweig et al. (1961a). Fibrin clots formed in the presence of these fractions were extensively washed to free them of all protein not firmly incorporated in the coagulum. Subsequently, these clots were dissolved in 5.0 M urea. Ultracentrifugal analysis of these redissolved clots revealed two peaks, one with a sedimentation constant of 8.0 corresponding to that of fibrinogen, and one with a constant of 5.25 corresponding to that of fraction D. It was, therefore, concluded that fraction D (termed the 5.25 segment by Alkjaersig et al. 1962) was identical with the "polymerization inhibitor", although the smaller protein fraction E could not be excluded as playing a contributory role. Significant amounts of fraction D seemed to be incorporated in the clot in this process. It was observed throughout the investigations of Fletcher et al. (1959a, 1962) that the clots formed in the presence of high concentrations of fibrinogen breakdown products exhibited abnormal physical properties; they were less homogeneous and more friable than normal fibrin clots and often showed a flocculate appearance.

Electron microscopic studies (Bang, 1961; Bang et al. 1962a; Bang, 1967) provide evidence that fibrin clots formed in the presence of small quantities of fraction D exhibit strikingly abnormal ultrastructural features. The physical properties of the "defective" fibrin are different from those of normal fibrin. A clot which finally forms in the presence of fraction D has a peculiar flocculate appearance. It is friable and its tensile strength is considerably less than normal.

Additional electron microscopic observations and ancillary physical-chemical data (Bang, 1967) have provided a hypothesis for the mechanism of "defective" fibrin formation. Normally, monomeric fibrin units line up to form string-shaped "intermediate polymers". These intermediate macromolecules in turn will aggregate laterally and longitudinally to form the fibrin network gel. The development of "defective" fibrin can be explained from evidence which would so far indicate that fraction D is capable of reacting with fibrin monomer to form abnormal fibrin polymers. A sizable amount of available fibrin monomer is tied up in these abnormal macromolecules and residual monomer although capable of forming fibers is so depleted that a solid homogeneous network is never formed. It is conceivable that "defective" fibrin may be functionally inadequate in vivo. The hemorrhagic diathesis associated with the administration of fibrinolytic agents may be worsened because fibrin when it finally form will constitute a poor "hemostatic plug".

Nussenzweig et al. (1961a) originally pointed out that an intermediate breakdown product of large but at the time undetermined molecular weight appeared temporarily in a plasmin fibrinogen incubation mixture prior to the appearance of the final fragments D and E. This early intermediate was designated fraction D-E by Nussenzweig et al. (1961a). Latallo et al. (1964) and Triantaphyllopoulos and Triantaphyllopoulos (1965) isolated this early large molecular weight intermediate fragment and evaluated its biological properties. Both of these groups of workers agreed that the large fragment D-E possess both antithrombin and antipolymerase activity as well as thromboplastin inhibitory activity. In addition, Kowalski and co-workers (1964) observed that this the "early fibrinogen breakdown products" is an inhibitor of platelet function; it inhibits the thrombin and adenosine diphosphate induced aggregation of platelets.

However, from later, carefully controlled experiments by Larrieu and co-workers (1967) it appears that the large molecular weight fibrinogen breakdown products possess inhibitory activity only in thrombin induced platelet aggregation, whereas the large molecular fragments exert no inhibitory function when ADP, collagen or epinephrine are used to initiate the aggregation reaction. For these latter reactions the inhibitory effect remains after heating the crude degradation products at 60° C or even 100° C for thirty minutes, whereas the inhibitory effect was impaired after dialysis. The role of low molecular weight peptide fragments is strongly suggested by these experiments since neither partially purified fragments D or E nor the early intermediate products D-E induced these modifications. Fletcher et al. (1966) and Fisher et al. (1967) have further contributed to the understanding of the sequential changes in the course of plasmin proteolysis in fibrinogen and the possible role of these abnormal fibrinogen fragments in pathologic states through biophysical measurements of individual isolated fibrinogen fragments. Fletcher and coworkers (1966) established that approximately 10 percent peptide material is cleaved off initially producing a fibrinogen derivative with a molecular weight estimated at 265,000 with a sedimentation constant identical to that of fibrinogen but with a significantly higher diffusion constant and, hence, an altered molecular configuration and axial ratio. This, the largest molecular weight fibrinogen derivative although it is still 100 percent clottable by thrombin, clots at a slower rate and presumably results in an abnormal polymer.

Following the release of an additional 5–10 percent low molecular weight peptides another fragment emerges with a sedimentation constant significantly lower than fibrinogen; this new class of intermediate breakdown products are still partially clottable by thrombin. This the second type of intermediate is probably identical to the fraction D-E intermediate described by Nussenzweig et al. (1961a). Only after extended incubation did three classes of plasmin resistant fragments emerge which were identified as identical to fraction D, E and A-B of Nussenzweig et al. (1961a). It was constantly noted throughout these experiments that a fast sedimentating peak appeared early during the early stages of incubation suggesting to the authors that significant polymer formation occurred as a consequence of random cleavage of arginine-glycine bonds in fibrinogen by plasmin.

Subsequent work by Fisher et al. (1967) provided evidence for the presence in the plasma of patients with pathologically enhanced fibrinolysis of both early intermediate and "late" breakdown products of fibrinogen.

When the clinical condition is mild the 265,000 MW fragment seems to prevail and only in more severe clinical states are fragments D and E clearly demonstrated.

Electron microscopical observations (Bang, 1967) would tend to support the contention that early intermediate products substantially contribute to the development of defective fibrin polymerization. When a cruder preparation of fibrinogen split products containing significant quantities of fraction D-E and/or higher intermediates was utilized the quantities of protein necessary for the electron microscopical demonstration of abnormal clot structure were substantially less than when an immunochemically pure preparation of fraction D was added.

Mosesson et al. (1957) succeeded in isolating from normal human plasma a fibrinogen fraction which differed significantly from highly purified human fibrinogen as prepared by Blombäck and Blombäck (1956) in terms of solubility characteristics.

This new fraction possessed a relatively higher solubility and was designated fraction I-8. The biophysical characteristics of this fraction from which a molecular weight of approximately 269,000 could be calculated made it seem likely to Mosesson and co-workers (1957) that their fraction I-8 might be identical to the first intermediate degradation product as described by Fletcher et al. (1966). Most recently this hypothesis was convincingly and elegantly confirmed by Sherman et al. (1968). Utilizing radioisotope-labelled infusions of fraction I-4 into experimental animals these authors successfully demonstrated the appearance of labelled fraction I-8 in these animals' plasmas. These latter observations provide an impressive albeit still indirect proof for the existence of a physiologic fibrinogenolytic mechanism active in the removal of fibrinogen and perhaps in part responsible for the high turnover rate of this protein.

V. Fibrinolysis in Normal Physiology

As indicated repeatedly in previous sections a more complete understanding of the normal physiological role of the fibrinolytic enzyme system would depend in large measure on the development of assay systems of sufficient specificity and sensitivity to accurately register the subtle variations arising as a consequence of differences in normal physiologic states. The large majority of assay procedures utilized in investigations of physiologic fibrinolysis do not fulfill any strict criteria for specificity and sensitivity. Although investigations into fibrinolysis in normal physiology have produced a number of provacative and attractive hypotheses of wide-ranging consequences the final and exact delineation of the role of this important enzyme to a large degree depends on the confirmation of a number of key observations through better assay systems than those currently available. In this section we shall attempt to cover only briefly a limited number of references from the extensive literature emphasizing in this selection hypotheses for which substantial and confirmed experimental support is available.

A number of stimuli which occur in various physiologic situations such as physical exercise and mental stress, notably acute anxiety produce enhancement of circulating fibrinolytic activity of varying intensity in different subjects (MacFarlane, 1937; Biggs et al. 1947). The latter authors also demonstrated that the injection of adrenaline regularly induced enhanced fibrinolytic activity, which led them to suggest that the fibrinolytic activity arising after physical and mental stresses is mediated through adrenaline release. Tagnon et al. (1946) first observed the rather consistent development of increased plasma fibrinolysis in clinical states associated with hypoxia and shock. Large doses of acetyl choline administered intravenously was also observed to elicit a potent fibrinolytic response (Soulier and Koupernik, 1948). Kwaan and co-workers in a series of papers (Kwaan et al. 1957a, b, c and 1958; Kwaan and Mc Fadzean, 1956) established that local ischemia is a potent mechanism for release of fibrinolytic activity. Kwaan and co-workers in the course of these investigations presented convincing arguments in their attempts to elucidate the mechanism for release of plasminogen activator into the circulation.

When arterial blood supply to the forearm was arrested and subsequently re-established after varying time intervals fibrinolytic activity developed. When the blood pressure cuff was inflated to produce only venous occlusion no fibrinolytic activity ensued.

The local production of fibrinolytic activity appeared to be the most intense in capillaries as previously noted by Mole (1948) but significant fibrinolytic activity was elaborated by veins and arteries as well.

A central role for the autonomic nervous system in the regulation of fibrinolytic activity was strongly suggested by the observations of Kwaan and co-workers (1957a) demonstrating that the local paravenous injection of epinephrine, acetyl choline, histamine and serotonin all resulted in enhanced fibrinolytic activity. Not only was plasminogen activator activity demonstrable locally in the vein adjacent to the injection site but fibrinolytic activity was elaborated from the entire venous circulation of the ipsilateral and frequently from the contralateral limb.

Kwaan et al. (1957c) believed that vasoconstriction of the vasa vasorum produces ischemia of the vein wall which in the final analysis is responsible for the release of fibrinolytic activity in veins. Later these authors (Kwaan et al. 1958) suggested a similar effector mechanism to regulate plasminogen activator release from arteries; this effector mechanism may be inhibited by exercising.

Kwaan (1964) using a histochemical technique "the fibrinolytic autograph" developed by Todd (1959) for thin frozen tissues slices was able to further pinpoint the localization of plasminogen activator in vein walls; his studies suggested that the vascular endothelium may serve as a labile pool for the activator.

In collaboration with Astrup (Kwaan and Astrup, 1967), he extended his observations to indicate that fibrinolytic activity in tissues exist as plasminogen activator in the vascular intima but not in all vessels. It appears more commonly in capillaries than in large vessels and more consistently in vessels of organs with high metabolic activity such as the myocardium, brain, renal medulla and functioning endocrine glands.

Fibrinolytic activity also is high in vessels of hyperplastic organs such as the uterine endometrium during the proliferative phase but is minimal or absent in atrophic tissue such as the uteri of castrated animals. In wound healing young capillaries migrating into young fibrous tissue are extremely rich in plasminogen activator which disappears as healing is completed. Such a pattern is also observed in the resolution of intravascular thrombi, atheromatous plaques and in tissue repair in a variety of pathologic lesions such as a myocardial infarction and ulcerative colitis during remission. The occurrence of high levels of plasminogen activator in newly established fibrous scar tissue as seen during the evolution of the acute myocardial infarction had been noted earlier by Fischer et al. (1959).

Holemans (1963) confirmed the central role of vasoactive compounds in mediating the release of plasminogen. A wide variety of vasoactive substances including epinephrine, norepinephrine, isopropyl norepinephrine, methoxamine, angiotensin, pitressin, vasopressin, oxytocine, bradykinin and tyramine all produced substantial increases in plasma fibrinolytic activity upon intravenous injection in dogs.

The demonstration that fibrinolytic activity in a variety of normal physiologic situation is due to plasminogen activator and that plasmin contributes insignificantly if any was furnished by Sherry et al. (1959b). These authors conclusively demonstrated enhanced levels of plasminogen activator following exercise, ischemia, pyrogens, electroshock, adrenaline and acetylcholine utilizing techniques which were sensitive and specific for plasminogen activator. No free plasmin was demonstrable. It should have been mentioned, however, that inherent difficulties in any assay system for the demonstration of free plasmin activity make this latter observation open to question.

The positive identification of a fibrinogen derivative (Sherman et al. 1968), the result of plasmin proteolysis, as a constituent of normal plasma infers that trace quantities of plasmin activity indeed plays a role in normal fibrinolytic regulation although assay systems are inadequate for its direct demonstration.

A question that is as important as the source and mechanisms underlying the release of plasminogen activator is the mechanisms responsible for the removal or degradation of these substances. Fletcher et al. (1964) presented evidence which indicated that the liver plays an important role in the clearing mechanism of plasminogen activators. Following such stimuli of fibrinolytic activity as the intravenous injection of nicotinic acid or electroshock individuals with normal liver function rapidly cleared activator from the circulation and a half-life for plasminogen activator of thirteen minutes in the phase of normal liver function was established while the clearance of activator from the circulation in patients with advanced liver disease was markedly prolonged. The normal controls as well as the patients were shown to have almost identical levels of plasma inhibitors.

Before concluding this section an extremely important area of future investigation should be emphasized. Plasmin aside from serving its vital fibrinolytic function has also been demonstrated to cause the release of bradykinin from kininogen (Eisen, 1964) and it, therefore, appears that the fibrinolytic enzyme system may serve a second important physiologic function in vasomotor control. Recently the development of improved methodology for the study of the exact phylogic role of fibrinolysis as a mediator of bradykinin and perhaps other vasoactive peptides was reported by Colman et al. (1969a, b) and this development may well have opened up an important new chapter in our understanding of the plasminogen-plasmin system in human physiology.

VI. Pathological Fibrinolysis

Fibrinolytic and proteolytic activity in plasma is frequently encountered in diseases of widely different origin. However, in many of these instances the pathogenesis of the hemorrhagic diathesis is complex and can certainly not be explained solely on the basis of a "fibrinolytic" coagulation defect. The coagulation anomaly that is our major concern here should, therefore, be considered only a possible contributory factor in fibrinolytic hemorrhagic states. The special problems arising from the frequent occurrences of pathologic fibrinolysis in conjunction with diffuse intravascular coagulation are discussed by Maki and Beller on page 404. Reviews have been furnished by Albrechtsen (1959). Sherry et al. (1959a), and Bang et al. (1964).

Fibrinolysis occurs clinically in the following conditions.

Obstetrical complications such as abruptio placentae (Dam et al. 1941), placenta prae-

via (Ratnoff et al. 1955), intrauterine retention of a dead fetus (Weiner et al. 1950), and amniotic fluid infusion (Albrechtsen et al. 1955); moreover, fibrinolysis seems to be a rare complication in placenta accreata, toxemia of pregnancy, Caesarian section, abortion, hydatid mole, extrauterine pregnancy, forceps deliveries, and sometimes in relation to otherwise perfectly normal deliveries (cited by Albrechtsen, 1959; and Beller, 1964).
Following major surgery, particularly pulmonary surgery and open surgery of the heart (von Kaulla and Swan, 1958; Mathey et al. 1950; Meyers et al. 1957).
Neoplastic disease, particularly cancer of the prostate (Dillard and Chanutin, 1949).
Cirrhosis of the liver (Goodpasture, 1914).
Miscellaneous diseases: Boeck's sarcoid (Nilsson et al. 1957), polycythemia vera (Björkman et al. 1956), and leukemia (Giraud et al. 1954).
In patients undergoing thrombolytic therapy with streptokinase (Fletcher et al. 1959b).
The syndrome of fibrinolytic hemorrhagic diathesis may be of dramatic intensity with fatal outcome. In the extreme cases it presents itself with complete afibrinogenemia and severe hemorrhage. However, it has been pointed out (Sherry et al. 1959c) that symptoms of lesser intensity and of a different nature -- purpuric manifestation and/or persistent mild hypofibrinogenemia in medical patients may be due to enhanced plasma fibrinolytic activity. Two mechanisms have been proposed to explain the uncontrolled plasma fibrinolytic activity. The first possibility is a release of an activator of plasminogen into the blood stream. The activated protease plasmin, capable of digesting both fibrinogen and fibrin and other coagulation moieties, could therefore be responsible for the development of a coagulation defect. The second possibility is a release of thromboplastic material resulting in diffuse intravascular clotting, leading to a direct depletion of coagulation moieties and presumably followed by a secondary fibrinolytic response. The present assay techniques do not always allow a distinction between these two possibilities as discussed by Maki and Beller (p. 404); moreover, evidence is mounting that a high percentage of cases of fibrinolytic hemorrhagic diathesis arise as a consequence of both these mechanisms (Bang et al. 1964).
The observations in patients with pathological fibrinolysis are probably not directly comparable with observations in patients receiving massive doses of the plasminogen activator streptokinase. However, an examination of the results obtained in the latter type of investigation provided a clue to the understanding of the fibrinolytic coagulation defect (Fletcher, 1960, Fletcher et al. 1962; Alkjaersig et al. 1962).
The infusion of large doses of streptokinase is accompanied by a rapid conversion of the inactive proenzyme plasminogen into the active protease plasmin. Plasmin eventually becomes neutralized by specific inhibitors present in plasma; however, this inhibition takes place at a rather slow and constant rate. Sufficiently rapid administration of sufficiently high doses of streptokinase are therefore, associated with a temporary state of hyperplasminemia.
In regard to coagulation moieties other than fibrinogen, different results have been obtained in experiments with plasmin and with purified coagulation factors. Alagille and Soulier (1956) reported that plasmin incubated with human plasma in vitro will destroy several procoagulants. Niewiarowski and Latallo (1957) and Donaldson (1960) also found that incubation of plasma or purified coagulation factors with plasmin resulted in their apparent degradation.
Fletcher et al. (1959b) and Fletcher (1960) summarized the coagulation anomalies encountered during infusion of streptokinase in those cases where a complete conversion of all available plasminogen led to a severe temporary hyperplasminemia:

1. A fall in plasma fibrinogen levels to 50–75% of the pretreatment values.
2. Delayed thrombin clotting time.
3. A prolongation in the one-stage prothrombin time; normal two-stage prothrombin time (Ware and Seegers, 1949).
4. Development of plasma "antithrombin activity", i.e., small amounts of the patients' plasma prolonging the clotting time of normal plasma.

5. Decrease in plasma Ac-globulin (factor V) levels to about 50 % of pretreatment values.
6. No significant alterations in other coagulation moieties when suitable modifications of routine assay techniques were utilized (Fletcher et al. 1962).

It soon became obvious that neither the moderately reduced fibrinogen levels nor the decrease in Ac-globulin (factor V) levels could adequately explain the coagulation defect. These observations were the starting point for an extensive biochemical investigation of an anomaly that appeared to involve the last phase of the coagulation of the blood, the fibrinogen-fibrin conversion.

An account for the development of our understanding of the exact nature of this coagulation defect is given in section IV.

Of major clinical importance is the perplexing problem of differentiating between bleeding states arising as a result of diffuse intravascular coagulation and the bleeding states occurring in association with pathological fibrinolysis. An exhaustive description of these problems will be given by Beller in chapter XI and Maki and Beller on page 404.

The discussion of pathologic fibrinolysis is not complete without reference to the scattered but extremely interesting cases reported in the literature where severe and recurrent thromboembolism occurs in association with enhanced levels of inhibitors of fibrinolysis. One such case report has already been referred to in section III, 4, a. In this case, reported by Nilsson and co-workers (1961), high levels of plasmin as well as an inhibitor of plasminogen activation were found. Similar findings in the patient's mother suggested the hereditary nature of this abnormality.

In another reported case (Naeye, 1961) high levels of plasmin inhibitors as well as activator inhibitors were also demonstrated. Significant but not striking elevations of blood antiplasmin levels have been observed in some cases of venous and arterial thrombosis and myocardial infarction as well as disease states such as uremia, pulmonary edema, familial hyperlipedimia, thyrotoxicosis, malabsorption syndromes (Correll and Sjoerdsma, 1962).

It should be emphasized that although thrombogenesis as a consequence of suppression of normal fibrinolysis by abnormally enhanced inhibitors constitutes an attractive hypothesis the paucity of data in the literature in support thereof would suggest that this mechanism if directly responsible for thrombosis is quite rare.

VII. Therapeutic Fibrinolysis

The development and clinical evaluation of fibrinolytic agents have received intensive interest in recent years. It has been unequivocally demonstrated that number of "fibrinolytic" enzyme preparations will dissolve preformed human plasma clots in vitro (Christensen, 1945) and experimentally induced intravascular thrombi in animals (Johnson and Tillet, 1952). The recent demonstration of successful dissolution of experimentally produced superficial venous thrombi in human volunteers by certain fibrinolytic agents (Johnson and McCarty, 1959; Johnson and McCarty, 1961; and Johnson et al. 1964a) has further stimulated interest. A number of fibrinolytic agents have undergone extensive clinical trials, and many preliminary reports often reflecting the enthusiasm of individual investigators claim striking results for such therapy. The efficacy of enzymatic treatment in thromboembolic disease in general has not been clearly proved in a large and well-controlled clinical series. A number of factors contributing to the present state of affairs can be enumerated.

The natural course of thromboembolic disease shows great variation from patient to patient. To date it has been impossible, with the diagnostic tools available, to establish standardized and exact criteria allowing continuous evaluation of either peripheral or central vascular occlusion.

A number of difficulties during the first years of clinical trials can be ascribed to the lack of complete understanding of the basic principles involved in the biochemistry and pharmacology of thrombolytic agents. Uncertainty about the standardization of available preparations has further complicated the issue. Individual investigators and individual pharmarceutical companies have introduced their own "fibrinolytic units" and only recently has the U.S. National Institutes of Health taken steps to create a uniform standard for this group of therapeutic agents (Sherry et al. 1964).

Many of the available preparations to date have produced marked allergic and pyrogenic side effects. Because of this, it has been necessary in many instances to stop therapeutic trials in patients long before adequate doses of the enzymes have been administered.

Although there are several reports on the use of fibrinolytic enzymes in the treatment of patients with thromboembolic diseases, it is impossible to assess the efficacy of fibrinolytic enzyme therapy on this basis, because the published reports deal with small scale and incompletely controlled clinical trials.

For want of sound and conclusive clinical data, the present section will deal mainly with the biochemistry, physiology, and pharmacology of enzymatic treatment in thromboembolic disease. It will present our current knowledge of the principles, the limitations, and the hazards involved in such therapy.

A variety of fibrinolytic agents have been suggested and tried clinically.

Purified Proteolytic Enzymes

Trypsin

Crystalline trypsin preparations administered intravenously have been evaluated therapeutically in rather extensive clinical series (Innerfield et al. 1952). Although the initial results were encouraging, this approach was soon abandoned because (1) no demonstrable fibrinolytic activity was present in vivo during such treatment, (2) multiple intravascular thromboses occasionally complicated the treatment, and (3) a serious local chemical thrombophlebitis frequently developed at the site of infusion.

Aspergillin-O

This enzyme, derived from the mold *aspergillus oryzae,* and having fibrinolytic and proteolytic properties, has been suggested as a therapeutic agent for thromboembolic disease (Stefanini and Marin, 1958). The published animal experiments and preliminary clinical data, however, have not demonstrated specific fibrinolytic activity for this enzyme. It appears to be a broad-spectrum proteolytic enzyme with no special advantages over trypsin.

Plasmin

From a theoretical standpoint, the use of the proteolytic enzyme plasmin purified from human or bovine plasma would seem to be an unfortunate choice. First, plasmin in concentrations less than the total plasmin inhibitor capacity in the blood, would produce little, if any, therapeutic benefit. Second, plasmin in excess of the total antiplasmin capacity, might be therapeutically effective but could produce a serious severe hemorrhagic diathesis secondary to uninhibited plasmin proteolysis of coagulation moieties necessary for hemostasis.

Johnson and McCarty (1961) recently provided a much needed clinical experimental confirmation of these theoretical considerations. They produced experimental superficial thrombophlebitis in the arm veins of human volunteers and found that the subsequent intravenous infusion of a plasmin preparation, free of plasminogen activators, did not result in the lysis of these experimental thrombi in a single instance. At the same time, a severe coagulation defect was found in those of the volunteers receiving plasmin in doses corresponding to or slightly exceeding plasmin inhibitor capacity.

Streptokinase

Streptokinase (SK) preparations of varying degrees of purity have been used extensively in clinical trials. The most highly purified batches of SK marketed for experimental use are prepared from actively growing Lancefield's group C streptococci. They contain 600 Christensen units of SK activity per microgram of nitrogen. Highly purified SK is homogeneous in biophysical assays, but it displays minor impurities on immunochemical analysis (Sherry et al. 1959a). As discussed in previous sections, the intravenous infusion of SK leads to enhanced levels of fibrinolytic activator activity and temporary hyperplasminemia. Through a continual intravenous infusion of SK, it has been possible to induce and maintain evidence of fibrinolytic activator activity of two to three hundred times the normal values for hours and days (Fletcher et al. 1959a, b). Lysis of experimentally induced thrombi in human volunteers has been demonstrated with such a regimen by Johnson and McCarty (1959).

There is one principal disadvantage of SK therapy. Streptokinase is antigenic in man and human blood contains SK-neutralizing antibodies in amounts varying greatly from person to person (Fletcher et al. 1958). The total amount of antibody contained in plasma of different individuals can neutralize from 5000 to many million units of SK. The most frequently observed titer for SK antibody equals 50,000–100,000 units of SK (Johnson et al. 1957). Moreover, the titer of SK-neutralizing antibody may show considerable variation over a period of time in the same person. Recent streptococcal infections and previous treatment with SK may produce enormous increases in antibody titer. SK antibody will immediately neutralize all SK during the initial phases of the infusion; only after sufficient amounts of SK have been administered to exhaust the total pool of SK antibody will subsequent SK infusion cause an activation of the plasmin-plasminogen system. It is necessary to determine the level of SK-neutralizing antibody in all patients prior to SK treatment and to gauge the initial doses accordingly. A rational thrombolytic therapy with SK did not become feasible until a simple and reproducible laboratory technique (Johnson et al. 1957) made it possible to assay SK antibody accurately.

In practice, the administration during the first hour of treatment of SK in amounts corresponding to the total SK antibody and the subsequent administration of 33–66 percent of the initial dose per hour during the following hours will produce a sustained and marked elevation of fibrinolytic activator activity throughout the infusion. This will produce a fall in circulating plasminogen to about 33–50 percent of the pretreatment level, with significant changes in the coagulation moieties but without hemorrhagic complications. Activator activity in plasma will return to normal levels within 1–2 hours and plasminogen and coagulation factors will return to pretreatment levels within 12–24 hours after the SK infusion is discontinued (Fletcher et al. 1959).

Urokinase (UK)

There are only a few reports dealing with the intravenous administration of UK, a plasminogen activator, purified from human urine to patients with thromboembolic disease (Hansen et al. 1961; McNicol et al. 1963; Fletcher et al. 1965). UK and SK exert principally the same effect on the fibrinolytic enzyme system in blood. However, UK has two theoretical advantages over SK: (1) It is not antigenic in man, as previously mentioned, and (2) in vitro observations strongly suggest that the fibrinolysis/fibrinogenolysis ratio is higher for UK than for SK (Sawyer et al. 1960b). The biochemical basis for this observation is not understood, but it may mean that the administration of UK will cause a more rapid lysis of intravascular thrombi with less nonspecific plasma proteolytic activity and less danger of hemorrhagic complications than is the case with SK administration. Until recently UK preparations were available in very small quantities, and in a number of instances complications of UK therapy were reported. This was related to the difficulty in separating UK completely from a urine thromboplastin-like material which limited the usefulness of the drug. The occasional development of thrombosis in patients receiving UK led most investigators to abandon this interesting fibrinolytic agent.

With a more highly-purified UK now being tried experimentally, clinical thromboembolism has not yet occurred and the clinical effectiveness of this material seems to be equal to that of SK (Johnson et al. 1964a); Fletcher et al. 1965).

Pharmacologic Activators

A wide variety of drugs of different origin, such as heparin (Schmitthauser et al. 1952) pyrogenic polysaccharides of bacterial origin (Meneghini, 1962; Stamm, 1962) irgapyrin (Sigg, 1952), and nicotinic acid (Weiner et al. 1958; Beller and Sellin, 1961), have been shown to cause an increase in fibrinolytic activator activity when administered to man or to experimental animals. The mechanism of action of these drugs is not known, but many of them, most notably nicotinic acid, have undergone clinical trial. The rationale for such therapy seems doubtful since the effect of all these drugs on the fibrinolytic enzyme system is brief, and since the measured activator activities constitute only a small fraction of the effect that can be obtained with SK.

SK-Plasmin Mixture ("Human Fibrinolysin")
The administration of SK-activated human plasminogen has been used in thrombolytic therapy by numerous investigators. Both the commercially available fibrinolytic agents, Actase® (Ortho) and Thrombolysin® (Merck, Sharp & Dohme) contain SK and free plasmin in varying ratios. The potency of both preparations is given in "fibrinolytic units", a term without clear and uniform definition. The two preparations exhibit great individual variation in their content of SK and plasmin. Fletcher et al. (1961) found that 50,000 "fibrinolytic units" of Actase contain approximately 6400 units SK and 5 caseinolytic units of plasmin. The recommended standard dose of Actase is 100,000–200,000 fibrinolytic (Actase) units, which corresponds to 12,000–24,000 SK units and 10–20 caseinolytic plasmin units.

It has been found that free SK and SK administered in mixtures with plasmin will be neutralized at the same rate by SK antibody; thus, the streptokinase concentration in 200,000 Actase units will be less than the total SK antibody in most patients. The plasmin contained in the same amount of Actase will be completely neutralized by the antiplasmins contained in 2–4 ml of human plasma.

It is easy to understand why Fletcher et al. (1960) failed to demonstrate enhanced levels of fibrinolytic activator activity in the blood following the administration of the recommended doses of Actase.

We have obtained in vitro evidence to indicate that highly purified plasmin as well as plasminogen activators in a narrow range of low concentrations may initiate and accelerate blood coagulation (Bang et al. 1962b).

Fletcher et al. (1961) also showed that 25,000 "fibrinolytic units" of Thrombolysin contain approximately 12,500 units SK and 50 caseinolytic units of plasmin. The recommended standard doses of 50,000–200,000 "fibrinolytic" units would contain sufficient amounts of SK to overcome the SK antibody in a number of patients, but not in all. It would also contain substantial amounts of free plasmin.

If patients with high titers of SK antibody were to be adequately treated with Thrombolysin, it would be necessary to administer this preparation in amounts far exceeding the recommended doses, and the amount of free plasmin given during such a regimen might result in a severe coagulation defect. There is no clear rationale for such combination therapy.

Side Effects of Fibrinolytic Therapy
Pyrogenic reactions, which are still encountered frequently during streptokinase and streptokinase-plasmin therapy, have features similar to those of other pyrogenic reactions. The mild reactions usually occur late, 6–8 hours after the start of the infusion, and consist of a temperature rise to 100–102° F, malaise, vomiting and leukopenia. Severe reactions usually occur rapidly after the start of the infusion, and are characterized by chill and frequently by hypotension, which may require administration of norepinephrine.

Allergic-Anaphylactic Reactions
Although immunologic reactions to SK or SK-Plasmin mixtures were previously claimed to be exceedingly rare, it is now apparent that with more widespread use of these drugs immediate allergic-anaphylactic reactions as well as delayed hypersensitivity reactions occur, particularly in patients who have received previous treatment with SK. There are some well documented cases of acute anaphylactic shock during an infusion of SK (Balstrup et al. 1962); skin eruptions are common.

Edema
In two patients reported recently (McNicol and Douglas, 1964) a 48–72 hour SK infusion successfully removed peripheral arterial thrombi. As soon as the artery became patent acute "wooden" edema developed in the pre-

viously ischemic extremity. The edema subsided within two–three days.

Laboratory Control of Therapeutic Fibrinolysis

Careful laboratory control of patients undergoing fibrinolytic therapy is necessary to assure that the therapy is effective, that the patient's plasma is capable of lysing fibrin clots, and that the therapy does not result in dangerous side effects.

The importance of these two principles is not generally recognized. The value of determining the individual variations in SK antibody before administration of SK or SK-plasmin preparations has been previously emphasized, but the necessity for performing a dose prediction test has unfortunately been widely ignored.

It is evident that the over-all fibrinolytic capacity of a patient's blood is determined by changes in a balance of activators, active enzyme, and inhibitors. The logical approach to the in vitro evaluation of the efficacy of fibrinolytic therapy is an assay which demonstrates that the patient's undiluted plasma is capable of dissolving a standardized preformed fibrin substrate. The fibrin plate technique designed by Astrup provides an adequate test system (Astrup and Müllertz, 1952). Its clinical usefulness is limited because it is time-consuming and insensitive to small variations in plasma fibrinolytic activity. Tests, utilizing the rate of lysis of preformed standardized ^{131}I-labelled fibrin clots incubated with the patient's plasma (see p. 380) have several theoretic advantages. They have proved useful in investigational work with fibrinolytic agents, but the use of such tests is limited to hospitals in which equipment for isotope work is available. A number of rapid and simple tests for a quantitative estimate of plasma fibrinolytic activity have been suggested as reliable laboratory assays. All these "bedside tests" (Milstone, 1941; Fearnley and Lackner, 1955) depend on measuring the combined activities of plasminogen activator and plasmin after their complete or partial separation from plasma inhibitors. Such assays do not reflect with accuracy the effective plasma fibrinolytic capacity and correlate poorly with the techniques which measure fibrinolytic activity in whole plasma. Their clinical use is not recommended.

A coagulation defect developing during therapy can be detected if repeated assays of the one-stage prothrombin time or plasma thrombin clotting time are performed. Either of these tests will constitute an adequate control of the patient's coagulation status, and may also provide a rough quantitative estimate of the severity of nonspecific plasma proteolytic activity. Plasmin activity in plasma is difficult to estimate accurately, since plasmin is partly inactivated during the assay procedure. Repeated measurements of plasma fibrinogen concentrations are desirable but not absolutely necessary as the rate of proteolytic breakdown of fibrinogen is reflected by the rise in the one-stage prothrombin time and the thrombin clotting time.

Indications for Fibrinolytic Therapy

Sufficient clinical data is not available to outline accurately the indications for fibrinolytic therapy and its limitations in thromboembolic disease. Extensive experimental work in animals permits a delineation of the factors which may determine the response to fibrinolytic agents in the clinical situation.

In animal experiments (Freiman et al. 1960) and also in a small clinical series (Johnson et al. 1964a), it has been shown that effective lysis of intravascular thrombi becomes impossible if the therapy is instituted 48 hours or more after for formation of the thrombus. Since organization and fibroblast invasion of the thrombus do not take place until after the first week following its formation, there is no good explanation for this early increase in resistance to enzymatic attack. It is possible that the clinical effect of enzymatic therapy noted in older peripheral vascular thrombi is related to a more recent extension of the original thrombus.

Animal experiments (Freiman et al. 1960) provide evidence that experimentally induced non-inflammatory phlebothrombosis responds more readily to enzymatic treatment than thrombophlebitis with severe vascular and perivascular inflammation.

Central or peripheral thrombosis and venous or arterial thrombi seem to respond equally well to treatment (Freiman et al. 1960). Whether these observations made in dogs without atherosclerotic vascular changes can be compared directly with the clinical situations in man is doubtful.

The plasminogen concentration in the fibrin clot, or rather the fibrin to plasminogen ratio, is of crucial importance in determining its resistance to enzymatic attack. There are animal experiments which suggest that fibrin clots formed at high fibrinogen levels respond poorly to therapy (Bang et al. 1959).

Experimentally induced thrombi formed during alimentary lipemia in dogs have been found to be greatly resistant to the action of fibrinolytic enzymes (Bang and Cliffton, 1960; Bang, 1962). The mechanism of this phenomenon is not clear. It was first assumed that the low-density beta lipoproteins found in these lipemic thrombi acted as specific plasmin or activator inhibitors. However, studies with the electron microscope have suggested a different explanation. It was shown that low-density beta lipoproteins display a strong affinity for fibrin, and it could be demonstrated visually that these fat macromolecules form a thick coat around the individual fibrin strands, thus seriously limiting the possibilities for contact between enzyme and substrate. These observations may prove important in determining the clinical response to enzyme therapy (Bang, 1967).

The state of the collateral circulation is important in determining the amount of enzyme delivered to the thrombus. Animal experiments (Freiman et al. 1960) have supported this contention.

VIII. Summary and Conclusions

The study of the fibrinolytic enzyme system like the study of the coagulation system has been in a state of extremely rapid development in recent years. The adaptation of methodological tools to specific problems in this kind of research from the fields of biochemistry, biophysics and immunochemistry have produced an impressive clarification of many issues. Development of specific and sensitive assay methods have permitted the use of refined experimental models; but with increasing sophistication and increased understanding of isolated reactions the complexities of this system maintained in a delicate homostatic balance also becomes increasingly more apparent. Emphasis on methodology, the continued question of the validity of "established" techniques and the continued search for improved methodology is essential for any further advances to be made in this field.

References

Ablondi, F. B., and Hagan, J. J. (1960). "The Enzymes". Academic Press. New York.

Ablondi, F. B., Hagan, J. J., Philips, M., and De Renzo, E. C. (1959). *Arch. Biochem. Biophys. 82,* 153.

Alagille, D., and Soulier, J. P. (1956). *Semaine Hop. Paris 32,* 355.

Albrechtsen, O. K. (1957a). *Brit. J. Haematol. 3,* 284.

Albrechtsen, O. K. (1957b). *Acta Physiol. Scand. 39,* 284.

Albrechtsen, O. K. (1959). *Acta Physiol. Scand. Suppl. 165,* 47.

Albrechtsen, O. K., Storm, O., and Trolle, D. (1955). *Acta Hematol. 14,* 309.

Ali, S. Y. (1967). *Biochem. J. 104,* 1P.

Ali, S. Y., and Lack, C. H. (1965). *Biochem. J. 96,* 63.

Alkjaersig, N. (1964). *Biochem. J. 93,* 171.

Alkjaersig, N., Fletcher, A. P., and Sherry, S. (1958). *J. Biol. Chem. 233,* 86.

Alkjaersig, N., Fletcher, A. P., and Sherry, S. (1959a). *J. Clin. Invest. 38,* 1086.

Alkjaersig, N., Fletcher, A. P., and Sherry, S. (1959b). *J. Biol. Chem. 234,* 832.

Alkjaersig, N., Fletcher, A. P., and Sherry, S. (1962). *J. Clin. Invest. 41,* 917.

Alkjaersig, N., Fletcher, A. P., and Sherry, S. (1965). *J. Lab. Clin. Med. 65,* 732.

Ambrus, C. M., and Markus, G. (1960). *Am. J. Physiol. 199,* 491.

Amris, C. J. (1964). *Abstracts of the 10th Congress of Hematology, Stockholm,* 1964.

Amris, C. J. (1965). *Scand. J. Haemtol. 3,* 19.

Amris, C. J., and Hilden, M. (1968). *Ann. N. Y. Acad. Sci. 146,* 612.

Anderer, F. A. (1965). *Z. Naturforsch. 20b,* 462.

Andersson, L. (1962). *Acta Chir. Scand. 124,* 355.

Andersson, L., and Nilsson, I. M. (1961). *Acta Chir. Scand. 121,* 291.

Andersson, L., Nilsson. I. M., Colleen, S., Granstrand, B., and Melander, B. (1968). *Ann. N. Y. Acad. Sci. 146,* 642.

Astrup, T. (1956a). *Blood 11,* 781.

Astrup, T. (1956b). *Lancet 2,* 565.

Astrup, T. (1958). *Thromb. Diath. Haemorrhag. 2,* 347.

Astrup, T. (1959). *In:* "Connective Tissue, Thrombosis and Atherosclerosis" (I. H. Page, ed.), p. 223. Academic Press. New York.

Astrup, T., and Alkjaersig, N. (1952). *Nature 169,* 314.

Astrup, T., and Kok, P. (1965). *Thromb. Diath. Haemorrhag. 13,* 587.

Astrup, T., and Müllertz, S. (1952). *Arch. Biochem. Biophys. 40,* 346.

Astrup, T., and Olesen, E. S. (1957). *Danish Med. Bull. 4,* 159.

Astrup, T., and Permin, P. M. (1947). *Nature 159,* 681.

Astrup, T., and Sterndorff, I. (1952). *Proc. Soc. Exptl. Biol. Med. 81,* 675.

Astrup, T., and Sterndorff, I. (1956), *Acta Physiol. Scand. 36,* 250.

Bachmann, F., Fletcher, A. P., Alkjaersig, N., and Sherry, S. (1964). *Biochemistry 3,* 1578.

Baker, W. J., Bang, N. U., Nachman, R. L., Raafat, F., and Horowitz, H. (1964). *Ann. Int. Med. 61,* 116.

Balstrup, F., Bang, N. U., and Iversen, K. (1962). *Ugeskrift Laeger 124,* 532.

Bang, N. U. (1961). *In:* "Thrombolytic Activity and Related Phenomena" (I. S. Wright, F. Koller and F. Strueli, eds.), p. 262. Friedrich-Karl Schauttauer-Verlag, Stuttgart.

Bang, N. U. (1962). *Thromb. Diath. Haemorrhag. 6,* 262.

Bang, N. U. (1965). *Modern Treatment 2,* 93.

Bang, N. U. (1967). *In:* "Blood Clotting Enzymology" (W. H. Seegers, ed.), p. 487. Academic Press, New York.

Bang, N. U., and Cliffton, E. E. (1960). *Thromb. Diath. Haemorrhag. 4,* 149.

Bang, N. U., Freiman, A. H., and Cliffton, E. E. (1959). *Clin. Res. 2,* 214.

Bang, N. U., Fletcher, A. P., Alkjaersig, N., and Sherry, S. (1962a). *J. Clin. Invest. 41,* 935.

Bang, N. U., Todd, M. E., and Wright, I. S. (1962b). *Thromb. Diath. Haemorrhag. 9,* 237.

Bang, N. U., Harpel, P. C., and Strueli, F. (1964). *Clin. Obstet. Gynec. 7,* 286.

Barg, W. F., Boggiano, E., and De Renzo, E. C. (1965). *J. Biol. Chem. 240,* 2944.

Barnett, E., and Baron, S. (1959). *Proc. Soc. Exptl. Biol. Med. 102,* 308.

Barnhart, M. I., and Riddle, J. M. (1963). *Blood 21,* 306.

Baumgarten, W., Cole, R., Richard, M. N., and Smith, F. B. (1957). *Science 125,* 604.

Beck, E., Schmutzler, R., and Duckert, F. (1963). *Thromb. Diath. Haemorrhag. 10,* 106.

Beller, F. K. (1964). *Clin. Obstet. Gynec. 7,* 372.

Beller, F. K., and Sellin, O. (1960). *Arzn. Forsch. 10,* 758.

Bergstrom, K. (1963). *Arkiv Kemi 21,* 517.

Bernik, M. B., and Kwaan, H. C. (1967). *J. Lab. Clin. Med. 70,* 650.

Bernik, M. B., and Kwaan, H. C. (1968). *Fed. Proc. 27,* 272.

Bickford, A. F., Taylor, F. B., Jr., and Sheena, R. (1964). *Biochem. Biophys. Acta 92,* 328.

Biggs, R., Mac Farlane, R. G., and Pilling, J. (1947). *Lancet 1,* 402.

Björkman, S. E., Laurell, C. B., and Nilsson, I. M. (1956). *Scand. J. Clin. Lab. Invest. 8,* 304.

Blombäck, B., and Blombäck, M. (1956). *Arki Kemi 10,* 415.

Brakman, P., and Astrup, T. (1964). *Sangre 9,* 46.

Carroll, H. J., and Tice, D. A. (1966). *Metabolism 15,* 449.

Celander, D. R., and Guest, M. M. (1959). *Am. J. Physiol. 197,* 391.

Celander, D. R., Langlinais, R. P., and Guest, M. M. (1955). *Arch. Biochem. Biophys. 55,* 286.

Chakrabarti, R., Birks, P. M., and Fearnley, G. R. (1963). *Lancet 1,* 1288.

Christensen, L. R. (1945). *J. Gen. Physiol. 28,* 363.

Christensen, L. R. (1946). *J. Gen. Physiol. 30,* 149.

Cliffton, E. E., and Downie, G. R. (1950). *Proc. Soc. Exptl. Biol. Med. 73,* 559.

Colgan, J., Gates, E., and Miller, L. L. (1952). *J. Exptl. Med. 95,* 531.

Colman, R., Mattler, L., and Sherry, S. (1969a). *J. Clin. Invest. 48,* 11.

Colman, R., Mattler, L., and Sherry, S. (1969b). *J. Clin. Invest. 48,* 23.

Cooperberg, A. A., and Neiman, G. M. G. (1955). *Ann. Int. Med. 42,* 706.

Correll, J. T., and Sjoerdsma, A. (1962). *Proc. Soc. Exptl. Biol. Med. 111,* 274.

Crawford, T., and Wolf, N. (1960). *J. Pathol. Bact. 79,* 221.

Dam, H., Larsen, J., and Plum, P. (1941). *Ugeskrift Laeger 103,* 257.

Davidson, F. M. (1960). *Biochem. J. 76,* 56.

Davies, M. C., Englert, M. E., and De Renzo, E. C. (1964). *J. Biol. Chem. 239,* 2651.

De Lee, J. B. (1901). *Am. J. Obstet. 44,* 785.

De Renzo, E. C., Barg, W., Boggiano, C., Engler, M. E., and Davies, M. C. (1963). *Biochem. Biophys. Res. Commun. 12,* 105.

De Renzo, E. C., Boggiano, E., and Hummel, B. C. W. (1965). *Fed. Proc. 24,* 260.

De Renzo, E. C., Boggiano, E., Barg, W. F., and Buck, F. F. (1967). *J. Biol. Chem. 242,* 2428.

Dillard, G. H. L., and Chanutin, A. (1949). *Cancer Res. 9,* 665.

Doleschel, W., and Auerswald, W. (1967). *Med. Pharmacol. Exp. 17,* 254.

Donaldson, V. H., (1960). *J. Lab. Clin. Med. 56,* 644.

Duguid, J. B. (1946). *J. Pathol. Bact. 58,* 207.

Duguid, J. B. (1959). *In:* "Connective Tissue, Thrombosis, and Atherosclerosis" (J. H. Page, Ed.), p. 13. Academic Press, New York.

Ehrenpreis, S., Laskowski, M., Jr., Donnelly, T. H., and Scheraga, H. A. (1958). *J. Am. Chem. Soc. 80,* 4255.

Eisen, V. (1964). *Brit. Med. Bull. 20,* 205.

Fantl, P., and Simon, S. E. (1948). *Austr. J. Exptl. Biol. Med. Sci. 26,* 521.

Fearnley, G. R. (1965). *In:* "Fibrinolysis". Williams and Wilkins Co, Baltimore.

Fearnley, G. R., and Lackner, R. (1955). *Brit. J. Hematol. 1,* 189.

Fearnley, G. R., Balmforth, G., and Fearnley, E. (1957). *Clin. Sci. 16,* 645.

Fibrinolysis (1964). *Brit. Med. Bull. 20,* 171.

Fischer, H., Brueckner, H., Fritzsche, W., and Becker, H. (1956). *62nd Cong. Verhdlg. Dtsch. Ges. Int. Med.,* Bergmann Muenchen

Fischer, S., Albrechtsen, O., and Bang, N. U. (1959). *Thromb. Diath. Haemorrhag. 3,* 554.

Fisher, A. (1946). *Nature 157,* 442.

Fisher, S., Fletcher, A. P., Alkjaersig, N., and Sherry, S. (1967). *J. Lab. Clin. Med. 70,* 904.

Fishman, J. B., and Kline, D. L. (1963). *Proc. Soc. Exptl. Biol. Med. 113,* 944.

Fletcher, A. P. (1960). *In:* "Proceedings of the Conference on Thrombolytic Agents" (H. R. Roberts and J. D. Geratz, Eds.), p. 148. University of North Carolina Press, Chapel Hill, North Carolina.

Fletcher, A. P., Alkjaersig, N., and Sherry, S. (1958). *J. Clin. Invest. 37,* 1306.

Fletcher, A. P., Alkjaersig, N., and Sherry, S. (1959a). *J. Clin. Invest. 38,* 1096.

Fletcher, A. P., Sherry, S., Alkjaersig, N., Smyrniotis, F. E., and Jick, S. (1959b). *J. Clin. Invest. 38,* 1111.

Fletcher, A. P., Alkjaersig, N., Sawyer, W. D., and Sherry, S. (1960). *J. Am. Med. Assoc. 172,* 912.

Fletcher, A. P., Alkjaersig, N., and Sherry, S. (1961). *J. Lab. Clin. Med. 57,* 620.

Fletcher, A. P., Alkjaersig, N., and Sherry, S. (1962). *J. Clin. Invest. 41,* 896.

Fletcher, A. P., Biederman, O., Moore, D., Alkjaersig, N., and Sherry, S. (1964). *J. Clin. Invest. 43,* 681.

Fletcher, A. P., Alkjaersig, N., Sherry, S., Genton, E., Hirsh, J., and Bachmann, F. (1965). *J. Lab. Clin. Med. 65,* 713.

Fletcher, A. P., Alkjaersig, N., Fisher, S., and Sherry, S. (1966). *J. Lab. Clin. Med. 68,* 780.

Freiman, A. H., Bang, N. U., and Cliffton, E. E. (1960). *Circulation Res. 8,* 409.

Gans, H., and Krivit, W. (1962). *Ann. Surg. 155,* 268.

Geiger, W. B. (1952). *J. Immunol. 69,* 597.

Gerheim, E. B., Ferguson, J. H., Travis, B. L., Johnston, C. L., and Boyles, P. W. (1948). *Proc. Soc. Exptl. Biol. Med. 68,* 246.

Giraud, G., Gazal, P., Latour, H., Izorn, P., Levy, A., Bargon, P., and Ribstein, M. (1954). *Sang 25,* 628.

Gitlin, D., and Craig, J. M. (1957). *Am. J. Pathol. 33,* 267.

Gitlin, D., Landing, B. H., and Whipple, A. (1953). *J. Exptl. Med. 97,* 163.

Gitlin, D., Craig, J. M., and Janeway, C. A. (1957). *Am. J. Pathol. 33,* 55.

Goldhaber, B., Cornman, I., and Ormsbee, R. (1947). *Proc. Soc. Exptl. Biol. Med. 66,* 590.

Goodpasture, E. W. (1914). *Bull. Johns Hopkins Hosp. 25,* 330.

Grob, D. (1949). *J. Gen. Physiol. 33,* 103.

Grossi, C. E., Moreno, A. H., and Rousselot, L. M. (1961). *Ann. Surg. 153,* 383.

Guest, M. M., and Celander, D. R. (1960). *Physiologist 3,* 69.

Guest, M. M., Daly, B. M., Ware, A. G., and Seegers, W. H. (1948). *J. Clin. Invest. 27,* 793.

Hansen, P. F., Jorgensen, M., Kjeldgaard, N. O., and Ploug, J. (1961). *Angiology 12,* 367.

Hayashi, T., and Mackawa, S. (1954). *Jap. J. Exptl. Med. 24,* 287.

Hedin, S. G. (1903). *J. Physiol. 30,* 195.

Hjort, P. F., and Hasselback, R. (1961). *Thromb. Diath. Haemorrhag. 6,* 580.

Holemans, R. (1963). *Med. Exptl. 9,* 5.

Holmberg, C. G. (1944). *Arkiv Kemi 17a,* 28.

Horowitz, R. E., Stuyvesant, V. W., Wigmore, W., and Tatter, D. (1965). *Arch. Pathol. 79,* 238.

Hummel, C. W., Buck, F. F., and De Renzo, E. C. (1966). *J. Biol. Chem. 241,* 3474.

Iatridis, S. G., and Ferguson, J. H. (1962). *J. Clin. Invest. 41,* 1277.

Innerfield, I., Schwarz, A., and Angrist, A. (1952). *J. Clin. Invest. 31,* 1049.

Jackson, H. D., and Mertz, E. T. (1954). *Proc. Soc. Exptl. Biol. Med. 86,* 827.

Jacobsson, K. (1953). *Acta Chem. Scand. 7,* 430.

Johansson, F. (1913). *Ztschr. Physiol. Chemie 85,* 72.

Johnson, A. J., and McCarty, W. R. (1959). *J. Clin. Invest. 38,* 1627.

Johnson, A. J., and McCarty, W. R. (1960a). *In:* "Proceedings of the Conference on Thrombolytic Agents" (H. R. Roberts and J. D. Geratz, eds.), p. 173. University of North Carolina Press, Chapel Hill, North Carolina.

Johnson, A. J., and McCarty, W. R. (1960b). *Am. J. Cardiol. 6,* 487.

Johnson, A. J., and McCarty, W. R. (1961). *Thromb. Diath. Haemorrhag. 5,* 391.

Johnson, A. J., and Tillett, W. (1952). *J. Exptl. Med. 95,* 449.

Johnson, A. J., Fletcher, A. P., McCarty, W. R., and Tillett, W. (1957). *Ann. N. Y. Acad. Sci. 68,* 201.

Johnson, A. J., McCarty, W. R., Tillett, W. S., Tse, A. O., Skoza, L., Newman, J., and Semar, M. (1964a). *In:* "Blood Coagulation, Hemorrhage and Thrombosis: Methods of Study" (L. M. Tocantins and L. A. Kazal, eds.), p. 449. Grune, New York.

Johnson, A. J., McCarty, W. R., Newman, J., and Lakner, H. (1964b). *J. Clin. Invest. 43,* 1265.

Kaplan, E. H. (1955). *Proc. Soc. Exptl. Biol. Med. 85,* 142.

Kaplan, E. H. (1944). *Proc. Soc. Exptl. Biol. Med. 57,* 40.

Kassell, B., Radicevic, M., Ansfield, M. J., and Laskowski, M., Sr. (1965). *Biochem. Biophys. Res. Comm. 18,* 255.

Kjeldgaard, N. O., and Ploug, J. (1957). *Biochem. Biophys. Acta 24,* 289.

Kline, D. L., and Fishman, J. B. (1961). *J. Biol. Chem. 236,* 2807.

Kocholaty, W., Ellis, W. W., and Jensen, H. (1952). *Proc. Soc. Exptl. Biol. Med. 80,* 36.

Kowalski, E., Budzynski, A., Kopec, M., and Murawski, K. (1960). *Blood 15,* 164.

Kowalski, E., Kopec, M., and Wegrzynowicz, Z. (1964). *Thromb. Diath. Haemorrhag. 10,* 406.

Kucinski, C., and Fletcher, A. (1966a). *Fed. Proc. 29,* 194.

Kucinski, C., and Fletcher, A. (1966b). *Fed. Proc. 29,* 647.

Kwaan, H. C. (1964). *Am. J. Clin. Pathol. 41,* 604.

Kwaan, H. C., and Astrup, T. (1967). *Lab. Invest. 17,* 140.

Kwaan, H. C., and Fisher, S. (1965). *Fed. Proc. 24,* 2.

Kwaan, H. C., and McFadzean, A. J. S. (1956). *Clin. Sci. 15,* 245.

Kwaan, H. C., Lo, R., and McFadzean, A. J. S. (1957a). *Clin. Sci. 16,* 241.

Kwaan, H. C., Lo, R., and McFadzean, A. J. S. (1957b). *Clin. Sci. 16,* 255.

Kwaan, H. C., Lo, R., and McFadzean, A. J. S. (1957c). *Brit. J. Haematol. 4,* 51.

Kwaan, H. C., Lo, R., and McFadzean, A. J. S. (1958). *Clin Sci. 17,* 361.

Lack, C. H. (1948). *Nature 161,* 559.

Larrieu, M. J., Inceman, S., and Marder, U. (1967). *Nouv. Rev. France d'Hematol 7,* 691.

Lassen, M. (1958). *Biochem. J. 69,* 360.

Latallo, Z., Fletcher, A. P., Alkjaersig, N., and Sherry, S. (1962a). *Am. J. Physiol. 202,* 675.

Latallo, Z., Fletcher, A. P., Alkjaersig, N., and Sherry, S. (1962b). *Am. J. Physiol. 202,* 681.

Latallo, Z., Budzynski, A. Z., Lipinski, B., and Kowalski, E. (1964). *Nature 203,* 1184.

Lendrum, A. C. (1961). *Ned. T. Geneesk. 105,* 1359.

Lepow, I. H., Pillemer, L., and Ratnoff, O. D. (1953). *J. Exptl. Med. 98,* 277.

Lesuk, A., Terminiello, L., and Traver, J. H. (1965). *Science 147,* 880.

Lesuk, A., Terminiello, L., Traver, J. H., and Groff, J. L (1967). *Thromb. Diath. Haemorrhag. 18,* 293.

Lewis, J. H., and Ferguson, J. H. (1951). *Am. J. Physiol. 166,* 594.

Lewis, J. H., and Ferguson, J. H. (1952), *Am. J. Physiol. 170,* 636.

Lohmann, K., Markwardt, F., and Landmann, H. (1964). *Thromb. Diath. Haemorrhag. 10,* 424.

Loomis, E. C., George, C., Jr., and Ryder, A. (1947). *Arch. Biochem. 12,* 1.

Lorand, L., and Mozen, M. M. (1964). *Nature 201,* 392.

MacFarlane, R. G. (1937). *Lancet 1,* 10.

Maki, M., and Beller, F. K. (1966). *Thromb. Diath. Haemorrhag. 16,* 668.

Marchal, G., Samama, M., Auvert, J., Duhamel, G., and Yver, J. (1961). *Semaine Hop. Paris 37,* 1700.

Markus, G., and Ambrus, C. M. (1960). *J. Biol. Chem. 235,* 1673.

Mathey, J., Daumet, P., Soulier, J. P., LeBolloch, A. G., and Fayet, H. (1950). *Mem. Acad. Chir. 76,* 764.

McNicol, G. P. (1962). *Scot. Med. J. 7,* 266.

McNicol, G. P., and Douglas, A. S. (1964). *Brit. Med. Bull. 20,* 233.

McNicol, G. P., Fletcher, A. P., Alkjaersig, N., and Sherry, S. (1961a). *J. Lab. Clin. Med. 58,* 34.

McNicol, G. P., Fletcher, A. P., Alkjaersig, N., and Sherry, S. (1961b). *J. Urol. 86,* 829.

McNicol, G. P., Fletcher, A. P., Alkjaersig, N., and Sherry, S. (1962). *J. Lab. Clin. Med. 59,* 15.

McNicol, G. P., Gale, S. B., and Douglas, A. S. (1963). *Brit. Med. J. 1,* 909.

Meneghini, P. (1950). *L'Informatore Med. Sec. Sci. 4,* 139.

Meneghini, P. (1962). *Thromb. Diath. Haemorrhag. 6,* 217.

Meyers, W. M., Burdon, K. L., and Riley, M. N. (1957). *J. Lab. Clin. Invest. 49,* 377.

Mikata, I., Hasegawa, M., Igarashi, T., Shirakura, N., Hoshida, M., and Toyama, K. (1959). *Keio J. Med. 8,* 279.

Milstone, H. (1941). *J. Immunol.* 42, 109.

Mirsky, I. A., Perisutti, G., and Davis, N. C. (1959a). *J. Clin. Invest. 38,* 14.

Mirsky, I. A., Perisutti, G., and Davis, N. C. (1959b). *Endocrinology 64,* 992.

Mole, R. H. (1948). *J. Pathol. Bact. 60,* 413.

Moltke, P. (1958). *Proc. Soc. Exptl. Biol. Med. 98,* 377.

Morris, R. H., Vassalli, P. M. D., Beller, F. K., and McCluskey, R. T. (1964). *Obstet. Gynec. 24,* 32.

Mosesson, M. W., Alkjaersig, N., Sweet, B., and Sherry, S. (1957). *Biochemistry 6,* 3279.

Müllertz, S. (1953). *Proc. Soc. Exptl. Biol. Med. 82,* 291.

Müllertz, S. (1955). *Biochem. J. 61,* 424.

Müllertz, S. (1957). *Ann. N. Y. Acad. Sci. 58,* 38.

Müllertz, S., and Lassen, M. (1953). *Proc. Soc. Exptl. Biol. Med. 82,* 264.

Naeye, R. L. (1961). *New Eng. J. Med. 265,* 867.

Nanninga, L. B., and Guest, M. M. (1964). *Arch. Biochem. Biophys. 108,* 542.

Niewiarowski, S., and Kowalski, E. (1957). *Trans. 6th Cong. European. Soc. Hematol., Copenhagen,* 1957 Karger, Basel.

Niewiarowski, S., and Kowalski, E. (1958). *Rev. Hematol. 13,* 320.

Niewiarowski, S., and Latallo, Z. S. (1957). *Bull. Acad. Polon. Sci. Classe (II) 2,* 219.
Nilsson, I. M., Skanse, B., and Gydell, K. (1957). *Acta Med. Scand. 159,* 463.
Nilsson, I. M., Skanse, B., and Gydell, K. (1960a). *Rev. Hematol. 15,* 451.
Nilsson, I. M., Sjoerdsma, A., and Waldenstrom, J. (1960b). *Lancet 1,* 1322.
Nilsson, I. M., Krook, H., Sternby, N. H., Soderberg, E., and Soderstroem, N. (1961). *Acta Med. Scand. 169,* 323.
Nordström, S., Blombäck, B., Blombäck, M., Olsson, P., and Zetterqvist, E. (1968). *Ann. N. Y. Acad. Sci. 146,* 701.
Norman, P. S. (1958). *J. Exptl. Med. 108,* 53.
Norman, P. S., and Hill, B. M. (1958). *J. Exptl. Med. 108,* 639.
Nussenzweig, V., and Seligman, M. (1960). *Rev. Hematol. 15,* 451.
Nussenzweig, V., Seligman, M., Pelmont, J. and Grabar, P. (1961a). *Ann. Inst. Pasteur 100,* 377.
Nussenzweig, V., Seligman, M., and Grabar, P. (1961b). *Ann. Inst. Pasteur 100,* 490.
Okamoto, S., and Okamoto, U. (1962). *Keio J. Med. 11,* 105.
Okamoto, S., Nagasawa, K., Takagi, K., Tsukada, H., Koyoi, W., and Sato, S. (1957). Mitsubishi Kasei Kogyo Kabushiki Kaisha Company.
Olesen, E. S. (1957). *Acta Physiol. Scand. 41,* 187.
Painter, R., and Charles, A. (1962). *Am. J. Physiol. 202,* 1125.
Pechet, L. (1965). *New Eng. J. Med. 273,* 966.
Permin, P. M. (1949). *Fibrinolytiske Enzyme (thesis).* Copenhagen: Store Nordiske Videnskabsboghandel.
Pillemer, L., Ratnoff, O. D., Blum, L., and Lepow, I. H. (1952). *J. Exptl. Med. 97,* 573.
Ploug, J., and Kjeldgaard, N. O. (1956). *Arch. Biochem. Biophys. 62,* 500.
Ploug, J., and Kjeldgaard, N. O. (1957). *Biochim. Biophys. Acta 24,* 278.
Ratnoff, O. D., Pritchard, J. A., and Colopy, J. E. (1955). *New Engl. J. Med. 253,* 63.
Remmert, L. F., and Cohen, P. (1949). *J. Biol. Chem. 181,* 431.
Rifé, U., and Shulman, S. (1963). *Thromb. Diath. Haemorrhag. 10,* 133.
Robbins, K., Summaria, L., Hsieh, B., and Shah, R. J. (1967). *J. Biol. Chem. 242,* 2333.
Ronwin, E. (1962). *Canad. J. Biochem. Physiol. 40,* 57.
Sawyer, W. D.- Fletcher, A. P., Alkjaersig, N. A., and Sherry, S. (1960a). *J. Clin. Invest. 39,* 426.
Sawyer, W. D., Alkjaersig, N. A., Fletcher, A. P., and Sherry, S. (1960b). *Thromb. Diath. Haemorrhag. 5,* 149.
Schmitthauser, K., Kopp, M., and Eichenberger, E. (1952). *Experientia 8,* 354.
Schneck, S. A., and von Kaulla, K. N. (1961). *Neurology, 11,* 960.
Schulz, F. H., and Knobloch, H. (1954). *Muenchn, med. Wschr. 96,* 1534.
Schulz, F. H., and Knoblock, H. (1954). *Muenchn. Med. Wschr. Thromb. Diath. Haemorrhag. 18,* 302.
Schultz, F. H., and Knoblock, H. (1954). *Muenchn. Med. Wschr. 96,* 1534.
Schwick, H. G., Heimburger, N., and Haupt, H. (1967). *Thromb. Diath. Haemorrhag. 18,* 302.
Scott, E. U. Z., Matthews, W. F., Butterworth, C. E., and Frommeyer, S. B. (1954). *Surg. Gynec. Obstet. 99,* 679.
Seegers, W. H., Levine, W. G., and Vandenbelt, J. M. (1945). *Arch. Biochem. Biophys. 6,* 85.
Sherman, L. A., Fletcher, A. P., and Sherry, S. (1968). *Fed. Proc. 27,* 693.
Sherry, S. (1965). *Series Haematologica 7,* 70.
Sherry, S., and Alkjaersig, N. (1957). *Thromb. Diath. Haemorrhag. 1,* 264.
Sherry, S., Fletcher, A. P., and Alkjaersig, N. (1959a). *Physiol. Rev. 39,* 343.
Sherry, S., Lindemeyer, R. I., Fletcher, A. P., and Alkjaersig, N. (1959b). *J. Clin. Invest. 38,* 810.
Sherry, S., Fletcher, A. P., Alkjaersig, N., and Sawyer, W. D. (1959c). *Trans. Assoc. Am. Physicians 72,* 62.
Sherry, S., Alkjaersig, N., and Fletcher, A. P. (1964). *J. Lab. Clin. Med. 64,* 145.
Shulman, N. R. (1952). *J. Exptl. Med. 95,* 605.
Shulman, S., Alkjaersig, N., and Sherry, S. (1958). *J. Biol. Chem. 233,* 91.
Sigg, B. (1952). *Praxis 41,* 1072.
Sjoerdsma, A., and Nilsson, I. M. (1960). *Proc. Soc. Exptl. Biol. 103,* 533.
Skoza, L., Tse, A. O., Semar, M., and Johnson, A. J. (1968). *Ann. N. Y. Acad. Sci. 146,* 659.
Slotta, K. H., and Gonzalez, J. D. (1964). *Biochem. 3,* 285.
Smyrniotis, F. E., Fletcher, A. P., Alkjaersig, N., and Sherry, S. (1959). *Thromb. Diath. Haermorrhag. 4,* 257.
Sobel, G. W., Mohler, S. R., Jones, N. W., Dowdy, A. B. C., and Guest, M. M. (1952). *Am. J. Physiol. 171,* 768.
Soulier, J. P., and Koupernik, C. (1948). *Sang 19,* 362.
Soulier, J. P., Mathey, J., LeBolloch, A. G., Daumet, P., and Fayet, H. (1952a). *Rev. d'Hematol. 7,* 30.
Soulier, J. P., Petit, P. F., and LeBolloch, A. G. (1952b). *Rev. d'Hematol. 7,* 48.
Soulier, J. P., Bernard, J., Bousser, J., Dreyfus, B., Hamburger, J., and Pequignot, H. (1964). *Presse Med. 72,* 167.
Stamm, H. (1962). *Thromb. Diath. Haemorrhag. 6,* 227.
Stefanini, M., and Marin, H. (1958). *Proc. Soc. Exptl. Biol. Med. 99,* 504.
Steichele, D. F., and Herschlein, H. J. (1961). *Med. Welt 112,* 2170.
Tagnon, H. J. (1942). *J. Lab. Clin. Med. 27,* 1119.
Tagnon, H. J., Levenson, S. M., Davidson, C. S., and Taylor, F. H. L. (1946). *Am. J. Med. Sci. 211,* 88.
Taylor, F. B., and Staprans, I. (1966). *Arch. Biochem. Biophys. 114,* 38.
The Fibrinolysin System (1966). *Fed. Proc. 25,* 28.
Thrombolytic Activity and Related Phenomena (1961). Wright, D., Koller, F., and Strueli, F., eds. Friedrich-Karl Schattauer-Verlag, Stuttgart.
Tillett, W. S. (1935). *J. Bacteriol. 29,* 111.
Tillett, W. S. (1938). *Bact. Rev. 2,* 161.
Todd, A. S. (1959). *J. Pathol. Bacteriol. 78,* 281.
Triantaphyllopoulos, D. C. (1958). *Can. J. Biochem. Physiol. 36,* 249.
Triantaphyllopoulos, D. C., and Triantaphyllopoulos, E. (1965). *Am. J. Physiol. 208,* 521.
Troll, W., and Sherry, S. (1955). *J. Biol. Chem. 213,* 881.
Ungar, G. (1952). *Lancet 2,* 742.
Ungar, G., and Mist, S. (1949). *J. Exptl. Med. 90,* 39.
von Kaulla, K. N. (1954). *J. Lab. Clin. Med. 44,* 944.
von Kaulla, K. N. (1956). *Acta Hematol. 16,* 315.
von Kaulla, K. N. (1963). *In* "Chemistry of Thrombolysis: Human Fibrinolytic Enzymes" (I. N. Kugelmass, ed.). C. Thomas, Springfield, Illinois.
von Kaulla, K. N., and Schneck, S. A. (1963). *In* "Chemistry of Thrombolysis: Human Fibrinolytic Enzymes" (I. N. Kugelmass, ed.). C. Thomas, Springfield, Illinois.
von Kaulla, K. N., and Swan, H. (1958). *J. Thoracic Surg. 36,* 519.
von Kaulla, K. N., Swan, H., and Paton, B. (1960). *J. Thoracic Cardiovasc. Surg. 40,* 260.
Walton, P. (1967). *Biochem. Biophys. Acta 132,* 104.
Ware, A. G., and Seegers, W. H. (1949). *Am. J. Clin. Pathol. 19,* 471.
Weiner, A. E., Reid, D. E., and Raby, C. C. (1950). *Am. J. Obstet. Gynec. 60,* 379.
Weiner, M., Redisch, W., and Steele, J. M. (1958). *Proc. Soc. Exptl. Biol. Med. 98,* 755.
White, W. E., Barlow, G. H., and Mozen, M. M. (1966). *Biochemistry 5,* 2160.
Williams, J. R. B. (1951). *Brit. J. Exptl. Pathol. 32,* 530.

Fibrinolytic Activity in Whole Blood, Dilute Blood, and Euglobulin Clot Lysis Time Tests

Henner Graeff and Fritz K. Beller

I. Introduction

The lysis time of blood clots in vitro exceeds 24 hours under normal conditions. The results are of value only if short lysis times are observed. In view of its lack of specificity, the usefulness of this technique is limited.

The lysis time shortens considerably if inhibitors are removed from plasma. This can be achieved either by dilution or by dilution and acidification to the isoelectric point (euglobulin precipitation). Although either the dilution or the euglobulin precipitation offer considerable practical advantages, their relevance to human biology is still controversial. It should be clearly understood that both techniques provide a means of measuring fibrinolytic activity following the separation of plasminogen activator and plasmin from the naturally occurring plasma inhibitors.

II. Blood Clot Lysis Time

Principle: Blood is clotted in a test tube and observed for lysis.

Material and reagents: Siliconized glass tubes 15×100 mm, 37° C water bath.

Procedure: Two ml of whole blood are allowed to clot either spontaneously or through the addition of thrombin (3 U/ml of blood). The tubes are incubated at 37° C and observed for 24 hours. If no lysis has occurred they are discarded and the test is regarded as negative.

Comment: Lysis times shorter than 24 hours indicate activator or plasmin activity. Contamination by microorganisms is avoided by sterilizing the glassware. The area of air gel interphase is of importance, and test tubes have to be identical in diameter (Marx, 1955). This rather insensitive test can be made somewhat more quantitative by measuring the clot by weight or by estimating its tyrosine content (Halse, 1948). The usefulness of the whole blood clot lysis test is limited by a number of additional factors. Any coagulation defect producing an inadequate clot may in this test system be misinterpreted as evidence of fibrinolysis. In clinical fibrinolytic states low fibrinogen levels and the presence of high levels of fibrinogen breakdown products may occur without concommitant elevation of plasminogen activator. The defective fibrin clot which forms under these circumstances may give the spurious impression of ongoing brisk fibrinolysis. It is therefore important to carefully watch and record the rate of clot formation as well as the lysis rates. Conversely, the whole blood clot lysis may appear entirely negative in brisk fibrinolytic states. The rate of lysis depends on both the level of plasminogen activator and the amount of plasminogen entrapped in the clot. When circulating plasminogen levels are reduced to zero, as seen in severe fibrinolysis, whole blood clot lysis can not take place. The demonstration of a fibrinolytic state under these circumstances depends upon the lysis of an extraneous plasminogen rich fibrin substrate such as the fibrin plate or a radioiodine labelled fibrin clot.

III. Diluted Blood Clot Lysis Time (Fearnley et al. 1957)

Principle: Dilution of blood or plasma decreases the inhibitor activity leaving plasminogen activator and/or plasmin free to cause lysis.

The assay is performed either by diluting the specimen and determining the lysis time, or by preparing serial dilutions, and determining after a fixed incubation period, which tubes are lysed. Lysis will proceed from the lowest to the highest concentration. Both procedures appear to be equally sensitive, but the latter might possibly be more convenient because of the fixed incubation period.

Material and reagents: Diethylbarbiturate buffer, pH 7.4, ionic strength 0.154, with merthiolate 1:10,000.
Thrombin solution, 40 U/ml.
Siliconized or polystyrene plastic tubes 12 × 75 mm.
Pipettes, 2,0 ml, 1,0 ml.
Waterbath at 37° C.

Procedure: 1) Diluted blood or diluted plasma clot lysis time, using one dilution (Fearnley et al. 1957; Lackner and Goosen, 1959): 2 ml of blood are drawn with a cold plastic syringe (two-syringe technique), and transferred into a test tube. One ml of blood is diluted with 9 ml of cold buffer solution. Two ml aliquots of the blood buffer mixture are pipetted into test tubes, each containing 0.1 ml thrombin solution. Final blood dilution is 9.5 %. Clots are set up in triplicate. If the blood was drawn at the bedside, it may be further stored for 30–60 minutes in melting ice. The tubes are covered with parafilm and incubated at 37° C. Lysis time is recorded by observing the samples or by using an automatic camera which takes pictures every half hour (Lackner and Goosen, 1959). Fearnley (1965) described a similar observation technique. If plasma is used, processing of the specimen and centrifuging for platelet poor plasma must be done at 4° C using a correction factor based on an estimated hematocrit of 45 % and a 1:10 dilution with citrate, 0.6 ml of plasma is added to 9.4 ml of buffer solution. 2) Diluted blood or diluted plasma clot lysis time using serial dilutions (Amery et al. 1962; Chakrabarty and Fearnley, 1962). Ten test tubes are placed in melting ice, numbers 2–9 each contain 2 ml of diethylbarbiturate buffer. Two ml of blood are added to tube number 1 and a dilution series is established by adding sequentially 2 ml aliquots from one tube to the next. The last 2 ml are discarded. A dilution range from 1:1 to 1:128 is achieved. A 0.2 ml aliquot of the thrombin solution is added, the tubes are covered with parafilm, inverted once, and incubated at 37° C. The test is read after 12, 24 or 48 hours. Higher fibrinolytic activity is indicated by lysis in a greater number of tubes. The lysis starts in the most diluted tubes.
Platelet poor plasma processed in the cold may also be assayed. The protein dilution for plasma differs somewhat from the one for whole blood, as no correction is done for hematocrit and trisodium citrate addition.

Comment: The processing of the specimen must be carried out in the cold or in ice water. Plasma samples have longer lysis times than whole blood. Fibrinolytic activity of the thrombin solution used is of significance. Isotonic buffers are preferable to buffers of low ionic strength as dilution fluids.

IV. Euglobulin Clot Lysis Time

Principle: Precipitation of the euglobulin fraction is attained by lowering the ionic strength and by acidification (Hedin, 1904; Milstone, 1941; MacFarlane and Pilling, 1946; Kowarzyk and Buluk, 1950; von Kaulla and Schultz, 1958). The precipitate is redissolved, clotted with thrombin or calcium and lysis time recorded.

Material and Reagents:
Polystyrene plastic tubes 16 × 100 mm, 12 × 75 mm;
Pipettes: 10.0 ml, 0.2 ml;
Refrigerated centrifuge;
Water bath (37° C);
Vortex mixer;
0.016 % acetic acid; 3.2 ml of 1 %acetic acid diluted up to 200 ml with distilled water pH 3.75 (Milstone, 1941);
Thrombin solution, 40 NIH U/ml;
Phosphate buffer, pH 7.3–7.5, ionic strength 0.154.

Procedure: Citrate blood (1:10 in 3.8 % trisodium citrate) is stored in ice water and centrifuged at 1,000 × G for 20 min. (+ 4° C). The platelet poor plasma is diluted with 12.5 ml Milstone reagent resulting in a pH varying between 5.2 and 5.6, depending on the buffer capacity of the plasma. The pH can easily be adjusted if desired, by diluting the plasma with 12.6 ml cold distilled water and adding drops of 0.5 % acetic acid under constant stirring (MacFarlane and Pilling,

1946). Precipitation with CO_2 is achieved by bubling the gas via a capillary tube through the diluted plasma sample for 2 min, resulting eventually in a pH of 5.6 (von Kaulla and Schultz, 1958). The tubes are kept in the ice bath for 20 min., after which time they are centrifuged at 1,000 × G for 15 min. The supernatant is decanted, the tubes inverted for 1 min. on absorbent paper and the remaining drops wiped off. The precipitate is dissolved in 0.7 ml phosphate buffer with a polystyrene plastic rod. A 0.5 ml aliquot is transferred into plastic tubes (12×75 mm), 0.05 ml thrombin solution is added, and mixed by Vortex mixer and the specimen is incubated at 37° C. In this test, the end point of lysis is taken at the time when the last bubbles enclosed in the fibrin gel arrive at the surface of the solution.

In cases of low fibrinogen levels or of high fibrinolytic activity, 0.2 ml of a 0.5 % fibrinogen solution may be added to 0.7 ml of the redissolved precipitate.

Comment: Plasminogen is largely isoelectrically precipitated at pH 5.2–5.4 (Norman, 1957; Kowalski et al. 1959; Blix, 1961). The ionic strength of the buffer used for redissolving the precipitate is 0.15. Lower salt concentrations around ionic strength 0.05 shorten the lysis time (Buckell and Truscott, 1959; Weiner, 1959). Merthiolate can be added in a concentration of 1:10,000.

Fibrinogen, factors V, VIII, XII, XIII and plasminogen remain in the precipitate in concentrations of 50–100 % of the original plasma values depending on ionic strength and pH. The yield of fibrinogen is highest at pH 5.4–6.4. Adding fibrinogen to the redissolved precipitate may therefore be helpful and is mandatory if euglobulins are prepared from serum. The yield of activity in serum euglobulin fractions is generally reduced.

Storage of the euglobulin fraction results in decline of activity, with increasing temperatures; loss of activity at 4° C takes place in a few hours (at –20° C within 1–2 days). It is essential to prepare the euglobulins in the cold or in ice water. Surface activation is substantially reduced by using polystyrene plastic tubes and siliconized pipettes.

The temperature optimum for the euglobulin lysis time is at 37° C. Contact activation with glasswool, kaolin, bentonite or celite results in shortened lysis times. This is not observed when Hageman deficient plasma is used (Sherry et al. 1959; Niewiarowski and Prou-Wartelle, 1959; Iatridis and Ferguson, 1961; Graeff, 1967).

Calcium can be used for clotting the precipitate. However, calcium retards or enhances the clot lysis depending on the activator activity of the precipitate (Ratnoff, 1952; Helle, 1967).

Euglobulin fractions can be prepared from whole blood (Johnson et al. 1964b). The correction factor for this method is based on an estimated hematocrit of 45 %. A 1.3 ml aliquot of citrated blood is added to 13.5 ml of cold distilled water and perfused with CO_2. Alternatively, 1.3 ml of blood is added to 13.5 ml of distilled water containing 0.22 ml of 1 % acetic acid. A slight increase of activator, possibly derived from the erythrocyte stroma may shorten the euglobulin clot lysis time (Kotschy and Jacobsen, 1964; Johnson et al. 1964a; Künzer and Haberhausen, 1963).

V. Discussion

Commercial thrombin preparations all contain large quantities of plasminogen, occasional batches may contain substantial quantities of plasmin-like activity and most batches possess low grade fibrinolytic activity when used in large quantities. Even highly purified thrombin preparations may possess fibrinolytic activity (Voss, 1965; Schulte, 1965; Brakman et al. 1964; Seegers et al. 1960). Purified thrombin in low concentrations sufficient for clotting fibrinogen reveals no lytic activity. It is therefore preferable to use low amounts of rather purified thrombin preparations.

The whole blood clot lysis time is insensitive and is therefore rarely used. The diluted blood clot lysis time is more sensitive and is considered of value as a screening technique. The observed activity is believed to derive from the separation of an activator-inhibitor complex. Therefore, "diluting out inhibitors" might be related to changes in the dielectric properties of the solution (Olesen, 1957). The diluted clot lysis time varies from day to day and from patient to patient. In addition, it differs considerably from species to species. It can be debated whether shorter lysis times reflect an increased activator activity or a decreased inhibitor activity, and it is not clarified whether enzyme substrate interactions in these complex systems are influenced by dilution. The extent to which apparent fibrinolytic activity in vitro reflects in vivo fibrinolysis is largely unknown. It is gratifying to note that a good correlation was found between the fibrinolytic activity as measured by the Fearnley dilution technique and by an assay measuring plasminogen activator in undiluted human plasma incubated with ^{131}I labeled plasma clots (Sherry et al. 1959).

The euglobulin lysis time is an artificial test system and primarily an activator-plasmin assay (Johnson et al. 1964b). The resulting fibrinolytic activity in vitro does not necessarily imply fibrinolysis in vivo. It is therefore not surprising that there is no constant correlation with different and more specific assays (von Kaulla, 1963; Beller et al. 1967).

Oxalated plasma has a longer euglobulin lysis time than citrated plasma. The yield of activator activity at pH 5.3 is higher in the presence of citrate (Blix, 1961; Buckell, 1958).

Fibrinolytic activity of the euglobulin fraction is greatly influenced by the precipitation procedure, pH, ionic strength, and by protein concentration. Differentiation between activator and plasmin activity can be achieved by adding EACA to the precipitate (Johnson and McCarthy, 1960). That interactions of a nonspecific nature influence the precipitation of activators and inhibitors, may be demonstrated by adding anionic polyelectrolytes (e.g. heparin, hyaluronic acid, dextran sulphates, bile acid compounds, purified peptone, metaphosphate etc.) (Olesen, 1957, 1965; Brakman and Astrup, 1964). The addition of hexametaphosphate at pH 5.9 induced an additional enzyme activity corresponding to C'1-Esterase activity, which differed from activator activity or plasmin (Harpel, 1967).

References

Amery, A., Vermylen, J., Maes, H., and Verstraete, M. (1962). *Thromb. Diath. Haemorrhag. 7,* 70.

Beller, F. K., Douglas, G. W., Morris, R. H., and Johnson, A. J. (1968). *Am. J. Obstet. Gynecol. 101,* 587.

Blix, S. (1961). *Scand. J. Clin. Lab. Invest. 13, Suppl. 58,* 3.

Brakman, P., and Astrup, T. (1964). *Sangre 9,* 46.

Brakman, P., Klug, P., and Astrup, T. (1964). *Thromb. Diath. Haemorrhag. 11,* 234.

Buckell, M. (1958). *J. Clin. Pathol. 11,* 403.

Buckell, M., and Truscott, M. (1959). *Nature 183,* 1268.

Chakrabarty, R., and Fearnley, G. R. (1962). *J. Clin. Pathol. 15,* 228.

Fearnley, G. R. (1965). "Fibrinolysis". William and Wilkins Co., Baltimore.

Fearnley, G. R., Balmforth, G., and Fearnly, E. (1957). *Clin. Sci. 16,* 645.

Graeff, H. (1967) unpublished data.

Harpel, P. (1967). *Federation Proc. 26,* 487.

Hedin, S. C. (1904). *J. Physiol. 30,* 195.

Helle, T. (1967). *Scand. J. Haematol. 4,* 21.

Iatridis, S. G., and Ferguson, J. H. (1961). *Thromb. Diath. Haemorrhag. 6,* 411.

Johnson, A. J., and McCarthy, W. R. (1960). "Experimental Thrombolysis in Man". *In:* Proc. Conf. Thrombolytic Agents. p. 173.

Johnson, A. J., Semar, M., and Skozal, L. (1964a). *Proc. 10th Congr. Intern. Soc. Hematol.,* Stockholm, 76.

Johnson, A. J., Semar, M., and Newman, J. (1964b). *In:* "Blood Coagulation, Hemorrhage and Thrombosis" (L. M. Tocantins and L. A. Kazal, eds.), pp. 465—467. Grune and Stratton, New York.

Kaulla, von K. N. (1963). "Chemistry of Thrombolysis: Human Fibrinolytic Enzymes". Charles C. Thomas, Springfield, Ill.

Kaulla, von K. N., and Schultz, R. L. (1958). *Am. J. Clin. Pathol. 29,* 104.

Kowalski, E., Kopec, M., and Niewiarowski, S. (1959). *J. Clin. Pathol. 12,* 215.

Kowarzyk, H., and Buluk, K. (1950). *Postepy Hig. Med. Doswjadczalnej 2,* 1.

Kotschy, M., and Jacobsen, C. D. (1964). *Scand. J. Clin. Lab. Invest. 16,* 55.

Künzer, W., and Haberhausen, D. (1963). *Klin. Wochschr. 16,* 831.

Lackner, H., and Goosen, C. G. (1959). *Acta Hematol. 22,* 58.

MacFarlane, R. G., and Pilling, J. (1964). *Lancet 2,* 562.

Marx, R. (1955). *In:* "Thrombose und Embolie", pp. 108. Karger, Basel.

Milstone, H. (1941). *J. Immunol 42,* 109.

Norman, Ph. S. (1957). *J. Exptl. Med. 106,* 423.

Niewiarowski, S., and Prou-Wartelle, D. (1959). *Thromb. Diath. Haemorrhag. 3,* 593.

Olesen, E. S. (1957). *Acta Physiol. Scand. 41,* 187.

Olesen, E. S. (1965). "Activation of the Blood Fibrinolytic System by Nonspecific Influences in Vitro." Munksgaard, Copenhagen.

Ratnoff, O. D. (1952). *J. Exptl. Med. 96,* 319.

Schulte, W. (1965). *Thromb. Diath. Haemorrhag. 13,* 561.

Seegers, W. H., Landaburu, R. H., and Johnson, J. F. (1960). *Science 131,* 726.

Sherry, S., Lindemeyer, R. I., Fletcher, A. P., and Alkjaersig, N. (1959). *J. Clin. Invest. 38,* 810.

Voss, D. (1965). *Klin. Wochschr. 43,* 935.

Weiner, M. (1959). *Nature 184,* 1937.

The Fibrin Plate Method for Assay of Fibrinolytic Agents*

Pieter Brakman and Tage Astrup

I. Principle

In the fibrin plate method measured amounts of fibrinolytically active solutions are placed as drops on the surface of a layer of fibrin followed by incubation and determination of the areas of the lysed zones produced. In principle, the assay is based on findings made in early work on tissue cultures, in which tissue fragments were observed to liquify the plasma or fibrin clot used as the solid support for cultivation. Tissue fragments, cell suspensions, as well as solutions, can be applied to the fibrin layer. The high sensitivity of the fibrin plate method, its accuracy, and its relative simplicity, which lends itself well to mass routine assays, led to its application in the assay of several proteases (Astrup and Alkjaersig, 1952), and to efforts to make it adequately standardized (Astrup and Müllertz, 1952). Experience gained in numerous applications over the following years (Astrup, 1966), made a need apparent for further standardization with particular reference to sensitivity and reproducibility. These studies have now been completed (Brakman, 1967).

Because the bovine fibrinogen used is rich in plasminogen, the regular fibrin plate assay does not discriminate between proteases and activators of plasminogen. However, fibrin plates in which the plasminogen has been destroyed by heating (Lassen, 1952) or in which plasminogen-free fibrinogen has been used (Brakman, 1965), are susceptible to proteases only.

II. Reagents

Reagent grade chemicals are used when not otherwise mentioned.

Potassium oxalate, 0.10 M (1.8 % w/v); 18.4 g neutral potassium oxalate, monohydrate, is dissolved in distilled water and diluted to 1000 ml.

Calcium phosphate, tribasic ($Ca_3(PO_4)_2$) precipitated (N. F. grade; Merck).

Ammonium sulfate ($(NH_4)_2SO_4$) a saturated solution is prepared at room temperature.

Physiological saline, 0.15 M (approx. 0.9 % w/v); 8.78 g NaCl is dissolved in distilled water and diluted to 1000 ml.

Fibrin plate buffer: In a volumetric flask 20.62 g sodium barbital (N. F. grade; Merck) are dissolved in 1350 ml distilled water and 500 ml 0.1 N HCl and 100 ml "salt solution" (see below) are added. The pH is adjusted to 7.75 with 0.1 N HCl and distilled water added to 2000 ml.

Salt solution: In a volumetric flask 4.89 g calcium chloride, dihydrate, ($CaCl_2 \cdot 2H_2O$) and 2.79 g magnesium chloride, hexahydrate, ($MgCl_2 \cdot 6H_2O$), and 109.12 g sodium chloride are dissolved in distilled water and diluted to 1000 ml. The purpose of this addition is to improve clot structure and to make lysed zones clearly demarcated.

Saline barbital buffer with gelatine: In a volumetric flask 5.85 g sodium chloride and 10.31 g sodium barbital (N. F. grade; Merck) are dissolved in 725 ml of distilled water and 250 ml 0.1 N hydrochloric acid. 2.5 g gelatine (bacteriological grade) are added and dissolved. The pH is adjusted to 7.75 with 0.1 N hydrochloric acid and distilled water added to 1000 ml.

Plasminogen activator is prepared from pig heart tissue and its strength estimated in units of a standard preparation (Astrup and Albrechtsen, 1957). A solution containing 3 to 4 Astrup and Albrechtsen (A & A) units per ml is prepared in saline barbital buffer with gelatine.

Bovine thrombin, 20 NIH U/ml in saline. Thrombin from Parke, Davis and Co., Detroit, or Leo Pharmaceuticals, Copenhagen,

* Supported by the U.S. Public Health Service, National Institutes of Health, National Heart Institute (Grant HE – 05020).

are only slightly contaminated with fibrinolytic activator of plasminogen (Brakman et al. 1964), and can usually be used without further purification.

III. Preparation of Fibrinogen

The ammonium sulfate precipitation procedure of Astrup and Darling (1942) and Astrup and Müllertz (1952) was modified as follows (Brakman, 1967): Bovine blood, collected in 0.1 vol. of the potassium oxalate solution, is centrifuged within a few hours of collection. The separated plasma is stirred for 20 min with 60 g tricalcium phosphate per liter to adsorb prothrombin. A good grade of calcium phosphate should change only slightly the pH of the plasma. The bulk of the tricalcium phosphate is separated in a refrigerated centrifuge (International PR 2, Head No. 276, 1350 × G, 30 min), the remainder being removed in a Sharpless supercentrifuge using a 1-H standard clarifier rotor at 25,000 r.p.m. The adsorbed plasma is stored overnight at 4° C, then slowly stirred at room temperature until it reaches 10°–15° C and filtered through glasswool. For fibrinogen precipitation one volume of the filtered plasma is diluted with 0.5 volume of cold distilled water. All volumes mentioned refer to the original volume of plasma used in each batch. The diluted plasma is stirred slowly in the cold room (4° C) while 0.6 volume of cold, saturated ammonium sulfate is added dropwise to the solution through a glass tube with its tip below the surface to avoid splashing and foaming. The solution, now 0.286 saturated with ammonium sulfate, is centrifuged at 1350 × G in the refrigerated centrifuge for 5 min and the precipitate redissolved at room temperature by addition of 0.5 volume of 0.15 M NaCl. After dilution with 1 volume of cold, distilled water 0.6 volume of cold, saturated ammonium sulfate is added as described. The mixture is centrifuged for 20 min at 1350×G, the supernatant discarded and the walls of the beakers wiped with paper tissue to remove excess fluid. The sediment is redissolved in 0.2 volume of distilled water at room temperature, the pH being cautiously brought to between 7.0 and 7.5 with 0.1 N sodium hydroxide. After final adjustment of pH to 7.50, the solution is filtered through glasswool. To determine the ionic strength of the fibrinogen solution its electrical conductivity is measured and the result read on a curve obtained by determining the conductivities of solutions of known concentrations of ammonium sulfate at controlled temperature (Brakman, 1967). The solution is stored overnight at 4° C, filtered through glasswool, and the fibrinogen concentration determined as fibrin by a gravimetric method. The coagulability is estimated from the UV absorbency at 280 mμ before and after removing fibrinogen as fibrin. The final solutions contain on an average 1.5 % fibrinogen and from 80 to 90 % clottable protein. They can be stored at –20° C for several years, or at 4° C for a few weeks. A precipitate forms during storage and should be removed by filtration through cotton or glasswool and centrifugation. Before accepted for routine use each batch of fibrinogen is controlled for clot quality and susceptibility to pig heart tissue activator.

IV. Technique of Assay

A. Regular Plasminogen–Rich Fibrin Plates

Solutions are prepared with a final fibrinogen concentration of 0.1 % and an ionic strength of 0.15. As an example, 200 ml of such a solution are obtained from a 1.6 % stock solution with an ionic strength of 0.45 as follows:
The 0.2 g fibrinogen required to produce 200 ml of a 0.1 % solution is contained in 12.5 ml of the 1.6 % stock solution. To bring this 12.5 ml to an ionic strength of 0.15, requires 25 ml water. First, 162.5 ml of fibrin plate buffer is added followed by 25 ml water to bring the final volume up to 200 ml. The fibrin is formed in disposable plastic Petri dishes (100 × 15 mm), especially selected for flatness (Lab-Tek Plastics, or Optilux Petri dishes Falcon Plastics). It is important that the fibrin layer is of even thickness. Previously, molded glass dishes were used but they require extensive cleaning. The actual inside diameter of the dishes is 8.4 cm. To each Petri

dish is added 6 ml of the fibrinogen solution by means of a Cornwall continuous pipetting outfit. The dishes are then placed on a horizontal glass plate (70 × 42 cm) mounted approximately 4 cm above a black table top. To each dish 0.2 ml thrombin solution is added with an automatic syringe. For complete mixing of the thrombin and fibrinogen solutions, the dishes are moved perpendicularly, followed by a circular movement. Mixing should be complete within 5–10 seconds. The dishes are covered and left for at least 30 min on the horizontal glass plate for clot formation. Clot thickness is 1.1 mm. The horizontal glass plate ensures a level, evenly clotted fibrin layer, facilitates evaluation of the freshly prepared fibrin plate, and makes easy the reading of the lysed areas. Later the dishes can be placed on top of each other and left at room temperature until used the same day. Special circumstances may require a change in thickness or of fibrin concentration.

For assays exactly 30 μl of the active solution is placed as a small drop on the surface of the fibrin layer with a 0.1 ml pipette graduated in 0.01 ml (Corning 7064-A, long tip). Test solutions should preferably have an ion composition and a pH similar to that of the fibrin clot. Usually, the activities are determined in triplicate on each plate. The dish is then incubated for 17 hours at 37° C. Shelves in incubators should be level glass plates. A water container with a large surface keeps the air in the incubator humid. The area of the lysed zones produced after 17 hours of incubation is a measure of the activity. This is arbitrarily expressed as the product in square millimeters of two perpendicular diameters, the mean value of the areas of the triplicate being determined. Readings are made with an accuracy of 0.5 mm and zones must be nearly circular in shape. Diameters are best measured with a micrometer caliper with a dial indicator gauge. For this purpose two metal needles are mounted on the micrometer.

B. Heated Fibrin Plates

The plasminogen present in the fibrin clot prevents the distinction between true proteolytic enzymes and activators of plasminogen. Nearly all fibrinolytic assays are complicated by this fact which has been a source of much confusion. To determine whether lysis is produced directly by a protease, or is caused indirectly by an activator of plasminogen, a fibrin clot without plasminogen is required. In an effort to overcome this problem, Lassen (1952) destroyed plasminogen in the fibrin plate by heat treatment which, however, left a denatured fibrin less sensitive to plasmin. Heated fibrin plates are made as follows:

Regular fibrin plates are prepared in glass Petri dishes, or in the disposible Optilux dish, which can withstand heating. After completion of clot formation the plates are placed in an oven preheated to 80° C. To avoid an uneven distribution of temperature, bimetallic thermometers are placed on each shelf and the plates are placed in single layers and are not stacked. The length of the heating period (60 min) is measured from the moment when the temperature on every shelf has again reached 80° C. A container with water and a small fan ensure saturation with water vapor in the oven. When the heated dishes are removed they are left uncovered during the period of cooling to avoid inside condensation of water. In each assay using the heated fibrin plate the absence of plasminogen is checked by placing 30 μl of urokinase solution (4 to 10 Ploug units per ml) in the center of the fibrin layer. If lysis occurs, these plates are discarded.

C. Plates from Plasminogen–Free Fibrinogen

Because heat treatment makes the fibrin less sensitive to plasmin, it would be better to use plasminogen-free fibrinogen to prepare fibrin plates sensitive only to proteases. However, most of the methods used to remove plasminogen from fibrinogen are cumbersome. Recently, adsorption on bentonite provided a simple means to remove the plasminogen, Brakman (1965). Briefly, the procedure is as follows:

To 100 ml of a regular fibrinogen solution, prepared as described and with a concentration above 1.2%, are gradually added 3 g bentonite (U.S.P. grade, Fisher) and the mixture slowly stirred for 20 min at room temperature. After centrifugation, the bentonite treatment is repeated leaving from 50 to 70% of the fibrinogen with little change in coagulability. Fibrin plates prepared from bentonite treated fibrinogen should not show lysis after application of drops containing 250 CTA units (200 Ploug units) of urokinase per ml.

V. Comments

A. General

To obtain satisfactory fibrin plates it is important that the described procedures are precisely followed. The quality of the fibrinogen is of greatest importance. The fibrin clot prepared as described is urea-insoluble.

The fibrin plate method is a convenient, accurate, and sensitive assay method. Urokinase solutions containing as little as 0.1 Ploug units per ml can easily be assayed. The concentration range which can be estimated is quite large (200 times). The amount of solution required for one assay is small (0.1 ml for a triplicate assay). For these reasons the fibrin plate method is an excellent and practical tool for biological assays, as well as a convenient screening test in column chromatography and gel filtration. Proteases, activators, and inhibitors can easily be detected and assayed with the fibrin plate method, and more than a hundred fractions may be handled daily. Data obtained in the assay of tissue activator have recently been reviewed, Astrup (1966). Activities of euglobulins precipitated from normal human plasma were reported (Brakman et al. 1966a). Assayed on different batches of fibrinogen, normal euglobulin activities were found to range from 50 to 318 square millimeters (Brakman et al. 1966b).

B. Other Fibrinogen Preparations

The large scale preparation of fibrinogen is inconvenient in laboratories lacking the necessary equipment, facilities and experience. Hence, commercially available fibrinogen preparations have been used by many investigators for preparing fibrin plates. We have compared several such preparations with the fibrinogen prepared as described above. Most of these preparations could not be recommended for use in the fibrin plate method.

Some fibrinogen preparations contain citrate which enhances activator activity (Müllertz, 1954). The presence of more than a trace of citrate should therefore be avoided in the regular fibrin plate method. All but one (Behringwerke, Marburg, Germany) of the different fibrinogens investigated contained too little plasminogen to assay activator in low concentrations. Other preparations were heavily contaminated with inhibitors causing deviations in the curves obtained in the double logarithmic graph. Additional problems encountered were the spontaneous clotting of fibrinogen solutions, or the contamination with fibrinolytically active compounds causing spontaneous lysis of the fibrin plates. Difficulties were sometimes caused by a softness of the fibrin clot, or because the active solutions tend to splash when applied to the fibrin surface, or by a glass-like appearance of the clot, which impeded measurement of lysed areas. The properties of some commercial fibrinogen preparations are described in detail elsewhere (Brakman, 1967). In regard to sensitivity, though not in other properties, the Behringwerke fibrinogen is at least equal to the regular fibrinogen described here. Fibrin plates prepared from Kabi human fibrinogen, though low in plasminogen, can be used in the assay of plasma euglobulins provided the plasma sample has a normal plasminogen concentration. Careful consideration should be given to the use of different fibrinogens in the fibrin plate method. Sometimes for special purpose it is possible to use other fibrinogen preparations than those here described.

C. Fibrinogen for the Fibrin Slide Technique

A modification of the fibrin plate method by which plasminogen activator in tissues can be demonstrated and localized at the cellular level was described by Todd (1959, 1964). This histochemical fibrin slide technique has been further improved (Kwaan and Astrup, 1963, 1967). The method requires a firm and solid fibrin layer free of particles disturbing microscopic evaluation. The ions present should not interfere with the various staining procedures. A fibrinogen solution with a concentration of 0.7 % and an ionic strength of 0.15 is needed. This fibrinogen is prepared from the regular fibrinogen described above by concentrating the solution by means of a LKB 6300 A Ultrafilter to a final concentration of above 2.2 %. The fibrinogen solution is then dialyzed twice in the cold (4° C) against at least forty times its volume of a phosphate buffer of 0.17 M with a pH of 7.75 (ionic strength of 0.30). After the second dialysis the concentration of the fibrinogen is determined and adjusted to 2.1 % with phosphate buffer of the same composition as used for dialysis. The solution is filtered through glasswool, centrifuged for 30 min at 10,000 to 15,000 rpm and stored in vials containing 0.5 ml. Before use the fibrinogen is thawed, diluted with 0.5 ml saline (0.15 M sodium chloride) and 0.5 ml distilled water added (adjusted the ionic strength to 0.15). This fibrinogen preparation has been successfully employed in the fibrin slide technique for the past years (Kwaan, 1966; Kwaan and Astrup, 1967).

References

Astrup, T. (1966). *Federation Proc. 25,* 42.
Astrup, T., and Albrechtsen, O. K. (1957). *Scand. J. Clin. Lab. Invest. 9,* 233.
Astrup, T., and Alkjaersig, N. (1952). *Arch. Biochem. 37,* 99.
Astrup, T., and Darling, S. (1942). *Acta Physiol. Scand. 4,* 45.
Astrup, T., and Müllertz, S. (1952). *Arch. Biochem. 40,* 346.
Brakman, P. (1965). *Ann. Biochem. 11,* 194.
Brakman, P. (1967). "Fibrinolysis. A Standardized Fibrin Plate Method and a Fibrinolytic Assay of Plasminogen." Scheltema and Holkema, Amsterdam.
Brakman, P., Klug, P., and Astrup, T. (1964). *Thromb. Diath. Haemorrhag. 11,* 234.
Brakman, P., Albrechtsen, O. K., and Astrup, T. (1966a). *Brit. J. Haematol. 12,* 77.
Brakman, P., Mohler, E. R., Jr., and Astrup, T. (1966b). *Scand. J. Haematol. 3,* 389.
Kwaan, H. G. (1966). *Federation Proc. 25,* 52.
Kwaan, H. C., and Astrup, T. (1963). *Arch. Pathol. 76,* 595.
Kwaan, H. C., and Astrup, T. (1967). *Lab. Invest. 17,* 140.
Lassen, M. (1952). *Acta Physiol. Scand. 27,* 371.
Müllertz, S. (1954). *Proc. Soc. Exptl. Biol. Med. 85,* 326.
Todd, A. S. (1959). *J. Pathol. Bact. 78,* 281.
Todd, A. S. (1964). *Brit. Med. Bull. 20,* 210.

The Purification of Profibrinolysin and Fibrinolysin

Paul J. Heberlein and Marion I. Barnhart

I. Introduction

In 1794 Hunter observed the inclottability of blood, in some cases of sudden death. The interim period has resulted in description of "fibrinolysis" (Dastre, 1895), correlation of fibrinolytic activity with blood globulins (Hedin, 1903), and recognition of a profibrinolytic protein in the plasma euglobulin fraction (Kaplan, 1944; Christensen, 1945; and Christensen and MacLeod, 1945). Barnhart and Riddle (1963) have demonstrated by immunofluorescence that one site for synthesis of profibrinolysin (PFL) is the eosinophil in bone marrow.

Purification of profibrinolysin (PFL), as any other protein, depends on available technology. The first attempt was made by Milstone (1941) and was an isoelectric precipitation from dilute serum. Since then other investigators have tried to improve on the final product. A significant advance was made by Remmert and Cohen (1949). Their procedure, like others to follow, was greatly aided by the Cohn et al. (1946) alcohol fractionation technique for plasma proteins. Certain features of the proenzyme noted by Remmert and Cohen (1949) continue to annoy the investigator who seeks highly-purified PFL. For example, the marked facility of PFL to coprecipitate with/or adsorb on other precipitating proteins, especially at alkaline pH, has slowed the ultimate isolation of PFL.

However, judicious use of physical properties of a molecule, gained simultaneously with its purification, can be exploited for further purification. Thus, the solubility, stability, protein-protein interactions and electrical properties can be used to advantage. Improved separation of PFL from its contaminants has resulted with ion exchange chromatography and gel fractionation. If one strictly adheres to the biochemical definition of "isolation" (a homogenous population of discrete molecules free of any accessory protein and solvent molecules), the isolation of PFL is still a future event. However, PFL has been purified to a high degree by various methods.

The ultimate goals of any purification scheme are biologic activity, high purity, excellent yields, stability and molecules similar to or identical with the "native" state. Compromise is more common than full achievement of these goals. Even so the final products of the various purification schemes provide molecules with special values for the objectives of the individual investigator.

The purpose of this chapter is to describe purification techniques for PFL and make a critical evaluation of their final products. No attempt is made to have a complete recital of the many purification procedures in the literature. Selection is made to provide contrasting ways to achieve a good quality PFL with well-defined properties. Information is provided to aid the investigator in deciding which of these protocols best suits his individual needs and is reasonable for his experience, laboratory facilities and time allotment.

II. Physicochemical Characteristics

Integration of the physical, chemical, biological and pharmacological properties is requisite for a complete understanding of the fibrinolytic system. Some of these properties of PFL and fibrinolysin (FL) are briefly discussed as they are pertinent to the purification schemes.

A. Native Profibrinolysin

The manipulations of purification alter to some degree the physicochemical state of any protein molecule away from that it assumed in its natural biosphere. Any purification method offers only a temporary route to a better way of obtaining the protein of interest. Each purification procedure contains some novelty which provides reagents that differ with respect to activity, purity, solubility, stability and size which are indicators of changes in three-dimensional structure. The degree of alteration of conformation is never known with certainty.

Until 1960, most PFL preparations were obtained by procedures (variations on the 1954 Kline method) that selectively denatured inert protein by extraction in dilute mineral acids and base, spanning a pH range of 2-11. The final product represented a several hundred-fold concentration over serum, but the PFL was highly insoluble and unstable at physiological pH. These characteristics were considered by some investigators as evidence for discrete conformational changes involving secondary and teritary structure (Slotta and Gonzalez, 1964, and Alkjaersig, 1964). Consequently, methods were developed which did not involve extremes in pH and resulted in a highly purified reagent, completely soluble and stable at physiologic pH. The molecules so obtained were termed "native profibrinolysin" (Slotta et al. 1962) or "euglobulin profibrinolysin" (Hink and McDonald, 1963), whereas the proenzyme molecule produced by acid and base extraction was termed "pseudoglobulin profibrinolysin". Differences in their properties will be noted later.

B. Electrical Properties

According to Derechin et al. (1962), purified PFL migrates as a β_2 globulin on paper electrophoresis. Hink and McDonald (1963) confirmed this and reported that fibrinolysin behaves as a β_1 globulin.

The isoelectric point of human pseudoglobulin PFL was reported by Shulman et al. (1958) as 5.6 while that of fibrinolysin was 6.2. Davies and Englert (1960) stated that the relative insolubility of pseudoglobulin PFL only permitted determination of a range of minimum solubility as pH 5.5 to 6.0. Alkjaersig (1964) showed that the electrophoretic properties of acid extracted human PFL were similar to nonacid extracted PFL. Heberlein and Barnhart (1967) reported an isoelectric point for canine euglobulin PFL as pH 5.25 (ionic strength = 0.1 phosphate).

C. Molecular Weight

Shulman et al. (1958) reported a molecular weight of 143,000 for human acid-treated PFL based on a sedimentation constant of 4.28–0.41 c and a diffusion constant of 2.92×10^{-7} cm^2 sec^{-1}. A molecular weight of 108,000 was estimated for glycerol-activated FL based on a sedimentation constant of 3.56–0.74 c. The molecular weight of FL was dependent upon the activating agent; streptokinase and urokinase activations gave higher molecular weight values for fibrinolysin. Davies and Englert (1960) reported a diffusion constant for purified pseudoglobulin PFL of 4.31×10^{-7} cm^2 sec^{-1}, resulting in a revision of the molecular weight to 83,800.

The dependence of conformation and sedimentation data on purification techniques and solvents (i.e., epsilon aminocaproic acid) was eloquently demonstrated by Alkjaersig (1964). Another revision of "monomer" molecular weight seems possible.

D. Solubility in Organic Solvents

1. Ethanol

One of the primary reagents for the precipitation of PFL is ethanol. During World War II, the need for concentrated plasma components led Cohn et al. (1946) to develop a fractionation technique involving variations of ionic strength, pH, temperature and ethanol content. This fractionation technique results in about 20 subfractions of plasma. The fraction III-3, contains a high concentration of PFL. At physiologic pH, PFL is insoluble in a 20 percent ethanol solution at –5° C, ionic strength of 0.005. In our experience, fraction III yields 40 percent of the plasma PFL.

The Cohn fractionation technique, particularly fractions III and its subfraction, III-3, is used in almost all of the purification processes. Heberlein and Barnhart (1967) have recently devised a modified Cohn fraction as the primary starting material in their purification process.

2. Diethyl Ether

This solvent has found limited use in the fractionation of plasma proteins (Kekwick et al. 1955). First, the solubility of ether in aqueous mixtures (up to 18.5 volumes percent below 0° C) is restrictive. Second, peroxide contamination makes it especially deleterious to proteins. The ether fractionation technique of Kekwick et al. (1955) produces a fraction, G.2 which corresponds, roughly, to the Cohn fraction III-3. Only Derechin et al. (1962) have utilized ether fractionation for purification of PFL.

3. Methanol

Methanol was found of some use for the precipitation of PFL (Wallen, 1962a; Heberlein and Barnhart, 1967). With a higher dielectric constant than ethanol, methanol is somewhat less precise as a specific precipitant but we find it less deleterious to PFL than ethanol. When methanol replaces ethanol fractionation the plasma proteins distribute themselves differently among the basic fractions (Pillemer and Hutchinson, 1945). In view of its toxicity, methanol may be considered a poor reagent for clinical fractionation.

4. Rivanol (Diamine-ethoxyacridine Lactate)

Rivanol has been used extensively for the preparation of γ-globulin (Horejsi and Smetana, 1948) and for β-metal combining globulins (Boettcher et al. 1958), ceruloplasmin (Steinbuch and Quentin, 1959), and thrombin (Miller, 1959). Recently, Steinbuch and Niewiarowski (1960) described the precipitation of a Rivanol-ceruloplasmin complex from Cohn fraction III. This complex could be dissociated at pH 4.0 in 50 percent ethanol.

The ceruloplasmin was precipitated with ethanol leaving a supernate of highly concentrated PFL, soluble at neutral pH.

5. Epsilon Aminocaproic Acid (E-ACA)

Perhaps the observation which has served most to advance the art of PFL purification was the E-ACA was a solvent that increased the solubility of PFL (Alkjaersig et al. 1959; Hagan et al. 1960). It was knownt hat E-ACA, at sufficient concentration, was an inhibitor of FL (Kaisha, 1957). More recently, E-ACA was shown to be a powerful competitive inhibitor of PFL activation (Alkjaersig et al. 1959; Ablondi et al. 1959).

The ability of E-ACA to increase the solubility of PFL and FL in neutral solutions probably is due to dissociation of protein complexes. In any event, many investigators have utilized this solvent in their purification process to obtain a highly purified fraction of PFL without resorting to extremes in pH. E-ACA has been used as an extraction medium (Wallen, 1962a; Bergstrom, 1963; Alkjaersig, 1964; Heberlein and Barnhart, 1967) or as an elution agent on various ion exchange resins (Bergstrom, 1963; Wallen, 1962b; Hink and McDonald, 1963).

6. Lysine and Other Amino Compounds

Hagan et al. (1960) found that lysine and lysine ethyl esters were also effective solubilizing agents for PFL and fibrinolysin. Lysine has advantages over E-ACA in not exhibiting the inhibitor qualities of E-ACA. Indeed, certain concentrations of lysine decrease the activator requirement for PFL (Kline and Fishman, 1964). Lysine has found particular use as an elution agent for PFL from ion exchange resins such as: (1) DEAE-cellulose or Sephadex (Wallen and Bergstrom, 1959, 1960; Derechin et al. 1962; Robbins et al. 1965); (2) TEAE-cellulose (Wallen, 1962b); (3) Carboxymethyl cellulose (Wallen, 1962b); or (4) tricalcium phosphate (Slotta and Gonzalez, 1964).

Finally, 3-amino propanol and 2-amino ethanol were reported by Norman (1960) to be effective elution agents for PFL from columns of DEAE-cellulose.

E. Solubility in Inorganic Solvents

1. Phosphate Salts

Limited success has occurred when phosphate salts were used for the fractionation of plasma proteins (Rane and Newhouser, 1954). Many plasma proteins form complexes with phosphate under appropriate conditions of pH and temperature. Accordingly, some use has been made of the phosphate precipitation of PFL (Kline, 1954; Kline and Fishman, 1961; Robbins and Summaria, 1963; and Richard et al. 1959). Cole and Mertz (1961) have shown that the yield of precipitated PFL was inversely proportional to the final molarity of phosphate. They achieved maximum purification and yield at a final phosphate concentration of 0.02 M. In view of this, it is interesting to speculate on the mechanisms involved in column chromatography of PFL which employs elution with gradient phosphate concentrations.

2. Cations

Heavy metal-protein complexes have been shown to be associated with many structural groups within the protein molecule, such as carboxyl, imidazole, alpha- and epsilon-amino, phenolic-OH and guanidine.

One of the divalent cations, Zn^{++}, combines specifically and reversibly with the proteins of plasma, primarily with the imidazole groups. A scheme of differential precipitation with barium and zinc sulfate led Surgenor (1952) to describe a fractionation of plasma. Three subgroups of plasma resulted, one of which contained PFL precipitated in 20 mM Zn^{++}, at pH 7.2. This precipitating agent has not found any widespread use for the purification of PFL.

Rybak (1959) reported that fibrinolysin forms a specific complex with magnesium ions. He utilized Kline-type PFL that was activated and complexed with 5 mM Mg^{++}. This complex was stable and active.

F. Stability

1. Euglobulin PFL

In our experience, we have found "native" PFL to be a highly stable proenzyme. At neutral pH, solutions stored at 32° C showed no deterioration for two weeks; at 4° C the solution was stable for several months, while a frozen solution (–70° C) retained 100 percent activity for over one year. The first indication of PFL deterioration is the appearance of spontaneous proteolytic activity. The amount of spontaneous activity reaches a maximum value, but always some amount of activatable PFL remains.

Repeated freezing and thawing or lyophilization were deleterious to the stability of the PFL molecule.

2. Pseudoglobulin PFL

Pseudoglobulin PFL, in contrast to euglobulin PFL, is relatively unstable at neutral pH. Its maximum stability is at pH 2–3 (Müllertz, 1955). Below pH 5, pseudoglobulin PFL is resistant to heat. When brought to 100° C at pH 2 and cooled, pseudoglobulin PFL retains 90 percent of its original activity (Troll and Sherry, 1955). E-ACA and glycerol increase the stability of PFL at neutral pH.

3. Fibrinolysin

The stability of euglobulin fibrinolysin is strikingly different from its proenzyme. At room temperature and neutral pH, 25 percent of the original activity may be lost in eight hours. The stability of the active principle is greatly dependent upon the enzyme concentration, solvent, temperature and pH. Fibrinolysin undergoes a rapid autodigestion (Norman, 1957) which is maximal at neutral pH. Agents such as E-ACA or glycerol stabilize both the proenzyme and fibrinolysin. Urea and methylamine inhibit the autodigestion of fibrinolysin (Norman, 1957). Fibrinolysin obtained from pseudoglobulin PFL is unstable at neutral pH.

G. Solubility

Euglobulin and pseudoglobulin PFL have different solubility characteristics. In our laboratory, dilute, neutral salt solutions of euglobulin PFL have been acquired which contain 40 mg/ml of purified PFL. No problems of solubility were experienced with "native" PFL unless lyophilized. In this case, up to one-half of the activity and protein were lost as insoluble components. Solutions of purified euglobulin PFL exhibit a very sharp range of minimum solubility at pH 5.0 to 5.7.

Pseudoglobulin PFL has only limited solubility in neutral aqueous solutions and is significantly soluble only at pH values below 5 and above 9 (Sherry et al. 1959). For these reasons, all physiochemical experiments performed on pseudoglobulin PFL require extreme pH conditions. Most of the physical data reported for PFL was obtained with acid solutions of pseudoglobulin PFL. Recent reports on comparative biophysical measurements of euglobulin and pseudoglobulin indicate large differences in the derived molecular parameters (Slotta et al. 1962; Slotta and Gonzalez, 1964; Alkjaersig, 1964). The investigator should be aware that these differences likely relate to conformational changes evoked by the purification steps.

H. Protein Associations

Remmert and Cohen (1949) first described the tendency of PFL in neutral solutions to coprecipitate with many of the plasma proteins. Attempts to selectively precipitate inert proteins, leaving PFL in solution, give low and erratic yields. PFL is discarded in the inert fractions with each step of the purification process, resulting in a large percentage loss. In our experience with five different methods, fibrinogen appeared to be a common contaminant.

If, however, the purification process is designed so that PFL is normally present as the precipitated component, then yields can be significantly increased (Nitschman et al. 1962; Shamash et al. 1964; and Heberlein and Barnhart, 1967). PFL is adsorbed to fibrin (Ablondi and DeRenzo 1959). In our laboratory we found that canine PFL could be adsorbed and desorbed from fibrin under special conditions. When the fibrin-PFL complex was carried in the purification process as long as possible, the final product had consistently high yields (at least 70 percent of the PFL assayable in a protamine precipitate of canine plasma). This purified material was devoid of spontaneous proteolytic activity and had the highest specific activity yet reported in the literature.

I. Surface Reactivity

We have observed an affinity of purified PFL and fibrinolysin for glass surfaces. To avoid loss from surface adsorption or denaturation, we perform all quantitative assays, activation and dilution, but not clot lysis, in siliconized glassware.

III. Methods for the Purification of Profibrinolysin

There are about twenty-five published methods for the purification of PFL and FL. As a full description of each is unreasonable, the difficult task of selection was necessary. We found four basic strategies were followed in the purification of PFL: (1) selective denaturation by acid and base extraction; (2) primarily chromatographic techniques; (3) extraction with ε-aminocaproic acid or lysine; and (4) the use of protein association phenomenon. The following were selected to represent each strategy: (1) the method of Kline and Fishman (1961); (2) the method of Alkjaersig (1960, 1964); (3) the method of Wallen (1962a, b); and (4) the method of Heberlein and Barnhart (1967). The other published methods are variants of these four and may receive brief mention.

A. Method of Kline and Fishman (1961)

The original description of PFL purification by Kline (1953, 1954) is based upon the observation by Christensen and Smith (1950) that PFL is stable in acid solutions. Kline also found PFL stable for up to 3 minutes in basic (pH 11) solutions. Further purification of the acid and base extracted PFL was realized by precipitation of the active component in the presence of phosphate salts and then extraction in lysine. Fig. 1 presents an abbreviated protocol.

1. Preparation of Cohn Fraction III

The starting material for the Kline and Fishman (1946) procedure is Cohn Fraction III. The technique followed in this laboratory was that described for the Cohn methods 6 and 9.

Fresh or frozen citrated (0.32 percent) plasma is cooled with stirring in a salt/ice bath to 0°. A sodium acetate-acetic acid buffered solution of 53.3 percent ethanol is added dropwise to make a final ethanol concentration of 8 percent at pH 7.2 ± 0.2. One ml of buffer (0.8 M sodium acetate buffered to pH 4.0 with glacial acetic acid) is added per liter of plasma. During addition of ethanol, the temperature of the solution is allowed to fall to −3°. A heavy precipitate (Fraction I) appears which consists primarily of fibrinogen. The precipitate is removed by centrifugation at −3° and discarded.

Supernate I is increased in ethanol content by the addition of sufficient 53.3 percent ethanol to make a 25 percent final concentration. The ethanol contains sufficient sodium acetate buffer for pH 6.9. Each liter of supernate requires 601 ml of 53.3 percent ethanol, 0.88 ml of 10 M acetic acid, 0.44 ml of 4 M sodium acetate and 2.30 ml of 95 percent ethanol. The precipitate (Fraction II and III) contains PFL and beta- and gamma-globulins.

Precipitate II + III (1 kg) is suspended in 2 liters distilled water at 0°. This mixture is diluted with 3 liters of cold, distilled water containing 112 ml of 0.5 M disodium phosphate (pH 9.2). The suspension is stirred to complete homogeneity at 0° before dilution to 26 liters with distilled water. Stirring is continued for one-half hour. The pH should be 7.2 ± 0.2. Next, ethanol (53.3 percent) is added to achieve a 20 percent ethanol concentration. The temperature is allowed to drop to −5°. After alcohol addition stirring is continued for 2–3 hours at −5°. The resulting Precipitate II + IIIW, is collected by centrifugation at −5°.

Precipitate II + IIIW (1 kg) is completely suspended in 2 liters cold, distilled water. Then 2 liters of cold water containing 0.35 moles of sodium acetate, is mixed in. For each kg of Precipitate II + IIIW 1 liter of cold acetate buffered distilled water is added to

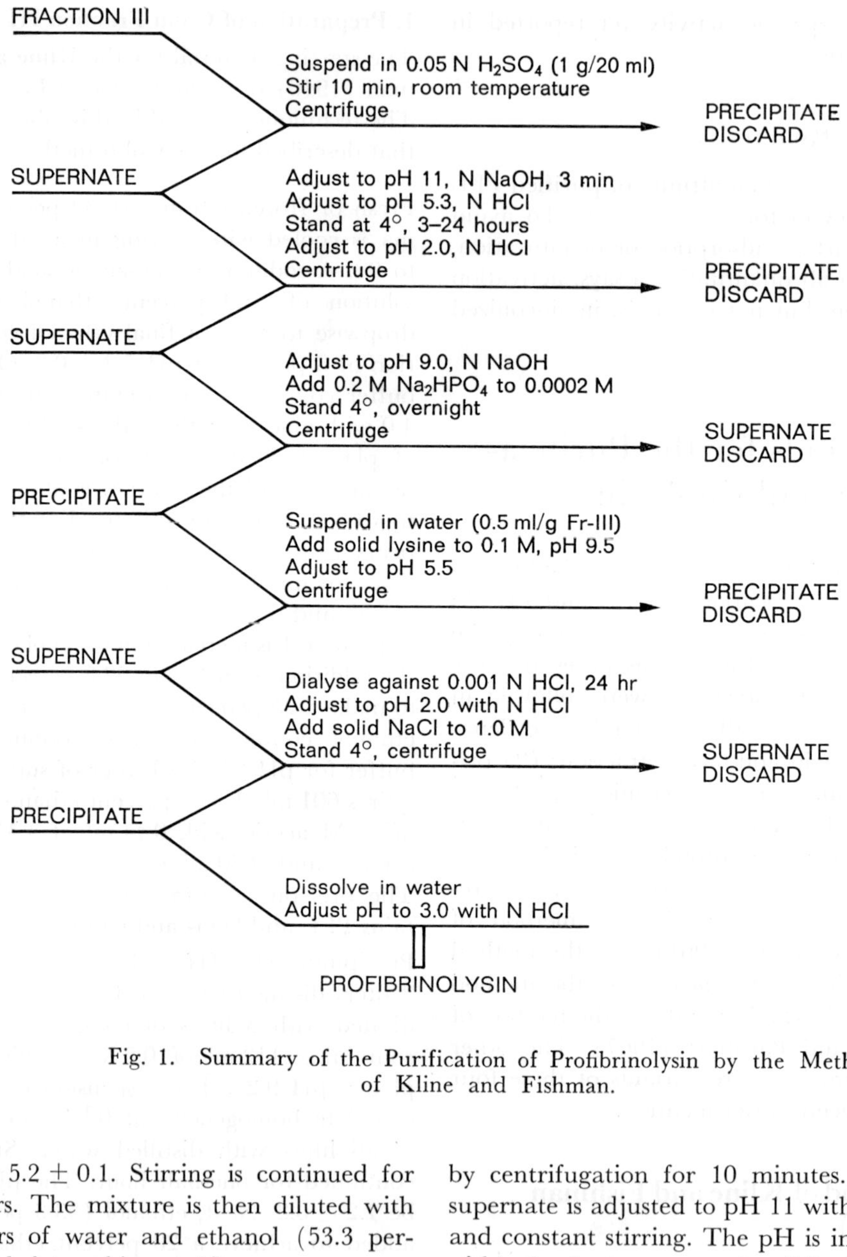

Fig. 1. Summary of the Purification of Profibrinolysin by the Method of Kline and Fishman.

give pH 5.2 ± 0.1. Stirring is continued for 2–3 hours. The mixture is then diluted with 13.5 liters of water and ethanol (53.3 percent) added to achieve a 17 percent concentration. The temperature is progressively lowered to –6°. After stirring for one-half hour, Precipitate III is collected by centrifugation at –6°.

2. Acid and Base Extraction of Fraction III

Fraction III paste is suspended in 0.05 N H_2SO_4 at a final concentration of 1 g/20 ml and stirred for 10 minutes at room temperature. The precipitated proteins are removed by centrifugation for 10 minutes. The acid supernate is adjusted to pH 11 with N NaOH and constant stirring. The pH is immediately within 3 minutes, returned to 5.3 with N HCl. The mixture is kept at 4° for a minimum of 3 hours or preferably overnight. Readjustment to pH 2.0 is made and the inert proteins removed by centrifugation for one hour.

3. Phosphate Precipitation

The clarified supernate, containing PFL, is then carefully adjusted to pH 9.0 with N NaOH and the final volume noted. A solution of 0.02 M disodium phosphate, pH 8.5, is then added to a final concentration of 0.0002 M. The precipitate containing the proenzyme, is allowed to mature overnight at 4°.

The precipitate is collected by centrifugation and redispersed in 0.5 ml of distilled water per gram of starting Fraction III. For complete solution a few drops of N HCl are added.

4. Extraction with Lysine

Solid L- or DL-lysine monohydrochloride is added next to give a final concentration of 0.1 M. The pH is momentarily adjusted to 9.5, then immediately returned to 5.5. After a few minutes of stirring at room temperature, the insoluble components are removed by centrifugation. The clarified solution is dialyzed overnight versus 0.001 N HCl to remove lysine.

PFL is precipitated from the dialysate by adjustment of the pH to 2.0 with N HCl and the addition of solid NaCl to a final concentration of 1.0 M. The collected precipitate (PFL) is redissolved in distilled water at pH 3.0.

5. Modifications of the Kline Method

Numerous attempts have been made to modify the original Kline (1953, 1954) and the Kline and Fishman (1961) procedures. These modifications were attempted primarily to increase the yields and solubility of PFL. The interested reader may refer to Norman (1960), Hagan et al. (1960), Richard et al. (1959), Robbins and Summaria (1963), and Roberts (1960).

The PFL product of Sgouris et al. (1960) merits special attention as it is a quality product with excellent stability. The method of Sgouris and associates employs Cohn fraction III prepared as previously described. The paste is extracted in a solution of 0.2 M sodium acetate, 0.01 M disodium phosphate, pH 7.7. Further purification is by isoelectric precipitation at pH 5.4. Inert protein is removed by selective denaturation in acid and base by a modified Kline (1953) procedure. The soluble proenzyme is precipitated at the isoelectric point and redissolved in water, pH 4.0. More inert protein can be removed by heat denaturation, carried out at 60° for 10 hours. Adjustment to pH 2.0 precipitates inert proteins which are removed by centrifugation. The purified proenzyme is dissolved in 0.1 M sodium phosphate, pH 7.7 and an equal volume of 99.5 percent glycerol is added.

Pseudoglobulin PFL and FL are many times more soluble in 50 percent glycerol near neutral pH than in buffers without glycerol. Glycerol also serves to stabilize FL during activation and storage. Finally, glycerol is nontoxic, bacteriostatic, possibly bactericidal and further increases stability of the active molecule and usefulness for in vivo studies.

Reagents produced by Sgouris at the Michigan Department of Health are used in many laboratories and by the American Red Cross as reference standards for fibrinolytic tests.

B. Method of Wallen (1962a, b)

PFL preparations contain some spontaneous proteolytic activity which increases considerably with time during the purification process. PFL is converted to FL by the presence of this proteolytic activity (Alkjaersig et al. 1958a). Wallen designed his purification technique to remove this spontaneous activity early in the process. This was accomplished by extraction of Cohn Fraction II + III with E-ACA. The resulting fraction (B-2) contained only trace amounts of spontaneous proteolytic activity (less than 0.5 percent).

The method involves isoelectric precipitation of Cohn Fraction II + III, extraction of inert proteins at pH 5.3 in 0.08 M sodium acetate (Edsall et al. 1944), extraction with E-ACA and, finally methanolic fraction of the E-ACA extract. Further purification may be achieved by column chromatography. A summary of this scheme is presented in fig. 2.

1. Isoelectric Precipitation of Fraction II + III

The source of crude PFL is the Cohn Fraction II + III (section III–A1). One kg of II + III paste is suspended in 2 liters of 0.1 M NaCl at 0°. After complete solution, the pH is adjusted to 5.3–5.4 with M acetic acid. A heavy white precipitate results which contains PFL. This precipitation is allowed to

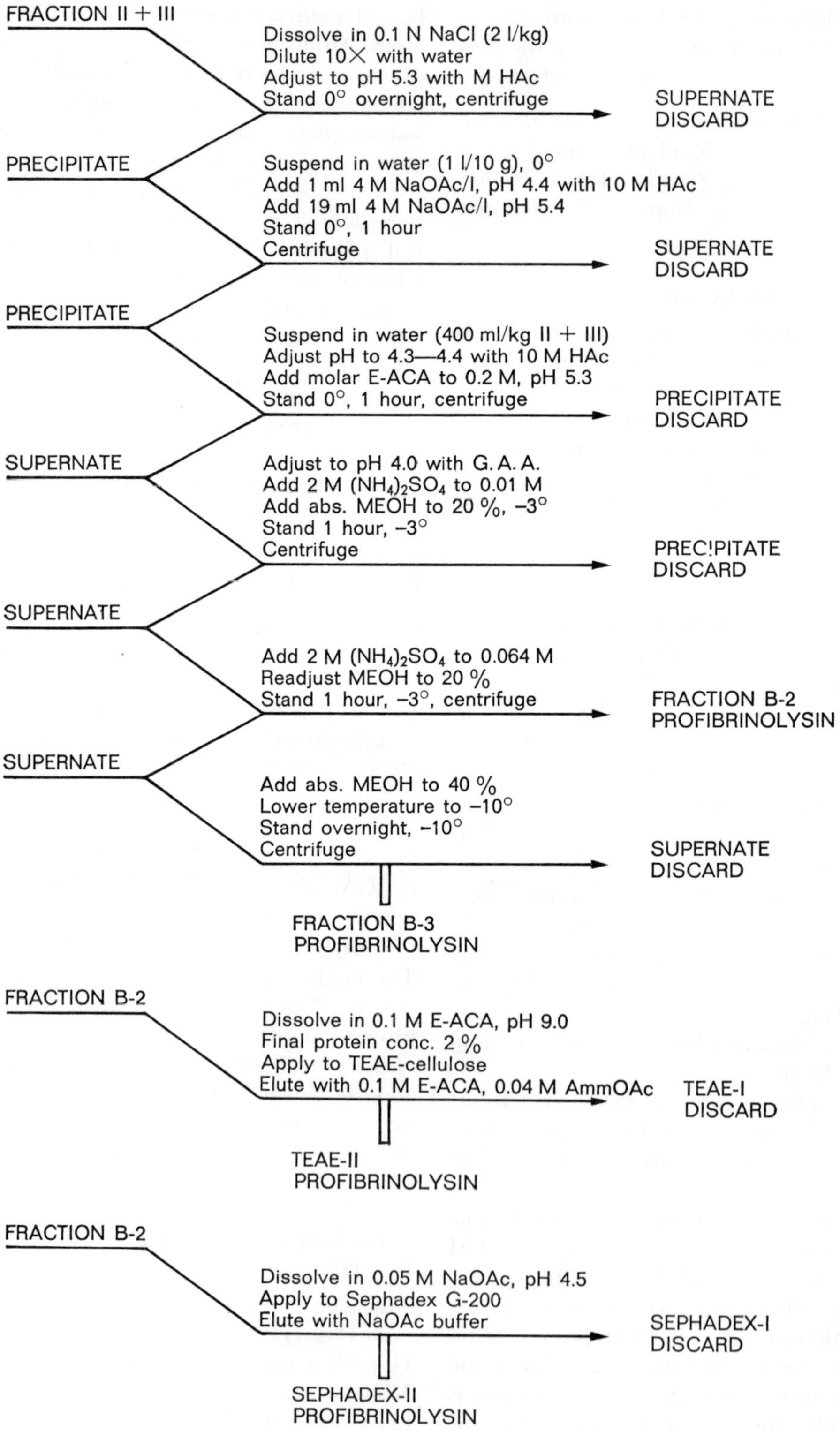

Fig. 2. Summary of the Purification of Profibrinolysin by the Method of Wallen

mature and settle for at least 3 hours (preferably overnight).

2. Sodium Acetate Extraction

After siphoning off most of the supernate, the isoelectric precipitate is centrifuged down and suspended in cold distilled water (100 ml/g). Complete suspension is required. Four M sodium acetate is added to this in the ratio of 1:1000. The pH is adjusted to 4.3–4.4 with 10 M acetic acid. After stirring for 10 minutes most of the protein dissolves. Again 4 M sodium acetate is added to a final concentration of 0.8 M with respect to the sodium ion. The pH rises to 5.3–5.4 as a heavy white precipitate forms. Stirring continues for one hour at 0°. The precipitated protein is collected by centrifugation.

3. Epsilon-Aminocaproic Acid Extraction

The precipitate is suspended in 40 ml of distilled water per gram of paste. The temperature is adjusted to 0° and pH 4.4 by addition of 10 M acetic acid (need about 2.25 ml/liter). Stirring for 10 minutes dissolves most of the protein. Molar epsilon-aminocaproic acid is then added by pipette, with stirring, to obtain a final concentration of 0.2 M. The pH rises to 5.3–5.4 and a white precipitate appears. Inert proteins, precipitated during stirring for one hour at 0°, are removed by cold centrifugation.

4. Methanol Fractionation

Subfraction continues with methanol and ammonium sulfate. Near pH 4.0 there is a difference in solubility of PFL and FL. Lowering the pH below this value does not significantly increase the separation from FL and possibly has deleterious effects upon the proenzyme molecule.

The E-ACA extract, at 0°, is adjusted to pH 4.0 with glacial acetic acid. For each liter, 5 ml of 2 M ammonium sulfate are added. Next 250 ml of absolute MEOH (measured at room temperature), precooled to about –60°, are added to a final methanol concentration of 20 percent. The final concentration of ammonium sulfate is 0.008 M.

The methanol must be precooled during its introduction to the E-ACA solution. In our laboratory, this is accomplished by placing a 200 ml glass funnel inside a second, stemless, 800 ml glass funnel. The stem of the inner funnel is passed through a rubber cork, held firmly in the exit of the larger funnel. Thus, the space between the inner and outer walls of the two concentric funnels holds a dry ice/ethanol bath which cools the methanol, during addition, to about –65°.

The temperature of the E-ACA alcohol mixture is allowed to decrease to –3°. The precipitate (fraction B-1) which forms during addition of the methanol is allowed to mature for one hour and discarded. The supernate is saved.

The concentration of ammonium sulfate in the supernate is adjusted to a final concentration of 0.064 M by the addition of 2 M ammonium sulfate. The concentration of methanol is retained by the addition of absolute methanol (35 ml of 2 M ammonium sulfate and 10 ml of absolute methanol per liter of supernate).

Fraction B-2 is salted out and matures for one hour at –3°. The purified PFL, collected by centrifugation for 45 minutes at –3°, contains the majority of the proenzyme with only traces (less than 0.5 percent) of spontaneous proteolytic activity. This material is dissolved in distilled water, stored frozen or lyophilized. In our hands the lyophilized material is difficult to redissolve and activity was lost so we avoided this manipulation.

A final fractionation of the E-ACA extract is possible and yields fraction B-3 which contains about one-third of the total proenzyme of the E-ACA extract but also has 2–10 percent spontaneous fibrinolytic activity.

5. Chromatography on TEAE-Cellulose

Fraction B-2 can be improved by chromatography on TEAE-cellulose columns. The ion exchanger is sedimented 2–3 times in 0.1 M NaOH and then several times in distilled water to remove fines. The slurry is poured into a column and the bed developed. The column, before use, is equilibrated overnight with 0.01 M epsilon-aminocaproic acid, pH 9.0 (adjusted with ammonia).

Fraction B-2 is dissolved in 0.1 M E-ACA, pH 9.0, to a final concentration of 2 percent. One gram of protein is applied to 10 g of ion exchange resin. This protein is washed into the column with the equilibration buffer. Elution with this buffer is continued until no more protein appears in the eluate.

The proenzyme is eluted from the column by a solution of 0.1 M E-ACA and 0.04 M ammonium acetate at pH 9.0. The fraction appearing with this solvent is called TEAE-II and contains the major portion of the proenzyme. In most cases, the spontaneous proteolytic activity is increased over the starting material, B-2.

6. Gel Filtration on Sephadex G-200

Gel filtration provides an alternate method for further purification of Fraction B-2. Sephadex G-200 is suspended in 0.05 M sodium acetate, pH 4.5 (50 ml/g) and allowed to swell at least 48 hours. After swelling, the Sephadex is sedimented several times to remove fines. The slurry is poured into a column to form a bed 3×85 cm and the column is washed overnight against the acetate buffer to stabilize the bed. A hydrostatic pressure greater than 15 cm of water on the gel bed is to be avoided.

Fraction B-2 (300 mg) is dissolved in 4.5 ml of 0.05 M sodium acetate, pH 4.5 and applied to the column. Elution is performed with acetate buffer. Fractions of 10 ml are collected every 30 minutes. This elution results in two, well separated peaks (Sephadex I and II). The most active fractions are pooled and precipitated by the addition of cold (–60°) ethanol to a final concentration of 25 percent. The precipitated protein (PFL) is sedimented at –15°, the paste is redissolved in buffer or water and stored frozen.

7. Modification of the Wallen Method

a. *Bergstrom (1963)* purified bovine PFL essentially according to Wallen except for a significant modification of the methanol fractionation. Fraction B-1 is precipitated in 20 percent MEOH, 0.016 M ammonium sulfate at 0°. Fractions B-2 and B-3 are precipitated together with 40 percent MEOH and 0.04 M ammonium sulfate at –15° and further purified by chromatography on carboxymethyl cellulose. Bovine PFL preparations were found to contain little or no spontaneous proteolytic activity. It was, therefore, unnecessary to separate the B-2 and B-3 fractions.

b. *Robbins et al. (1965)* reported purification of human PFL by extraction of Cohn Fraction $III_{2,3}$ at 4° in 0.05 M tris –0.1 M NaCl, containing 0.2 M lysine at pH 9.0. Chromatography followed on DEAE-Sephadex with Tris-lysine buffers for elution of the PFL. Over 3 percent of the activatable fibrinolytic activity could be accounted for by spontaneous proteolytic activity.

C. Method of Alkjaersig

Alkjaersig (1960) presented preliminary results on the purification of Human PFL by DEAE-cellulose chromatography, avoiding extremes in pH. Later Alkjaersig (1964) presented a full description of two methods for the purification: one utilizing the solvent effects of E-ACA, the other not. Both methods yield fractions which are further purified by chromatography on DEAE-cellulose or DEAE-Sephadex. The resulting PFL products had equivalent purity but differed significantly in yields. A summary of these procedures are presented in Figures 3.

1. Method 1: Preparation of Euglobulin Fraction

One liter of plasma is defibrinated by the addition of 300 NIH units of thrombin and calcium chloride to a final concentration of 25 mM. This serum is diluted 20-fold with distilled water and the pH adjusted to 5.3 with 10 percent acetic acid. Isoelectric precipitation is allowed to proceed overnight at 2° and the precipitated euglobulin collected by centrifugation.

The precipitate is dissolved in 250 ml of 0.01 M Na_2HPO_4, pH 8.5 (adjusted with N HCl). After overnight dialysis against 6.25 liters of the same buffer, the insoluble material is removed by high speed centrifugation (33,000 g) and filtration through Whatman No. 2 paper. This crude euglobulin PFL is chromatographed on DEAE-cellulose.

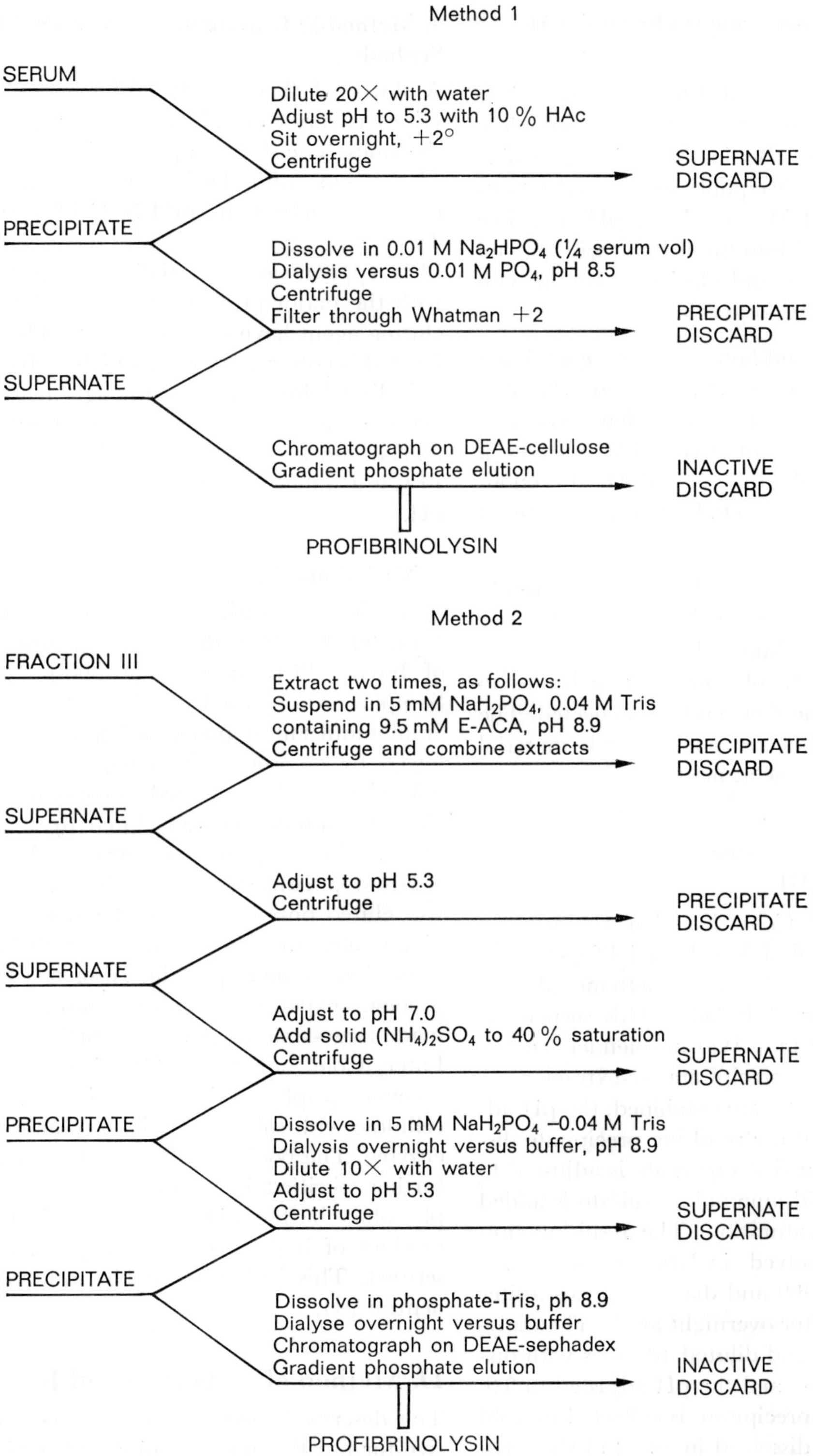

Fig. 3. Summary of the Purification of Profibrinolysin by the Method of Alkjaersig.

2. Method 1: Chromatography on DEAE-Cellulose

The crude PFL is applied to a column (2.5 × 40 cm), containing 16 g of DEAE-cellulose (Brown and Co., Berlin, N.H., USA) which has been previously equilibrated with the starting buffer, 0.01 M phosphate, pH 8.5. The sample is washed into the column with 250 ml of starting buffer and elution is begun with buffer concentration gradients.

A one liter round-bottom flask, containing starting buffer, serves as the mixing chamber and is connected to a 500 ml Erlenmeyer flask containing a limit buffer of 0.3 M NaH_2PO_4, pH 6.5 (adjusted with 2 N NaOH). Fractions (10–20 ml) are collected at a flow rate of 60 ml/hour.

The initial effluent fractions contain protein but little PFL. PFL begins to emerge after about 640 ml of buffer has passed through. The main portion of inert protein begins to emerge when one liter has been collected. The most active tubes are pooled. This material is soluble and stable at neutral pH.

3. Method 2: Pretreatment of Cohn Fraction III

Forty grams of Cohn Fraction III are suspended in 800 ml of 5 mM NaH_2PO_4 –0.04 M tris (hydroxymethyl) amino methane, pH 8.9, containing 1.0 g of E-ACA. This suspension is homogenized in a Waring blender, centrifuged and the precipitate re-extracted as above. The extracts are combined, the pH adjusted to 5.3 and the resulting precipitate discarded. The clarified supernate is adjusted to pH 7.0 and solid ammonium sulfate is added to 40 percent saturation. The resulting precipitate is dissolved in 100 ml of 5 mM NaH_2PO_4, pH 8.9 and dialyzed versus 5 liter of the same buffer overnight at 4°. The dialysate is clarified and diluted 10 times with distilled water at 0° and the pH adjusted to 5.3. The isoelectric precipitate is collected by cold centrifugation, dissolved in 50 ml of the Tris-phosphate buffer, pH 8.9 and, again, dialyzed overnight at 4°. The clarified supernate is ready for DEAE-Sephadex.

4. Method 2: Chromatography of DEAE-Sephadex

A slurry of 25 g of DEAE-Sephadex, G-50 (fine) is very carefully decanted to get rid of the fines. The slurry is poured into a column (4 × 40 cm) and the bed allowed to equilibrate overnight with 5 mM NaH_2PO_4 –0.16 M Tris.

PFL appears as a partially confluent peak with the major protein after about 440 ml of eluting agent have passed through. The yields from this column are not as high as from the DEAE-cellulose column, although the specific activities are comparable. The peak tubes are pooled and assayed. This purified fraction of PFL is a stable and soluble product at neutral pH.

5. Variations of the Alkjaersig Methods

Coincidentally with Alkjaersig's description, Dalby et al. (1960) described the purification of bovine PFL on calcium phosphate gel. Samples are prepared for chromatography by ammonium sulfate precipitation of serum, followed by an isoelectric precipitation at pH 5.3. The sample is applied to columns of calcium phosphate gel and eluted by step-wise increases in phosphate concentration. Although a 5-fold purification was achieved, the PFL was eluted only over a broad range of phosphate concentration, making difficult further resolution of inert protein. Also, mechanical problems experienced with calcium phosphate made large-scale preparations difficult.

Later, Cole and Mertz (1961) reported on chromatography of bovine PFL on DEAE-cellulose with substantial yields of active pro-enzyme. The pooled, active fractions could be further purified by precipitation on 0.02 M phosphate buffers, pH 7.4, to give a final active product of high specific activity (170 times serum). This PFL was soluble and stable at neutral pH.

D. Method of Heberlein and Barnhart

The described methods were not very effective for purification of canine PFL which we wanted. Following a different route we developed a method which gave high yields of good quality canine PFL.

It was observed by Nitschmann et al. (1962) that PFL would coprecipitate with fibrinogen. Shamash et al. (1964) similarly made use of this fact in their method for the purification of human PFL. Further, Ablondi and DeRenzo (1959) observed the adsorption of PFL to fibrin clots. We have found that under certain conditions, fibrin-adsorbed PFL could be eluted, quantitatively with E-ACA. We utilized this phenomenon in hopes of increasing yield and also, paying attention to the observations of Blix (1961), took advantage of the fact that FL is apparently more strongly adsorbed to the fibrin than PFL so preferential elution of PFL becomes possible. Also, the methanol fractionation of a E-ACA extract, as described by Wallen (1962a), was used to further separate PFL from spontaneous proteolytic activity.

Combination of these approaches gave a highly purified PFL, devoid of spontaneous proteolytic activity, soluble at neutral pH, stable and with excellent yields. The overall purification is comparable to any other procedure described but γ-globulin was detected by immunology and ultracentrifugation techniques. This contaminant is easily removed by chromatography on hydroxyapatite, which has a higher specific adsorbance for γ-globulin than for the β-globulin, PFL. Our procedure provides a product of PFL of the highest purity (averaging 714 times plasma) with <0.1 percent spontaneous proteolytic activity and representing at least 68 percent of the plasma proenzyme. Furthermore, this method is adaptable to canine, bovine and equine plasmas without modification.

The total procedure involves recalcification of the plasma, alcohol and isoelectric precipitation, extraction with sodium acetate and E-ACA, methanol precipitation and chromatography on hydroxyapatite. A schematic summary is presented in fig. 4.

1. Recalcification and Ethanol Precipitation

Fresh or frozen citrated (0.32 percent) plasma (1000 ml) is placed in a 4 liter stainless steel beaker containing 1000 ml of cold distilled water. The mixture is quickly cooled to 0° and 53.3 percent ethanol added by drops to a final concentration of 3 percent. The temperature is decreased to $-^1/_2$°. $CaCl_2$ (4 M) is then added by pipette to a final concentration of 25 mM/l plasma. Stirring is increased to a rate just below foaming of the plasma. Formation of fibrin proceeds to completion and requires two hours. The completeness of recalcification is determined by the failure of a sample of the supernate to form a clot on addition of thrombin at 37°. The fibrin is easily seen as finely suspended particles.

The fibrin-serum mixture is increased in ethanol content by addition of 53.3 percent ethanol to a final concentration of 25 percent. The temperature is dropped to –5°. Stirring is continued for 10 minutes after ethanol addition and the pH adjusted to 5.4 with 10 M acetic acid. This mixture is stirred for one hour at –5°.

The precipitate is collected by centrifugation for 10 minutes at –5° and is stored frozen, or used immediately in the next step. For each liter of plasma, about 200 g of paste is obtained.

2. Isoelectric Precipitation

The 200 g of paste is suspended in 400 ml of 0.1 M NaCl, cooled immediately to 0° and stirred until complete suspension. The mixture is then diluted to 4.2 liters by the addition of 3.6 liters of cold distilled water. The pH is readjusted to 5.4, if necessary, and stirring continued for two hours at 0°. The isoelectric precipitate is collected by centrifugation for 10 minutes. The paste can be stored frozen or used immediately in the next step.

3. Sodium Acetate Extraction

The paste is suspended in 1000 ml of cold distilled water and stirred to complete homogeneity. Next 1.0 ml of 4 M NaOAc is added and the pH adjusted to 4.4 with 10 M acetic acid with stirring for 10 minutes. Again, 4 M NaOAc is added to a final concentration of 0.08 M (19 ml/liter). The pH is observed to rise to 5.4 ± 0.1 along with the appearance of a heavy precipitate. The extraction is allowed to continue for 45–60 minutes at 0° and the precipitate collected by centrifugation for 10 minutes at 0°. The paste obtained is

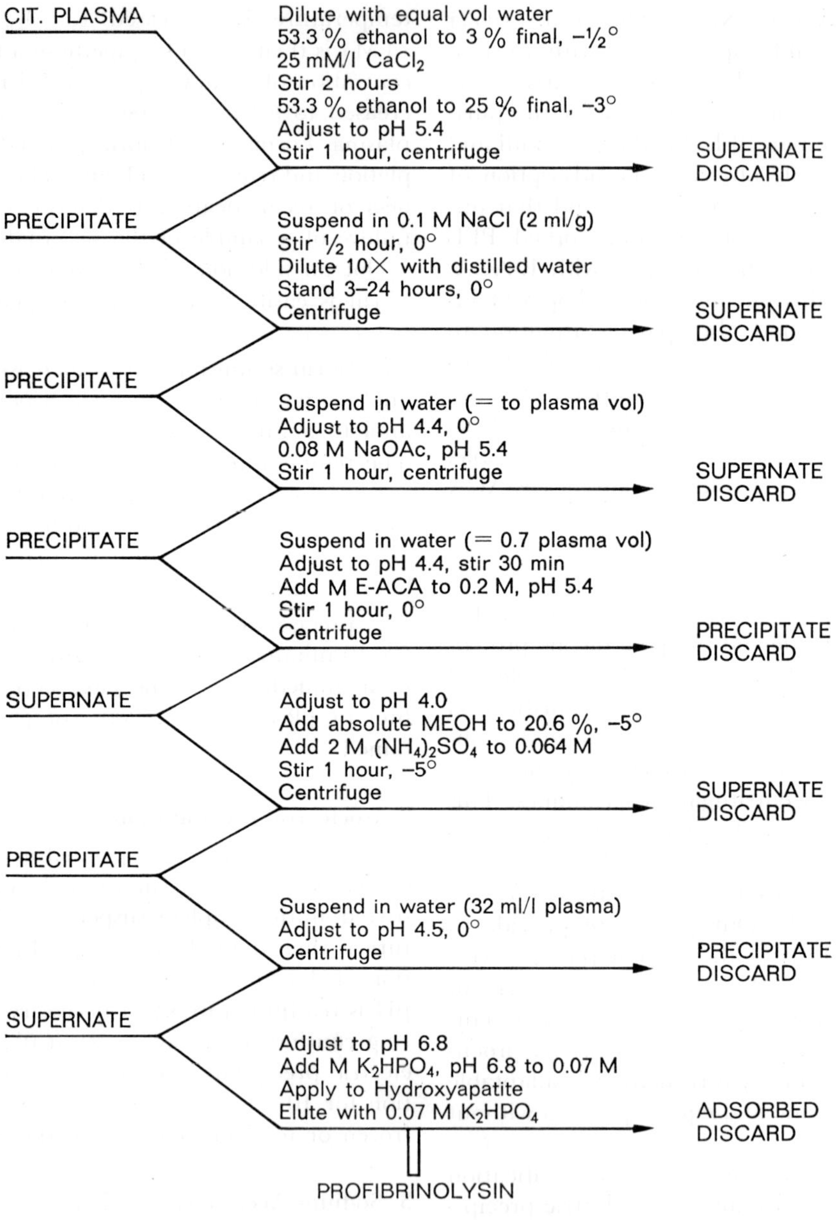

Fig. 4. Summary of the Purification of Profibrinolysin by the Method of Heberlein and Barnhart.

stored frozen or used immediately in the following step.

4. Epsilon Aminocaproic Acid Extraction

The precipitate is suspended in 700 ml of cold distilled water and the pH adjusted to 4.4 with 10 M acetic acid. Stirring is continued for 20 minutes during which time most of the protein is seen to dissolve. Then 175 ml of M E-ACA is added and the pH rises to 5.4 ± 0.1 as a heavy precipitate appears. Extraction is continued with stirring for 45–60 minutes. Inert, precipitated proteins and fibrin are removed by centrifugation at 0° for one-half hour. The clarified supernate is fractionated immediately.

5. Precipitation of Crude Profibrinolysin

The E-ACA extract is cooled to 0° and the pH adjusted to 4.0 with glacial acetic acid. The volume is noted and cold (–60°) absolute methanol (section III-B) is added to a final concentration of 20.6 percent. During addition of the alcohol (260 ml/liter, measured at room temperature) the temperature is decreased to –5°. Next 2 M ammonium sulfate is added, by pipette, to a final concentration of 0.064 M. A fine, white precipitate results which is allowed to mature at –5° for 45–60 minutes. This crude proenzyme is collected by centrifugation for 30 minutes at –5°, drained of excess supernate by inverting the centrifuge in a freezer (–30°), and the paste dissolved in distilled water (32 ml/liter plasma). The pH of the solution is adjusted to 4.5 with N NaOH and the solution stored overnight at 4°. The precipitate is discarded after centrifugation. The clarified supernate contains partially purified PFL and is stored frozen or further purified.

6. Chromatography on Hydroxyapatite

The PFL solution is cooled to 4° and the pH adjusted to 6.8 with N NaOH. Molar K_2HPO_4, pH 6.8 (adjusted with glacial acetic acid) is added to attain a final phosphate concentration of 0.07 M.

A slurry of 50 ml of hydroxyapatite (Bio-Rad Co., Richmond, Calif.) and 50 ml of Whatman cellulose powder is decanted of fines and poured into a column to produce a bed 2.5× 40 cm. The column is equilibrated overnight with one liter of 0.07 M phosphate, pH 6.8. Then 32 ml of sample, containing 160 mg of protein, is placed on the column and washed in. The chromatogram is developed by continued washing with 0.07 M phosphate. Fractions (8–10 ml) are collected at a flow-rate of 60 ml/hour. The highly purified PFL begins to emerge after one column volume of buffer has passed through. The tubes are assayed for protein (Biuret) and activity (Celander and Guest, 1959). Those tubes which contain over 10 percent of the applied activity are pooled and labeled as HT-PFL. This product is stable, indefinitely, when stored at –70°.

IV. Purification of Fibrinolysin

The active enzyme, fibrinolysin, is relatively unstable when compared to its precursor, PFL. Usually purified FL is obtained by activating purified proenzyme. Thus, any of the previously described PFL procedures may be utilized to obtain an equally purified fraction of fibrinolysin.

A. Spontaneous Activation

Spontaneous activation in 50 percent glycerol may be achieved as described by Alkjaersig et al. (1958b). Kline PFL is dissolved in 0.05 M phosphate, pH 7.6, in the presence of 50 percent glycerol. Activation occurs at 30° (an adequate compromise between rate of activation and stability). Complete activation of PFL takes five days. The conversion is essentially quantitative, as compared to streptokinase activation. Completeness of activation is not dependent on the initial concentration of proenzyme, although the rate of activation is materially influenced within a protein range of 0.03 to 1 percent.

The optimum pH for spontaneous activation in 50 percent glycerol is at 7.6. Stability is excellent in 50 percent glycerol with 80 percent of the original activity retained for 20 months at room temperature.

If a dry preparation is desired it may be lyophilized from a solution of the activated enzyme which has been dialyzed against 0.01 N HCl. The lyophilized product is soluble in acid distilled water. At neutral pH, the solubility of "Kline" fibrinolysin is similar to its inactive precursor. Maximum solubility in saline occurs near 1 mg percent but, 50 percent glycerol increases the solubility to 350 mg percent at pH 7.6.

B. Activation with Urokinase

Kjeldgaard and Ploug (1957) reported that Kline PFL was optimally activated at pH 9.0 in 0.5 M tris (hydroxymethyl) aminomethane buffers which contain 150 Ploug units of urokinase/ml.

Alkjaersig et al. (1958a) reported maximal activation with urokinase at pH 7.6, utilizing 255 Ploug units of urokinase/ml.

Sgouris et al. (1960) described conditions for activation of their PFL with urokinase. A solution of PFL in 50 percent glycerol is incubated at 32° with 0.52 units of heat-treated (10 hours at 60°) urokinase/ml. Complete conversion of the proenzyme is attained in six days. Faster activation occurs with larger amounts of urokinase. The FL is filtered through a Seitz-type filter to give a water clear, sterile solution.

C. Activation with Streptokinase

A third means of activation is described by Blatt et al. (1964). To Kline PFL (amount of product obtained from 8–10 liters of serum) is added 250,000 units of streptokinase, (Varidase, Lederle Laboratories) at pH 7.2. After stirring for 30 minutes the pH is adjusted to 3.0. The solution is dialyzed against 0.001 N HCl for 24–48 hours at 4°. The dialysate is adjusted to a protein concentration of 0.3 percent and fractionated by the addition of solid NaCl to a final concentration of 4 percent. The precipitated, inert proteins are removed by centrifugation and the supernate adjusted to a concentration of 10 percent by the addition of sufficient solid NaCl. This precipitated fibrinolysin can be collected by centrifugation, dissolved in appropriate buffers or lyophilized to a dry powder.

V. Evaluation of the Profibrinolysin Reagents

It is possible to compare products on the basis of physiochemical measures of homogeneity and properties of solubility, sedimentation and kinetics. A rough comparison can be made of the total concentration from the starting material, plasma or serum.

A. Assay Comparisons

It is unfortunate that a standardized assay and unit definition has not been adopted. Numerous assays describe the purity of products. As FL has o broad specificity, the natural substrate, fibrin, casein, gelatin and synthetic molecules are used. Activity on foreign or synthetic substrates, while helpful, do not inform about intensity of action on natural protein substrates that FL may encounter in the body. Until reactivity on a standard substrate in a standard assay is widely adopted, it remains difficult to accurately compare PFL products derived by different purification schemes.

B. Total Concentration from Plasma or Serum

In many instances the data is readily available in the original description of the method. Where these figures were not given, we have derived a figure from the reported data.

To express purification of the final product, in terms of specific activity (unit/mg) of the "total profibrinolysin" in plasma or serum, a method of quantitative precipitation must be employed to eliminate the effect of plasma inhibitors. Precipitation with protamine sulfate (Celander and Guest, 1959) is considered to be quantitative (Guest, 1954) and is our routine assay for total plasma PFL. Also, we found the precipitation of the euglobulin components, by acidification (pH 5.3) of a 20-fold dilution of plasma at 0°, yields 90–95 percent of the total plasma PFL when compared to a protamine sulfate precipitate.

The specific concentration of the proenzyme from plasma or serum is quite variable and dependent upon the procedure and species (Table 1). With our new procedure from canine plasma, the total concentration was comparable to others but almost doubled after chromatography on hydroxyapatite. Each laboratory claims reproducibility, however, application of a procedure in other laboratories is seldom as successful as the original.

C. Yield

Yield is another gauge to compare purification processes (Table 2). High yields in relation to high purity are not the experience.

Three factors have roles in obtaining high yields of quality PFL: (1) the solvent action of basic amino acids (E-ACA or lysine); (2) exploitation of the coprecipitation tendencies of PFL with fibrin; and (3) careful handling.

Table 1: A Comparison of Total Purification of Profibrinolysin from Plasma and Serum.

Method	Specie	Source	Purification
Kline and Fishman	Human	Cohn Fraction III	400
Wallen	Human	Cohn Fraction II + III	
Sephadex-II			425
TEAE-II			450
B-3			91*
Alkjaersig	Human		
Method 1		Euglobulin	400
Method 2		Cohn Fraction III	471*
Heberlein and Barnhart			
	Canine	Plasma	730**
	Equine	Plasma	740**
Bergstrom	Bovine	Plasma	479*

* Derived inferentially from data
** Produced in the authors' laboratory

Table 2: Comparison of Yields of Profibrinolysin from Plasma.

Method	Specie	Yields from Plasma (%)
Kline and Fishman	Human	12*
Wallen	Human	
TEAE-II		4.5*
Sephadex-II		3.4*
B-3		3.8*
Alkjaersig	Human	
Method 1		57*
Method 2		8.5*
Heberlein and Barnhart		
	Canine	56**
	Equine	56**
Bergstrom	Bovine	4*

* Derived inferentially from data
** Obtained in the authors' laboratory

D. Solubility and Stability

Differences in solubility and stability of the euglobulin and pseudoglobulin PFL have been discussed (section II). It follows that the euglobulin PFL produced by the methods of Wallen or Alkjaersig or Heberlein and Barnhart, cannot be exposed to extremes in pH without partial or complete conversion to molecules exhibiting the physical properties of the pseudoglobulin type (Hink and McDonald, 1963; Slotta et al. 1962; and Alkjaersig, 1964). Freeze-drying also results in greatly decreased solubility of the active components.

E. Spontaneous Activity

The presence of spontaneous proteolytic activity is a major concern. All PFL products contain some amount of spontaneous activity. Detection depends on the sensitivity of the assay system (Chapter X). With active enzyme present, the proenzyme is slowly converted to compromise stability.

The amounts of spontaneous proteolytic activity resulting from the four basic methods are expressed as a percentage of the total activable material of the final product (Table 3).

Table 3: Comparison of Proteolytic Activity Present in purified Profibrinolysin

Method	Specie	Percent Spontaneous Activity
Kline and Fishman	Human	2.1
Wallen	Human	
TEAE-II		1.17
Sephadex-II		?
B-3		6.6
Alkjaersig	Human	
Method 1		0
Method 2		0
Heberlein and Barnhart		
	Canine	<0.1
	Equine	<0.1
Bergstrom	Bovine	<0.1

F. Ultracentrifuge Studies

Analysis by this method demonstrates that the product derived by the method of Kline and Fishman is a single sedimenting component with a Svedberg unit of $S^{\circ}_{20,w}$ 3.2.

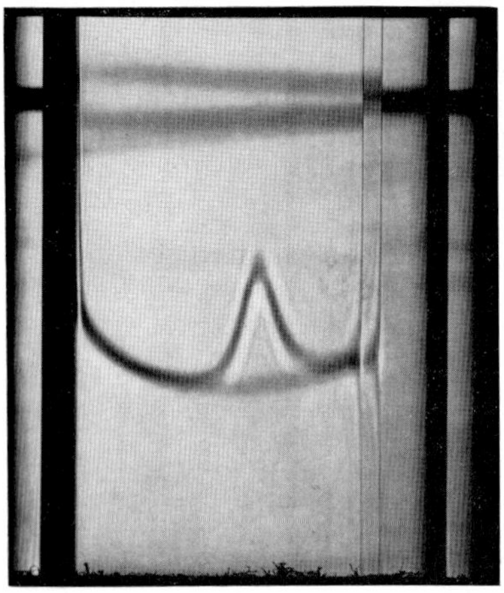

Fig. 5. Ultracentrifuge pattern of canine HT-profibrinolysin obtained by the method of Heberlein and Barnhart. 10 mg/ml concentration in 0.1 M KCl. Rotor speed 59,760 rpm. Temperature 20 ± 0.01°. Picture taken at 60 minutes. Sedimentation is to the left.

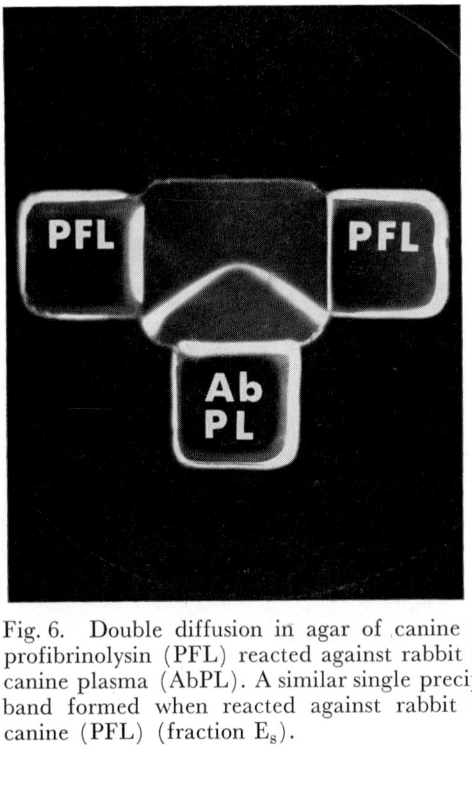

Fig. 6. Double diffusion in agar of canine HT-profibrinolysin (PFL) reacted against rabbit anti-canine plasma (AbPL). A similar single precipitin band formed when reacted against rabbit anti-canine (PFL) (fraction E_s).

Data presented by Alkjaersig indicated the product obtained by Method 2 had a symmetrical Schlieren pattern with a sedimentation constant of 4.9, at zero concentration. Further, Alkjaersig reported that exposure of this euglobulin PFL to acid, below a critical value of pH 4.5, or in solutions containing 10 mM E-ACA decreased the sedimentation coefficient toward that reported by Kline and Fishman. Thus, the sedimentation behavior of purified PFL is fairly complex and related to the method of purification, solvents and pH.

Wallen has not reported ultracentrifugal analysis of his most purified fractions of PFL. Finally, the material produced by the method of Heberlein and Barnhart was viewed in the ultracentrifuge (Fig. 5). As can be seen, a single sedimenting component was produced, with a sedimentation constant of $S^{\circ}_{20,w}$ 5.25. The PFL exhibited the customary concentration dependent regression line, which was calculated to be 5.25–0.12 c.

G. Immunochemical Analysis

One of the more sensitive indicators of homogeneity is provided by immunodiffusion of the purified PFL against a potent polyvalent antiserum (Chapter X). The shape and number of resulting precipitin bands are indicative of purity, relative to the specificity of the antibody.

Immunochemical data was not available to the authors for the Kline and Fishman or Wallen materials. Alkjaersig reported that immunoelectrophoresis of material purified by Method 2, had two bands which blended rather than crossed. She suggests that this may represent a reaction of identity of electrophoretically separated PFL aggregates. This is further demonstrated by electrophoresis of the purified fraction on polyacrylamide gel followed by exposure to the antiserum. Only a single precipitin band resulted.

Finally, immunodiffusion of the canine PFL produced by Heberlein and Barnhart, resulted in the appearance of a single precipitin band when diffused against a potent polyvalent canine antiplasma (Fig. 6).

H. Electrophoretic Analysis

Electrophoresis on starch or polyacrylamide gels provide another powerful tool for the analysis of homogeneity of a purified component. The PFL products are compared for their behavior on these media.

Mertz and Chan (1963) reported the electrophoresis of Kline and Fishman PFL on starch gels at pH 2.5. One major and three minor bands were observed. They suggested that these components represented degraded PFL molecules produced during purification.

Wallen reported that electrophoresis of Fraction TEAE-II, on starch gels at pH 4.0, presented two major and two minor protein bands. Sephadex-II Fractions had one major and two minor bands. Several of these components contained activity.

Alkjaersig subjected highly purified PFL from her method 2 to polyacrylamide gel electrophoresis at pH 8.1 and reported at least four stained bands. All of these, when eluted, had activity when activated. Alkjaersig suggested that the separate bands represented different PFL polymers rather than discrete electrophoretic entities.

The PFL of Heberlein and Barnhart in starch gel electrophoresis (pH 8.65) showed four distinct stained bands of protein (Fig. 7). To ascertain which band(s) contained the proenzyme, a novel, in situ, analysis was devised. With this assay any artifacts produced by cutting and elution of the bands were avoided.

1. In situ Assay of Profibrinolysin and Fibrinolysin

The assay consists of exposure of unstained, electrophoresed protein bands to the substrate, fibrin. To assay PFL, the fibrin contains an appropriate activator. The fibrin is presented to the electrophoretic medium (starch gel, cellulose acetate or polyacrylamide) as a component in the matrix of a cellulose acetate strip. This fibrin-acetate strip is laid over the area of protein migration and activation and lysis allowed to proceed. The fibrin-acetate strip is then washed of its soluble lytic products while the unlysed fibrin, still present in the cellulose acetate strip, is stained to show discrete zones of lysis. Details of the assay follow.

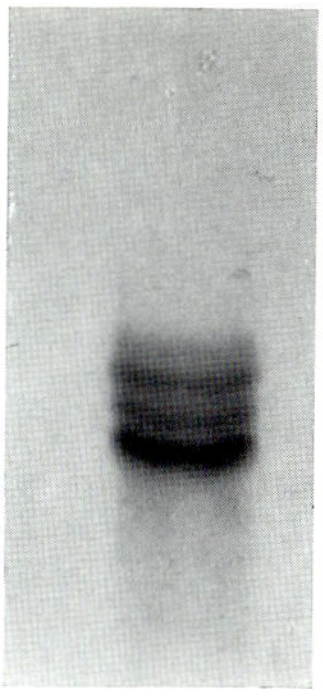

Fig. 7

Fig. 8

Fig. 7. Starch-gel electrophoresis of canine HT-profibrinolysin 250 VDC for six hours at room temperature. Stained with Napthol Blue Black.

Fig. 8.

a. Strips of Cellulose acetate (2.5 × 10 cm, Oxo, Ltd., London) are hydrated in a Tris buffered solution (pH 8.65) of 0.2 percent bovine fibrinogen for five minutes. The strips are blotted.

b. The blotted strips are soaked for 10 minutes in a Tris buffered solution of thrombin (20 Iowa units/ml) to polymerize the fibrinogen present in the cellulose acetate matrix.

c. After blotting, the strips are sandwiched between two glass microscope slides which are taped securely together. The strip is heated for 15 minutes in the Tris buffer at 85° to destroy any spontaneous proteolytic activity.

d. When electrophoresis is complete, the gel is sliced horizontally to expose an inner surface. The top slide is stained for protein. To the bottom slice is applied the fibrin-acetate strip, which has been previously soaked in a solution of urokinase (0.93 M.A.U./ml). If the assay is for FL, no activator is necessary. The strip is applied directly over the area of electrophoresis, extending from the origin to the saltfront. Care is taken to avoid trapping air bubbles beneath the fibrin-acetate strip. The strip is not covered while diffusion and lysis proceeds at room temperature. Usually 10–20 minutes gives optimum lysis but it varies with the purity and load of the proenzyme.

e. When lysis is complete, the fibrin-acetate strip is removed and washed for five minutes with constant motion in a saline solution. The unlysed fibrin in the strip is stained in a solution of Ponceau S (0.2 percent in 3 percent TCA) for five minutes. The excess stain is cleared by repeated washing of the strip in 5 percent acetic acid.

2. Results

Application of this new assay to the electrophoresed PFL of Heberlein and Barnhart, clearly demonstrated that all four bands were proenzyme and capable of activation (Fig. 8). Zones of lysis did not appear unless activator was present. No other protein zones were visible on the gel except those which exhibited proenzyme activity.

There was a relationship between the intensity of the stained band and the degree of lysis produced which suggests that the specific activity of each moiety is approximately equivalent.

The mobility of each component was calculated relative to the movement of albumin (Table 4). The regular interval between each

Table 4: Relative Mobilities and Concentration of the Multiple Reactive Components of Canine Profibrinolysin.

Profibrinolysin Component	R_f*	ΔR_f**	Percent of Component In Total Pattern
Alpha	0.476	0	10
Beta	0.447	.029	20
Gamma	0.391	.056	20
Delta	0.370	.021	50

* Relative to albumin
** Difference in R_f of component from preceeding component

component, as well as the closeness at which they migrate, suggests a family of related molecules rather than aggregates.

The relative concentration of each band was calculated by measurement of the band area (Table 4). It is interesting to acknowledge the relationship between mobility and concentration of the bands.

These multiple reactive components cannot be resolved when the purified proenzyme contains more than 0.5 percent spontaneous proteolytic activity, instead only a broad smear results. Even traces of the active enzyme probably partially degrade the proenzyme, resulting in a loss of resolution between the multiple reactive bands.

Multimolecular forms of enzymes are not unusual today so multimolecular forms of proenzyme (isoproenzymes) also may exist. The data presented by Wallen (1962b), Alkjaersig (1964) and by Mertz and Chan (1963), Robbins et al. 1963), and Slotta and Gonzalez (1964) do not provide a firm case for the existence of isoproenzymes. Multimolecular forms of fibrinolysin have been hypothesised by Markus and Ambrus (1960).

Whether the phenomenon of multiple reactive components of PFL is due to complexes between PFL and inert protein, or to alteration of the PFL molecule during the purification process, or whether there truely exists isoproenzymes cannot be answered without further attempts to isolate and characterize these separate reactive components.

V. Conclusions

Of the several methods for the purification of PFL, four methods have been fully described as representative of the current strategies for the purification of PFL. Each technique results in a reagent possessing unique qualities in terms of solubility, stability, homogeneity and yield. From these representative methods, the investigator may wish to choose that process which best suits his needs with regard to the requirements of the experiment.

The chemistry of fibrinolysis can be more accurately studied with reagents approximating the native molecule. Whether any of the described methods produces such a reagent is controversial. The existence of multiple reactive components may be viewed as evidence that none of the existing purification processes produce a molecule which is not altered, on the other hand, isoproenzymes may indeed exist in plasma.

Acknowledgement

This study was aided by the National Institutes of Health Grants 1-FL-GM-33, 527-01 and HE 04712, U.S. Public Health Service.

References

Ablondi, F. B., and DeRenzo, E. C. (1959). *Proc. Soc. Exptl. Biol. Med. 102,* 717.

Ablondi, F. B., Hagain, J. J., Philips, M., and DeRenzo, E. C. (1959). *Arch. Biochem. 82,* 153.

Alkjaersig, N. (1960). *Federation Proc. 19,* 58.

Alkjaersig, N. (1964). *Biochem. J. 93,* 171.

Alkjaersig, N., Fletcher, A. P., and Sherry, S. (1958a). *J. Biol. Chem. 233,* 86.

Alkjaersig, N., Fletcher, A. P., and Sherry, S. (1958b). *J. Biol. Chem. 233,* 81.

Alkjaersig, N., Fletcher, A. P., and Sherry, S. (1959). *J. Biol. Chem. 234,* 832.

Barnhart, M. I., and Riddle, J. M. (1963). *Blood 21,* 306.

Bergstrom, K. (1963). *Biochim. Biophys. Acta 77,* 673.

Blatt, W. F., Segal, H., and Gray, J. L. (1964). *Thromb. Diath. Haemorrhag. 11,* 393.

Blix, S. (1961). *Scand. J. Clin. Lab. Invest. 13,* 16.

Boettcher, E. W., Kistler, R., and Nitschmann, H. (1958). *Nature 181,* 490.

Celander, D. R., and Guest, M. M. (1959). *Am. J. Physiol. 197,* 391.

Christensen, L. R. (1945). *J. Gen. Physiol. 28,* 363.

Christensen, L. R., and MacLeod, C. M. (1945). *J. Gen. Physiol. 28,* 559.

Christensen, L. R., and Smith, D. H., Jr. (1950). *Proc. Soc. Exptl. Biol. Med. 74,* 840.

Cohn, E. J., Strong, L. E., Hughes, W. L., Jr., Mulford, D. J., Ashworth, J. N., Milin, M., and Taylor, H. C. (1946). *J. Am. Chem. Soc. 68,* 459.

Cole, E. R., and Mertz, E. T. (1961). *Can. J. Biochem. Physiol. 39,* 1419.

Dalby, A., Cole, E. R., and Mertz, E. T. (1960). *Can. J. Biochem. Physiol. 38,* 1029.

Dastre, A. (1895). *Arch. Physiol. Norm. Pathol. 7,* 408.

Davies, M. C., and Englert, M. E. (1960). *J. Biol. Chem. 235,* 1011.

Derechin, N., Johnson, P., and Szuchet, S. (1962). *Biochem. J. 84,* 336.

Edsall, J. T., Ferry, R. M., and Armstrong, S. H., Jr. (1944). *J. Clin. Invest. 23,* 557.

Guest, M. M. (1954). *J. Clin. Invest. 33,* 1553.

Hagan, J. J., Ablondi, F. B., and DeRenzo, E. C. (1960). *J. Biol. Chem. 235,* 1005.

Heberlein, P. J., and Barnhart, M. I. (1967). To be published in *Thromb. Diath. Haemorrhag.*

Hedin, S. G. (1903). *J. Physiol. 38,* 195.

Hink, J. H., and McDonald, J. K. (1963). *Vox Sanguinis 8,* 103.

Horejsi, I., and Smetana, R. (1948). *Acta Med. Scand. 2,* 550.

Hunter, J. (1794). "Treatise on Blood, Inflammation and Gunshot Wound". G. Nicol, London.

Kaisha, M. K. K. K. (1957). Patent Specification 770, 693 London, England, The Patent Office, October 21, 1954, p. 9. Granted, 1957.

Kaplan, M. H. (1944). *Proc. Soc. Exptl. Biol. Med. 57,* 40.

Kekwick, R. A., MacKay, M. E., Nance, M. H., and Record, B. R. (1955). *Biochem. J. 60,* 671.

Kjeldgaard, N. O., and Ploug, J. (1957). *Biochim. Biophys. Acta 24,* 283.

Kline, D. L. (1953). *J. Biol. Chem. 204,* 949.

Kline, D. L. (1954). *Yale J. Biol. Med. 26,* 365.

Kline, D. L., and Fishman, J. B. (1961). *J. Biol. Chem. 236,* 3232.

Kline, D. L., and Fishman, J. B. (1964). *Thromb. Diath. Haemorrhag. 11,* 75.

Markus, G., and Ambrus, C. M. (1960). *J. Biol. Chem. 235,* 1673.

Mertz, E. T., and Chan, J. Y. S. (1963). *Can. J. Biochem. Physiol. 41,* 1811.

Miller, K. D. (1959). *Nature 134,* 450.

Milstone, H. (1941). *J. Immunol. 42,* 109.

Mullertz, S. (1955). *Biochem. J. 61,* 424.

Nitschmann, H., Schlunegger, U., and Schneider, C. (1962). *Vox Sanguinis 7,* 641.

Norman, P. S. (1957). *Proc. Soc. Exptl. Biol. Med. 96,* 709.

Norman, P. S. (1960). *Federation Proc. 19,* 62.

Pillemer, L., and Hutchinson, M. C. (1945). *J. Biol. Chem. 158,* 299.

Rane, L., and Newhouser, L. R. (1954). *U.S. Armed Forces Med. J. 5,* 368.

Remmert, L. F., and Cohen, P. O. (1949). *J. Biol. Chem. 181,* 431.

Richard, M. N., Rose, C. B., Smith, W. E., and Baumgarten, W. (1959). *Vox Sanguinis 4,* 126.

Robbins, K. C., and Summaria, L. (1963). *J. Biol. Chem. 238,* 952.

Robbins, K. C., Summaria, L., Elwyn, D., and Barlow, G. H. (1965). *J. Biol. Chem. 240,* 541.

Roberts, P. S. (1960). *J. Biol. Chem. 235,* 2262.

Rybak, M. (1959). *Clin. Chim. Acta 4,* 310.

Sgouris, J. T., Inman, J. K., McCall, K. B., and Anderston, H. D. (1960). *Vox Sanguinis 5,* 357.

Shamash, Y., Rimon, A., Megged, A., and Aviram, I. (1964). *Vox Sanguinis 9,* 191.

Sherry, S., Fletcher, A. P., and Alkjaersig, N. (1959). *Physiol. Rev. 39,* 343.

Shulman, S., Alkjaersig, N., and Sherry, S. (1958). *J. Biol. Chem. 233,* 91.

Slotta, K. H., Michl, H., and Santos, B. G. (1962). *Biochim. Biophys. Acta 58,* 459.

Slotta, K. H., and Gonzalez, J. D. (1964). *Biochem. 3,* 285.

Steinbuch, M., and Niewiarowski, S. (1960). *Nature 186,* 87.

Steinbuch, M., and Quentin, M. (1959). *Nature 183,* 323.

Surgenor, D. M. (1952). *Quart. Rev. Intern. Med. Dermatol. 9,* 145.

Troll, W., and Sherry, S. (1955). *J. Biol. Chem. 213,* 881.

Wallen, P. B. (1962a). *Arkiv. Kemi. 19,* 451.

Wallen, P. B. (1962b). *Arkiv. Kemi. 19,* 469.

Wallen, P. B., and Bergstrom, K. (1959). *Acta Chem. Scand. 13,* 1464.

Wallen, P. B., and Bergstrom, K. (1960). *Acta Chem. Scand. 14,* 217.

Caseinolytic Techniques*

Daniel L. Kline

I. Introduction

Caseinolysis was first used for the measurement of plasmin and plasminogen by Remmert and Cohen (1949). Modifications of the original procedure have been applied to the estimation of plasminogen activators, such as streptokinase (SK) and urokinase (UK).
The principle of the method involves the hydrolysis of casein by plasmin and the estimation of fragments soluble in trichloroacetic acid by chemical analysis or, more commonly, ultraviolet absorption. In the method described below, the original procedure of Remmert and Cohen (1949) has been modified as follows: (1) commercially available Hammersten casein is purified to procedure a uniform substrate, (2) in the conversion of plasminogen to plasmin, the high potency SK now available permits the elimination of a 10-minute pre-incubation period, (3) the concentration of casein has been reduced to eliminate a lag period which occurs at concentrations above 2%.

II. Plasminogen

A. Reagents

1. *Casein (modified from Müllertz (1955)):* Suspend 9 g of "Hammersten" casein (Nutritional Biochemicals, Cleveland) in 300 ml of 0.15 M phosphate buffer, pH 8.0 and dissolve by placing in boiling water for 15 min with occasional stirring. Cool. Adjust to pH 2 with 1 N HCl. Add 450 ml of 0.17 M perchloric acid. (May be refrigerated overnight at this point if desired.) Centrifuge in two 250 ml bottles at 2,000 rpm for 10 minutes. Resuspend precipitate in each bottle in 200 ml of distilled water. If precipitate is *carefully* dispersed as a very fine suspension, two washes with water are sufficient. If supernate after two washes is not almost opaque, wash one or more additional times. This is important to obtain low blanks. Dissolve precipitate in 300 ml of 0.15 M phosphate buffer, pH 8.0. The pH at this point should be about 7. Adjust to pH 7.5 with 1 N NaOH. Filter through glass wool, bottle in 10 ml portions and keep frozen until use. Remains stable indefinitely.

2. *Perchloric acid:* Stock solution, 1.7 M: 75 ml of 70% perchloric acid plus 425 ml distilled water. To 50 ml of 1.7 M perchloric acid, add 450 ml of water to make 0.17 M solution.

3. *Phosphate buffer, 0.15 M, pH 8.0:* For preparation of casein: Dissolve 1.5 g $NaH_2PO_4 \cdot H_2O$ and 20.5 g Na_2HPO_4 (anhydrous) in 900 ml water. If necessary, adjust to pH 8 with 1 N HCl or NaOH. Make up to 1 liter.

4. *Phosphate buffer, 0.15 M, pH 7.5:* For plasmin assay: As above but adjusted to pH 7.5. (1 ml of 1:10,000 merthiolate per 100 ml of buffer can be added as a preservative.)

5. *Streptokinase:* Bottle content dissolved in sufficient buffer, pH 7.5, to make 20,000 U/ml.

B. Procedure (modified Remmert & Cohen)

Materials *(in order of add'n)*	Volume in assay tube *(Total Volume 6 ml)*
plasminogen solution	up to 2.5 ml
phosphate buffer, pH 7.5	to bring vol. to 2.95 ml
casein solution	3.00 ml
streptokinase	0.05 ml

Mix. Place in water bath at 37° C. At 2 min, remove 2 ml and blow into 3.0 ml of 10% TCA. Shake gently. Let stand 15 min (room temperature). Centrifuge in 15 ml plastic tubes about 2,500 rpm for 10 min. Transfer su-

* The Committee on Thrombolytic Agents has published recommended procedures and Units in Thrombosis Diath. Haemorrh. 30 (1969), 259.

pernatant to a clean tube by means of a Pasteur pipette (fitted with a rubber bulb) whose tip has been wrapped with absorbent cotton. Read in Beckman spectrophotometer at 280 mμ or estimate tyrosine with Folin-Ciocalteau reagent. At 62 min, remove 2 ml and treat similarly.

C. Calculations

By definition, 1 R. & C. unit* equals the liberation of 450 μg of tyrosine equivalents per hour. From a standard tyrosine curve, with 6% TCA as the solvent, the factor to convert optical density to μg tyrosine/ml is determined. This should be close to 150 for a 10 mm light path in the Beckman spectrophotometer at 280 mμ.

$$\frac{\text{O. D.} \times 150 \times 3 \times 1\ \text{hr.} \times 5}{450} = \text{units in sample.} \quad (1)$$

The 3 and 5 in the calculations are corrections for dilution. In simplified form:

$$\text{O. D.} \times 5 = \text{units in sample}$$

$$\frac{\text{O. D.} \times 5 \times 1\ \text{ml}}{\text{ml used}} = \text{units/ml sample.} \quad (2)$$

Note: The actual conversion factor is 153. By using 150 for simplicity of calculation, an error of 2% is introduced. Direct comparison with results obtained by the original R. & C. procedure indicates that this unit times 0.9 equals the original R. & C. unit. As prepared above, the casein solution is close to 1.6% giving a final concentration of 0.8% in the assay. No lag phase occurs but the hydrolysis of casein is not linear above an optical density of about 0.35. The range for optimal results is 0.5–1.5 units per assay. Perchloric acid (PCA) (0.5 M) can be used in place of TCA. The standard tyrosine curve must be determined with 0.3 M PCA as solvent and gives a factor for conversion of O. D. to μg tyrosine/ml of about 137 at 275 mμ, or O. D. × 4.6 = units in sample. PCA solutions are more stable and have a lower blank than TCA.

* 1.1 R. and C. unit = 1 Michigan State Department of Health unit = 1 CTA unit. Therefore, a solution containing 22 R. and C. units contains 20 Michigan State Department of Health or CTA units.

III. Plasmin

To measure plasmin, the procedure is identical except for the omission of SK and the substitution of an equal volume of buffer. To estimate spontaneous plasmin in plasminogen, at least 1.5 ml of plasminogen solution should be used.

Plasminogen or plasmin may be measured in plasma or serum after destruction or removal of antiplasmin. To destroy antiplasmin, the plasma or serum sample is adjusted to pH 2.0 with 1 N HCl, let stand for 15 min, readjusted to pH 7.5 and assayed against casein as described (Alkjaersig et al. 1959). Plasmin and plasminogen may be separated from antiplasmin by precipitation of euglobulins. The sample is diluted with 19 parts of water and is then adjusted to pH 5.3 with 2% acetic acid (v/v). The precipitate is collected after 10 min and is redissolved to the original plasma or serum volume in the buffer used in the casein assay. Normal human plasma contains about 2 R. & C. units per ml. The values obtained by the two procedures agree closely (Kline, 1966).

IV. Plasminogen Activators

Caseinolytic assays for streptokinase and urokinase may be carried out by pre-incubating the activator with 10 potential units of plasminogen and then determining the amount of plasmin formed. Bovine plasminogen whose activity has been measured in a preliminary analysis after activation with UK (1000 units per casein unit) or human plasminogen with not more than 2% spontaneous plasmin activity, are suitable substrates. Activation of human plasminogen by SK is almost instantaneous. When UK is used, a preliminary activation, 10 min at 37° C, is recommended before casein is added to measure the plasmin formed. It is important to note that an excess of plasminogen is present, and when the activator is UK, the formation of plasmin continues during the assay. It is recommended that a curve of approximately 2, 4, 6, 8 and 10 units of UK or SK be obtained in parallel with a curve in which a standard activator solution is used.

At present, the Committee on Thrombolytic Agents, NIH, is investigating a new substrate, α-casein, which is more sensitive than Hammersten casein. If α-casein becomes commercially available, suggestions will be made by the Committee for its use and a new unit will be defined (Johnson et al. 1969).

References

Alkjaersig, N., Fletcher, A. P., and Sherry, S. (1959). *J. Clin. Invest. 38,* 1086.
Kline, D. L. (1966). *Proc. Soc. Exptl. Biol. Med. 121,* 184.
Müllertz, S. (1955). *Biochem. J. 61,* 424.
Remmert, L. F., and Cohen, P. P. (1949). *J. Biol. Chem. 181,* **431.**
Johnson, A. J., Kline, D. L., and Alkjaersig, N. (1969). *Thromb. et Diath. Haemorrh.*

Plasminogen Assays Using Fibrin as a Substrate

Henner Graeff and Fritz K. Beller

I. Introduction

The methods presented can be used for assaying plasminogen in plasma as well as in biological fluids or purified systems. For plasma the plasminogen assay requires three basic steps: 1) removal or reduction of inhibitors, 2) activation of plasminogen, 3) the determination of the generated activity on a suitable fibrin substrate.

The following methods are used to separate plasminogen from plasmin inhibitors: a) acidification to a pH of 2–3 (Alkjaersig et al. 1959) b) lowering the ionic strength and acidification to pH 5.2–5.4 (Milstone, 1941; von Kaulla and Schultz, 1958) c) treatment with acetone (Brakman, 1967) d) adding a cationic polyelectrolyte like protamine sulphate and adjusting to pH 9 (Celander and Guest, 1959) e) dilution (Johnson and Tillet, 1962). Plasminogen can be assayed 1) by forming a streptokinase plasmin complex or 2) by the direct formation of plasmin.

Fibrinogen, fibrin, casein or synthetic esters are used as substrates. Fibrin as substrate was shown to have higher sensitivity than fibrinogen, casein or synthetic esters (Celander and Guest, 1959; Maki, 1962; Moser and Frey, 1966). Esterolytic procedures are described by Troll and caseinolytic techniques by Kline in this volume.

II. Method of Johnson and Tillet (1952); (Johnson and Tse, 1967):

Principle: Plasma, biological fluids, or purified plasminogen solutions are diluted 1:100 and higher. Thus inhibitors are diminished. Adding streptokinase forms a streptokinase-plasmin complex which activates bovine plasminogen to plasmin. The lysis time of fibrin clots is directly related to the plasminogen content of the test solution.
The original method (Johnson and Tillet, 1952) has recently been modified using N-Tris (hydroxymethyl) methyl-2 amino methanesulfonic acid (TES) buffer (Johnson and Tse, 1967).

Materials and reagents:

TES buffer, pH 7.5, ionic strength 0.15 (see Chapter II, p. 62).
Gel-buffer, pH 7.5, ionic strength 0.2: 5.0 g gelatine (purified calfskin gelatine, Amend Drug and Chemical Co. New York, N.Y.) are dissolved in 500 ml distilled water and TES buffer is added to a total volume of 1 liter.
Streptokinase (Behring Werke, Marburg and American Hoechst Inc., Cincinnati, Ohio) or Varidase, (American Cyanamid, Lederle Div., Pearl River, New York): 3,000 units/ml, dissolved in Gel-buffer.

Fibrinogen: Bovine fibrinogen, fraction I (Armour Pharmaceutical Co., Kankakee, Ill.): 5 mg/ml, dissolved in TES-buffer.
Thrombin: 20 units/ml, dissolved in TES-buffer.
Waterbath 37° C.
Vortex mixer.
Pipettes: 0.2 ml, 1 ml, 5 ml.
Glass test tubes: 12 mm × 75 mm (Falcon, Fisher Scientific, New York). Plastic tubes: 16 mm × 100 mm.
Stop watches.

Procedure: Test solution and reagents are stored in plastic tubes or siliconized glassware. Clot lysis is assayed in regular glass tubes. Test tubes containing between 0.45 to 0.6 ml of TES buffer (Table 1) are placed in an ice bath. Varying amounts of diluted plasma (1:100 diluted in TES buffer), or biological fluids or purified human plasminogen are added as indicated in Table 1. If the mean lysis times are not in the range of 4–20 min, a more dilute system may be employed.

Table 1: Composition of Plasminogen Assay System with Serial Plasma Dilutions.

Reciprocal of the dilutions of plasma	TES buffer ml	Sample 1:100 diluted ml	SK ml	Fibrinogen ml	Thrombin ml
713	0.45	0.14	0.1	0.2	0.1
1,000	0.50	0.10	0.1	0.2	0.1
1,500	0.50	0.066	0.1	0.2	0.1
2,000	0.60	0.050	0.1	0.2	0.1
2,700	0.60	0.037	0.1	0.2	0.1
4,000	0.60	0.025	0.1	0.2	0.1
5,500	0.60	0.018	0.1	0.2	0.1
7,130	0.60	0.014	0.1	0.2	0.1
10,000	0.60	0.010	0.1	0.2	0.1

0.1 ml streptokinase solution, 0.2 ml fibrinogen solution and 0.1 ml thrombin solution are added.
Thrombin is added quickly. Immediately after the addition of thrombin the individual tubes are swirled on a Vortex mixer for 5 sec and placed at constant temperature of 37° C. A stopwatch is started upon completion of preparation of the last tube. It is of considerable importance to carry out all the above mentioned procedures as rapidly as possible. Air bubbles, produced by swirling, are trapped in the forming clot. When clot lysis occurs, the air bubbles rise, depending on the state of liquefaction. Endpoint is taken as the time, when the last air buble has reached the meniscus.

Calculations:
A graph is constructed on double log paper recording lysis time on the abscissa and plasma dilution on the ordinate (Fig. 1). Deviation from a straight line relationship for the lower plasminogen dilution can be attributed to the presence of inhibitors.
One unit of plasminogen in this system is arbitrarily defined as the amount of plasminogen producing a lysis time of 10 min. As seen in fig. 1, the calculation of plasminogen activity per ml of plasma can be accomplished by drawing a vertical line going through the ten minutes point on the abscissa and establishing the intercept with the straight line part of the plasminogen dilution curve. The construction of the graph permits a direct reading of plasminogen activity per ml on the

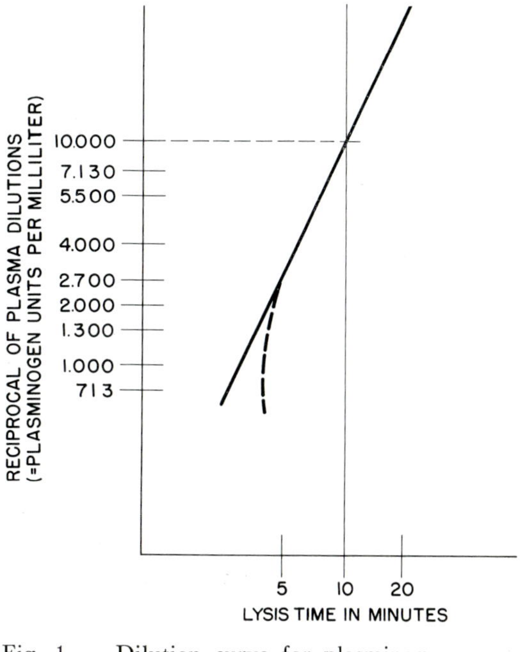

Fig. 1. Dilution curve for plasminogen assay. Time versus reciprocal of dilutions. Note the deviation from straight line relationship at lower plasma dilutions indicating the presence of inhibitors.

ordinate by connecting the point of intercept to the ordinate with a horizontal line. Normal range of plasminogen activity in human plasma is 5,000–7,000 units per ml.

Comment: In Johnson's method a standardized clot is made from commercially available fibrinogen (Armour fraction I) resulting in 0.45 mg clottable protein. One unit of plasminogen is the amount of plasminogen which lysis a one ml clot consisting of a 0.1 % bovine fibrinogen solution buffered with isotonic TES buffer at 37° C in 10 min. Compared to esterolytic assays the technique is more sensitive and plasminogen values below 100 U/ml test solution can be assayed.

Under the above conditions, 300 U SK per assay tube were sufficient to form the SK-plasmin complex. No plasmin activity was found if fibrinogen free of plasminogen was used. The lysis time of the control (without plasma or fluid) should extend 24 hours. Therefore, contamination of bovine fibrinogen or thrombin with plasmin should be ruled out. Armour fibrinogen contains large amounts of citrate which increases fibrinolytic activity, (Blix, 1961; Brakman, 1967). If different commercial fibrinogen preparations are used, different activities will be obtained for one and the same plasma. The plasminogen content of the following fibrinogen preparations was found to be adequate for this assay: Armour, Behring, Poviet (de Vreker, 1965). Lyophylized fibrinogen has to be kept dry at all times. In addition, even variations in fibrinogen batches may give different activities for one and the same plasma. Thus, the one serious potential source of error utilizing commercially available fibrinogens is the significant variation of plasminogen from batch to batch. This factor can be in part eliminated by establishing the intrinsic plasminogen concentration for each batch of fibrinogen used in the laboratory. With the advent of reproducible techniques for removing plasminogen from fibrinogen (see Chapter VI, p. 247) the use of plasminogen free fibrinogen in combination with known quantities of plasminogen is now replacing the use of commercial fibrinogen. The assay as outlined above involving hypertonic TES buffer solutions gives shorter lysis times and increased reproducibility.

III. Method of Brakman

Principle: Plasma is treated with acetone. The resulting precipitate, containing only weak inhibitor activity is redissolved, activated with urokinase and assayed on plasminogen free fibrin plates.

Materials and reagents:

Trisodium citrate solution 3.2 %.

Saline solution, 0.15 M.

Saline citrate solution; 9 parts saline and 1 part citrate solution.

Acetone, reagent grade.

Ethyl ether, anhydrous.

Saline barbital buffer with 0.25 % gelatine: 5.85 g sodium chloride and 10.31 g sodium barbital are dissolved in 725 ml of distilled water and 250 ml 0.1 N hydrochloric acid, 2.5 g gelatine (bacteriological grade) are added and dissolved. The pH is adjusted to 7.75 with 0.1 N hydrochloric acid and the solution is diluted up to 1000 ml with distilled water.

Urokinase solution for activation (20 Ploug units per ml) in saline barbital buffer with gelatine.

Procedure: Platelet poor citrated plasma obtained by centrifugation at 2000 × G for 30 min is stored at –20° C. Prior to use, the sample is thawed at room temperature and 1 ml is pipetted into a 16 × 100 mm glass tube. Acetone (cold, 4° C) totalling 4 ml is added, the first 2 ml drop by drop, while the tube is gently shaken. The solution is centrifuged for 5 min at 250 × G. The supernatant is discarded. Four ml of ice cold acetone are added, the mixture stirred with a stainless steel spatula and again centrifuged for 5 min at 250 × G. The supernatant is discarded, 4 ml of cold ethyl ether are added to the precipitate, the mixture is stirred, centrifuged as above and the supernatant is discarded. The remaining precipitate is stirred with a spatula while the tube is kept in hand at an angle of about 30°. After the ether has evaporated a white powder should remain. Several tubes may be processed under a stream of warm air. When the powder is dry, 1.1 ml saline citrate solution is added and the powder is redissolved. One ml of the solution is pipetted into a 10 × 75 mm tube in the ice water bath. A 0.5 ml aliquot of saline citrate solution is added to each of 4 tubes and serial dilutions are prepared by transferring 0.5 ml at each step, thus achieving dilutions down to 6.25 %. The last 0.5 ml are discarded. To each tube 0.5 ml urokinase solution is added, and from each tube 3 drops (0.03 ml) are placed on plasminogen free plates. The fibrin plates are incubated for 17 hours at 37° C. Simultaneously a pooled normal frozen control plasma (from at least 10 donors) is also assayed. For preparation of the plasminogen free fibrin plates see p. 247 ff.

Calculations: The activity of the solution is recorded as the diameter product in square mm. A graph is plotted on double logarithmic paper. Straight line plots for normal and test solutions should be parallel. The 100 % solution on the standard curve is used as reference and the concentration of the test sample is expressed in per cent of this concentration.

Comment:
The plasminogen is assayed as plasmin and this assay is therefore somewhat less sensitive than the activator assay. Acetone treatment of the plasma has to be done very slowly, otherwise larger precipitates will result which still contain inhibitor activity. These precipitates are difficult to dissolve. After evaporation of the ether the powder has to be redissolved rapidly. Large numbers of samples can be processed at one time. The disadvantages are the long incubation time and the fact that a plasma pool is used for normal reference.

IV. Method of Celander and Guest (1959); (Guest, 1954)

Principle: Plasma is treated with protamine sulfate, diluted, the precipitate redissolved and activated with Staphylokinase. The resulting activity is assayed on bovine fibrin clots.

Material and reagents:
Bovine fibrinogen in a 0.2 % solution (Ware et al. 1947), see Chapter VI, p. 241.
Protamine sulfate (Eli Lilly Comp. Indianapolis, Ind.): 0.8 % solution in 0.9 % saline.
Staphylokinase, prepared from freshly isolated cultures of staphylococcus aureus as described by Lewis and Ferguson (1951). For use, the lyophilized powder is dissolved in saline to a final concentration of 4–8 mg/ml.
Imidazole buffer, pH 7.25, is prepared by dissolving 1.72 g imidazole in 8.0 ml of 0.1 N HCl, adjusting the desired pH and diluting to 100 ml.

Procedure: Citrated platelet poor plasma (2 ml) obtained by centrifugation at 2,000 × G for 30 min are mixed with 0.5 ml protamine sulfate solution. The pH is adjusted to 9 with 0.1 N NaOH and kept at 28° C for 1 hour. The pH is then returned to 7.0 by adding 0.1 N HCl. The mixture is diluted 1:40 with distilled water. After 15 min. the tubes are centrifuged at 1,500 × G for 10 min at 20° C. The supernatant is discarded. To the precipitate is added sequentially 0.8 ml of 0.9 % saline, 0.9 ml of imidazole buffer and 0.1 ml of staphylokinase solution. The tube is incubated at 28° C. After 20 min. and every 15 min. thereafter, 0.2 ml of the incubation mixture is removed and diluted with imidazole buffer. Diluted aliquots are added to 0.2 ml bovine fibrinogen solution and the mixture is clotted by the addition of thrombin. The incubation is continued until two successive aliquots results in identical lysis time (after 90–120 min.). Dilution versus lysis times are plotted on double logarithmic paper. The dilution factor for aliquots of incubation mixture must be established empiricly. The dilution chosen for each aliquot is one which produces a lysis time between 5 and 20 min. One unit is defined as that amount of activity which lyses 0.4 ml of a 0.1 % fibrin clot in 300 seconds at 37° C. Alternatively, the precipitate may be redissolved in isotonic buffer and assayed by the methods described above. Instead of staphylokinase, streptokinase (1500 U) can be used (Guest, 1954).

Comment: The method was elaborated for the plasminogen assay in canine plasma. Canine plasma fractions treated with staphylokinase do not convert bovine plasminogen to plasmin. Therefore, only the amount of plasmin formed is measured. The use of staphylokinase preparations from freshly isolated staphylococcus aureus is stressed by the authors. The yield of plasminogen after protamine precipitation is higher than after euglobulin precipitation (Celander and Guest, 1959; Heberlein and Barnhart, see p. 337 ff). For plasminogen assays depending on plasminogen to plasmin conversion, the use of urokinase is recommended since neither streptokinase nor staphylokinase consistently produce plasminogen activator in different animal species.

Discussion: The original plasminogen assays in plasma used Quick's concept of the prothrombin time to assay the precursor of the enzyme. Streptokinase, as well as thrombin, was added to plasma and the lysis of the fibrin clot measured. This technique does not result in a quantitative plasminogen assay, mainly because of the large amount of inhibitors in plasma.

Guest and Celander (1956) and Blix (1961) described assay systems by which human plasma was diluted and activated with large amounts of streptokinase. The resulting activity was assayed using bovine fibrin clots rich in plasminogen. The authors assumed that prokinase or proactivator was determined. Witte and Dirnberger (1954) described a similar technique in which the precipitate was formed by precipitation at 30% ammonium sulfate saturation.

Recent data have indicated that the sequence of events in this type of assay is as follows: by adding streptokinase to human plasminogen in equimolar or higher concentrations, a streptokinase-plasmin complex is formed. It should be emphasized that very high concentrations of streptokinase (> 10,000 U/ml) inhibit fibrinolytic activity (Siegel and Clifton, 1956; Beller and Reinhardt, 1958; Abe and Deutsch, 1959). The streptokinase-plasmin complex activates bovine and human plasminogen (Kline and Fishman, 1961; Ling et al. 1965; Hummel et al. 1965, 1966; De Renzo et al. 1966). Plasminogen can also be assayed by direct activation to plasmin with urokinase which requires fibrinogen free of plasminogen, or by estereolytic assays. This approach was utilized by Brakman by determining the resulting activity on fibrin plates.

The amount of plasminogen is not only dependent on the amount of recovered plasminogen, but also on the residual inhibitors. The elimination of inhibitors is achieved either by dilution, by acetone treatment, by acidification, or by adding protamine sulfate. The highest yield of plasminogen is achieved by the dilution method (Berg et al. 1966). In the euglobulin fraction the plasminogen content varies depending on the pH choosen for precipitation, and some inhibitors may still remain. Acetone treatment only reduces inhibitor activity and the resulting yield of plasminogen is lower than after dilution. Protamine sulfate treatment in canine plasma results in a higher recovery rate of plasminogen than the euglobulin fraction (see p. 336) (Heberlein and Barnhart). In rabbit plasma the inhibitor concentration is high and the plasminogen content low. Under this condition the dilution technique does not result in diminished inhibitor activity. Either treatment with acetone, protamine sulfate or acidification is required (Graeff and Beller, 1967).

De Vreker (1965) described a dilution technique similar to that of Johnson and Tillet (1952), whereby the fibrinogen solution was adjusted so that one unit of human plasminogen produced clot lysis in 30 min. The disadvantage lies in the fact that pooled plasma was taken as a reference point assuming that normal human plasma contains 5,000 units of plasminogen.

Johnson and Tse (1967) have recently standardized the plasminogen assays, on behalf of the Committee on Thrombolytic Agents. TES buffer was introduced into the test system and the activity expressed in units. One unit corresponds to the activity resulting in lysis of a standard clot in 10 min (TES buffer, ionic strength 0.15, 37° C, 1 mg fibrinogen per ml clot).

References

Abe, T., and Deutsch, E. (1959). *Wien. Z. Inn. Med. Grenzg.* *40*, 52.
Alkjaersig, N., Fletcher, A. P., and Sherry, S. (1959). *J. Biol. Chem.* *234*, 823.
Beller, F. K., and Reinhardt, U. (1958). *Blut 4*, 367.
Berg, W., Korsan-Bengsten, K., and Ygge, J. (1966). *Thromb. Diath. Haemorrhag.* *16*, 1.
Blix, S. (1961). *Scand. J. Lab. Clin. Invest.* *13*, Suppl. 58, 3.
Brakman, P. (1967). Fibrinolysis, Scripta Medica 8, Scheltema & Holkema, Amsterdam.
Celander, D. R., and Guest, M. M. (1959). *Am. J. Physiol.* *197*, 391.
Graeff, H., and Beller, F. K. (1967). Unpublished data.
Guest, M. M. (1954). *J. Clin. Invest.* *33*, 1553.
Guest, M. M., and Celander, D. R. (1956). *Am. J. Physiol.* *187*, 602.
Hummel, B. C., Schor, I. M., Buck, F. F., Boggiano, E., and de Renzo, E. C. (1965). *Anal. Biochem.* *11*, 532.
Hummel, C. W., Buck, F. F., and de Renzo, E. C. (1966). *J. Biol. Chem.* *241*, 3474.
Johnson, A., and Tillet, W. S. (1952). *J. Exp. Med.* *95*, 449.
Johnson, A. J., and Tse, A. O. (1967). Personal communication.
Kaulla, K. N. von, and Schultz, R. L. (1958). *Am. J. Clin. Pathol.* *29*, 104.
Kline, D. C., and Fishman, J. B. (1961). *J. Biol. Chem.* *236*, 2807.
Lewis, J. H., and Ferguson, J. H. (1951). *Am. J. Physiol.* *166*, 594.
Ling, Ch. M., Summaria, L., and Robbins, K. C. (1965). *J. Biol. Chem.* *240*, 4213.
Maki, M. (1962). *Tohoku J. Exptl. Med.* *78*, 264.
Milstone, H. (1941). *J. Immunol.* *42*, 109.
Moser, K. M., and Frey, M. B. (1966). *Thromb. Diath. Haemorrhag.* *15*, 252.
Renzo, E. C., de, Boggiano, E., Barg, W. F., Jr., and Buck, F. F. (1966). *J. Biol. Chem.* *242*, 2428.
Siegel, M., and Clifton, M. (1956—57). *J. Gen. Physiol.* *40*, 377.
Vreker, R. A., de, (1965). *Acta Haematol.* *34*, 305.
Ware, A. G., Guest, M. M., and Seegers, W. H. (1947). *Arch. Bioch. Biophys.* *13*, 231.
Witte, S., and Dirnberger, P. (1954). *Klin. Wochschr.* *32*, 133.

The Esterase Assay of Enzymes of Blood Clotting and Lysis

Walter Troll

Glossasy

α-acetyl-L-arginine methyl ester	AAMe
α-benzoyl-L-arginine methyl ester	BAMe
α-benzoyl-L-arginine	BA
α-tosyl-L-arginine methyl ester	TAMe
α-tosyl-L-arginine	TA
L-lysine methyl ester	LMe
α-acetyl-L-lysine methyl ester	ALMe
α-acetyl-glycine-L-lysine methyl ester	AGLMe
α-benzoyl-L-lysine methyl ester	BLMe
α-tosyl-L-lysine methyl ester	TLMe

I. Introduction

The use of esters of amino acids for the assay of proteolytic enzymes grew out of the unexpected observation that these substances happen to be the most sensitive substrates for these enzymes. If their proteolytic and other biological properties had not been known by the time esters of amino acids were used as substrates, these enzymes would have been described as amino acid esterases with some low activity on other substrates such as: proteins or fibrinogen. The use of esters of amino acids as substrates for trypsin and chymotrypsin was introduced by Schwert et al. (1948) and Neurath and Schwert (1950). The field of proteolytic enzymes was widened by the observations of Sherry and Troll (1954) and Troll et al. (1954) that TAMe and LEe were substrates for plasmin, and TAMe was a substrate for thrombin. Sherry et al. (1965) have pointed to the advantages of the use of esters, not only for assay purposes, but also for the distinction of specific enzymes such as: urokinase, thrombin from bovine and human sources, and thrombokinase. The use of these esters as both substrates and specific inhibitors of enzymes has also been suggested. The methods specific for thrombin in the presence of plasmin by the use of lysine methyl ester (LMe) as an inhibitor with TAMe with the methyl group tritium labelled has been developed (Troll et al. 1969). This type of assay offers the opportunity of determining thrombin in a mixture of enzymes which may include, in addition to plasmin, other TAMe esterases which have been observed in blood plasma.

Some of the experimental methods which have been proposed are described in the next section followed by a discussion of the general usefulness of these types of studies.

II. Experimental Methods for Assaying Esterase Action

The hydrolysis of esters can be followed by a variety of methods: 1) The disappearance of the ester substrate measured colorimetrically, 2) the differential UV absorption of the ester and the formed acid, 3) the appearance of acid and 4) the measurement of the alcohol formed.

A. Disappearance of Ester Substrate Method

Principle: The colorimetric determination of esters due to a hydroxylamine ferric complex has been proposed by Hestrin (1949) for acetylcholine esters. This method depends on the conversion of the ester by an alkaline hydroxylamine solution to a hydroxamate and the color formation of this compound with ferric chloride in acid.

Material and Methods: 1) 2 M hydroxylamine hydrochloride, 2) 3.5 M sodium hydroxide, 3) concentrated hydrochloric acid, 1 part + 2 parts water, 4) 0.37 M ferric chloride in 0.1 M hydrochloric acid.

Procedure: One ml of the solution to be analyzed, which would contain from 5×10^{-3} M to 1×10^{-2} M ester, are added to 2 ml of an equal mixture of reagents 2 M hydroxylamine hydrochloride and 3.5 M sodium hydroxide (this mixture can be prepared ahead of time and is stable for several hours). The solution is allowed to react for 10 min which is sufficient time for most esters except for TAMe, where this mixture is allowed to stand for 3 hours at 37° C. Then 1 ml of ferric chloride reagent is added. If a precipitate forms due to proteins, the solution is centrifuged then 1 ml of ferric chloride reagent is added. The color is determined at 540 mμ in a colorimeter; a blank is run by reversing the order of addition of reagents, that is, the hydrochloric acid plus 2 parts of water are added first to the test solution, then the hydroxylamine alkaline mixture, followed by ferric chloride reagent. Under these circumstances no hydroxamate is formed and the color due to the solution of the test sample is determined.

Comment: This method is a universal method for quantitative investigation of esterase action. It can be applied directly to blood plasma with the centrifugation step indicated. This test has the advantage of ease and is useful for assaying a variety of esters as possible substrates for enzymatic activity. For quantitation it suffers from the disadvantage that it is frequently not possible to use the assay at optimum concentration of the ester since one is dealing with a small difference in two large numbers.

B. Esterase Activity Measured by the Differential UV Absorption of the Ester and the Acid

Principle: This method which was introduced by Schwert and Takenaka (1955), and expanded by Hummel (1959), depends on the different absorption spectra exhibited by esters such as TAMe, BAMe, and the hydrolysis products of BA and TA.

Material and Reagents: 1) 0.05 M Tris buffer, pH 8.1, containing 0.01 M calcium chloride. 2) TAMe is used as a substrate at 1.04×10^{-3} M, thrombin is used in the concentration of 10 to 50 mg/ml. Two cuvettes are employed. The blank cuvette contains tosyl arginine methyl ester at 1.04×10^{-3} M with water added and the sample solution contains the same concentration of substrate with the enzyme added. 3) Beckman spectrophotometer with thermo spaces maintained at 30° C. 4) Absorbance is measured at 247 mμ.

Comment: A linear absorbance increase was noted proportional to the amount of enzyme used in the range of 10 to 50 mg of purified thrombin. This method which can be applied

with variation to all amino acid esters containing aromatic groups has the advantage that the kinetics of the assay are continuously and readily determined, but it suffers from the limit of the concentration of substrate (TAMe) employed. In our hands, this method has worked out well with purified enzyme but gave unreliable results with biological solutions containing much UV absorbing material. Blank ultraviolet absorption was much increased and turbidity changes with proteins during the assay gave incorrect values.
The UV assay offers the opportunity of using aliphatic amino acid esters such as: lysine methyl ester (LMe) as competitive substrates. Since these esters do not offer either a blank or any change of absorption during the assay, the influence can be studied separately. We had developed an assay specific for thrombin initially based on using TAMe with an excess of lysine methyl ester. We have perfected such a system with the assay described in the last section using radioactive substrate.

C. Measurement of Esterase Action by Formation of Acid

This method is probably the most widely used and can be used at any beginning substrate concentration. Schwert et al. (1948) and Neurath and Schwert (1950) applied it by maintaining the pH during an incubation with the electrodes of a pH-meter inserted, using a burette with 0.01 M sodium hydroxide. This method was also used by Ronwin (1957) with TAMe as a substrate and thrombin as the enzyme. It is of some advantage to use a low concentration of buffer, e. g. 10^{-3} M Tris buffer, to obtain a smooth curve of titration. The availability of automatic instruments such as a radiometer pH-stat which plots the amount of alkali added on a graph has made this method of choice for esterase assays. The only disadvantage of this method is that only one sample at a time can be determined and it is difficult to routinize in a clinical laboratory.

The formol titration method based on the observations of Iselin and Niemann (1950), and used by Troll and Sherry (1955), is most readily applicable to esters in which the amino group is substituted. For example, we have used 0.1 M TAMe in 0.2 M Tris buffer pH 8 incubated with 0.5 ml of enzyme which could be either plasmin, thrombin, streptokinase activated plasminogen, etc., at 37° C in a total volume of 5 ml. One ml samples were withdrawn at various times into 1 ml of 37 % formaldehyde, maintained at pH 8 and back titrated to pH 8 with 0.01 M sodium hydroxide using phenol red as an indicator. For a blank we have set up a sample using no enzyme. Samples were withdrawn simultaneously from the blank mixture as well as from the enzyme mixture. This corrects for spontaneous hydrolysis of the ester which has been pointed out by Ronwin (1957) to be a source of error in these assays. Results are expressed as μM acid formed per 10 min during the zero order portion of the esterase action.

III. Methods Depending on the Alcohol Liberated

Principle: Two methods depending on methanol release have been employed. One is based on the colorimetric estimation of methanol originally described by Siegelman et al. (1962). The other depends on titrium labelled methanol (Troll et al. 1969).

The colorimetric method was recommended by Sherry et al. (1964) for BAMe, AAMe, TAMe, BLMe and TLMe, pointing to the advantage for being able to carry our multiple assays. A typical assay as applied to thrombin is given:

Material and Reagents: 1) Thrombin; 2) 0.015 M substrate (BAMe, AAMe, etc.); 3) phosphate buffer containing 0.9 % sodium chloride, pH 7.6 for the substituted esters, and pH 6.5 for LMe; 4) potassium permanganate, 2 % aqueous; 5) sodium sulfite in a 10 % solution; 6) chromotropic acid (mixing 200 ml of cold water, 100 ml of 2 % solution of 4,5-dihydroxy-2, 7-anphthalene sulfuric acid disodium salt and 600 ml of cold concentrated sulfuric acid and making the volume up to 100 ml with water; 7) waterbath; 8) spectrophotometer.

Procedure: A 0.3 ml aliquot of thrombin is added to 3 ml of 0.015 M substrate in 0.1 M phosphate buffer and incubated at 37° C in a waterbath. To stop the reaction after 10 min to one hour, 0.1 ml of a 10% solution of sodium sulfite was added to each to decolorize them. This was followed by 4.0 ml of chromotropic acid. The solution was heated in a boiling water bath for 50 min, made up to 5 ml and read at 580 mμ. A standard solution of methanol was used to determine the μM of methanol released.

Comment: This method is applicable to all methyl ester substrates and has led to the best identification of substrate activity of the variety of enzymes involved in blood clotting.

IV. Radioactive Methanol Method

Principle: The desirability to use one ester as a substrate with another ester as a comparative has led to the radioactive methanol method. Competition experiments of synthetic esters with natural substrates, has from the start, been the decisive evidence that esterase activity against TAMe and clotting of fibrinogen is carried out at the same enzyme center. The competition between esters for the clotting site of fibrinogen reveals striking differences between esters which show no such inhibition. This is not directly related to their ability to be split by these enzymes. Thus, several lysine esters such as TLMe, are good substrates for thrombin, yet do not effectively inhibit the clotting of fibrinogen as competitors. It appeared to us then, that we could develop specific assays for a variety of enzymes by using one ester as a substrate with labelled methanol and a second as a competitive inhibitor with unlabelled methanol.

An example for such an assay for thrombin which could be applied in the presence of plasmin, is described below.

Material and Reagents: 1) TAMe with labelled methanol was prepared from a solution of 3.2 g TAMe in 10 ml methanol, tritium labelled, containing from 1 to 5 mc, from New England Nuclear. The solution was cooled in an ice bath and dry HCl gas bubbled through it for one min. It was then stoppered and maintained for 24 hours at room temperature. The tritium labelled methanol was distilled off and the TAMe crystals washed with ether.

The tritium labelled methyl esters of TAMe, ALMe, and AGLMe are now commercially available from Cyclo Chemicals Corp., California. The radioactive esters are dissolved in dimethyl formamide in sufficient quantity so that 5 micro liters of the solution will contain from 10 to 20,000 CPM. 2) 0.1 molar of the cold ester employed is dissolved in dimethyl formamide. 3) Toluene scintillant containing 5 g of PPO (2,5-Diphenyloxazole) and 0.3 g Dimethyl POPOP (1,4-bis-2-(4-methyl-5-Phenyloxazoly)-Benzene per liter of toluene. 5) 1 M LMe in water. 6) Enzyme solution, thrombin, plasmin, etc. 7) Trypsin solution 1 mg/ml. 8) Scintillation counter.

Procedure: 5 ml of the radioactive ester, 10 ml of the cold ester in dimethyl formamide, 100 ml of the 1 M tris buffer, and up to 100 micro liters of enzyme solution are placed in a counting vial, 10 ml of toluene scintillant is added and the solution is shaken immediately. A count is taken in the scintillation counter and this count is called the zero count of the enzyme digestion. The vessel is incubated at 37° C and after 30 min, 1 hour, 2 hours, and 3 hours, the vessel is re-shaken and counted in the scintillation counter. Finally, 10 μg of trypsin is added in 10 μl, the container is incubated for 10 min and re-shaken. Count of this incubated sample is called the 100% count. Percent hydrolysis is calculated at each time by subtracting the zero count from the counts obtained at the various time intervals and dividing by the 100% count minus the zero count. From this, one obtains the percent hydrolysis of the ester being analyzed. Spontaneous hydrolysis is determined employing a tube in which the enzyme is omitted.

Comment: The water: toluene distribution coefficients of TAMe, ALMe and AGLMe in this system is sufficiently different from that of methanol so that the percent hydrolysis can be readily calculated from the method described above. The system is very sensitive and is capable of assaying $^1/_{10}$ micro gram of trypsin. In addition, if one desires to assay thrombin separately from other proteolytic enzymes, 1 molar LMe is added. Activity of trypsin, plasmin, and urokinase are inhibited while the thrombin activity remains the same. This method then offers the opportunity of measuring thrombin in the presence of plasmin or trypsin.

V. Discussion

The observation of the esterase action for enzymes involved in blood clotting and lysis, such as thrombin, plasmin, thrombokinase and urokinase has led to a number of generalizations. All these enzymes appear to be trypsin-like in being able to split only substrates with the basic amino acids arginine and lysine. The general similarity of these enzymes was further brought out by the observation that at least thrombin reacts with an analogous mechanism to that of trypsin and chymotrypsin in that it forms an acyl intermediate (Lorand, 1965). This was established with the use of carbobenzoxy-L-tyrosine-p-nitrophenyl ester where it was possible to demonstrate bursts of release of nitrophenyl groups.

The greatest interest found in these enzymes, however, is not their general properties, but their specificity of action. Thrombin only splits a single arginine-glycine bond, of all those available in a large molecule like fibrinogen, the liberate fibrinopeptide, leaving behind a protein destined to become fibrin (Lorand, 1965). Thus, this is an example of limited and purposeful proteolysis. Similarly, thrombokinase will activated prothrombin, but will not react with fibrinogen (Milstone et al. 1963). Attempts to rationalize these specificities of action in terms of esterase activity have as yet not been entirely successful, but the specificity of preferences of these enzymes for definite and different substrates has supported the notion that the preferentially split ester will lead you to the peptide bond that is being split. The difficulty of the dissection of the essential nature of enzyme specificity is not unlike the problems of deciphering the recognition site of antibodies with the aid of haptenic groups. This is particularly apparent when the TAMe enzyme, thrombin, from two species, human and bovine, are compared (Sherry et al. 1965). Both thrombins have virtually the same avidity for TAMe and BAMe, with a Michaelis constant of 5.5×10^{-3} and 1.2×10^{-3} respectively. However, they differ by a factor of 20 in their avidity for TLMe, the values for the bovine enzyme being 2.5×10^{-2}, and for the human, 5.3×10^{-3}. They are essentially alike in all other substrates, e. g., they show very low activity against LMe. Coupled with the observation that TAMe is a powerful inhibitor of clotting of fibrinogen, while TLMe is not, we can conclude that the main requirement of thrombin is an arginine ester with an aromatic substituent on the amino group. To confirm this hypothesis, more experiments will have to be performed which measure avidity of the capability of binding these substrates with the enzymatic sites with greater accuracy.

Perhaps the most different enzyme from thrombin, in clotting and lysis actions, is urokinase, which shows the greatest avidity for ALMe (Sherry et al. 1964) and AGLMe (Walton, 1967). Substitution of a tosyl group into the amino group of lysine has relatively little effect on the substrate activity of these esters against urokinase. The acetyl substituted lysine esters are excellent compared to the substrates for the activation of plasminogen by this enzyme. The essential nature of this enzyme can then be defined as requiring the amino acid lysine, with the preference of an aliphatic substituent on the alpha amino group.

It is relatively easy to interpret the amino acid in the preferential substrate used by these two enzymes. Thus, it has been shown that it is an arginine-glycine bond that is broken by thrombin (Lorand, 1965). There has been earlier evidence that lysine splitting is related to activation of plasminogen by other activators (Troll and Sherry, 1955), and this is indeed the amino acid link which appears to be involved in the activation of trypsinogen (Davie and Neurath, 1953). The substituent of the alpha amino group cannot be so readily rationalized since such substitutions do not occur in the natural protein substrates. They represent accidental good fits into the enzymatic site which cannot be translated at present into protein structure, but they are of help in characterizing these enzymes. The remainder of the enzymes involved in blood clotting, in fact of all proteolytic enzymes in the trypsin group, lie somewhere between the extremes of thrombin and urokinase (Sherry et al. 1965). In order to develop specific methods, several of these esters will have to be pitted against each other with additional help from inhibitors such as the soybean trypsin inhibitor. The main advantage of the esterase assay of enzymes involved in blood clotting and lysis remains the case of quantitation and precise kinetic analysis. With the aid of radioactive substrates it may well become the most sensitive assay as well.

References

Davie, E. W., and Neurath, H. (1953). *Biochim. Biophys. Acta 11*, 442.
Hestrin, S. (1949). *J. Biol. Chem. 180*, 249.
Hummel, B. C. W. (1959). *Can. J. Biochem. Physiol. 35*, 1393.
Iselin, M. B., and Niemann, C. (1950). *J. Biol. Chem. 182*, 821.
Lorand, L. (1965). *Federation Proc. 24*, 784.
Milstone, J. H., Oulianoff, N., and Milestone, V. K. (1963). *J. Gen. Physiol. 47*, 315.
Neurath, H., and Schwert, G. W. (1950). *Chem. Rev. 46*, 69.
Ronwin, E. (1957). *Can. J. Biochem. Physiol. 35*, 743.
Schwert, G. W., and Takenaka, Y. (1955). *Biochim. Biophys. Acta 16*, 570.
Schwert, G. W., Neurath, H., Kaufman, S., and Snoke, J. K. (1948). *J. Biol. Chem. 172*, 221.
Siegelman, A. M., Carlsen, A. S., and Robertley, T. (1962). *Arch. Biochem. Biophys. 97*, 159.
Sherry, S., and Troll, W. (1954). *J. Biol. Chem. 208*, 95.
Sherry, S., Alkjaersig, N., and Fletcher, A. P. (1964). *J. Lab. Clin. Med. 64*, 145.
Sherry, S., Alkjaersig, N., and Fletcher, A. P. (1965). *Amer. J. Physiol. 209*, 577.
Troll, W., and Sherry, S. (1955). *J. Biol. Chem. 213*, 881.
Troll, W., Sherry, S., and Wachman, J. (1954). *J. Biol. Chem. 208*, 85.
Troll, W., Roffman, S., and Sunocka, U. (1968). Manuscript in preparation.
Troll, W., Roffman, S., and Sanocka, U. (1969). *Fed. Proc. Vol. 28*, 2.
Walton, P. L. (1967). *Biochim. Biophys. Acta 152*, 104.

Assay of the Plasminogen Activator in Tissues*

Tage Astrup, Pia Glas and Preben Kok

I. Principles

The firm binding of the tissue plasminogen activator to structural cellular proteins delayed its extraction, isolation, and quantitative assay until it was found that the activator could be brought in solution by strong potassium thiocyanate (Astrup and Stage, 1952), and be recovered after acid precipitation (Astrup and Sterndorff, 1956). A quantitative assay was developed (Astrup and Albrechtsen, 1957). Solutions containing the activator are applied to plasminogen-rich fibrin plates (Astrup and Müllertz, 1952), and the areas of the lysed zones are used as measures of fibrinolytic activity. When graphed in a double logarithmic plot, a linear relation between concentration and activity emerges. Concentrations are obtained by comparison with a standard. The accuracy of the determination of the concentration in a solution, expressed as the coefficient of variation, is 7% or less. The exclusion of protease activity can be ensured by the absence of lysis after application to fibrin plates in which plasminogen has been destroyed by heating (Lassen, 1952), or which have been prepared from plasminogen-free fibrinogen (Brakman, 1965).

Because of its high sensitivity, the fibrin plate method is suited particularly to the assay of

* Supported by the U.S. Public Health Service, National Institutes of Health, National Heart Institute (HE-05020).

plasminogen activator in tissues. When purified and concentrated solutions of activator are available the lysis time method may be used. However, because of the large volume of substrate relative to the test volume applied, and because clot formation takes place in absence of the test solution, the fibrin plate method is influenced less by compounds contaminating the active solutions, especially such as would interfere with clot formation.

Several improvements have been introduced in the technique of the fibrin plate method in order to secure reproducibility and to standardize the method (Brakman, 1967; see p. 333). The use of strong thiocyanate solution in the tissue activator assay requires additional precautions and modifications. Data on the plasminogen activator concentrations in animal and human tissues have recently been reviewed (Astrup, 1966).

II. Reagents and Materials

Unless otherwise stated, reagent grade chemicals (American Chemical Society) are used.

A. Potassium Thiocyanate Solutions

1. *Potassium thiocyanate, 2 M:* 194.4 g KSCN is dissolved in water and diluted to 1000 ml in a volumetric flask. Daily, before use, an appropriate amount is adjusted to pH 7.75 with solid sodium bicarbonate.

2. *Potassium thiocyanate, 1 M, with 0.25% gelatine:* Gelatine ("bacteriological", 0.5 g) is dissolved in 100 ml water heated to 70–80° C under mechanical stirring and added to 100 ml 2 M KSCN solution. This solution should not be used for more than a week. Daily, an appropriate amount is adjusted to pH 7.75 as above.

B. Fibrin Plate Buffer

Barbital buffer (0.05 M) containing 0.09 M sodium chloride, 0.0017 M calcium chloride, and 0.0007 M magnesium chloride, pH 7.75, total ionic strength 0.15 (see p. 332).

C. Fibrinogen

Bovine fibrinogen is prepared as described by Astrup and Müllertz (1952), and modified and improved by Brakman (1967) see p. 333. The commercially available fibrinogen preparations were found less satisfactory and some of them contain large amounts of citrate, which make the clots susceptible to the strong solutions of KSCN required in the tissue activator assay. The final solution is adjusted to 0.1 % fibrinogen and ionic strength 0.15 in fibrin plate buffer and is freshly prepared each day as described on p. 333.

D. Thrombin

The thrombin, prepared with 20 NIH units of bovine thrombin per ml 0.15 M NaCl solution, must be practically free from contaminating fibrinolytic agents (Brakman et al. 1964; Schulte, 1965) (see also p. 335).

E. Preparation of a Standard for Tissue Activator Assays

A plasminogen activator standard is prepared from pig hearts as described by Astrup and Albrechtsen (1957) and its potency determined by comparison with our reference standard. Briefly described, the procedure is as follows:

Fresh pig hearts are cleaned and cut into pieces of heart muscle, which are then thoroughly ground in a meat grinder (10 times or more). One kg ground muscle is suspended in 10 liters of 0.15 M sodium chloride at room temperature and stirred mechanically for 15 min with 50 ml of toluene added. The tissue is separated by centrifugation and resuspended in 5 liters of 0.15 M sodium chloride (25 ml of toluene added) and stirred overnight in the cold room. Next day the tissue is separated and treated twice with 5 liters of 0.15 M sodium chloride and 3 times with 5 liters of distilled water followed by 3 treatments with 0.5 liters of acetone. The dehydrated powder is suspended in 0.5 liters of dry ether, filtered through coarse filter paper, washed with dry ether, and dried in the air by manual treatment with a spatula (Precaution: A dry atmosphere is required for this latter procedure. Humid air will produce a condensation of water on the powder during drying, ruining the preparation). The light, grayish tissue is ground thoroughly in a mortar. It is stable when stored away from light, heat, and moisture. The yield is about 100 g per kg heart muscle. The standard preparation is made from an extract obtained from this powder by treatment for 2 hours with 100 ml 2 M KSCN per 10 g powder, followed by centrifugation. The supernatant, diluted with 7 volumes of distilled water, is adjusted to pH 1 with 1 M HCl and centrifuged for at least 15 min at 1400 × G. After wiping off remaining fluid from the walls of the container, the sediment is redissolved to the original volume in saline-barbital buffer (0.05 M sodium barbital, 0.10 M sodium chloride, pH 7.75) by mechanical stirring for 15 min. After centrifugation the clear supernatant is lyophilized. The yield is about 20 g per 100 g of heart powder. The lyophilized powder, which should be completely soluble in 1 M KSCN, is distributed in sealed vials and stored at –20° C in a closed container over silica gel. Its activity varies from 0.5 to 2 tissue activator units (Astrup and Albrechtsen units) per mg. For assays a solution containing between 10 and 20 Astrup and Albrechtsen (A and A) units per ml is prepared in 1 M KSCN with gelatine. It was found, Astrup and Kok (1965), that one A and A unit equals approximately 0.1 CTA unit of urokinase (as defined by the Committee on Thrombolytic Agents, advisory to the National Heart Institute) but the comparison in units is valid only within certain limits because tissue activator and urokinase are chemically different.

F. Glassware

Because of the ease with which tissue activator is adsorbed to glass, all pipettes and other glassware, which have been exposed to the active solutions should be carefully cleaned afterwards, either by treatment in chromic acid-sulfuric acid solution or by soaking in 0.5 M NaOH, followed by thorough rinsing. Glassware used to prepare active solutions should be kept separate.

III. Preparation of Fibrin Plates

Fibrin plates are prepared as described on p. 332, using disposable, plastic Petri dishes with inside diameter 84 mm. The volume of fibrinogen solution was raised to 9 ml and clotted with 0.3 ml thrombin solution yielding a fibrin layer about 1.7 mm thick. This 50 % increase in substrate volume diminishes the influence of the concentrated KSCN test solution in the assay (see below).

To test for protease activity, heated fibrin plates or plates made from plasminogen-free fibrinogen are prepared as described on p. 333, using the revised amounts mentioned above to maintain otherwise identical conditions.

IV. Isolation of Tissue Activator

A. Tissue Samples

Fresh tissue samples are washed free from blood and excess fluid removed by blotting with filter paper. The samples are weighed and, if not immediately assayed, placed in small, tightly closed tubes and kept at –20° C. Storage for a few weeks causes no measurable decrease in activator content. By prolonged storage the activity decreases slowly.

B. Homogenization and Extraction

Tissue samples, cut into small pieces, are treated in a Potter-Elvehjem homogenizer (cooled in ice water) with 2 M KSCN solution freshly adjusted to pH 7.75 with solid $NaHCO_3$, using 3.0 ml of KSCN solution per 100 mg of tissue. When only small amounts of tissue are available (20–30 mg) the relative extraction volume can be increased somewhat without significantly affecting the results (Astrup et al. 1965). During homogenization, which requires a variable period of time depending upon the structure of the tissue, overheating of the tissue suspension should be avoided. After homogenization, the suspension is slowly shaken mechanically for one hour at room temperature.

C. Acid Precipitation

1. Regular Procedure

After centrifugation of the tissue suspension at 2900 × G for 10 min, an aliquot (usually 1.0 ml) of the supernatant ("crude extract") is diluted with 7 volumes of distilled water followed by addition of 1 M hydrochloric acid to pH 1. At this pH acid labile activators originating from the blood or present in the tissue are destroyed. The precipitate contains the stable tissue activator while inhibitory agents, if present, mostly remain in the supernatant. After 30 min at room temperature the mixture is centrifuged, and the sediment redissolved in an amount of the 1 M KSCN solution identical with the original volume of the aliquot (usually 1.0 ml) by neutralization with solid $NaHCO_3$. This solution is referred to as the "stock solution" of the sample.

2. Modified procedure for special tissues

Some acid supernatants remain turbid even after prolonged centrifugation at high speed, and in these activator activity can be demonstrated after neutralization. In such cases complete separation of the tissue activator can be accomplished by co-precipitation with a tissue extract free from demonstrable activator activity. We have used a crude extract prepared from skeletal muscle of rabbit. The modified procedure is as follows: To one volume of the crude extract of the tissue sample are added 6 volumes of water and one volume of the rabbit muscle extract. The mixture is then acidified to pH 1 and the procedure completed as before.

V. Assay on Fibrin Plates

A. Technique

To increase the accuracy of the determinations and to make sure that activities can be compared in terms of concentrations, serial dilutions of the stock solutions are assayed and the results plotted in a double logarithmic graph (see below). The dilutions are made with freshly neutralized 1 M KSCN solution containing gelatine. A standard tissue activator preparation is dissolved in 1 M KSCN (containing gelatine) and serially diluted to obtain a reference curve.

Of each dilution exactly 30 µl are placed (in triplicate) on the fibrin plate. The plates are incubated at 37° C for 15 to 18 hours. For details see p. 332. The area of a lysed zone is

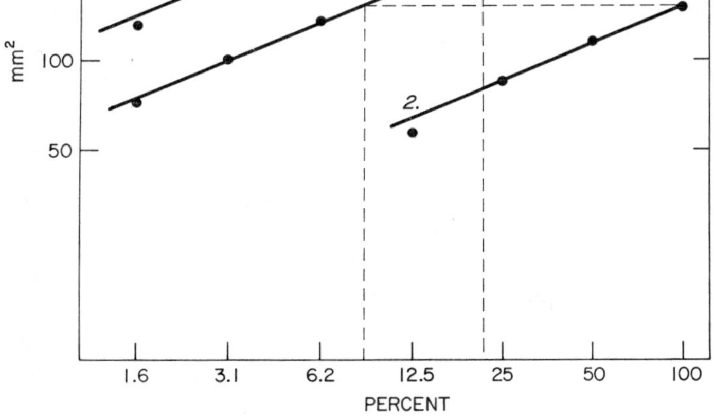

Fig. 1. Assay of Plasminogen Activator in Human Brain Tissue.
Abscissa: Concentration of test solutions in percent of stock solution (logarithmic).
Ordinate: Activity in mm² as product of perpendicular diameters (average of triplicate, logarithmic).

recorded as the product in mm^2 of two perpendicular diameters. The averages of triplicates are plotted in a double logarithmic graph (see Fig.) with the concentrations in percentages of the stock solution as abscissa and the activities, recorded as diameter products, as ordinate. To provide a basis for interpolation the curves should be linear and parallel with the standard curve simultaneously estimated. Accurate determinations require that the diameter products should be in the range from 100 to 800 mm^2. Downward deflections may occur at the high concentrations, probably caused by traces of inhibitors contaminating the samples. Likewise, deflections occurring at low concentrations could be due to a decreased susceptibility to lysis caused by traces of inhibitor in the fibrinogen. In such cases, straight lines parallel to the standard curve are drawn through intermediate values. Interpolation on the standard curve converts the recorded activities to concentrations of plasminogen activator expressed in units per ml. The final results are reported in units per gram fresh tissue. The estimation of plasminogen activator in human brain tissue is illustrated in the figure.

The *standard curve* was obtained from a stock solution containing 10.0 A and A units per ml. *Curve 1* was from a stock solution (10.8 ml) prepared from 359 mg of pia mater. Interpolation shows the standard solution (100%) to correspond in activity to 21.5% of the test sample equalling

$$\frac{10.0 \times 100}{21.5} \text{ units per ml.} \qquad (1)$$

Since 359 mg tissue yielded 10.8 ml extract, this gives a concentration of

$$\frac{10.0 \times 100 \times 10.8 \times 1000}{21.5 \times 359} = 1400 \qquad (2)$$

A and A units per gram fresh tissue. *Curve 2* represents an assay of 162 mg tissue from the dentate nucleus in 4.9 ml. The solution (100%) yields the same activity as 7.6% of the standard stock solution. Hence, the concentration of plasminogen activator in the test sample is

$$\frac{10.0 \times 7.6}{100} \text{ units per ml.} \qquad (3)$$

The amount (4.9 ml) obtained from 162 mg tissue gives

$$\frac{10.0 \times 7.6 \times 4.9 \times 1000}{100 \times 162} = 23 \qquad (4)$$

A and A units per gram fresh tissue.

B. Evaluation and Comments

The tissue plasminogen activator is firmly bound to structural proteins of the cell and cannot be completely extracted with the usual aqueous solvents. We have confirmed our earlier finding that 2 M KSCN is an excellent solvent. It is important to simultaneously assay dilutions of a reference standard prepared with the diluent used in the sample. Some discrepancies in the literature could probably be explained by a disregard of this condition. The 3-step extraction procedure originally used to ensure complete extraction (Astrup and Albrechtsen, 1957), could in most comparative assays be replaced by the less time consuming procedure here described without significant loss in accuracy.

Since the volume of the fibrin substrate in the plate is 100 times larger than the volume of the 3 drops of the test sample applied to the fibrin surface, the overall composition of the substrate is not significantly changed by compounds present in the drops. However, local deviations may be caused by the high salt concentrations in the drops. Thus, the 2 M KSCN solution has a marked delaying effect on lysis during the first few hours. Hence, in the test solution the concentration was decreased to 1 M KSCN. Gelatine was added to prevent adsorption of active agents to glass. Concentrations in different tissues usually range from 0 to 3000 A and A units per gram yielding stock solutions containing 100 A and A units per ml or less. The fibrin plate method described here is about 100 times more sensitive to plasminogen activators than the clot lysis time method and a wide range of activator concentrations can be assayed. A concentration of 0.1 A and A unit per ml can still be measured. Commercially available fibrinogen preparations, because of their deficiency in plasminogen, usually yield fibrin more resistant to activators. Frequently, however, they are sensitive to the concentrated KSCN solutions because of the presence of citrate. Phosphate buffer also makes the fibrin sensitive to KSCN. On regularly prepared fibrin plates, drops of a 1 M KSCN solution produce no lysis but give rise to a clarification of the fibrin layer around the drop immediately after its application. The addition of dextran or agar to the fibrinogen to obtain a more solid clot should be avoided, since the development of clear zones might be caused by the salt effects mentioned and not by true lysis. When the fibrinogen is made according to our descriptions such additions are unnecessary.

VI. The Clot Lysis Time Method

Tissue plasminogen activator can be assayed by the lysis time method when high concentrations are available. The lowest concentration in a sample solution which can be measured varies from 10 to 100 A and A units per ml depending upon the concentration of plasminogen in the fibrinogen. The lysis time method is more accurate than the fibrin plate assay, the coefficient of variation being about 1 %. Since high salt concentrations interfere with clot formation and clot lysis, use of the lysis time method is limited to the comparison of relatively concentrated activator preparations which are soluble in saline or buffers (Bachmann et al. 1964; Kok and Astrup, 1969). The principle used by Lassen (1958) gives a high accuracy of end-point determination. Briefly described, the technique is as follows:

An activator stock solution (100 to 2000 A and A units per ml) is prepared in saline barbital buffer containing 0.5 % gelatine (0.05 M sodium barbital, 0.1 M NaCl, pH 7.75) and serial dilutions are made with the same buffer. In a glass tube, 10 × 75 mm, exactly 1.0 ml activator solution and 0.1 ml thrombin solution (40 NIH units per ml in 0.15 M NaCl) are mixed and incubated at 37° C for exactly 3 minutes. At zero time 1.0 ml of a 0.5 % fibrinogen solution in saline-barbital buffer, preheated at 37° C for a few minutes, is added to the mixture. Clotting occurs in about 30 seconds and small air bubbles appear. The lysis time is the interval between zero time and the moment when the rising air bubbles pass the middle of the clot volume in the tube. Lysis times are read in seconds and plotted in a double logarithmic graph with the activator concentration in percentages of the stock solution as abscissa and the lysis time or its reciprocal as ordinate. Interpolation on a standard curve yields the activator concentration.

It should be noted that Lewis and Ferguson (1950) were able to determine low concentrations of the tissue activator by the lysis time method by performing the assay in the cold room and extending the lysis period over several days.

References

Astrup, T. (1966). *Federation Proc. 25*, No. 1, 42.

Astrup, T., and Albrechtsen, O. K. (1957). *Scand. J. Clin. Lab. Invest. 9*, 233.

Astrup, T., Beller, F. K., Glas, P., and Rasmussen, J. (1965). *Obstet. Gynec. 25*, 853.

Astrup, T., and Kok, P. (1965). *Thromb. Diath. Haemorrhag. 13*, 587.

Astrup, T., and Müllertz, S. (1952). *Arch. Biochem. Biophys. 40*, 346.

Astrup, T., and Stage, A. (1952). *Nature 170*, 929.

Astrup, T., and Sterndorff, I. (1956). *Acta Physiol. Scand. 36*, 250.

Bachmann, F., Fletcher, A. P., Alkjaersig, N., and Sherry, S. (1964). *Biochemistry 3*, 1578.

Brakman, P. (1965). *Anal. Biochem. 11*, 149.

Brakman, P. (1967). "Fibrinolysis. A Standardized Fibrin Plate Method and a Fibrinolytic Assay of Plasminogen." Scheltema and Holkema, Amsterdam.

Brakman, P., Klug, P., and Astrup, T. (1964). *Thromb. Diath. Haemorrhag. 11*, 234.

Kok, P., and Astrup, T. (1969). *Biochemistry 8*, 79.

Lassen, M. (1952). *Acta Physiol. Scand. 27*, 371.

Lassen, M. (1958). *Scand. J. Clin. Lab. Invest. 10*, 384.

Lewis, J. H., and Ferguson, J. H. (1950). *J. Clin. Invest. 29*, 1059.

Schulte, W. (1965). *Thromb. Diath. Haemorrhag. 13*, 561.

Assay Methods for Individual Fibrinolytic Components – Urokinase and Streptokinase

Milton M. Mozen

I. Introduction

Human plasminogen, a proenzyme constituent of plasma may be activated to the proteolytic enzyme plasmin in a variety of ways. The two most widely studied activators of plasminogen are streptokinase, a protein produced by hemolytic streptococci, and the human urinary enzyme, urokinase. Although both of these activators generate plasmin activity from plasminogen, their mechanisms of action are different. Whereas urokinase can directly activate the plasminogen of a variety of species, streptokinase must first interact with a human proactivator substance, believed to be plasmin (Zylber et al. 1959; Kline and Fishman, 1961; Roberts, 1962; Blatt et al. 1964; Ling et al. 1965). The product of this interaction, activator, can then generate plasmin activity from plasminogen of nonhuman origin.

Assay methods for urokinase and streptokinase largely depend on the activation of plasminogen under conditions where streptokinase or urokinase are the rate limiting reagents, and then quantitating the active plasmin evolved. The assay of activator thus becomes essentially a plasmin assay. A wide variety of substrates susceptible to proteolysis have been used for this purpose including; fibrin (Loomis et al. 1947), fibrinogen (Müllertz, 1952; Nanninga and Guest, 1964), casein (Remmert and Cohen, 1949), Azocasein (Hummel et al. 1965), protamine-heparin complex (Kjeldgaard and Ploug, 1957; Greig and Cornelius, 1963), and synthetic esters of lysine and arginine (Troll et al. 1954; Hagen et al. 1956; Lassen, 1958; Roberts, 1958; Kline and Fishman, 1961; Ronwin, 1961).

Urokinase, in contrast to streptokinase, can directly catalyze the hydrolysis of synthetic amino acid esters. Kjeldgaard and Ploug (1957) demonstrated the hydrolysis of α-N-p-toluenesulfonyl-L-arginine methyl ester and L-lysine ethyl ester by relatively high concentrations of partially purified urokinase. Lorand and Mozen (1964) found that the catalytic activity of urokinase preparations of varying degrees of purity on the hydrolysis of p-nitrophenyl carbobenzoxy-L-tyrosinate paralled fibrinolytic activity with purified fractions. The kinetics of hydrolysis of various α-N-acyl amino acid esters was described by Sherry et al. (1964). Of the substrates tested, α-N-acetyl-L-lysine methyl ester was the most rapidly hydrolyzed and was utilized in developing a quantitative assay for urokinase. The substrate α-N-acetylglycyl-L-lysine methyl ester has been found by Walton (1967) to be sensitive to urokinase activity, and to offer advantages over those esters previously described. Chief among these are its availability in purified crystalline form, its sensitivity to low concentrations of urokinase, and its relatively high degree of specificity.

Ester hydrolysis catalyzed by urokinase can be estimated in a number of ways. The liberated amino acid may be titrated directly with alkali, (Sherry et al. 1964; Walton, 1967), by formol titration (Troll et al. 1954), or precipitated with solvent and determined turbidometrically (Kjeldgaard and Ploug, 1957). Alternatively the disappearance of ester substrate may be measured colorimetrically after reaction with alkaline hydroxylamine and subsequent ferric complex formation (Hestrin, 1949; Alkjaersig et al. 1958). With methyl ester substrates the release of methanol can be quantitated colorimetrically utilizing the chromotropic acid reaction (Siegelman et al. 1962; Sherry et al. 1964).

The general principles described here for the assay of urokinase and streptokinase have been utilized, with individual variations, by many investigators. It would be superfluous to attempt to detail all of the methods and modifications which have been used. Therefore procedures which have proved successful over many years of use by commercial firms will be described below.

II. Urokinase Assay

A. Definition of Urokinase Unit

The unit of urokinase activity which has become generally accepted is termed the CTA unit. A CTA unit refers to the standard activity unit adopted by the Committee on Thrombolytic Agents of the National Heart Institute. This unit is based on the activity of standard urokinase preparations (supplied by Abbott Lab, North Chicago, Ill. and Sterling Winthrop, Albany, N. Y.) which were independently assayed in several laboratories, and by various assay procedures. Utilizing the ability of urokinase to directly catalize the hydrolysis of α-N-acetyl-L-lysine methyl ester (ALMe), Sherry et al. (1964) defined the CTA unit in kinetic terms. One CTA unit of urokinase activity releases from ALMe 46.2×10^{-3} μM of methanol in one hour at 37° C. Conversion factors for commonly used urokinase units are: 1 CTA unit is equivalent to 2 Abbott, 12 Sterling-Winthrop (SWRL) or 0.7 Ploug-Kjeldgaard units.

B. Fibrin Tube Method (White et al. 1966)

Principle: Urokinase added to a buffered solution of bovine fibrinogen, containing plasminogen, and clotted with thrombin, results in an amount of lysis of the formed fibrin clot which is proportional to the urokinase concentration. By maintaining a constant incubation time, and varying the amount of added urokinase, a level of urokinase activity is estimated which results in 50% lysis of the fibrin clot.

Reagents: Human serum albumin: Human serum albumin (0.1%) is used for diluting urokinase samples. It is prepared fresh daily by dissolving 1 mg/ml of Human Albumin Fraction V (Pentex, Inc., Kankakee, Illinois) in distilled water.

Thrombin: Bovine Thrombin Topical 10,000 N.I.H. units/vial (Parke, Davis and Co., Detroit, Michigan) is diluted with distilled water to 16.7 N.I.H. units/ml and kept frozen in small portions. A fresh bottle is thawed daily, and is not reused.

Sodium Barbital Buffer (0.05 M): 10.3 g Barbital Sodium, N. F. powder is dissolved in about 950 ml distilled water, adjusted to pH 7.6 with 1 N HCl, and diluted to 1 liter.

Fibrinogen: Armour's Bovine Fraction I (containing 40–50% sodium citrate) is dissolved at 16 mg/ml in the sodium barbital buffer. This fibrinogen solution is freshly prepared just prior to use.
Because commercial lots of bovine fibrinogen may vary considerably in plasminogen content, it is frequently necessary to select a suitable batch from a number of samples tested. In general a lot is satisfactory if it fulfills the following criteria: 1) The clot formed after the addition of thrombin, and in the absence of urokinase, remains firm with no evidence of lysis after 16 hours incubation at 37° C. 2) Under conditions of the assay to be described, 50% clot lysis occurs with urokinase at a level of about 0.2–2.0 CTA units per tube.

Assay Procedure: 1) Dilute a urokinase standard and each sample to be run with 0.1% human serum albumin to about 2 CTA units per ml. The standard should be of known potency which has been compared against the CTA standard, e.g. Abbott Urokinase Assay Standard Lot No. 2021–209, 2100 CTA units per vial. Standards are best preserved in the lyophilized state since solutions, even though frozen, lose activity at an appreciable rate. 2) A series of 10 tubes, 13×100 mm, is used for each sample and standard to be assayed. Pipette into these tubes graduated amounts of the diluted urokinase solution, e.g. 0.09, 0.10, 0.11, 0.12, 0.13, 0.14, 0.15, 0.16, 0.17, 0.18 ml/tube. 3) Add 0.3 ml thrombin solution to each, followed immediately by 1 ml fibrinogen solution, and shake to insure good mixing. A firm fibrin clot forms within 30 sec. 4) Incubate at 37° C for 16 hours in a constant temperature water bath. 5) Visually estimate to the nearest 10% the fraction of clot remaining in each tube. 6) Calculate from the standard, the amount of urokinase which will produce a 50% clot. Do this by direct examination or interpolation of 2 adjacent tubes in the series. 7) By comparison to the standards and known dilution factors, calculate the amount of urokinase in the original sample.

$$\frac{\text{Units of Std. in 50\% Clot Tube}}{\text{Volume of Sample in 50\% Clot Tube}} \times \text{sample dilution} = \text{units urokinase/ml original} \quad (1)$$

Comments·
With each assay group, the standard is run with a series of 10 tubes both at the beginning and at the end of the run. The average of the 50% clot point concentration is used for calculating potency of the samples.
When diluting urokinase to the desired concentration, it is preferable to add the urokinase solution to the diluent to minimize glass adsorption losses.
In contrast to many other urokinase procedures, this one allows for the determination of very low concentrations of urokinase such as that found in whole urine.
To maintain fibrinogen for an extended period, the stock bottles should be kept dry (over P_2O_5) and at refrigerated temperatures.

In our laboratory, a single operator can carry out as many as 40 determinations plus 2 standards in a single assay series.
Statistical analyses of a series of assays performed on assay standards indicated an estimated error of ± 24% from the mean for a single assay at the 95% probability level. If three separate assays are carried out on the same sample, the estimated error is reduced to about ± 16%.

III. Streptokinase Assay

A. Christensen (1949) Modified Fibrinolytic Method*

Principle: Plasmin, liberated from plasminogen by streptokinase, is measured by its ability to lyse a standard fibrin clot. One Christensen unit of streptokinase is that amount which will completely lyse a standard clot in 10 min under the conditions of the assay.

Reagents: Borate Buffer: Dissolve 11.1 g boric acid, 7.0 g sodium borate ($Na_2B_4O_7 \cdot 10H_2O$) and 9.0 g NaCl in distilled water and dilute to 1 liter. Adjust to pH 7.4–7.5 with 5 N HCl and store in the cold.

Gelatin Diluent: (For diluting streptokinase solutions) Dissolve 5 g of a purified gelatin in a small amount of warm distilled water followed by 13.6 g KH_2PO_4, 10 g NaCl, and 10 ml of a 1:100 dilution of sodium ethylmercurithiosalicylate (thimerosal). Dilute to near 1 liter with distilled water, adjust to pH 7.4–7.5 with 10 N NaOH, and dilute to one liter.

Bovine Fibrinogen: Dissolve Armour's Bovine Fraction I (dried and maintained over P_2O_5) in borate buffer to 0.25%, e.g. 90 mg in 36 ml.

Plasminogen: Prepare a paste of human fraction III (dried and maintained over P_2O_5) with a small quantity of borate buffer and dilute to a 0.25% suspension with borate buffer, e. g. 90 mg in 36 ml. Keep in an ice bath until ready for use and use only for four hours.

Thrombin: Prepare a working solution of thrombin by diluting in borate buffer to a concentration of 20 N.I.H. units/ml.

Assay Procedure
1) Prepare a 2 fold dilution series (gelatin diluent) of the sample to be tested and an appropriate standard, labeled in Christensen units. An example of a suitable range would be 50, 25 and 12.5 Christensen units/ml.
2) Add to 75 × 10 mm glass Wasserman tubes (one tube for each streptokinase dilution) the following reagents in rapid succession: 0.1 ml streptokinase dilution, 0.4 ml fibrinogen solution, 0.5 ml plasminogen suspension, and

* This is the procedure employed by the Lederle Laboratories and the Division of Biologics Standards. Details were generaously furnished by Mr. Gordon R. Personeus, Lederle Laboratories, Pearl River, New York.

0.1 ml thrombin. Shake each tube after the addition of plasminogen, and after the addition of the thrombin.

3) Place the tubes immediately in a 37° C water bath and observe when clotting occurs (usually within 30 sec) at which time the timer is set.

4) After a 5 min incubation period, examine the first tube of each series every 30 sec for 10 min by lifting the tube vertically out of the water bath. Examine one tube at a time until the clot is lysed, then examine the next tube in the same manner. Lysis of the clot is complete when all bubbles have disappeared.

5) Record the lysis time for each streptokinase dilution. Readings of three tubes are used in calculating the end-point. To be a satisfactory assay, lysis in the first tube must occur between 6.0–7.5 min, in the second tube, 9.0–10.5 min and in the third, 12.0–15.0 min.

Calculations

Plot the results of the test (three readings) for each sample on log-log graph paper; lysis time along the ordinate against dilution on the abscissa, and draw the best straight line. Read as the end point dilution from the abscissa the point of intersection of the drawn line with the 10 minute line. By a direct comparison of the end-point of the sample with that of the standard (in Christensen units) and multiplying by appropriate dilution factors, the concentration of streptokinase in the test solution can be determined. For example, streptokinase in units per ml of unknown equals:

$$\frac{\text{Dilution factor of unknown at 10 min line}}{\text{Dilution factor of standard at 10 min line}} \times \text{Streptokinase units/ml std} \qquad (2)$$

Comments

Human fibrinogen is not used since it usually contains plasminogen which may be activated by streptokinase. Also significant levels of anti-streptokinase may be present.

When selecting a plasminogen preparation, it is important to consider the large variability in specific activity from batch to batch as well as variations in the anti-streptokinase content.

When this assay is carried out by an experienced operator, an estimated error of ± 10% to 15% at the 95% probability level can be anticipated. Through replicate assays the estimated error may be reduced.

References

Alkjaersig, N., Fletcher, A. P., and Sherry, S. (1958). *J. Biol. Chem.* *233,* 86.

Blatt, W. F., Gray, J. L., and Jensen, H. (1964). *Thromb. Diath. Haemorrhag.* *11,* 85.

Christensen, L. R. (1949). *J. Clin. Invest.* *28,* 163.

Greig, H. B. W., and Cornelius, E. M. (1963). *Biochim. Biophys. Acta* *67,* 658.

Hagen, J. J., Ablondi, F. B., and Hutchings, B. L. (1956). *Proc. Soc. Exptl. Biol. Med.* *92,* 627.

Hestrin, S. (1949). *J. Biol. Chem.* *180,* 249.

Hummel, B. C. W., Schor, J. M., Buck, F. F., Boggiano, E., and DeRenzo, E. C. (1965). *Anal. Biochem.* *11,* 532.

Kline, D. L., and Fishman, J. B. (1961). *J. Biol. Chem.* *236,* 2807.

Kjeldgaard, N. O., and Ploug, J. (1957). *Biochim. Biophys. Acta* *24,* 283.

Lassen, M. (1958). *Biochem. J.* *69,* 360.

Ling, C., Summaria, L., and Robbins, K. C. (1965). *J. Biol. Chem.* *240,* 4213.

Loomis, E. C., George, C. Jr., and Ryder, A. (1947). *Arch. Biochem.* *12,* 1.

Lorand, L., and Mozen, M. M. (1964). *Nature* *201,* 392.

Müllertz, S. (1952). *Acta Physiol. Scand.* *26,* 174.

Nanninga, L. B., and Guest, M. M. (1964). *Arch. Biochem. Biophys.* *108,* 542.

Remmert, L. F., and Cohen, P. P. (1949). *J. Biol. Chem.* *181,* 431.

Roberts, P. S. (1958). *J. Biol. Chem.* *232,* 285.

Roberts, P. S. (1962). *Can. J. Biochem. Physiol.* *40,* 1203.

Ronwin, E. (1961). *Acta Haematol.* *26,* 21.

Siegelman, A. M., Carlson, A. S., and Robertson, T. (1962). *Arch. Biochem. Biophys.* *97,* 159.

Sherry, S., Alkjaersig, N., and Fletcher, A. P. (1964). *J. Lab. Clin. Med.* *64,* 145.

Troll, W., Sherry, S., and Wachman, J. (1954). *J. Biol. Chem.* *208,* 85.

Walton, P. L. (1967). *Biochim. Biophys. Acta* *132,* 104.

White, W. F., Barlow, G. H., and Mozen, M. M. (1966). *Biochemistry* *5,* 2160.

Zylber, J., Blatt, W. F., and Jensen, H. (1959). *Proc. Soc. Exptl. Biol. Med.* *102,* 755.

Assay for Plasminogen Activators with Labelled Fibrin Substrates

Nils U. Bang

I. Introduction

The process of in vivo clot dissolution commonly referred to as thrombolysis is complex and not completely elucidated. According to the prevalent theory formulated by Sherry and co-workers (1959), thrombolysis is mediated through the activation of plasminogen entrapped in in vivo fibrin deposits as well as in vitro fibrin clots. Activation of plasminogen contained in fibrin results from plasminogen activators adsorbing onto or diffusing into fibrin. Activation of in situ entrapped plasminogen and breakdown of the fibrin clot from within provides the only rational explanation for the rapid disintegration of fibrin clots under assault of plasminogen activators. In vitro experiments in Sherry's laboratory (Alkjaersig et al. 1959) demonstrated convincingly that the rate of lysis of a preformed fibrin clot increases in parallel with both the quantity of plasminogen entrapped in the clot and the concentration of plasminogen activator in the surrounding medium.

Plasma thrombolytic activity is of major physiological and pathological significance but most routinely employed techniques for the quantitation of this activity suffer from serious theoretical as well as technical shortcomings. Assays involving determination of whole blood or plasma clot lysis are valuable for detecting markedly enhanced thrombolysis but are inadequate for detecting low levels of thrombolytic activity because of the very long lysis times involved and because of lack of a concisely defined end point. Most techniques developed to increase the sensitivity of the thrombolytic assay involve procedures which aim at separating activators and active plasmin from activator inhibitors and plasmin inhibitors. Although assays of this nature such as dilute plasma clot lysis times (Fearnley et al. 1952) or euglobulin lysis times (Milstone, 1941) have in many instances provided results of potential significance for the understanding of the physiology and pathology of human fibrinolysis such results can always be subjected to the valid criticism that a complex balance between individual plasma components has been disrupted making their true biological relevance open to question.

Assay procedures involving the use of labelled fibrin were introduced by several authors in order to circumvent these theoretical limitations without sacrificing the sensitivity of the assay procedure. All assays for plasma thrombolytic activity involving labelled fibrin substrates test freshly drawn unaltered plasma. In principle the method involves the determination of "label" released from tagged human plasma clots immersed in unaltered plasma. These use of unaltered plasma and preformed clots mimics in vivo conditions and permits the collection of data of greater physiologic significance than data from test systems involving isolated plasma components.

II. Radioiodine-Labelled Fibrin

A. Labelling of Fibrinogen with ^{131}I and ^{125}I

The method for iodinating fibrinogen to be described is essentially that of Eisen and Keston (1949) as modified by Alkjaersig et al. (1959) and Fletcher (1964).

Principle: Alkaline solution of carrier-free radioactive iodide (^{131}I or ^{125}I) is mixed with a known quantity of KI, evaporated to a small volume and acidified. The iodide is subsequently oxidized to free iodine by the addition of $NaNO_2$, the excess nitrous acid destroyed by ammonium sulphamate and the pH of the solution brought to 8–9. The fibrinogen solution is immediately admixed with the iodine solution; under these conditions iodination of the protein takes place within a minute or two. Excess unbound radioiodine is removed by ion exchange on an Amberlite IRA-400 column.

Reagents: 20 mc of ^{131}I or ^{125}I, IRA-400 (Cl) Amberlite resin, Potassium iodide (0.02 M), Hydrochloric acid (2 N), Sodium hydroxide (2 N), Sodium nitrite (1 M), Ammonium sulphamate (1 M), Borate buffer (0.1 M, pH 8.0). Phosphate buffer with 0.9 percent NaCl, Bovine fibrinogen (92–98 percent tyrosine clottable by thrombin).

Sodium nitrite is unstable and must be made up fresh on each occasion. Bovine fibrinogen is freshly dissolved on each occasion in 0.1 M borate buffer. Four ml of 5 percent solution is prepared. A 1 × 30 cm chromatography column is used for the IRA-400 resin. A 20 cm column is formed in the usual manner and is equilibrated with the phosphate saline buffer.

Procedure: Using remote handling equipment, 20 mc of ^{131}I is transferred to a small beaker. Approximately 1 ml of water is added to the original container and the washings added to the beaker. One hundred microliters of 0.02 M KI is added. The pH of the mixture is tested (sample withdrawn with a small Pasteur pipette and tested on pH paper), which should be alkaline; if not, a small quantity of 1 N NaOH is added until this is achieved.

The beaker is heated gently on an electric hot-plate until the volume is reduced almost to dryness; the beaker is then removed from hot-plate and allowed to cool.

Sufficient 2 N HCl is added to bring the pH to below 2. This usually requires 150–200 microliters. The pH is tested on pH paper.

Exactly 50 microliters of 1 M sodium nitrite is added. The solution turns brown.

Fifty microliters of 1 M ammonium sulphamate is slowly added. Gas is evolved.

Sufficient 2 N NaOH to bring pH to between 7 and 8 is added. This usually requires 150–200 microliters.

Four ml fibrinogen solution is added from pipette with bulb and rapidly mixed by withdrawing the solution from beaker into the pipette and expelling it back several times.

The test pH should be approximately 8. Wait 15 minutes.

Note: Each step should be completed by mixing of the reacting substances for 30–60 seconds.

The fibrinogen-iodine mixture is then passed 4 times through the IRA-400 resin column at maximum feasible flow rate without application of positive pressure. As the effluent is collected in a beaker it is immediately withdrawn by a pipette and re-applied to the top of the column. Care must be exerted to keep the liquid level above the top of the resin bed at all times. About 8 ml of phosphate saline buffer is used as a wash.

Heparin, 0.2 ml is added (1 mg/ml) to the solution which is stored in a lead container at 4° C.

The fibrinogen solution is assayed for percentage radioactivity and percentage tyrosine clottable by thrombin according to Ratnoff and Menzie (1951).

This method should be attempted only by persons trained in the use of isotopes. Minimum equipment required is lead shielding, fume cupboard, isotope storage and disposal facilities, simple remote handling apparatus, survey meter and badge service. In addition, a well-type gamma scintillation detector and a suitable gamma spectrometer with a single-channel pulse height analyzer is required.

B. Preparation of in vivo ^{75}Se-Labelled Fibrinogen according to Gans et al. (1967)

In vitro labelled proteins as a rule exhibit faster turnover rates than in vivo labelled material and differences in physiologic clearance rates of in vitro and in vivo labelled proteins have also been demonstrated (Armstrong et al. 1955; Berson et al. 1953; and Gabrielli et al. 1954). On the other hand, the in vivo labelled material has significant shortcomings in that it requires large amounts of amino acids to produce high specific activity material since the injected labelled precursors may be lost in the urine or removed by organs which do not contribute to plasma protein synthesis. Under usual circumstances tagged proteins are diluted substantially by unlabelled proteins from intra and extravascular pools. The following procedure was designed specifically to enhance production of high specific activity labelled fibrinogen at the lowest possible expense in terms of injected labelled precursors.

Principle: A high intensity gamma emitter ^{75}Se as seleno methionine is used as the labelling precursor. ^{75}Se has the added advantage of a 120-day half-life.

Enhancement of fibrinogen synthesis and incorporation of the labelled amino acid at greater rate and concentration is accomplished by artificial defibrination.

Urinary loss of the radioactive amino acid is prevented by nephrectomizing the injected animals.

In order to provide a labelled amino acid pool during the entire period of new fibrinogen formation a constant infusion of seleno methionine is preferred.

An in vivo labelled gamma-emitting fibrinogen of relatively high specific activity and with a long half-life can thus be harvested by conventional purification procedures (see chapter VI).

Materials and Methods: Mongrel dogs and retired Holtzman breeder rats are used for all experiments. The rats are fed Purina rat chow and the dogs a Standard laboratory formulation.

Surgical Procedures: Bilateral nephrectomies are carried out under Nembutal anesthesia through small midline incisions.

Defibrination: Defibrination of the rats is obtained by a single injection of 2500 units of bovine thrombin into the peritoneal cavity. Defibrination in the dogs is accomplished through a two-hour constant I.V. infusion of 2500 units of bovine thrombin.

Labelling Material: L-^{75}seleno-methionine is used as the labelled amino acid in all procedures. Material of a specific activity of 1.0 to 1.9 mc/mg methionine is recommended. Prior to its use, radioactivity of this material is determined in a well counter. Amounts used in the rat range from 50–200 microcuries per animal, and in the dog 900 microcuries are used. Slow, continuous infusions are carried out with the use of a Harvard infusion pump.

Determination of Radioactivity: Radioactivity of 1 ml aliquots of each blood sample is determined in a well counter with a single-channel-analyzer unit. Each sample is counted to a total of 5000 counts and background is subtracted. This results in a counting error of $\pm$ 1.4 percent at one standard deviation.

Expected Results in Typical Experiments: According to Gans et al. (1967), the slow intravenous infusion of a hundred μc ^{75}Se methionine over a 17-hour period into four nephrectomized thrombin-defibrinated rats resulted in a fibrinogen prepared from the plasma of these animals exhibiting an average of 7,715 counts per minute per mg of fibrinogen. The range of counts was 7,000–8,120. Two animals similarly prepared received 200 μc. ^{75}Se methionine each. The specific activity of the fibrinogen prepared from the plasma of these animals was 13,220 and 20,762 counts per minute per mg fibrinogen. The authors also established that identical procedures in non-nephrectomized animals resulted in considerably lower specific activity of the fibrinogen prepared from their plasma; the average activity of the fibrinogen being 4,691 counts per minute per mg.

Results obtained with flash labelling were compared with those obtained with the continuous infusion of the labelled amino acids. When 100 μc of ^{75}Se methionine was administered as a single intraperitoneal injection to two nephrectomized defibrinated rats the activity of the fibrinogen prepared from the plasma of these animals was 5,929 and 6,103 counts per mg fibrinogen.

In all experiments where thrombin defibrination and nephrectomy had been carried out the ratio of fibrinogen specific activity over total plasma protein specific activity was high; the average value being around 2.0 indicating selective incorporation of labelled seleno methionine into fibrinogen under these experimental conditions.

Comments: The technique as outlined provides an important research tool for the study of the turnover rates of fibrinogen and fibrin in a variety of physiologic and pathologic states. The theoretical advantages of producing a less altered, more natural fibrinogen through this technique are obvious. However, the procedures as outlined are cumbersome and the specific activity of the fibrinogen, although improved considerably by nephrectomy and thrombin defibrination in the animal, are still far below the specific activities readily achieved with in vitro labelling procedures. The use of in vivo labelling technique can therefore not be recommended for the labelling of fibrinogen to be used in vitro test systems.

C. The Preparation of ^{131}I or ^{125}I labelled Clots

Principle: Trace radioiodine labelled plasma fibrin clots are immersed into plasma or other biological fluids or solutions to be assayed for plasminogen activator activity. After incubation at 37° C for specified time periods the remnants of the labelled clot are removed and the radio-activity of the test solution measured. The radio-activity released from the labelled clot is directly proportional to the concentration of plasminogen activator activity in the test fluid. A known plasminogen content of the labelled clots can be maintained by incorporating known quantities of plasminogen purified according to Kline (1953). This plasminogen, insoluble at neutral pH, will remain in the tagged clots during the washing procedures necessary for removal of non-clottable tagged protein from the clots prior to their use. The sensitivity of the substrate clots can be increased within limits by increasing the amount of plasminogen, by decreasing their volume and by decreasing plasma protein and antiplasmin content according to the method of Sawyer et al. (1960a, b; see section C, 2).

Conversely, plasminogen-poor clots can be prepared from regular plasma clots without plasminogen added following extensive washing which effectively removes the majority of soluble plasminogen content in the clot. Plasminogen-poor clots can be utilized for plasmin assays since they retain their sensitivity for plasmin while losing their sensitivity for plasminogen activator. Two procedures for preparing clots are outlined below; the first by Alkjaersig et al. (1959) is suitable for the preparation of the large number of clots sufficiently sensitive to pick up high levels of plasma thrombolytic activity encountered in patients during the administration of streptokinase or urokinase for therapeutic purposes.

Clots prepared by the second method (Sawyer et al. 1960a, b) exhibit considerably greater sensitivity to plasminogen activator, the sensitivity being sufficient to quantitate the low levels of thrombolytic activity normally present in resting man.

1. Method of Alkjaersig et al. (1959)

Materials: ^{131}I or ^{125}I labelled fibrinogen prepared as outlined in section A.

A pool of several units of out-dated blood bank plasma. Freshly-drawn plasma is not suitable for the preparation of substrate fibrin clots due to the presence of sufficient plasminogen activator activity in most fresh plasmas to cause significant spontaneous lysis of the substrate clots. The standard plasma is frozen in small aliquots and stored frozen until use.

Plasminogen purified according to Kline (1953).

Nichrome or other suitable metal wires coiled into spirals at the lower ends.

A well-type gamma scintillation counter and scaler with pulse height analyzer.

Procedures: ^{131}I or ^{125}I labelled fibrinogen, 1–4 μl in 1–2 percent solution and 1 caseinolytic unit of plasminogen contained in less than 0.1 ml volume are admixed into 0.5 ml volume are admixed into 0.5 ml of plasma in an 8 by 80 mm serologic tube. The quantity of added radioactivity is calculated to give approximately 100,000 counts per minute per plasma clot. A metal spiral wire is inserted into the tube and five units of thrombin contained in a 0.1 ml volume is added. Clotting is allowed to go to completion in 1–2 hours at 37° C and the formed clots withdrawn from the tubes by means of the wire. In order to reduce blank radioactivity, the clots are immersed into a large volume of normal saline and washed overnight at 4°C. If the clots are prepared in bulk and if the initial mixing of reagents (plasma iodinated fibrinogen and plasminogen) is performed in a single beaker prior to distribution into individual tubes, it is essential to stir the contents of the beaker well and continuously since otherwise the plasminogen suspension at the pH of the plasma will be unevenly distributed between the tubes.

2. Method of Sawyer et al. (1960a, b)

Materials: In addition to the materials and equipment described in section C, 1 the following additional equipment is needed.

A geared electrical motor.

Glass tubing (OD approximately 7 mm).

Five ml capicity Buchner-type funnels fitted with medium porosity central glass discs.

Procedure: Sufficient radioiodine labelled fibrinogen to give 100,000 counts per minute per clot is admixed with a 0.2 ml volume of pooled plasma and 0.4 caseinolytic units plasminogen contained in a volume of no greater than 0.05 ml. Clotting is induced with one unit of thrombin contained in 0.1 ml. The clots are formed in suitable lengths of glass tubing sealed at one end; as coagulation is taking place, the tube is placed in the chuck of the electric motor and rotated in the horizontal plane at approximately 350 rpm. The clots formed under these circumstances are small compact completely synerized and have largely expelled entrapped plasma. Such clots contain extremely low levels of antiplasmins, a critical feature for their enhanced sensitivity. When the clot is fully formed it is floated from the tube with phosphate buffered saline (0.1 M PO_4, pH 7.6, in 0.9 percent NaCl) and washed overnight in this buffer under continuous gentle agitation.

Single clots are drained of the wash fluid and immersed in 0.2 ml of the patient's plasma or other test fluid. Incubation is continued for two hours at 37° C; the clot remnants are separated from the surrounding fluid by filtration through the small Buchner funnel using an additional 2 ml of isotonic saline as a wash. The total filtrate is assayed for radioactivity. Blank values are obtained by incubating labelled substrate clots in 0.2 ml of saline and additional substrate clots in 0.2 ml of aged plasma.

The Buchner funnels prior to reuse have to be carefully cleaned using soaking in papaine and suitable resin containing detergents.

3. Calculations

The same calculations can be applied for the methods of Alkjaersig et al. (1959) and Sawyer et al. (1960a, b). After correction of background counts the results can be calculated as follows:

$$\frac{\text{Specimen count}}{\text{Completely lysed count}/\mu\text{g fibrin in clot}} = \mu\text{g fibrin lysed by plasma specimen}$$

Figures for completely lysed clot count are obtained by averaging the counts for three standard substrate clots completely hydrolyzed in 1 cc of 2.5 normal NaOH at boiling water temperature for 10 minutes. When measuring high activities according to Alkjaersig et al. (1959) it is usually sufficient to express the results as percentage clot lysis:

$$\frac{\text{Specimen count}}{\text{Completely lysed clot}} = 100$$

4. Normal Levels

The normal levels by the tagged clot assay according to Sawyer et al. (1960a) has been established to lie between 2.7–8.9 μg of fibrin lysed per two hours for a group of normal young unstressed human subjects. However, significant corrections have to be applied due to the spontaneous lysis of clots incubated in saline or aged plasma (averaging respectively, 2.0 and 3.6 μg fibrin lysed per 2 hours); applying these correction factors the average value for plasma thrombolytic activity was given as 1.4–3.0 μg fibrin lysed per 2 hours. This method is quite adequate for the detection of pathologic fibrinolytic states where values of 2–20 fold increases over normal levels may be encountered (Sawyer et al. 1960a). However, the low levels of normal activity do not permit an adequate analysis of subtle variations under normal physiologic conditions nor will this technique reliably quantitate lower than normal levels of thrombolytic activity in disease states where this has been suggested as a possible etiologic factor.

The values for thrombolytic activity during intensive streptokinase therapy as measured by the technique of Alkjaersig et al. (1959)

has been reported to lie between 100–1,000 μg of fibrin lysed per 30 minutes (i. e., values several hundred fold the resting level) (Fletcher et al. 1959).

III. Fluorochrome Labelled Fibrin

A variety of techniques for labelling fibrinogen and fibrin with fluorescent substances have been reported in the literature and the use of fluorochrome labelled fibrin has been suggested as a substitute for radioiodine labelled fibrin for laboratories where the special equipment needed to perform radioisotope counting is unavailable. The principle features and advantages of fluorescent labelled fibrin techniques are identical to those mentioned for iodinated fibrin. The only equipment needed to establish a fluorochrome fibrin thrombolytic assay is a suitable fluorometer. When appropriate steps are taken to reduce the background fluorescence produced by normal plasma the sensitivity of fluorescein fibrin techniques is as good as the sensitivity of radioiodine fibrin assays.

A. Preparation of Fibrinogen Labelled with Lissamine Rhodamine B 200

The following technique is based on the method described by Chadwick et al. (1958) as modified by Lüscher and Käser-Glansmann (1961).

Preparation of Thionylchloride from Lissamine Rhodamine B 200: One gram of the dried dye is intimately mixed with 2.0 g of dry PCl_5 by grinding for five minutes in a mortar. Ten ml of dried acetone are added. The mixture is stirred occasionally and after five minutes it is filtered. The dark purple-colored solution contains the thionylchloride of the dyestuff. All operations are carried out under a hood at room temperature. The product is immediately used for conjugation with the protein.

Conjugation of Dye with Fibrinogen: Purified human fibrinogen with a clottability of 90 percent or above is prepared according to the method of Blombäck and Blombäck (1956; see Chapter VI, p. 222). To a solution containing about 1.5 percent of protein is added the same volume of carbonate buffer (0.5 M, pH 9.0) and the solution is gently stirred in an ice bath. The solution of the thionylchloride is added dropwise at a ratio of 0.1 ml/ml of protein solution. The addition of the reagent should be completed within 15 minutes. Stirring is then continued for another 15 minutes; the pH is controlled and if necessary brought to about 8.0. Activated charcoal is then added to 0.5 g per ml of the solution and the mixture is gently agitated at room temperature for another 60 minutes. The adsorbent is then removed by centrifugation. The purple-colored protein solution, which contains no free dyestuff, is dialyzed overnight at 10° C against buffered saline in order to restore physiological pH and ionic strength. The concentration of the final product is brought to 5 mg protein/ml either by dilution or by dialysis against polyethyleneglycol (Kohn, 1959). The yield of fluorescent fibrinogen varies from 60–70 percent.

Determination of Fibrinolytic Activities: A 0.4 ml aliquot of the solution containing fibrinolytic activity (i. e., plasmin, plasminogen, serum) is pipetted into each of four clean test tubes. These solutions are made up in 0.05 M phosphate buffer of pH 7.4. A 0.1 ml aliquot of plasminogen activator (or 0.9 percent saline, if activation is unnecessary) are added, followed by 0.4 ml of fluororescent fibrinogen as a 0.5 percent solution. This mixture is brought to 37° C and immediately clotted by addition of 0.1 ml of a thrombin solution in saline containing 64 μ/ml. As a control, the same incubation mixture, containing 0.4 ml of phosphate buffer instead of the test solution is prepared. The fluorescent clots are incubated at 37° C. After suitable time intervals, which will depend on the fibrinolytic activity present (for instance 5, 10, 15 and 25 minutes for diluted, activated serum), the contents of the test tubes are brought to 5 ml by addition of cold, 0.9 percent saline. The remaining clots are squeezed out, the diluted incubation mixture is filtered through a small cotton pad and its fluorescence is immediately measured in a suitable fluorometer. The sample is irradiated with a mercury arc, using the bands from 405 to 436 mμ, and a secondary filter is used for the elimination of radiation below 560 mμ.

Comments: According to Lüscher and Käser-Glansman (1961) this technique gives a constant value of fluorescence even without incubation; this can be accounted for by small amounts of soluble fluorescent material contaminating all fibrin preparations. The removal of trace contaminants of soluble fluorescence resulted in a greatly lowered yield of labelled fibrinogen. However, impurities were found to be constant for a given preparation and it was therefore not considered necessary to remove them quantitatively. According to the authors this technique is sensitive and specific and proved well suited for kinetic studies in purified systems although no data is given for the performance of this test system in quantitating thrombolytic activity in human plasma.

B. Preparation of Fluorescein Isocyothiocyanate-Labelled Fibrin

Several authors have reported on methods for labelling fibrinogen with fluorescein isocyothiocyanate. The method to be described was first reported by Rinderknecht (1960) and modified by Pappenhagen et al. (1962). Suitable modifications were introduced by Strässle (1962) and further elaborated by Genton et al. (1964) to adapt this technique for the quantitation of plasma thrombolytic activity. Specific data and conditions enumerated in the following are those reported by Genton et al. (1964).

Materials: Bovine fibrinogen 95 percent clottable by thrombin prepared by the method of Blombäck and Blombäck (1956) (see Chapter VI, p. 222) is used for labelling. Bovine thrombin (Parke-Davis & Co.) diluted with 50 percent glycerol to a concentration of 100 NIH units per ml is stored in small aliquots at –20° C; prior to use it is diluted to 5 NIH units per ml with 0.3 M sodium chloride in 0.1 M sodium phosphate pH 7.6, designated "saline phosphate buffer".

"Human plasma" refers to a single large pool, stored in small aliquots at –20° C until used. Human plasminogen (containing 90 to 100 caseinolytic units per ml) is prepared by the method of Kline (1953) from human Cohn fraction III. Fluorescein isocyothiocyanate (FITC) is used in the celite-absorbed form (10 percent on celite).

Procedure: Four hundred mg of fibrinogen (50 percent sodium chloride by weight) is dissolved at 25° C in 4 ml distilled water. One hundred mg celite-adsorbed FITC suspended in 0.5 M bicarbonate buffer (pH 9.0) is added with stirring, the pH being maintained at 9.0 with 0.1 N sodium hydroxide. After a 30 minute equilibration period followed by centrifugation, the supernatant is filtered through a 3.5 cm diameter Sephadex G 50 column (12 gm dry Sephadex equilibrated with saline phosphate buffer, column height 14 cm). Freedom of the eluate from unbound dye is established by filtering an aliquot through an identical Sephadex column and determining that the dye/protein ratio remains unaltered.

The molar ratio of dye/protein in the conjugate is calculated after determination of solution absorbancy at 4,500 Å in 1 cm cells (OD) and protein concentration in mg/ml (C_p) by the following formula:

$$\text{molar ratio } \frac{\text{fibrinogen}}{\text{FITC}} = 3.5 \times 1.9 \frac{\text{OD}}{C_p}$$

the factor 3.5 being a function of fibrinogen molecular weight (350,000) and the factor 1.9 being derived from the molecular weight and extinction coefficient of FITC.

FITC-Labelled Substrate Clots: Four-tenths ml of a mixture containing nine volumes of plasma, one volume FITC-labelled fibrinogen, and one volume plasminogen is clotted with 0.1 ml thrombin (0.5 NIH units) in a 10 × 75 mm tube on a coiled 26 gauge wire made by nichrome or other suitable metal. Fully formed clots are suspended by means of the wire from the edge of a 1 liter beaker and washed overnight in buffered saline at 4° C. Individual clots are distributed into 10 × 75 mm tubes, filled with buffered saline, and stored at –20° C. Clots are calculated to contain 1.2 mg fibrin (of which 17 percent is labelled with FITC) and 3–4 caseinolytic units plasminogen; however, the clot-washing procedure removes a fraction of the entrapped plasminogen, and direct analysis of substrate clots show 0.5 to 1.0 caseinolytic unit plasminogen per clot.

FITC labelled fibrin clots, used for the experiment are prepared from 0.2 ml FITC labelled fibrinogen (3 mg/ml) and 0.1 ml thrombin (0.5 units).

Assay for Plasma Thrombolytic Activity: Oxalated blood (10 ml blood taken into 0.2 ml 20 percent potassium oxalate) is refrigerated on drawing and processed within a few minutes. Following centrifugation in the cold, 0.2 ml plasma is incubated for 30 minutes at 37° C with a single previously thawed substrate clot in a 10 × 75 mm tube. Buffered saline (1.5 ml) is added and after agitation of the clot by means of the wire both are withdrawn, any fibrin fragments being removed with an applicator stick. With a cotton-tipped pipette, a 1 ml sample is diluted to 6 ml with buffered saline, corresponding to a dilution of 1:51 with respect to the original plasma concentration.

Clot blank values are obtained by substituting buffered saline for the plasma sample in the procedure and plasma blank values by appropriate dilution of the original plasma sample. One hundred percent fluorescence values for fully lysed clots are determined by substituting 0.2 ml urokinase solution (100 to 200 CTA units) for plasma in the procedure and processing the lysed clot after 30 to 45 minutes of incubation.

Fluorescence measurements can be made in a Beckman ratio fluorometer equipped with Wratten 47B primary (Eastman Kodak) and Corning Nos. 4303 plus 3486 secondary filters and the number 4 reference balance rod, or in an Aminco-Bowman spectrophotofluorometer employing the number 4 slit arrangement and 4,900 Å excitation–5,300 Å emission setting.

With the sensitivity of the Backman ratio fluorometer set at 100 percent with a fully lysed substrate clot, 24 nonicteric plasma samples yielded plasma blank values of 3 to 5 percent scale deflection. The same plasma samples in the Aminco-Bowman spectrophotofluorometer gave readings rangig from 0.5 to 1.5 percent of the fully lysed substrate clot.

Tetracycline did not increase plasma blank values with either instrument, but grossly icteric plasma gave high values (15 to 30 percent scale deflections at a bilirubin concentration of 10 to 12 mg percent) on the ratio fluorometer, but not with the spectrophotofluorometer. Plasma samples showing hemolysis yielded blank values in the normal range and plasma blank values were unaltered in patients receiving thrombolytic therapy with urokinase. Sensitivity to plasminogen activators for labelled clots stored for up to 4 months remained unaltered.

Comments: The FITC labelled clot assay is simple requiring only an inexpensive filter fluorometer; it is rapid because results can be made available within 60–90 minutes after receipt of the sample and it is convenient because substrate clots may be prepared in large batches and stored without deterioration at –20° C for several months.

Genton et al. (1964) systematically investigated the correlation between ^{131}I labelled clot assays and FITC clot assays. At levels of substantially increased plasma thrombolytic activity as encountered in thrombolytic therapy a correlation between the FITC and ^{131}I labelled clot assays is excellent. With the simple Beckman filter ratio fluorometer plasma activity equivalent to 80–800 μg fibrin lysed per 30 minutes will yield fluorometer scale deflections of 10–70 percent for a plasma blank value of 3 percent since each 1 percent deflection on the instrument scale is equivalent to 12 μg fibrin lysed.

Sensitivity of the method may be enhanced by increasing the degree of FITC labelling and by prolonging incubation (up to 2 hours).

FITC conjugates are well suited to plasma assay as the excitation-emission wavelength (4,900 to 5,300 Å) will be unaffected by intrinsic protein-amino acid fluorescence (2,850 to 3,400 Å); these properties of the labelled fibrinogen suggest that the method might be readily adapted, by use of a spectrophotofluorometer rather than a filter fluorometer, to the assay of low-level plasma thrombolytic activity.

Although the author's have not as yet even with these modifications achieved sensitivity sufficient to determine plasma thrombolytic activity in the physiologic range (1–5 μg fibrin lysed pere 2 hours incubation), they suggest that suitable improvements in their technique could result in a sensitivity of the assay sufficient for this purpose.

Unlike the ^{131}I labelled fibrin assay, in which total clot radioactivity may be easily determined, the establishment of 100 percent fluorescence reference values for the FITC assay presents some difficulty. Conjugation of fluorochrome dyes with protein causes fluorescence quenching, and, similarly, degradation of the labelled protein with rupture of fluorescence bonding sites produces an increase of apparent solution fluorescence. In a typical series of experiments reported by Genton et al. (1964) the unclotted fibrinogen control read 2,500 fluorescence units in the Aminco-Bowman instrument, 2,814 fluorescence units (12 percent increase) after treatment with urokinase, and 3,580 fluorescence units (44 percent increase) after ficin treatment. By varying experimental conditions, these ratios could be substantially altered. With the procedure described, complete lysis of a substrate clot in 30 minutes by 0.2 ml urokinase (200 units) gives consistent 100 percent fluorescence reference levels approximately 12 percent higher than those of the native conjugate. The validity of establishing 100 percent fluorescence reference values in this manner is strongly supported by the data and theoretical considerations given in the publication by Genton et al. (1964).

IV. Summary and Conclusions

The availability of labelled fibrin clot assays has substantially added progress in understanding of the exact changes in the biochemical state of the fibrinolytic enzyme system induced by the infusion of plasminogen activators such as streptokinase and urokinase in man. The adoption of these techniques in clinical work has also provided useful information in respect to the rate and degree of activation of the fibrinolytic enzyme system in pathologic fibrinolytic states. In isolated studies these techniques have served to establish reliable values for normal baseline levels of thrombolytic activity in man.

But it should be re-emphasized as discussed earlier in this chapter that these techniques have not been developed to levels of sensitivity permitting the accurate quantitation of physiologic variations of thrombolytic activity in normal undiluted plasma nor do they permit estimation of depressed levels of plasminogen activator activity in pathologic states.

The further development of labelled fibrin assays possessing sensitivity sufficient to permit exacting studies in these areas must be considered a prime objective in continued research of the physiology and pathology of fibrinolysis in man.

References

Alkjaersig, N., Fletcher, A. P., and Sherry, S. (1959). *J. Clin. Invest. 38*, 1986.

Armstrong, S., Bronsky, D., and Hershman, J. (1955). *J. Lab. Clin. Med. 46*, 857.

Berson, S. A., Yalow, R. A., Schreiber, S. S., and Post, J. (1953). *J. Clin. Invest. 32*, 746.

Blombäck, B., and Blombäck, M. (1956). *Arkiv Kemi 10*, 415.

Chadwick, C. S., McEntegart, M. G., and Nairn, R. C. (1958). *Immunol. 1*, 315.

Eisen, H. N., and Keston, A. S. (1949). *J. Immunol. 63*, 71.

Fearnley, G. R., Revill, R., and Tweed, J. M. (1952). *Clin. Sci. 11*, 309.

Fletcher, A. P., Alkjaersig, N., and Sherry, S. (1959). *J. Clin. Invest. 38*, 1096.

Fletcher, A. P. (1964). *In:* "Blood Coagulation, Hemorrhage and Thrombosis" (Tocantins, L. M., and Kazal, L. A., eds.). Grune and Stratton, New York.

Gabrielli, E. R., Goulian, D., Kinersley, T., and Collet, R. (1954). *J. Clin. Invest. 33*, 136.

Gans, H., Mcleod, J., and Lowman, J. T. (1967). *Blood 29*, 517.

Genton, E., Fletcher, A. P., Alkjaersig, N., and Sherry, S. (1964). *J. Lab. Clin. Med. 64*, 313.

Kline, K. L. (1953). *J. Biol. Chem. 204*, 949.

Kohn, J. (1959). *Nature 183*, 1055.

Lüscher, E. F., and Käser-Glansmann, R. (1961). *Vox Sang. 6*, 116.

Milstone, H. (1941). *J. Immunol. 42*, 109.

Pappenhagen, A. P., Köppel, J. L., and Olwin, J. H. (1962). *J. Lab. Clin. Med. 59*, 1039.

Ratnoff, O. D., and Menzie, C. (1951). *J. Lab. Clin. Med. 37*, 316.

Rinderknecht, H. (1960). *Experientia 16*, 426.

Sawyer, W. D., Alkjaersig, N., Fletcher, A. P., and Sherry, S. (1960a). *Thromb. Diath. Haemorrhag. 5*, 149.

Sawyer, W. D., Fletcher, A. P., Alkjaersig, N., and Sherry, S. (1960b). *J. Clin. Invest. 39*, 426.

Sherry, S., Fletcher, A. P., and Alkjaersig, N. (1959). *Physiol. Rev. 39*, 343.

Strässle, R. (1962). *Thromb. Diath. Haemorrhag. 8*, 112.

Streptokinase Tolerance Test

W. Fischbacher

I. Introduction

The therapeutical activation of the fibrinolytic enzyme system by streptokinase (SK) is dependent upon a dose which is high enough to exceed the SK neutralizing antibodies normally present in plasma. The concentration varies in different individuals. Johnson et al. (1957) described a dose prediction test in whole blood which was subsequently modified by Fletcher et al. (1958), Deutsch and Fischer (1960) and Fischbacher (1960).

II. Predicted Dose Test (Fletcher et al. 1958) (modification Deutsch and Fischer, 1960)

Principle: SK is added to oxalated or citrated plasma or blood, and the clot lysis time is recorded. The amount of SK necessary for activation is multiplied by the plasma or blood volume in order to obtain the initial dose of SK necessary for thrombolysis.

Materials and methods
Citrated blood (one part 3.8% trisodium citrate solution and 9 parts of blood).
Barbital buffer pH 7.3, ionic strength 0.153.
Streptokinase solution: The test should be performed with streptokinase which is identical to the therapeutical preparations used. It is prepared in dilutions of 100, 200, 300, 400, 500, 750 and 1000 units per ml in barbital buffer.
Thrombin: 20 U/ml
Test tubes: 16 mm in diameter
Water bath, 37° C.
Technique: Barbital buffer (0.1 ml) is pipetted into the first tube. Into 7 additional tubes, 0.1 ml of barbital buffer containing decreasing concentrations of SK is added. The SK amount per tube is 0, 10, 20, 30, 40, 50, 75 and 100 units. An aliquot of 0.1 ml thrombin is added to each tube followed by 0.8 ml of the patient's citrated blood. The tubes are kept in the water bath at 37° C and the time of lysis recorded.

Results: The lysis time closest to ten minutes allows estimation of the SK antibody. The ten minute value obtained with 0.8 ml blood is multiplied by 5000 (Blood volume for patients of average weight). The result is the amount of streptokinase needed to overcome SK inhibition and to start initial fibrinolytic activation.

III. Streptokinase Tolerance Test Using the Thrombelastograph (TEG) Fischbacher 1960

Principle: Instead of observing lysis in the test tube, the TEG is used to determine the end point of lysis.

Materials and methods
Oxalated blood (1.34% 1:10) is centrifuged at 1800 rpm for 10 min. The platelet rich plasma is kept in ice water.
Streptokinase is added to one cuvette by drops using a tuberculin syringe to which an 18 gauge needle is attached and bent at a right angle. The SK solution is diluted so that one drop contains approximately 40 units. Samples of 0.2 ml can be kept in the deep freezer.
$CaCl_2$, 1.29% solution.
Thrombelastograph (see Chapter III).

Technique: Oxalated plasma (0.22 ml) is placed into one cuvette. One drop of SK containing 40 U is added and the sample is recalcified with 3 drops of $CaCl_2$ (approximately 0.05 ml). The sample is mixed by lowering the plunger three times into the cuvette. It is then covered with paraffin oil.

The second and third cuvettes are filled with 0.22 ml plasma to which one drop of streptokinase is added containing 20 and 10 units SK respectively. The lysis time (time from beginning of minimal amplitude of 1 mm until the amplitude has just disappeared) is then recorded on the scale or measured on the developed film.

If the amplitude increases in cuvette 1 (longer than 5 minutes), the SK tolerance will be over 40 U per cuvette and cuvettes 2 and 3 can be emptied and refilled with plasma to which 2 drops (80 units) and 3 drops (120 units) of SK respectively are added. If however, the cuvette content lyses immediately, the next SK concentration is diluted to 5 units and 2.5 units, respectively. The lysis times in the TEG are plotted against streptokinase concentrations on double logarithmic paper (Fig. 1) which results in a streptokinase dilution curve. The 10 minute sample indicates the SK tolerance per cuvette. Multiplication by a factor of 5 gives the SK tolerance per 1 ml plasma. Very high concentrations of

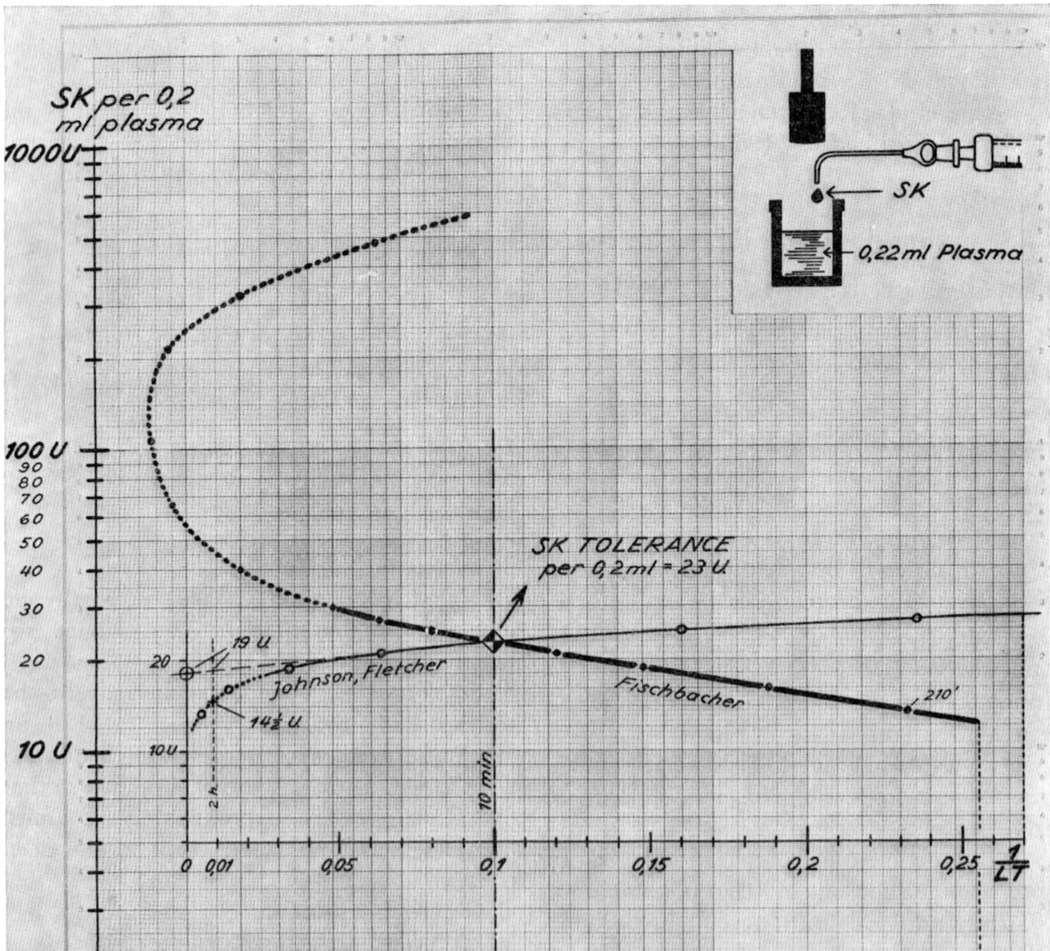

Fig. 1. Sample of plasma-SK-dilution curve: SK dose on the ordinate; lysis time (reciprocal lysis time respectively) on the abscissa.

streptokinase cause an inhibition of lysis which is indicated in the dilution curve by the deviating from the straight line.

IV. Comment

Basically the prediction test is satisfactory for the evaluation of the SK tolerance. The original test of Johnson et al. (1957) is satisfactory if a dry bath (metal block) is available. Test tubes containing the SK dilutions are prepared in advance to contain 60, 40, 25, 15, 10, 5 and 0 units of SK. At the bedside, 0.2 ml blood is added to each tube and after 10 min the lowest dose which achieves lysis (= SK tolerance per 0.2 ml blood) is used for calculation.

The reciprocal curve (Johnson et al. 1957; Fletcher et al. 1958) has its limitations since the plot is not a straight line throughout. Deviation from the straight line is to a certain degree unpredictable (see Fig. 1). The calculation of the initial dose differs among authors.

The following example is based on a patient whose blood volume is 6,000 ml of blood or 3,600 ml of plasma, respectively (Fig. 1).

Johnson et al. 1957 (2 hour lysis dose: for clot lysis in 2 hours 14.5 units of SK per 0.2 ml plasma are required. This corresponds with 72.5 units of SK per ml of plasma or 43.5 units SK per ml of blood. The doses calculated are therefore 43.5 × 6,000 = 260,000 units SK.

Fletcher et al. 1958 (20 minute lysis dose): According to the standard curve a dose of 20 units of SK per 0.2 ml plasma is required. Fletcher bases his calculation on 0.18 ml and not on 0.2 ml of plasma. The dose of SK would therefore be 18 units SK or 90 units per ml respectively. The calculated dose in his scheme would therefore be 18 × 5 × 3,600 = 324,000 units SK.

Deutsch and Fischer (1960) (10 minute lysis dose): SK tolerance corresponds to 23 units per 0.2 ml or 115 units per ml plasma and 69 units per ml blood. Deutsch and Fischer (1960) base their calculation on 50 units SK (corresponding to 0.72 ml blood). The dose is therefore 50 × 6,000 = 300,000 units SK.

Fischbacher (1960, 1961) (10 minute lysis dose): SK tolerance results in 23 units per 0.2 ml or 115 units per ml plasma. The dose calculated is therefore 115 × 3,600 = 415,000 units SK.

References

Deutsch, E., and Fischer, M. (1960). *Thromb. Diath. Haemorrhag. 4,* 482.

Fischbacher, W. (1969). "Beitrag zur Fibrinolyse", Dissertation Zürich.

Fischbacher, W. (1961). *Thromb. Diath. Haemorrhag. 6,* 547.

Fletcher, A. P., Alkjaersig, N., and Sherry, S. (1958). *J. Clin. Invest. 37,* 1306.

Fletcher, A. P., Alkjaersig, N., and Sherry, S. (1959). *J. Clin. Invest. 38,* 1096.

Johnson, A. J., Fletcher, A. P., McCarty, W. R., and Tillett, W. S. (1957). *Ann. N. Y. Acad. Sci. 68,* 201.

Determination of Inhibitors of Fibrinolysis

Clara M. Ambrus

I. Introduction

A. Physiological Role

The high level of antiplasmins in the circulation and their presence in most tissues (Albrechtsen, 1959) suggests that fibrinolytic inhibitors play an essential role in maintaining a balance among members of the fibrinolysin system; activators, plasminogen and plasmin. Norman (1958) and Norman and Hill (1958) described the existence of two types of inhibitors in the circulation, reversible and irreversible. Ambrus and Markus (1960) have shown that dissociation of plasmin from antiplasmin increased in the presence of a fibrin substrate. Plasmin then adsorbs selectively to fibrin and lyses it (Back et al. 1961). Thus, the physiological role of antiplasmins may be, on one hand, the prevention of excess fibrinolysis and thus bleeding; and on the other hand, the assurance of local fibrinolysis in the event of clot formation.

Inhibitors of the fibrinolysin system may theoretically act at various points. They may be inhibitors of activators, plasminogen or plasmin, or may interfere with the process of activation. Relatively little attention has been paid to inhibition achieved by interaction with the fibrin substrate resulting in increased resistance of the clot to fibrinolysis. Some of the synthetic plasmin inhibitors have been shown by Ambrus and associates (1968) to act in part by protecting fibrin from plasmin.

B. Naturally Occurring Inhibitors

1. Tissue Inhibitors

In addition to circulating antiplasmin, inhibitors of the fibrinolysin system have been demonstrated in several human and animal tissues (Macfarlane and Biggs, 1948; Lewis and Ferguson, 1950). In most tissues they occur concomitantly with fibrinolytic activators. Separation of the inhibitors from the activators has been achieved by different methods. Macfarlane and Biggs (1948) subjected saline extracts from tissues to isoelectric precipitation and separated out the inhibitors in the albumin fraction and the activators in the globulin fraction. Tagnon and Petermann (1949a and b) and Tagnon and Palade (1950) separated inhibitors from activators in the rat lung by differential centrifugation. An effective method of separation of activator and inhibitor was worked out by Astrup and Stage (1952) employing extraction with thiocyanate. Using this method in bovine tissues, an additional fibrinolytic inhibitor named pulmin was discovered in the lung (Albrechtsen, 1957) and uterus (Astrup and Albrechtsen, 1957), but not in other tissues or species. Pulmin differs from other tissue inhibitors in its solubility characteristics and in its spectrum of inhibition.

In the normal liver, activator activity was shown either to be absent or at very low levels (Albrechtsen, 1959). Inhibitor, however, is very high. Mattii and associates (1964) have shown in isolated perfused organ preparations that the liver is the main site of plasma antiplasmin production. Decrease of protein synthesis and thus antiplasmin production in the cirrhotic liver may unmask activator activity in this organ (Astrup et al. 1960). The platelets also contain antiplasmins (Johnson and Schneider, 1953, Alkjaersig, 1961, and Den Ottolander, 1968).

The methods employed in the studies quoted do not permit differentiation between activator inhibitors and plasmin inhibitors. Whichever is present in the tissues, the result will be local inhibition of fibrinolysis. The role of fibrinolytic activity in tissues as an essential component in the sequence of reparative processes after tissue injury was discussed at length by Astrup (1966). The tissue inhibitors of fibrinolysis may act as regulators of such processes.

2. Circulating Inhibitors

(a) Antiplasmins: It is well established that the inhibitory activity of plasma results from several distinct proteins. Early literature in this field did not always distinguish between antiproteolytic and specific antiplasmin activity. Several investigators have worked out methods of fractionation to separate these activities (Grob, 1949, Shulman, 1952, and Jacobsson, 1955). Ratnoff et al. (1954) described the presence of three or more different inhibitors of the fibrinolysin system in human serum. Norman (1958) and Norman and Hill (1958) described two distinct antiplasmins in human plasma. One is an alpha-2-globulin, which acts rapidly and forms an easily dissociable complex with plasmin. The other, an alpha-1-globulin, is slowly acting, and does not form a dissociable complex. The first inhibitor (alpha-2) is relatively heat stable and combines with plasmin independently of temperature. The second inhibitor (alpha-1) is heat labile and combines with plasmin at a rate dependent on temperature and the concentrations of both plasmin and inhibitor. It was estimated that there is sufficient alpha-1 globulin inhibitor in the plasma of an average individual to neutralize 30 times the amount of plasmin which may be generated by ac-

tivating all of the plasminogen in the circulation. Several methods have been described to isolate and characterize these inhibitors (Rybak and Rejnek, 1959; Mann et al. 1966; Rimon et al. 1966; Shamash and Rimon, 1964, 1965, 1966).

(b) Antiactivators: The existence of antiactivators in the circulation has been suggested (Lewis and Ferguson, 1950; Jacobsson, 1955). Antistreptokinase antibodies occur in the circulation as a result of streptococcal infection. Consequently their level shows high individual variation. In the therapeutic use of streptokinase or streptokinase activated plasmin this antibody level has to be taken into consideration (Fletcher et al. 1958) (see also p. 322). In addition to antibodies, Jacobsson (1955) described a substance in normal plasma which inhibits clot lysis by streptokinase. This is clearly different from antibody on the basis of electrophoretic mobility. Johnson and McCarty (1959) found naturally occurring streptokinase inhibitors to be quantitatively at least as important as antibody.

C. Synthetic Inhibitors

The recognition of fibrinolytic hemorrhage as a clinical entity (for review see Back and Ambrus, 1966; Porter, 1967) has renewed interest in plasmin inhibitors and has led to the synthesis of several compounds with antifibrinolytic activity (Symposium in Keio J. Med. *8*, 4, 1959; Okamoto et al. 1964; Melander et al. 1965). For further discussion see p. 322.

II. Methods of Determination

A. General Principles

Antiplasmin assays are based on the measurement of residual fibrinolytic activity after incubation of the test material with plasmin. When this is a biological specimen, plasma, serum or tissue, the inhibitory effect is determined in the presence of the other components of the fibrinolysin system contained in the specimen. The results therefore reflect the balance of these components rather than the actual level of antiplasmins. Simultaneous determination of plasminogen, plasmin, activator and antiplasmin will permit a more meaningful evaluation of the results than assay of either of these factors alone.

Determinations of antiactivators are based on modified antiplasmin assays. The test material is incubated first with an activator (usually streptokinase or urokinase), then the mixture added to plasminogen and the developing plasmin activity measured. This is compared to a control, where activation of plasminogen is achieved in the absence of the test material. If inhibition occurs, in our opinion it is difficult to ascertain whether the inhibitor acted against the activator or against the plasmin end product.

As discussed previously (I, B2), several proteins have been isolated that inhibit plasmin activity. The "reversible" and "irreversible" inhibitors of Norman (1958) can also be differentiated by their speed of action. The reversible inhibitor combines with plasmin instantaneously; inhibition by the irreversible antiplasmin progresses with time. Accordingly, antiplasmin activity of the same sample measured at various time intervals allows for a simplified differentiation of these two types of inhibitors.

In recent years several methods of protein separation have been applied to the isolation and purification of antiplasmins. These methods, however, while ideal for research purposes do not lend themselves at present for routine laboratory determinations.

It follows from the previous discussion that any fibrinolytic assay can be used for the determination of plasmin inhibitors. There are a few considerations, however, which apply peculiarly to the antiplasmin assay:

(1) *Choice of plasmin:* Plasminogen present in the assay material may convert to plasmin; this will increase residual fibrinolytic activity and thus show a falsely low level of inhibitor. Plasminogen conversion can be minimized by choosing plasmin preparations which have no activator activity. It follows that streptokinase or urokinase activated plasmins are not ideal for the antiplasmin assay. Bovine plasmin or

human plasmin activated in the presence of glycerol (as stabilizer) have no activator activity. Unfortunately, glycerol interferes with the fibrinolytic assay. Spontaneous activation of human plasminogen into plasmin can be achieved, under optimal conditions, without glycerol (Markus et al. 1958). Complete conversion of plasminogen to plasmin will occur in a few days. In the first day such a "spontaneous plasmin" may have activator activity; this, however, disappears with time, while fibrinolytic activity remains.

(2) *Choice of substrate:* Norman (1958) demonstrated that the fast acting inhibitor dissociates from plasmin as the concentration of the casein substrate is increased. Ambrus and Markus (1960) have shown that the degree of dissociation of an enzyme-inhibitor complex depends both on the substrate and the type of plasmin used in the assay. Fibrin as a substrate has a greater affinity for plasmin than casein in the presence of antiplasmin; UK-plasmin dissociates more readily than SK-plasmin, and this, in turn, better than "spontaneous plasmin". These findings should be kept in mind when choosing an assay and evaluating results.

(3) *Choice of temperature:* In general biological material collected for determination of components of the fibrinolysin system should be kept cold. Refrigeration is satisfactory for a few hours; for longer storage, freezing is preferred. In our experience, freezing does not change antiplasmin activity of serum or plasma. The antiplasmin assay involves incubation of a plasmin-antiplasmin mixture for a certain period of time. Since plasmin is heat-labile the temperature of incubation is critical. Some investigators incubate at 28° C to minimize the decomposition of plasmin; others, who prefer to use 37° C, add a plasmin stabilizer to the incubation mixture (e.g. methylamine or lysine – see II, C1).

Among the many assays available to measure fibrinolytic activity the caseinolytic assay and the fibrinolytic assay performed in tubes have been most often used for antiplasmin determinations. Several of these will be described in detail.

B. Antiplasmin Assays Based on Fibrinolysis

1. Method Using Human Fibrin as Substrate (Ambrus et al. 1969)

Principle: This method is essentially a modification of the assay described by Loomis et al. (1947). Plasmin activity is measured by the lysis time of a purified human fibrin clot incorporating the assay material at 45° C. For the determination of antiplasmin activity, serum is mixed with spontaneous plasmin for one hour at 28° C, then the mixture is assayed for residual plasmin activity.

Materials: Fraction I and crude human thrombin isolated by the method of Miller and Copeland (1962) are purified from plasminogen according to the method of Hink and McDonald (1962).

a) Preparation of Fibrinogen Free of Plasminogen

Buffers: *Sodium citrate 0.017 M sodium chloride 0.2 M buffer pH 6.4*
Sodium citrate 8.09 g
Sodium chloride 5.845 g
Add 475 ml distilled water. Adjust to pH 6.4 with 5% citric acid.
Adjust final volume to 500 ml with distilled water and recheck pH.

Acetate buffer 0.05 M pH 3.7
Sodium acetate 0.45 g
Add 980 ml distilled water. Adjust to pH 3.7 with glacial acetic acid (17 M). Adjust final volume to 1,000 ml with distilled water and recheck pH.

Sodium citrate buffer 0.019 M containing 4% dextrose pH 7.2
Sodium citrate 8.82 g
Dextrose 20.0 g
Add 450 ml distilled water. Adjust to pH 7.2 with 5% citric acid. Adjust final volume to 500 ml with distilled water and recheck pH.

Imidazole diluent
Imidazole buffer 0.05 M, pH 7.2–4.0 ml
Sodium chloride 0.85% – 96.0 ml

Fibrinogen: Twenty-five grams of human fibrinogen are dissolved in 330 ml 0.017 M trisodium citrate – 0.2 M sodium chloride buffer pH 6.4 at room temperature. Cool to 5° C and continue the steps below in the cold room. Use a refrigerated centrifuge. Add 330 ml 2% ethyl alcohol, let stand 15 minutes, and centrifuge for 20 minutes at 2,000 rpm. Discard precipitate and adjust supernatant to pH 3.8 with 2 M HCl. After standing for 15 minutes, centrifuge for 20 minutes at 2,000 rpm. Discard supernatant and dissolve precipitate in 985 ml 0.05 M acetate buffer pH 3.7 at room temperature. Cool to 5° C, add 79 ml 2.9 M NaCl, let stand 15 minutes and centrifuge again for 20 minutes at 2,000 rpm at 5° C. Repeat NaCl precipitation and dissolving in acetate buffer steps several times. The number of times required depends on quality of the starting fraction. Usually 6–7 precipitations are required to obtain a satisfactory purity. Do the last precipitation with 44.5 ml 2.9 M NaCl, let stand 15 minutes, centrifuge for 20 minutes at 2,000 rpm at 5° C to obtain precipitate 1. Remove supernatant and add to it 23 ml 2.9 M NaCl. Let stand 15 minutes and centrifuge 20 minutes at 2,000 rpm at 5° C to obtain precipitate 2. Discard supernatant. Dissolve precipitates 1 and 2 by suspending each in 200 ml 0.019 M sodium citrate buffer containing 4% dextrose pH 7.2 until a relatively homogenous suspension is formed. Adjust to pH 6.5 with 1 N NaOH. Remove to room temperature, and stir until suspension acquires room temperature. Adjust to pH 7.2 with 1 N NaOH. Keep stirring at constant room temperature maintaining pH 7.2 by adding additional 1 N NaOH until all particles appear to be in solution. Filter through glass wool and dialyze against 20 liters of imidazole diluent at room temperature for 24 hours changing the dialysis fluid at least three times. Freeze the final fibrinogen solutions in convenient aliquots.

Precipitate 1 usually yields a more dilute and less pure fibrinogen solution than precipitate 2. For the fibrinolytic assay the solution obtained from precipitate 2 is used. This has usually a protein concentration of 1.2–1.5% of which at least 90% is clottable protein.

Preparation of Plasminogen Free Thrombin:
Buffers: *Phosphate buffer 0.15 M pH 7.3*
$Na_2HPO_4 \cdot 7H_2O$ 32.16 g q. s. to 800 ml with distilled water.
$NaH_2PO_4 \cdot H_2O$ 6.21 g q. s. to 300 ml with distilled water.
Add 232 ml of 2) to 768 ml of 1) and check pH, which should be 7.3.

Thrombin: Use siliconized glassware at all times. Ten grams of crude human thrombin are suspended in 1,000 ml of cold phosphate buffer at 4° C. Stir for 30 minutes at 4° C. Add 20 g of calcium phosphate and stir for 30 minutes at 4° C. Add 200 g of $(NH_4)_2SO_4$ and stir for 30 minutes at 4° C. Let stand for 30 minutes at 4° C. Centrifuge for one hour at 7,000 rpm in Serval Centrifuge at 4° C in plastic bottles. Remove from bottles and filter supernatant through Whatman No. 2 Filter Paper at 4° C using a plastic or siliconized glass funnel. Dialyze overnight against 16 liters of distilled water at 4° C. Remove from dialysis bags. Freeze in convenient aliquots in siliconized tubes.

Plasminogen is purified according to the method of Kline (1953). Five hundred grams of human Fraction III (Plasminogen) are stirred for one hour in 10,000 ml of 0.05 N H_2SO_4 at room temperature. Filter through gauze at room temperature. Adjust pH which is approximately 2.2 to pH 11.0 with 1 N NaOH. After one minute at this pH, readjust to pH 5.3 with 1 N HCl. Let stand overnight at 4° C. Adjust pH to 2.0 with 1 N HCl. Centrifuge for 45 minutes at 9,000 rpm in Serval Centrifuge at 4° C. Put supernatant in one inch Cellulose Casing Bags (Visking Co.) and dialyze against running tap water overnight. Remove bags from tap water and dialyze against 16 liters of distilled water at 4° C overnight. Remove bags and pool together. Adjust to pH 5.3 with 1 N HCl. Let stand at 4° C until the precipitate has settled to the bottom, usually overnight. Siphon off and discard supernatant. Adjust the pH of the precipitate which contains some supernatant from 5.3 to pH 2.0, or if desired to pH 8.5; and freeze or lyophilize for storage.

Preparation of Spontaneous Plasmin Free of Activators:
Buffers: *Bicarbonate buffer 1.0 M pH 8.5*
$NaHCO_3$ 42.0 g q. s. to 500 ml with distilled water.

Na_2CO_3 10.6 g q. s. to 100 ml with distilled water.
To 500 ml of $NaHCO_3$ add 10.2 ml of Na_2CO_3 – pH 8.5.
Check with pH meter.

Phosphate buffer 1.0 M pH 7.2
$Na_2HPO_4 \cdot 7H_2O$ 26.814 g q. s. to 100 ml with distilled water (1).
$NaH_2PO_4 \cdot H_2O$ 13.805 g q. s. to 100 ml with distilled water (2).
To 72 ml of (1) add 28 ml of (2) – pH 7.2. Check with pH meter.

Procedure: Non-Activator Spontaneous Plasmin: Suspend 1 g of lyophilized purified human plasminogen powder (see above) in 7 ml of distilled water. Add 1.0 ml of 1.0 M bicarbonate buffer and 1.0 ml of 1.0 M phosphate buffer. Q. s. to 10.0 ml in a 10 ml volumetric flask. Let the resulting 10 % solution stand at room temperature for two days. After the two days at room temperature check the plasmin activity and the activator activity. If the preparation is high in plasmin activity and is devoid of activator activity it is suitable for use in the antiplasmin assay. Freeze in convenient aliquots and do a standard curve.

b. Tests Used to Check the Reagents
Assay for Plasminogen Contamination of Fibrinogen and Thrombin: :
Buffers: *Bicarbonate buffer 0.1 M pH 8.5*
$NaHCO_3$ 4.2 g q. s. to 500 ml with distilled water.
Na_2CO_3 1.06 g q. s. to 100 ml with distilled water.
To 500 ml of (1) add 10.2 ml of (2) – pH 8.5. Check with pH meter.

Imidazole buffer 0.05 M pH 7.2
Imidazole powder (Edcan Co.) 1.36 g q. s. to 100 ml with distilled water.
25 ml (1)
18.6 ml 0.1 N HCl
q. s. with distilled water to 100 ml. Check with pH meter.

Imidazole diluent as above
Procedure: Do a clottable protein biuret on the fibrinogen to determine the concentration and dilute with imidazole diluent to a final concentration of 0.6 %. Dilute the thrombin with imidazole buffer pH 7.2 so that it will give a 15 second clotting time at 45° C when mixed with 0.2 ml of imidazole buffer and 0.3 ml of 0.6 % fibrinogen.
Set up at 45° C and at 28° C the following mixtures:
0.1 ml imidazole buffer pH 7.2
0.1 ml streptokinase (1, 10, 100, 500, 1000, 2000 units/ml in 0.1 M bicarbonate buffer pH 8.5)
0.1 ml human thrombin (15 second clotting time)
0.3 ml human fibrinogen (0.6 %)

Control: Use 0.1 ml of 0.1 M bicarbonate buffer instead of the SK. Check daily for lysis. With ideal reagents, clots are stable for one day at 45° C and for three days at 28° C. The reagents are acceptable, however, if the clots placed at 28° C lyse after the first 24 hours.

c. Assay for Activator Activity of Spontaneous Plasmin: Set up the following tubes:
1) 0.1 ml spontaneous plasmin + 0.1 ml plasminogen
2) 0.1 ml spontaneous plasmin + 0.1 ml 0.1 M bicarbonate buffer
3) 0.1 ml plasminogen + 0.1 ml 0.1 M bicarbonate buffer
incubate each tube for 10 minutes at 28° C. Then add 0.1 ml thrombin diluted to give 15 second clotting time and 0.3 ml fibrinogen (0.6 %); place in 45° C water bath and check for lysis time. This is converted to units on the standard curve (see below). If activator activity is present, units in tube (1) will be greater than units obtained in tube (2) and (3) together. (Tube 3 will probably not lyse within several hours.) If the units are equal, the spontaneous plasmin preparation has no activator activity.

d. Measurement of Antiplasmin Activity
Equipment needed – Two water baths, for 28° C and 45° C respectively; 0.1 ml siliconized pipettes to be used only for delivering the thrombin; 0.2, 1.0, 5.0 and 10.0 ml serological pipettes; ice bath; siliconized test tubes for thrombin; 10 × 75 mm Kimax test tubes for the assay; interval timer; reset clock, with seconds division.
Reagents needed – Purified human fibrinogen diluted to 0.6 % with imidazole diluent and

kept at room temperature. Purified human thrombin diluted with imidazole buffer to give a 15 second clotting time when 0.1 ml is mixed with 0.3 ml fibrinogen (above) and 0.2 ml imidazole buffer. Thrombin is kept on ice.
Imidazole buffer 0.05 M pH 7.2.

Procedure – From the test solution kept on ice, 0.2 ml is pipetted into an assay tube. Put tube in 45° C water bath and immediately add 0.1 ml of thrombin with a siliconized pipette. Immediately after adding the thrombin, add 0.3 ml of fibrinogen, and at the same time start the reset clock, swirl two or three times. As the clot forms, bubbles are trapped in the fibrin mesh. When all of the bubbles suddenly rise to the top the clock is turned off and thus the lysis time is determined.

Note: When testing for plasmin in a sample which contains fibrinogen (e.g., plasma or euglobulin) reverse the order of the addition of thrombin and fibrinogen.

Preparation of Standard Curve:
Using the fibrinolytic assay, a standard curve is prepared with the spontaneous plasmin described before. At least 12 serial dilutions of plasmin (1:1, 1:2, 1:4, etc.) are set up using 0.1 M bicarbonate buffer pH 8.5 as diluent; and plasmin assay is performed on each as described. Plot on a log-log paper the per cent concentration of plasmin solution (undiluted or 1:1 = 100%) on the abscissa and the lysis time for each concentration on the ordinate axis. The line obtained should be shifted to have a 2-minute lysis time on the ordinate corresponding to one unit of plasmin on the abscissa. By definition, one Roswell Park Memorial Institute (RPMI) unit of plasma is that activity which will lyse the standard clot described above in two minutes at 45° C.

Antiplasmin Assay:
Spontaneous plasmin is diluted to have an activity of 5 RPMI units per ml. The test is set up as follows:

0.5 ml spontaneous plasma + 0.1 ml test solution – tube 1

0.5 ml spontaneous plasmin + 0.1 ml imidazole buffer – tube 2

Incubate each tube for 60 minutes at 28° C. Remove and put in ice bath. Do plasmin assay on 0.2 ml of each tube at 45° C.

Calculation (Units in 0.2 ml of tube 2 – units in 0.2 ml of tube 1) × 30 = units/ml of test solution.

Units: 1 RPMI unit of antiplasmin is that amount of antiplasmin that will inhibit 1 RPMI unit of plasmin in 60 minutes at 28° C.
Remarks – If antiplasmin activity is too high, no plasmin activity will be found in tube 1. The test material should then be diluted, the assay repeated, and calculations adjusted accordingly. In our experience, however, 3 U of spontaneous plasmin is usually adequate for the determination of average circulating antiplasmin levels. These have been found to be around 10 RPMI units per ml serum with considerable variation in both directions.
Incubation for 60 minutes measures total antiplasmin activity. Determination of fibrinolytic activity immediately after mixing serum with plasmin will permit an estimate of the immediate inhibitor.
Once the reagents are prepared the antiplasmin assay is simple and reproducible. The reagents are prepared in large quantities, sufficient for a year's supply, distributed in small aliquots and frozen. The same reagents are used for the determination of the other members of the fibrinolysin system (Ambrus et al. 1960, 1963).

2. Methods Using Bovine Fibrin as Substrate

a. Method of Guest (1964)
Principle: Antiplasmin activity is assayed by incubation of test material with bovine plasmin for 30 minutes at 28° C. Residual plasmin activity is measured by incorporating this mixture into a bovine fibrin clot and determining the time of clot lysis at 28° C, as compared to the lysis time of a clot containing plasmin alone. The method measures total inhibitory activity.

Materials
Fibrinogen – A relatively pure commercial bovine fibrinogen or crude bovine fibrinogen purified by the freezing-thawing technic (Ware et al. 1947) is stored in 0.5–2% con-

centration in imidazole diluent (Guest et al. 1948) at –20° C. Prior to use the fibrinogen solution is thawed at 40° C without agitation and diluted to 0.2% with saline. This solution is maintained at 40° C in a water bath during the assay procedures.

Thrombin – Topical thrombin (Parke, Davis and Company) is diluted with a solution of saline-glycerol (equal parts) to contain 1433 NIH units per ml.

Bovine Fibrinolysin is prepared according to the method of Loomis et al (1947) or obtained from Parke, Davis and Company. It is diluted with imidazole buffer pH 7.2 to contain 4 U per ml of plasmin activity when tested as described below. Such a solution is kept in an ice bath and used for not longer than three hours, after which time the activity starts to decrease.

Procedure

Standardization of fibrinolysin: The test tubes used in the assay are 50 mm × 8 mm I.D. They are placed in a 28° C water bath. Fibrinolysin 0.1 ml, and 0.1 ml of 0.9% NaCl are pipetted into the tube, then 0.2 ml of the 0.2% fibrinogen solution. A stop watch is started with the addition of the fibrinogen, and the mixture in the tube is stirred for 2–3 seconds with a 3–4 mm diameter glass rod previously immersed in the thrombin solution. In this manner clotting in the tube will occur in about 15 seconds. Lysis is checked by tipping of the tube at frequent intervals and marking the time when the content of the tube flows freely. The concentration of fibrinolysin is so adjusted to achieve lysis of the above clot in 120 ± 5 seconds, which corresponds to an activity of 0.4 units in the clot. One unit of fibrinolysin in this method is the activity which will lyse 1 ml of a 0.1 % fibrin clot in two minutes at 28° C, in an isotonic saline solution buffered with imidazole to pH 7.2. Since the above clot is 0.4 ml total volume instead of 1, the activity measured is only 0.4 units.

Measurement of Antiplasmin Activity

Citrated or oxalated plasma is diluted 1:5 or 1:10 with a solution made from 1 part of 0.9% NaCl and 2 parts of imidazole buffer pH 7.2. From this diluted plasma, 0.1 ml is added to 0.1 ml of fibrinolysin containing 0.4 U (see above). The tube is incubated for 30 minutes at 28° C. At the end of the incubation time, 0.2 ml of a 0.2% fibrinogen solution is added, a stop watch is started, and thrombin is added with the stirring rod. The tube is returned to the 28° C water bath and examined for lysis at frequent intervals. The end point is the complete dissolution of the clot.

Calculations

Five units of antifibrinolysin, within 30 minutes at 28° C and pH 7.2, will reduce the activity of one unit of fibrinolysin to 0.5 unit. To obtain a standard curve from which the units of antifibrinolysin can be estimated, it is necessary to plot a series of pooled plasma dilutions against the dissolving time of the standard clot. The 210-second lysis time should be determined accurately since this corresponds to an inactivation of one-half of the fibrinolysin added to the system. This point on the curve corresponds to 5 units of antifibrinolysin according to the definition of antifibrinolysin units, given above. Having found this point on the curve, the ordinate can then be divided into fractions and multiples of 5 units. When the lysis time of the standardized fibrin clot containing diluted plasma and fibrinolysin has been determined as described above, the number of units of antifibrinolysin are read on the ordinate of the graph. Since the plasma is diluted in preparation for the assay, an additional correction must be made. Thus, if 1 ml of anticoagulant were added to 7 ml of blood, 6 units of antifibrinolysin were read on the graph, the dilution of the plasma was made by adding 9 parts of saline to 1 part of blood, and the hematocrit was 40, the calculation would be:

$$A \times B \times C \times D = Ua \quad (1)$$

$$\frac{(1{:}00\text{–}0.40)8}{((1{:}00\text{–}1.40)8)\text{–}1} \times \frac{10}{1} \times 4 \times 6 = 273 \quad (2)$$

A = correction for dilution due to anticoagulant

B = dilution of plasma with saline

C = correction for 1 ml clot

This correction is arrived at as follows: Since 0.1 ml of diluted plasma is used to inactivate a certain fraction of the fibrinolysin in a 0.4 ml clot, 0.25 ml of plasma would be required to inactivate the same fraction of fibrinolysin in a 1.0 ml clot and 1 ml of plasma would contain four times as much antifibrinolytic activity as was obtained in the assay with a 0.4 ml clot.

D = units of antifibrinolysin which are read from the standard curve for the species being studied.

Ua = units of antifibrinolysin per ml plasma.

Normal Range of Values: Man: 55 to 100 units.

Remarks: 1) The assay is based on the inhibition of the enzyme, fibrinolysin. If inhibition of trypsin is used in the procedure, the results will be obtained in antitrypsin units and not antifibrinolysin units. 2) If a lysis time other than 120 ± 5 seconds is used for the standard fibrinolysin preparation (without added antifibrinolysin) in the assay, a new standard curve relating lysis times to antifibrinolysin units must be prepared. 3) It is convenient to prepare the fibrinolysin solution with a higher enzyme concentration than that which would be expected to give 120 seconds in the assay and make dilutions of this solution to bring its lysis time, when tested without added plasma, to 120 ± 5 seconds. 4) Bovine reagents are more readily available and cheaper than human reagents. In this method fibrin and fibrinolysin are bovine. When inhibitory activity of human plasma is measured, unknown factors of species specificity may enter. It was shown that dissociation of plasmin-antiplasmin complex increases in the presence of fibrin of the same species (Ambrus and Markus, 1960).

b. Method of Johnson et al. (1964)

Principle: Dilutions of inhibitor are preincubated at room temperature with glycerol-activated plasmin for a standard period of time. The mixture containing residual free plasmin is added to bovine fibrinogen, clotted and the lysis time noted. The reduction in plasmin activity is proportional to the amount of inhibitor. The total inhibitory content is measured.

Materials

Fibrinogen: Bovine fibrinogen or Fraction I is used (standard Lot No. 6211, Armour Pharmaceutical Company, Kankakee, Illinois, or Nutritional Biochemicals Corporation, Cleveland, Ohio); 12.5 mg are weighed and stored in test tubes in vacuum desiccators with anhydrous phosphorous pentoxide as the desiccant. Immediately before use, 0.5 to 1.0 ml of buffer, saline-phosphate buffer pH 7.5, is added to each tube, and a glass rod is pressed against the tube sides to wet the fibrinogen; more buffer is added to bring the volume to 2.5 ml. The solution is stored on ice until used.

Thrombin: Topical thrombin (Parke, Davis and Company, Detroit, Michigan) is dissolved in saline-phosphate buffer to contain 20 NIH units per ml. It should be kept on ice until needed.

Plasmin: Glycerol-activated human plasmin (prepared for the American National Red Cross by the Michigan State Department of Health) is stable for long periods of time under refrigeration. Immediately prior to each assay the plasmin is diluted to 10 units/ml with 25 per cent glycerol in saline-phosphate buffer, pH 7.5, and kept on ice.

Buffer: Saline (0.07 M)-Phosphate (0.06 M) Buffer pH 7.5

NaCl	4.092 g
Na_2HPO_4	7.156 g
KH_2PO_4	1.306 g
Merthiolate	10 mg

Dissolve in approximately 900 ml distilled water.

Adjust to pH 7.5 and bring to final volume of 1 liter.

Procedure: A dilution series of the assay material is prepared; of this, 0.5 ml is delivered into 12 × 75 mm test tubes. 0.15 ml plasmin (diluted with 25 per cent glycerol in saline-phosphate buffer to contain 1.5 units) and saline-phosphate buffer are added to a final volume of 0.7 ml. The tubes are pre-incubated at room temperature for 10 minutes, then placed in an ice bath. Two 1-unit and one $1^1/_2$-unit plasmin control, in which saline-phosphate buffer is substituted for the sample, are similarly incubated. Two-tenths ml bovine fibrinogen and 0.1 ml thrombin are added to each tube to form a standard clot. The tubes are agitated at once, placed in a 37.5° C water bath to clot, a stop watch is started, and the clots watched for lysis. Endpoint is the time when the air bubbles formed in the fibrin meshwork suddenly rise to the top.

Calculations

Lysis times are plotted against the reciprocals of the final dilutions of the sample on a log-log plot. The reciprocal of the dilution having a lysis time equal to that of a 1-unit control (as indicated by the intercept on the lysis time curve) is taken as the endpoint and represents the number of $^1/_2$ units/ml in the sample. Divided by 2, it gives the number of units/ml sample.

Remarks: The final concentration of glycerol in the tubes should not be more than about 5 %. High concentrations change the structure of the clot as evident from the transparency of the clot, and influence lysis times.

C. Antiplasmin Assays Based on Caseinolysis

1. Methods Using Casein as Substrate

a. Determination of Total Inhibitory Activity

Principle: Serum is incubated with spontaneous plasmin for 60 minutes at 28° C, then assayed for residual caseinolytic activity with the method of Remmert and Cohen (1949).

Materials

Casein (Nutritional Biochemical Corporation) was purified according to the method of Müllertz (1955). Three grams are dissolved in 100 ml distilled water by addition of 0.15 N NaOH to pH 8.0, heated at 100° C for 15 minutes and cooled. This solution is acidified by the dropwise addition of 2–3 ml N HCl with constant stirring. At the onset of precipitation 4 ml of N HCl are added quickly, bringing the pH to 2.0–2.2. In this way a massive isoelectric precipitation of slowly soluble casein is avoided. The clear solution (100 ml) is precipitated by the quick addition of 150 ml of 0.17 M perchloric acid and left suspended in the acid overnight at room temperature. It is then washed three times with distilled water, redissolved and diluted up to the original volume with 0.1 M phosphate buffer pH 7.4. The solution, designated as 3 % (W/v) casein, is stored in small aliquots at –20° C.

Spontaneous Plasmin – See B 1

Imidazole Buffer – See B 1

1.7 M perchloric acid

Procedure: Spontaneous plasmin is diluted to have an activity of 5 RPMI units per ml. The test is set up as follows:

Tube 1: 2 ml spontaneous plasmin + 0.4 ml test solutions

Tube 2: 2 ml spontaneous plasmin + 0.4 ml buffer

Incubate each tube for 60 minutes at 28° C. Remove and put in ice bath. For each mixture set up four tubes with 0.5 ml mixture + 0.5 ml 3 % casein, 2 of each to be precipitated with 2 ml 1.7 M perchloric acid immediately, and two of each to be precipitated after 30 minutes of incubation at 24° C.

The precipitated solutions are centrifuged at 9,000 rpm for 40 minutes, after which the supernates are pipetted off and their optical densities measured in a Beckman model DU spectrophotometer at 275 mμ. The difference in optical density between each pair of samples indicates the breakdown of casein during the 3-minute digestion period.

Calculations

The values obtained are multiplied four-fold and expressed as Δ O.D. per ml mixture in 60 minutes. Delta O.D. of 0.100 has been expressed as 1 caseinolytic unit of plasmin. The difference between Δ O.D. obtained with plasmin alone and plasmin-serum mixture corresponds to the plasmin inhibitory activity of the serum. Since, in 1 ml mixture, the amount of serum is only 0.82 ml the results have to be divided by 0.22 to obtain antiplasmin activity per ml of serum.

b. Determination of "immediate" and "slow" inhibitor

(Method of Norman, 1958, and Norman and Hill, 1958)

Principle: Residual caseinolytic activity immediately after mixing plasma with plasmin corresponds to the immediate inhibitor. For the slow inhibitor, plasma and plasmin are first incubated for 180 minutes at 25° C; only then is residual caseinolytic activity determined. Since during this incubation time plasmin may loose activity, a stabilizer is added to the plasma-plasmin mixture as well as to the control plasmin-buffer mixture. Norman uses methylamine as stabilizer; Shamash and Rimon (1964) use lysine.

Materials

Casein purified as described before (Cla) is prepared in a 4% solution in borate-saline buffer at pH 7.4. This solution is usable for one week if kept in the refrigerator at 4° C.

Buffers: Borate-Saline buffer

$Na_2B_4O_7 \cdot 10H_2O$	19.108 g	q.s. to 1000 ml with distilled water (1)
H_3BO_3	12.404 g	q.s. to 1000 ml
NaCl	2.925 g	with distilled water (2)

Mix (1) and (2) until pH 7.4 is obtained.

Dissolve 400 mg of human plasminogen (purified according to the method of Kline and Fishman, 1960) in 200 ml borate-saline buffer, pH 7.4, and add 3.0 mg streptokinase. After incubation for 30 minutes at 25° C, 200 ml 2 M NaCl is added and pH adjusted to 2.0 with N HCl. The resulting precipitate is separated by centrifugation, washed twice with 1 M NaCl at pH 2.0, and finally dried with alcohol and ether. The resulting white powder is stable at 5° C for at least a year. When a solution of plasmin in buffer is needed, first a concentrated stock solution is made in 0.0025 M HCl; this is then diluted with buffer at the beginning of the experiment to have approximately 40×10^{-3} caseinolytic units per ml.

Streptokinase: Varidase, a lyophilized mixture of streptococcal enzymes consisting of streptokinase, streptodornase, other proteins and phosphate buffer (Lederle Laboratories Division, American Cyanamid Company) contains about 4000 Christensen units of streptokinase per mg.

Methylamine: C.P. methylamine hydrochloride is dissolved in borate-saline buffer and the pH adjusted to 7.4.

Caseinolytic Assay

Procedures: Into 16 × 100 mm test tubes (set up duplicates) mix 0.5 ml plasmin, 0.5 ml borate-saline buffer and 1 ml casein. Incubate at 37° C for 30 minutes, then add 0.5 ml 15% trichloracetic acid. Tubes should stand overnight; then centrifuge for 60 minutes at 2700 rpm. The optical density of the supernatant solution is read in a Beckman DU spectrophotometer at 280 mμ.

Blanks are prepared in the following way. One ml casein, 0.5 ml borate-saline buffer and 0.5 ml 15% trichloracetic acid first, followed by 0.5 ml plasmin. From here on these blanks are handled the same way as the experimental tubes, and the optical density readings obtained are subtracted from the readings of the experimental tubes.

A *standard curve* should be prepared by determining the caseinolytic activity of a dilution series of plasmin as described above. Optical densities on the ordinate are plotted against dilutions of plasmin on the abscissa. One caseinolytic unit is the activity which increases 1 unit of optical density at 280 mμ per minute of digestion. Taking into account the 30-minute digestion time, and the concentrations of the dilution series it is possible to calculate the specific activity of the plasmin lyophilisate and express it in caseinolytic units per ml plasmin. The standard curve is then reconstructed having optical densities on the ordinate and caseinolytic units on the abscissa. For each new preparation of plasmin or casein a new standard curve should be prepared.

A *second standard curve* is prepared by repeating the above procedure in the presence of 0.1 M methylamine. In each tube of the plasmin dilution series, 0.4 ml 5 M methylamine is substituted for 0.4 ml borate-saline buffer resulting in a final concentration of

0.1 M methylamine. This standard curve will be used for calculations of the slow inhibitor.

Immediate-Inhibitor Assay
One-half ml plasma diluted 1:2 with borate-saline buffer pH 7.4 is mixed with 0.5 ml plasmin (approximately 16×10^{-3} units) and 1 ml 4 % casein in 16 × 100 ml tubes. Control tubes contain borate saline buffer instead of plasma. After 30 minute incubation at 37° C the assay is performed as described above. Optical densities are converted to units on the standard curve. The difference in optical densities between the tubes with and without plasma corresponds to the amount of inhibitor in the plasma. The total dilution of the plasma is eight-fold (2-fold originally, then 4-fold when mixed with plasmin and casein). Correcting for this dilution, inhibitory units can be expressed per ml plasma.

Slow Inhibitor Assay: Plasma diluted 1:5 or 1:10 with borate-saline buffer pH 7.4 is used. One-half ml of this plasma is mixed with 0.4 ml 5 M methylamine and 0.1 ml plasmin (containing approximately 80×10^{-3} units). Control tubes should contain additional 0.5 ml borate-saline buffer instead of plasma. After 180 minutes of incubation at 25° C, 0.2 ml is removed from the mixtures and added to 0.8 ml borate saline and added buffer and 1 ml 4 % casein. Duplicate sets are prepared. These sets are incubated at 37° C for 30 minutes and caseinolytic assays performed. Blanks, as before, are assembled by adding trichloracetic acid to the plasmin-methylamine-plasma mixture first and casein only second. Precipitation, centrifugation, and determinations of optical density of supernates are performed as in the regular caseinolytic assay. For the conversion of optical density to units the standard curve with methylamine is used. The final dilution of plasma is 100 or 200 depending on whether the initial plasma dilution is 1:5 or 1:10. Units are expressed as inhibition of plasmin units per ml undiluted plasma.

c. Modification of the method of Norman by Shamash and Rimon (1964)
Only those materials and steps are mentioned which differ from the method of Norman described above.

Buffers: Saline-phosphate buffer
1.34 g of K_2HPO_4 and 0.9 g of NaCl are dissolved in 80 ml of distilled water; the pH is adjusted to 7.4 and the final volume is brought to 100 ml.

Lysine-phosphate buffer
2.2 g of lysine hydrochloride are dissolved in 100 ml of saline-phosphate buffer, and the pH is corrected to 7.4. Fresh buffer is always used.

Procedure: Two caseinolytic units of plasmin in 0.4 ml lysine-phosphate buffer, various amounts of plasma and enough lysine-phosphate buffer to make a total volume of 2 ml are mixed and incubated at 37° C; 0.5 ml samples are withdrawn from these mixtures at 0 time, and after 1 and 2 hours of incubation, added to 1 ml of 3 % casein solution in saline-phosphate buffer and further incubated for 30 minutes. The residual caseinolytic activity is then assayed. Control tests are performed using plasmin and lysine-phosphate buffer alone. For evaluation, standard curves are prepared with dilution series of plasmin and plasmin with lysine.

2. Method Using Azocasein as Substrate (Markus and Werkheiser, 1964)

Materials
Azocasein prepared according to Charney and Tomarelli (1947): Dissolve 50 grams of casein (Nutritional Biochemical Comp.) in 1000 ml distilled water, add 10 grams of sodium bicarbonate and boil to dissolve (this takes approximately 15 minutes); then cool down in an ice bath to approximately 3° C. In a separate beaker in an ice bath, dissolve 5 grams of sulfanilamide in 30 ml 1 N NaOH and 120 ml distilled water, add 2.2 grams $NaNO_2$ and let cool. Add 13 ml 5 N HCl (the mixture will turn yellow) and stir for five minutes. Add this mixture dropwise to the casein keeping the pH at 8.5 with 1 N NaOH (the solution will turn red), and stir for about 30 minutes while in an ice bath. Dialyze against running *cold* tap water overnight, then against distilled water at 4° C for one day.
The azocasein should be diluted to 1–2 % so that it is in 0.1 M borate buffer pH 8.5 and

that when used in the azocasein assay will give an optical density reading between .100 and .150 for a blank when read in the spectrophotometer at a wave length 390 mμ.

Buffers: Borate buffer 0.1 M pH 8.5
Dissolve 3.09 g boric acid in about 100 ml distilled water, add 1 N NaOH until pH 8.5 and all boric acid is in solution, q.s. to 500 ml with distilled water. Recheck pH. It is not advised to make a dilution of a more concentrated buffer to get one of a lower molarity as it will result in a buffer with a pH which is higher than 8.5.

Procedure: The method described for the caseinolytic assay can be modified using azocasein instead of casein. The set up is the same as under the procedure described before (Cla). Enzyme inhibitor and enzyme buffer containing tubes are set up as before, incubated for 60 minutes at 28° C, then mixed with azocasein in a 1:1 ratio in duplicates and incubated again for 30 minutes at 24° C. At the end of the second incubation 1.12 M perchloric acid is added to each of the tubes which are then centrifuged at top speed for 15 minutes in an International clinical centrifuge. The supernatants are subsequently pipetted off and recentrifuged. The optical densities of the final supernatants are determined at 390 mμ in a Beckman model DU spectrophotometer. The absorption maximum of the azo dye at acid pH values is in the ultraviolet; the wave length chosen provides sufficient sensitivity without interference from the absorption of the aromatic residues of the peptides present in the supernatants. Since protein fragments, other than the split products of azocasein, do not absorb at this wave length, blanks may contain only buffer in place of the enzyme solution.

References

Albrechtsen, O. K. (1957). *Acta Physiol. Scand. 39,* 284.
Albrechtsen, O. K. (1959). *Acta Physiol. Scand. 47,* Supplement 165.
Alkjaersig, N. (1961). *In* "Blood Platelets" (S. A. Johnson, R. W. Monto, J. W. Rebuck and R. C. Horn, eds.), p. 329. Little Brown and Company.
Ambrus, C. M., and Markus, G. (1960). *Am J. Physiol. 199,* 491.
Ambrus, C. M., Weintraub, D. H., Dunphy, D., Dowd, J. E., Pickren, J. W., Niswander, K. R., and Ambrus, J. L. (1963). *Pediatrics 32,* 10.
Ambrus, C. M., Weintraub, D. H., Niswander, K. R., and Ambrus, J. L. (1965). *Pediatrics 35,* 91.
Ambrus, C. M., Ambrus, J. L., Lassman, H. B., and Mink, I. B. (1968). *Ann. N. Y. Acad. Sci. 146,* 430.
Ambrus, C. M., Ambrus, J. L., and Lassman, H. B. (1969). Unpublished.
Ambrus, J. L., Ambrus, C. M., Sokal, J. E., Markus, G., Back, N., Stutzman, L., Razis, D., Ross, C. A., Smith, B. H., Rekate, A. C., Collins, G. L., Kline, D. L., and Fishman, J. B. (1960). *Am. J. Cardiol. 6,* 462.
Astrup, T. (1966). *Federation Proc. 25,* 42.
Astrup, T., and Albrechtsen, O. K. (1957). *Scand J. Clin. Lab. Invest. 9,* 233.
Astrup, T., and Stage, A. (1952). *Nature 170,* 929.
Astrup, T., Rasmussen, J., Amery, A., and Poulsen, H. E. (1960). *Nature 185,* 619.
Back, N., and Ambrus, J. L. (1966). *In* "Surgical Bleeding" (S. Gollub and A. W. Ulin, eds.), pp. 309—409. McGraw Hill Book Company, New York.
Back, N., Ambrus, J. L., and Mink, I. B. (1961). *Circ. Res. 9,* 1208.
Charney, J., and Tomarelli, R. M. (1957). *J. Biol. Chem. 171,* 501.
Den Ottolander, G. J. H., Leijnse, B., and Cremer-Elfrink, H. M. J. (1968). *Thromb. Diath. Haemorrhag. 18,* 404.
Egeblad, K., and Astrup, T. (1966b). *Scand. J. Clin. Lab. Invest. 18,* 567.
Fletcher, A. P., Alkjaersig, N., and Sherry, S. (1958). *J. Clin. Invest. 37,* 1306.
Grob, D. (1949). *J. Gen. Physiol. 33,* 103.
Guest, M. M. (1964). *In* "Blood Coagulation, Hemorrhage and Thrombosis" (L. M. Tocantins and L. A. Kazal, eds.), pp. 280, 286. Grune and Stratton, New York.
Guest, M. M., Daly, B. M., Ware, A. G., and Seegers, W. H. (1948). *J. Clin. Invest. 27,* 785.
Hink, J. H., Jr., and McDonald, K. (1962). *Nature 194,* 1080.
Jacobsson, K. (1955). *Scand. J. Clin. Lab. Invest. 7,* Supplement 14, 55.
Johnson, A. J., and McCarty, W. R. (1959). *J. Clin. Invest. 38,* 1627.
Johnson, A. J., Tse, A. O., and Newman, J. (1964). *In* "Blood Coagulation, Hemorrhage and Thrombosis" (L. M. Tocantins and L. A. Kazal, eds.), pp. 481—482. Grune and Stratton, New York.
Johnson, S. A., and Schneider, C. L. (1953). *Science 117,* 229.
Kline, D. L. (1953). *J. Biol. Chem. 204,* 949.
Kline, D. L., and Fishman, J. B. (1960). *Am. J. Cardiol. 6,* 387.
Lewis, J. H., and Ferguson, J. H. (1950). *J. Clin. Invest. 29,* 1059.
Loomis, G. C., George, C., Jr., and Ryder, A. (1947). *Arch. Biochem. 12,* 1.
Macfarlane, R. G., and Biggs, R. (1948). *Blood 3,* 1167.
Mann, R. D., Cotton, S., and Jackson, D. (1966). *J. Clin. Pathol. 19,* 185.
Markus, G., and Ambrus, C. M. (1960). *J. Biol. Chem. 235,* 1673.
Markus, G., and Werkheiser, W. C. (1964). *J. Biol. Chem. 239,* 2637.
Markus, G., Ambrus, C. M., Wissler, F., and Woernley, D. L. (1958). *Federation Proc. 17,* 104.
Mattii, R., Ambrus, J. L., Sokal, J. E., and Mink, I. (1964). *Proc. Soc. Exptl. Biol. Med. 116,* 69.
Melander, B., Gliniecki, G., Granstrand, B., and Hanshoff, G. (1965). *Acta Pharmacol. Toxicol. 22,* 340.
Miller, K. D., and Copeland, W. H. (1962). *Proc. Soc. Exptl. Biol. Med. 111,* 512.
Müllertz, S. (1955). *Biochem. J. 61,* 424.
Norman, P. S. (1958). *J. Exptl. Med. 108,* 53.

Norman, P. S. (1966). *Federation Proc. 25,* 63.
Norman, P. S., and Hill, B. M. (1958). *J. Exptl. Med. 108,* 639.
Okamoto, S., Sato, S., Takada, Y., and Okamoto, U. (1964). *Keio J. Med. 13,* 177.
Porter, G. H. (1967). *Med. Clin. No. Amer. 51,* 1061.
Ratnoff, O. D., Lepow, I. H., and Pillemer, L. (1954). *Johns Hopkins Hosp. Bull. 94,* 169.
Remmert, L. R., and Cohen, R. P. (1949). *J. Biol. Chem. 181,* 431.
Rimon, A., Shamash, Y., and Shapiro, B. (1966). *J. Biol. Chem. 241,* 5102.
Rybak, M., and Rejnek, J. (1959). *Clin. Chim. Acta 4,* 364.
Shamash, Y., and Rimon, A. (1964). *Thromb. Diath. Haemorrhag. 12,* 119.
Shamash, Y., and Rimon, A. (1965). *Vox Sanguinis 10,* 599.
Shamash, Y., and Rimon, A. (1966). *Biochim. Biophys. Acta 121,* 35.
Shulman, N. R. (1952). *J. Exptl. Med. 95,* 593.
Special Issue on the Studies Concerning the Actions of Epsilon Amino-caproic Acid and Blood Plasmin (1959). *Keio J. Med. 8,* 4.
Tagnon, H. J., and Palade, G. E. (1950). *J. Clin. Invest. 29,* 317.
Tagnon, H. J., and Petermann, M. L. (1949a). *Proc. Soc. Exptl. Biol. Med. 70,* 359.
Tagnon, H. J., and Petermann, M. L. (1949b). *J. Clin. Invest. 28,* 814.
Taylor, F. B., Jr., Allen, L. W., and Bickford, A. M., Jr. (1964). *Arch. Biochem. Biophys. 104,* 277.
Ware, A. G., Guest, M. M., and Seegers, W. H. (1947). *Arch. Biochem. 13,* 231.

Differentiation Between Intravascular Coagulation and Intravascular Proteolysis

M. Maki and F. K. Beller

I. Introduction

Disseminated intravascular coagulation (DIC) has been confirmed to occur in a variety of disease states (see Chapter XI, p. 514). In a number of patients, a significant element of enhanced fibrinolysis is also demonstrable. It is, therefore, important to evaluate which of these juxtaposed mechanisms prevails. The development of laboratory criteria to aid us in making this judgment is of major concern not only from the standpoint of obtaining a more complete understanding of the pathophysiology involved, but also in practical therapeutical terms.

II. Methods for Differentiation

An examination of the data enumerated on Table 1 will make it apparent that this differentiation is impossible to establish by most classical laboratory criteria. In disseminated intravascular coagulation levels of fibrinogen, factors V and VIII are low because these procoagulants are consumed in the process of coagulation, whereas the levels of factors VII, IX and X remain unchanged or slightly elevated. Not very well understood is the occasional finding of low factor VII levels (Mc Gehee et al. 1967, Beller et al. 1968). In pathological fibrinolysis (fibrinogenolysis) fi-

Table 1: Coagulation Factors and Components of the Fibrinolytic Enzyme System in Disseminated Intravascular Coagulation (A) and Fibrinolysis (B).

	A	B
Fibrinogen	low	low
Prothrombin (2-stage)	low*	normal
Factor V	low	low
Factor VII–X	normal**	normal
Factor VIII	low	low
Platelets	low	normal
Thrombin clotting time (Patient's plasma)	long	long
Thrombin clotting time (Patient's + normal plasma)	normal	long
Plasminogen	normal to low	low
Plasminogen activator	absent	present (?)
Plasmin inhibitor	normal	low
TEG r value	normal	long
TEG ma value	low***	low
Fibrin(ogen) breakdown prod.	absent or pres.	present
Antithrombin III	low	normal

* No agreement between several authors.
** Although from a theoretical point it is supposed to be normal; cases have been found which were low in factor VII.
*** Result of low fibrinogen, low platelets.

brinogen and factors V and VIII are also low since all are readily hydrolized and irreversibly inactivated by plasmin. The levels of factors VII, IX and X resist enzymatic digestion by plasmin. Measurement of any of these clotting factors is therefore useless for this kind of differentiation.

Measurement of prothrombin by two-stage methods could be expected on theoretical grounds to comprise a useful tool since prothrombin is consumed during coagulation but resists plasmin proteolysis. Although prothrombin measurement has been found to provide useful guidance in many cases (Mammen, 1967), it may be somewhat limited in view of some other well documented cases of DIC where prothrombin levels have been found to be normal (Baker et al. 1964).

Systemic assays of the components of the fibrinolytic enzyme system might provide more information. The measurement of plasminogen is limited. Plasminogen is low in "pure" fibrinolytic states such as encountered during infusion of streptokinase (Johnson and McCarthy, 1959) since plasminogen is converted to plasmin which subsequently combines with inhibitors to form inactive complexes. The same holds true for idiopathic primary pathological fibrinolysis (Merskey et al. 1967). On the other hand plasminogen is usually substantially decreased in clinical states where disseminated intravascular coagulation predominates. The mechanism for this phenomenon is not completely understood but it can be explained probably by the well publicized propensity for plasminogen to become entrapped in the meshwork of fibrin deposits in biological fluids.

Assays of antiplasmin levels in our hands have proven quite reliable and useful in that a significant activation of the plasminogen-plasmin system is always associated with a fall in plasmin inhibitor levels, whereas normal inhibitor levels are encountered when the fibrinolytic component is insignificant. The direct measurement of fibrinolytic activity in blood, plasma or euglobulin fractions which is in precise terms the measurement of plasminogen activator is paradoxically one of the more unreliable criteria. The plasminogen activator is quite labile and its exact quantitation provides therefore a problem; moreover abnormal plasma proteolysis is frequently transient in nature. Plasminogen activator may increase suddenly and may return to normal within a few hours or a few days. However, the consequences of plasma proteolysis i.e. proteolytic degredation of procoagulants and a significant decrease of plasminogen and plasmin inhibitors may persist considerably longer. It is therefore feasible to encounter clinical cases of pathological fibrinolysis with normal or seemingly normal levels of fibrinotytic activity. Only extremely short euglobulin lysis times, e. g. less than 30 minutes are indicative of in vivo pathological fibrinolysis. The kinase inhibitor (Johnson et al. 1964) is reduced in cases with intravascular coagulation as well as with pathological fibrinolysis (Merskey et al. 1967, Graeff and Beller, 1968). Thrombin clotting time measurements reflecting the levels of fibrinogen degradation products with anticoagulant properties can be of significant help. A prolongation of the thrombin clotting time in a test system which contains equal parts of the patient's plasma and normal plasma or in the presence of human fibrinogen amounting to several seconds above normal values reliably establishes a significant component of abnormally enhanced fibrinolysis. If on the other hand, the thrombin clotting time is significantly prolonged in a test system containing patient's plasma only but is fully corrected by the addition of normal plasma or fibrinogen, this would indicate intravascular coagulation of considerable severity. The test system fails where intravascular coagulation produces only a moderate decrease in fibrinogen levels since it requires a reduction in plasma fibrinogen to less than 100 mg% in order to produce a prolongation of the thrombin clotting time. It was recently shown by von Kaulla and von Kaulla (1968) that antithrombin III activity is reduced in intravascular coagulation.

The recent demonstration (Beller and Maki, 1967) that differentiation between fibrinogen and fibrin split products can be accomplished in vitro by heat treatment, might provide the development of specific test systems. In our limited experience, they seem to be of value in differentiating pathological states where fibrinogenolysis prevails, as opposed to a situation where intravascular coagulation and subsequent fibrinolysis is of major importance (Fig. 1).

The specific demonstration of fibrinolysis breakdown products by immunological techniques is winning wide acceptance. Simplified techniques (immuno radial diffusion) allow quantitation of split products and can be developed in routine laboratories. The tanned red cell hemagglutination inhibition immune assay (Merskey et al. 1966) (see later) seems to be the most sensitive technique for the quantitative detection of fibrinolysis breakdown products. However, the technique is difficult to perform.

In a final analysis platelet counts by phase microscopy or through automated techniques provide an as valuable a guide line as any of the techniques discussed above. There is ample evidence in the literature that the platelet count in pure fibrinolytic states as exampled by streptinokinase therapy remains normal and the registration of a significant fall in platelet count would therefore be a strong argument in factor of diffuse intravascular coagulation. The thrombelastogram is of some value. The presence of breakdown products whether from fibrinogen or fibrin, produce a prolongation of the r and k values and a decrease in the amplitude under experimental condition (Maki et al. 1964; Hirsch et al. 1965). A lytic phenomenon in the presence of

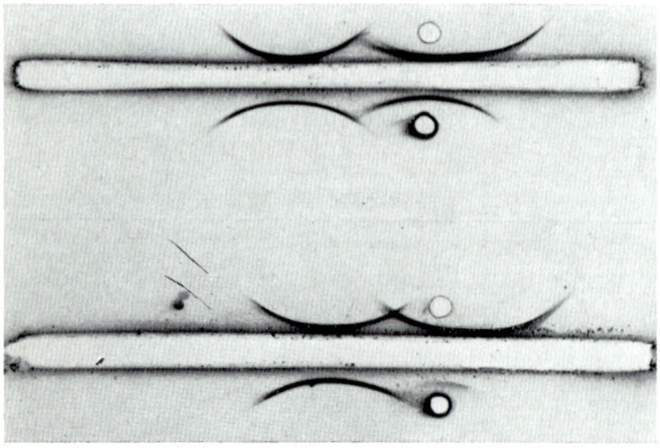

Fig. 1. Patterns of immunoelectrophoresis of fibrinogen degradation products: upper well: split products after fibrinolysis, lower well after fibrinogenolysis. A = before and B = after heating. Note the disappearance of fraction D after heating of fibrinogenolysis products.

a normal amplitude excludes the presence of large quantities of breakdown products. A normal or shortened r value with a strongly reduced amplitude (ma) indicates a severe reduction in fibrinogen and is indicative for intravascular coagulation. Additional technical details can be found in (Chapter XI, p. 514).

From this discussion it is apparent that platelet count and possibly prothrombin determination (2-stage) may allow differentiation between intravascular coagulation and proteolysis at the present time. These tests completely fail after massive blood replacement. A battery of tests including at least one of the immunological methods might provide more evidence for a certain disease mechanism but final proof is very difficult to establish.

III. Techniques for Assay of Split-Products

In the following certain quantitative and semiquantitative techniques will be enumerated which have proven useful diagnostic tools in clinical situations for the demonstration of split products of fibrinogen or fibrin. For additional information concerning techniques for quantitating fibrinogen related products, the reader is referred to p. 407 of this Chapter, and Chapter X, p. 470.

A. Simple Radial Immunodiffusion (Mancini et al. 1964)

1. Principle

The diameter of a circle of immune precipitate formed around a well cut in the agar containing antiserum, is directly proportional to the concentration of antigen tested. The differentiation between fibrinogenolysis and fibrinolysis products is made by comparing the diameters of the circles before and after heating of the test material (Beller and Maki, 1967).

2. Equipment

Plastic petri dishes of 8 cm diameter.

Cutter for preparing a well of 2 or 5 mm diameter.

Water baths thermoregulated at 48° C, 56° C, and 60° C.
Capillary tube attached to vacuume pump.
Pipettes; 10 ml calibrated to 0.1 ml subdivision.
Micropipettes; 0.1 ml calibrated to 0.01 ml subdivision.
Test tube rack and test tubes in various sizes.
Equipment for photography.

3. Reagents

Sodium barbital acetate buffer (Oxoid BR 11 G, pH 8.6) is prepared by adding 16.5 g of granules to one liter of distilled H_2O.
Two percent purified agar (Behringdiagnostic, American Hoechst, New York) dissolved in buffer is prepared and 100 mg of sodium azide or 10 μg of merthiolate per 100 ml of the solution is added as a perservative.
Rabbit antiserum against human fibrinogen.
Normal saline.

4. Procedure

Five ml of antiserum dilution (2–3 ml antiserum is diluted with the buffer to a total volume of 5 ml or higher depending on the titer of the antiserum) and 10 ml of agar solution dissolved previously in a boiling water bath are kept at 48° C for 10 min. The antiserum and the agar are combined and the mixture is poured into a prewarmed (60° C) petri dish. After about 30 minutes, wells of equal size (2 or 5 mm) are cut into the solidified agar gel and the centers are removed by aspiration with a capillary tube attached to a vacuum pump. The test solution (0.02 ml for 2 mm diameter well and 0.05 ml for a 5 mm diameter well) is dispensed with a micropipette. The agar gel plate is allowed to stand on a level surface for 24 hours at room temperature. The diameter of precipitate circle formed around the well is measured by placing the plate on top of a ruler.

5. Recording

The result obtained can be copied directly onto contact photographic paper at a one to one scale. It is, however, recommended that it be copied only after repeated washing of the plate with 0.5% amidoblack in order to obtain a better contrast. The stained agar plate can also be dried slowly at room temperature. The resulting film can then be peeled from the petri dish, covered with a commercial plastic wrapping paper and preserved for later reference.

6. Calculation and Interpretation

The concentration of split products is expressed as mg% fibrinogen calculated from a standard curve (Fig. 2). Since the diameter of immune circle is influenced by various factors such as titer of the antiserum, temperature, and molecular weight of the antigen, fibrinogen standard solutions in various concentrations should be tested simultaneously. Fibrinogen assayed by the radial immunodiffusion technique results in a linear relationship between the logarithmic expression of fibrinogen concentration and the diameter of the circle.

7. Comment

Petri dishes are covered and can then be stored at 4° C for 2–3 days before use.
A minimum concentration of fibrinogen which could be detected on this method is approximately 2 mg%.

B. Tanned Red Cell Hemagglutination Inhibition Immune Assay (TRCHII) (Merskey et al. 1966)

1. Materials

Latex particles coated with antifibrinogen antibody (Fi-test) (Hyland Laboratories, Los Angeles, Calif.).
Microcapillary tubes (1.4–1.6 mm O. D.) (Yankee-Microhematocrit tubes A 2931. Clay-Adams, Inc. N. Y.).
Sheep red blood cells (SRBC) 1–14 days old in Alsever's solution.
Formalin (3 percent in normal saline (0.85% w/v); pH adjusted to 7.0–7.5 with 0.1 N NaOH.
Acid buffer: 0.15 M sodium phosphate dibasic –0.35 volume; 0.15 M potassium phosphate monobasic –0.65 volume; 0.15 M sodium chloride —1.0 volume; pH adjusted to 6.4.

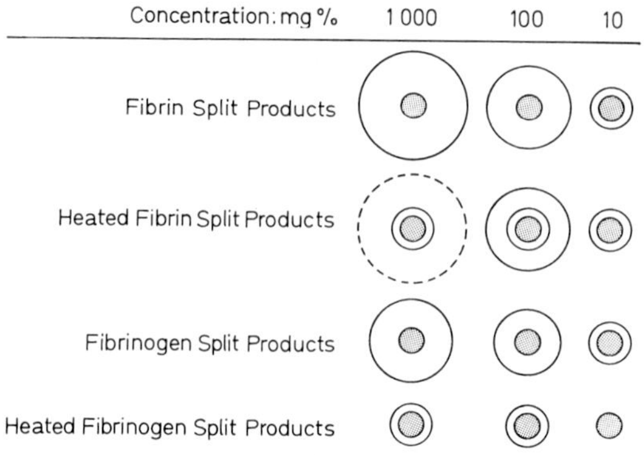

Fig. 2. Radial immune diffusion technique. Decreasing concentration of fibrinogen and fibrinogen split products.

Citrate buffer; same concentrations as acid buffer except that 0.1 M sodium citrate is substituted for sodium chloride; pH adjusted to 6.4.

Sodium azide stock solution 100 mg/ml in water.

Tannic acid, 10 mg/ml in water is diluted 1:400 in acid buffer.

Bovine thrombin. (Thrombin Topical, Parke, Davis & Co., Detroit, Michigan).

Glycerol-activated human plasmin, 165 units/ml (Prepared by the Michigan State Department of Health, Lansing, Mich., for the American National Red Cross).

Kunitz pancreatic trypsin inhibitor, 1.0 mg/ml (each mg is equivalent to 3100 Christensen units of plasma) (Worthington Biochemical Co., Freehold, N. J.).

Normal horse serum adsorbed with SRBC. Five parts serum to one part SRBC is incubated 15 min at 37° C and centrifuged at 1000 × G for 10 min after which the cells are discarded. The adsorbed serum is diluted 1:250 in citrate buffer.

Normal human plasma: Blood is collected from healthy donors and $^1/_{10}$ volume of 3.8 % trisodium citrate and Trasylol (Preparation A 128; proteinase inactivator. Farbenfabriken Bayer A. G., Leverkusen, Germany; is added immediately. Plasma is obtained by centrifuging the mixture at 1,200 × G for 15 min at 4° C.

Normal human serum: Blood from healthy donors is mixed with Trasylol (100 units/ml) allowed to clot for 8 hours at 37° C, and the serum separated. Other normal serum samples were aged for 24 hours at room temperature, lyophilized and used for antiserum adsorption.

Antifibrinogen serum: Rabbits were immunized with highly purified, plasminogen poor fibrinogen. Such fibrinogen preparations usually showed one component in the ultracentrifuge, on immunoelectrophoresis, and in starch gel electrophoresis. Clottable protein, 250 μg, in Freund's complete adjuvant was injected into the foot pads and neck muscles. Two weeks later 100 μg of clottable protein in 0.25 ml of aluminum hydroxide (Aluminum hydroxide suspension, Cutter laboratories, Berkely, Calif.) was injected intravenously. Intramuscular injections were repeated at 10–14 days intervals until high titer antiserum was obtained. The antiserum was adsorbed three to six times with lyophilized, aged human serum (1.0–2.0 mg/ml) at 37° C for 4 hours, then at 4° C for 12–18 hours. The stock antiserum with 1.0 mg/ml sodium azide added, was stored at –60° C, and the working antiserum for daily use was stored at 4° C. When tested against normal human plasma or purified plasminogen, only one precipitin band could be demonstrated by either immunodiffusion or immunoelectrophoresis. When the antiserum was mixed with an equal volume of plasma in a microcapillary tube, a heavy flocculation was observed within 3 min, but the precipitate was negligible in 18 hours when a similar mixture was made with normal human serum. Commercial antisera (Hyland Laboratories, Los Angeles, Calif.; Behringwerke, Marburg-Lahn, Germany) are suitable for TRCHII and immunodiffusion in agar gel but may produce insufficient precipitate for use in the microcapillary precipitin test. Results in the TRCHII were similar whether antisera against fibrin (Hyland Laboratories, Los Angeles, Calif.) or human fibrinogen or the split products resulting from the in vitro digestion of the fibrinogen by plasmin were used. While the authors have not fully evaluated all these antisera in the TRCHII against pathologic plasma or serum, no striking differences are apparent to date.

2. Methods

Precipitin test: A microcapillary tube was filled with fibrinogen antiserum to a depth of 2.0 cm and an equal volume of test material added, the tube sealed with heat, and the mixture incubated for 18 hours at 37° C. The amount of precipitate was observed periodically and after 18 hours measured in mm. The capillary tubes were then centrifuged at 11,000 rpm for 5 min (Micro-capillary centrifuge. International Equipment Co., Boston, Mass.) and the deposit measured with 40 × magnification.

Fi-test: The sample was diluted in 0.1 M glycine buffer containing 1.0 % NaCl, pH 8.2. One drop of diluted sample was mixed with two drops of Fi-test reagent on a glass slide, and the mixture was observed for agglutination. Macroscopic or microscopic evidence of agglutination within 120 seconds was considered a positive reaction.

Immunodiffusion and Immunoelectrophoresis: Immunodiffusion was performed in agar gel on microslides by the method of Ouchterlony and immunoelectrophoresis by the method of Scheidegger.

Tanned Red Cell Hemagglutination Inhibition Immunoassay (TRCHII): Sheep red blood cells (SRBC) were washed four times in 50 volumes of saline.

One volume of 8 % SRBC in saline was mixed with one volume of 3 % formalin in saline (pH 7.0–7.15).

Cells were agitated gently for 18–24 hours at 37° C with a magnetic stirrer.

Formalin SRBC were washed four times with 50 volumes of distilled water containing 1.0 mg/ml of sodium azide. Cells could then be stored at 4° C for months.

Sensitization Procedure: One volume of red cells was centrifuged (1000 × G for 5 min) washed 3 times with 50 volumes of acid buffer, and a 2 % suspension was made in acid buffer.

One volume of these cells was mixed with one volume of freshly mixed tannic acid (1:40,000) and incubated at 56° C for 60 min with occasional stirring.

The mixture was centrifuged (1000 × G for 5 min); the cells were washed 3 times in 50 volumes of acid buffer and a 4 % suspension was made in citrate buffer.

The red cell suspension was then divided. Four-fifth volume was sensitized by adding an equal volume of 1:250 diluted normal plasma, or alternatively purified fibrinogen, 1.0 μg/ml of clottable protein. A similar proportion of aged normal serum was added to the remaining one-fifth volume as a control. The cell suspensions were incubated at 37° C rather than 56° C since fibrinogen denatures at the higher temperature. As indicated above, the cells were coated with either purified fibrinogen of plasma; serum is used as a control since it does not sensitize the cells. The amount of antigen used for cell suspension is not critical, for no significant differences with plasma dilutions ranging from 1:100 to 1:5000 or approximately 25 μg to 0.5 μg of fibrinogen/ml were found. The cells were centrifuged (1000 × G for 5 min), washed three times in 50 volumes of citrate buffer, and a 2.5 % suspension was made in citrate buffer with 1:250 adsorbed horse serum and 1.0 mg/ml sodium azide. The final concentration of cells was checked by microhematocrit.

Dilution technic: Citrate buffer containing 0.4 % of adsorbed horse serum was used as a diluent buffer throughout the test. Reagents mixed in round bottomed test tubes provide readable settling patterns but a microtitration kit (Microtiter, Cooke Engineering Co., Alexandria, Va.) is much more convenient, yielding accurate results more quickly and requiring very small quantities of reagents.

Antiserum titration: Antiserum was diluted serially in the buffer (doubling dilutions). One volume of sensitizied (or control) cells and one volume of buffer were added to one volume of diluted antiserum. Results were read after storage at 4° C for 12–18 hours. A dilution of 1:2000 is used for the inhibition test. A positive reaction is shown by the formation of a coarse agglutinate or loosely stipple mat at the bottom of the tube, and a negative reaction by a button or doughnut shaped ring at the bottom of the tube.

Adsorption of serum or other test material: Ocassionally, samples of serum or thrombin-treated plasma showed a non specific agglutination up to a titer of 1:8 which could usually be reduced to 0 or 1.0 by prior adsorption of the sample for 2 hours at 4° C with $^1/_5$ volume (or more) of fresh of formalinized washed, packed SRBC.

Inhibition assay: Doubling dilutions of adsorbed normal plasma or other test material were made in citrate buffer and an equal volume of diluted antiserum was added to each tube. After standing at 4° C for 10 min, one volume of cold (4° C) cell was added. The tubes were shaken, left at 4° C for 12–18 hours, then read. The last negative tube was regarded as the end point. Suitable controls with each assay included dilutions of normal plasma, serum or other test material with sensitizied and control cells but no antibody, as well as control cells with antibody.

Cells: SRBC maintained their reactivity for at least 21 days after sensitization. If not used within two hours of washing, they should be rewashed three times in fresh buffer.

Buffers: Citrate buffer was used exclusively to prevent clot formation, a possibility when acid buffer is used with plasma or fibrinogen.

Heparin and Thrombin: Heparin (±20 units/ml) or thrombin (100 NIH units/ml) did not inhibit specific hemagglutination of sensitized cells.

Sensitivity and precision: Dilute antiserum improved the sensitivity of the assay but too high a dilution made the end point difficult to define. The assay's precision was increased by using additional intermediate dilutions. The concentration of red blood cells in the final mixtures must be similar in all tubes.

Reproducibility: The inhibition assay yielded more sensitive and consistent results when performed at 4° C. There are variations produced with a standard normal plasma tested 3–5 times a week over a period of 2 months with a constant dilution (1:5000) of antiserum. The use of standard control plasmas permitted control of the daily tests results.

3. Comment

This method is most sensitive, however, the technique is extremely difficult to perform and contains manifold sources of error. It cannot be considered a routine assay. The technique does not allow for differentiation between split products derived from fibrinogen or fibrin.

C. Tyrosine Technique for the Assay of Split Products (Nanniga and Guest, 1967)

1. Principle

This method allows for the assay of split products of fibrinogen or fibrin without an immune assay.

2. Technique

Fibrinogen is removed by precipitation with 25% saturated neutralized ammonium sulfate at room temperature (23° C). To 1 ml of plasma 6.5 ml saline are added in a graduated centrifuge tube and mixed; 2.5 ml saturated and neutralized ammonium sulfate is added; the precipitate is removed by centrifugation. The supernatant solution is transferred to another graduated centrifuge tube (volume transferred = A). The split product is precipitated by heating; the tube containing the supernatant solution is heated for 30 min at 58° C, then centrifuged at 3,000 × G; the precipitate is washed twice with saline. Tyrosine in the precipitated split products is determined. The precipitate containing the digestion product is dissolved in 2 ml of 2.5% NaOH and digested at 100° C for 30 min; water is added to 2.5 ml and the tyrosine is estimated in 1 ml samples, in duplicate.

The concentration of split products is calculated on the equation

$E_{640} \times f \times 2.5 \times 10/A$ mg/ml

where f is the factor transferring the extinction into split product concentration.

3. Comment

The test can be done in plasma, since only fibrinogen and split products precipitate at 56° C. After removal of the fibrinogen with ammonium sulfate precipitation, split products are the only factor potentially present in plasma with precipitates at 56° C.

References

Baker, W. G., Bang, N. U., Nachman, R. C., Farow, R., and Horowitz, H. (1964). *Ann. Int. Med. 61,* 116.

Beller, F. K., and Maki, M. (1967). *Thromb. Diath. Haemorrhag. 17,* 114.

Beller, F. K., Maki, M., and Epstein, M. D. (1968). *Am. J. Obstet. Gynecol. 101,* 587.

Graeff, H., and Beller, F. K. (1968). *Thromb. Diath. Haemorrhag. 20,* 420.

Hirsch, J., Fletcher, A. P., and Sherry, S. (1965). *Am. J. Physiol. 209,* 415.

Johnson, A. J., and McCarthy, W. R. (1959). *J. Clin. Invest. 38,* 1627.

Johnson, A. J., Tse, A. O., and Newman, J. (1964). *In* "Blood Coagulation, Haemorrhage and Thrombosis" (L. M. Tocantins and L. A. Kazal, eds.), pp. 479—481. Grune and Stratton, New York.

McGehee, G., Rapport, S. I., and Hjort, P. T. (1967). *Ann. Int. Med. 67,* 250.

Maki, M., Kikuchi, I., and Murakimi, A. (1964). *Tohoku J. Exptl. Med. 84,* 201.

Mancini, S., Vaerman, J. P., Carbonara, D., and Heremans, J. F. (1964). *Proc. 11th Coloquium Protides of the Biological Fluids, Brugge 1963,* 370.

Mammen, E. F. (1967) personal communication.

Merskey, C., Kleiner, G. J., and Johnson, A. J. (1966). *Blood 28,* 1.

Merskey, C., Johnson, A. J., Kleiner, G. J., and Woil, H. (1967). *Brit J. Haematol. 13,* 528.

Nanninga, L. B., and Guest, M. M. (1967). *Thromb. Diath. Haemorrhag. 17,* 440.

von Kaulla, K. N., and von Kaulla, E. (1968). *Abstr. XIIth Congr. Intern. Soc. Hematol. 184,* TT 14.

CHAPTER IX

Hemostasis

HERBERT I. HOROWITZ and ARTHUR R. SPIELVOGEL

I. Introduction

A. The Scope of Hemostasis

Whenever a blood vessel is injured a series of reactions are called into play designed to arrest the loss of blood. The sum total of these responses are encompassed by the term hemostasis. How much blood is lost in a given period of time is in part determined by the type of injury, the size of the vessel and its ability to contract; by the ability of supporting tissues to limit blood loss; by the flow and pressure properties of the blood itself. The cessation of bleeding, however, is ultimately due to platelet function. The blood platelets form a mass or plug which initially halts the loss of blood. The platelets further interact with protein coagulants to provide more permanent hemostasis through clot formation. This chapter will be concerned with current knowledge as to the mechanisms by which platelets perform these functions. This is an area of recent intensive investigations which have provided a framework upon which many details remain to be added.

B. Definitions

As with so many rapidly expanding fields, problems of terminology have led to some needless confusion. The Subcommittee on Haemostasis of the International Committee on Hemostasis & Thrombosis (Roskam, 1966) has recently defined some of the important terms in hemostasis. Their recommendations are summarized below.

Stopping the loss of blood from a site of vascular injury is achieved first by a mass of densely packed platelets, called the *hemostatic platelet plug*. That initial cessation of bleeding results from platelet function is attested to by the prolonged bleeding time consistently associated with thrombocytopenia; this is equated with defective *primary hemostasis*. Primary hemostasis (and the primary bleeding time) are normal in hemophilic patients with severe deficiencies of one or another of the protein clotting factors. These patients however have abnormal *total hemostatic plugs* since their hemostatic platelet plugs are not reinforced by normal fibrin formation. They are subject to *rebleeding*, the phenomenon of again bleeding after initial hemostasis is achieved, and are considered to have defective *secondary hemostasis*.

In the process of formation of the hemostatic plug, platelets *adhere* to the edges of the injured blood vessel. Adhesion refers to the sticking of a platelet to a surface other than that of another platelet. When platelets stick one to another they are aggregating. (Platelet *agglutination* is reserved for the antibody-mediated immunological response.)

Platelet viscous metamorphosis (VM), a term originally used by Eberth and Schimmelbusch (1885) to describe changes in single platelets, has been used in many different contexts by different investigators. The Subcommittee on Haemostasis proposes a restricted definition (Roskam, 1966). "Viscous metamorphosis circumscribes the sum of the morphological, biochemical and functional changes undergone by platelets in the course of formation of a hemostatic plug. Although it has been used to define various phases of this process, strictly it is intended to indicate the platelet reactions to thrombin in the presence of calcium ions."

The phrase, *platelet release reaction* has been used (Grette, 1962) to describe the transfer of intraplatelet constituents, including adenine nucleotides, biologically active amines, amino acids, potassium ions, proteins and platelet clotting factors, to the sourrounding media during viscous metamorphosis. Table 1 lists those substances commonly included in this expression, table 2 lists those substances capable of eliciting all or part of the release reaction, and table 3 describes the morphological features of viscous metamorphosis. The release reactions may proceed in more than one phase, so that when the phrase is used accuracy demands that the user describe fully what is measured. *Degranulation* is another component of VM and refers to the disappearance of electron-dense particles as seen by electron microscopy.

II. Phylogenetic Aspects of Hemostasis

This subject has been extensively reviewed by Heilbrunn (1961). Unicellular organisms are capable of preserving their intracellular fluid by a surface precipitation reaction (SPR) which has surprising similarity to mammalian blood coagulation. SPR requires calcium to develop; in calcium-free media minute injuries to cells result in complete loss of intracellular fluid. However, in the presence of calcium an activity forms within the cells which is comparable to thrombin, in that once formed, it can induce SPR in the absence of calcium. In some cells SPR is visualized as gel formation, but in others vacuolization and formation of fibrils are evident. In some organisms the reaction can be inhibited by dilute heparin solution (e. g., the giant amoeba, Chaos chaos).

SPR is common to most, if not all, types of protoplasm and can be looked upon as hemostasis on the cellular level. As organisms became more complex they required circulatory systems of even greater complexity for their survival. Hemostatic mechanisms comparable to, and perhaps elaborated from, SPR, have been incorporated into the circulating hemolymph or blood. Three types of reactions have been found in crustaceans by Tait (1911) and indicate the divergent pathways in which hemostasis has developed. The first type, considered to be the most primitive and essential device for arresting bleeding, consists of aggregation of the blood corpuscles without any subsequent jellying of the plasma. Levin and Bang (1966a, b) have studied this mechanism thoroughly in the horseshoe crab, Limulus. A clotting protein analogous to fibrinogen is present in the hemocytes, or nucleated thrombocytes, of the Limulus. Aggregation of hemocytes may be inhibited by the sulfhydril inhibitor, NEM which also inhibits aggregation of mammalian blood platelets (Bryan et al. 1964; Robinson et al. 1963). The second type of reaction includes aggregation of cells as a first step, followed by jellying (clotting) of the plasma. In the third type, cell aggregation is relatively insignificant, though special "explosive corpuscles" (Hardy, 1892) cause localized clots followed by generalized plasma coagulation. The analogy of these cellular and plasma hemostatic mechanisms to hemostatic platelet plug formation and secondary hemostasis dependent on fibrin formation in mammalian species is evident.

The response of mouse liver cells and of cells of the lime mold Dictogostetium discordeum to ADP and ATP offers additional evidence of a common phylogenetic pattern in cellular and blood reactions (Jones and Wooley, 1967).

III. Platelet Adhesion - the Interaction of Platelet with Surfaces other than those of other Platelets

Primary hemostasis involves the construction of an intraluminal dam to bridge over any loss in continuity of an injured blood vessel. This dam must be anchored to some portion of the injured vessel. Of the components of the blood vessel wall, Bounameaux (1959), Hugues (1960), Hugues and Lapiere (1964) found that platelets adhere only to collagen.

Zucker and Borrelli (1962) have shown that this reaction is specific for collagen and can be inhibited by preincubating connective tissue with the enzyme collagenase. The reaction between collagen and platelets is extremely rapid (Spaet and Zucker, 1964), occurring in seconds even in the absence of ionic calcium. Since some ionic calcium is needed for further platelet aggregation reactions, use of platelet-rich ethylene diaminetetraacidic acid (EDTA) plasma permits the study of adhesion without further platelet-platelet interaction (Spaet et al. 1967). Using this technique they have shown that platelets on contact with collagen degranulate transfering sizable amounts of adenine nucleotides (largely ADP) to the surrounding media.

Mustard and his coworkers (1967) have made an important contribution to our understanding of the interaction of platelets with other surfaces. In addition to collagen, platelets adhere to latex particles. Here again adhesion and subsequent platelet aggregation can be distinguished. If the latex is uncoated by plasma proteins only adhesion takes place, but latex particles which have adsorbed plasma proteins bring about release of adenine nucleotides and platelet aggregation. The protein constituent responsible for inducing release of platelet constituents and for aggregation is gamma globulin. Antigen-antibody complexes are also competent to induce both adhesion and aggregation.

The adhesion reaction to collagen is a phenomenon peculiar to blood platelets. The nature of this reaction is not known. It does not appear to be electrostatic since both platelets and collagen fragments have a net negative charge (Spaet and Zucker, 1964). Platelets can phagocytose particulate material, including collagen fragments (Mustard et al. 1967). However, lysed platelets and platelet debris following sonic disruption still adhere to collagen (Spaet et al. 1967), thus making it unlikely that adhesion is the result of an attempt of the platelet to engulf the collagen. In sharp contrast to platelet aggregation, platelet adhesion to collagen is irreversible (Spaet and Zucker, 1964).

The first steps of hemostasis which ensue when a blood vessel is ligated, leading to adhesion of platelets to exposed collagen, are depicted in fig. 1 and 2. Fig. 3 is a low power electron micrograph showing platelets which have degranulated on contact with collagen.

IV. Platelet Aggregation

Observations of blood flowing through tissues of experimental animals have shown that platelets aggregate following initial adhesion. Aggregates propagated to form permeable masses of platelets which in some instances broke off and separated in the flowing blood. This aggregation was reversible. The growth of the hemostatic platelet plug thus results from circulating platelets sticking to those which have originally adhered to denuded collagen (Zucker, 1947, 1961; Berman, 1961).

The pioneer studies by Hellem (1960) indicated that a heat stable factor was extractable from red cells ("factor R") and was capable of aggregating platelets. Gaarder and her associates (1961) subsequently identified this substance as adenosine 5'diphosphate (ADP). A large number of investigations have

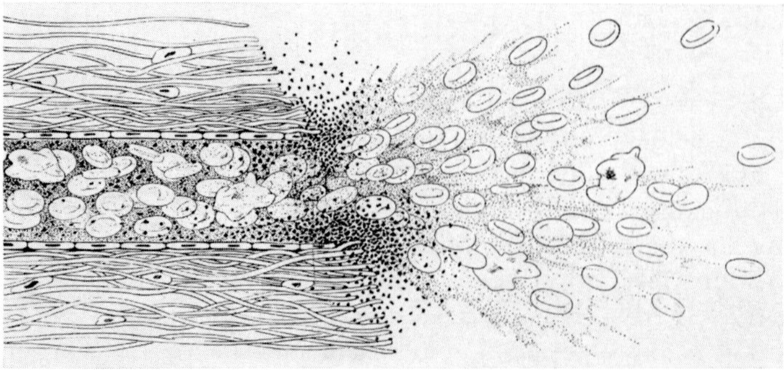

Fig. 1. Within seconds of an injury to a blood vessel platelets selectively adhere to the exposed collagen fibers, thereby initiating hemostasis. (We are indebted to the Editors of Hospital Practice and to Dr. T. H. Spaet for permission to use figures 1, 2, 4, 5 and 7 and to Dr. R. B. Erickson for figure 3.)

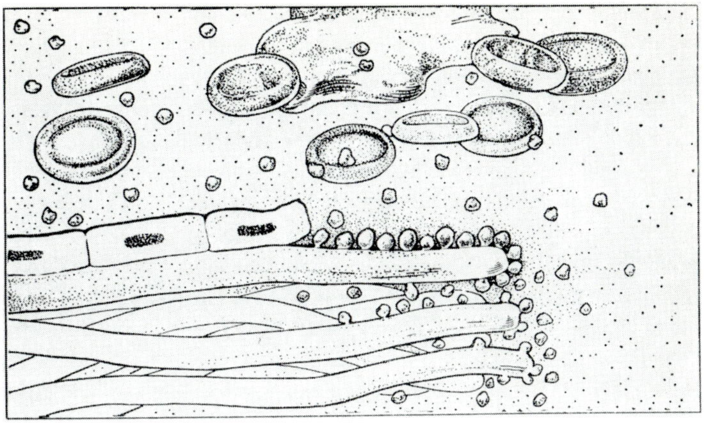

Fig. 2. A single layer of platelets is depicted coating the exposed collagen at a higher magnification of figure 1.

firmly established that ADP is the substance responsible for platelet aggregation and the growth of the hemostatic platelet plug. These studies are extensively reviewed by Marcus and Zucker (1965).

A. Source of ADP for Early Platelet Plug Formation

The platelets themselves are the probable source of the ADP leading to platelet aggregation. The ATP content of platelets is quite high – 23.6 μ moles per gram of wet weight, according to Schmitz et al. (1962) – and is readily broken down to ADP. When platelets adhere to collagen they release considerable ADP (Spaet et al. 1967; Hovig, 1963). Although no one has yet measured the concentration of ADP at the platelet surface in the course of in vivo hemostasis, calculation of the amounts of ADP released from the platelet and the concentration of ADP needed for in vitro platelet clumping square with the platelets-collagen reaction being sufficient source of the required ADP (Mitchell and Sharp, 1964).

ATP being a constituent of all cells, ADP required for platelet plug formation could be derived from any of the damaged tissues. Johnson et al. (1965) have assigned the red cells an important role in hemostasis, presenting evidence of red cell hemolysis and ADP release early in experimental cuts in the rats. Similarly, tissue injury could lead to ADP release into blood vessels in certain circumstances. Nonetheless, the bulk of evidence points to the platelet as the sole and sufficient source of adenine nucleotides necessary for aggregation.

B. Propagation of the Platelet Plug

It is unlikely that sufficient ADP is released from the platelets by the initial adhesion to collagen to account for the slow build up of the platelet plug. In animal preparations (Berman, 1961) one may observe several stages

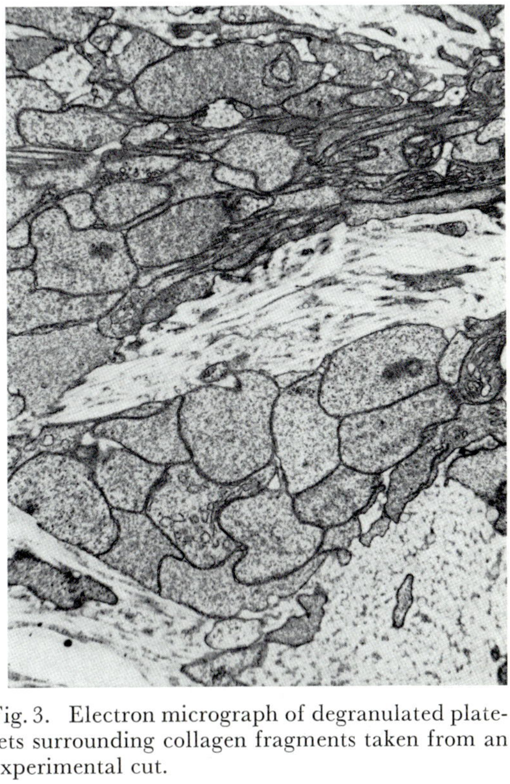

Fig. 3. Electron micrograph of degranulated platelets surrounding collagen fragments taken from an experimental cut.

of platelet aggregates form at the initial site of vessel injury, then break off to be swept downstream, as new platelets begin to form a new and more effective plug. Thus, investigators have looked for other ways in which aggregating platelets can release further ADP and in this way propagate the hemostatic plug.

An obvious candidate has been readily at hand in thrombin. Thrombin in low concentrations causes platelets to aggregate (Lüscher, 1956; Zucker and Borrelli, 1959). This action can be blocked by substances which inhibit ADP or remove it from plasma, indicating that thrombin aggregates platelets by inducing release of ADP. Assigning thrombin a role in these early stages of hemostasis implies that coagulation reactions are activated. The evidence for this concept is conflicting. Johnson and her colleagues (1965) find very early evidence of fibrin formation in experimental cuts. On the other hand, Mustard's group (1967) (among many others) have failed to find such early fibrin. In addition, severe hemophiliacs have normal bleeding times, implying normal hemostatic plug formation, though obviously they have great trouble in elaborating thrombin.

A more likely agent for propagating the platelet plug is ADP. In vitro studies have shown that sufficient exogenous ADP induces release on endogenous platelet nucleotides, predominantly ADP. The effect of ADP on platelets has been studied by following changes in optical density in continuously agitated platelet-rich plasma (O'Brien, 1962, 1963, 1964; Born and Cross, 1963; Murphy et al. 1964). As platelets aggregate to form larger and larger clusters more light is transmitted through the initially opalescent platelet-rich plasma, resulting in a decrease of optical density. As aggregates disperse optical density again increases. After a latent period of about 30 seconds, low concentrations of ADP (10^{-6} to 10^{-5} M) produce a smooth, monophasic curve when optical density is plotted against time. Aggregation reaches a maximum at one to two minutes, then dispersal of aggregates causes the optical density to return towards baseline values. Higher concentrations of ADP (above 10^{-4} M) give a biphasic response. Again there is a latent period, with initial aggregation occurring as with lower ADP concentrations. However, instead of the dispersal of aggregates, after a short plateau further aggregation with even more decrease of optical density follows (MacMillan, 1966). Platelet aggregation is no longer reversible. The initial aggregation seen with both low and high concentrations of ADP has been interpreted as being due to the aggregating action of the exogenous ADP. The second phase of aggregation seen with higher concentrations of ADP may be the result of release of endogenous platelet nucleotides.

C. Requirements for ADP-induced Platelet Aggregation

In contrast to platelet adhesion to collagen, platelet aggregation by ADP has an absolute requirement for divalent cation. ADP will aggregate platelets in citrated, heparinized and

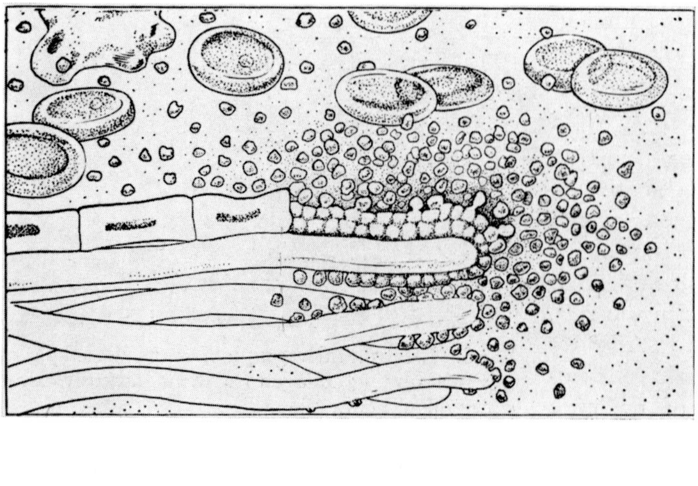

Fig. 4. In the next phase of hemostasis platelets aggregate on to those already adherent to collagen. ADP, released from the platelets, is believed to be responsible for this aggregation.

native plasmas (Born and Cross, 1963; Spaet et al. 1967), but aggregation may be reversed by added citrate (Mitchel and Sharp, 1964). No platelet aggregation occurs with ADP in EDTA plasma (Born and Cross, 1963); the inhibitory effect of this chelating agent can, however, be overcome with additional calcium (Cuthbertson and Mills, 1963). In studies using carefully washed platelets, potassium and calcium were found to be essential to ADP-clumping; magnesium could substitute only partially for calcium.

A plasma factor has been found to be essential for ADP-induced platelet aggregation (Born and Cross, 1964; McClean et al. 1964). Washed human platelets suspended in isotonic buffer solutions will not aggregate with ADP but aggregating ability is restored by small amounts of plasma. Highly purified fibrinogen can substitute completely for plasma (Cross, 1964; Haslam, 1964). However, platelets from patients with "afibrinogenemia" aggregate normally with ADP (Rodman and Mason, 1967). These patients do have small amounts of platelet and plasma fibrinogen, however, so that absolute requirements for small amounts of fibrinogen at the level of the platelet membrane are not ruled out by these observations. Deykin (1967) has indicated that a plasma protein distinct from fibrinogen is also required for ADP-induced platelet aggregation. Stages in ADP-induced platelet aggregation leading to the propagation of the hemostatic platelets plug are represented in fig. 4 and 5. Fig. 6 is an electron micrograph of a small clump of platelets aggregated by thrombin in vitro.

D. Summary of Experimental Findings Related to ADP-induced Platelet Aggregation

Some of the features of platelet aggregation by ADP have already been described but will be briefly summarized at this point.

1. The reaction is specific for ADP, it is inhibited by ATP, AMP or adenosine.
2. It requires divalent cations, which likely complex with ADP to make the active compound.
3. Fibrinogen is essential; another plasma protein may also be required.
4. At low concentrations platelet aggregation is reversible.
5. It may be inhibited by removal of calcium, or fibrinogen.
6. Inhibition by ADP breakdown products (AMP and adenosine) is competitive.
7. The inhibition by adenosine initially increases with time suggesting that adenosine is incorporated into platelets (Born, 1967). Studies of ADP derivatives radioisotopically labelled with either P^{32} or C^{14} confirm this suggestion and also indicate that ATP, ADP, or AMP must be broken down to adenosine before they can again entry into platelets (Salzman et al. 1966).
8. Enzymes capable of rapidly degrading AMP to adenosine are present in plasma and on the platelet surface (Spaet et al. 1967).

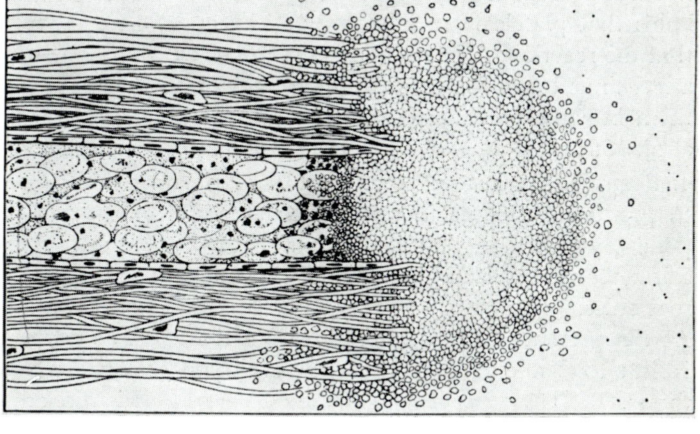

Fig. 5. Primary hemostasis is now complete. A platelet plug has occluded the cut vessel; no bleeding is observed. The events depicted in Figures 1, 2, 4 and 5 are those which occur during the "bleeding time" determination.

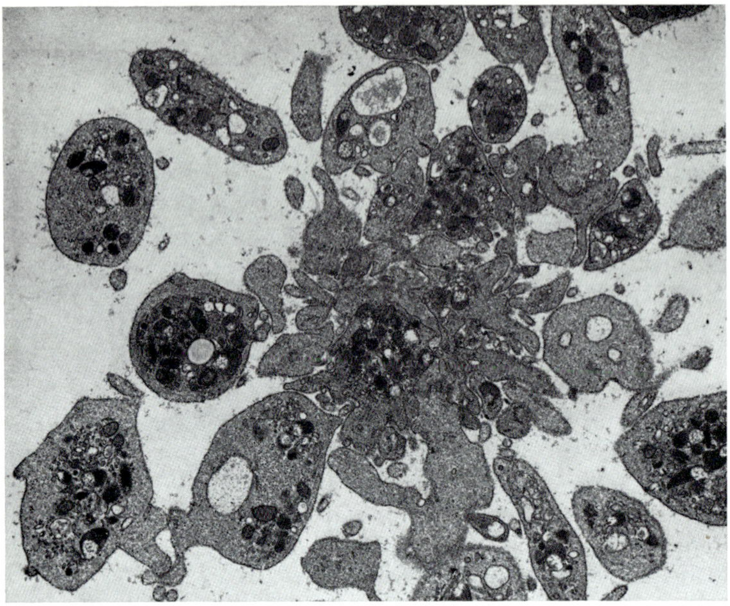

Fig. 6. Electron micrograph of small clumps of platelets in citrated plasma. Aggregation in this case was induced by concentrations of thrombin too low to cause clotting.

E. Mechanism of ADP-induced Platelet Aggregation

Four theories have been proposed as to the mechanism of ADP-induced platelet aggregation.

1. Calcium, some plasma protein, and ADP have been viewed as forming a stable bridge between platelets (Hellem and Owren, 1964). The absence of ADP incorporation as such into platelets and platelet aggregates makes this hypothesis untenable.
2. The conversion of ADP to AMP by the platelet membrane is postulated as providing energy for some as yet unidentified aggregating reaction (Spaet and Lejnieks, 1966; Spaet et al. 1967).
3. An ingenious theory proposed by Salzman holds that platelets are inherently sticky and that the reaction, ATP → ADP, is required as a continued source of energy to maintain them in a non-sticky configuration (Salzman et al. 1966).
4. Born (1967) has proposed that ADP acts to produce a change in some platelet component which then permits formation of disulfide bonds between platelets and fibrinogen molecules.

At the present state of our knowledge there is little to choose amongst the last three hypotheses.

V. Consolidation of the Platelet Plug

A. Relationship of Plasma Coagulation Factors to Platelets

The platelet's "plasmatic atmosphere" has been assigned a special role in coagulation and hemostasis (Roskam, 1923). All plasma procoagulants are found in good concentration in packed platelets, but fibrinogen (Salmon and Bounameaux, 1957; Seligman et al. 1957), factor V (Hjort et al. 1955), and factor XI (Horowitz and Fujimoto, 1965) appear to bear a special relationship to the platelet.

Platelet fibrinogen has been found in granule as well as membrane fractions of platelets (Nachman et al. 1964). Though it has many properties in common with plasma fibrinogen, certain immunological properties and response to proteolytic digestion suggest that the two may be different molecular species (Davey and Lüscher, 1966). Fibrinogen has been found immunologically in megakaryocytes and may be formed by these cells as well as by hepatic cells (Goksen and Yunis, 1964). The role of fibrinogen as a co-factor for ADP-induced platelet aggregation has already been mentioned.

Factor V is avidly adsorbed from plasma by platelets (Hjort et al. 1955) and is likely responsible for the activity known as platelet factor I. It remains associated with platelets through many successive washes (Bounameaux, 1957; Horowitz and Fujimoto, 1965). According to Esnouf (1965) factor V functions in coagulation when adsorbed to particulate platelet factor 3. Its presence in high concentration on the platelet membrane would thus facilitate coagulation.

Iatrides and Ferguson (1965) found "surface factor" closely adsorbed to the platelet; we (Horowitz and Fujimoto, 1965) have shown this activity to be due to factor XI; like factor V it is avidly adsorbed by deficient platelets and persists with the platelet through many successive washings. Factor XII, however, is readily removed from platelets by a single washing. The close association of platelets and factor XI may be important for the initiation of coagulation reactions following primary hemostasis.

Roskam (1923) has proposed that platelets are surrounded by their own plasmatic atmosphere, one in which coagulation reactions would be favored. According to this concept, thrombin would generate in small amounts quite early and in direct relationship to the platelet membrane. Thus thrombin could be assigned an important role in the "firming-up" of the primary hemostatic plug, in concentrations insufficient to clot fibrinogen and at a time when plasma coagulation reactions have barely been initiated.

B. Further Interaction of Platelets and Coagulation – Activation of Platelet Factor 3

Most authors agree that the primary hemostatic plug is insufficient for long term hemostasis in the absence of efficient coagulation and fibrin clot formation. Many feel that thrombin is essential to induce clot retraction, thereby "firming-up" the primary hemostatic plug. We have already seen how small amounts of thrombin could evolve locally in the platelets' plasmatic atmosphere. For fuller evolution of thrombin and clot formation it is likely that platelets must play an additional role.

Fantl and Ward (1958) first pointed out that the platelet factor 3 of intact blood platelets is present in a masked form, not immediately available to participate in thromboplastic reactions. Platelet factor 3 measurement is described elsewhere in this book (Chapter IX, p. 436); the activity has been identified with isolated phosphatides of serine and ethanolamine but is believed to be present in platelets as a phospholipoprotein.

Considerable controversy exists as to the physical state of platelet factor 3 as it enters coagulation reactions. Material with platelet factor 3 activity may be derived from platelet granules, membrane fragments, and soluble material from the top layer following isopycnic centrifugation of disrupted platelets (Marcus et al. 1966). Each of these subcellular platelet fractions has been proposed as the source of active platelet factor 3.

Johnson et al. (1965) find that intact granules leave structurally intact platelets early in the course of coagulation as observed by electron microscopy. White et al. (1966) on the other hand, see the early appearance of unusual electron-dense particles in their electron micrographs of clotting platelets and interpret them to be phospholipid micelles. These structures are believed to be derived from platelet granules and are seen to emerge from otherwise intact platelets as coagulation proceeds. These findings have been challenged as being artefacts of fixation. Marcus and his coworkers (1966) determined that the platelet factor 3 activity of membrane fragments was greater per mg of nitrogen than that of granule fragments. The shortest times in the Russell's viper venom test (Stypven time) or in the thromboplastin generation test could be obtained only with membrane fragments, which on the whole most closely resembled the coagulant activity of disrupted platelets. He inferred that significant platelet factor 3 activity was primarily a platelet membrane function, the lesser activity of the granules being an incidental concomitant of tissue phospholipoprotein, and not important for hemostasis. Since Marcus' starting material consisted of disrupted washed platelets, it is uncertain whether soluble or readily soluble platelet factor 3 material was lost in the processing. Lüscher (personal communication) using technics similar to those of Marcus, was able to separate granules into two fractions; one of these had even greater activity than did the membranes.

Findings that the most active platelet factor 3 is anatomically localizable to platelet membranes do not exclude a role for soluble or granule platelet factor 3 in hemostasis. Horowitz and Papayoanou (1967) have confirmed previous observations (O'Brien, 1955; Alagille and Soulier, 1957; Shinowara, 1961) that serum derived from blood or plasma containing platelets has an activity lacking in serum obtained from thrombocytopenic blood or plasma. This activity is identical to platelet factor 3 in prothrombin consumption and Stypven time tests. It is non-sedimentable in high centrifugal fields (175,000 × G for 2 hours) and resists denaturation at 60° C. Although the greater fraction of available platelet factor 3 activity appears to remain with particulate platelet fractions during coagulation, 5 to 25 % appears to be released in non-sedimentable form to interact with coagulation factors in plasma (Horowitz and Papayoanou, 1967).

Electron micrographs of coagulating blood have demonstrated fibrin deposition beginning both in close approximation to platelet membranes, and in plasma unrelated to membranes (White et al. 1966; Mustand et al. 1967). Prothrombin activation induced by membrane platelet factor 3 would account for the former, whereas soluble or microparticulate "non-sedimentable" platelet factor 3 released from platelets would explain the latter.

C. Mechanism of Activation of Platelet Factor 3

During the reactions of hemostasis platelets change from inert to active sources of platelet factor 3. The mechanism and physical or chemical intermediates which bring about this activation have received attention.

Denuded collagen fibers, the candidates for initiation of primary hemostasis, are also capable of activating platelet factor 3 (Niewiarowski et al. 1965). This activation may be important in leading to early evolution of thrombin, which is also a potent activator of platelet factor 3 even in sub-clotting concentrations (Horowitz and Papayoanou, 1968). The list of platelet factor 3 activators can be extended to include many of the agents which induce platelet aggregation; such a list would include ADP, epinephrine, serotonin, trypsin, kaolin or celite, endotoxins, and latex particles (Horowitz and Papayoanou, 1968).

Since kaolin or celite, which massively activate factors XII and XI, are potent platelet factor 3 activators, one could conclude that activation is accomplished through the action of the contact factors. However, platelet factor 3 activation by celite occurs readily and completely in plasmas from patients with congenital deficiencies of factors XII, XI, and also factor VIII, X, and V. On the other hand, activated factor XI eluted from celite fails to activate intact platelets. Thus contact activation does not activate platelets (Horowitz, 1964; Horowitz and Papayoanou, 1968).

D. The Platelet Release Reaction

Our studies (Horowitz and Papayoanou, 1967) and those of Hardisty and Hutton (1966) suggest that platelet factor 3 activation (and release) takes place as part of a generalized platelet release reaction. The substances released from platelets (or altered in their activity) in response to a variety of stimulants are listed in Table 1. Some substances capable of eliciting all or part of the "release reaction" are listed in Table 2. While the situation in in vivo hemostasis is a complex one, with many activities capable of activating platelet factor 3 being present, viz, collagen, ADP, biologically active amines, and thrombin, the role of ADP in this reaction appears to be a central one.

There is some indication that the release reaction may occur in two phases, the first being associated with reversible ADP-induced aggregation. If this stimulus is sufficiently strong then there is release of large amounts of endogenous ADP (Macmillan, 1966). Most platelet factor 3 activation appears to occur during this second, irreversible phase. Many of the agents appearing in Table 1 also appear in Table 2 providing a setting where self perpetuating reactions leading to primary and secondary hemostasis can take place.

E. Clot Retraction and Thrombosthenin

Bettex-Galland and Lüscher (1960, 1961) extracted a protein fraction from human platelets with properties strikingly similar to muscle actomyosin. This protein comprises 15% of total platelet protein and is very likely responsible for consolidation of the hemostatic platelet plug. Thrombosthenin has been identified as acting on a system of microtubulus under the platelet membrane (White et al. 1966) and has also been found in the platelet membrane. It has ATP-ase activity which is calcium and magnesium dependent. Antibodies to thrombosthenin specifically inhibit clot retraction (Nachman and Marcus, 1966). Thrombosthenin contraction is believed to result from high concentrations of thrombin and thus takes place after the loose primary hemostatic plug has arrested initial bleeding, probably at or shortly before the time that sufficient thrombin has evolved to induce fibrin clot formation.

VI. Morphological Aspects of Hemostasis

A. Ultrastructure of the Platelet

Platelets are small disc-shaped fragments of megakaryocyte cytoplasm, usually 2–4 μ in diameter and thus the low resolving power of the light microscope does not permit adequate visualization of their internal structure. Recent studies with the electron microscope, both by shadow casting (Rebuck et al. 1960) and ultra-thin sectioning (Rodman and Mason, 1967) have defined platelet morphology. Each platelet is surrounded by a limiting membrane, and contains mitochondria, vacuoles, glycogen particles, and dense granules. Serotonin has been identified in the darkly staining granules (Tranzer et al. 1966). A series of microtubules circumvent the platelet (White et al. 1966). These structures may play a role both in clot retraction and in centralization of granules in response to ADP and clot formation (Rodman and Painter, 1967).

B. Morphology of Platelet Plug Formation

By examining experimentally damaged blood vessels, Zucker (1947) has established the importance of the platelet plug in primary hemostasis. Light microscopic observations of microincised mesenteric vessels have demonstrated initial local vasoconstriction, followed by rapid formation of a platelet plug at the site of injury. Using similar techniques, Hugues (1962) and Bounameaux (1957) demonstrated that platelets initially adhere to traumatized mesenterial fibers, which have subsequently been shown by electron microscopy to have the characteristic cross-striations of collagen (Kjaerheim and Hovig, 1962). Platelets in contact with collagen lose their internal structure (degranulation), while their limiting membranes remain intact. These changes occur in 1% EDTA PRP indicating independence from calcium ions.

Platelet aggregation follows platelet adhesion to collagen and results in vessel occlusion. Platelets clumped by lows doses of ADP appear to have intact membranes and a full complement of granules, suggesting that ADP clumped platelets do not undergo the release of additional ADP (fig. 7). High doses of ADP cause large platelet aggregates which are tightly packed and appear degranulated in some areas (fig. 8). However, other cross-sections of the same platelet aggregates show areas of concentrated granules and mitochondria, and marked pseudopod formation. Thus degranulation may be only apparent and represent sections through platelet pseudopods.

A similar morphologic picture is seen in the center of an in vivo hemostatic plug even 45 seconds after injury (Kjaerheim and Hovig, 1962). Platelet clumps produced by low doses of thrombin (Rodman and Mason, 1962) also have a similar structure. Thus there is suggestive morphologic evidence that the platelet plug may be propagated by ADP release from aggregating platelets. The platelet plug 30 minutes after injury has a homogeneous appearance by light microscopy, which was interpreted as platelet fusion. Electron microscopy of this mass (Kjaerheim and Hovig, 1962), reveals that although platelets are degranulated, they have not fused and indeed plasma membranes are intact. In vitro studies with thrombin-treated platelet-rich plasma suggest that these morphologic changes are a result of thrombin action and may be the last step in achieving primary hemostasis.

C. Platelet-fibrin Interactions

Secondary hemostasis is achieved by blood coagulation and fibrin formation in the static column of blood behind the hemostatic platelet plug. Light microscopy reveals erythrocytes, leucocytes and platelets diffusely enmeshed in a fibrin network (Zucker, 1947), a picture similar to that found when whole blood is allowed to clot in a test tube. Organization of the sealed vessel then occurs with fibrous tissue forming the permanent seal.

D. Morphology of Clot Retraction

Following in vitro blood coagulation, the clot retracts and serum is expressed. The function of clot retraction is not clear and Budtz-Olsen

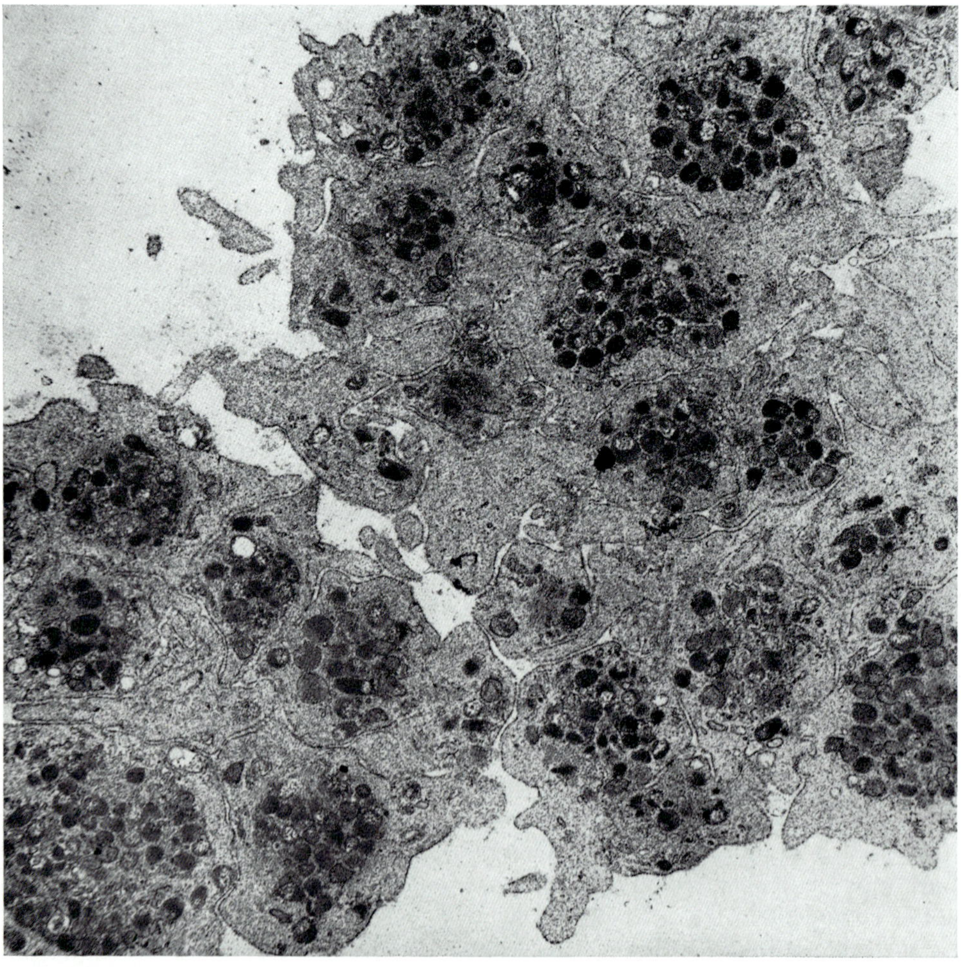

Fig. 7. Aggregation of platelets in citrated plasma with 10^{-5} M ADP. Aggregates are small and individual platelets appear to posses intact granules.

(1951) suggests that it may be a phylogenetic relic which has been maintained in spite of the development of more complicated and more efficient hemostatic mechanisms. Light microscopic examination of stained sections of retracting clots led Budtz-Olsen to conclude that platelets adhere to fibrin strands and to each other via cytoplasmic pseudopods. Clot retraction was felt to be a result of contraction of these cytoplasmic strands as platelets appeared to pull together in the retracting clot. Contraction of fibrin strands was never seen.

Ultrastructural studies suggest that platelets adhere to fibrin particles. White et al. (1966) find fibrin in close association with platelet microtubules and suggest that these organelles may play a role in clot retraction. The ultrastructure of isolated thrombosthenin, the contractile platelet substance, is quite similar to microfilaments within platelets (Zucker-Fränklin et al. 1967).

VII. Summary and Conclusion

There is general agreement as to the broad outlines of the hemostatic scheme, though interpretation of the mechanisms and sequence of specific events will remain in dispute pending further work in this active area of experimentation. In response to injury the body calls upon systems of cellular and fluid hemostasis which have evolved in repeating

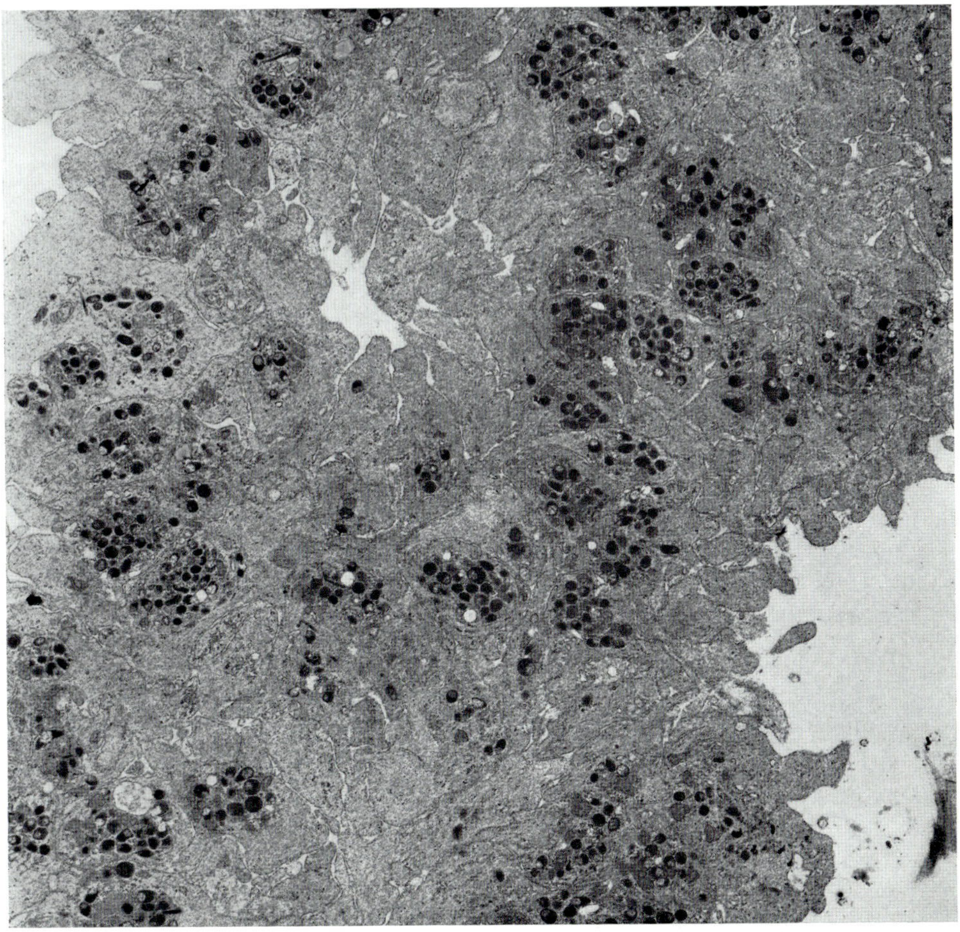

Fig. 8. Aggregation of platelets in citrated plasma with 2×10^{-4} M ADP. Aggregates are larger and in some areas platelets appear to be degranulated. This may be a false impression resulting from pseudopod formation. See text for full discussion.

patterns throughout the phylogenetic tree. These systems borrow activities and substances freely from each other, so that a complex web of interactions is to be anticipated.

Denuded collagen is now believed to trigger the sequence. Platelets rapidly adhere, perhaps in an attempt to engulf this foreign substance. In so doing, they degranulate, releasing a bundle of active agents (Table 1). While relatively few platelets may be involved in the initial adhesion, the released material, particularly ADP, is itself capable of inducing massive platelet aggregation. Up to this stage the reaction is potentially reversible. However, sufficiently high concentrations of ADP may lead to the second phase of platelet release, including additional nucleotides and platelet factor 3. Alternatively, small amounts of thrombin may evolve in the platelet plasmatic atmosphere and contribute to irreversible platelet changes. The platelet plug propagates to occlude any bleeding tear; primary hemostasis is achieved. In the now stagnant plasma behind the primary plug coagulation factors are activated and interact with the available platelet factor 3, both at the platelet surface and in the plasma. Prothrombin is activated to give large amounts of thrombin which in turn initiates the contraction of thrombosthenin and consolidation of the primary plug, and in addition leads to the development of the supporting fibrin clot.

Table 1. Substances and Activities Released by Platelets in Response to Thrombin and Other Agents.

1. Biologically active amines
   a. Serotonin
   b. Adrenaline
   c. Noradrenaline
   d. Histamine
2. Adenine nucleotides
   a. ATP
   b. ADP
   c. AMP
3. Amino acids
4. Potassium ions
5. Proteins
   a. Acid phosphatase
6. Platelet factor 3
7. Platelet factor 4

Table 2. Substance Capable of Eliciting All or Part of the Platelet Release Reaction.

1. Collagen
2. Biologically active amines
   a. Serotonin
   b. Adrenaline
   c. Noradrenaline
   d. Histamine
3. Proteolytic enzymes
   a. Thrombin
   b. Trypsin
   c. Reptilase
4. Aggregated gamma globulin
5. Latex particles
6. Celite or kaolin
7. ADP
8. Bacterial endotoxins
9. Antigen-antibody complex

Table 3. Morphological Aspects of Viscous Metamorphosis.

1. Platelet swelling – transformation of discs to spiny spheres
2. Concentration of granules to the central part of the platelets
3. Aggregation and enlargement of aggregates
4. Degranulation – loss of granular structure
5. Tight packing of aggregated platelets with mosaic formation
6. Loss of external platelet membranes and ballooning

References

Alagille, D., and Soulier, J. P. (1957). *Rev. Franc. Etudes Clin. Biol. 2,* 231.

Berman, H. J., (1961). *In:* "Anticoagulants and Fibrinolysis". (R. L. MacMillan and J. F. Mustard, eds.), p. 35, Lea and Febiger, Philadelphia.

Bettex-Galland, M., and Lüscher, E. F. (1960). *Thromb. Diath. Haemorrhag. 4,* 178.

Bettex-Galland, M., and Lüscher, E. F. (1961). *Biochim. Biophys. Acta 49,* 536.

Born, G. V. R. (1967). *Federation Proc. 26,* 115.

Born, G. V. R., and Cross, M. J. (1963). *J. Physiol. 168,* 178.

Born, G. V. R., and Cross, M. J. (1964). *J. Physiol. 170,* 397.

Bounameaux, Y. (1957). *Rev. Franc. Etudes Clin. Biol. 2,* 52.

Bounameaux, Y. (1959). *C. R. Soc. Biol. 153,* 865.

Bryan, F. T., Robinson, C. W., Gilbert, C. F., and Langdell, R. D. (1964). *Science 144,* 1146.

Budtz-Olsen, O. E. (1951). "Clot Retraction". Blackwell Scientific Publications, Oxford, England.

Cross, M. J. (1964). *Thromb. Diath. Haemorrhag. 12,* 524.

Cuthbertson, W. F. J., and Mills, D. C. B. (1963). *J. Physiol. 168,* 29.

Davey, M. G., and Lüscher, E. F. (1966). *In:* "Platelet Protein". Proc. of Federation of European Biochem. Soc. 3rd Meeting, Warsaw. In press.

Deykin, D. (1967). *New Eng. J. Med. 276,* 622.

Eberth, J. C., and Schimmelbusch, C. (1885). *Virchows Arch. 103,* 39.

Esnouf, P. (1965). *Thromb. Diath. Haermorrhag. Suppl. 17,* 103.

Fantl, P., and Ward, H. A. (1958). *Austral. J. Exptl. Biol. 36,* 499.

Gaarder, A., Jonsen, J., Laland, S., Hellem, A., and Owren, P. A. (1961). *Nature (London) 192,* 531.

Goksen, M., and Yunis, E. (1964). *Nature 200,* 590.

Grette, J. (1962). *Acta Physiol. Scand. Suppl. 56,* 195.

Hardisty, R. M., and Hutton, R. A. (1966). *Brit. J. Haematol. 12,* 764.

Hardy, W. B. (1892). *J. Physiol. 13,* 165.

Haslam, R. J. (1964). *Nature 202,* 765.

Heilbrunn, L. V. (1961). *In:* "Functions of the Blood". (R. G. Macfarlane and A. T. H. Robb-Smith, eds.), pp. 283—301. Academic Press, New York.

Hellem, A. J. (1960). *Scand. J. Clin. Lab. Invest. Suppl. 12,* 51.

Hellem, A. J., and Owren, P. A. (1964). *Acta Haematol. 31,* 230.

Hjort, P. F., Rapaport, S. I., and Owren, P. A. (1955). *Blood 10,* 1139.

Horowitz, H. I. (1964). *Thromb. Diath. Haemorrhag. Suppl. 17,* 243.

Horowitz, H. I., and Fujimoto, M. M. (1965). *Proc. Soc. Exptl. Biol. Med. 119,* 487.

Horowitz, H. I., and Papayoanou, M. F. (1967). *J. Lab. Clin. Med. 69,* 1003.

Horowitz, H. I., and Papayoanou, M. F. (1968). *Thromb. Diath. Haemorrhag. 19,* 18.

Hovig, T. (1963). *Thromb. Diath. Haemorrhag. 9,* 264.

Hugues, J. (1960). *C. R. Soc. Biol. 154,* 866.

Hugues, J. (1962). *Thromb. Diath. Haemorrhag. 3,* 177.

Hugues, J., and Lapiere, C. M. (1964). *Thromb. Diath. Haemorrhag. 11,* 322.

Iatrides, P. G., and Ferguson, J. H. (1965). *Thromb. Diath. Haemorrhag. 13,* 114.

Johnson, S. A., Balboa, R. S., Pederson, H. J., and Buckley, M. (1965). *Thromb. Diath. Haemorrhag. 13,* 65.

Jones, P., and Wooley, D. A. (1967). *Nature.* In press.

Kjaerheim, A., and Hovig, T. (1962). *Thromb. Diath. Haemorrhag. 7,* 1.

Levin, J., and Bang, F. B. (1966a). *Federation Proc. 28,* 497.

Levin, J., and Bang, F. B. (1966b). *Blood 28,* 985.

Lüscher, E. F. (1956). *Vox Sang. 1,* 133.

Macmillan, D. C. (1966). *Nature 211,* 140.

Marcus, A. J., and Zucker, M. B. (1965). "The Physiology of Blood Platelets". Grune & Stratton, New York.

Marcus, A. J., Zucker-Franklin, D., Safier, L. B., and Ullman, H. L. (1966). *J. Clin. Invest. 45,* 14.

McLean, J. R., Maxwell, R. E., and Huller, D. (1964). *Nature 202,* 605.

Mitchel, J. R. A., and Sharp, A. A. (1964). *Brit. J. Haematol. 10,* 78.

Murphy, E. A., Hegardt, B., Rowsell, H. C., and MacMillan, R. L. (1964). *J. Lab. Clin. Med. 64,* 548.

Mustard, J. F., Glynn, M. F., Nishizawa, E. F., and Packham, M. A. (1967). *Federation Proc. 26,* 106.

Nachman, R. L., and Marcus, A. J. (1966). *J. Clin. Invest. 45,* 1051.

Nachman, R. L., Marcus, A. J., and Zucker-Franklin, D. (1964). *Blood 24,* 853.

Niewiarowski, S., Bankowski, E., and Rogowicka, I. (1965). *Thromb. Diath. Haemorrhag. 14,* 387.

O'Brien, J. R. (1955). *Brit. J. Haematol. 1,* 223.

O'Brien, J. R. (1962). *J. Clin. Pathol. 15,* 452.

O'Brien, J. R. (1963). *J. Clin. Pathol. 16,* 223.

O'Brien, J. R. (1964). *J. Clin. Pathol. 17,* 275.

Rebuck, J. W., Riddle, J. M., Johnson, S. A., Monto, R. W., and Sturrock, R. M. (1960). *Henry Ford Hosp. Med. Bull. 8,* 273.

Robinson, C. A., Mason, R. G., and Wagner, R. H. (1963). *Proc. Soc. Exptl. Biol. Med. 113,* 857.

Rodman, N. F., and Mason, R. G. (1967). *Federation Proc. 26,* 95.

Rodman, W. F., and Painter, J. C. (1967). *Federation Proc. 26,* 320.

Roskam, J. (1923). *Arch. Intern. Physiol. 20,* 241.

Roskam, J. (1966). *Thromb. Diath. Haemorrhag. Suppl. 22,* 317.

Salmon, J., and Bounameaux, Y. (1957). *Arch. Intern. Physiol. Biochem. 65,* 632.

Salzman, E. W., Chambers, D. A., and Neri, L. L. (1966). *Thromb. Diath. Haemorrhag. 15,* 52.

Schmitz, H., Schliepen, T., and Gross, R. (1962). *Klin. Wochschr. 40,* 13.

Seligman, M., Goudemand, B., Jonin, A., Bernard, J., and Grabar, P. (1957). *Rev. Hematol. 12,* 302.

Shinowara, G. Y. (1961). *Acta Haematol. Jap. 24,* 716.

Spaet, T. H., and Lejnieks, I. (1966). *Thromb. Diath. Haemorrhag. 15,* 36.

Spaet, T. H., and Zucker, M. B. (1964). *Am. J. Physiol. 206,* 1967.

Spaet, T. H., Erickson, R. B., and Spielvogel, A. R. (1967). *In:* "Physiology of Hemostasis and Thrombosis" (S. A. Johnson and W. H. Seegers, eds.) pp. 154—178. Charles C. Thomas, Springfield, Ill.

Tait, J. (1911). *J. Marine Biol. 9,* 191.

White, J. G., Silver, M. J., and Krivit, W. (1966). *Blood 28,* 984.

Tranzer, J. P., Da Prada, M., and Phetscher, A. (1966). *Nature 212,* 1574.

Zucker, M. B. (1947). *Am. J. Physiol. 148,* 275.

Zucker, M. B. (1961). *Sci. Am. 204,* 58.

Zucker, M. B., and Borrelli, J. (1959). *J. Appl. Physiol. 14,* 575.

Zucker, M. B., and Borrelli, J. (1962). *Proc. Soc. Exptl. Biol. Med. 109,* 779.

Zucker-Franklin, D., Nachman, R. L., and Marcus, A. J. (1967). *Federation Proc. 26,* 705.

Bleeding Time Techniques

Christian F. Borchgrevink

I. Introduction

Normal hemostasis in small vessels depends on the building of hemostatic plugs composed of platelets. The bleeding time which is an expression of hemostasis in such vessels measures all the factors necessary for the formation of efficient platelet plug. These factors have been thoroughly discussed by Horowitz in the preceeding section on p. 412.

Several methods have been introduced to determine the bleeding time in man. The majority are variations of the Duke, of the Ivy, or the immersion methods and only these will be described in some detail.

II. Methods

A. Method of Duke

In 1910, Duke described his method for measuring the bleeding time which has since been universally adopted. He made a small cut in the lobe of the ear, without mentioning the depth of the cut or the instrument he used. The blood was carefully adsorbed onto a filter paper every 30 seconds. The bleeding during the first half of a minute should make a blot of 1–2 cm in diameter. Normal bleeding time was less than 3 minutes. He stated that within certain limits the time did not depend on the size of the cut.

Dishoeck and Jongkees (1940) considered that the adhesion of the lips of the incision might prevent bleeding. By pressing a thin metal plate with a hole 4 mm in diameter against the ear, part of the skin protruded through the hole and could be cut off by a razor blade. Thus an open wound was produced. The mean normal bleeding time in 450 determinations was 3 minutes and 25 seconds. No range was given.

Although it is generally stated that the size of the cut is of little importance, this is probably not correct when estimating small deviations from the normal. It is therefore recommended that a puncture 3 mm deep be made in the lobe with a spring lancet or another sharp instrument. The blood should be blotted with a piece of filter paper every 15–30 seconds without touching the surface of the ear. A normal bleeding time is considered to be less than 3 to $3^1/_2$ minutes.

B. Method of Ivy

Ivy et al. (1941) felt that variations in the capillary tone might influence the bleeding time and make the test less suitable in certain pathological conditions. They therefore developed the following method: A blood pressure cuff was placed on the upper arm and inflated to 40 mm Hg. With a mechanical stylet set at a uniform depth ($2^1/_2$ mm, or 3 mm) a puncture was made on the forearm near the elbow over the pronator muscles. Blood was removed every 10 seconds with a filter paper. A second puncture was made 5 minutes after the first puncture had stopped bleeding. If the first puncture did not bleed, no bleeding time was recorded. The test was repeated until 3 punctures had bled. The average was recorded as the person's bleeding time. The upper normal limit was 240 seconds. However, several recordings longer than 125 seconds were considered pathological.

Hjort and Stormorken (1957) introduced a modification. Instead of using a stylet, they used a new surgical blade and made 3 horizontal cuts 2 cm apart, 1 mm deep and 3–4 mm long. The mean bleeding time was 6.2 minutes with a range of 2–$12^1/_2$ minutes.

C. "Immersion" Method

The concept behind the immersion method is to maintain a constant temperature on the skin and in the environment. The hand is immersed for a few minutes into a beaker containing normal saline at 37° C. A wound is made on the tip of the finger 6 mm deep and 2 mm wide (Copley and Lalich, 1942), or 4 mm deep in the hypotenar eminence (Adelson and Crosby, 1957). In the latter method a blood pressure cuff inflated to 40 mm Hg on the upper arm was used, and normal bleeding time was less than 7 minutes. Values more than $8^1/_2$ minutes were definitely abnormal. With the method of Copley and Lalich (1942) the normal value was less than 3 minutes, and more than 6 minutes was definitely prolonged.

D. Aspirin Tolerance Test

Quick (1966) observed that the Duke bleeding time in many normals became prolonged 2 hours after the intake of 1.3 gm of aspirin. He suggested that this was due to a depression of a plasma factor necessary for normal hemostasis in small vessels. In patients with mild von Willebrand's disease even 0.65 gm of aspirin significantly prolonged the bleeding time. Quick feels that the ingestion of 0.65 gm aspirin 2 hours prior to performing the bleeding time test increases its sensitivity and consequently its usefulness.

E. Blood Loss During the Bleeding Time

The skin bleeding time test may yield other information in addition to the duration of bleeding. Several authors have shown that not only a prolonged bleeding time but also the intensity of the bleeding and the total blood loss may be of value in distinguishing between normal individuals and patients with hemorrhagic diathesis. In the immersion method Adelson and Crosby (1957) hemolysed the red cells with saponin and measured the hemoglobin content in the beaker. Knowing the patients' hemoglobin value and the amount of saline in the beaker, the blood loss could be calculated.

De Nicola and Candura (1961) in a modified Duke test let the blood be sucked into capillary tubes 1 mm in diameter and 90 mm long every 30 seconds, or during intense bleeding every 15 seconds. The tubes were placed vertically on plasteline.

Willoughby and Allington (1961) used the Ivy bleeding time, eluted the blood from the filter paper and measured the hemoglobin. Knowing the hemoglobin of the test person, blood loss could be calculated.

F. Resistance of the Hemostatic Plug

After bleeding has stopped in a standard bleeding time test a new bleeding may sometimes be provoked by applying pressure. Lewalle et al. (1959) tested the bleeding time in the forearm without pressure. Three minutes after arrest of bleeding 40 mm of stasis was applied. Copley and Lalich (1942) used a pressure of 100 mm Hg 30 seconds to 50 minutes after arrest of bleeding.

There was no correlation between the bleeding time and the resistance of the hemostatic plug.

G. Secondary Bleeding Time

The fact that patients with severe clotting defects have a normal bleeding time but a tendency to profuse and prolonged late bleeding, was the basis for the secondary bleeding time test of Borchgrevink and Waaler (1958). The modified Ivy bleeding time is carried out as described by Hjort and Stormorken (1957) (section B), the cuts being slightly longer, about 10 mm long and 1 mm deep. Twenty-four hours later the crusts are gently removed without cutting new vessels, and a new bleeding is provoked. This is measured in the same way as the primary bleeding time.

In normal persons the secondary bleeding time was always shorter than the primary with a median value about $2^1/_2$ minutes and an upper limit of 6 minutes. The secondary bleeding time was prolonged in patients with defects in their intrinsic clotting system and was proportional to the clotting defect.

The test is clinically of limited value in differentiating between hemorrhagic disorders, since more sensitive tests are at hand. Its importance, however, lies in underlining the difference between the primary and the secondary hemostatic mechanism, the former being independent and the latter dependent on plasma clotting.

III. Comments

The bleeding time test had for a long time the reputation of being of little value because many variables would interfere with the result, i. e. the thickness of the skin, the surrounding temperature, the instrument used and the depth of the cut or the puncture. Nevertheless, in experienced hands, the bleeding time is remarkable stable from day to day in one individual. Occasionally a single cut may unexplainably give a prolonged time in normals. It is therefore recommended to use three cuts.

The bleeding time is a test for platelet function, being prolonged when there are too few or too many platelets; when they are qualitatively defective (thrombasthenia); when there is a defect in release of platelet factor 3 (thrombocytopathia); when the surface of the platelets is coated with protein as in multiple myeloma or foreign material (dextran). In addition, there is good evidence that a plasma factor is necessary for normal primary hemostasis, and when this factor is lacking (von Willebrand's disease?) the bleeding time is prolonged. It may be prolonged in uremia, leucemia, cirrhosis of the liver and other serious diseases.

It is slightly prolonged in anemia, and it has been postulated that red cells are necessary for normal hemostasis (Hellem et al. 1959). It is slightly longer in females than in males, which may, however, only reflect the difference in hemoglobin value between the two sexes.

It is normal in clotting defects and during anticoagulant treatment and in non-thrombocytopenic purpura. Large doses of heparin will prolong it (Hjort et al. 1960).

The methods of choice for clinical application are the Duke or the Ivy bleeding time, or one of their modifications. They are both reliable and easy to carry out. In patients with hemorrhagic disorders applying local hemostasis may create a problem when using the Duke bleeding time. The Ivy bleeding time, preferred in this laboratory, is probably more sensitive and this may or may not be an advantage. In patients with von Willebrand's disease it is possible to normalize the Duke bleeding time by fresh plasma or plasma concentrates with only a small reduction of the Ivy bleeding time (Borchgrevink et al. 1963). There is evidence that such patients do not bleed excessively after operations (Nilsson et al. 1963), and if this is so, the prolonged Ivy bleeding cannot be considered a useful guide in preoperative evaluation.

Both tests are sensitive to technical variations. It is recommended that each investigator or laboratory determine their normal range rather than rely on the values given in the literature.

It is likely that measuring the amount of blood loss during the bleeding time test will yield valuable information in doubtful cases of hemorrhagic disorders. It may also be useful when evaluating new hemostatic drugs. It is possible that making the test more sensitive by using aspirin or other drugs may be of importance in selected cases, but so far there is no real evidence for this conjecture.

The resistance of the hemostatic plug and the secondary bleeding time probably have no place in the clinical diagnosis of bleeding disorders.

References

Adelson, E., and Crosby, W. H. (1957). *Acta Haematol. 18,* 281.

Borchgrevink, Chr. F., and Waaler, B. A. (1958). *Acta Med. Scand. 162,* 361.

Borchgrevink, Chr. F., Egeberg, O., Godal, H. Chr., and Hjort, P. F. (1963). *Acta Med. Scand. 173,* 235.

Copley, A. L., and Lalich, J. J. (1942). *J. Clin. Invest. 21,* 145.

Dishoeck, H. A. E. V., and Jongkees, L. B. W. (1940). *Klin. Wochschr. 19,* 1216.

Duke, W. W. (1910). *J. Amer. Med. Assoc. 55,* 1185.

Hellem, A. J., Borchgrevink, Chr. F., and Ames, S. B. (1961). *Brit. J. Haematol. 7,* 42.

Hjort, P., and Stormorken, H. (1957). *Scand. J. Clin. Lab. Invest. 9, Suppl. 29,* 86.

Hjort, P., Borchgrevink, Chr. F., Iversen, O. H., and Stormorken, H. (1960). *Thromb. Diath. Haemorrhag. 4,* 389.

Ivy, A. C., Nelson, D., and Bucher, G. (1941). *J. Lab. Clin. Med. 26,* 1812.

Lewalle, J., Bounameaux, Y., and Roskam, J. (1959). *Thromb. Diath. Haemorrhag. 3,* 165.

Nicola, de, P., and Candura, M. D. (1961). *Hemostase 1,* 113.

Nilsson, I. M., Magnusson, S., and Borchgrevink, Chr. F. (1963). *Thromb. Diath. Haemorrhag. 10,* 223.

Quick, A. J. (1966). *Am. J. Med. Sci. 252,* 265.

Willoughby, M. L. N., and Allington, M. J. (1961). *J. Clin. Pathol. 14,* 381.

Tests for Capillary Fragility and Resistance

Christian F. Borchgrevink

I. Introduction

Tests for capillary fragility or capillary resistance have gained little popularity over the years and not without reason. Few, if any, of the tests for the hemostatic function are influenced by so many uncontrollable variables. Little is known of the role which small vessels have in normal hemostasis and even less of their role in hemorrhagic disorders. This lack of deeper understanding and knowledge is reflected in the lack of enthusiasm in accepting methods available for testing capillary fragility.

Two principally different methods, with many modifications, are in common use, and they show good correlation (Kramar, 1962).

II. The Pressure Method (Torniquet Test, Rumpel-Leede, Gothlin, Hess)

The principle of the method is to increase the intracapillary pressure for a period of time. This may lead to leakage of red cells from the vessels either in form of rhexis bleeding or diapedesis through "intact" vessel walls.

Procedure

A blood pressure cuff is placed on the upper arm and inflated to a certain pressure. In the various published methods the pressure applied has varied from midway between systolic and diastolic pressure to a prefixed level usually 90 or 100 mm of Hg. According to different authorities, the time of pressure application also varies from a few minutes to 15 minutes. A 1–5 cm circle is drawn on the volar side of the forearm. The pressure is released and after waiting from 2 to 15 minutes, the number of petechiae within the circle are counted.

In our laboratory employing 90 mm of Hg of pressure, 5 minutes of pressure time, a 5 cm circle and a recirculation time of 5 minutes the normal value is less than 10 petechiae. More than 20 petechiae are considered abnormal.

Not only the number of petechiae, but also their size should be noted. Petechiae of more than 1 mm in diameter are usually not seen in normal patients (Stavem, 1965).

III. The Suction Method

The principle of the method is to observe the appearance of petechiae when a negative pressure is applied on a certain area of the skin. The pressure at which petechiae start to appear (the critical pressure) is an expression of the capillary resistance. Several different types of apparatus have been designed for the purpose (resistometer, petechiometer). The test may be carried out in different areas of the skin, but as the capillary resistance varies from area to area, it is recommended that the volar side of the forearm be employed.

A suction cup, 2 cm in diameter (Brown, 1949), is placed a few cm below the bend of the elbow and a suction of 100 mm Hg is applied for 1 minute. If no petechiae appear, the pressure is released, the cup is placed on an adjacent area of the skin and a negative pressure of 200 mm Hg is applied. If this does not result in the appearance of petechiae, the procedure is repeated at 300 mm Hg. The "critical pressure", i. e. the negative pressure necessary to produce petechiae in normals has been estimated at 142.5 mm.

Gough (1962) utilized the interscapular area with a suction time of 30 seconds.

Smith (1958) used progressively increasing negative pressure starting with 100 mm Hg, and increments of 25 mm Hg. The suction bell was $2^1/_2$ cm in diameter and the pressure time 15 seconds. Below 100 mm Hg decrements of 20 mm Hg were applied on adjacent skin areas. The normal value for appearance of petechiae in 76 persons was 197 mm Hg ± 7 mm Hg.

In an extensive review, Kramar (1962) recommended the proximal volar aspect of the forearm as a testing area employing a transparent suction cup of 7 mm in inner diameter with a 1 minute suction time starting at 150 mm Hg and increasing or decreasing the pressure.

IV. Comments

Capillary resistance falls during menstruation. If tested at other times during the menstrual cycle, the capillary resistance of females seem not to be different from that observed in males. Diurnal variations have been described and the resistance may decrease as the day advances. Most workers find no change with age, except for a high capillary resistance in infants. However, Gough (1962) showed convincingly a rectilinear decrease with age from 380 mm Hg at the age of 20, to 150 mm Hg at the age of 75 years. He employed the interscapular area, while the majority of investigators preferred the forearm.

Capillary resistance is decreased in vitamin C deficiency whereas it is increased with steroids, oestrogens and bioflavinoids.

The tests for capillary fragility are of little value. They are applied in clinical medicine for the diagnosis of hemorrhagic disorders. The test can be positive in thrombocytopenia and in qualitative platelet defects, von Willebrand's disease, non-thrombocytopenic purpura, anaphylactic purpura and fibrinolytic states.

The pressure method is simple but sometimes uncomfortable to the patient. It is crude, and the results cannot easily be quantitatively recorded.

The suction method is slightly more complicated since a suction device is needed. It has the advantage that several areas can be tested at the same or nearly the same time. Changes in capillary resistance are more easy to follow with the suction method than with the pressure method since a distinct critical pressure value is recorded. In tense and nervous people there may be spasm of the arterioles resulting in a falsely high resistance particularly in the first test, which therefore should be regarded with suspicion if a particularly high value is found. For experimental work the suction method is definitely superior to the pressure method.

References

Brown, E. E. (1949). *J. Lab. Clin. Med. 34,* 1714.
Gough, K. R. (1962). *Brit. Med. J. 1,* 21.
Kramar, J. (1962). *Blood 20,* 83.
Smith, A. F. (1958). *Acta Med. Scand. 164,* 341.
Stavem, P. (1965). *Scand. J. Clin. Lab. Invest. 17,* 607.

Platelet Count Techniques, Platelet Adhesiveness and Aggregation Tests

J. R. O'Brien

I. Introduction

Routine tests are carried out in a hospital laboratory because they are useful to the clinician but the distinction between a routine test and a research investigation is imprecise and depends upon the clinical importance of the information and on the acceptance of the test which includes such things as fashion, cost and complexity. There is an increasing awareness of the clinical importance of platelet function and at present, adhesiveness tests are more than research exercises and less than universally accepted routine tests.

The concept assumed in all platelet adhesiveness tests is simple, obvious and attractive. In both haemostasis and thrombosis platelets stick to the relevant site and pile up i. e. stick to platelets already stuck; this mass becomes consolidated and plays a vital part in the clinical event. A closer look reveals at once a great lack of precise information about these events. To what kind of surface in the body do platelets stick? What forces hold platelets to the vessel wall or to each other? Does the microenvironment a few hundred Angstroms from a platelet bear any relation to that in the general circulation? What is the contribution of red cells and of plasma to these events? How great a part does the local hydrodynamic situation play? If the systemic platelets are abnormal during a thrombotic episode, is this abnormality permanent, or only episodic? The list of unanswered questions is endless and it is not appropriate to discuss these problems further here, but without answers the design of tests is bound to be largely empirical. So it is proposed to enumerate a few of the tests at present available, to describe some of these in some detail, to consider the mechanism they may be measuring and their possible usefulness both to the clinician and to the research worker.

II. Platelet Count Techniques

Since platelet counting is an essential part of many platelet tests, it will be considered first. This enumeration is more difficult and less dependable than, for example the white cell count, and no agreed technique has emerged. The details of blood collection and techniques, as well as observer error, will all affect the result. In the author's laboratory, platelet counts, usually in duplicate, are performed as follows: One part of blood is diluted into 19 parts of Feissly and Lüdin's fluid (1949) (3 gm cocaine hydrochloride, 0.2 gm NaCl in 100 ml water) using a white cell bead pipette (it might be better, but more expensive, to use a bulk dilution technique). After allowing an hour for haemolysis, the pipettes are shaken and a counting chamber filled. This is put in a moist atmosphere (e.g. Petri dish with wet blotting paper) for 30 minutes for the platelets to settle. Using phase contrast illumination at least 200 platelets are counted and from the area counted the number per cmm is worked out. Whenever possible the pipettes are coded and muddled so that the counter cannot know which pipette he is counting. The advantage of this method is that the platelets are swollen and sphered and the red cells lysed.

Nygaard (1933) separates the platelets from the red cells by sedimentation in the diluent but uses 1 ml of blood. Brecher and Cronkite (1950) use ammonium oxalate as a haemolytic agent and Rees and Ecker (1923) use citrate and formaline and dye but the red cells are not haemolysed. Electronic counting is also possible. A special Coulter particle counter (Bull et al. 1965) and the Celloscope probably give reliable results on patients' blood but counting platelets after various manipulations such as passage through a glass column may well prove less reliable. There are many difficulties in electronic counting. The small size of the platelet requires special modifications to exclude too large and too small particles and the use of a small aperture in the Coulter Counter; thus the true platelet signals are differentiated from "noise" in the circuit and small contaminating particles in the diluting fluid. The greatest problem, however, involves the separation of the platelets from the red cells. This can be done by gravity, or by centrifugation of either the blood or preferably a dilution of the blood. The counts obtained then have to be adjusted for the volume of red cells displaced, and this is not a simple relation to the packed cell volume. Methods are considered by Dacie & Lewis (1968). The author uses Bull's (1965) method but he additionally swells the platelets in cocaine.

III. Platelet Adhesiveness Tests

A. Borchgrevink's in Vivo Adhesiveness Test (1960)

Principle: Platelet counts are made from venous blood and from blood issuing from superficial bleeding time cuts. If the count

from the cuts is lower than the venous count, then the difference is presumably due to loss of platelets by adhesion to the lips of the cut.
Method: With a sphygmomanometer inflated on the upper arm to 40 mm Hg two or more cuts 10 mm long and 1 mm deep are made on the volar aspect of the forearm. Two platelet counts are taken from freshly issuing blood during the first two minutes of bleeding. The percentage difference between the mean of the skin cut counts and venous counts is called the "percentage of adhesive platelets".
Critique: This method emphasises the part that platelets play in haemostasis but in the author's experience as well as in Borchgrevink's see his Fig. 1) the percentage is usually proportional to the bleeding time. This test is probably poorly reproducable and thus usually adds no further information to that obtained from a simple bleeding time.

B. The Wright Rotator Method (1942)

Principle: Heparinized blood is rolled round a small flask for 20 or more minutes; the difference between the mean platelet counts before and after this treatment expressed as a percentage of the initial count, i.e. the percentage of platelets lost, is taken as a measure of adhesiveness.
Method: All surfaces are siliconized except the flasks. Five ml of blood are heparinized, final concentration 4 units/ml and a 2 ml aliquot is delivered into each of two special flasks clipped onto a wheel rotating at 3 rpm. Two initial pre-treatment platelet counts are taken and after 20 minutes two counts are taken from each flask carefully sampling the middle of the pool of blood. Further counts may be taken up to 80 minutes but add little further information. The flask must be thoroughly, identically and ritualistically cleaned. The details are probably unimportant providing the surface has exactly the same treatment each time. If "I" is the initial count and "F" the final count then the percentage of platelets lost i. e. the "adhesiveness" $= \frac{I-F}{I}$ 100.
Critique: This test is probably useful since it has been reported to be abnormally high in thrombotic conditions such as post-operative patients (Wright 1942), myocardial infarction (McDonald and Edgill, 1957) and homocystinuria (McDonald et al. 1964). There is however, considerable overlap between abnormals and the normals and this test is claimed to distinguish only between the two groups and usually cannot identify abnormal individuals. Studies of decreased adhesiveness are few and this test is normal in von Willebrand's Disease (O'Brien, 1967b).
Some of the platelets lost stick to the wall of the flask and many more stick to those already stuck and some platelets will form aggregates. The presence of red cells undoubtedly contributes to this result increasing the number of platelets lost. The red cells on contact with glass may liberate factor R (Hellem, 1960) which is adenosine diphosphate (ADP) thereby enhancing the "stickiness" of the platelets; alternatively red cells may be relatively inert particles but since they occupy half the total blood volume they must greatly influence the hydrodynamic situation. Clearly, glass is a totally unphysiological surface and hence while the results of all tests involving glass contact may be useful they may not directly indicate the nature of a disturbance of physiology. Further theoretical disadvantages of this method are the large blood air interface, which may "activate" platelets, and the long contact time. In vivo platelets flowing past a wound stick within 1–2 seconds (Hughes, 1957) thus events evolving in 20 minutes in 2 ml of "captive" anti-coagulated blood may bear little relation to in vivo events. All methods depending on the difference between two counts, since the enumeration of platelets is relatively inaccurate, must have a considerable experimental error.

C. Hellem's Glass Bead Column Method (1960)

Principle: Anti-coagulated blood (or plasma) is pushed through a column of glass beads i. e. over a large surface, and the percentage of platelets lost in transit is estimated by counting the platelets before and after the passage.
Method: The column contains 5 mg of glass beads of 0.5 mm diameter held in a plastic

tube of 5 mm bore by a silk-covered plug at each end. The time for the leading edge of the blood to cross the column, i. e. the transit time, is 30 seconds. Ten ml of citrated blood is transferred to two 5 ml syringes that are fitted onto a pump that delivers 1 ml of blood in 23.5 seconds. From the first syringe 1 ml is collected directly for the control platelet count. Then a column of glass beads is connected and exactly 1 ml of blood forced through the column and into the counting fluid – the final count. The second syringe is then treated similarly and the results averaged and "percentage of platelets lost" is calculated as in the Wright technique (1942). Nygaard's (1933) platelet counting technique is used.

Critique: This method has been used to study platelet glass reactions and is grossly abnormal in thrombasthenia, a condition in which most platelet stickiness tests are abnormal; but it has not been extensively used in studies of thrombosis and is not abnormal in von Willebrand's Disease, so its clinical value remains to be established.

1. Modification by O'Brien

O'Brien (1961) reported a similar method except he used native blood which seems a more physiological material to study in preference to citrated blood. The transit time was 30 seconds. He, like Hellem, studied experimental conditions that influenced the test but did not report any abnormal results since the coagulopathies studied were all normal.

2. Modification by Hellem et al.

Hellem et al. (1963) modified his test by adding a small critical concentration of ADP before passage through the column. This test has now been shown to be normal in von Willebrand's Disease (Cronberg et al. 1966) and its clinical usefulness has yet to be established. The situation is complex enough in these glass columns (vide infra) without the addition of ADP. It is not known how rapidly the ADP is metabolised at various temperatures by the red cells, platelets and plasma, nor is it known to what extent ADP enhances platelet-to-glass and platelet-to-platelet adhesion nor whether aggregates form of such a size that they are mechanically restrained.

D. Salzman Glass Bead Column Technique (1963)

Principle: Native blood is sucked directly from a venipuncture through a column of glass beads into a small vacuum tube, containing anticoagulant. The percentage of platelets lost on passage through the column is determined by the difference between counts taken before and after passage.

Method: This method consists of collecting blood directly into a vacuum tube for a control platelet count; then a second venipuncture is performed and the double ended needle is connected to a standard column of glass beads through which the blood is sucked into a vacutainer. About six ml of blood must be delivered in 40–50 seconds, otherwise the test is unsatisfactory.

Critique: This method has been extensively used and is useful since there are a number of reports that it clearly distinguished between normals and patients with von Willebrand's Disease (e. g. Strauss and Bloom, 1965) with little overlap between these two populations (although a few people seem unable to confirm these findings). It is also abnormally low in uraemia (Salzman and Neri, 1966).

It has the advantage that native blood is exposed immediately to glass and, apart from the first drop, is not exposed to air. It is rapid and easy to perform and if standardized columns of beads become available commercially, this will lead to comparability of results in different laboratories. It has the disadvantage that the speed of flow through the column cannot be identical for all runs and this must influence the results. It may be a theoretical disadvantage that the speed decreases as the vacuum decreases as the vacutainer fills.

1. Modification by O'Brien and Heywood

O'Brien and Heywood (1967) modified the original test so that the speed of flow through the column was fast; the leading edge of the blood takes 3.5 sec to traverse the column which is 7 cm long. With this modification this test is useful since it clearly distinguishes between most von Willebrand patients and normals and like Salzman's method, gives low figures in uraemia (O'Brien, 1967). This test is slightly more cumbersome than that of Salzman since a pump is necessary to force the blood through the bead column. It is performed on native blood collected into a plastic syringe which fits into the pump. It has the theoretical advantage that the blood is forced through the column at a constant speed. For research purposes it may have a further advantage that the effluent blood can be sampled serially.

Most reports of abnormal platelet adhesiveness have employed methods involving glass yet any connection between platelet-glass interactions, which are poorly understood, and events in the body might be coincidental. A number of general points relevant to glass have already been mentioned under the different tests. Platelets in the presence of one or more proteins and sufficient calcium ions stick to and then spread on the glass surface. At some stage they liberate ADP. The surface of a stuck platelet changes since other platelets preferentially stick to those already stuck. Most of the platelets emerging from the bead columns are in small clumps, thus mechanical retention of clumps could occur. Under some circumstances it can be shown that glass makes platelets change their shape to become more spherical (O'Brien and Heywood, 1966). Contact with glass can also sphere red cells possibly due to a pH change and the contribution of red cells either as a source of ADP or mechanically has been mentioned. Since changing the temperature of blood from 37° C to 4° C is apparently without effect on two column methods, it seems unlikely that new enzyme activity develops during the passage through a column. However, speed of flow must greatly influence the events in these columns. The methods of Hellem (1960) and O'Brien (1961) with slow transit times do not give abnormal results in von Willebrand's Disease and the results are parallel to the Wright method (Hirsch et al. 1966). Yet the methods of Salzman (1963) and O'Brien and Heywood (1967) with fast transit times distinguish von Willebrand's Disease from normal, and O'Brien's (1967a) method has no correlation with the Wright results, (Reber & Struder 1965; O'Brien 1967), but Sjögren et al. (1969) found other correlations.

IV. Chandler's Tube Technique (1958)

Sufficient native or anticoagulated blood is put into a plastic tube, the two ends of which are then joined to make a ring with the pool of blood filling the bottom one third. This ring is slowly rotated so that the pool of blood stays at the bottom but a film of blood is lifted up from one side and transferred round to the other side. A "white body" histologically resembling a fresh thrombus, forms where the film joins the pool. Various parameters can be measured and this method has proved a valuable research tool but it does not seem applicable to routine use.

V. Quantitative Platelet Aggregation Tests

Principle: It is assumed that ADP or another aggregating agent plays a major part in platelet activation during haemostatic or thrombotic events in the body. This technique measures how "sticky" platelets become on adding ADP etc. It depends on the observation that little light passes through a finely dispersed "milky" suspension of particles (platelets) but that more light will pass if the particles coalesce (aggregate). Born (1962) and O'Brien (1962) reported that if platelet-rich plasma is placed in a photometer and stirred and an aggregating agent added, then the optical transmission increases as the platelets aggregate.

Method: There are a number of machines that are suitable. The size and shape of the cuvette and of the stirrer, the speed of stirring, the anticoagulant, the age and temperature of the plasma must all be standardized, as well as the nature, the amount, the concentration and the speed of adding the aggregating agent. The aggregometer made by Bryston Manufacturing*, Ltd., coupled to a Bausch and Lomb Model VOM 5 pen recorder is

* Bryston Manufacturing Ltd., Hamilton, Ontario, Canada; Chrono-Log Corporation, 2583 West Chester Pike, Broomall, Pa., U.S.A.

suitable. Cuthbertson and Mills (1963) have reported a micro method. O'Brien and Heywood (1966) have described the use of an adjusted EEL (Evans Electroselenium, Ltd.) titrator coupled to a Honeywell 10 mV pen recorder; this latter will now be summarized. Citrated platelet-rich plasma is obtained by slow centrifugation of blood. Heparinized plasma can be used but is less stable. Two ml of plasma is warmed to 37° C, transferred to the cuvette and stirred and the signal of the pen recorder adjusted. An aggregating agent usually in sufficient concentration to give a moderate response is added and the tracing continued. The greatest slope of the tracing can be measured and is related to the maximal rate of aggregation. If disaggregation occurs, the total optical density change, the time till disaggregation begins and the slope of the disaggregation tracing can all be measured. Aggregation patterns can also be obtained following the addition of appropriate concentrations of serotonin, thrombin, adrenaline, collagen and glass beads. Other methods of measuring the change in opacity and in adjusting for the platelet count have been devised (Emmons and Mitchell, 1965).

Critique: Under these experimental conditions each aggregating agent presumably stimulates a comparatively small number of enzymatic steps resulting in a membrane change which is monitored second by second and recorded as a rate of aggregation. While a given decrease in the optical density of the plasma indicates some degree of platelet aggregation, the exact number of single platelets, of dimers, of clumps of ten or a hundred platelets at any one time is unknown. Nevertheless and not unexpectedly these methods have been successfully and intensively used in the study of the pharmacology and dynamics of platelet aggregation. It is probable that ADP, either the intrinsic platelet ADP liberated under some circumstances, or extrinsic ADP appearing from outside, plays a central role in platelet physiology in the body, but the clinical use of this type of test is not proven. Furthermore, the red cells and conceivably even some specially sticky platelets are discarded in the preparation of the plasma. Nevertheless, these tests are abnormal in Glanzman's Disease and would be ideal for revealing a single enzyme defect in rare haemorrhagic diseases. While each individual has his own characteristic response to each of these aggregating agents and his own degree of variability from day to day (O'Brien 1967a) it has not yet been firmly established whether any of these tests are consistently abnormal in the more common disease like venous thrombosis or uraemia (but see Emmons and Mitchell, 1965, and Castaldi et al. 1966). Nevertheless, these methods test precise attributes of the platelets and should be persued.

VI. Platelet Electrophoresis

Platelet adhesion almost by definition must involve electrostatic forces; so it would be of interest to know the net charge and distribution of charges over the platelet surface. Hampton and Mitchell (1966a) showed that the electrophoretic mobility (ζ potential) of platelets was decreased by exposure to glass. The mobility increased fifteen minutes after the addition of a critical small concentration of an aggregating agent, while it decreased with larger concentrations. These authors (1966b) report an increased sensitivity to aggregating agents in acute illness. This test is not likely to be used as a routine test and its relevance to in vivo events is obscure, but it remains an intriguing research observation.

VII. General Conclusions

At the present time while the contribution of platelets to haemostasis and thrombosis is acknowledged (Mustard et al. 1967) the details of the processes involved are obscure. The mechanisms tested by the present platelet stickiness tests are also to varying extents ill-understood. Accordingly, until more is known of platelet physiology and of platelet tests, it seems wise to use a wide battery of tests. At present the author is using the following tests on a more or less research basis: The bleeding time, the Wright (1942), O'Brien and Heywood (1967) glass column and aggregation by ADP, 5-H.T., adrenaline, thrombin, collagen and glass beads. The normal ranges of the various tests must be established locally since, as in so many aspects of surface chemistry, a tiny change in technique can greatly alter the result. It should be re-emphasised that many other kinds of test exist and the selection of tests is to some extent arbitrary, e. g., the thromboelastogram and see Holdrinet et al. (1969). The value of some of these in thrombosis has recently been reviewed (Hampton, 1969; O'Brien, 1969). In addition, other platelet functions e. g., Platelet Factor 3 and Platelet Factor 4, are likely to be of great physiological importance.

It seems that we are still at the stage to testing our tests. Further refinements in existing tests will undoubtedly occur. With increasing knowledge some current tests will be discarded and others designed to test significant mechanisms or just plain but empirical tests will emerge. In anc case this type of test is here to stay.

References

Borchgrevink, C. F. (1960). *Acta Med. Scand. 168,* 157.
Born, G. V. R. (1962). *Nature 194,* 927.
Brecher, F., and Cronkite, E. P. (1950). *J. App. Physiol. 3,* 365.
Bull, B. S., Schneiderman, M. A., and Brecher, G. (1965). *Am. J. Clin. Pathol. 44,* 678.
Castaldi, P. A., Rozenberg, M. C., and Stewart, J. H. (1966). *Lancet II,* 66.
Chandler, A. B. (1958). *J. Lab. Invest. 7,* 110.
Cronberg, S., Nilsson, I. M., and Silver, J. (1966). *Acta Med. Scand. 180,* 43.
Cuthbertson, W. F. J., and Mills, D. C. B. (1963). *J. Physiol. 168,* 29.
Dacie, J. V., and Lewis, S. M. (1968). *Practical Haematology. 4th Ed.,* p. 73. J. & A. Churchill, London.
Emmons, P. R., and Mitchell, J. R. A. (1965). *Lancet I,* 71.
Feissly, R., and Lüdin, H. (1949). *Rev. Hematol. 4,* 481.
Hampton, J. R. (1969). *Brit. J. Hosp. Medicine 3,* 1504.
Hampton, J. R., and Mitchell, J. R. A. (1966a). *Nature 209,* 470.
Hampton, J. R., and Mitchell, J. R. A. (1966b). *Brit. Med. J. 1,* 1078.
Hellem, A. J. (1960). *Scand. J. Clin. Lab. Invest. 12, Suppl.* 51.
Hellem, A. J., Odegaard, A. E., and Skalhegg, B. A. (1963). *Thromb. Diath. Haemorrhag. 10,* 61.
Hirsh, J., McBride, J. A., and Wright, H. P. (1966). *Thromb. Diath. Haemorrhag. 16,* 100.
Holdrinet, A., Ewals, M., and Haanen, C. (1969). *Thromb. Diath. Haemorrhag. 32,* 174.
Hugues, J. (1957). *Thromb. Diath. Haemorrhag. 3,* 177.
McDonald, L., and Edgill, M. (1957). *Lancet II,* 457.
McDonald, L., Bray, C. L., Field, C., and Love, F. (1964). *Lancet I,* 745.
Mustard, J. F., Packham, M. A., Rowsell, H. C., and Jorgensen, L. (1967). *Thromb. Diath. Haemorrhag. Suppl. XXVI,* 261.
Nygaard, K. K. (1933). *Proc. Mayo Clin. 8,* 365.
O'Brien, J. R. (1961). *J. Clin. Pathol. 14,* 140.
O'Brien, J. R. (1962). *J. Clin. Pathol. 15,* 446.
O'Brien, J. R. (1967a). *Coagulation 1,* 311.
O'Brien, J. R. (1967b). Unpublished.
O'Brien, J. R., and Heywood, J. B. (1966). *Thromb. Diath. Haemorrhag. 16,* 752.
O'Brien, J. R., and Heywood, J. B. (1967). *J. Clin. Pathol. 21,* 56.
O'Brien, J. R. (1969). *J. Roy. Coll. Phycns. Lond. 3,* 193.
Reber, K., and Struder, A. (1965). *Thromb. Diath. Haemorrhag. 13,* 428.
Rees, H. M., and Ecker, E. E. (1923). *J. Am. Med. Assoc. 80,* 621.
Salzman, E. W. (1963). *J. Lab. Clin. Med. 62,* 724.
Salzman, E. W., and Neri, L. L. (1966). *Thromb. Diath. Haemorrhag. 15,* 84.
Sjögren, A., Böttiger, L. E., and Biörck, G. (1969). *Acta Med. Scand. 185,* 127.
Strauss, H. S., and Bloom, G. E. (1965). *New Engl. J. Med. 273,* 171.
Wright, H. P. (1942). *J. Pathol. Bacteriol. 54,* 461.

Assays for Platelet Factors

Erwin Deutsch

I. Introduction

Platelet factors are defined as substances or activities which are located inside of the thrombocytes and which are involved in the clotting mechanism. These substances may be found in other cells as well. Plasma factors of the coagulation system are adsorbed to the platelet surface (Atmosphère Plasmatique according to Roskam), and it is sometimes difficult to evaluate whether a certain activity is adsorbed onto the surface or whether it is derived from the thrombocytes. Platelet factor 1 is nothing more than adsorbed plasma factor V. The entity should therefore no longer be called a platelet factor. Platelet factors 2, 3 and 4, however, seem to be substances located in the cell. Fibrinogen seems to be partially adsorbed from plasma and partially located in platelets. Finally, for the fibrin stabilizing factor it was suggested that this substance is derived from platelets (Loewy, 1967).

Intact platelets are not active in coagulation. Platelet factors are partially released in vivo and in vitro by platelet aggregating agents, e. g. thrombin, and totally be freezing and thawing, exposure to ultrasound, or hypotonic solutions.

II. Preparation of Platelet Suspensions

Blood is drawn by the 2 syringe technique whereby the second syringe containing 0.1 ml of 0.1 M EDTA is filled up to 1.9 ml with blood. Siliconizing of glassware is mandatory. The blood is centrifuged for 10 minutes at 300 × G. The platelet rich plasma is taken off with siliconized pipettes in siliconized or plastic tubes, and spun for 30 minutes at 3,000 × G. The plasma is pipetted off and the precipitate suspended with a solution of 0.1 ml 0.1 M EDTA and 1.9 ml of a 0.9 % NaCl.

The platelet suspension is then centrifuged for 20 minutes at 3,000 × G and resuspended as above. This procedure is repeated 3 times. After the last washing the platelets are suspended in a small volume of 0.9 % NaCl. Knowing the initial platelet count the final suspension can be made up to any desired platelet count through appropriate dilution of the platelet button.

The centrifugation procedure is done at room temperature or under refrigeration. However, the temperature should not be below 10° C.

Comment: The platelets do not remain completely intact even under utmost care.

III. Platelet Factor 1

A. Principle

The activity is identical to that of plasma factor V. It can be assayed by a one stage technique using congenital or artificial factor V deficient plasma (Owren, 1947), a two stage assay based on the thromboplastin generation test (Deutsch, 1955), or by using the two stage prothrombin assay according to Seegers (Deutsch et al. 1955).

B. Comment

The activity of lysed platelets may be less than that of intact ones.

IV. Platelet Factor 2

A. Principle

Platelet factor 2 accelerates the conversion of fibrinogen to fibrin in the presence of thrombin. The assay technique is therefore based on a modified thrombin clotting time (Deutsch et al. 1956).

B. Material and reagents

1. 1 % bovine fibrinogen (Behring Werke, Marburg, Germany; American Hoechst, New York).
2. Platelet suspension with different platelet concentrations.
3. Thrombin solution adjusted to give a clotting time in this test system of 20 seconds.
4. Veronal buffer pH 7.3–7.4 (Owren, 1947).

C. Procedure

To 0.2 ml of the fibrinogen solution, and 0.1 ml of buffer (blanc) or the platelet suspension, 0.1 ml thrombin solution is added and the coagulation time determined.

D. Comment

The shortening of the thrombin clotting time is proportional to the concentration of platelet factor 2.

V. Platelet Factor 3

Principle of the methods: Platelet factor 3 is the lipoprotein derived from platelets. It can be assayed by 5 different techniques:

1. One stage assays based on a modification of the partial thromboplastin time. The ad-

vantage lies in using platelet rich plasma and avoiding the time consuming preparation of platelet suspensions (Stapp, 1959; Husom, 1961; Egli, 1961).
2. One stage techniques based on stypven time assay, a technique which is not very specific since the method is influenced by lipids without platelet factor 3 activity.
3. Two stage technique based on the thromboplastin generation test (Soulier et al. 1955; Winckelmann and Walther, 1964).
4. Two stage technique using purified prothrombin (Alkjaersig et al. 1955).
5. Thrombelastographic techniques (Sokal, 1959). In the following only the techniques 1 and 3 are discussed.

A. One Stage Technique According to Husom (1961)

1. Material and reagents

1. 35 mM $CaCl_2$ in distilled water.
2. Celite powder (Speedex).
3. Cephalin suspension (Hjort et al. 1955) or Tachostyptest diluted 1:50 (Hormon Chemie, Munich, Germany).
4. Diluting solution I (Hjort et al. 1955): 100 ml 0.1 M trisodium citrate and 600 ml 0.9% NaCl.
5. Diluting solution II (Hjort et al. 1955): 200 ml Veronal buffer (Owren) pH 7.4 and 200 ml 25.66 mM trisodium citrate and 600 ml 0.9% NaCl.
6. Adsorbed platelet free bovine plasma: 9 parts bovine blood and 1 part 2.5% potassium oxalate monohydrate are mixed, centrifuged for 30 minutes at 1,300 x g at 4° C. The plasma is filtered through a 20% and then a 50% Asbestos filter (1.5–2 Kg pO_2/cm^2, change filter after each 300 ml). The filtered plasma is dialized over night at 4° C against 0.9% NaCl and spun in the ultracentrifuge for 60 minutes at 4° C at 144,700 x g. The supernatant is frozen and stored in small amounts. For the test, the plasma is diluted 1:4 with diluting solution II.
7. Platelet free human substrate plasma: Citrated blood is centrifuged for 30 minutes at 1,700 x g and 4° C. The plasma is separated and centrifuged for 60 minutes at 144,700 x g and 4° C. The supernatant plasma is recovered with a needle and a syringe avoiding both the surface layer and the precipitate and frozen in small amounts. For the test, the plasma is activated with 30 mg/ml Celite at room temperature for 10 minutes.
8. Test plasma: Citrated blood is centrifuged for 30 minutes at 70 x g at 4° C. The number of platelets is counted. Samples of 0.2 ml are frozen 2 times and thawed and diluted with solution I and II to the desired platelet number (100 to 4,000/mm^3).

2. Procedure

0.2 ml activated platelet poor human plasma, 0.2 ml diluted adsorbed bovine plasma and 0.2 ml test plasma are mixed and incubated for 3 min at 37° C. Than 0.2 ml $CaCl_2$ are added and the coagulation time determined.

3. Graphic evaluation

The results are related to normal platelets based on a dilution curve with normal platelets or a partial thromboplastin (e. g. Tachostyptest, Hormon Chemie, Munich, Germany).

B. Two Phase Method Based Upon the Thromboplastin Generation Test (Biggs and Douglas, 1953)

The technique is identical to the thromboplastin generation test as described in Chapter III, p. 86. As a source for platelets two suspensions are used:
1. Intact platelets 100,000/mm^3.
2. The same solution after freezing and thawing. The normal values for "intact" platelet suspension are 19.9 seconds (18.3–21.5 sec), for disrupted platelets 10.0 seconds (8.4–11.6 sec) (Winckelmann and Walther, 1964).

C. Platelet Factor 3 Availability Test (Spaet and Cintron, 1965) modified (Lechner, 1967)

1. Material and reagents

1. Intact patient platelet rich plasma prepared by centrifugation of citrated blood in siliconized tubes at 300 x g for 10 min.
2. Platelet poor patient plasma obtained by centrifugation of the platelet rich plasma for 30 min at 3,000 x g.

3. Intact platelet free normal citrated plasma.
4. Kaolin suspension 10 mg/ml in 0.9 % NaCl.
5. Russell's Viper Venom (Stypven, Borough and Welcome) 10 μg/ml in 0.9 % NaCl.
6. 0.05 M $CaCl_2$ solution.

2. Procedure

First platelets are counted in the patient's platelet rich plasma and adjusted to three concentrations: 200,000; 100,000 and 50,000 platelets/mm³ with platelet free patient plasma. Exactly 90 min after drawing the blood, 1.0 ml standardized platelet rich plasma and 1.0 ml Kaolin suspension are mixed in a glass tube at 37° C. Immediately, and following 30 min of incubation, 0.1 ml of the described mixture is added to 0.1 ml normal plasma and 0.1 ml Stypven. After adding 0.1 ml $CaCl_2$ the clotting time is measured.

3. Results

Clotting time of the mixture measured prior to incubation is approximately 40–50 sec with substantial variations from individual to individual. This value is influenced by the lipid concentration of the plasma.
After 30 min incubation the normal clotting time is:

for 200,000/mm³ suspension	15–23 sec
for 100,000/mm³ suspension	15–30 sec
for 50,000/mm³ suspension	19–32 sec

This value reflects the amount of platelet factor 3 available, but gives only a rough quantitative measurement. It is important whether the 30 minute-value is shorter than the initial one or not. The availability of platelet factor 3 is missing in thrombasthenia, and decreased in uremia and paraproteinemia. The result depends primarily on the ability of the platelets to adhere to kaolin particles.

D. Comment

Only traces of platelet factor 3 are present in the circulating blood. This can be shown for instance by comparing the Stypven time of platelet free plasma with that of intact platelet rich plasma; these times are identical. Washed platelet suspensions contain fragments of platelets and therefore free platelet factor 3. It is of special significance to determine whether platelet factor 3 is low in absolute terms or whether the substance is not released properly in a given patient. When platelet factor 3 is assayed in "intact" platelet rich plasma in a one stage system with short coagulation times (e. g. with stypven or activated plasma or serum) the release of platelet factor 3 by thrombin during the reaction is low. The release increases in a system with long reaction times, and is pronounced in a two stage system. This means that in all test systems with socalled "intact" platelets, the result is influenced to a certain extent by the release of platelet factor 3 by thrombin. The absolute amount of platelet factor 3 can only be assayed after destroying platelets. Special tests for the detection of release defects are methods for the determination of the osmotic resistance (Ulutin and Karaca, 1959), as well as the platelet factor 3 availability test (see Section V, C).

VI. Platelet Factor 4 (Deutsch, 1959)

A. Principle

Platelet factor IV neutralizes heparin. For the assay a test system is used consisting of heparin, heparin cofactor, fibrinogen and thrombin. The result is expressed in μg heparin which is neutralized by a suspension of 100,000 platelets (Deutsch, 1959) or in equivalents of protamin sulfate (Poplawski and Niewiarowski, 1965). Sokal (1959) described a thromboelastographic method.

B. Material and reagents

1. 1 % fibrinogen solution (Behring Werke, Marburg, Germany; American Hoechst, New York).

2. Thrombin (Topostasin, Hoffmann La-Roche, Basel). The substance of one ampule containing 3,000 units is dissolved in 3 ml 50 % glycerol and stored at –20° C. The stock solution is prepared by adding 0.1 ml thrombin solution to 4.9 ml distilled water.

3. Heparin co-factor: 9 parts of bovine blood are added to 1 part 1.33% sodium oxalate; centrifuged platelet free plasma is stored in small quantities at –20° C. Material which is thawed cannot be used further.
4. Heparin: Stock solution with 10 and 15 units per ml. This solution preserves activity at 4° C for 1–2 weeks. For the test, solutions are prepared containing 0.75, 1.0, 1.25 and 1.5 units/ml.
5. Platelets: The patient's blood is withdrawn in siliconized equipment (1:10 trisodium citrate) and spun for 10 min at 300 × G. The platelet rich plasma is divided into two parts. One part is centrifuged at high speed (40 min at 3,000 × G) for platelet poor plasma; a platelet count is performed on the other part of the platelet rich plasma and the PRP diluted with the platelet poor plasma to the desired concentration of 100,000 and 150,000/mm³. The platelet rich plasma is tested "intact" and after freezing and rethawing.
6. Veronal buffer pH 7.4 (Owren, 1947).

C. Procedure

1. Incubation

Dilution curve	*Test system*
0.2 ml fibrinogen	0.2 ml fibrinogen
0.2 ml bovine plasma	0.2 ml bovine plasma
0.1 ml platelet free patient plasma	0.1 ml platelet rich patient plasma with different platelet concentrations
0.1 ml veronal buffer or heparin in different concentrations	0.1 ml chosen heparin solution
0.1 ml thrombin solution	0.1 ml thrombin solution

2. Dilution curve

Platelet poor plasma, buffer and different heparin solutions are tested and plotted on semilogarithmic paper (log clotting time in sec against heparin concentration in units). For the test, the heparin concentration which produces clotting times between 60 and 90 sec is used.

3. Assay

The chosen heparin concentration is used with platelet rich plasma instead of platelet poor plasma. The assay should be done with at least two platelet concentrations.

4. Calculations

It can be appreciated from the dilution curve, how much heparin is left after the reaction with platelets. The difference between the heparin concentration used and the remaining amount in the incubation mixture, gives the amount of heparin inactivated by the platelet suspension.

5. Evaluation

The normal value obtained for 10^7 intact platelets (100 μl) was 0.025–0.05 units heparin; for 10^7 destroyed platelets (100 μl) 0.045–0.07 units heparin.

D. Comment

A defect of platelet factor 4 release is diagnosed if the activity of the intact platelet suspension is reduced, with normal activity of the lysed platelets. An absolute deficiency is only diagnosed if a decrease is demonstrable in the test sample utilizing destroyed platelets.

VII. Platelet Fibrinogen

The quantitative assay of platelet fibrinogen is based on immunochemical methods with antifibrinogen serum.

VIII. Fibrin Stabilizing Factor

The method of Loewy (1967) is preferred.

References

Alkjaersig, N., Abe, T., and Seegers, W. H. (1955). *Am. J. Physiol. 181,* 304.
Biggs, R., and Douglas, A. S. (1953). *J. Clin. Pathol. 6,* 23.
Deutsch, E. (1955). *Wien. Z. Inn. Med. 36,* 355.
Deutsch, E. (1959). *Thromb. Diath. Haemorrhag. 4,* 93.
Deutsch, E., Johnson, S. A., and Seegers, W. H. (1955). *Circ. Res. 3,* 110.
Deutsch, E., Wawersich, E., and Franke, G. (1956). *Proc. 6th Internat. Congr. Haematol., Boston,* p. 477. Grune & Stratton, New York.
Egli, H. (1961). *Thromb. Diath. Haemorrhag. 6,* 533.
Hjort, P., Rapaport, S. I., and Owren, P. A. (1955). *J. Lab. Clin. Med. 46,* 89.
Husom, O. (1961). *Scand. J. Clin. Lab. Invest. 13,* 609.
Lechner, K. (1967). Unpublished.
Loewy, A. G. (1968). *Thromb. Diath. Haemorrhag. Suppl. 28,* 1.
Owren, P. A. (1947). "The Coagulation of Blood." Oslo.
Poplawski, A., and Niewiarowski, S. (1965). *Thromb. Diath. Haemorrhag. 13,* 149.
Sokal, G. (1959). *Rev. Belg. Pathol. Med. Exptl. 27,* 103.
Soulier, J. P., Larrieu, M. J., and Wartelle, O. (1955). *Acta Haematol. 14,* 160.
Spaet, T. H., and Cintron, J. (1965). *Brit. J. Haematol. 11,* 269.
Stapp, W. F. (1959). VII. Kongr. der Europ. Ges. f. Haemat., London 1959, Mittlg. Nr. 208.
Ulutin, O. N., and Karaca, M. (1959). *Brit. J. Haematol. 5,* 302.
Winckelmann, G., and Walther, C. (1964). *Folia Haematol. 9,* 2.

Clot Retraction

M. Bettex-Galland

I. Introduction

The ability of a normal blood clot to contract spontaneously under expulsion of serum largely results from specific functions of blood platelets. The historical aspects and the basic experimental results have been reviewed and critically analyzed by Budtz-Olsen (1951) and by Benthaus (1959). Reference is also made to the review chapters by Biggs and MacFarlane (1962) and to the more recent book of Marcus and Zucker (1965).
The formation of the hemostatic plug proceeds in three steps:
Adherence of the platelets to collagen, formation of the platelet aggregate and consolidation of the platelet aggregate.
Clot retraction is an essential part of platelet aggregate consolidation, i. e. the contraction phase of viscous metamorphosis. Therefore, the study of clot retraction permits a quantitative assessment of one of the important functions of platelets.

II. Methods

Retraction can be measured in whole blood, in platelet rich plasma and in purified systems. For clinical purposes where the test should be simple and rapid, whole blood or platelet rich plasma are preferable. On the other hand, purified systems are chosen, when individual factors influencing clot retraction are under study.

A. Measurement of Clot Retraction Using Whole Blood (Method of MacFarlane, 1939)

a. Material: Graduated centrifuge tubes with a scale marked in 0.1 ml divisions. The tubes should be perfectly clean and unscratched. Glass rods which are about $^1/_2$ inch longer than the tube and have a small "button" like expansion formed about $^1/_2$ inch from the end. Corks to fit the tubes with a bore to receive the rod in an easy sliding fit.

b. Performance of the Test: Blood (a little more than 5 ml) without anticoagulant is obtained by venipuncture and transferred to the centrifuge tube up to the mark 5.0 ml. The assembly of glass rod with cork stopper is immersed into the blood. The tube is placed in a water bath at 37° C. One hour after clotting, the glass rod with the attached retracted clot is removed. The volume of the fluid remaining in the tube is measured using the tube graduation marks. Retraction is expressed as percentage of the remaining fluid in relation to the total fluid (e. g. if 5 ml blood express 3 ml of fluid, retraction is 60 %).

c. Normal Values: The average value for healthy persons is 54 %, the normal range is 48 % to 64 %.

d. Comments: Whole blood clot retraction methods reflect not only platelet count and function, but are also influenced by hematocrit and fibrinogen concentration. However, this type of assay more closely simulates in vivo conditions. The fall-out phenomenon, i. e. the release of erythrocytes from the retracting clot is readily observed.

B. Measurements of Clot Retraction Using Platelet-Rich Plasma

1. Method of Bettex-Galland and Lüscher (1960)

a. Material and Reagents: Siliconized glassware is used for the preparation of platelet-rich and platelet-poor plasma. Test tubes (10 × 0.8 cm) of high melting point glass and of high and constant quality should be used. They must be cleaned with chrome sulfuric acid and thoroughly rinsed with distilled water. Shortly before use, their lower parts 3–4 cm) are made evenly red-hot by rotation over a Bunsen burner, producing a surface from which the clot will detach spontaneously or upon light shaking one or two minutes after its formation (Fonio, 1953).

Platelet-rich plasma: Blood is taken by clean venipuncture and immediately mixed with $^1/_4$ volume ACD in siliconized centrifuge tubes. The blood is immediately centrifuged for 10 min at about 150 x g at room temperature to remove the red and white cells. After centrifugation the platelet-rich plasma is pipetted off and diluted with platelet-poor plasma of the same individual to a concentration of 300,000 platelets/cmm.

Platelet-poor plasma is prepared by centrifugation of the platelet-rich plasma at 700 x g for 20 min at room temperature.

0.2 M Imidazole-HCl buffer, pH 7.4.
0.1 M Glucose in 0.15 M NaCl.
0.1 M $MgCl_2$ or $CaCl_2$.
Thrombin (commercial preparation) 60 U/ml in 0.15 M NaCl.

b. Performance of the Test: 0.6 ml platelet-rich plasma (300,000 platelets/cmm), 0.3 ml imidazole-HCl buffer, 0.1 ml glucose are pipetted into the test tube. Then 0.1 ml $CaCl_2$ or $MgCl_2$ is added together with 0.1 ml thrombin. After short mixing the test tube is placed in a water bath of 37° C.

c. Estimation of the Clot Retraction: The extent of clot retraction is given by the length of the retracted clot as compared to the total length of the clot at zero time. For a rough estimation it is sufficient to measure the final result of clot retraction after 60 min of incubation at 37° C. More information is gained by following the time course of the retraction process. Measurements may be performed after 5, 15, 30 and 60 min respectively (Fig.

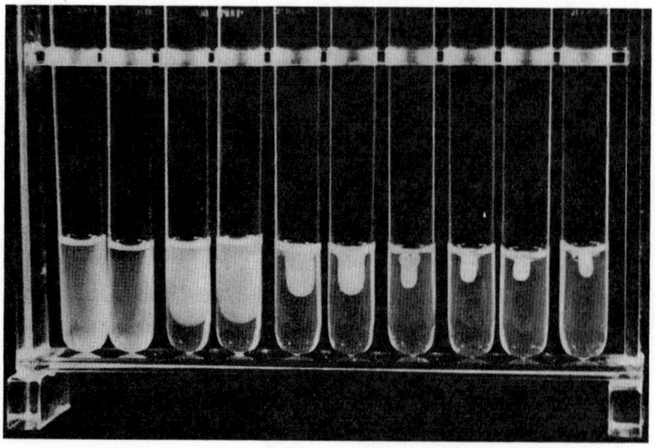

Fig. 1. Clot retraction in platelet-rich plasma prepared from human ACD-blood. Test tubes on left side of pairs contain Mg^{++}, those on the right side Ca^{++}. Time intervals after the addition of thrombin were (from left to right) 0, 5, 15, 30, and 60 minutes. Method of Bettex-Galland and Lüscher (1960).

1). Percent clot retraction versus time may be plotted graphically, as illustrated in Fig. 2.

2. Method of Benthaus (1959)

a. Material and Reagents: Siliconized centrifuge tubes are used for the preparation of the platelet-rich plasma. The test is performed in glass tubes (1.4 × 12 cm) with a graduation of 100 scale units each corresponding to 0.1 ml.

Platelet-rich plasma: 1.0 ml 3.8 % trisodium citrate solution is mixed with 4 ml patient's venous blood in a siliconized centrifuge tube. Platelet-rich plasma is obtained either by spontaneous sedimentation of the red cells or by centrifugation 10 min (150 x g) at room temperature.

Tissue thromboplastin: Any preparation suitable for prothrombin times may be used.
0.1 M $CaCl_2$.
0.85 % sodium chloride solution.

b. Performance of the Test: Reagents are pipetted into the graduated glass tube in the following sequence: 0.5 ml of 0.1 M $CaCl_2$, 2–3 drops tissue thromboplastin and 0.85 % saline to a total volume of 9.0 ml. Then 1.0 ml platelet-rich plasma is added and mixed by inverting three time. After clotting of the mixture (about 2 min) the tube is turned around quickly to detach the clot from the tube wall. Then the clot is incubated at 37° C. An exact vertical position of the tube is important.

c. Estimation of Clot Retraction: After 12 hrs the length of the clot is measured using the graduation of the glass tube. The volume of the clot is calculated according to the formula:

$$V = a^3 \times 10^{-5}$$

(V = volume of the retracted clot in ml, a = length of the clot after retraction in scale units of the test tube. For details of the derivation of this equation see Benthaus, 1959). Since the total volume is 10 ml, the volume of the expressed fluid is 10 ml minus clot volume (V). Retraction is expressed as percentage of the expressed fluid from the total volume.

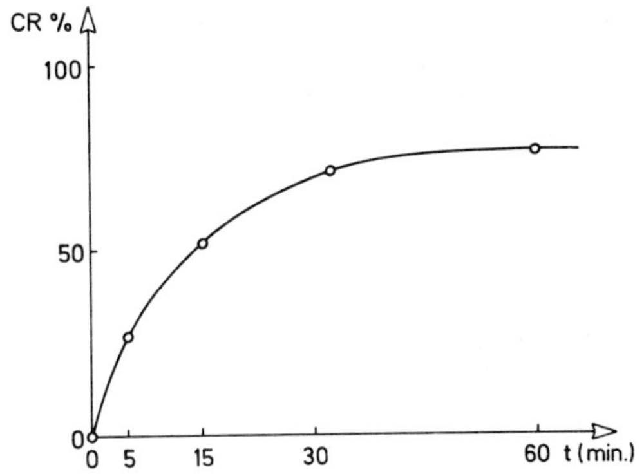

Fig. 2. Clot retraction in platelet-rich plasma prepared from human ACD-blood, plotted versus time. Method of Bettex-Galland and Lüscher (1960).

d. Normal Values: Average retraction with this method is 98 %, the lower limit being 91 %.

e. Comments: More accurate results are obtained by keeping platelet count in the platelet-rich plasma constant by appropriate dilutions with platelet-poor plasma of the same patient as described above (section II, B, 1, a).

C. Measurement of Clot Retraction in a Purified System (Bettex-Galland and Lüscher, 1960)

a. Material and Reagents: Same glassware as in method B 1.

Washed Platelets: 4 parts blood and 1 part ACD solution are mixed in siliconized tubes or plastic containers. Platelet-rich plasma is obtained by centrifugation at 150 x g for 10 min at room temperature; the platelet-rich plasma is submitted to a second centrifugation at 700 x g for 20 min at room temperature. The platelet pellet thus obtained is resuspended in 0.15 M saline containing 0.1 % EDTA. Now the suspension is cooled to 1–4° C, centrifuged and the washing is repeated. Then the platelets are suspended in cold saline solution. The presence of a few red or white cells in these preparations does not affect the result. The suspension is adjusted to a platelet count of 600,000/cmm by dilution with saline. The first part of this procedure should be carried out at room temperature because platelets undergo changes in shape in the cold and tend to aggregate (Zucker and Borelli, 1960), a process which may become irreversible in whole blood or in plasma; tests should be carried out within 24 hours after collection of the blood. Storage of the platelets in the cold is essential.

Fibrinogen: Cohn fraction I (Cohn et al. 1946) or highly purified fibrinogen according to Blombäck and Blombäck (1956) may be used. A solution of 12 mg/ml in 0.15 M NaCl is prepared. Since fibrinogen preparations are best stored at higher salt concentrations it is essential to adjust their ionic strength to 0.15 before the experiment;

0.2 M Imidazole-HCl buffer, pH 7.4.
0.1 M Glucose in 0.15 M NaCl.
0.1 M $MgCl_2$ or $CaCl_2$.
Thrombin (commercial preparation) 60 U/ml in 0.15 M NaCl.

b. Performance of the Test: A 0.3 ml suspension of washed platelets (600,000/cmm), 0.5 ml imidazole-HCl buffer, 0.1 ml fibrinogen (12 mg/ml) and 0.1 ml glucose are mixed in the test tube. Then 0.1 ml $CaCl_2$ or $MgCl_2$ and 0.1 ml thrombin (60 U/ml) are added together. The mixture is incubated at 37° C and the retraction measured in the same way as in method B 1 (Fig. 3).

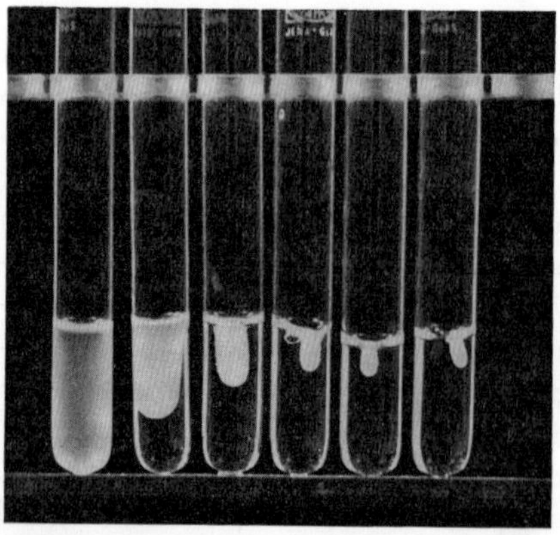

Fig. 3. Clot retraction in a purified system. Human platelets prepared from ACD-blood; fibrinogen prepared according to Blombäck and Blombäck (1956); Ca^{++}. From left to right time intervals were 0, 5, 15, 30, and 60 minutes after the addition of thrombin. Method of Bettex-Galland and Lüscher.

III. Comments

Reduction or complete absence of clot retraction is found in thrombasthenia (Glanzmann, 1918). In a small group of patients a defect in the glycolytic system of the platelets and low levels of ATP in the platelets has been found which explains the inability for clot retraction of these platelets (Löhr et al. 1961). In the majority of cases however the nature of the platelet defect is still obscure. The poor clot retraction in macroglobulinemia is due to the coating of platelets with paraproteins (Pachter et al. 1959).

Clot retraction is also reduced in pronounced thrombocytopenia. By measuring the clot retraction antibodies against platelets may be recognized. If normal platelets are incubated with plasma or serum containing antibodies, the platelets are "injured" and clot retraction is impaired (Retraction-inhibition test; Lüscher, 1956). Serum is less suitable for this test because it often contains traces of thrombin due to the delayed prothrombin consumption in thrombocytopenic blood.

Several agents are known to inhibit clot retraction:

a. EDTA is a chelating agent which binds Ca^{++} and Mg^{++}. This inhibition is reversed by adding Ca^{++} or Mg^{++}.

b. Sulfhydryl-blocking agents such as mercurials and monoiodoacetate are powerful inhibitors of clot retraction in low concentrations. In contrast, other metabolic poisons, as for instance NaCN and NaF, are effective only at high concentrations (Marcus and Zucker, 1965, Øllgaard, 1951). The same holds for Salyrgan, in spite of the fact that it is a most powerful inhibitor for thrombosthenin, the contractile protein of the actomyosin type, isolated from blood platelets (Bettex-Galland and Lüscher, 1965).

c. Certain synthetic antihistamins (Tephorin and Diparcol) also inhibit clot retraction. Their mode of action remains yet to be elucidated.

References

Benthaus, J. (1959). *Thromb. Diath. Haemorrhag. 3,* 311.
Bettex-Galland, M., and Lüscher, E. F. (1960). *Thromb. Diath. Haemorrhag. 4,* 178.
Bettex-Galland, M., and Lüscher, E. F. (1965). *Adv. Prot. Chem. 20,* 1.
Biggs, R., and MacFarlane, R. G. (1962). "Human Blood Coagulation and Its Disorders". Blackwell, Oxford.
Blombäck, B., and Blombäck, M. (1956). *Arkiv Kemi 10,* 415.
Budtz-Olsen, O. E. (1951). "Clot Retraction". Blackwell, Oxford.
Cohn, E. J., Strong, L. E., Hughes, W. L. Jr., Mulford, D. J., Ashworth, J. N., Melin, M., and Taylor, H. L. (1946). *J. Am. Chem. Soc. 68,* 469.
Fonio, A. (1953). *Ergeb. Inn. Med. Kinderheilk. 4,* 1.
Glanzmann, E. (1918). *Jb. Kinderheilk. 88,* 113.
Löhr, G. W., Waller, H. D., and Gross, R. (1961). *Deut. Med. Wochschr. 86,* 897.
Lüscher, E. F. (1956). *Vox Sang. 1,* 133.
MacFarlane, R. G. (1939). *Lancet I,* 1199.
Marcus, A. J., and Zucker, M. B. (1965). "The Physiology of Blood Platelets". Grune & Stratton, New York.
Øllgaard, E. (1951). *Acta Haematol. 6,* 220.
Pachter, M. R., Johnson, S. A., Neblett, T. R., and Truant, J. R. (1959). *Am. J. Clin. Pathol. 31,* 467.
Zucker, M. B., and Borrelli, J. (1960). *Thromb. Diath. Haemorrhag. 4,* 424.

Electron Microscopic Techniques for Blood Platelets Fibrinogen and Fibrin

J. J. Sixma

I. Introduction

In view of the regular use of morphological data in the study of hemostasis, it seems desirable that a laboratory manual on methods of investigation in the field of blood coagulation and thrombosis should pay attention also to the manner in which data on the ultrastructure of blood platelets are obtained.

The question arises whether it would be sufficient, in this respect, to refer to a manual on electron-microscopic histological techniques. The basic information for morphological studies of blood platelets can indeed be found in such a manual, but there are sufficient "variations on the theme" to justify a separate discussion in the context of this book. Deviations from conventional techniques mainly concern fixation and the isolation of the platelets also merits special attention. The creation of optimal conditions requires more precautions than are generally necessary in electron microscopy.

Although the great interest in blood platelets and their morphological changes during the hemostatic process actually does not date back further than the past decade, platelets happened to be among the first biological objects studied with the electron microscope. This resulted from the fact that platelets characteristically spread on a surface and become so thin that a beam of electrons can pass through them.

After the first studies by Wolpers and Ruska (1939), Bessis et al. (1950) made extensive use of electron microscopy to study blood platelets. The full thickness technique was used also by such authors as Bloom (1954) and Köppel (1958); but they concerned themselves more with the dynamic processes of coagulation. The data obtained by this method are reviewed by Rebuck et al. (1960).

When suitable techniques of ultra-thin sectioning were later developed, many more details in blood platelet ultrastructure were disclosed (Kautz and DeMarsh, 1955; Rinehart, 1955). Comprehensive data can be found in David-Ferreiras's review (1964).

The principal ultrastructural features of blood platelets are briefly reviewed in the following; the data included here will provide the frame of reference for the subsequent discussion on fixation techniques. As we know from light microscopic investigations, circulating blood platelets are disc-shaped. Their diameters range from 2 μ to 5 μ. The shape of fixed blood platelets is largely dependent on the technique of fixation. After osmium tetroxide fixation (the conventional technique in earlier electron microscopy work), blood platelets are usually spherical, with a few pseudopodia.

Blood platelets possess a membrane about 75 Å thick consisting of two dark layers separated by a light layer. A number of structures are found in the cytoplasmic matrix known collectively as "granulomere" in light microscopy literature. They are dense granules (α-granulomere), mitochondria (β-granulomere), translucent vacuoles and tubules, vacuoles containing ferritin, and glycogen accumulations. The cytoplasm also contains microtubules and fibrils. One blood platelet contains some 50–80 dense granules with a diameter of 2000–3000 Å. They are enveloped by a well-defined membrane and often show an eccentric dark spot.

The mitochondria (β-granulomere) are small (1600–2200 Å) and usually spherical. No more than three mitochondria are found per platelet section. Only two or three cristae are visible in each mitochondrion. The platelet also contains larger and smaller translucent sacs which, according to their dimensions, are called vesicles (down to the smallest distinguishable) or vacuoles (larger). These structures are sometimes referred to collectively as "elements clairs" (γ-granulomere). These systems are probably of triple origin. They are believed to originate in part from the Golgi system; they may arise, in part, from the endoplasmic reticulum of the megakaryocyte and they may form during pinocytosis and phagocytosis. The vesicles containing ferritin are known as siderosomes (or δ-granulomere). Blood platelets can also phagocytize other particles such as quartz (Bloom, 1954), thorium dioxide (David-Ferreira, 1961), latex particles (Glynn et al. 1965), fat (Schulz and Wedell, 1962) and virus particles (Danon et al. 1959). The ε-granulomere are granules of 180–200 Å with a substructure of 30 Å. These granules are found scattered among the dense granules, but usually in groups of a few hundred. Experience gained with other tissues has taught us that such granules contain glycogen (David-Ferreira and David-Ferreira, 1962). Making use of enzyme digestion of ultra-thin sections, Jean and Gautier (1961) demonstrated that this applies also to the ε-granulomere of blood platelets.

After the introduction of glutaraldehyde fixation, two new structures were described. Bessis and Breton-Gorius (1965) found bundles of fibrils of 60 Å diameter radiating into the pseudopodia, and microtubules of 230 Å diameter encircling these granules which, by their technique, were localized in the center of the blood platelet. These structures were found in blood platelets which were first allowed to spread on glass and then subsequently fixed, dehydrated, embedded and sectioned. Examination of platelets retaining their disc-shape has shown that the microtubles form an annular arrangement in the periphery of the disc (Behnke, 1965; Haydon and Taylor, 1965; Sandborn et al. 1966; Sixma and Molenaar, 1966). Fibrils are most in evidence in the pseudopodia but there are indications suggesting that they are situated in a criss-cross arrangement beneath the membrane (Sixma and Molenaar, 1966; Bull, 1966).

II. Isolation of Blood Platelets

A. Collection of Blood

In isolating blood platelets, use is generally made of a siliconized needle and siliconized glassware or other non-wettable surfaces. The use of non-wettable material has the disadvantage that more blood platelets adhere to these surfaces than to glass, but on the other hand, the activation of clotting factors by glass must affect the blood platelets. In order to prevent activation of clotting factors due to contamination of the blood by tissue thromboplastin, it is our custom to collect the first few ml blood obtained at venipuncture in a separate receptacle; this blood is not used. The effect of tissue thromboplastin on platelet morphology is uncertain, but it is little trouble to take this extra precaution.

B. Anticoagulants

The anticoagulants most commonly used are ethylenediaminetetra-acetic acid (EDTA), sodium citrate, heparin and (sodium) oxalate. Oxalate has found little use in morphological studies, since oxalate interferes with the isolation of platelets. During centrifugation the platelets collect in the buffy coat, and few remain in the supernatant plasma (Barkhan, 1957).

The use of EDTA as an anticoagulant has the disadvantage that it changes the shape of the blood platelets from disc-shaped to spherical (Zucker and Borelli, 1954). Also EDTA is unsuitable as an anticoagulant in the study of platelet aggregation because platelet aggregation always requires the presence of ionized calcium. On the other hand, EDTA can be used for work with washed blood platelets because platelets can be readily re-suspended in EDTA plasma. Yet even in this respect the use of EDTA is probably inadvisable because there are indications that EDTA causes membrane lesions. We have personally observed the rapid occurrences of membrane lesions after repeated washing of blood platelets in a 1 percent EDTA solution. EDTA is commonly used in the form of the disodium salt, and sometimes in the form of the dipotassium salt. The final concentrations employed vary from 0.06 percent to 0.2 percent. Nine parts blood are generally collected in one part anticoagulant. The use of buffered EDTA is probably of little value since plasma in itself has sufficient buffer capacity.

Relatively little use is made of heparin as an anticoagulant. It exerts no distinct influence on the morphology of blood platelets, but spontaneous platelet aggregation tends to occur in heparinized plasma. Heparin is, therefore, a suitable anticoagulant only when blood platelets can be fixed immediately for morphological study. The usual final heparin concentrations range from 5 to 1000 U/ml. One disadvantage of heparin as an anticoagulant is that most coagulation studies cannot be made in heparinized blood, or only after neutralization with protamine sulphate.

The anticoagulant most widely used is sodium citrate (trisodium citrate dihydrate at a concentration of 3.8 percent), of which 1 ml is added to 9 ml blood. In addition to aggregation experiments, various experiments concerning the physiology of coagulation can be carried out in this way. The principal advantage of trisodium citrate is that it induces little or no change in the shape of blood platelets. An acid citrate dextrose (ACD) mixture e. g., as used by Aster and Jandl (1964) is probably as suitable for platelet work as is sodium citrate.

C. Isolation

Differential centrifugation is commonly used in isolating blood platelets. For this purpose the blood is centrifuged at about 135 x g in order to obtain platelet-rich plasma for 10–15 minutes. The blood platelets are isolated from the supernatant, usually by centrifugation at 625 x g for 15 minutes. Caps placed on the centrifuge tubes protect the pellet against carbon or metal particles from the centrifuge, which may produce scratchmarks in the sections. Theoretically, blood platelets can be isolated with the aid of a Millipore filter, but this method has proven impractical because it causes pronounced mechanical distortion of the platelets.

D. Temperature

The temperature at which blood platelets are isolated is dependent on the specific requirements of the experiment. If the experimental arrangement calls for fixation of platelets immediately after isolation then the optimal temperature is 37° C since over short time periods the least change in shape occurs at that temperature (Zucker and Borelli, 1954). On the other hand, enzymatic degradation is markedly enhanced at 37° C. Most notably, autodigestion by lysosomal enzymes occurs readily at 37° C (Firkin et al. 1965). If blood platelets are to be stored for some time before fixation or must be otherwise processed then isolation is best performed at 4° C. We personally isolate platelets at room temperature, by way of compromise between these two possibilities.

III. Fixation

A. Criteria of good fixation

Before discussing various fixation techniques, it is of importance to consider the criteria of good fixation. While there are no absolute criteria, some general guidelines can be established. The conventional starting-point in evaluating fixation is a good correlation between morphological detail and adequacy of fixation. A well-fixed cell presents the appearance of structural complexity; the cytoplasm in particular displays a delicate structure and shows no coarse floccular precipitation. The cell membrane must be complete. Mitochondria and the endoplasmic reticulum are sensitive indicators in evaluating the quality of fixation. When fixation is poor, the mitochondria are swollen, empty and spherical. The endoplasmic reticulum consists of flat cisterns usually of equal width, dilated cisterns often represent an artefact of fixation. The possibility of shrinking or swelling of the entire cell must be kept in mind when platelets as well as other cells are fixed in suspension. Even under optimum conditions for fixation there is no guarantee that the entire tissue or all cells of a suspension have been adequately fixed. During fixation, a different microclimate may have existed in certain parts of the tissue or of the suspension.

This variability of fixation can cause serious problems in investigations where conclusions about the action of a drug are made from morphological changes occurring after exposure to the agent in question. Since inadequate fixation also causes changes in morphological features, a large material and a number of observations large enough to permit statistical analysis will be required. This is hardly attractive in view of the time-consuming nature of electron microscopic studies. Fortunately, in study of blood platelets these factors are of minor importance since one is confronted with numerous sections through the same type of cell, of small dimensions.

B. Osmium fixation

Until a few years ago osmium tetroxide fixation was the technique most commonly used in electron microscopy. In recent years, however, the aldehydes (particularly glutaraldehyde) have begun to replace osmium tetroxide as *primary* fixative. As a general fixative, osmium tetroxide gives good results.

We used a 1 percent osmium tetroxide solution buffered according to Zetterqvist (1956) (Table 1). The presence of calcium ions was found not to influence the fixation. We obtained similar results with more conventional buffering according to Palade (1952), with our without addition of sucrose (34–45 mg/ml); (Table 2).

Table 1. Osmium Tetroxide Buffered According to Zetterqvist (1956).

Solution A	sodium veronal	14.7 gm
	sodium acetate	9.7 gm
	distilled water up to	500 ml
Solution B	sodium chloride	40.0 gm
	potassium chloride	2.1 gm
	calcium chloride	0.9 gm
	distilled water up to	500 ml
Solution C	0.10 N-HCl	

The buffered fixative is obtained by mixing

Solution A	10,0 ml
Solution B	3.4 ml
Solution C (approximately)	11.0 ml

with 0.5 gm osmium tetroxide in 25.0 ml distilled water. The pH is adjusted to 7.2–7.4 with the HCl.

Table 2. Osmium Tetroxide Buffered According to Palade (1952).

Solution A	sodium veronal	2.89 gm
	sodium acetate	1.90 gm
	distilled water up to	100 ml
Solution B	2 % osmium tetroxide solution in distilled water	
Solution C	0.1 N-HCl	
Solution D	distilled water	

The final buffered fixative is prepared by mixing

Solution A	5.0 ml
Solution B	2.5 ml
Solution D	2.5 ml
Solution C	±5.0 ml
	(to pH 7.3–7.5)

The addition of 45 mg sucrose/ml is the modification according to Caulfield (1957).

A pellet of blood platelets is fixed by pouring off the supernatant plasma and replacing it immediately by the buffered osmium tetroxide solution. The fixation is carried out at 4° C. The duration of fixation is 1–2 hours, dependent on the thickness of the pellet (osmium tetroxide only slowly pervades a tissue or pellet). The remaining osmium tetroxide is then washed out with 0.9 percent NaCl for 2 × 30 minutes. The pellet is dehydrated, divided into small fragments and embedded, making sure that only well-fixed fragments are embedded. These are characterized by a pronounced black colour. In general, osmium fixation of blood platelets centrifuged to a

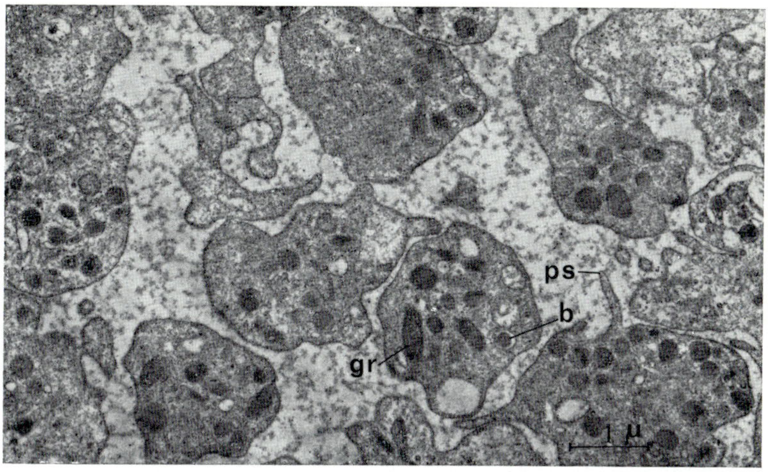

Fig. 1. Osmium fixation according to Feissly et al. (1957). Staining by uranyl acetate and lead citrate. Dense granules (gr) and a bull's eye granule (b) are clearly visible. There are several pseudopodia (ps) present.

pellet gives poor results. Numerous pseudopodia form, and extraction of cellular constituents readily occurs.

Fixation of blood platelets in suspension generally yields better results. According to one conventional fixation technique (Feissly et al. 1957) 1 ml of a 1 percent buffered osmium tetroxide solution was added to the anticoagulant per 8 ml blood. The blood platelets were isolated from the blood by differential centrifugation, whereupon the pellet was further fixed with 1 percent buffered osmium tetroxide as described above (Fig. 1). At the first centrifugation, it was generally found desirable to keep centrifuge speeds slightly below the conventional because all blood cells had become heavier as a result of fixation.

This fixation according to Feissly can also be used if an experiment is to be carried out with the platelets in PRP prior to fixation. Feissly's original technique has the disadvantage that is doesn't leave the shape of the platelets entirely unchanged. The platelets become spherical instead of disc-shaped, and a few pseudopods are generally visible. By adding larger volumes of buffered osmium tetroxide one ensures better fixation of the blood platelets in the shape they have in vivo. The differences in contrasts between different parts of the platelet are often less marked, possibly because less material has been extracted. The plasma membrane is sometimes ruptured and, surprisingly, there is often no staining of glycogen – which normally stains intensively with a lead compound. In this way good results can be obtained for generation of aggregates (Fig. 2) as they react more as a tissue.

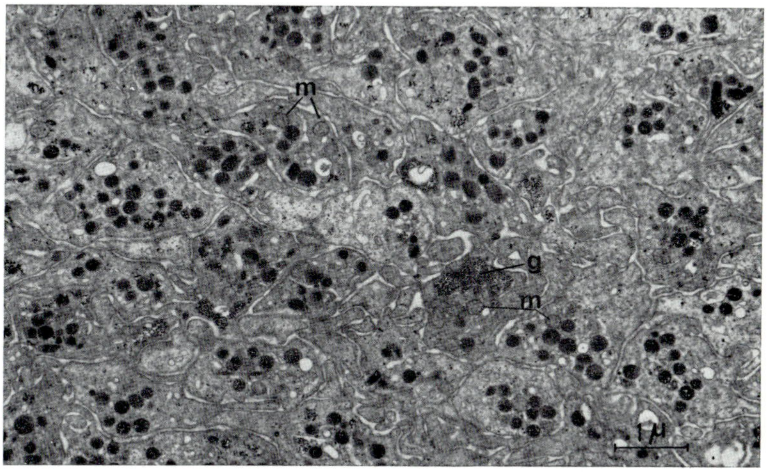

Fig. 2. Osmium fixation with higher osmium concentration (2 ml osmium tetroxide to 0.2 ml PRP). Staining by uranyl acetate and lead citrate. Aggregation caused by epinephrin. The platelets are closely packed and have retained their granules. Two mitochondria (m), recognizable by their double membrane, are clearly distinguishable. Glycogen (g) is very conspicuous.

C. Glutaraldehyde fixation

Fixation of a pellet can be achieved with a 1–5 percent glutaraldehyde solution buffered with 0.10 M phosphate buffer or cacodylate buffer at pH 7.4 (Sabatini et al. 1963). The rate and degree of fixation in the case of blood platelets is probably independent of temperature, and can therefore be carried out at room temperature. After fixation for 1 hour, the remaining glutaraldehyde is washed out with 0.10 M phosphate or cacodylate buffer containing 0.20 M sucrose. The pellet is kept in this buffer at 4° C until further processing starts. Because the contrast of blood platelets fixed exclusively with glutaraldehyde is low, post-fixation with osmium tetroxide is necessary. This is done with 1 percent osmium tetroxide buffered at pH 7.4. The duration of fixation is 60 minutes. It is carried out at 4° C. The osmium tetroxide is subsequently washed out with 0.9 percent NaCl for 2 × 30 minutes, whereupon the tissue is further dehydrated and embedded. The results obtained in this way are superior to those of osmium tetroxide fixation of a pellet. The blood platelets still have pseudopodia, but there is less extraction of material during fixation.

For fixation of platelets in suspension it is impossible to use the same glutaraldehyde concentration because, unlike a pellet, a suspension does not react as a tissue reacts. At glutaraldehyde concentrations exceeding 2 percent, marked gel formation occurs in blood or plasma and impedes further processing. This can be avoided by using glutaraldehyde concentrations of 2 percent or less, or by collecting a small quantity of blood or plasma in a large amount of buffered glutaraldehyde solution, ensuring a degree of dilution at which fixation of plasma proteins causes no gel formation. Even so, fixation according to Sabatini et al. (1963) gives poor results. The blood platelets prove to contain numerous vacuoles and dilated cisterns (sometimes they show a "Gruyère cheese" aspect). Due to the marked dilation of cisterns the cytoplasm seems dense and shrunken (Fig. 3). The cause of this phenomenon has not so far been systematically studied.

A number of efforts have been made to achieve optimal fixation. Brief fixation with glutaraldehyde buffered with cacodylate can be followed by post-fixation with osmium tetroxide. This prevents dilation of cisterns but seems to entail extraction of material in particular of the cytoplasmic matrix. By using a fixative at a lower pH than normal, dilation of cisterns can likewise be prevented. We carried out this type of fixation by adding 1 ml of a 2 percent glutaraldehyde solution buffered with 0.1 M phosphate citrate pH 3.7 to 9 ml blood with anticoagulant, analogous to the technique of Feissly et al. (1957); this gave a final pH of about 5.4. After differential centrifugation the pellet was further fixed with the same fixative at pH 3.7. Reasonable results can be obtained in this way, although

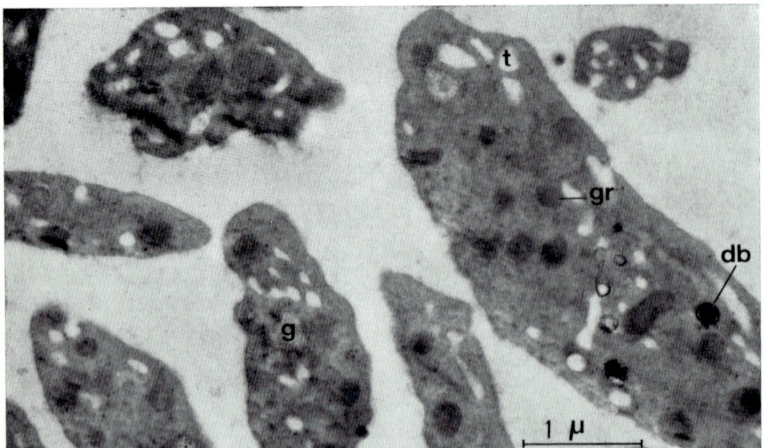

Fig. 3. Glutaraldehyde fixation in suspension with 2 % glutaraldehyde buffered with 0.10 M phosphate buffer at pH 7.40. Postfixation with osmium tetroxide. Staining by uranyl acetate. Widened tubules and vacuoles, or better perhaps, cisterns (t) are scattered throughout. Dense bodies (db) and glycogen (g) can be observed.

this fixation technique probably is less than ideal due to the extraction which it entails and the variation of the pH.

Minute changes in the molarity of the buffer proved to have little effect on the above described fixation artefacts, but at distinctly lower molarity dilations of the tubular system disappeared. However, other artefacts occurred in these cases. The blood platelets assumed a swollen appearance with occasional empty, blisterlike evaginations of the membrane. By slightly increasing molarity it is possible to achieve a point in which dilated tubules are no longer observed while swelling artefacts do not yet occur. Optimum conditions were achieved when 8 ml 1 percent glutaraldehyde in 0.07 M phosphate buffer (pH 7.4) was added to 2 ml blood or plasma (Fig. 4).

The ultimate osmolarity of the buffered glutaraldehyde solution was about 280 mosmol. After fixation for 1 hour at room temperature the blood platelets were centrifuged off. The pellet was washed with and kept in 0.9 percent NaCl buffered with one-tenth 0.10 M phosphate buffer pH 7.4. An investigation of the importance of the contribution of the glutaraldehyde to the osmolarity of the fixation mixture and a study concerning the use of other buffers are still in progress.

D. Other fixatives

In 1956, Luft introduced potassium permanganate as fixative especially suitable for fixation of the membrane systems of the cell. Many other cell organelles are so affected as to be virtually unrecognizable and this severely limits the application of this fixative. It has seldom been used in blood platelet studies. Hovig (1965) used this fixation to study membrane changes following exposure to enzymes, and David-Ferreira and David-Ferreira (1962) demonstrated the presence of glycogen in blood platelets with the aid of this agent.

Aldehydes other than glutaraldehyde can also be used in fixation of blood platelets. Formaldehyde may well have been underestimated as a fixative (Pease, 1964). Preliminary personal experience with buffered formaldehyde has shown that it is probably useful in the fixation of blood platelets. Fibrillar structures in the cytoplasm, however, had a distinctly more coarse appearance than in glutaraldehyde-fixed material.

Of the remaining aldehydes, only hydroxyadipaldehyde has actually been used. This is known to be a poor fixative, but it has the advantage that it exerts a less marked influence on enzyme activity in histochemical experiments (Sabatini et al. 1963).

IV. Dehydration and Embedding

For dehydration we have used the scheme shown in Table 3. This applies to the use of epon or araldite as embedding agent. Some authors, however, recommend a brief period of dehydration because extraction of material

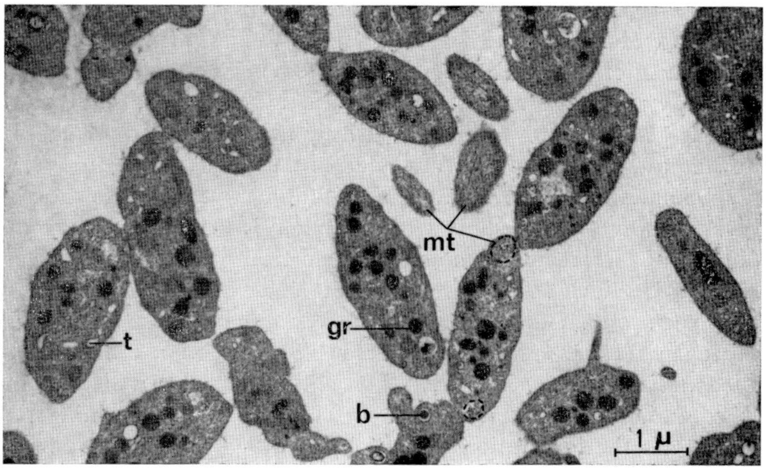

Fig. 4. Glutaraldehyde fixation in suspension by addition of 8 ml 1 % glutaraldehyde buffered with 0.07 M phosphate buffer pH 7.4 to 2 ml blood. Postfixation with osmium tetroxide. Staining by uranyl acetate and lead citrate. Note the microtubules (mt) in cross-section and sectioned longitudinally.

can still occur during this procedure (Pease, 1964).

Table 3. Dehydration and Embedding.

ethanol 30%	15 minutes
ethanol 50%	15 minutes
ethanol 70%	overnight
ethanol 90%	30 minutes
"ethanol 100%"	30 minutes
pure ethanol	60 minutes
pure ethanol	60 minutes
propylene oxide	60 minutes
propylene oxide	60 minutes
propylene oxide + embedding mixture (1:2)	60 minutes
embedding mixture	minimum 3 hours

Propylene oxide is stored in the presence of $MgSO_4$ to keep it dry. It is filtered before use.

The epon mixture used for embedding is indicated in Table 4. Table 5 provides similar data for araldite. Polymerization is effected at 35° C (12 hours), 45° C (12 hours) and 60° C (24 hours). During this process constant relative humidity must be ensured in the room in which embedding takes place, because in the case of epon this affects the cutting characteristics of the plastic.

Table 4. Epon.

Epon 812	4.30 gm
Dodecenyl succinic anhydride (DDSA)	1.40 gm
Methyl nadic anhydride (MNA)	1.40 gm
Dimethyl amino methyl phenol (DMP 30)	0.15 gm

Table 5. Araldite.

Araldite M (CY 212)	5.50 gm
Dodecenyl succinic anhydride (DDSA)	5.50 gm
Dibutyl phthalate	0.10 gm
Dimethyl amino methyl phenol (DMP 30)	0.20 gm

Several embedding media other than the above-mentioned plastics have been used in the study of blood platelets. The butylmethylmethacrylate mixture almost exclusively used in the past, cannot be recommended because it sublimates in the electron beam. By adding divinylbenzene, a cross-linked methacrylate is obtained which remains stable in the electron beam (Kushida, 1961). Good results have also been obtained with Vestopal W and Maraglas (Ryter and Kellenberger, 1958; Freeman and Spurlock, 1962).

The fundamental factor in all types of embedding is the infiltration of the plastic monomer into the tissue. Especially with a viscous monomer, this infiltration is of crucial importance if a readily cut plastic is to be obtained. In view of this, it is generally necessary to use a transitional solvent between absolute alcohol and the embedding media, e. g., propylene oxide, in epon and araldite embedding. It is also of great importance to use small tissue fragments and long periods of infiltration.

V. Staining

In order to intensify contrast in electron microscopic images, an electron-dense stain can be added either before or after embedding i. e., one "stains" the non-embedded block of tissue or the ultra-thin plastic section. In the former case, one usually employs phosphotungstic acid at a concentration of 2 percent in absolute alcohol. During dehydration this is added as an extra step after the absolute alcohol. A 1 percent $KMnO_4$ solution has also been used frequently. The disadvantage of these techniques is on the one hand that part of the stain is extracted during embedding, and on the other hand that the stain can influence the quality of embedding. Since good techniques have been developed for post-embedding staining, techniques requiring staining of the non-embedded block have largely been abandoned.

For post-embedding staining, use is made of uranyl acetate, lead compounds, vanadium salts, $KMnO_4$, phosphotungstic acid and impregnation with an ammoniacal silver solution. Most conventional techniques depend on lead compounds (e. g., lead citrate, lead tartrate or lead hydroxide) and uranyl acetate. Since our experience is most extensive with lead salts and uranyl acetate, these are the staining techniques to be discussed here.

For uranyl acetate staining, a saturated solution of uranyl acetate in water is used (Watson, 1958). The section, already mounted on a grid, are stained by allowing them to float on a drop of uranyl acetate placed on a layer of dental wax in a Petri dish. For epon sections, staining times required vary from 30–60 minutes; for araldite sections they range from 45 to 60 minutes. After staining the uranyl acetate is washed off with distilled water. This staining is especially well-suited for studying the dense granules in the blood platelets.

Among the lead salt stains we prefer the lead citrate technique according to Reynolds (1963) (cf Table 6). Measures must be taken to prevent contamination of the sections by lead carbonate. As a general purpose stain, lead gives a better contrast than uranyl acetate; the membranes and glycogen in particular are well contrasted. At greater magnifications, however, lead staining is less suitable in that the tissue assumes a granular character. The use of lead salts is therefore not advisable if instrument magnifications exceeding 15,000 diameters are employed. Staining time for epon is 5–20 minutes and for araldite somewhat longer.

Table 6. Lead Staining According to Reynolds (1963).

1. Prepare lead citrate by mixing	
lead citrate	1.33 gm
sodium citrate	1.76 gm
distilled water	30 ml
2. Shake this suspension vigorously for 1 minute and allow it to stand for 30 minutes with intermittent shaking.	
3. Add	
sodium hydroxide N	8.0 ml
distilled water up to	50.0 ml

The lead citrate dissolves. The solution is centrifuged before use till it is clear. It is stable for six months.

Since uranyl acetate and lead citrate supplement each in contrasting different tissue components in the study of blood platelets, the two stains can be combined to good advantage.

VI. Other Techniques in the Study of Blood Platelets

To study the reaction of blood platelets to a surface, use can be made of full thickness techniques which, prior to 1955, were the sole means of studying the ultrastructure of blood platelets. A glass slide is immersed in a 1 percent solution of formvar in chloroform so that a coating of formvar forms on the slide. The slide is placed in blood or PRP. After a period of incubation the slide is washed and then placed in a fixative, e. g., buffered 1 percent osmium tetroxide solution. After a brief period of fixation the layer of formvar is removed from the slide and transferred to grids. Examination with the electron microscope then discloses only the contours of the blood platelet; nothing of its internal structure is visible. It is possible in this way to distinguish the various transformations of blood platelets known also in light microscopy, viz.: the round form, the dendritic form (with many pseudopods), the transitional form and the spread-out form, i. e., the blood platelet spread completely over the surface.

Bessis and Breton-Gorius (1965) described a technique of studying the internal structure of blood platelets adhering to a surface. A carbon-coated slide was placed in plasma. After incubation, the blood platelets were fixed in situ, dehydrated and embedded by placing capsules filled with epon upside-down on the slide. After polymerization, the capsules were detached from the glass surface by applying abrupt changes of temperature.

Bull (1966) used the adhesion technique in effecting negative staining of structures localized below the platelet membrane. One drop of PRP was brought into contact with a carbon-coated grid. After 3 minutes the drop was removed with filter paper, the blood platelets remaining attached to the grid. A drop of phosphotungstic acid (neutralized with KOH to pH 6.8) was twice applied to the grid and immediately removed. The grid was then air dried. The platelets were made susceptible to staining by rendering the membrane permeable to the stain; this was achieved by creating, in the PRP, circumstances which caused the occurrence of viscous metamorphosis.

VII. Histochemical Studies

Histochemical studies of blood platelets have so far been relatively scarce. The various investigations will be briefly reviewed.

Gautier and his co-workers studied the influence of various enzymes on ultra-thin sections of blood platelets embedded in Vestopal W. They succeeded in localizing glycogen with the aid of amylase digestion (Jean and Gautier, 1961). By exposing the sections to the effect of pepsin, they demonstrated that the dense granules have a high protein concentration (Falcão et al. 1964). For localization of enzymes, only techniques using lead as capturing agent have so far been employed. White and Krivit (1965), studied the localization of ATP-splitting enzymes in this manner. The phosphate groups released from ATP react with the lead ion of the incubation medium and enable the investigator to localize the enzyme because they precipitate in the tissue as insoluble and electron dense lead phosphate. These investigations are carried out in tissue fixed with one of the aldehydes, e. g., hydroxyadipaldehyde, for the cell membrane must be permeable to the incubation medium, and the enzyme must be fixed without losing its action. According to Behnke (1966), techniques based on demonstration of enzyme localizations with lead ions, may be of very limited nature in the study of blood platelets due to the nonspecific adherence of lead particles to this tissue. We have personally had disappointing experiences in localizing ATPase with lead as capturing agent in blood platelets fixed with glutaraldehyde.

Electron microscopic localization of proteins in blood platelets is feasible in principle with aid of labelled antibodies. White et al. (1965) made use of ferritin-labelled antifibrinogen to localize fibrinogen in blood platelets during viscous metamorphosis. Since this labelled antifibrinogen had been added to PRP, platelets were actually labelled with immune complexes consisting of fibrinogen and the labelled antibody. Blood platelets whose membranes had been rendered permeable by repeated washing, showed a diffuse distribution of the labelled agent.

We personally found that fibrinogen was no longer demonstrable on the blood platelet membrane after washing twice in 0.9 percent NaCl. We were able to localize fibrinogen in blood platelets by incubating ultra-thin sections with labelled antifibrinogen. The dense granules and the vacuoles (somewhat swollen in our fixation technique) proved to contain no fibrinogen. The fibrinogen was found localized in the cytoplasmic matrix.

Besides fixation, it is especially embedding and polymerization that are important for maintaining the antigenic structure of the molecule to be localized by immuno-electron microscopy in ultra-thin sections. Moreover, removal of non-specifically absorbed protein molecules is difficult but essential. For this purpose we designed a micro-electrophoresis apparatus. Non-specific absorbed protein was removed from the ultra-thin sections by submitting it to free electrophoresis (Sixma, 1966). Adequate control studies are essential for immuno-electron microscopy. The elaborateness of the procedure and the difficulty of obtaining pure antibodies exclude large-scale use of this fertile histochemical technique.

For localization of serotonin in blood platelets, Davis and Kay (1965) used an autoradiographic technique adapted to electron microscopy. They localized serotonin both in the granules and in the cytoplasm. The applicability of electron microscopic autoradiography is limited by the poor resolution which characterizes this technique. Around every silver granule observed in the ultimate image, one should imagine a circle with a radius of $\pm 0.2\,\mu$, indicating the area within which the radioisotope is localized. Given the minute dimensions of the various blood platelet organelles, this means that accurate localization is virtually an illusion.

VIII. Fibrinogen and Fibrin

A. Fibrinogen

Fibrinogen has been studied with the aid of shadow casting and negative staining. It consists of nodules which are often encountered in chains of three individuals (Hall and Slayter, 1959). The size of these nodules has been reported as ranging from 60 to 220 Å. The majority of authors maintain that the nodules are spherical. Köppel (1967) believes that the bovine fibrinogen molecule consist of nodules of 220 Å which correspond to his model of a pentagonal dodecahedron. The peptide chains of the fibrinogen molecule are believed to

form the facets of this model as double alpha helices.
Shadow casting is best done with platinum or platinum carbon shadowing. Further details about these techniques can be found in various manuals on electron microscopic technique (Kay, 1965). Negative staining of fibrinogen can be achieved without difficulty by the conventional technique, using 1–2 percent phosphotungstic acid (PTA) buffered to pH 6.0–7.4 with drops of 1 N KOH. The fibrinogen solution is applied to the surface of the phosphotungstic acid solution and allowed to spread. After about 1 minute one drop is placed on the grid by touching the grid to the surface. The excess of PTA is removed with the aid of a filter paper. An alternative possibility is to spray a mixture of fibrinogen solution and PTA solution onto the grid. Negative staining can also be carried out by placing a drop of the fibrinogen solution on the grid, followed by the blotting of excess liquid onto filter paper, repeating the procedure with the PTA solution. The highly variable results obtained in studies of the fibrinogen molecule suggest that some parameters in these studies have not yet been sufficiently controlled.

B. Fibrin

Fibrin in the electron microscopy presents the appearance of a fibrous network with characteristic periodical electron-dense cross striations. Wyllie (1964) pointed out that fibrin does not invariably show this cross striation. The pH at which fibrin forms and the rate of fibrin formation are believed to be determinants of this striation. The periodicity is usually about 220 Å. Köppel (1967) in addition described a periodicity of 165 Å associated with cross striation obliquely to the longitudinal axis of the fibrin fibers. The cause of the periodicity of the fibrin structure is to be sought in the arrangement of the fibrinogen molecules. A number of structural models have been suggested. Hall and Slayter (1959) maintain that the fibrinogen molecule, 475 Å long and consisting of a strand of three nodules, shortens to about 50 percent of its original length. The periodicity results from the formation of linear aggregates of fibrinogen molecules parallel to the longitudinal axis of the fibrin fiber, with the terminal nodules touching. Bang, (1964, 1967) proposed a model based on direct electron microscopical observation and measurements of individual fibrinogen molecules and intermediate polymer macromolecules. This model proposes the formation of intermediate fibrin polymers to occur through staggered overlapping of individual monomeric units and fiber formation through staggered overlapping of several intermediate macromolecular chains. This model is in agreement with observed hydrodynamic data for fibrinogen and intermediate polymer dimensions and does not preclude shortening of fibrinogen during the transition to fibrin monomer, an assumption which was made by Hall and Slayter (1959). The concept of fibrin formation through staggered overlapping of monomeric and intermediate polymeric units was supported by low angle x-ray diffraction data (Stryer et al. 1963).
Laki (1962) accepts the fibrinogen model of Hall and Slayter (1959) in principle, but believes that the molecules are perpendicular to the longitudinal axis of the fibrin fiber. Köppel (1967) believes that the periodicity is explained by a side-by-side arrangement of the fibrinogen molecules, each the shape of a pentagonal dodecahedron. The size of the fibrinogen molecule (about 220 Å) thus determines the periodicity. The electron-dense bands are the edges of the fibrinogen molecules, formed by double peptide chains.

References

Aster, R. H., and Jandl, J. H. (1964). *J. Clin. Invest. 43,* 843.
Bang, N. U. (1964). *Thromb. Diath. Hemorrhag. Suppl. 13 12,* 73.
Bang, N. U. (1967). *In* "Blood Clotting Enzymology" (W. Seegers, Ed.). Acad. Press, New York.
Barkhan, P. (1957). *J. Clin. Path. 10,* 26.
Behnke, O. (1965). *J. Ultrastr. Res. 13,* 469.
Behnke, O. (1966). *J. Histochem. and Cytochem. 14,* 432.
Bessis, M. (1950). *Blood 5,* 1083.
Bessis, M., and Breton-Gorius, J. (1965). *Nouv. Rev. Franc. d'Hematol. 5,* 657.
Bloom, G. (1954). *Ztschr. Zellforsch. 40,* 222.

Bull, B. S. (1966). *Blood 28,* 901.
Danon, D., Jerushalmy, Z., and de Vries, A. (1959). *Virology 9,* 719.
David-Ferreira, J. F. (1961). *Ztschr. Zellforsch. 55,* 89.
David-Ferreira, J. F., and David-Ferreira, K. (1962). *Ztschr. Zellforsch. 56,* 789.
David-Ferreira, J. F. (1964). *Intern. Rev. Cytol. 17,* 99.
Davis, R. B., and Kay, D. (1965). *Nature 207,* 650.
Falcao, L., Gautier, A., Lombardi, L., Jean, G., and Probst, M. (1964). *J. Microscopie 3,* 519.
Feissly, R., Gautier, A., and Marcovici, I. (1957). *Rev. d'Hematol. 12,* 397.
Firkin, B. G., O'Neill, B. J., Dunstan, B., and Oldfield, R. (1965). *Blood 25,* 345.
Freeman, J. A., and Spurlock, B. O. (1962). *J. Cell. Biol. 13,* 437.
Glynn, M. F., Movat, H. Z., Murphy, E. A., and Mustard, J. F. (1965). *J. Lab. Clin. Med. 65,* 179.
Hall, C., and Slayter, H. S. (1959). *J. Biophys. Biochem. Cytol. 5,* 11.
Haydon, G. B., and Taylor, D. A. (1965). *J. Cell. Biol. 26,* 273.
Hovig, T. (1965). *Thromb. Diath. Hemorrhag. 13,* 84.
Jean, G., and Gautier, A. (1961). *Compt. Rend. Acad. Sci. 253,* 2247.
Kautz, J., and DeMarsh, G. B. (1955). *Rev. d'Hematol. 10,* 314.
Kay, D. (1965). "Techniques for Electron Microscopy", Blackwell Scient. Publ., Oxford.
Köppel, G. (1958). *Ztschr. Zellforsch. 47,* 401.
Köppel, G. (1967). *Ztschr. Zellforsch. 77,* 443.
Kushida, H. (1961). *J. Electronmicros. 10,* 197.
Laki, K. (1962). *Sci. American 206,* 60.
Luft, J. H. (1961). *J. Biophys. Biochem. Cytol. 9,* 409.
Luft, J. H. (1956). *J. Biophys. Biochem. Cytol. 2,* 799.
Palade, G. E. (1952). *J. Exptl. Med. 95,* 285.
Pease, D. C. (1964). *In* "Histological Techniques in Electron Microscopy". Acad. Press, New York.
Rebuck, J. W., Riddle, J. M., Johnson, S. A., Monto, R. W., and Sturrock, R. M. (1960). *Henry Ford Hosp. Med. Bull. 8,* 273.
Reynolds, E. S. (1963). *J. Cell. Biol. 17,* 208.
Rinehart, J. F. (1955). *Amer. J. Clin. Pathol. 25,* 605.
Ryter, A., and Kellenberger, E. (1958). *J. Ultrastr. Res. 2,* 200.
Sabatini, D. D., Bensch, K., and Barnett, R. J. (1963). *J. Cell. Biol. 17,* 19.
Sandborn, E. B., LeBuis, J. J., and Bois, P. (1966). *Blood 27,* 247.
Schulz, H., and Weddell, J. (1962). *Klin. Wochenschr. 40,* 1114.
Sixma, J. J. (1966). Thesis, Utrecht.
Sixma, J. J., and Molenaar, I. (1966). *Thromb. Diath. Hemorrhag. 16,* 153.
Stryer, L., Cohen, C., and Langridge, R. (1963). *Nature 197,* 793.
Watson, M. L. (1958). *J. Biophys. Biochem. Cytol. 4,* 475.
White, J. G., Krivit, W., and Vernier, R. L. (1965). *Blood 25,* 241.
White, J. G., and Krivit, W. (1965). *Blood 26,* 554.
Wolpers, C., and Ruska, H. (1939). *Klin. Wochenschr. 18,* 1077, 1111.
Wyllie, J. C. (1964). *Exptl. Mol. Pathol. 3,* 468.
Zetterqvist, H. (1956). Thesis, Stockholm.
Zucker, M. B., and Borelli, J. (1954). *Blood, 9,* 602.

CHAPTER X

Immunologic Techniques

MARION I. BARNHART

I. Introduction

Blood coagulation and clot lysis require a number of plasma proteins that possess distinctive properties of chemistry, activity and immunology. Their unique immunologic features can be exploited in laboratory assays to provide valuable information of physiologic alterations or of pathologic states. With specific antisera the various plasma proteins can be identified on a basis other than biologic activity, quantitated, and in some cases localized to cells (Barnhart, 1967). In addition, detection of autoantibodies, formed by an individual responding abnormally to his own body constituents, becomes possible.

Successful application of immunologic techniques depends upon the discriminative ability of the developed immune serum. A broad spectrum antiserum has advantage in certain tests but is worthless in others. A highly selective antiserum may be required for exact identification. It is the unique structural features as well as distinct chemical groupings of molecules that are responsible for their immunogenicity (Kabat and Mayer, 1961). Development of specific antisera for the distinctive antigenic determinants permits either qualitative or quantitative evaluation of molecules bearing similar determinants. Thus "native" and biologically active proteins can be measured as can their degradation products providing they retain the prerequisite determinant groups.

A variety of immunochemical tests are available for assay of clot promoting or lysing proteins in body fluids (blood, extravascular fluids or extracts from cells and tissues). Immunologic techniques based on precipitin reactions, or complement fixation, or passive cutaneous anaphylaxis or fluorescence provide a wide range of sensitivity. Selectivity relates to the characteristics of the developed antisera employed in the respective tests. Most of these test are relatively easy to perform in a reasonable time, require small samples, and are reproducible. Extra care and time may be necessary in the work preliminary to the actual immunologic test. For the most selective and sensitive procedures special attention must be given to purification of the protein antigen, antibody production and immunologic characterization of the antiserum.

Finally, the fluorescent antibody technique has special advantages for cellular studies (Coons, 1956). These are no better than the selectivity of the antibody employed. Also, cellular concentration of the protein antigen limits the technique. Under optimal conditions specific immunofluorescence marks a cellular localization or sites of synthesis and storage or degradation depots of proteins concerned in clot formation or lysis (Barnhart, 1967).

II. Antibody Production

Proteins possess the requisite properties to elicit an immune response and develop circulating antibodies. Several methods are practical to provoke antibody formation and are detailed in most standard immunology texts (Kabat and Mayer, 1961) and in other publications (Cohn, 1952; Goodman et al. 1957; Barnhart, Anderson and Baker, 1962). Selection among these should be determined by requirements of the test system and the objectives of the investigator. The most powerful antisera are elicited by multiple injections of relatively large amounts of the desired antigen in conjunction with an adjuvant. This procedure is useful in preparing broad spectrum antisera. For example, antiplasma produced as described is especially valuable in immunoelectrophoresis to mark the numerous protein constituents of test plasma. However, microgram quantities of protein are sufficient to provoke circulating antibodies which are highly selective and frequently powerful (Barnhart et al. 1962). This method minimizes the immune response to trace contaminants so that univalent antibody of limited reactivity results.

A. Immunogenicity

Several proteins that are functional in blood coagulation and clot lysis have proved to be immunogenic (Table 1). Specific antisera were evoked by quality products of any one of the following purified proteins: accelerator globulin (Barnhart et al. 1963); antihemophilic globulin (Berglund, 1962a, b; McLester and Wagner, 1964; Barnhart, 1967); autoprothrombin II and autoprothrombin C (Barnhart, 1967); fibrin and fibrinogen and their lysis products (Nussenzweig and Seligman, 1960; Nussenzweig et al. 1961; Barnhart and Anderson, 1962; Berglund, 1962b; Lewis and Wilson, 1964; Hirsh et al. 1965; Barnhart, 1967); fibrinolysin (Barnhart, 1967; Back et al. 1965); fibrinopeptides (Barnhart, 1963; Berglund and Blombäck, 1965; Barnhart, 1967); Hageman factor (Barnhart et al. 1967); platelet factor 3 (Barnhart and Walsh, 1966); plasmin inhibitor (Schwick, 1964); prethrombin (Barnhart et al. 1967); profibrinolysin (Barnhart et al. 1962; Riddle and Barnhart, 1965; Back et al. 1965; Robbins et al. 1965); prothrombin (Halick and Seegers, 1956; Miller, 1958; Schwick and Schultze, 1959; Barnhart, 1960; Barnhart et al. 1962; Berglund, 1962a; Anderson and Barnhart, 1964a); thrombin (Halick and Seegers, 1956; Schwick and Schultze, 1959; Berglund, 1962a; Barnhart, 1967); and trypsin inhibitor (Schwick, 1964).

In general our experience has been that plasma proteins are exceptionally good antigens;

Table 1. Immunogenicity of Coagulation and Lytic Proteins.

Product[a]	Rabbits Injected	Dose mg/kg body wt	Precipitin Titer (reciprocal of dilution)[b]
Ac-globulin, Bovine	12	0.5–5.0	512–4096
Auto-prothrombin C, Bovine	8	0.1–1.0	256–512
Auto-prothrombin II, Bovine	6	1.0–3.0	2048–4096
Fibrin, Human	4	1.3–3.8	128–512
Fibrinogen			
Bovine	28	0.1–50.0	1024–8192
Canine	44	0.001–5.0	1024–16384
Equine	3	1.0–10.0	2048
Guinea Pig	4	0.3–0.5	4096–8192
Human	99	0.1–2.0	1024–16384
Rat	9	0.5–10.0	4096–8192
Fibrinolysin			
Bovine	3	0.5–1.0	256–2048
Human	7	0.5–1.0	512–2048
Fibrinopeptides			
Bovine A	1	1.0	256[c]
Bovine B	1	1.0	128[c]
Human A	1	1.0	256[c]
Human B	2	1.0	256[c]
Hageman Factor, Bovine	8	0.1–1.0	64–4096
Platelet Cofactor I			
Bovine	11	0.1–11.0	512–4096
Human	14	0.1–1.0	2048–8192
Platelet Factor 3			
Canine	3	1.0–3.0	1[d]
Bovine	2	–	16
Prethrombin, Bovine			
Prothrombin			
Bovine	23	0.01–3.0	16–4096
Canine	12	0.3–5.0	512–4096
Human	17	0.01–8.0	256–4096
Profibrinolysin			
Canine	30	0.1–1.0	64–4096
Equine	5	0.1	64–2048
Human	62	0.1–1.0	8–4096

[a] Highly purified products.

[b] Stock, 1% purified protein used for immunization, diluted as indicated.

[c] Titered against purified fibrinogen. No reaction against fibrinopeptide.

[d] Platelet agglutination a better index of strength and a good reaction occurred.

this may relate to their molecular weights exceeding 10,000. But proteins derived from prothrombin or fibrinogen were less immunogenic than the parent as the number of antigenic determinant groups was reduced by the limited proteolysis. Also, chemical manipulations such as acetylation alter the immunogenic power of molecules. For example, acetylated thrombin was not an effective antigen (Barnhart et al. 1962) although thrombin was weakly antigenic in comparison to prothrombin (Barnhart, 1967).

Other important considerations for demonstrating the immunogenicity of a molecule are the sensitivity of various animal species to the injected material, the route of administration, the dosage, the reagents included with the antigen as adjuvants, the number of injections and the time of collection of the antiserum. In our work we prefer New Zealand white rabbits. Dutch rabbits appear more suitable for multiple injection procedures and large doses of antigen. Chickens are good reactors to the plasma proteins (Goodman et al. 1957), however, the high salt content of the antiserum can be troublesome. Commercial sources frequently prefer the larger animals, horse, goat, and sheep, as antibody producers. The horse produces flocculating antibody which is characterized by a broad equivalence zone. All the other favored species produce precipitating antibodies which exhibit a narrow equivalence zone but form insoluble antigen-antibody complexes in excess antibody. Guinea pigs are better suited for hypersensitivity responses than as sources of antibody for ex vivo study.

B. Immunization Procedures

Precipitating antibodies can be elicited in mammals and birds by any route of injection, especially when the antigen is given with adjuvant. Each laboratory has its own preferred immunization schedule and the bias is largely dictated by previous success. Combination of the antigen with some carrier, Freund's adjuvant or aluminum hydroxide, provides the opportunity for slow release of antigen and repeated stimulation of the immune mechanism after only a single injection. With weak antigen and small molecular weight peptides is may be advisable to use plastic particles coated with the material of interest. Berglund and Blombäck (1965) prepared potent anti-fibrinopeptide B by coating acrylic plastic particles with fibrinopeptide B (molecular weight near 1400).

Multiple injections are favored when a polyvalent antiserum is desired as there is repeated opportunity for minor components of the antigen preparation as well as the major constituent to evoke an immune response. A single injection of an antigen emulsion can provide an effective stimulus to the immune mechanism and favor antibody production against the major constituent of the antigen.

The amount of antigen injected is an important determiner of the antibody response. Relatively large doses of purified proteins (3–100 mg/kg rabbit) are costly and even trace contaminants may be present in amounts sufficient to provoke their own antibody response. Smaller doses of highly purified proteins (0.1–2 mg/kg rabbit) are more realistic and favor production of antibody to the major constituent. Even smaller amounts of immunogenic material can be effective. As little as 0.1 μg of typhoid O antigen can elicit an excellent antibody response in rabbits (Grabar and Oudin, 1947). Fibrinogen is also very immunogenic and a dose of 1 μg/kg rabbit evoked a recognizable antibody response (Barnhart et al. 1962). Profibrinolysin and prothrombin in doses as low as 10 μg/kg rabbit elicited precipitating antibodies after our single injection technique. One or more of these 3 plasma proteins are trace contaminants of many purified plasma proteins. For reasons of economy and selectivity in our laboratory we prefer microgram doses of highly purified protein mixed with $Al(OH)_3$ and given only once intramuscularily. This schedule favors good antibody production for the major component while keeping trace contaminants so low that they may not stimulate an immune response.

An attractive solution to the problems of blocking antibody response to known contaminants is use of animals made tolerant to the contaminant. Immunologically tolerant animals can be prepared by injecting newborns with massive doses of a material or by injecting adult animals with puromycin and large doses of the desired material. Berglund (1963) produced fibrinogen tolerant rabbits by injecting newborns with fibrinogen. Schwartz and Dameshek (1963) produced albumin tolerant rabbits with the puromycin procedure in adults. Theoretically a colony of fibrinogen tolerant rabbits offer advantages but practically the cost in time and testing may offset these.

Technical details for immunization of rabbits follow. Several steps are preliminary to injection of the antigen. Healthy young adult New Zealand rabbits are weighed and their weight recorded (we prefer rabbits near 2 kg). The rabbits should be test bled from either blood vessels of the ear (marginal vein or median artery) or by cardiac puncture using sterile technique. After cardiac puncture 1–2 days pass before immunization to be sure the animal was not harmed by the procedure.

1. Test Bleeding and Harvesting Technique

The selected area is shaved, washed if necessary and wiped with 70% ethyl alcohol. The ear is vigorously rubbed with a pad soaked in xylene to dilate the blood vessels. The blood vessel is punctured with a sterile 22 gauge needle which directs the immediately flowing blood into centrifuge tubes. The needle is removed, bleeding stopped by pressure and the area washed with soap and water. A fine description of the procedure for cardiac bleeding appears in the text of Campbell and associates (1964). The collected blood is permitted to clot and is stored overnight in a refrigerator. The clot can be cut once prior to centrifugation (Servall Refrigerated Centrifuge, 4000 RPM for 10 min). The clear serum is labeled and stored in a deep freeze at –20° C.

2. Preparation and Injection of Antigen

The dose is calculated in terms of the body weight for the selected rabbit.

a. Aluminum Hydroxide and Single Intramuscular Injection. The required amount of antigen is placed in solution in no more than 2 ml of sterile saline (0.9%). This is mixed with an equal volume of aluminum hydroxide suspension (Wyeth Amphojel is a convenient and satisfactory preparation). The 2–4 ml $Al(OH)_3$ suspension of antigen is drawn into a 5 ml sterile syringe and injected in 2 ml amounts into the high muscle of 1 or both hind legs.

b. Freund's Adjuvant and Multiple Subcutaneous Injections. Freund's adjuvant is prepared by mixing in the small metal container of a Waring blender, 8.5 vol of sterile light mineral oil with 1.5 vol of sterile mannide mono-oleate (Arlacel A, Atlas Powder Co., Wilmington, Del.) to provide an emulsion (when suitable a drop applied to water should not spread but retain its shape). To this emulsion is added 10 mg heat-killed Mycobacterium tuberculosis or butyricum (Difco, Detroit) per 100 ml and the required amount of antigen in saline (0.9%). The selected rabbit is given 1–2 ml of the antigen preparation subcutaneously with sterile technique. One or several injections can be placed along each side of the vertebral column and if desired repeated at daily or longer intervals.

3. Harvesting

From 9–14 days after the $Al(OH)_3$ injection or 6–8 weeks after the Freund's procedure the rabbit is test bled. A microring precipitin test (Section II, A) on this serum as well as the rabbit's own preimmunization serum establishes the effectiveness of the immune response and rules out nonspecific reaction of the animal. The immunized rabbit can be exsanguinated by cardiac puncture at any convenient time over the next several months.

III. Antibody Characterization

After the antiserum has been developed it is essential to assay individual antisera for their strength and specificities. These qualities cannot be assumed. Fortunately considerable information can be gained from small samples. Such knowledge permits a decision either to exploit the special characteristics of that serum or to pool it with other antisera for a broad spectrum reagent. Some immunochemical tests require such multivalent antisera while other tests require highly selective univalent antisera. The objectives of the investigator dictate the prerequisites for antibody quality.

A few of the techniques for establishing the strength and specificity of the antisera are described in this section.

A. Microring Precipitin Test

This is a rapid qualitative indicator of precipitating antibody. We use this test routinely to assess the effectiveness of immunization in our rabbits. Serial dilutions of the soluble antigen (1% in saline) are layered over the undiluted antiserum or preimmunization serum placed in very small test tubes (sealed fine glass tubing, internal diameter 3 mm). The end point is the highest dilution of antigen to give a barely detectable ring at the interface with the specific antibody. With care as little as 0.1 μg of protein will form a visible ring. Long tipped micropipetes deliver 0.25 ml of the reagents (clear solutions) into the tubes. A brass or plastic rack holds 12–15 tubes upright. The ring formation at room temperature is recorded at 1, 2, 4 and 24 hrs. The most significant reactions occur early. Rings can be graded at 1–4 plus in terms of their size or density. Antisera of good potency give rings to tube 10 (antigen dilution 1/1024 or 2.5 μg present). More powerful antisera show reactions to tube 15 (antigen dilution 1/32728 or 0.08 μg present).

If desired the precipitin can be sedimented by centrifugation and the supernatants tested for remaining antigen or antibody. Thus the position of the equivalence zone (quantitative combination of antigen and antibody) can be established for a future quantitative precipitin analysis.

B. Gel Diffusion

Precipitin reactions also occur in semisolid media, i. e. agar or acrylamide gels. Although the analysis takes longer than the microring test it is more sensitive and provides information on the relative heterogeneity of the developed antiserum. As different molecules seldom diffuse at identical rates, there is opportunity for several antigen-antibody systems to show their presence by discrete and separate precipitin band formation. Immunodiffusion can be useful in identification of partially degraded proteins when antigenic determinant groups are retained that react with antibody to the parent molecule. Also, interrelationships or divergence of protein can be studied between species.

Under carefully controlled conditions much useful information can be gained on the characteristics of antibody or antigen. However, several limitations are intrinsic and need be considered. First, the method cannot detect soluble antigen-antibody complexes. Second, even when the system is capable of insoluble complexes, a sufficient concentration of the two reactants must be present to form a visible precipitin band. Third, care must be exercised to avoid artifacts due to bacterial contamination, temperature variation or evaporation of the sample.

1. Diffusion Plates

The equipment and procedure for double diffusion in agar will be described. Several variants of Ouchterlony plates were designed by Wilson (1958, 1959) and Goodman (1962). These plates (Fig. 1) are specially constructed of lucite (Grafar Corporation, Detroit) with lantern slide glass tops (Fig. 1, Parts 14 and 16) and bottoms to aid in observation and photography. Plates similar to the original Ouchterlony design permits study of 5–7 different materials in the same plate (Fig. 1; plates 6 and 8). Other plate variants have larger or smaller wells placed at different angles with respect to one another to increase resolving power (Fig. 1; plates 11, 12, and 13) or encourage more rapid precipitin band formation (Fig. 1; plates 3, 4, 5, 9, and 10). One plate (Fig. 1; Plate 2) has six parallel reaction sites permitting comparison while quantitive studies and resolving power are excellent. All the plates rest on a brass or lucite rim (Fig. 1; Part 7) to protect the bottom from scratches.

Small samples (0.02–0.2 ml) placed in wells that are cut out of the agar, diffuse into agar and ordinarily show precipitin bands within 6–24 hrs. Plates may be observed and photo-

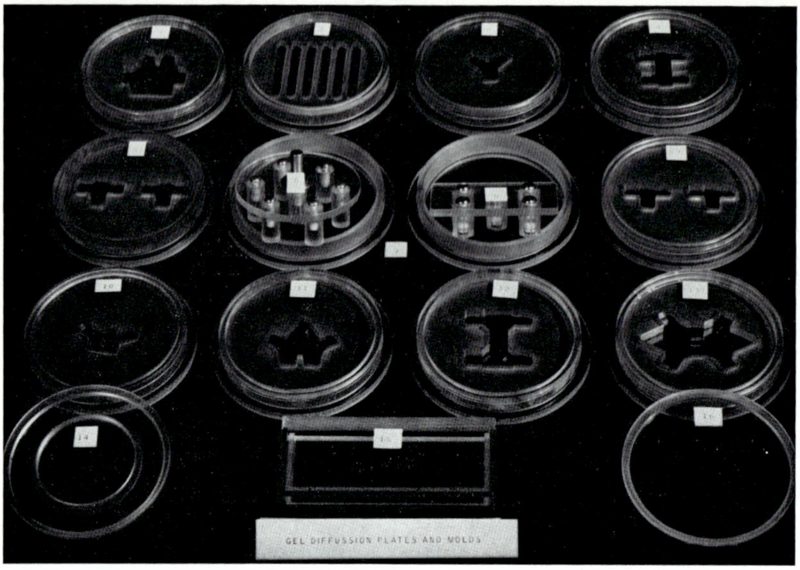

Fig. 1. Various Wilson type and Ouchterlony type plates for gel diffusion.

graphed at any time. As the plates have closely fitted lids and are taped, evaporation is minimized so reactions develop without artifact over several days.

2. Preparation of Gel

Agar (Bacto-Agar Certified, Difco, Detroit) is placed in solution in phosphate buffered saline (9 vol saline to 1 vol 0.01 M buffer) by heating in a flask in boiling water. The agar (0.75 %) has merthiolate added to a concentration of 0.01 % to retard bacterial growth. If preferred, Chloromycetin (0.005 %) can be used for the same purpose.

Also suitable for immunodiffusion are gels prepared from 0.85 % Ionagar (Consolidated Laboratories Inc., Chicago Heights, Illinois), 1.5 % Noble Agar (Difco), 0.75 % Agarose (Marine Colloid Inc., distributed by Baush and Lomb) or 3.5 % Acrylamide (Canal Ind. Corp., Bethesda). Acrylamide gel plates require longer for precipitin band formation but fine precipitins stand out in sharp contrast against the water clear acrylamide gel.

3. Charging Plates

The clean (washed in a mild detergent and thoroughly rinsed in distilled water) dry plate is coated with a thin layer of hot dilute agar (0.37 %) by a brief exposure. These plates can be dried in a 37° C incubator or vacuum dessicator overnight or they may be charged with more hot agar (0.75 %) for immediate use. The hot agar is added to the analysis chamber until the agar reaches but does not overflow the top. As the agar cools and hardens the agar should shrink and become level with the top of the chamber.

When the gel has hardened, a sharp knife that fits the space exactly is used to cut out the wells which will hold the sample and antisera. Care must be exercised not to separate the main gel from the plate. The wells are coated and resealed to the main block of agar by addition of 0.1 ml hot dilute agar. The lid is replaced and the plate sealed with masking tape. These plates can be used or refrigerated in an inverted position for several days. Before use plates should be brought to room temperature and checked for cracks in the agar.

Samples (0.02–0.2 ml) are pipetted into the wells. If desired either 0.01 ml of merthiolate (0.01 %) or a drop of Chloromycetin (0.005 %) can be added to the wells. Ordinarily the merthiolate contained in the agar is adequate to prevent bacterial growth. Daily drawings are made to illustrate the exact position of the precipitin bands.

4. Interpretation

The number of precipitin bands formed is a measure of the number of antigen-antibody systems present (Fig. 2, 3). This number may represent only a minimum of the systems on hand. However, the method can provide a criterion of purity when well characterized antisera are employed with various dilutions of a test protein.

The positions of the bands with respect to the antigen and antibody wells give information on the relative concentrations of the 2 reactants (Fig. 3B). Near the equivalence ratio the precipitin band is immobile and positioned midway between the reactant wells. With either antigen or antibody in excess the precipitin band is displaced toward the weaker reactant.

The density of the precipitin band provides a relative gauge of the potency of the antiserum. Weaker antisera react to form finer precipitin bands. Such antisera can be concentrated for more acceptable reagents. Also the concentration of the antigen relates to the density of the band.

The pattern of the precipitin band formation can be most instructive. Molecules with similar antigenic determinant groups will exhibit complete fusion of their precipitin bands (Fig. 2 A, C). Molecules that have some antigenic groups in common but others that are unique will show a spur; i.e. one band pro-

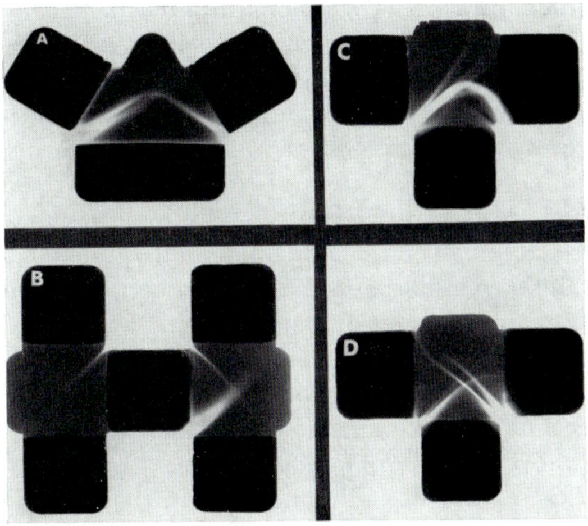

Fig. 2. Interpretation of immunodiffusion patterns. A. Pattern illustrates 2 reactants in left well with 1 identical with the molecules in the right well. Nonidentity of the second component in the left well is shown by the faint lower precipitin band intersecting the fused precipitin band of identity. Antiplasma is in the lower well. The left well contains a mixture of purified fibrinogen and prothrombin. The right well contains prothrombin. B. Pattern illustrates a single reactant (left pattern) with antifibrinogen (human) located in the central well. The right pattern shows spur formation and indicates some but not all of the molecules in lower right well have similar or identical antigenic determinant groups to those of molecules in upper right well. Various species plasmas were in the upper and lower wells. C. Multicomponent systems in both right and left wells reacted against antiplasma in lower well. Note heavy fusion band for molecules that are immunologically similar. Note 3 bands intersecting fused band. There are at least 6 components in the left well and 3 components in the right well. D. Multicomponent systems with reactions of nonidentity especially prominent by intersecting lines.

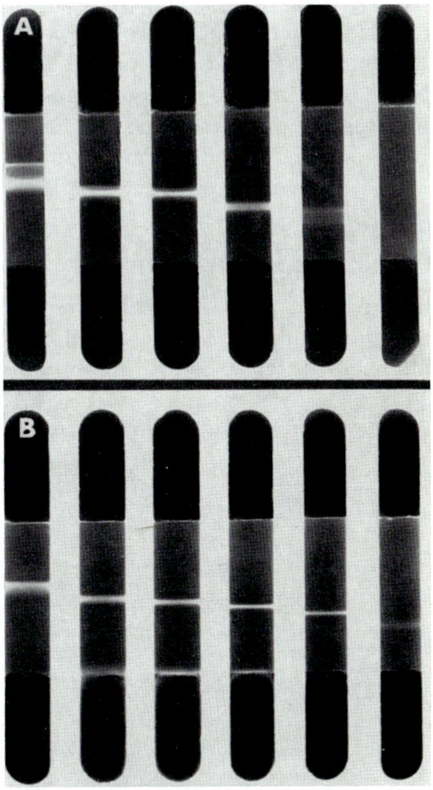

Fig. 3. Immunodiffusion patterns in Wilson comparative analysis plates. A. Illustrates a multicomponent system with antibody above and various dilutions of antigen in the lower wells. B. Shows a single component system with antifibrin in upper wells reacted against fibrin (5, 3, 1.5, 0.75, 0.36, and 0.18 mg/ml in lower wells).

jecting beyond the other (Fig. 2 B). Molecules with dissimilar antigenic groups will show complete intersection of their precipitin bands (Fig. 2 D). If the precipitin lines do not reach each other, no judgement can be made on the similarity or dissimilarity of the 2 molecules from different sources.

5. Photography

The precipitin bands are best viewed over an illuminator box (Grafar Corp., Detroit) which provides a dark background and fluorescent illumination from the sides. A camera support permits photography of the bands from above.

Another satisfactory method to record the precipitin bands makes use of a condensor type enlarger (Bessler). The plates are first rinsed with distilled water using care to avoid distortion of the gel. The wells are filled with distilled water. The plates are positioned on the negative carrier and placed between the condensor lens and enlarger lens. With illumination a print is made on Kodabromide (F5) paper. Any enlargement desired can be made with this simple direct method.

C. Immunoelectrophoresis

This method permits a triple characterization of a substance in terms of its electrophoretic mobility, its diffusion, its immunochemical specificity and sometimes its biologic reactivity. The agar gel procedure was introduced by Grabar and Williams (1953). Many valuable details on the method and its application appear in the book by Grabar and Burtin (1964). Several proteins concerned in blood coagulation and clot lysis are easily separated by immunoelectrophoresis without any prior treatment (Fig. 4). The method also has utility in identification and characterization of protein degradation products, i. e. fibrinogenolytic products (Fig. 5).

Advantages of the method are that minute samples of single substances or mixtures are processed under mild conditions and show their presence by precipitin arc formation. The method is extremely specific and sensitive. Trace impurities show up with concentrations near 0.1 % when a good quality antiserum is used. With a univalent antiserum immunologic relatives of the original antigen can be identified even though mobilities may be atypical. With care and high quality reagents valuable information can be gained on the homogeneity or heterogeneity of purified products, or of multicomponent biological systems such as blood and synovial fluid. The technique also permits recognition of abnormal proteins in pathologic states.

Disadvantages of the method are that soluble antigen-antibody systems cannot be identified, the reactants must be soluble in the buffer

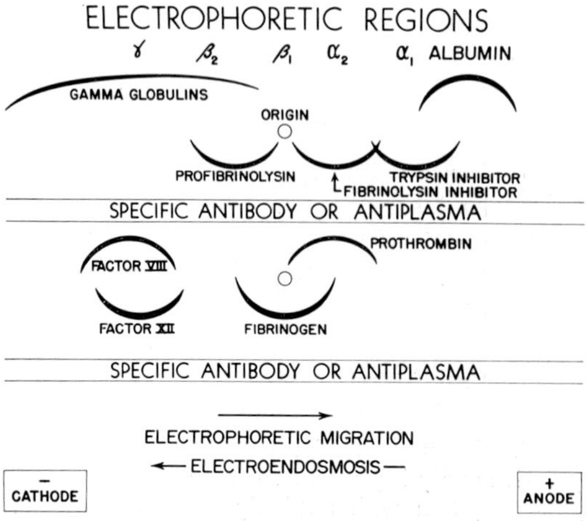

Fig. 4. Diagram of immunoelectrophoretic patterns for several proteins concerned in clot formation or lysis.

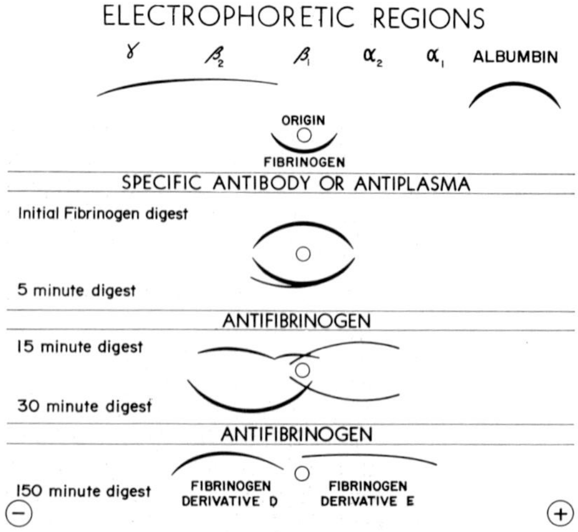

Fig. 5. Diagram of immunoelectrophoretic positions of fibrinogen and several of its split products resulting from digestion with fibrinolysin.

system, and well-characterized antisera are required for the most discriminating studies.

The technique applied to microscope slides will be briefly described as used in our laboratory.

1. Preparation of Agar

A 4% agar solution is prepared by dissolving 8 gm in 200 ml distilled water by heating in a hot water bath. An equal vol of Barbital buffer (0.2 M, pH 8.2 and 0.1 ionic strength) is added through a funnel containing glass wool. Buffers more acid than pH 6.5 favor nonspecific precipitation while buffers more alkaline than pH 8.2 reverse or inhibit precipitin formation. The agar can be stored in 20 ml quantities and melted down when needed.

2. Preparation of Slides

Dry slides, precleaned with alcohol, are placed on a level surface. With a pipet gently applied to the middle of the slide, 2.5 ml of hot agar (2%) is released. Usually an even film distributes over the slide. After 15–30 minutes the gel hardens. Then a special cutter is used for cutting holes and troughs in the gel. The agar is removed from the antigen holes by a needle attached to a water aspirator. Slides should be used immediately although they can be stored overnight in the humidifying chamber.

3. Sample Application and Electrophoresis

The electrophoresis apparatus is filled with Barbital buffer and Whatman filter paper 1 used as barriers against electrolyte decomposition products.

The test antigen is added with a micropipet to the holes in the agar. The slides are placed on the rack in the electrophoresis cell. After 3–5 minutes for absorption to occur, a drop of hot agar is placed on the hole to seal it. Whatman filter paper (2 × 9 inch) provides the wicks to the buffer. Care is taken to insure a wet connection exists between the agar and the buffer. The assembly is covered and the electric leads attached. The voltage is set at 40 volts, equivalent to about 6 volts/cm. The duration of the run is 30–45 minutes depending on the separation desired.

4. Diffusion

The slides are removed from the electrophoresis chamber. The pre-cut troughs are now removed with the aid of a capillary pipet attached to a water aspirator. The trough is filled by capillary pipet with the antiserum. Small pieces of filter paper are placed on the ends of the slides and moistened with distilled water. The rack and slides are placed in a humidifying chamber overnight at room temperature.

5. Drying and Staining

The rack and slides are placed in a washing tray. Saline (0.9%) is gently added with care not to dislodge the agar film. Washing with repeated changes of saline continues for 4 hrs. Distilled water is next added with several changes before permitting the slide to remain overnight in the water.

The rack of slides is removed the next day and strips of moist filter paper applied to each slide. The rack is placed in a 37° C incubator for drying.

Slides are stained in Ponceau S (0.2%) for about 5 min. A tap water bath is used with a gentle rocking motion to remove excess dye without dislodging the agar film. Occasional slide removal and blotting with filter paper speeds dye extraction and keeps the agar film flattened on the slide. Air drying completes the process.

6. Interpretation

Individual antigen-antibody systems will show as precipitin arcs or lines at various positions in the agar gel. These positions are specific for each protein and depend on the degree of its ionization (number of electric charges), on the value of the electric field and on the size, shape, and molecular weight of the protein (Fig. 4, 5).

With electrophoresis in an alkaline environment, the proteins are negatively charged and move through the gel toward the anode (positive electrode). The slowest moving or stationary proteins will move toward the cathode (negative electrode) as electroendosmosis occurs. This serves to nullify or reverse the anodic migration because the liquid in the agar gel assumes a positive charge and carries the soluble proteins along. The final position of any protein is characteristic for the specific conditions of the test. Thus mobilities can be compared and electrophoretic groups identified.

The shape and position of the arc relative to the antiserum trough can be instructive. The curvature of the precipitin arcs relates to the diffusion coefficients rather than the concentrations. When the antigen diffuses more slowly than the antibody the arc curves away from the antibody. When both antigen and antibody diffuse at the same rate a straight precipitin line will form. The precipitin arc or line will form nearer the weaker reactant.

When the antiserum contains antibodies against all of the antigens in a multicomponent system and proportions are adequate, the number of arcs truely indicate the heterogeneity of the mixture. A quality univalent antibody can be useful to show the degree of contamination in purification work especially when different dilutions of reagents are employed.

IV. Immunochemical Tests – Qualitative

A. Identification of Coagulant Factors

Several plasma proteins important in blood coagulation can be identified with the aid of specific antisera in diffusion plates or after immunoelectrophoresis. Examples are given of double diffusion in agar plates with Fig. 2A illustrating prothrombin-antiprothrombin, while Fig. 2C shows fibrinogen-antifibrinogen. With immunoelectrophoresis the mobilities of prothrombin, fibrinogen, platelet cofactor I (Factor VIII) and Hageman factor (Factor XII) can be related to γ globulin and albumin (Fig. 4). Schwick et al. (1967) have identified natural antithrombin as well as other natural antiproteases by immunoelectrophoresis.

A fluorescent assay can be used to identify prothrombin associated with subcellular structure (Anderson and Barnhart, 1964b). The fluorescent reagent is specific antiprothrombin complexed with rhodamine (see section VI B). Aliquots of various subcellular fractions, prepared by differential centrifugation of cell homogenates in sucrose, are mixed with the fluorescent antiprothrombin. If prothrombin is contained in the cell organelles it will fix the fluorescent antibody to the structure. After incubation near 25° C the mixture is centrifuged and the supernatant is assayed for the remaining fluorescence using a fluorometer (Turner). Controls are supernatants obtained from the cell fraction either subjected to a similar procedure except not exposed to fluorescent antiprothrombin or treated with fluorescent γ globulin devoid of antiprothrombin. With knowledge of the dye-protein ratio of the fluorescent antiprothrombin, the amount of antiprothrombin fixed by the cell organelles can be calculated. An idea on the amount of prothrombin contained in the cell organelles can be gained by comparison with the amount of fluorescent antibody removed from solution when measured amounts of purified prothrombin are added under controlled conditions. At best this method is only semi-quantitative.

Fibrinogen can be determined with the semi-quantitative Hyland Laboratory *Fi* test. Hirsh et al. (1965) have compared this method with others for fibrinogen and found it to be rapid and reliable even when fibrinolytic products are present. The *Fi* test employs latex particles coated with rabbit anti-human fibrinogen. Agglutination of the *Fi* reagent occurs when fibrinogen in glycine buffer is added to the system. Comparison of the speed of the agglutination and its size with reactions produced by purified fibrinogen permits a rough quantitation.

The inert particle test theoretically can provide rapid semi-quantitative information for any protein of interest. Several types of particles (polystyrene latex, collodion, bentonite and modified erythrocytes) can be coated with any purified protein. Thus one can obtain a measure of antibody with antigen-coated particles or antigen when the coating is a specific antibody. The test can be extremely sensitive and detect as little as 0.02 μg of protein (Carpenter, 1965).

B. Identification of Fibrinolysis Factors

Profibrinolysin and fibrinolysin can be identified in diffusion systems and immunoelectrophoresis by precipitin reaction with immune sera to profibrinolysin and fibrinolysin. The proenzyme reacts equally well with antibody to itself or to the activated molecule, fibrinolysin. Profibrinolysin is a β globulin of slow mobility (Fig. 4).

Natural inhibitors for fibrinolysin exist in plasma and serum and have been identified by immunoelectrophoresis (Schwick, 1964b). A fibrinolysin inhibitor is an α_2 macroglobulin while a trypsin inhibitor with general protease blocking power is an α_1 globulin (Fig. 4).

Degradation products of fibrinolysis react with antibody to fibrinogen, the parent molecule. Several investigators Nussenzweig and Seligmann, 1960; Berglund, 1962b; Lewis and Wilson, 1964; Fletcher, 1965, Hirsh et al. 1965; Barnhart and associates, 1967; have used electrophoresis on either agar, cellulose acetate or acrylamide coupled with immunologic identification. The electrophoretic mobilities of the various proteolysis products change with the time permitted for digestion (Fig. 5). The major proteolysis product, fibrinogen derivative D, is a β globulin which develops progressively slower mobilities or becomes more electropositive than fibrinogen. The minor product, fibrinogen derivative E, is an α globulin which has faster mobilities or becomes more electronegative than fibrinogen during digestion.

The "Fibrin Degradation Flocculation Test" described by Ferreira and Murat (1963) is a simple, rapid and sensitive test with promise for clinical use. Specific anti-human fibrin is placed in cavity plates preferably or capillary tubes and mixed with serum containing the fibrin degradation products. The container is gently rotated for 5–8 min and then examined against a dark background to see if flocculation has occurred. Using serial dilutions of fibrinogen derivative D or derivative E a rough quantitation can be made. The authors suggest that as little as 15 μg of fibrinogen or derivative will flocculate the antifibrin.

C. Detection of Autoantibody

The evidence that immune mechanisms may underlie or contribute to certain diseases in man is accumulating. Auto-immune processes have been suggested for such diseases a thyroiditis, uveitis, rheumatoid arthritis, lupus erythematosus, pernicious anemia, multiple sclerosis, and myasthenia gravis (Roitt and Doniach, 1967).

Thrombophlebitis migrans also may have an auto-immune component with fibrin as the stimulating agent (Mammen et al. 1967). It is interesting that a number of the possible auto-immune diseases have during their course episodes of acute inflammation. Fibrin formation and destruction during resolution of inflammation is a natural defense mechanism. The sequence of events in our patient with thrombophlebitis migrans provided strong circumstantial evidence for development of auto-antifibrin as a pathogenetic factor in the thrombosis that followed. A pneumonia that responded to treatment preceeded the thrombotic state. Fibrinous exudates and fibrinolysis occur in pneumonia. Certainly the pneumococcus organisms stimulate the immune mechanism and could have served as adjuvants to promote antibody formation to altered fibrin or fibrinogen. Circulating antifibrinogen was demonstrated in this patient during the thrombosis phase but finally disappeared.

The lesions in these various diseases may relate to circulating auto-antibody, to delayed hypersensitivity reactions or may not have an auto-immune basis. The solution for current problems in part resides in methodology but testing times also limit correlation of laboratory findings with the disease state. No further mention of tests for delayed hypersensitivity will be given. A brief discussion of methods of value in detecting circulating autoantibodies follows.

1. Immunoelectrophoresis

When auto-immune disease is suspected the patient's plasma or serum can be used as the antibody source and reacted against various purified proteins. Development of a precipitin band indicates the presence of a circulating antibody in the patient. A diagram of results obtained with immune sera reacted against purified fibrinogen is compared with the pattern of response obtained when plasma or serum of a patient with auto-antifibrin is reacted with purified fibrinogen or plasma (Fig. 6). Normal plasma or serum does not form a precipitin with purified fibrinogen.

The demonstration of auto-antibody was especially prominent when Bacto-Agar (Difco) was used. Neither Agarose nor Noble Agar were suitable. Details for slide preparation and immunoelectrophoresis were previously described (Section III C).

2. Coated Particles

Rheumatoid factor may be an auto-antibody against altered γ globulin (IgG). Several tests making use of particles coated with IgG have been used to measure rheumatoid factor. The test of Schoenfeld and Epstein (1965) employs sheep erythrocytes coated with proteolysis products of normal γ globulin. Coated latex particles have also been used. The end point is agglutination of the treated particles when patient plasma or serum is added. A positive response does not necessarily signify rheumatoid arthritis as several other diseases also give positive tests.

V. Immunochemical Tests – Quantitative

These have their basis in either the precipitin reaction, complement fixation or local passive cutaneous anaphylaxis. This ranking also illustrates the order of sensitivity of these tests with passive cutaneous anaphylaxis about 1000 × more sensitive than complement fixation which is about 100 × more sensitive than precipitin tests. However, precipitin tests are easier to do, frequently require less time and permit detection of as little as 0.1 μg under controlled conditions. Neither complement fixation nor passive cutaneous anaphylaxis will be described further although they have proved useful in evaluating prothrombin relatives and species kinships of fibrinogen (Barnhart, 1967).

Several investigators (Boyden et al. 1947; Goodman et al. 1951; Schultz and Schwick, 1959; Goodman and Vulpe, 1961; Hawkins, 1964) have shown the value of turbidometric or nephelometric determination of the formed precipitin. In turbidometric assays samples are small, the reaction time relatively short and a photometer provides the measure of antigen-antibody complexing. Within seconds after mixing the reagents turbidity begins and proceeds to a maximum ordinarily by 30–60 min. A relatively steady state persists for sometime before the turbidity begins to decline as larger aggregates of the antigen-antibody form and settle out. The maximum turbidity corresponds well with the amount of material that can be precipitated in the system. Antigen can be most accurately measured when there is excess antibody present. There is reasonably good agreement with the quantitative precipitin test of Heidelberger and Kendall (1932). In regions of antigen excess the turbidometric method is not accurate because the precipitin complex redissolves. In the region of antibody excess near the equivalence zone there is a constant relationship between the turbidity developed and the amount of material precipitated. The turbidometric method is most instructive when several dilutions of the test fluid containing the antigen are reacted with a fixed amount of antibody so that the peak response can be determined (Table 2).

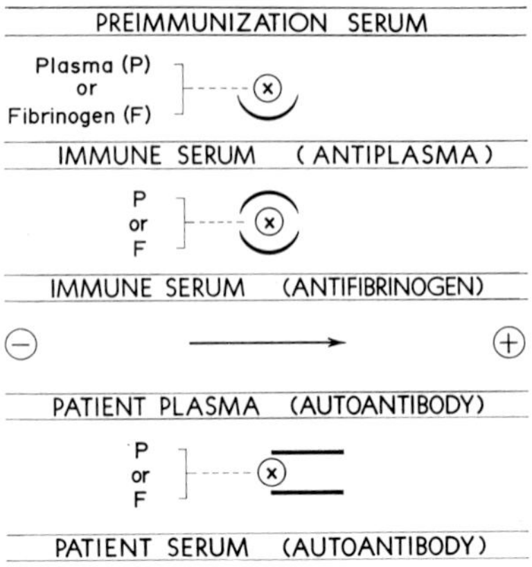

Fig. 6. Diagram of immunoelectrophoretic design contrasting induced immunity and auto-immunity. Only 1 reactant in plasma has been shown although many precipitin bands would react with immune serum (antiplasma).

Table 2. Turbidometric Analysis of SFRM Illustrating Reactions with Antigen Excess and Antibody Excess.

Sample (Reciprocal of dilution)	Quantitative Precipitin Test (mg/ml)	
	Normal Serum	Pathologic Serum[a]
10	0.15	0.25
20	0.20	0.40
40	0.20[b]	0.80
80	0	1.20[b]
160	0	0.80
320	0	0

[a] From a patient with cerebrovascular thrombosis.
[b] Most accurate value in antibody excess.

There is a limitation inherent to the immunologic method in that all molecules with similar antigenic determinant groups will react with the antibody. This means that metabolic breakdown products, if present, as well as biologically active proteins will form precipitins and be measured together. Sometimes it is possible to separate the various types of immunologic relatives and obtain an independent measure of each.

A. Coagulation Parameters

The turbidometric assay has proved useful in quantitating prothrombin, the plasma thrombin inhibitor (antithrombin III) and fibrinogen.

1. Prothrombin

Prothrombin can be determined in plasma defibrinated with thrombin (Barnhart, 1967). Serial dilutions ($^1/_{10}$ to $^1/_{100}$) of plasma are mixed with specific antiprothrombin. The antiprothrombin reagent may be improved by adsorbing with either serum or dicoumarolized plasma. The developed turbidity relates to the prothrombin-antiprothrombin complex formed in the incubated mixture. Conversion of the turbidity readings to amounts of prothrombin are made by reference to a standard curve prepared with known amounts of purified prothrombin. Another approach to quantitation compares turbidity readings of known samples with a reference curve which relates turbidity to the number of prothrombin units determined as present in several dilutions of control defibrinated plasma. For accurate measurements of prothrombin the antiprothrombin must be present in excess. Verification of the removal of prothrombin activity from the test samples can be made by application of the quantitative 2-stage prothrombin procedure to the supernatants left after sedimenting the precipitins formed during the 1–4 hrs incubation. More details for our turbidometric test follow in section V B.

2. Antithrombin III

The quantitative precipitin test with turbidometric evaluation was used by Schwick et al. (1967) to measure antithrombin III in human plasma. This test requires an antibody formed against purified human antithrombin III. Using specific antisera, human plasma has about 40 mg% antithrombin III.

3. Fibrinogen

The quantitative precipitin test has been used by Schultze and Schwick (1959) and also in our laboratory to measure human plasma fibrinogen. Schultze and Schwick report values from 310–730 mg%; in general they find agreement between their immunologic test and that for thrombin-clottable fibrinogen. In our experience the immunologic amount (320–970 mg%) usually is higher than thrombin-clottable fibrinogen. An average of the 20 normals studied immunologically gives 560 mg% while thrombin-clottable fibrinogen in normals has rarely exceeded 300 mg%. Differences between our fibrinogen values may relate to some differences in assay procedures but also could relate to dietary or metabolic differences between the German and American subjects used in the 2 studies. As the data from both laboratories are still very limited, the differences may disappear as more data are collected.

Complete details for our turbidometric assay are given in section V B but a few points of concern in the fibrinogen assay are presented here. To insure that we operate in a region of antibody excess the plasma is serially diluted. Ordinarily we find maximal turbidity and the most accurate measure of fibrinogen with dilutions in the range of $^{1}/_{80}$ to $^{1}/_{640}$. To the diluted sample (0.1 ml) are added antifibrinogen (0.3 ml) and saline to make a total volume of 5 ml. The mixture is incubated at 37° for 1 hr. The developed turbidity is measured and converted to μg of fibrinogen by reference to a standard curve prepared for the species fibrinogen of interest (Fig. 7). Purified fibrinogen (Barnhart and Forman, 1964) is diluted with saline (0.9% sterile) to the desired concentrations. The diluents, water or saline (Sherman Laboratories, Detroit) all have a low particle content and are especially suited for nephelometry. Note in Fig. 7 that the linear relationship between the turbidity and the amount of fibrinogen is lost when more than 10–15 μg of fibrinogen (antigen excess) is present in the system.

It is important to recognize that this immunologic test on plasma actually measures more than thrombin-clottable fibrinogen. In fact all molecules bearing the special antigenic determinant groups of fibrinogen react with the antifibrinogen. While the developed turbidity is produced predominantly by thrombin-clottable fibrinogen, other fibrinogen related molecules derived metabolically or from proteolytic action on fibrin are measured at the same time. In normal individuals these nonclottable fibrinogen relatives represent only a small fraction of the clottable fibrinogen. However, they do account for some of the precipitin. Thus this immunochemical test is best termed a measure of "total fibrinogen-related molecules" or "plasma fibrinogen-related molecules". It might be abbreviated tFRM or pFRM.

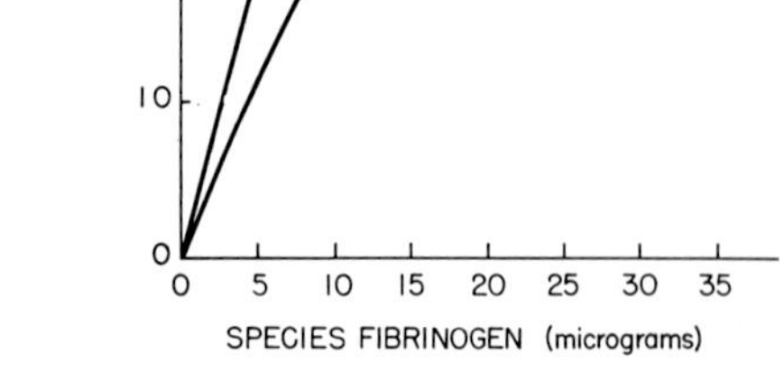

Fig. 7. Calibration curves for quantitative turbidometric assay of fibrinogen-related molecules from either human or canine fluids.

B. Fibrinolytic and Fibrinogenolytic Products

The turbidometric precipitin analysis can be used to measure degradation products of either fibrin or fibrinogen. First thrombin-clottable fibrinogen must be removed from the system by either recalcifying plasma or adding thrombin. Heat defibrinogenated plasma of normal subjects can be used but not when the patient is suspected or has increased plasma proteolytic activity. The turbidity that develops when diluted serum is reacted with univalent antifibrinogen can be related to fibrinogen (Fig. 7). It is true that fibrinogen derivates contain fewer antigenic determinant groups than fibrinogen and are not likely to bind as much antifibrinogen. However, purified fibrinogen provides a more reproducible standard for comparison than attempting to relate to isolated fibrinogen derivatives. Furthermore the fibrinogen and fibrin proteolysis products are several and may exist together in varying proportions dependent upon the duration and extent of the proteolysis. Preparation of either a mixed antibody or an antigen standard that would more accurately measure the proteolysis products is presently unrealistic.

The test works equally well with either canine or human systems. The only special requirements are specific species antifibrinogen and purified species fibrinogen. Although some degree of cross reaction occurs between canine and human materials, the greatest amount of species antigen is fixed by the antifibrinogen of the same species.

The turbidometric test for the described nonclottable molecules is a measure of "serum fibrinogen-related molecules" or abbreviated to sFRM. The procedure used in our laboratory follows.

1. Instrumentation and Glassware

The Turner Fluorometer-Nephelometer (Turner, Palo Alto, Calif.) is used to measure the turbidity of any formed antigen-antibody complexes. The range is set at X3 and the sensitivity dial at 2. The primary filter (No. 22) passes light of 578 mμ. The secondary filter is of clear glass. A reagent blank is used to zero the instrument so that direct readings for turbidity of the precipitin results.

Matched square cuvettes of special glass are cleaned by warming for 10 min in 50% nitric acid solution. Do not boil or the cuvettes will etch and be optically damaged. Cuvettes are rinsed thoroughly in distilled water. A final rinse is made in distilled water of low particle content (Sherman Lab., Detroit). We store the clean cuvettes in 0.9% saline (Sherman Lab.) until needed. Cuvettes can be reused during a test if thoroughly rinsed with saline. The outsides of the cuvettes are dried with paper for optical glass (Kim Wipes, Kimberley Clark, Neenah, Wisconsin) prior to inserting in the nephelometer.

2. Standardization of Antiserum

At first we use an individual antiserum to prepare a calibration curve relating turbidity to fibrinogen content. Each time the antifibrinogen reagent ran out we had to prepare a new curve and results were slightly different. Experience encouraged us to select sera for a pooled reagent which we adjusted to match our best calibration curves. Thus greater volumes of specific antibody were prepared and the results from time to time were more comparable.

Select several antifibrinogen sera of good strength that have been previously characterized as single component by immunoelectrophoresis or double diffusion in agar. Centrifuge each separately unless they are already clear. Hemolyzed antisera are not suitable. Modify a small amount of each antiserum with saline to provide several concentrations (i. e. 100%, 75%, 67%, and 50%). React 0.3 ml of each antiserum with purified fibrinogen in microgram amounts (i. e. 5, 10, 20, and 30) and with saline (0.9%) added to make a total volume of 5 ml. These mixtures are incubated at 37° for 1 hr. The developed turbidity is read on the nephelometer. From these data various antifibrinogen sera can be selected and combined in the proper dilution for the pooled reagent. Weak antisera can be concentrated and may be suitable for the pool. The final pooled antifibrinogen is retested against purified fibrinogen and the slope of the curve should approximate the reference curve (Fig. 7). This pooled antibody is used undiluted in the test system.

3. Test for Fibrinogen Related Molecules

Plasma (0.3 ml) is reacted with 0.06 ml $CaCl_2$ (1.3%). A firm clot ordinarily forms but if not, 0.06 ml of thrombin (400 Iowa U/ml) is added. After 30 min at 37° with occasional pressure on the clot, the preparation is centrifuged for 5 min at 1300 g. The supernatant contains nonclottable fibrinogen related molecules. Serial dilutions ($^1/_{10}$–$^1/_{320}$) are made with saline. To test tubes containing 4.6 ml saline are added 0.1 ml of the serum dilutions and 0.3 ml of standardized antifibrinogen. A reagent blank is also prepared by mixing the antifibrinogen with saline. These tubes are thoroughly mixed and incubated at 37° for 1 hr. The mixtures are then poured into clean cuvettes for determination of turbidity.

4. Interpretation

The turbidity readings are converted to equivalents of fibrinogen by reference to a standard curve (Fig. 7). In normal serum the peak response usually is achieved with dilutions $^1/_{40}$–$^1/_{80}$. The merit of testing several dilutions is that the peak response stands out from the region of antigen excess where the measurement is inaccurate because of resolubilization of the precipitin complex (Table 2). Experience with our test on 72 normal humans gave 0.2 to 0.6 mg/ml serum with an average value of 0.3. Most of the results fall in the range of 20–40 mg%. It is interesting that the data of Schultze and Schwick (1959) on 8 subjects ranged from 27–44 mg%.

Values for sFRM above 60 mg% have not been found in the normal series and reflect increased proteolysis of fibrin or fibrinogen. We have found sFRM values as high as 640 mg% in patients enduring cerebrovascular thrombosis, with or without therapeutically induced fibrinolysis and in extracorporeal circulation (Barnhart, 1967). Schwick and associates (1963) reported an increase in serum fibrinolytic products following administration of streptokinase. We have found elevated sFRM in patients with myocardial infarction and some patients with hereditary connective tissue diseases. In contrast, the sFRM was in the normal range in 32 patients with various types of arthritis even when local fibrinolysis was evident in the synovial fluid of inflammed joints (Barnhart et al. 1967a).

C. Fibrinolytic Potential

The turbidometric precipitin test can be used to quantitate the plasma proteins, profibrinolysin and fibrinolysin. These molecules contain similar antigenic determinant groups and both react with immune serum prepared with either purified profibrinolysin or fibrinolysin. We prefer to use antibody against profibrinolysin in the test because it has more reactive sites than immune antifibrinolysin. For reasons previously emphasized the turbidometric test must be run with antibody excess. The developed turbidity is measured with a nephelometer and converted to either units or mg of profibrinolysin by reference to a standard graph. The reference graph was prepared by reacting immune antiprofibrinolysin and various amounts of purified human profibrinolysin (Michigan Dept. of Health, courtesy of Dr. J. Sgouris and the American Red Cross, courtesy of Dr. J. Pert). When it was necessary to employ a new antiserum a new calibration curve was run and the antibody either diluted or concentrated to give results matching the original standard curve. Linear relationships in antibody excess were not found above 200 μg (0.56 casein units) of profibrinolysin. The test is sensitive, reproducible and requires only 0.1 ml of plasma which is diluted ($^1/_{50}$ to $^1/_{200}$) before mixing with a good quality immune antiprofibrinolysin. The test measures total fibrinolytic capacity of the plasma to represent both profibrinolysin and fibrinolysin content.

Details and precautions for the assay follow those presented in section V B except 1 ml of the dilute plasma was mixed with 3.7 ml saline and 0.3 ml of the specific antiserum.

As the assay depends upon the immunologic features of the molecules and not their enzymatic activity on natural or synthetic substrates, it is not necessary to do the test immediately. Repeat assays on plasma were made immediately and after storage in the frozen state for months without significant loss of immunologic reactivity. There was loss of reactive material if the plasma was recalcified as fibrin adsorbs some of the protein with fibrinolytic potential. Activation of the plasma with streptokinase or urokinase did not modify results much although most of the protein was converted to fibrinolysin.

The assay has been used in a limited number of normal humans (40) (Table 3). It also was used in following the responses of 40 patients with progressive cerebrovascular thrombosis during their treatment by the Wayne State University School of Medicine, Cerebrovascular Unit under the direction of Dr. J. Sterling Meyer. Some representative data of our experience are given (Table 4). The most prominent feature in our cerebrovascular

Table 3. Fibrinolytic Protein by Quantitative Immunoprecipitin Analysis.

Normal Females	Caseinolytic Equivalents U/ml	Normal Males	Caseinolytic Equivalents U/ml
1	2.05	1	2.93
2	2.20	2	2.56
3	2.40	3	2.85
4	1.93	4	3.00
5	1.82	5	3.08
6	2.28	6	3.31
7	2.11	7	3.00
8	2.48	8	2.94
9	2.14	9	2.85
10	2.17	10	2.22
11	2.20	11	2.22
12	2.34	12	2.14
13	2.42	13	2.51
14	1.91	14	2.56
15	2.05	15	2.51
16	2.31	16	2.70
17	1.82	17	2.80
18	2.08	18	3.85
19	2.34	19	3.40
20	2.05	20	1.94
Mean	2.16 ± .14		2.76 ± .46

Table 4. Fibrinolytic Protein in Normal and Pathologic Plasmas

Condition	Fibrinolytic Protein (Caseinolytic Equivalents U/ml) Specimens								
	1	2	3	4	5	6	7	8	9
Normals[a]									
1 F	2.05	1.97	1.94	2.05	1.99	1.97	2.11	1.99	1.71
2 F	2.31	2.28	2.05	2.25	2.36	2.34	2.14	2.31	2.34
3 F	1.82	1.80	1.71	1.77	2.25	2.06	1.97	1.71	2.40
4 F	2.34	2.05	2.00	1.71	1.94	1.85	1.71	1.77	1.97
Improved CVT[b]									
1 F	2.82	3.11	1.40	2.60	2.46	3.22	3.45		
2 F	1.82	1.40	1.71	1.71	1.91				
3 F	2.79	2.64	2.85	2.79	2.79	3.00			
4 F	1.48	2.34	2.62	2.42	2.22	2.48			
1 M	2.09	2.04	2.09	2.48	3.42				
2 M	1.80	2.56	2.48	2.19	1.91	2.56	2.94	3.14	
3 M	1.31	2.11	2.28	2.11	1.88				
4 M	3.06	2.32	3.06	2.70	2.61	4.22	3.82	4.62	3.28
5 M	2.80	2.60	2.65	2.48	3.14	2.80	2.85		
6 M	4.05	1.62	3.51	3.28	2.22				
Deteriorated CVT[b]									
1 F	2.08	2.02	2.02	2.30	2.20				
2 F	2.51	2.14	2.14	2.19	2.11	2.51			
3 F	2.65	1.51	1.91	1.70	2.16	2.05			
4 F	2.27	2.44	2.57	2.66	2.90				
1 M	2.85	2.82	2.90						
2 M	2.05	1.85	2.05	1.71	1.85	1.85	1.91		
3 M	2.65	2.54	2.76	2.65	2.54	2.76			
4 M	1.85	2.05	1.71	1.91					

[a] Normal Females (F) studies over 3 months.

[b] Cerebrovascular Thrombosis Patients on anticoagulants or general supportative care. Samples taken from pre-treatment through 72 hr. M designates Males.

thrombosis series was that the fibrinolytic potential varied considerably and increased especially in those patients with some clinical improvement. In some patients this correlated well with profibrinolysin activity measured on a standard fibrin clot. Other patients showed a decline in fibrinolytic potential and this may reflect the continued thrombi formation with its adsorption of the profibrinolysin and fibrinolysin from plasma. A few patients with unfavorable responses to their disease showed low levels of fibrinolytic potential which were not appreciably modified during treatment.

The major deterrent to more widespread use of this method is the necessity for a highly screened specific antibody. With the recent improvements in purification and yield of profibrinolysin (Chap. VIII) and the fact that minute quantities of the purified protein elicit antibody formation the immunologic assay may be viewed more favorably. It is not unrealistic to expect the results of our turbidometric assays within 3 hrs of drawing blood from the patient. This is a reasonable expectation when the laboratory is ready to perform with a good quality antibody and a calibration curve on hand.

D. Protease Inhibitors

The quantitative precipitin test has been applied by Schultze and associates (1963) to measure either the α_1 antitrypsin or the α_2 antiplasmin activity in human plasma. Schwick et al. (1967) report on 2 other protease inhibitors, α_1 antichymotrypsin and inter-α-trypsin inhibitor. Each of these natural protease inhibitors require their specific immune serum. Turbidometric assay provided the following results for normal human plasma: 210–500 mg% of α_1 antitrypsin, 14–35 mg% of α_1 chymotrypsin, 10–30 mg% of inter-α-trypsin inhibitor, and 220–380 mg% of α_2 antiplasmin. The α_1 antitrypsin may be identical with the "slow reacting antiplasmin" described by Norman. Antithrombin III also inhibits trypsin and plasmin (fibrinolysin).

VI. Fluorescent Antibody Technique

This method, introduced by Coons and associates (1942), combines the selectivity and sensitivity of immunology with the precise cellular localizations of microscopy. Since the technique was made practical by further studies of Coons and Kaplan (1950), by Riggs and associates (1958), by Chadwick, McEntegart and Nairn (1958) and by Nairn (1962) it has received wide attention.

The immunofluorescent technique has practicality in the clinical laboratory. Numerous microorganisms (bacteria, protozoa, helminths, fungi) and viruses can be identified on the basis of possessing certain unique antigens. Auto-immune diseases can be detected with laboratory tests revealing the presence of antitissue components such as nuclear or thyroid auto-antibodies. The cellular uptake of protein degradation products resulting from natural or induced proteolysis can be studied. An example of this is the uptake of fibrinolytic products by the liver reticuloendothelial cells (Barnhart and Cress, 1966). The phagocytosis of native protein aggregates formed in vivo can be followed. Illustrations of this last function are the phagocytosis of fibrin by neutrophils during disseminated microthrombosis (Barnhart, 1965a), and in acute inflammation (Riddle and Barnhart, 1964).

Immunofluorescence has value in basic physiologic, pharmacologic and pathologic studies. The fate of certain injected materials (foreign or native) can be followed. Foreign proteins usually localize in the reticuloendothelial system (Coons, 1954). Cellular localizations of native proteins such as enzymes and hormones (Marshall, 1954), γ globulin (Coons and associates, 1955), accelerator globulin (Barnhart et al. 1963), and platelet cofactor I (Barnhart, 1967) may represent sites for biosynthesis. Unless the rate of synthesis can be modified experimentally with serial evaluations made on cells and extracellular fluids, the immunofluorescent response may only indicate stored protein. Such an experimental design has been successful in revealing liver parenchymal cells as sites for synthesis of fibrinogen (Barnhart and Forman, 1963) and of prothrombin (Anderson and Barnhart, 1964b; Barnhart, 1965).

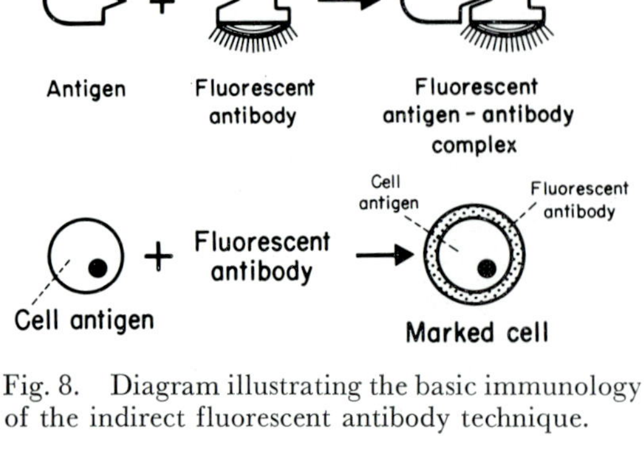

Fig. 8. Diagram illustrating the basic immunology of the indirect fluorescent antibody technique.

A. Basic Principles: Advantages and Limitations

The immunologic basis for the fluorescent antibody technique is presented schematically. The direct method employs a specific antibody complexed with fluorescent dye (Fig. 8). Any responding cell will attract fluorescent antibody and emit light when exposed to ultraviolet or blue wave lengths. Controls support the belief that nonspecific adsorption of protein is minimal. Success is achieved because the antisera for the blood coagulation proteins are powerful and not much reduced by the conjugation with fluorescent dye. The direct method is our standard procedure.

The indirect method or sandwich technique (Fig. 9) is valuable with weak antisera as it is about 10 × more sensitive than the direct method (Coons, 1956). More antibody combining sites are made available in this procedure so that more fluorescent antibody will adhere to the cell. In practice the unlabeled antibody specific for the antigen of interest is applied to cells. Then a fluorescent antibody against γ globulin is layered over the preparation. If the unlabeled antibody for the selected cell antigen was prepared in rabbits, then the fluorescent tool must be labeled anti-rabbit γ globulin. This reagent reacts with the cell coating of rabbit γ globulin which was attracted by the cell antigen and the cell fluoresces. Some investigators prefer this method because only one fluorescent antibody is necessary to follow several different proteins providing their antibodies were made in the same species. Also, the method has great value in detection of auto-antibodies.

Immunocytology can be exquisitely sensitive and most specific but is no better than the antibody employed. With availability of a quality fluorescent antibody and adequate controls run concurrently, the test is rapid, economical and discriminative. It has advantage in histochemistry and cytochemistry as the antigen is precisely identified and may be localized to specific cell structure. The intensity of specific fluorescence permits a qualitative idea of the cellular concentration of the antigen. Of course, an adequate antigen concentration is necessary to bind enough antibody to show fluorescence. A most striking demonstration of the sensitivity and selectivity of the method results when a few cells in a heterogeneous population fluoresce vividly while their neighbors remain dully auto-fluorescent (Fig. 10).

Limitations also exist for the fluorescent antibody technique. Establishing the specificity of the fluorescent response is an obligation of the investigator. Specificity should not be imagined it must be tested. Even the demonstration that the fluorescent antibody reacts only with a highly purified antigen does not rule out the cellular reaction or extracellular response being with immunologic relatives of antigen. Supplemental procedures may be necessary to establish the significance of the fluorescent reaction for native or biologically active molecules as contrasted to degradation products. Association of the antigen to or in cell structure may permit discrimination between a site of synthesis, a storage depot or a digestive vacuole (phagosome or lysosome).

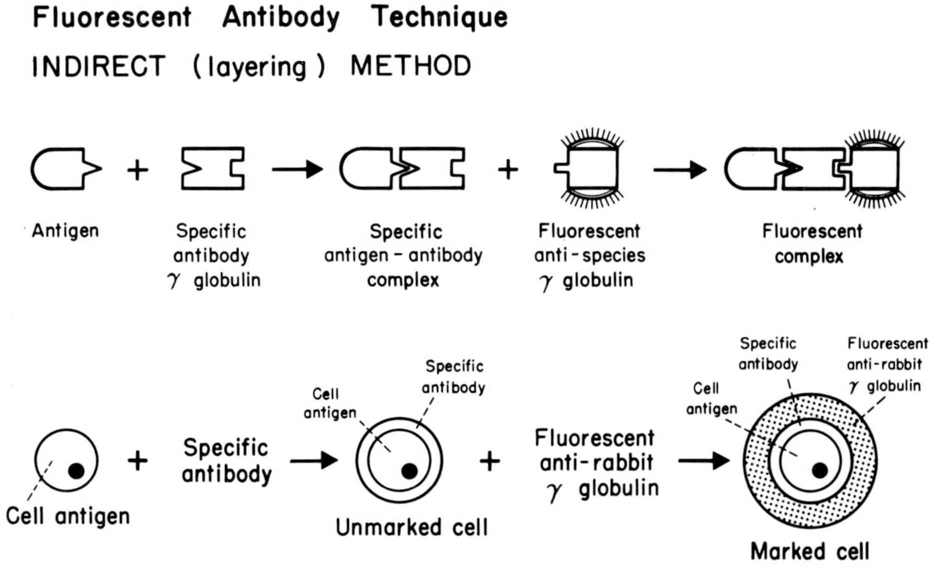

Fig. 9. Diagram illustrating the immunologic basis of the direct fluorescent antibody technique.

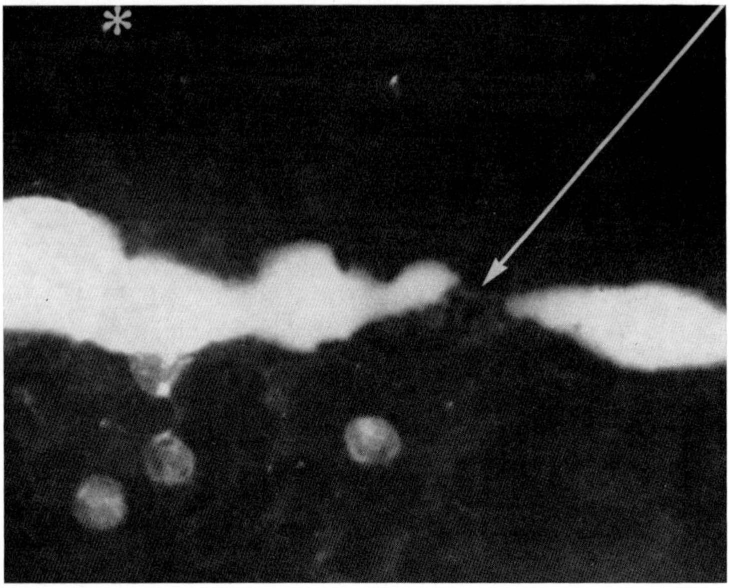

Fig. 10. Fluorescent photomicrograph of a canine blood smear following experimental microthrombosis. The broad white demarkation across the center divides the smear into an autofluorescent area (*) above and a region below that was exposed to fluorescent antifibrinogen. Of the many cells on the smear only neutrophils bound the fluorescent antibody. As the upper area of the smear was covered with nonfluorescent antifibrinogen regions of complete and partial block exist near the center of the slide. Note the neutrophil (arrow) that exhibits this blocked reaction. Tri × film, mag. × 800.

Thus prompt fixation of the cell reactant with limitation of diffusion and suppression of auto-fluorescence is desired. The perfect fixative has not been found yet. Quantitation of the antigen by microcytofluorometry (Goldman and Carver 1961) poses many problems which have not been satisfactorily resolved. Selected technical details of our laboratory experience with some critical discussion follow.

B. Preparation of Fluorescent Antibody

A well-characterized good quality rabbit antiserum is selected. The γ globulin is separated from the other serum proteins and chemically complexed to a fluorescent dye (rhodamine or fluorescein). The fluorescent antibody is separated from any free dye by either dialysis or gel filtration. The potency of the fluorescent antibody should be determined to be sure it was not lost during conjugation. The dye-protein ratio of the conjugate provides a reliable index of the tissue response (Barnhart, 1960). The fluorescent antibody is stable in the frozen state for months, even years. Following long storage the potency and presence of free dye should be checked. Free dye can be eliminated as before. The potency can be improved if necessary by concentration against Carbowax 6000 (25% Union Carbide and Carbon Co., New York) or in a similar mild manner.

1. Separation of γ Globulin

A 2-step procedure provides γ globulin that is at least 99% pure. Ethodin (also known as Rivanol; Winthrop Laboratories, Special Chemical Division, New York) is used as a 0.4% solution adjusted to pH 7.4–7.6 with sodium carbonate. The procedure is essentially one of those proposed by Horejsi and Smetana (1956). The reaction is run near 1–4° C. For 1 vol of antiserum (usually 20–30 ml) 3 vol of Ethodin is added dropwise from a funnel with attached Pasteur pipet. The mixture is slowly stirred for 30 min. A heavy yellow precipitate forms which is the albumin, α globulin and most of the undesired β globulin. The slightly yellow supernatant contains γ globulin and is decanted. This supernatant is decolorized by addition of a small amount of activated charcoal with slow stirring. The mixture is filtered through premoistened Whatman 41 H filter paper. Usually the charcoal procedure must be repeated for complete decolorization. The described γ globulin concentrate is further purified with ethanol to eliminate trace contaminants. Cold ethanol (53.3%) is added dropwise to provide a final concentration of 25%. The temperature is dropped to –4 or –5° C and the mixture is slowly stirred for 15 min. The γ globulin is precipitated and collected after centrifugation in the cold for 10 min at 2520 g. The γ globulin is redissolved in about 3 ml of saline (0.9 %). Protein is determined by the biuret reaction (Robinson and Hogden, 1940). The volume of the solution is adjusted to about 10 mg protein/ml. The γ globulin concentrate can be frozen until needed.

2. Preparation of Rhodamine Sulfonyl Chloride

This reagent is prepared according to Chadwick et al. (1958) and requires a fume hood to protect the chemist who should wear gloves to avoid burns and stains. Lissamine rhodamine B-200 (Imperial Chemical Industries, Ltd., England) is ground for 5 min in a mortar. For 1 g of rhodamine 2 g of phosphorous pentachloride is added and ground for another 5 min in the hood. To the mixture is added 10 ml acetone (dried over calcium sulfate or choride) and thoroughly mixed. The mixture is filtered through Whatman 41 H paper. The residue on the paper is carefully scraped away and mixed with another 10 ml acetone. This acetone extract is filtered through the original filter paper. The procedure is repeated until 12–15 ml of acetone extract is collected. The acetone extract contains rhodamine sulfonyl chloride (RSC), and should be tightly capped and stored in the cold.

The dye concentration is determined from serial dilutions ($^1/_{500}$–$^1/_{3000}$) of the acetone extract. The optical density of the saline diluted samples is read in a spectrophotometer at 560 mμ. These readings are compared with a standard curve for μg rhodamine. With appropriate correction for dilution the RSC concentration ranges from 12 to 48 mg/ml. The dye concentration is unsuitable for the conjugation procedure with less than 12 mg/ml.

3. Complexing RSC with Purified Antibody

Our procedure deviates from that of Chadwick et al. (1958) and Nairn (1962) by using specific amounts of dye and protein in the conjugation procedure. We obtain an adequately labeled antibody when 25–850 μg dye/mg protein is reacted. Essentially complete recovery of the labeled antibody occurs with concentrations of dye from 250–500 μg/mg protein. Most of our conjugates are prepared with 419 μg RSC/mg protein.

The γ globulin concentrate is thawed at 37° C and an equal vol of carbonate buffer (pH 9; 4 ml 0.5 M $NaCO_3$ + 46 ml 0.5 M $NaHCO_3$ + 150 ml distilled water) is added. The temperature is dropped near 1° C while slowly stirring. RSC is added very slowly dropwise (about 1 drop/30 sec) to avoid denaturation. After the dye addition the mixture near 1° C is slowly stirred for 4–6 hrs but no longer. The mix is then centrifuged at 2,500 g for 15 min to remove insoluble particles.

4. Complexing FITC with Purified Antibody

Fluorescein Isothiocyanate (FITC; Baltimore Biological Laboratory, Baltimore, Md.) was used with 0.05 mg FITC/mg protein in carbonate buffer. Conditions were similar to those described with the duration limited to 4–6 hrs. Essentially this is the procedure of Riggs and associates (1958). Good quality fluorescent antibodies were obtained but the yield and dye-protein ratios were seldom as high as with RSC.

5. Removal of Free Dye

Dialysis offers a simple and mild method to eliminate free dye from that complexed to protein. The procedure described requires 3–7 days with frequent changes of dialysis fluid but can be shortened considerably by using a Seegers dialyzer (Grafar Corp., Detroit) and keeping the dialysis fluid in motion. A dye-protein mixture is placed in $^1/_4$ inch dialysis tubing (cellulose; Arthur H. Thomas Co., Philadelphia). The partially filled dialysis casing is placed in a stainless steel bucket containing about 8 liters of phosphate buffered isotonic saline near pH 7 (the phosphate buffer comprises 10 % of the saline). A magnetic stirring bar is placed in the bucket and the dialysis fluid is kept in constant slow motion. Dialysis is best done in the cold to minimize denaturation. The dialysis is considered adequate when the dialysis fluid shows an optical density of less than 0.01 when checked in a spectrophotometer at 560 mμ. Gel filtration offers an efficient fast means for separating free from complexed dye. Time is taken though in preparation of the column and there may be some fluorescent antibody retained on the column. Sephadex 25 or 50, medium particle size (Pharmacia, Piscataway, N. J.) is satisfactory. Best results in our laboratory are with Bio-Rad P 20 (Bio-Rad Lab., Richmond, Calif.) prepared in phosphate buffered saline pH 7.2. After decanting the fines, the swollen beads are poured as a slurry into a column and equilibration achieved by passing at least 2 bed volumes of buffered saline. The clear red or green antibody solution (10 ml) is placed on the column (100 ml bed vol) and allowed to percolate over the beads. Phosphate buffered saline is then added to give a convenient flow rate.

The first colored band to emerge from the column is the dye-protein complex. This is collected and frozen for storage. The free dye ultimately is washed off the column and discarded. The clean column can be reused several times.

6. Dye-Protein Ratios of the Fluorescent Antibody

Experience has shown that dye-protein ratios greater than 4×10^{-3} indicated preparations suitable for immunocytology (Barnhart, 1960). Reasonable approximations of the protein and dye concentrations can be made with a Beckman DU spectrophotometer. The specific absorption of the tyrosine and tryptophane constituents of the protein are gained at 280 mμ. Absorption at 480 mμ gives a measure of FITC. Absorption at 560 mμ gives a measure for RSC. Reference to appropriate standard curves permits the calculation of a dye-protein ratio. Most of our RSC antibodies have ratios near 10×10^{-3} and give excellent specific staining of cells.

7. Removal of Undesired Components in Fluorescent Antibody

Ordinarily antibodies evoked by minute amounts of highly purified protein are specific for just one protein. Immunologic testing provides the base for assurance of the univalence or multivalence of the antibody. Fluorescent univalent antibody does not require further treatment before applying as the immunocytology tool.

When a second antibody is known to exist in the fluorescent antibody and its presence is troublesome, adsorption can be used to eliminate it. Small amounts (0.1–1.0 mg) of purified material can be added to the fluorescent antibody and slowly mixed for 1 hr in the cold. However, the adsorbed antibody must be tested immunologically to be certain that the undesired antibody is completely removed.

When the fluorescent antibody is thought to be specific for a plasma protein which does not exist except in minute amounts in serum, adsorption with dried serum protein may remove some undesired antibodies. Again proof of the effectiveness lies in immunologic testing of the adsorbed antibody.

C. Cell Preparations

It is essential for immunofluorescent cytology that the cell specimens be placed on absolutely clean slides. Fixation in cold solutions must be prompt. A low intensity of autofluorescence aids evaluation of specific fluorescence.

1. Processing of Slides

Even precleaned microscope slides obtained from a supplier are cleaned again to eliminate any fluorescent substances from their surfaces. The slides are soaked at least 18 hrs in acid-alcohol (5 ml concentrated HCl made up to 1 liter with 95% ethanol). Slides are dried with clean gauze and stored in a closed container to avoid lint and dust contamination.

2. Cell Specimens

Several kinds of cell preparations are suitable for immunofluorescence. Blood, bone marrow or inflammatory exudate smears are made of moderate thickness with care to leave a feather edge. Smears are rapidly air dried.

Cells imprints provide intact whole cells (Fig. 11). This is a favored preparation in our laboratory because the cell antigen is more concentrated than in cell sections and highly autofluorescent connective tissue does not adhere to the slide. Background autofluorescence is minimized as adhering blood is ultimately washed away in later processing. Cell imprints are prepared by pressing a clean slide gently against a fresh evenly cut surface of an organ biopsy obtained surgically. The intact whole cells are transferred from the organ surface to the slide and rapidly air dried.

Frozen sections (1–3 μ thick) are prepared in a cryostat at –18° C from frozen blocks of tissue. The tissue was previously quick-frozen on removal from the individual by dipping in petroleum ether precooled to –90° C. The thin section is transferred with aid of a fine brush to a cold slide which is immediately removed from the cryostat and warmed by applying the finger to the undersurface of the slide. This warming helps the thin section spread and adhere to the clean glass surface. The slide is thoroughly air dried before storing in a covered container to protect from dust. These preparations are useful when the total tissue architecture needs study. Information can be gained on extracellular structures as well as the organization of immunofluorescent cells within the organ. Serial sections are desirable for the controls that accompany specific staining.

Paraffin sections (3–5 μ thick) have limited usefulness. Serial sections are valuable for controls and studies of cell organization within the tissue. After fixation, the tissue blocks are embedded in low melting point paraffin (48–52° C) with infiltration for no longer than 2 hrs. Xylol and alcohol dehydration are made as rapidly as possible. These modifications in conventional paraffin procedure minimize protein denaturation and were successful in preserving some of the prothrombin in liver cells (Barnhart, 1960).

Polyethylene glycol (Carbowax) sections (3–5 μ thick) are suitable for some studies of tissue architecture. Following freeze-substitution, the blocks are embedded in Carbowax 400 which is molten near 37° C. When cooled to near 20° C the block is hard enough to section. Mounting of the section is aided by a drop of ethanol on a clean slide. After drying, store as described.

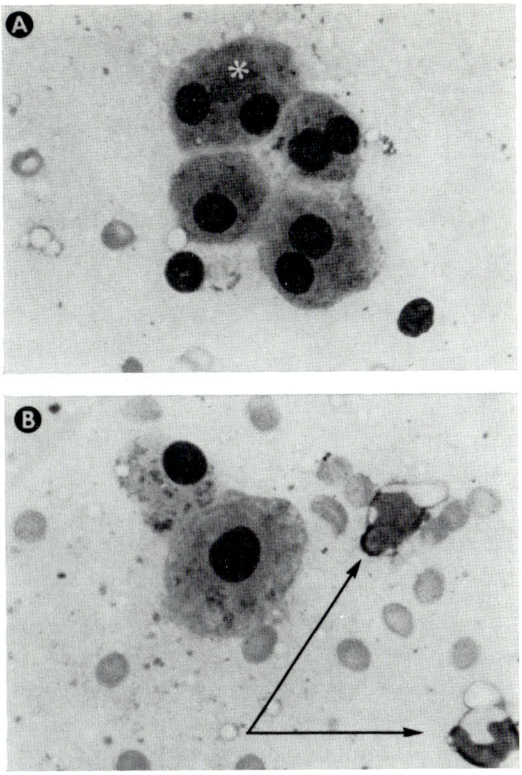

Fig. 11. Photomicrographs of human liver cell imprints stained with Leishmans stain for 15 min. A. A clump of hepatocytes with a binucleate parenchymal cell shown (*). Erythrocytes are the faint staining small, round or oblong elements. The 2 dark round objects are nuclei from ruptured hepatocytes. Mag. × 1280. B. Note the macrophages at arrows. Mag. × 2580.

3. Fixation

Selection of a fixative which suppresses autofluorescence is absolutely necessary. We prefer cold Wolman and Behar (1952) fixative (19 part absolute ethanol + 1 part glacial acetic acid). All of our cell preparations are fixed for 10 min at –18° C.

A number of different fixatives have been used over the years. These are formalin (10%, buffered or fumes), Bouin solution, Hemperl solution, Carnoy no. 1, absolute ethanol, 95% ethanol, Wolman and Behar methyl alcohol, and acetone. The least intense autofluorescence was achieved with ethanol, acetone, and Wolman and Behar which was best and especially suppressed the autofluorescence of blood cells.

D. Fluorochroming Procedure

Only the direct method will be described. A potent and specific fluorescent antibody is selected and should be particle free. The dye concentration is controlled by diluting the stock fluorescent antibody with saline (0.9%) to provide a solution with an optical density near 0.20. For RSC conjugates the spectrophotometer is set at 560 mμ in contrast to 480 mμ used for FITC conjugates. This adjustment ordinarily provides a dye-antibody complex with a dye concentration from 20–80 μg/ml. Several drops of fluorescent antibody are applied to cover the cell specimen. Care is taken to avoid evaporation and uneven staining.

Staining times are varied to suit the cell preparation. In general adequate specific fluorescence results with staining times varied from 10–45 min. Liver imprints and frozen sections require about 20 min. Blood smears, inflammatory exudates and bone marrow smears require about 45 min.

Fluorescent antibody that is not bound by cell imprints and smears is removed by careful rinsing with cool tap water poured from a beaker. The procedure is repeated numerous times for about 2 min before drying. Usually cover slips are not applied. Frozen sections are rinsed in phosphate buffered saline, pH 7 and mounted in buffered glycerol (9 parts low or nonfluorescent glycerol plus 1 part buffered saline). The cover slip is sealed with melted polyethylene glycol (Carbowax 1540). There is very little deterioration for about 3 months. Slides sealed with paraffin last longer. Fluorochromed slides are stored in covered boxes.

Controls and tests for specificity of the cell response should be run at the same time as the cell specimen is treated with fluorescent antibody. Thus the exact amount of autofluorescence and the specificity can be evaluated.

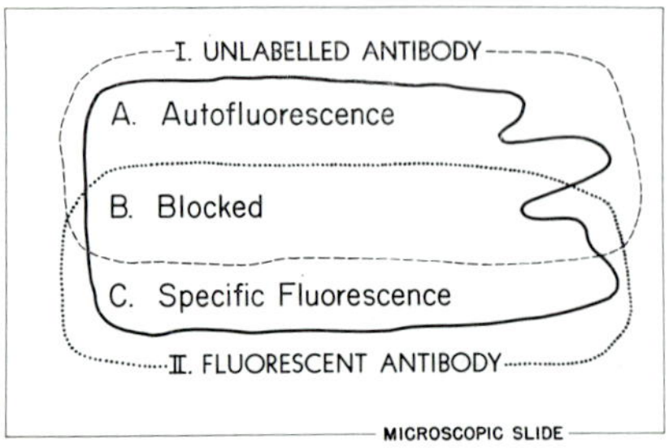

Fig. 12. Schematic diagram of a staining procedure to illustrate specificity. The blood smear edges are indicated by the heaviest line. The sequence of application of antibodies is indicated. Note that there is intentional overlap of the 2 antibodies.

E. Establishing Specificity

The following considerations help evaluate the specificity of the fluorescent reaction.

1. Autofluorescence

This is a natural property of cells and tissues. The intensity of autofluorescence varies with the type and age of the cell or tissue and also the fixative. Always observe either untreated or saline treated cells or those treated with either nonimmune serum or unlabeled antibody. Compare the degree of control fluorescence with that in the fluorochromed preparation (Fig. 10). With cell smears this comparison is easy because the smear can be subdivided (Fig. 12). One region is treated with unlabeled antibody carefully rinsed and dried to provide the autofluorescent area. Another region is treated with fluorescent antibody and permitted to overlap the autofluorescent area so that a blocked region is on the same slide. The slide is carefully rinsed and dried. The specimen is then examined with the fluorescent microscope and the intensities of fluorescence compared.

2. Free Dye

Use free dye in the appropriate concentration. This is a good control with frozen sections as they do not take on dilute free dye. Smears and imprints are stained to some extent by free dye. Thus it is important to have all the dye conjugated in the fluorescent antibody product.

3. Fluorescent Normal Rabbit γ Globulin

This reagent is prepared from nonimmune γ globulin. The fluorescent agent is adjusted to the same dye concentration as the specific fluorescent antibody. Little or no staining results when fluorescent normal rabbit γ globulin is applied to cells.

4. Blocking Experiments

This procedure makes use of unlabeled specific antibody to cover the antibody combining sites of cell antigens. When specific fluorescent antibody is next applied there are fewer or no combining sites left. Consequently, the specific fluorescence is reduced or abolished when compared to cytofluorescence achieved with only the fluorescent antibody (Fig. 10–12).

5. Adsorption Experiments

The specific fluorescent antibody can be treated with any purified protein desired and then applied to cell specimens. The cytofluorescent response should be reduced or lost when the fluorescent antibody is adsorbed with the antigen used to originally elicit the specific antibody. Adsorption of the fluorescent antibody with unrelated proteins should not alter the fluorescent response to the treated antibody. Adsorption of fluorescent antibody with various tissue powders or activated charcoal may reduce undesired background staining but also removes some of the specific antibody.

6. Double Tagging

With suitable cell specimens a double fluorochroming procedure may be rewarding. This is especially true when 2 different proteins of interest are packaged in separate cell structures. Such a partitioning occurs in phagocytic cells in inflammatory exudates (Barnhart et al. 1967b). A smear is roughly subdivided into several areas (Fig. 13). The RSC antibody (red) is applied in one area, and then carefully rinsed away without contacting the other cells of the specimen. The slide is dried for 30 min. Next the FITC antibody (green) is applied to a different area of cells but some overlapping of the red area is intentional. Again the slide is rinsed carefully and dried. When this preparation is exposed to ultraviolet or blue light the cell inclusions that have attracted the RSC antibody will fluoresce red while those that reacted with FITC antibody will fluoresce green. In the area of stain overlap one may see both red and green regions within the same cell and thus identify 2 different proteins. If the 2 proteins exist together in a single phagosome, then the fluorescent response will be yellow. On the same slide regions of autofluorescence and block can be present for comparison with specific fluorescence.

F. Microscopic Observation and Photography

Any properly equipped fluorescent microscope can be used. Our observations and photography are with a Zeiss Photomicroscope and fluorescent accessories. The light source is an Osram HBO 200 mercury lamp. We prefer the darkground condenser (Zeiss Ultra Z) as dark backgrounds make cell evaluations easier. The exciter filter is either a BG 12 alone or combined with a BG 38. The following barrier filters or photographic filters are useful; OG 1, OG 4, OG 5 and the narrow band filters in wave lengths of 470–530 mμ are equally good.

Quenching of fluorescence on exposure to ultraviolet light is more troublesome with FITC fluorochrome than with RSC antibody. The RSC preparations usually regain much of their fluorescence after removal from the light activation.

For black and white photography, Eastman Tri X film is suitable. Exposure times of

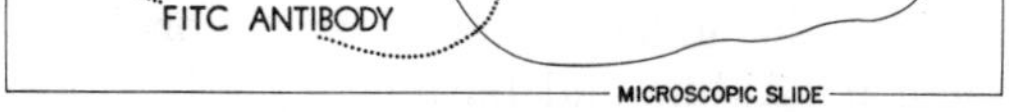

Fig. 13. Schematic diagram of a staining procedure to illustrate double fluorescent tagging. Either the RSC or FITC antibody can be applied as step II with the remaining one used as step III. For best results, drying between steps is recommended. Note in the area of overlap between C and D cells may stain red or green or yellow depending on the proteins contained.

1–15 min are satisfactory and depend upon the fluorescent intensity. With short exposures, 1–2 min, forced development (about 10 min in Eastman Dektal 76) is necessary.

Color photography on the daylight type of Eastman High Speed Ektachrome or Anscochrome 200 gives fairly true reproductions of the fluorescent colors. Exposures of 6–15 min permit standard commercial development and color reproduction is good. Shorter exposure requires special development and colors seldom match the original.

G. Neutrophil Fluorescence in Thrombosis and Bleeding Disorders

Neutrophilic leucocytes appear to be an important thrombolytic mechanism according to specific immunofluorescence (Barnhart, 1965, 1967). In normal individuals peripheral blood neutrophils do not contain significant amounts of fibrinogen-related molecules. Following diffuse microthrombosis some of the circulating neutrophils accumulate fibrinogen-related material (Fig. 10). A similar pick-up of fibrinogen-related material is a frequent response of neutrophils in patients with progressive cerebrovascular thrombosis (Barnhart, 1963, 1967). Two possible explanations could account for these findings. First, the neutrophils are mobile phagocytic cells and could enter thrombi and phagocytize fibrin. Second, the neutrophils could ingest fibrinolytic products as some degree of fibrinolysis may accompany thrombosis. Until recently we could not select between these explanations. It is now clear that soluble fibrinolytic products are not ingested by neutrophils but are removed from the circulation by reticuloendothelial cells of the liver (Barnhart et al. 1967). In other studies we demonstrated by immunofluorescence and electron microscopy that extravascular neutrophils do indeed phagocytize fibrin and digest it (Riddle and Barnhart, 1964). These findings strongly support the view that neutrophil fluorescence during or following thrombosis reflects phagocytosis of fibrin from the thrombi. At present we do not know the full clinical significance of this observation. However it seems reasonable that the fibrinogen-related fluorescence of neutrophils in patients with thrombosis signals that there is some traffic through the thrombi. Immunofluorescent testing of peripheral blood smears from patients during acute and recovery phases of their thrombotic disease might be some aid in prognosis or evaluating the effectiveness of therapy.

Fibrinolytic bleeding is a problem of increasing concern. Unfortunately an acceptable method for establishing the underlying cause has not been found. A favored therapy for fibrinolytic bleeding has been to give such agents as episilon amino caproic acid or Trasylol (Farbenfabriken Bayer AG, Leverkusen, Germany) which inhibit the fibrinolytic enzyme system. However, primary fibrinolysis (over activity of fibrinolysin) is not the only basis for these bleeders. Secondary fibrinolysis is no longer a rare event but is now recognized as complicating such diverse syndromes as traumatic shock, afibrinogenemia, transfusion reactions, septicemia, heat stroke, anaphylaxis, acute renal insufficiency and may cause death after open heart surgery. Selection of therapy is critical. If the fibrinolysis is a compensatory response to generalized microthrombosis, the thrombosis should be halted rather than eliminate the defense mechanism of fibrinolysis. In secondary thrombosis, early and effective treatment with heparin may be life saving as the thrombosing tendency is controlled. Obviously, the clinician needs laboratory support to aid his diagnosis and select the correct therapy promptly to avoid a fatal outcome.

Immunocytology on peripheral blood neutrophils may offer an acceptable means of differentiating between secondary and primary fibrinolysis. As previously stated neutrophils from subjects with generalized microthrombosis show a positive response with fluorescent antifibrinogen to signal a contact with a fibrin deposit. In contrast neutrophils do not show specific fluorescence during or after primary fibrinolysis. Thus, the presence or absence of fibrinogen-related molecules in circulating neutrophils may be a key to the underlying cause of fibrinolytic bleeding.

An immunofluorescent test on blood smears is practical, rapid, sensitive and reliable. The test requires clean slides, a fluorescent microscope, and a good quality fluorescent antifibrinogen (commercial reagents may be suitable and when polyvalent can be improved by adsorption with serum). Blood smears are air dried and fixed in Wolman and Behar fixative as previously described. Controls can be run on the same slide with the specific fluorescent reaction (Fig. 12). A comparison smear of normal blood should be processed with the patient smear as a test on glassware and reagents. Estimated time from smear to test result is about 3 hrs. A positive response in the neutrophils suggests the patient has or is resolving thrombi. A negative response in a bleeding patient is compatible with but not pathognomonic of primary fibrinolysis. Such information plus the clinical history and accessory laboratory data may permit a more reasoned judgement on the underlying cause for the bleeding problem and may aid in selection of therapy.

VII. Conclusion

Immunochemical procedures have utility in both the research and clinical laboratory. Depending upon the objectives, tests can be selected that are specific, sensitive, reliable, rapid and economical. Such procedures should complement and not replace already established tests. For some situations the immunochemical approach is the only one feasible.

With experience these tests are not more difficult than other laboratory methods. Much of the effort required is preparatory for the actual test on an unknown specimen. The immunochemical test is no better than the antibody employed.

With attention to the problems and limitations of immunology, the unique advantages can be exploited in advancing both our basic knowledge and gaining appreciation for the natural history of disease and its correction.

Acknowledgement

This study was aided by grants from the National Institutes of Health, U.S. Public Health Service and the Michigan Heart Association. Gratitude is expressed to Arlys Vettraino, Olga Sufritz, John Rogers, Barry Smiler and Walter Farris for their competent technical assistance.

References

Anderson, G. F., and Barnhart, M. I. (1964a). *Am. J. Physiol. 206,* 929.

Anderson, G. F., and Barnhart, M. I. (1964b). *Proc. Soc. Exptl. Biol. Med. 116,* 1.

Back, N., Hiramoto, R., and Ambrus, J. L. (1965). *Blood 25,* 1028.

Barnhart, M. I. (1960). *Am. J. Physiol. 199,* 360.

Barnhart, M. I. (1963). *Thromb. Diath. Haemorrhag. 10* (Supp. 13), 104.

Barnhart, M. I. (1965a). *Federation Proc. 24,* 846.

Barnhart, M. I. (1965b). *J. Histochem. Cytochem. 13,* 740.

Barnhart, M. I. (1967). *In:* "Blood Clotting Enzymology" (W. H. Seegers, ed.) Academic Press, New York.

Barnhart, M. I., and Anderson, G. F. (1962). *Proc. Soc. Exptl. Biol. Med. 110,* 734.

Barnhart, M. I., and Cress. D. C. (1966). *Proc. Intern. Sym. Atherosclerosis and the Reticuloendothelial System, Plenum Press, New York.*

Barnhart, M. I., and Forman, W. B. (1963). *Vox Sanguinis 8,* 461.

Barnhart, M. I., and Forman, W. B. (1964). *In:* "Blood Coagulation, Hemorrhage and Thrombosis" (L. M. Tocantins and L. A. Kazal, eds.), pp. 230—232. Grune and Stratton, New York.

Barnhart, M. I., and Riddle, J. M. (1963). *Blood 21,* 306.

Barnhart, M. I., and Walsh, R. T. (1966). *Federation Proc. 25,* 553.

Barnhart, M. I., Anderson, G. F., and Baker, W. J. (1962). *Thromb. Diath. Haemorrhag. 8,* 21.

Barnhart, M. I., Cress, D. C., and Vettraino, A. V. (1967). *Federation Proc. 26,* 538.

Barnhart, M. I., Cress, D. C., Henry, R. L., and Riddle, J. M. (1967). *Thromb. Diath. Haemorrhag. 17,* 78.

Barnhart, M. I., Ferar, J., and Aoki, N. (1963). *Federation Proc. 22,* 164.

Barnhart, M. I., Grammens, G., and Mammen, E. F. (1966). Unpublished observations.

Barnhart, M. I., Marciniak, E., and Seegers, W. H. (1967). Unpublished observations.

Barnhart, M. I., Riddle, J. M., and Bluhm, G. B. (1967a). *Ann. Rheumatic Diseases. 26,* 206.

Barnhart, M. I., Riddle, J. M., and Bluhm, G. B. (1967b) *Ann. Rheumatic Diseases 26,* 281.

Berglund, G. (1962a). *Brit. J. Haematol. 8,* 204.

Berglund, G. (1962b). *Intern. Arch. Allergy Appl. Immunol. 21,* 193.

Berglund, G. (1963). *Intern. Arch. Allergy Appl. Immunol. 22,* 65.

Berglund, G., and Blombäck, B. (1965). *In:* "Genetics and the Interaction of Blood Clotting Factors" (F. Koller and F. S. Streuli, eds.), p. 265. F. K. Schattauer-Verlag, Stuttgart.

Boyden, A., Bolton, E., and Gemeroy, D. (1947). *J. Immunol. 57,* 211.

Campbell, D. H., Garvey, J. S., Cremer, N. E., and Sussdorf, D. H. (1964). "Methods in Immunology". W. A. Benjamin, Inc., New York.

Carpenter, P. L. (1965). "Immunology and Serology". Saunders, Philadelphia.

Chadwick, C. S., McEntegart, M. G., and Nairn, R. C. (1958). *Immunology 1,* 315.

Cohn, M. (1952). *In:* "Methods Medical Research" (A. G. Corcoran, ed.), Vol. 5, p. 271. Year Book Pub., Chicago.
Coons, A. H. (1954). *Ann. Rev. Microbiol. 8,* 333.
Coons, A. H. (1956). *Intern. Rev. Cytol. 5,* 1.
Coons, A. H., and Kaplan, M. H. (1950). *J. Exptl. Med. 91,* 1.
Coons, A. H., Creech, H.J., Jones, R. N., and Berliner, E. (1942). *J. Immunol. 45,* 159.
Coons, A. H., Leduc, E. H., Connolly, J. M. (1955). *J. Exptl. Med. 102,* 49.
Ferreira, H. C., and Murat, L. G. (1963). *Brit. J. Haematol. 9,* 299.
Fletcher, A. P. (1965). *Federation Proc. 24,* 822.
Goldman, M., and Carver, R. K. (1961). *Exptl. Cell Res. 23,* 265.
Goodman, M. (1962). *Human Biol. 34,* 105.
Goodman, M., and Vulpe, M. (1961). *World Neurology 2,* 589.
Goodman, M., Wolfe, H. R., and Norton, S. (1951). *J. Immunol. 66,* 225.
Goodman, M., Ramsey, D. S., Simpson, W. L., Remp, D. G., Babinski, D. H., and Brennan, M. J. (1957). *J. Lab. Clin. Med. 49,* 151.
Grabar, P., and Burtin, P. (1964). "Immunoelectrophoretic Analysis". Elsevier Pub., New York.
Grabar, P., and Oudin, J. (1947). *Ann. Inst. Pasteur 73,* 627.
Grabar, P., and Williams, C. P. (1953). *Biochim. Biophys. Acta 10,* 193.
Halick, P., and Seegers, W. H. (1956). *Am. J. Physiol. 187,* 103.
Hawkins, J. D. (1964). *Immunology 7,* 229.
Heidelberger, M., and Kendall, F. E. (1932). *J. Exptl. Med. 55,* 555.
Hirsh, J., Fletcher, A. P., and Sherry, S. (1965). *Am. J. Physiol. 209,* 415.
Horejsi, J., and Smetana, R. (1956). *Acta Med. Scand. 155,* 65.
Kabat, E. A., and Mayer, M. M. (1961). *"Experimental Immunochemistry".* 2nd Edition, Thomas, Springfield, Illinois.
Lewis, J. H., and Wilson, J. H. (1964). *Am. J. Physiol. 207,* 1053.
Mammen, E., Schmidt, K. P., and Barnhart, M. I. (1967). *Thromb. Diath. Haemorrhag. 18,* 605.
Marshall, J. M. (1954). *Exptl. Cell Res. 6,* 240.
McLester, W. D., and Wagner, R. H. (1964). *Federation Proc. 23,* 576.
Miller, K. D. (1958). *J. Biol. Chem. 231,* 987.
Nairn, R. C. (1962). "Fluorescent Protein Tracing". Livingston Ltd., London.
Nussenzweig, V., and Seligmann, M. (1960). *Rev. Hematol. 15,* 451.
Nussenzweig, V., Seligmann, M., and Grabar, P. (1961). *Ann. Inst. Pasteur. 100,* 490.
Riddle, J. M., and Barnhart, M. I. (1964). *Am. J. Pathol. 45,* 805.
Riggs, J. L., Selwald, R. J., Burckhalter, J. H., Downs, C. M., and Metcolf, T. G. (1958). *Am. J. Pathol. 34,* 1081.
Robbins, K. C., Summaria, L., and Elwyn, D. (1965). *J. Biol. Chem. 240,* 541.
Robinson, H. W., and Hogden, C. G. (1940). *J. Biol. Chem. 135,* 707.
Roitt, I. M., and Doniach, D. (1967). *Brit. Med. Bull. 23,* 66.
Schoenfeld, L. S., and Epstein, W. V. (1965). *Vox Sanguinis 10,* 482.
Schultze, H. E., and Schwick, G. (1959). *Clin. Chim. Acta 4,* 15.
Schultze, H. E., Heimburger, N., Heide, K., Haupt, H., Störiko, K., and Schwick, H. G. (1963). *Proc. 9th Cong. European Soc. Haemat. Lisbon. Karger, New York,* p. 1315.
Schwartz, R. S., and Dameshek, W. (1963). *J. Immunol. 90,* 703.
Schwick, H. G. (1964a). *Thromb. Diath. Haemorrhag.* (Supp. *13)* 85.
Schwick, G. (1964b). *Behringwerke-Mitt. 44,* 103.
Schwick, G., and Schultze, H. E. (1959). *Clin. Chim. Acta 4,* 26.
Schwick, H. G., Heimburger, N., and Haupt, H. (1967). *Thromb. Diath. Haemorrhag. 18,* 302.
Schwick, H. G., Kranz, T. H., Schmidtberger, R., and Störiko, K. (1963). *Proc. 9th Congr. European Soc. Hematol. Lisbon. Karger, New York,* p. 1300.
Wilson, M. W. (1958). *J. Immunol. 81,* 317.
Wilson, M. W. (1959). Experimental Records 1957—1958 Medical Library, Wayne State University, Detroit, Michigan.
Wolman, M., and Behar, A. (1952). *Exptl. Cell Res. 3,* 619.

Immune Assay of Tissue Thromboplastin

E. Halberstadt

I. Introduction

Post-partum hemostasis is accomplished by two mechanisms: contraction of the uterus and blood coagulation. Whereas uterine contractility has always been considered a predominant factor, the importance of blood coagulation is only recently fully appreciated. How the coagulation process is so rapidly triggered in the maternal vessels remains still unclear.

From the results of Puder (1957) and Schwenzer (1960) and our own investigations, which showed a considerable higher content of tissue thromboplastin in placentas separated manually during cesarean sections than in normally separated placentas after delivery, it may be concluded that during normal separation of the placenta coagulation is started by tissue thromboplastin. Tissue thromboplastin may also enter the maternal circulation. Similar ideas have been postulated by Page et al. (1951) and Schneider (1959) to explain coagulation defects in the premature separation of a normally implanted placenta. Based on this hypothesis, we attempted to find tissue thromboplastin in the maternal blood using a hemagglutination inhibition test.

II. Hemagglutination Inhibition Reaction

The method is based on the hemagglutination inhibition reaction (Boyden, 1951; Stavitsky, 1964). Antiserum against human brain thromboplastin is prepared in rabbits. Sheep red blood cells are sensitized with the homologous antigen (tissue thromboplastin) and are agglutinated by the antiserum. The hemagglutination can be inhibited by serum, plasma or other fluids containing the chemically unidentified tissue thromboplastin.

A. Material and Reagents

Brain tissue thromboplastin (Deutsch et al. 1964).
Acetone.
Citrated plasma (1:9).
Rabbit serum.
Veronal-buffer pH 7.2 (see Chapter II, p. 62).

Freund's complete and incomplete adjuvant (Difco Laboratories, Detroit, Michigan).

Sheep red blood cells in Alsever's solution.

0.15 M phosphate-buffered saline pH 6.4 and 7.2.

(pH 7.2: 4.27 gm NaCl, 2.45 gm KH_2PO_4, 10.15 gm $NaHPO_4 \cdot 2\,H_2O$ in 1,000 ml of distilled water).

(pH 6.4: 4.27 gm NaCl, 6.94 gm KH_2PO_4, 3.4 gm $NaHPO_4 \cdot 2\,H_2O$ in 1,000 ml of distilled water).

0.85 percent saline.
Tannic acid.

1. Immunization of rabbits

As antigen, 40 mg tissue thromboplastin are dissolved in 2 ml of sterile 0.15 M saline and emulsified with 2.0 ml Freund's complete adjuvant. To immunize rabbits (young animals 2.5–3.0 kg body weight), 1.0 ml of the emulsion is injected i. m. at four different sites, preferably on both sides close to the shoulder girdle and in each gluteus maximus muscle. Before each injection and in weekly intervals thereafter about 5 ml of blood are obtained from the animals for titer measurement. The titer as measured by the hemagglutination test, shows a continous increase in antibody concentration. Before immunization no antibodies should be found. The injections are repeated after four weeks with Freund's incomplete adjuvant.

2. Preparation of the antiserum

After four weeks the antibody titer against brain thromboplastin is usually 1:20,480. At this time, 20–30 ml of blood are withdrawn from the animals. After coagulation, the blood is centrifuged at room temperature at 6,000 g. The serum is inactivated at 56° C for 30 min and absorbed with three times washed sheep red blood cells (SRBC); (0.3 ml of washed, packed SRBC to 1.0 ml antiserum). After 30 min, the mixture is centrifuged and the antiserum is stored in aliquot volumes at –28° C.

3. Homogeneity of the immunologic system and immunological identity of brain and placental thromboplastin

Gel-diffusion according to Ouchterlony is used. Because of the large size of the tissue thromboplastin molecules, Sepharose 2 B (Pharmacia Fine Chemicals, Uppsala) is required instead of agar. Five ml Sepharose, 8.5 ml of phosphate-buffered saline, pH 7.2, and 1.5 ml of 1:1,000 aqueous merthiolate (Eli Lilly and Co. Indianapolis, Ind.) are heated to 100° C and poured into Petri dishes 8 cm in diameter. After cooling, wells (one in the center, four in a distance of 2 cm) are cut. The antiserum (1:81,920) is placed in the central well. The peripheral wells are filled with 200 mg% acetone dried brain powder dissolved in normal citrated plasma or placental extracts (see below). The plates are covered and stored at room temperature. After some days the resulting antigen-antibody complex appears as a continous precipitation line, proving the purity of the system and the immunological identity of placental and brain thromboplastin. To obtain placental extract, fresh placentas are perfused with 0.85% NaCl through the umbilical vein. Membranes and adhesive blood clots are removed. The tissue of the basal plate is homogenized and 10 mg tissue are incubated with 10 ml inactivated normal citrated plasma at 37° C for one hour. The suspension is frequently shaken, centrifuged at 3,000 g for 15 min and the supernatant used for immunodiffusion.

4. Preparation of Sheep red blood cells (SRBC)

Two to three days old SRBC in Alsever's solution are washed three times in saline and a 2.5 % cell suspension in phosphate-buffered saline (PBS), pH 7.2, is prepared. One volume of cell suspension and one volume of tannic acid (1:10,000 in saline) are incubated at 37° C with occasional shaking for exactly 10 min. After the cells are washed three times in phosphate-buffered saline (PBS), pH 7.2, they are brought to a concentration of 2.5 % in PBS, pH 7.2. Five mg antigen (tissue thromboplastin) are dissolved in 40 ml of phosphate buffered saline (PBS), pH 6.4, and 10 ml of tanned cells are added. After storage for 10 min at room temperature the cells are precipitated by centrifugation, washed three times in PBS, pH 7.2, and resuspended to a concentration of 2.5 % with PBS, pH 7.2, containing $^1/_{250}$ normal rabbit serum. The final concentration is checked in a photometer at 578 mμ, in a dilution of 1:100 with PBS, pH 7.2. The extinction coefficient should be in a range of 0.96 ± 0.02. The sheep cells may be stored for several days at 4° C, but at the first appearance of hemolysis, they are discarded.

5. Preparation of normal rabbit serum

Normal rabbit serum is inactivated at 56° C for 30 min and adsorbed (0.3 ml coated SRBC for 1 ml of serum). The serum is centrifuged after 30 min (1,200 rpm, 10 min room temperature) and stored at –28° C.

B. Passive Hemagglutination Test

For the passive hemagglutination test the antigen is non-specifically adsorbed to tanned erythrocytes. In the presence of the homologous antibody, the red cells are agglutinated, merely serving as indicator of an antigen-antibody reaction. A set of 16 test tubes and 3 control tubes is prepared. The first test tube receives 0.9 ml, all other tubes including the controls receive 0.5 ml of PBS, pH 7.2, with $^1/_{100}$ volume of normal rabbit serum. Next, 0.1 ml (titer 1:20,480) of antiserum is pipetted into the first tube. After thorough mixing, a serial dilution is made by transferring 0.5 ml from one tube to the next tube. The last 0.5 ml are discarded. The control tubes contain no antiserum. Now 0.05 ml of the sensitized cells are added to each tube. All tubes are mixed well and incubated over night at 4° C. As titer, we consider the highest dilution of antiserum which still shows a clearly positive agglutination. Before each new titer measurement, the freshly prepared cell suspension is tested with the standard antiserum.

C. Hemagglutination Inhibition Test

Before adding the cell suspension, each tube receives 0.1 ml of plasma or serum to be tested. The plasma or serum is inactivated and absorbed once with washed SRBC prior to use. The tubes are stored at room temperature for 1 hour and to each tube is added 0.05 ml of sensitized cells.

III. Comments

Cohen and Chargaff (1940) observed that rabbits can be sensitized against human tissue thromboplastin. Shirakura et al. (1959) confirmed these results and demonstrated that there is no immunologic identity between tissue and plasma thromboplastin. If small amounts of antigen (tissue thromboplastin) are mixed with plasma or serum, inactivated and tested by the hemagglutination inhibition test, the titer drops according to the concentration of antigen. It makes no difference whether plasma or serum is used. Serum or plasma without thromboplastin do not inhibit the titer (Table 1).

During delivery measurable amounts of thromboplastin appear in the maternal circulation. The peak concentration is reached in the post-partum period. In some women, tissue thromboplastin can be detected up to 12 hours post-partum. The highest concentration is found in the retroplacental serum, but

Table 1. Sensitivity of the Hemagglutination Inhibition Test.

Serum (plasma) concentration of tissue thromboplastin mg%	μg/0.1 ml	titer
0	0	1:20,480
5	5	1:10,240
10	10	1:5,120
20	20	1:2,560
40	40	1:1,280
80	80	1:640

considerable amounts are also detectable in umbilical venous blood.

Since immunological identity exists between brain and placenta thromboplastin, it cannot be proven that the tissue thromboplastin found in the maternal circulation originates from the placenta. The presence of thromboplastic activity of placental tissue and the fact that there is thromboplastin in the blood of the umbilical vein makes this origin probable. The uterus could possibly serve as a further source of thromboplastin.

References

Boyden, S. U. (1951). *J. Exptl. Med. 93,* 107.

Cohen, S. S., and Chargaff, W. (1940). *J. Biol. Chem. 136,* 243.

Deutsch, E., Irsliger, K., and Lomoschitz, H. (1964). *Thromb. Diath. Haemorrhag. 12,* 12.

Page, E. W., Fulton, D. L., and Glendening, M. B. (1951). *Am. J. Obstet. Gynecol. 61,* 1116.

Puder, H. (1957). *In:* "Physiologie und Pathologie der Blutgerinnung in der Gestationsperiode" (H. Runge and I. Hartert, Eds.) p. 112. Schattauer Verlag, Stuttgart.

Schneider, C. L. (1959). *Ann. N. Y. Acad. Sci. 75,* 634.

Schwenzer, A. W. (1960). *Arch. Gynäkologie 195,* 114.

Shirkurat, T., Hasagawa, T., Sakai, T., and Mackawa, T. (1959). *Acta Haematol. 22,* 232.

Stavitzky, A. B. (1964). *In:* "Immunological Methods" (J. F. Ackroyd, Ed.), p. 363. Blackwell Scientific Publication, Oxford.

Chapter XI

Thrombosis*

Stanford Wessler and William E. Stehbens

I. Introduction

Thrombotic disease has become an increasingly important cause of disability and death as infectious diseases have responded to chemotherapeutic attack and as public health measures designed to control or eliminate noxious environmental factors have progressively become more effective. This apparent increase in thrombo-embolic phenomena is, in part, due to an increased awareness of the ubiquity of thrombosis. The problem is further compounded by the possibility that an absolute as well as a relative increase in thrombotic phenomena is being observed.

The scope of the problem can be appreciated when it is recalled that arterial thrombosis can initiate or aggravate myocardial infarction, cerebral vascular accidents, valvular heart disease, arrhythmias, congestive failure, shock, bowel necrosis, gangrene, and certain blood dyscrasias. Rarely, it complicates infections. Venous thrombo-embolism is also associated with heart disease. Moreover, it can complicate malignancy, a normal pregnancy, surgery, bodily trauma and simple immobilization. Finally, venous thrombo-embolism occurs in otherwise healthy young people.

An accurate estimate of the incidence of thrombosis is made difficult by the fact that there exists no satisfactory technique for the recognition of the incipient or active thrombotic state in man. Knowledge of the incidence of thrombo-embolism is based essentially on extensive statistical analyses of large groups of patients. DeBakey (1954) has described the deficiencies of this approach which in large measure is related to a dependence on inadequate criteria for the clinical diagnosis and classification of thrombo-embolic phenomena.

In this regard it must be recalled that only a small fraction of patients with thrombo-embolic episodes exhibits clinical manifestations. A recent study demonstrated antemortem pulmonary thrombo-emboli in more than 60 percent of all autopsies in a general hospital (Freiman et al. 1965). There is strong experimental evidence to support the view that the embolic traces observed at necropsy reflect only a small portion of the embolic material reaching the lung during life (Freiman et al. 1961; Wessler et al. 1961). Since many emboli undergo complete lysis, or eventually become incorporated into the vessel wall, the incidence of embolic episodes could well be greater than the 60 percent figure mentioned above.

II. Definition

When one considers its role as a possible etiological factor and as the major complication of atherosclerosis, the importance of thrombosis in human pathology cannot be overemphasized. The terms thrombosis and clot are often used synonymously but in recent times the difference, though perhaps only semantic, has been stressed.

Thrombosis is the formation of a solid or semi-solid mass from constituents of the blood anywhere within the heart or blood vessels during life. It can vary considerably in histological structure. Neoplastic permeation and

* This work was supported, in part, by Research Grant HE 1/470 from The National Institutes of Health, U.S. Public Health Service.

invasion of blood vessels, although frequently associated with thrombus formation, are excluded by definition. A mass formed from the constituents of the blood in vitro or within the cardiovascular system after death is a clot. However, semi-solid masses, morphologically similar to true thrombi, may be formed from blood in vitro by the Chandler technique (Chandler, 1958; Poole, 1959), and antemortem thombi can sometimes resemble postmortem clots microscopically. Thus, histological structure does not always provide an adequate means for differentiating between thrombi and clots.

III. Pathology of Human Thrombi

Because of the difficulties in distinguishing between a thrombus and a postmortem clot, it is essential that suspected thrombi be examined both macroscopically and microscopically at several different levels to ascertain with certainty the exact nature of the plug. Antemortem thrombi are usually attached to the vessel wall though relatively loosely if of recent formation. Thrombi are dry and tend to have a dull surface as has the underlying inner surface of the blood vessel wall in contrast to the normal shiny surface of the endothelium. In general the vessels are distended, do not collapse or retract and consequently are prone to pout or protrude from the cut surface. This phenomenon is readily seen when calf muscles containing thrombosed veins are cut transversely. The distended condition and the dark red-blue color of the exposed but unopened thrombosed vein is consistent with the antemortem nature of the coagulum. Though also a notable feature in thrombotic occlusion of the relatively thin walled cerebral arteries, it does not occur with non-occlusive mural thrombi. As a rule infected thrombi are softer, more friable and may be frankly purulent.

Postmortem clots frequently form loose casts which are moist, shiny, rubbery and readily removed. In general uniformly red and resembling red currant jelly, they simply represent coagulation of blood. If sedimentation of red cells occurs prior to coagulation, the clot, particularly in the heart and large vessels, will be dark red inferiorly and yellow in the upper segment with the line of demarcation often quite sharp.

In the gross, thrombi are usually described as having a white head comprised largely of platelets and a red tail consisting mainly of coagulated blood, constituting rapid and secondary propagation. Thrombi, therefore, are not infrequently classified according to color as white, red or mixed types, classification ultimately depending on the amount of red cell incorporation within the mass. Nevertheless, it is possible to find considerable variation in appearance in one thrombus with a segment resembling postmortem clot in color and histological structure. For this reason one must diligently search for pale mottling or striae of grey-white color which may be due either to fibrin or to the lines of Zahn composed of platelet masses. Histologically, such organization is confirmatory evidence for the diagnosis of a thrombus.

A. Venous and Arterial Thrombi

Venous thrombi are remarkable for their dark color, although mottling is still evident, and for their tendency to extensive propagation. Most of these thrombi occur in the veins of the lower limb especially in the deep veins. Emphasis has been placed on the role of stasis in the soleal venous sinuses and in the valvular sinuses of larger veins (Cotton et al. 1965).

Arterial thrombi are usually paler than those so frequently observed in the veins of the lower limb, and, as propagation does not occur to the same extent, involve a smaller segment of the artery. This latter manifestation is perhaps due to the more deleterious effects that follow arterial occlusion. In thick-walled arteries, the thrombus is not visible from the external surface and the frequent presence of severe atherosclerosis, often with calcification, makes localization of the thrombus technically more difficult than when veins or cerebral arteries are involved. For this reason thrombi are probably often overlooked in coronary arteries with gross atherosclerosis and indeed some pathologists have resorted to postmortem arteriography for their localization.

Occluding thrombi occur most frequently and more generally than is often realized in the main distributing arteries. The stimulus to search for these lesions depends ultimately on the collateral circulation and whether or not serious secondary effects ensue. The aorta and common iliac arteries are rarely occluded even when the atherosclerosis is so advanced that widespread gross ulceration of the vessel surface is present. The ulcerated areas are quite obviously blood stained and while adherent thrombi are to be seen, massive and occlusive thrombi are not prevalent. This could be due to hemodynamic factors which vary with the radius of the vessel. In large vessels such as the aorta, some mural thrombi appear to have formed as the result of localized dissection of the wall and these often resemble intramural hemorrhage. Occasionally they are responsible for distortion and narrowing of the lumen.

In arterial aneurysms thrombosis is commonly found and in large chronic sacs the thrombus exhibits the well-known laminated appearance of alternating light and dark zones. Dark red or recent thrombus may be seen external to the thick laminated thrombus. In large ruptured aortic sacs there may be extensive red thrombus and it may be difficult to differentiate between intra-aneurysmal thrombus and the hematoma following leakage. In small intracranial aneurysms serial sections have revealed that a considerable part of the sac wall can be infiltrated with or consist of fibrin-like material (Stehbens, 1963a). As yet little is known of the underlying changes in the aneurysm wall or of the hemodynamic factors which predispose the sac to thrombosis. The investigation of Black et al. (1960) has shown that thrombosis in the sac of experimentally produced aneurysms was dependent on the mathematical relationship between the volume of the sac and the dimensions of the orifice.

The distinction between thrombosis in situ and embolism is at times not easy to resolve but usually such circumstantial evidence as the source of embolism can be of the utmost assistance in deciding between the two possibilities.

B. Intracardiac Thrombi

Postmortem clots in the heart at autopsy can be easily recognized. They may be intermingled with the trabeculae carneae rather than attached to the heart wall and they can extend into and form a cast of the arteries, particularly the pulmonary arteries.

Agonal thrombi are alleged to be the most rapidly formed of all thrombi (Cappell, 1958). It is reported that they occur in either or both ventricles, that they are attached at the apex, and that they extend through into the pulmonary artery or less frequently into the aorta. Being yellowish or pink and of stringy consistency, they are described as consisting predominantly of fibrin separated out from the circulating blood in patients dying slowly, in the agonal state. Nevertheless, this variety of thrombus is a doubtful entity because postmortem clots in which sedimentation of red cells has occurred are sometimes labelled as agonal in type. Furthermore, there is no evidence to prove that agonal thrombi occur as rapidly as has been alleged and it is beyond conjecture why fibrin should separate out to form agonal thrombi in the heart and not elsewhere.

True thrombi in the heart occur principally in association with recent or old myocardial infarction, disease of the cardiac valves and auricular fibrillation. They can be quite large and are usually pale and mottled. Except for the presence of bacteria and an inflammatory reaction in the vegetations of bacterial endocarditis, these thrombi structurally resemble those found elsewhere and in most cases their nature is readily discernible.

Not infrequently overlooked are Lambl's excrescenses which are small filiform projections found individually or in tufts along the free border of the cardiac valves. They have been considered to be the end result of small tears of the subendothelial connective tissue and the small tags which then project from the valve surface have had small amounts of thrombus deposited on them. These in turn become endothelialized (Saphir, 1960). Mechanical factors have been invoked as playing a role in their pathogenesis (Rodbard, 1956; Saphir, 1960), though Magarey (1949) believed that they resulted from the organization of partially attached fibrin on the surface of the valve, and to them he attributed the gradual thickening of the cusps. However, it has not been explained why fibrin should be attached in filiform excrescences at this site and the underlying cause of the fibrin deposition remains obscure. Nonbacterial thrombotic endocarditis could have its origin in these excrescences.

IV. Experimental Thrombosis

A. Microcirculation

Following the early investigations of thrombosis and hemostasis in living animals, the platelet has been said to play a dominant role in this complex biological reaction to injury. In the main, investigations have involved the infliction of gross trauma of one sort or another after which it has been demonstrated repeatedly that platelets aggregate to form a "white" mass. The chemical mechanism underlying this platelet aggregation is still far from clear though it is now generally accepted that the release of adenosine diphosphate (ADP) is either an essential step or the "final common pathway" (Born et al. 1964; O'Brien, 1964). The adhesion of platelets to the vessel wall has been regarded as the first observable change in experimental thrombosis induced by injury (Bizzozero, 1882; Eberth et al. 1886; Welch, 1887; Welch, 1889; Zucker, 1947; Payling-Wright, 1958). However, it is frequently declared that, apart from preliminary vasomotor changes, the first tissue response in acute inflammation, produced by similar injurious agents, is the sticking of leukocytes to endothelium (Cohnheim, 1889; Cappell, 1958; Payling-Wright, 1958; Florey, 1962), and platelet sticking is not mentioned. This variation in response may be accounted for by a difference in the intensity of the injury (Silver et al. 1965a; Stehbens, 1965a), yet the gross discrepancy in the literature serves to indicate our ignorance of the essential differences in the behaviour of platelets, leukocytes and erythrocytes in vivo and there is need for further study of the very early stages of thrombosis to determine the exact sequence of events. As thrombi also contain leucocytes and erythrocytes, it is pertinent to discuss the behaviour of these cellular constitutents of the blood in vivo and their tendency to aggregate.

Transparent chambers inserted in rabbits' ears are admirably suited to the study of the behaviour of these blood constituents (Silver et al. 1965a; Stehbens, 1967a; Stehbens, 1967b; Stehbens, 1967c). In non-inflamed ear chambers, leukocytes do not adhere to the vessel wall nor are they visible in the stream in some vessels. The earliest observable stage is the momentary hesitation of a leukocyte in the stream as it comes into contact with the endothelium and the indication is that its velocity is less than that of the red cells which cannot be seen individually. In more prominent degrees of sticking, the leukocytes roll along the endothelium at an irregular rate, sometimes being washed free and adhering again downstream. When rolling, deformation in shape is observed for there is a wide area of attachment. In inflammation, leukocytes frequently remain fixed to the vessel wall in one place for long periods, then emigrate or are washed away. Rolling leukocytes appear to be as sticky to one another as to the endothelium itself. Individual leukocytes occasionally may become temporarily impacted in a capillary and in a severe inflammatory reaction, leucocyte sticking may reach such proportions that flow is considerably impeded.

Erythrocyte behaviour differs considerably from that of leukocytes. Red cells do not roll along endothelium but pass by at the speed of the stream (Silver, 1965a). In a fast flowing stream erythrocytes usually move so rapidly that individual cells cannot be distinguished except at the apex or crotch of a bifurcation. Momentarily they may be seen bent around a spike and only occasionally do they adhere to a leukocyte or to the vessel wall. In this latter instance, they usually remain fixed for a considerable length of time and have either a tear-drop outline with a very localized point of attachment, or are dumb-bell in shape if a portion of the cell projects through the endothelium. In contrast to leukocyte sticking, the localized point of attachment suggests mechanical fixation rather than a stickiness of opposing cell surfaces. Moreover, they are not sticky to passing cells. In stagnant vessels erythrocytes may form rouleaux. In a flowing stream mild red cell aggregation may be difficult to recognize and is most readily seen where red cells impinge on the apex of a bifurcation if the flow is sufficiently slow. If the red cells are adherent, they become distorted and elongated before being separated when they resume their normal shape. This course of events cannot be appreciated in a fast flowing stream though no doubt the adhesiveness could be demonstrated by high speed cinematography.

The detailed behaviour of platelets in the microcirculation other than the observation of aggregation in advanced thrombosis has to a large extent been overlooked until recent times. Mention has been made that occasional platelets adhere to endothelium (Florey, 1962) but more extensive observations have since been made using rabbit ear chambers (Silver et al. 1965a; Stehbens, 1967a; Stehbens, 1967b; Stehbens, 1967c). In non-inflamed ear chambers, platelets rarely adhere to the vessel wall and, contrary to popular belief, the presence of a platelet in the plasma zone is not necessarily an indication that it is about to stick to endothelium. When platelets adhere, they do so at very localized points of attachment and are easily washed away. Other platelets may adhere to those already fixed to the vessel wall, though they do not adhere to one another in the circulation nor in stagnant vessels. Platelets do not adhere to circulating erythrocytes but it is not unusual for one or two platelets to adhere to a leukocyte which is rolling along the vessel wall. However, not all leukocyte sticking is associated with this phenomenon.

These observations indicate the essential differences in behaviour of leukocytes, erythrocytes and platelets in the small vessels of rabbit ear chambers, with particular reference to their sticking to endothelium. It is remarkable that despite the intensive investigations of the microcirculation, the factors responsible for the stickiness of these cells either to endothelium or to one another, completely remain undetermined.

It has been observed in the microcirculation (Silver et al. 1965a) that following mild trauma, an accentuation of the tendency of platelets to adhere to leucocytes results in the gradual build-up of platelet-leukocyte thrombi which shed embolic fragments — the so-called thromboembolism. This process at times was observed to be quite localized, and even confined to a single vessel and the minimal nature of the trauma was stressed. Considering the innumerable small vessel injuries that must occur in man constantly, it seems reasonable to believe that such leukocyte-platelet aggregation must be reversible.

The experimental introduction of substances to increase platelet aggregation is accompanied to a varying degree by an accentuation of this platelet-leukocyte response, though in some instances massive red cell aggregation also occurs (Swank, 1958; Stehbens et al. 1960; Silver et al. 1965a; Silver et al. 1965b; Stehbens, 1967d). In these circumstances large red cell masses ("sludged blood") (Knisely, 1965) have been seen impeding or completely obstructing blood flow (Silver et al. 1965a; Stehbens, 1967d). By definition such red cell aggregates must also be considered as a type of thrombus.

The ultrastructure of early platelet aggregation has been investigated (Stehbens, 1967b; Stehbens et al. 1967) and in confirmation of the light microscopic findings, platelets initially exhibited no deformation in shape and the areas of contact between the platelets was limited. Subsequent changes indicated that the adjoining platelets gradually became applied to one another with consequent alteration in shape, but dendritic forms, degranulation and rearrangement of granulomere location were not observed in these early stages. The significance of the amorphous material surrounding the platelets in the aggregated state is not known and in view of the techniques used in the investigation (Stehbens et al. 1967), additional studies are needed. However, it is conceivable that the material could be concerned with the initial adhesion of platelet to platelet or platelet to leukocyte. It has been suggested that platelet aggregation might be induced by the adsorption of flocculated plasma proteins or possibly fibrin on to the platelet surface (Sharp, 1961). Trace amounts of thrombin might lead to clotting of plasma fibrinogen adsorbed on the platelet surface and it is pertinent that some materials which induce platelet clumping (Stehbens et al. 1960; Silver, 1965a; Stehbens, 1967d) are known to produce a fall in plasma fibrinogen (Swank, 1959; Spaet, 1963). In the aggregation of platelets and the formation of a tightly packed mass, it is now known that fusion of platelets does not occur. With electron microscopy it is seen that platelets ultimately form a tightly packed mosaic and it has been suggested that the close approximation of platelets to one another may be related to the known property of platelets to spread on a "foreign" surface – in this instance an altered platelet surface (Stehbens et al. 1967).

An additional important conclusion made from these studies of early in vivo changes was that pseudopod formation and dendritic forms can be artefacts induced by the separation and handling of the platelets prior to fixation for electron microscopy (Stehbens et al. 1967; Stehbens, 1967c). Therefore, if platelets have already undergone considerable morphological change as evidenced by many published electron micrographs of "normal" platelets separated prior to fixation, they may have also undergone considerable biochemical change due to the alteration in environment. In fact, these findings raise a serious question as to how germane in vitro observations on platelets are to the observed in vivo phenomena.

Another approach to the experimental study of early thrombosis has been to examine sheets of endothelium en face, because the underlying vessel wall is one of Virchow's triad of pathogenic factors. However, one of the difficulties encountered in this technique is artefact and it is not sufficiently appreciated how readily endothelium is damaged in the handling of vessels. Samuels and Webster (1952) believed that stigmata along the silverstained endothelial cell borders were platelet thrombi but electron microscopy has failed to substantiate this (Majno et al. 1961) and similar staining reactions can be induced in vitro in the absence of blood (Stehbens, 1965a). In a recent study of inflamed or damaged veins, platelets were found to adhere to severely damaged endothelium at the edge of areas of desquamation and where the endothelium had been denuded, but not to normal endothelium (Stehbens, 1965a). This was in agreement with Poole et al. (1963) who found thrombi adherent to amorphous remnants of endothelium or to basement membrane. There is also the possibility that in inflammation and trauma, platelets may adhere to subendothelial structures when endothelial cells separate in the formation of stomato (Stehbens, 1965a).

There is ample circumstantial evidence that stasis is of importance in thrombogenesis in man and this information is strongly supported by the experimental stasis thrombus. As mentioned previously some red venous thrombi may closely resemble clots histologically and the red thrombus which is believed to have been formed by rapid propagation is that which can lead to disability and death. It is also the red thrombus of the venous circulation that is the most amenable to therapy. The problem remains why these thrombi should propagate to such a remarkable extent in veins but it is possible that relative stasis may be responsible for propagation though not for initiation of thrombosis itself.

B. Macrocirculation

Most experimental thrombi in large blood vessels are developed on the basis of a vascular lesion. Many of these techniques have been reviewed by Henry (1962). In almost all experimental thrombi due to trauma, the platelet masses, although varying in size in relation to the degree of the stimulus, remain limited to the zone of injury. These thrombi, moreover, contain a relatively small amount of fibrin with entrapped erythrocytes when compared with the extensive venous thrombi often seen in man in which fibrin rather than the platelet constitutes a major component. Therefore, one of the key problems is to deduce what it is that facilitates the propagation of the red thrombus.

Because of the skepticism concerning the role of the coagulation thrombus itself in initiating intravascular coagulation and the lack of success in correlating causally in vitro alterations in clotting factors with overt thrombosis, a technique was devised for the production of coagulation thrombi in animals. It is dependent upon the induction of systemic hypercoagulability and localized retardation of blood flow (Wessler, 1955).

In this model system a segment of jugular vein is freed from its surrounding structures and its tributaries ligated. Aged homologous or heterologous mammalian serum, free of thrombin, is then infused into a distant systemic vein. If, seconds following the infusion, the previously freed jugular segment is gently isolated with clamps, a uniform red thrombus forming a cast of the occluded segment develops within minutes after vein isolation. Thrombi also form behind the distal clamp where stasis is incomplete, but nowhere else in the circulation. Neither the infusion of serum alone, vein clamping alone, nor the infusion of silicone-processed plasma followed by vein isolation produce such thrombi; overt intimal injury appears to be unnecessary, for thrombosis follows serum infusion, even if jugular vein blood flow is retarded by gentle digital pressure through the intact skin. Finally, the thrombus and its subsequent histopathologic evolution is similar to that observed in man and is initiated by a mechanism demonstrated to be operative in human subjects (Wessler, 1962).

A series of experiments were undertaken to establish the nature of the thrombus-inducing activity in human serum that was called Serum Thrombotic Accelerator, or STA, activity. Elaboration of STA activity was found to be dependent upon the presence in serum of the first three procoagulants (Hageman Factor (XII), PTA (XI), and Christmas Factor (IX)) involved in the formation of intrinsic thromboplastin (Wessler et al. 1960). Subsequently, it was shown that STA activity was dependent upon the presence in serum of the activated forms of PTA and Christmas Factor (Wessler et al. 1966a). Moreover, it was demonstrated in several laboratories that the liver has the capacity to discriminate between precursor and activated forms of clotting factors and to remove only the latter from the circulation (Spaet, 1962; Deykin, 1966; Wessler, 1966b). These observations emphasize that it is not so much the absolute quantity of circulating clotting factors that contributes to hypercoagulability, but rather the presence in the circulation of some of the coagulation factors in an activated form.

It can thus be suggested that if clotting factors, such as PTA or Christmas Factor, are circulating in an activated form, the blood may be considered hypercoagulable but not thrombotic. The role of stasis may be interpreted as a means whereby the activated products of coagulation are protected from the liver clearance mechanism that would normally remove them from the circulation before coagulation proceeded far enough to cause fibrin deposition.

In the animal model, the thrombotic trigger is the presence in the blood stream of an activated clotting factor. The injection of the precursor form has invariably failed to produce thrombosis in these experimental systems. Thus, from these studies evidence has been provided concerning the means whereby stasis may facilitate the deposition of this type of thrombus. These investigations have also permitted recognition of the mechanisms that exist either in circulating blood or in organs such as the liver for rapidly inactivating or removing activated clotting intermediates.

V. Etiology of Thrombosis

The factors initiating thrombosis in man are not known. Whether they are in part attributable to certain drugs, to relative immobilization, or to the high caloric or high fat content of the diet is undetermined. More than 100 years ago, Virchow crystallized the general principles of thrombosis, documented the concept of embolization and enunciated the series of hypotheses that are today referred to as Virchow's triad: namely, that local injury, stasis, and systemic alterations in coagulability are causative factors in intravascular coagulation. Virchow's observations were extended by his associates and students and were effectively summarized in a critical monograph by Welch (1899) at the turn of the century.

We have progressed little from Virchow's position, despite a remarkable acceleration of research in the areas related to thrombosis. Part of this acceleration is due to the newer knowledge gained from the unravelling of the hemorrhagic states, part from the development of potent anticoagulant and lytic agents, and part from the concurrent availability of sensitive clotting assays. The literature is rich in accounts of the coagulation mechanism, the chemistry of anticoagulant drugs and their application, whereas incisive treatises on the etiology and pathogenesis of thrombosis become significant by virtue of their scarcity.

Numerous aspects of thrombosis in man remain unexplained. Because venous thrombosis in the lower limbs is rare in the very young, it would suggest that there is an age dependent factor involved, but we do not even know whether this incriminates the vessel wall, the rate of blood flow or a change in the thrombotic tendency of the circulating blood.

To date there is no adequate explanation for coronary thrombosis. The underlying lesion is more than probably a form of damage to the endothelium or innermost part of the intima. The result of tearing, desquamation or sloughing of the intimal surface, atheromatous ulcers with dissection and thrombosis frequently occur in the aorta and similar lesions are found in the coronary arteries (Stehbens, 1963b). Drury (1954) said that thrombosis usually results from necrosis or rupture of the endothelium overlying an atheromatous plaque. Others (Benson, 1926; Clark et al. 1936; Leary, 1935; Horn et al. 1940) have drawn attention to the tearing of the overlying intima. Leary (1935) believed that the necrotic centents of atheromatous abscesses or cavities could rupture into the lumen. This view is now generally accepted and it has been extended to suggest that mechanical weakness or fragility of the atherosclerotic intima could account for the initial disruption of the intima (Stehbens, 1963b; Stehbens, 1965b).

The reason for the localization of bacteria in cardiac valve cusps in the production of bacterial endocarditis is not clear. It is known, however, that one of the primary functions of platelets is to clear the blood stream of foreign material including particulate matter and bacteria (Stehbens et al. 1960). Therefore, if there are small tears and areas of damage on the valve cusps as Magarey's (1949) study of Lambl's excrescences indicates, it is quite likely that platelets aggregated about bacteria would lodge at such sites and induce endocarditis. Alternatively the bacteria could adhere to platelet deposits already on the cusps. However, in view of the frequency with which gross arterial intimal defects occur in the aorta, one would expect bacterial arteritis to complicate advanced atherosclerosis, but such a complication is extremely rare.

The role of stasis in thrombus formation has been accepted for more than a century and there is much circumstantial and experimental evidence in support of this concept (Wessler, 1963). However, the manner in which stasis participates is not fully understood. The available evidence would cast doubt on the possibility that stasis alone could produce thrombosis. Certainly it is unlikely that it alone could produce massive venous thrombosis. Roentgenographic studies in man have demonstrated that in the deep veins of the leg retardation of blood flow can occur unassociated with thrombosis (Stanton et al. 1949; McLachlin et al. 1960). Animal data even more strongly suggest that stasis alone is incapable of producing thrombosis and that blood remains fluid within a normal intima isolated from the general circulation – an observation first described in 1771 by the now classic experiments of Hewson (1771), and amply confirmed by subsequent investigators. Taken together these observations indicate that profound retardation of blood flow can occur normally in man and that there is a remarkable intravascular resistance to coagulation of such a static column of blood. Some alteration, either in the endothelium or in the circulating constituents of the blood, must be present to initiate massive thrombosis.

Eddy currents are the other hemodynamic factor invoked as a predisposing cause though in the small blood vessels in the rabbit ear chamber, platelet deposition and aggregation do not seem to be associated with these flow disturbances (Stehbens, 1967a; Stehbens, 1967c) and the observation need not be pertinent to conditions prevailing in larger vessels. Nevertheless, the topography of platelet deposits seen in plastic flow chambers inserted in extracorporeal shunts has been thought to be governed by such hydraulic factors (Murphy et al. 1962). However, the nature of the lining material of such models complicates this theory. Further investigation of this aspect of thrombosis is certainly warranted.

Alteration in the blood itself is the third part of Virchow's triad and one wonders what role the circulating constituents of the blood, particularly the various clotting factors play in the initiation of thrombosis. The relationship between thrombo-embolic phenomena and the coagulation mechanism is difficult to evaluate. If fibrin is part of the thrombus, then the clotting system has been activated. The critical question, however, is at what point and in what manner does the coagulation mechanism participate in thrombogenesis? Is there such an entity as hypercoagulability and does it precede or follow thrombosis?

A distinction can be made between a hypercoagulable and a thrombotic state. Hypercoagulability can be defined as a state in which activated clotting factors normally absent from circulating blood are either released from tissues directly into the circulation or are formed intravascularly. The thrombotic state refers to the additional condition in which the active circulating products overcome the inhibitory capacity of the blood and the tissue clearance mechanisms to form a thrombus.

While animal studies have facilitated a definition of hypercoagulability and have shown how it may be potentiated or removed, they have so far failed to show how the trigger itself is formed. Unless the mechanisms responsible for the in vivo development of an activated clotting factor can be elucidated, the existence of a hypercoagulable state, as defined above, will remain unproven.

Clinically, the term systemic hypercoagulability has been used more loosely. If one searches for evidence of hypercoagulability among patients with venous thrombosis, one finds that support of the concept is marshalled from at least four areas: (1) the absence or relative rarity of phlebitis among patients with congenital deficiencies of specific clotting factors, (2) procoagulant plasma elevations in the immediate postpartum period, (3) recurrent phlebitis in patients with persistent elevations of specific clotting factors, and (4) the proven prophylactic efficacy of anticoagulant drugs.

Objections to accepting these arguments come readily to mind. The data on patients with congenital deficiencies are scanty and include few individuals in the older age group. Moreover, exceptions have been reported with thrombosis developing in patients with low levels of fibrinogen (Factor I), ac-globulin (Factor V), proconvertin (Factor VII), and antihemophilic factor (Factor VIII). Pregnant women in the third trimester have procoagulant elevations of the same order as that found in the post-partum period, yet there is a smaller incidence of phlebitis during pregnancy than is observed after delivery. Similarly, the thrombophilic patient with persistently increased circulating levels of a specific procoagulant has long periods free of intravascular coagulation during which the procoagulant is as elevated as during episodes of phlebitis. It might reasonably be expected that a several-fold increase in a circulating procoagulant would set the stage for a greater or more rapid explosion of enzyme coagulation kinetics. Here, however, the clinical data are in keeping with the experimental observations: namely, that the trigger (as defined by the experimental hypercoagulable state) is lacking in the system.

Many patients, of course, develop phlebitis without any detectable change in their clotting profile, whereas others show changes in clotting factors that appear to be consequent rather than causal to the thrombosis (MacFarlane, 1959; McDonald, 1957). Finally, in regard to anticoagulant therapy, the fact that interference with clotting reactions prevents venous thrombosis does not establish a priori that the basis of this effect is related to the prevention of any systemic hypercoagulability.

While attempts to prove the existence of systemic hypercoagulability remain unavailing, the possible role of local hypercoagulability in forehand that anticoagulant or fibrinolytic drugs will be effective agents to control this type of thrombus. A more thorough test of these agents would be additional evaluations of their effects on thrombi induced by other methods assuming different etiologies. For this purpose I have included methods based on mechanical trauma, perivascular applications of thrombosing substances, slowing of circulation, intravascular insertions of foreign bodies, electric currents, dietary regimen, and artificial in vitro procedures.

Mechanical trauma provides thrombogenic mechanisms arising from injury to blood vessel components not offered by other methods. The slowing of blood flow at the experimental thrombus location provides thrombogenic or thrombolytic mechanisms attributable to rates of blood flow, eddy currents, and settling and sedimentation of blood elements, among other considerations, which are not possible in methods involving isolated vascular segments by ligation. Flowing blood allows selective differential accumulation of thrombus components during its formation and contributes to natural mechanisms of thrombolysis. The combination of component additions to the thrombus and component subtractions from the thrombus will determine its incidence and size in time. If the rates of addition are greater than the rates of subtraction the thrombus will increase in size, propagate, and eventually involve mechanisms of organization. If the rates of subtraction are greater than the rates of addition, then obviously, resolution of the thrombus will result. That these mechanisms are occurring from the time of thrombus inducement should be recognized and considered when evaluating preventive or curative measures. The time of observation becomes an important consideration to establish incidence or thrombus size for any given method of experimental thrombus production.

Intravascular insertion of foreign bodies provides an opportunity to study the response of blood to given surfaces. Development of intravascular accumulations on these surfaces should be evaluated with regard to the particular substance composing the surface. Evaluation of measures to alter this response must be considered in like manner and should not be reduced to generalized concepts effective against all other types of thrombotic mechanisms.

Methods utilizing electric currents provides a controlled means to study bioelectric attractions of blood components to a given vascular location. The magnitude of current applied agrees with measurements of currents of injury. Results should be interpreted as the responce to electrical attractions. Thrombotic mechanisms such as blood coagulation may not be involved whereas other mechanisms such as blood flow dynamics and cellular enzyme release may be superimposed.

Methods for in vitro artificial thrombus production have been included here since they provide a possibility for the establishment of a rapid laboratory procedure to test for impending thromboembolic conditions. Results should not be considered identical to events occurring in vivo for reasons given in more detail in the section following the method description.

Controlled dietary regimen provides an opportunity to alter certain blood components. These methods are useful for chronic thrombotic responses to the alteration in the composition of the blood. Perhaps the methods would be more useful in the study of thrombosis when combined with one of several other methods. For instance, results from direct mechanical injury to blood vessels without dietary alterations in blood content can serve as control for comparison. In this regard, many of the other methods for experimental thrombus production can be combined to bring several sets of thrombogenic and thrombolytic mechanisms into play.

The incidence and size of thrombi produced by many experimental methods depends upon the time of observation or harvest. Except in the case of isolated vascular segments by double ligations, thrombogenic and thrombolytic mechanisms under conditions of flowing blood are occurring from the time of thrombus inducement. Early thrombotic masses may have already been resolved and removed from the experimental location by the time observation or harvest of the thrombus is executed. What is observed may be only a few minutes "old" even though inducement occurred hours earlier. Time is one of the more important considerations in the study of thrombosis and the effects of prevention or curative measures. In addition, care should be exercised in the removal of thrombi formed, especially when quantitative measurements are desirable.

Methods described in the categories below are selected, generally, for utilization of the dog as the experimental animal of choice. This does not imply that the dog is the better animal for study. Apparently rodents lend themselves better to those studies involving dietary controls in the production of experimental thrombosis. Many of the other methods can also be adapted to animal species other than the dog. Direct microvascular microscopic observations are more easily performed on smaller animals. The chemical and cellular composition of the blood should be considered in the selection of an animal to be used. Guidelines for certain physiologic parameters and differential cell counts can be obtained from Zweifach (1961).

Selection of a given method to induce experimental thrombosis depends on what the investigator wishes to accomplish. Complete evaluation of preventive or curative measures must involve their effectiveness against thrombosis resulting from alterations in vascular walls, alterations in blood content, and alterations in blood flow. Furthermore, some methods are designed to study early events in thrombosis. In some methods the early events may be based on the clotting of blood and in others on platelet sticking. The study of thrombus resolution or organization may require still different methods of thrombus development. Once again, results must be interpreted in view of the method of thrombus inducement used and do not necessarily apply to all types of thrombi. Indeed, the partial effectiveness of given preventive or curative measures is probably due to overlooking the possibility of other sets of mechanisms operating independently of the set being controlled. Appreciation of this point was emphasized by Mustard et al. (1964) in a review on platelets and atherosclerosis.

II. Categories of Methods to Produce Experimental Thrombosis and Specific Examples

A. Injections of Thrombosing Substances

1. Preliminary Comments

The most widely used concept for inducing experimental thrombosis is that of the injection or infusion of substances thought to alter a normal situation in a way occurring pathologically in nature. These methods necessarily are based on preconceived notions of the etiology and pathogenesis of thrombosis. Alterations in either the vascular wall or the clotting mechanisms have been the prime targets although partial or complete stasis of blood flow have been superimposed.

One of the earliest methods (Dietrich, 1941) attempted to produce thrombophlebitis by the injections of bacteria into isolated venous segments. The method was adequate for that purpose. Thromboembolic conditions and thrombosis superimposed upon emboli have been experimentally produced by the injections of broken-up and whole blood clots. Since blood coagulation underlies these procedures successful results from fibrinolytic agents should be attained. Embolic lesions have been produced in local situations such as ear veins of rabbits (Pryce et al. 1950), partal vein and liver of dogs (Robertson et al. 1954), pulmonary system of dogs (Jacques and Hyman, 1957), femoral arteries of dogs (Duffy and Furth, 1959), and mesenteric vessels of dogs (Lee et al. 1961). Useful techniques for follow-up study of thromboembolism produced by injecting clotted blood utilize radioactive tagging such as $Na_2Cr^{51}O_4$ for red cells (Duffy and Furth, 1959) and I^{131} fibrinogen to tag the fibrin formed (Ambrus et al. 1957; Back et al. 1958).

Injections of sclerosing agents have been used extensively for methods to induce experimental thrombosis for the primary purpose of studying anticoagulant and fibrinolytic effects of various substances. The sclerosing agents are believed to damage vascular endothelium.

Ether (Flexner, 1902; Loeb and Meyers, 1910), vaseline, paraffin, oil of turpentine, croton oil, olive oil, caster oil, carbolic acid (Yatsushiro, 1913), and saturated NaCl (Kojima, 1933) were among the chemicals used to study thrombosis before ready availability of anticoagulants or fibrinolytic agents. The effectiveness of heparin has been studied on thrombi produced by the injection of sodium ricinoleate (Murray et al. 1937; Solandt and Best, 1938), sodium morrhuate (Wright et al. 1952), and monoethanolamine oleate (Jewell et al. 1954). Dicumarol-like compounds have been studied on thrombi produced by monoethanolamine oleate (Bingham et al. 1941; Richards et al. 1942; Jewell et al. 1954). Sodium morrhuate, topical thrombin, and thromboplastin have been used to induce thrombosis to study the anticoagulant, fibrinolytic, and thrombolytic properties of trypsin (Innerfield et al. 1952). Effects of various fibrinolysin preparations have been evaluated on thrombi produced by the injections of sodium morrhuate (Johnson and Tillet, 1952; Cliffton et al. 1954; Grossi et al. 1954; Freiman et al. 1960; Kamiya and Fukuta, 1960; Nahum et al. 1960; Wilson, 1960; Marin et al. 1961) and thrombin (Grossi et al. 1954). Other substances used to induce thrombosis have included 50% glucose, acetic acid, silver nitrate, osmic acid, ferric chloride, calcium chloride, formaldehyde, ethyl alcohol, sulfuric acid, and many more. A more extensive survey of these methods can be found in an annotated bibliography by Henry (1962).

Injections of homologous or heterologous serum to induce experimental thrombosis was used early by several investigators (Flexner, 1902; Loeb et al. 1910; Feissly, 1925; Rabinovitch, 1929). Wessler (1953) gave impetus to methods utilizing serum by developing a more standard approach although his method was not significantly different from that of the Swiss investigator, Feissly (1925). Numerous studies have made use of this method to evaluate thrombolytic agents. The reader can consult the annotated bibliography by Henry (1962) for further references.

Trypsin (Eagle and Harris, 1937; Holden et al. 1949; Wessler, 1953) and thromboplastin (Copley and Stefko, 1947; Innerfield et al. 1952; McLetchie, 1952; Sherry et al. 1954; Boyles, 1958; Kudrjashov et al. 1961) have also been injected to induce experimental thrombosis. However, probably the most widely used substance has been thrombin. Warner et al. (1939) noticed intravascular thrombosis following the injection of purified thrombin. An extensive list of methods following these early observations can be found in the annotated bibliography by Henry (1962). Since the injection of thrombin to induce experimental thrombosis is the most widely used method representing this subcategory, I have elected to present the details of two methods here.

2. A Quantitative Method to Induce Radioactive Thrombi and Emboli (Ambrus et al. 1956)

a. Method. Dogs are anesthetized with sodium pentobarbital (25 mg/kg, i.v.) and sections of femoral or jugular veins or femoral arteries are isolated by arterial clamps placed on both the distal and proximal ends. All side branches except one are ligated. A fine polyethylene cannula is inserted into the remaining side branch. Most of the blood in an isolated segment is withdrawn through this cannula into a syringe containing 2.5 μc of P^{32} labeled sodium phosphate. The mixture is rapidly reintroduced through the cannula into the vein segment. Repeated withdrawing and reinjecting several times will insure thorough mixing. (Radioactive phosphorous is taken up by the red and white blood cells.) Thrombin (50 to 100 units in physiological saline) is then introduced into the segment. The polyethylene cannula is removed and the side branch ligated. The blood vessel is placed into the groove of a lead shield to which another shield containing a radioaction sensitive detector tube is attached. Radioactive counts can be made with a radiation rate meter and a suitable recorder. (Reference to specific models of such equipment is purposely omitted here subject to the investigators own preference in regard to modern apparatus.)

Aluminum wire is used to apply a semiconstricting ligature downstream from the induced clot before the segment isolation clamps are removed. If emboli are desired, no such partial ligatures are needed.

b. Precautions and Modifications. The above procedure can be performed without the injection of thrombin into the isolated vascular segment. Following mixing with radioactive material the blood can be allowed to clot spontaneously within the segment. In place of P^{32} labeled sodium phosphate, red cells can be tagged with Cr^{51}. Red cells must be incubated with Cr^{51} before being introduced into the segment. Ambrus et al. (1956), suggest that 10 ml of blood be removed from the animal and placed in a test tube containing sodium oxalate and 40 μc of Cr^{51}. The mixture is incubated for two hours at 37° C. The blood is then centrifuged at 2000 rpm and the red cells washed three times with Tyrode solution. Approximately 0.6 ml of the concentrated labeled red cells are then injected into a vascular segment containing blood and isolated as previously described. Thrombin is then injected as before to form the clot. I^{131} can also be used in a similar manner. Ambrus et al. (1956) suggest that the I^{131} fibrinogen be prepared according to the method of Mihalyi and Laki (1952).

Canalized clots can be produced by introducing a polyethylene rod through the segment where the clot is formed. Following coagulation of the blood within the segment the rod is removed and blood is allowed to flow through the clot when the isolation clamps are removed.

3. Inducement of Experimental Thrombosis to Simulate the Conditions of Mechanical Trauma Existing During Surgery of Small Arteries. Method of Deaton and Anlyan (1960)

a. Method. Common femoral arteries of dogs are exposed and dissected free over a 2 cm segment. All side branches are clamped, divided and ligated with fine silk. A no. 18 needle is placed parallel to and next to the artery and a No. 3–0 plain catgut ligature is tied around both the needle and artery distal to the experimental segment. The needle is then removed leaving a constricting but nonoccluding ligature around the artery. The 2 cm segment is isolated between bulldog clamps and the blood within the segment is aspirated (No. 24 needle) into a syringe containing 100 units of thrombin in 2 ml of saline. The mixture is rapidly reinjected into the segment. Two minutes later the bulldog clamps are removed. The wound is then closed for long term studies.

b. Precautions and Modifications. Obviously this method produces a 100% incidence of clotting type thrombin within several minutes. However, Deaton and Anlyan (1960) found this incidence to be reduced to 45% occlusive and 10% nonocclusive thrombi in three weeks. Since these blood clots are induced in the absence of blood flow, the chemical constitution and cytoarchitecture is limited to those blood elements in the isolated segment. Differential concentration of these elements does not have an opportunity to develop. Mechanical trauma to the arteries is limited to the surgical exposure, needle puncture, and ligations. Deaton and Anlyan found a greater incidence of thrombosis following chemical intimectomy with sulfuric acid. At least 75% of the arteries were thrombosed one to 14 days after inducement. In this procedure all blood was aspirated from the experimental segment and 0.1 normal sulfuric acid was injected to fill the segment. Two minutes later a second needle was introduced into the segment and the vessel was flushed with water for five minutes. All needles and clamps were then removed. Mechanical intimectomy with arteriotomy and a dental burr stripping gave a higher incidence of thrombosis in 24 hours indicating that mechanical manipulations enhanced the stimulus to thrombus formation compared to intimal destruction alone.

Qualitatively, results from the infusion of thrombin into isolated vascular segments are satisfactory from the point of view of reproducibility and 100% incidence. However, this method assumes that the underlying cause for thrombosis is that of blood clotting. Methods utilizing chemical or mechanical trauma are difficult to analyze since thrombogenic and thrombolytic mechanisms are operating from the time of thrombus inducement in the presence of blood flow. Incidence found will depend on the time observations are made and will vary considerably depending on the relative contributions made by thrombogenic and thrombolytic mechanisms. To evaluate the effects of drugs under these conditions would be difficult and perhaps misleading.

B. Mechanical Trauma

1. Preliminary Comments

Mechanical trauma to blood vessels was first used by Jones (1851) to induce experimental thrombosis. Methods involving damage to the entire vessel wall by crushing the vessels directly were extensively used by Eberth and Schimmelbusch (1888). Later these methods were used to study the effects of heparin (Murray et al. 1937) and Dicumarin (Dale and Jacques, 1942) on the incidence or extent of thrombi produced. A standard technique utilizing direct crushing blows to blood vessels was developed by Hirsch and Loewe (1946) and these investigators later tested the effects of anticoagulants on thrombosis (Loewe et al. 1947, 1948). Loewe's group used rabbits in their experimental studies. Their techniques were adapted for dogs by Wilson (1960) and this method is presented below to exemplify this category.

Many investigators feel that direct mechanical injury to blood vessels is the technique which most nearly resembles spontaneous in vivo thrombosis. The thrombi form under conditions of flowing blood, no additional variables are imposed as in the case of injecting thrombogenic substances, and the living viable cells are allowed to respond in a physiologic way as opposed to those techniques where sclerosing or fixing agents are applied. Not all methods, however, involve total vascular wall damage. Attempts have been made to damage only the endothelium of blood vessels or only the perivascular tissue. Zahn (1875) accomplished a separation of endothelial cells by forceful stretching of blood vessels. Thrombi were seen first to form at the lines of endothelial cell separation. This method was later used by Rabinovitch and Pine (1943, 1949) to study the effects of heparin and penicillin on venous thrombosis and thrombophlebitis. Nelson (1952) used the technique to study the effects of ACTH on venous thrombosis in dogs. A dental excavator was introduced to blood vessels of dogs by Welch (1887) to scrape the endothelium directly as a method to study the structure of "white thrombi" produced. This method was extended to human volunteers by Johnson and McCarty (1959) to test the effects of infused streptokinase on the thrombi formed. Endothelium plus intima was stripped away by a needle or dental burr in the thrombus inducing method investigated by Deaton and Anlyan (1960).

Perivascular tissue injury or injury to tissues at a distance from the thrombotic vascular site were used by Lutz et al. (1951) in the hamster, by Borgstrom and Gelin (1957) in rabbits and by Knisely et al. (1960) in frogs and amphiuma. These methods imply that substances are released by damaged tissues and have thrombotic effects at distant sites predisposing to adherence and deposition of thrombus constituents. Knisely (1960) showed that in amphibia blood cell aggregations and subsequent settling of these masses to gravitationally dependent portions of blood vessels at sites of slow flow led to thrombosis due to adherence of these masses at the points of settling.

2. Combination of Mechanical Trauma with Thrombin Injection to Induce Experimental Thrombosis

a. Method. Wilson (1960) observed thrombosis in mesenteric blood vessels of the dog following direct trauma. Since the thrombi were usually smaller than the size of the vessels occlusion of flow did not develop. The method described here combines mechanical trauma with thrombin injection.

A 4 to 5 cm segment of mesenteric vein is dissected free from surrounding tissue. The segment is collapsed between clamps and traumatized by striking it with an instrument handle against a flat ribbon retractor. Twenty units of thrombin (in 0.5 ml saline) is introduced into the segment with a No. 26 needle. The segment is allowed to fill with blood by removing the appropriate clamp and is then reclamped for 20 to 30 minutes. A semiconstricting ligature is placed downstream to prevent the clot from slipping away.

b. Precautions and Modifications. Thrombosis will occur with the mechanical trauma alone. The thrombi developed can be observed with transillumination and a microscope. That they are not always occlusive is not a drawback of the method. They are forming under the conditions of flowing blood and are developing in time in response to both thrombogenic and thrombolytic mechanisms. To add exogenous thrombin at this point insures that blood clotting will be the basis for the intravascular mass formed. Certainly fibrinolytic agents will be effective against these thrombi as was found by Wilson. He also observed, however, that rethrombsois occurred in these segments following fibrinolytic digestion of the original thrombus (blood clot) and postulated that this secondary thrombosis may have been due to vascular injury.

C. Perivascular Applications of Thrombosing Substances

1. Preliminary Comments

Most of the agents applied topically to blood vessels as a method to induce experimental thrombosis are tissue fixing agents with the exception of topical thrombin (Berman et al. 1954, 1955). Topical thrombin undoubtedly induces thrombi by way of clotting mechanisms by diffusion into the blood vessels. The fixing agents, however, are of questionable value since normal metabolism of the vascular wall cell components are disrupted or halted and normal response of cells contributing to the formation, dissolution, or organization of resulting thrombi may also be altered. Alcohol and osmic acid were topically applied to exposed omental vessels of the dog by Eberth and Schimmelbusch (1888). These investigators felt that stasis occurred before the stages of pathology in the formation of thrombi could develop. Blake et al. (1959) assayed for the antithrombic activity of anticoagulants on thrombi developed from the perivascular application of 10% formalin mixed volume for volume with 60% methyl alcohol. Ashwin and Jacques (1961) utilized this method to study the effects of P^{32}, dextran, reserpine, and stypturen on thrombus formation in rats. Rosenberg et al. (1959) utilized 10% to 40% formalin in a calibrated technique for experimental production of venous thrombosis in rabbits. This technique is presented here in detail.

Croton oil (Samuel, 1867; Lutz et al. 1951), ricinoleate (Solandt et al. 1939), ferric chloride (Reimann-Hunziker, 1944), and silver nitrate (Eberth and Schimmelbusch, 1888; Kristenson, 1921; Jansen and Tage-Hansen, 1949) have also been applied perivascularly to induce experimental thrombosis.

2. Perivascular Application of Formalin to Induce Experimental Thrombosis

a. Method. Rosenberg et al. (1959) developed the following procedure to produce standardized experimental thrombi. The abdomen of rabbits under open-drop ether anesthesia is opened through a midline incision. The infrarenal portion of the inferior vena cava is located and a small opening is made in the overlying peritoneum. A curved hemostat is introduced into the opening and a perivenous pocket is created by blunt dissection. A pursestring suture of fine silk is positioned around the opening. A measured solution of 10% to 40% formalin in introduced into the pocket by syringe and needle, taking care not to lacerate the vein. The needle is withdrawn and the suture is drawn taut and tied. The abdominal incision may now be closed for long term observations.

Rosenberg et al. (1959) found an incidence of thrombosis 24 hours later of 4 in 20 trials with 10% formalin, 15 in 20 trials with 20% formalin, 14 in 20 trials with 30% formalin, and 17 in 20 trials with 40% formalin. They reported these thrombi to be primarily composed of platelets and leukocytes.

b. Precautions and Modifications. This technique can be used for any animal species and for perivascular application of agents other than formalin. Undoubtedly, formalin induces platelet-type thrombosis in response to this kind of vascular injury. Since formalin is a known fixing agent certainly normal physiologic functions of cells of the blood vessel wall or within the accumulated mass are impaired or eliminated. Caution must be taken in regard to mechanisms of thrombus organization with this and similar methods. The incidence of thrombosis depends on the time of thrombus harvest and observation. Whatever time period is selected should be used throughout any set of experiments directed toward finding the effects of thrombolytic agents on these kind of thrombi. Care should be taken to consider a thrombus found 24 hours (for example) after inducement to be a 24 hour old thrombus. The animals own thrombolytic mechanisms are undoubtedly functioning under these conditions of flowing blood and in reality the major portion of a thrombus found at 24 hours may only be several minutes old.

Caution must be taken to evaluate the effects of enzymes and other agents for thrombolytic purposes since the experimental site is surrounded with a solution capable of destroying the very effects desired. That an agent is noneffective may not have anything to do with thrombosis but rather may result from the experimental design.

D. Slowing of Circulation

1. Preliminary Comments

Zielonko (1873) observed slowing of the blood flow, vascular dilation and accumulations of colorless blood cells in arteries, capillaries and veins gradually occluding these vessels following sciatic and crural nerve section in frogs. Gradual vascular occlusion was also accomplished by swelling of plastic vascular sleeves by Berman et al. (1956) and by Litvak and Vineberg (1959). In some preparations thrombi were found to contribute to the vascular occlusion.

Partial or complete occlusions of blood vessels with ligatures and clamps are common techniques either used alone to slow or stop the circulation (Pfitzer, 1879; Senftleben, 1879; Zahn, 1884; Eberth and Schimmelbusch, 1888; Potts and Smith, 1943; O'Neill, 1947; Mehrotra, 1953) or in combination with other techniques (Wessler, 1952; Samuels and Webster, 1952). The report of Mann et al. (1938) must be considered when thrombosis following partial ligations is attributed to slowing of the circulation. These investigators found that when a one cm length of the carotid artery of the dog was reduced in cross sectional area to 50% there was no change in flow volume. To get a 50% reduction in flow volume the cross sectional area had to be reduced by 90%. The diameter of a blood vessel (5 mm in diameter) could be reduced by 40% without a reduction in flow volume. The internal diameter had to be reduced by 70% to get a 50% reduction in flow volume.

Kiesewetter and Shumaker (1948) experimented with common carotid and femoral arteries, and external jugular and femoral veins of dogs. A method of placing partial penetrating ligatures of silk or 000 chromic catgut to narrow the lumen and at the same time leave a foreign body inside the intimal layer of veins was considered unreliable. These investigators also tested methods including: application of one Kelly clamp at full tension across an artery for 20 seconds; application of several Kelly clamps at full tension across an artery for 20 seconds; and double partial ligations with silk or catgut and application of multiple Kelly clamps at full tension across the intervening segment for 20 seconds. All of these methods were abandoned by Kiesewetter and Shumaker (1948) as ineffective or too variable. These conclusions must be evaluated in view of the findings by Mann (1938). In addition, care must be taken to insure that some flow of blood is permitted so that those blood elements eventually forming a thrombic mass in the experimental segment are allowed to reach the segment.

2. Gradual Vascular Occlusion with Occurrance of Experimental Thrombosis

a. Method. Litvak and Vineberg (1959), following reports by Berman et al. (1956) that casein plastic cylinders swelled in saline and were capable of occluding arteries, tested several sleeve designs and developed the following method for vascular occlusion. Only those sleeve designs resulting in thrombosis as a part of the vascular occlusion are presented here.

Casein plastic rods 12 mm in diameter and 50 cm in length are used[1]. Eight and 25 mm

[1] American Plastics Corporation, Bainbridge, New York.

lengths of these rods are drilled to form sleeves with 5 to 7 mm luminal diameters and encased in one mm thick stainless steel housings. A longitudinal slot is cut along the side of the housing and plastic sleeve to allow insertion of the blood vessel into the sleeve. Swelling of the casein plastic sleeve is directed toward the lumen and may be measured in vitro by immersion in normal saline at 38° C. Sleeves are stored in a dehydrating desiccator prior to use and sterilized in 1:1000 Zephiran solution.

Left and right femoral or carotid arteries are exposed under aseptic conditions over a distance necessary to position the casein plastic sleeves. The experimental sites are exposed again at given times for observation.

The following tests are made to determine occlusion: (1) palpation for arterial pulsations proximal and distal to the sleeve site; (2) transection of arteries distal to the sleeve to observe whether or not blood would pass through the sleeved segment; and (3) removal of the sleeved segments for tests of in vitro flow of saline through them at a constant pressure. Vascular segments can then be removed from the sleeves for histologic examination.

Reduction or absence of pulsations usually occurs by 27 to 36 days and reduction or absence of flow in vivo and also when tested in vitro usually occurs in about the same time. Microscopic examination usually reveals a fibroblastic response of the vascular walls and formation of intraluminal thrombi arising concentrically from the intima. In completely occluded vessels, thrombotic material is usually found to fill the lumen proximal and distal to the sleeve site.

b. Precautions and Modifications. This method is useful for the development of gradual vascular occlusion over a period of several weeks. Observations on the concurrent development of collateral circulation may be a special feature. The formation of thrombi at the experimental site may be incidental. That thrombotic material accumulates in the vicinity of these casein sleeves lends support to the usefulness of this method for the study of thrombogenesis or thrombolysis. Thrombi develop under conditions of flowing blood and over a relatively long period of time similar to some spontaneously occurring thrombi in human. Thrombi found 30 days after the sleeve application, however, may not be thrombi 30 days old. The material accumulated at the site may have been there only a few hours or a few minutes. Use of radioactive tracing systems may be helpful.

The application of vascular sleeves requires a certain degree of adventitial stripping. Since nutritional supply to larger blood vessels is primarily by way of vasa vasorum, it as interrupted or removed by adventitial stripping. A form of vascular injury is thereby introduced so that the only stimulus to thrombogenesis is not necessarily slowing of blood flow. In addition, swelling of the casein plastic sleeves may result in a form of pressure atrophy.

E. Intravascular Insertion of Foreign Bodies

1. Preliminary Comments

A number of methods designed to induce artificial pulmonary thromboembolism have been modified for experimental thrombosis techniques. Dunn (1920) injected potato starch emulsions into dogs, cats, goats, and rabbits and found thrombosis secondary to pulmonary embolism. Filter paper fibers alone or soaked in rabbits blood or human fibrin (Wartman, 1951) and autogenous or heterogenous fibrin sediment (Barnard, 1953) have been injected into rodents with similar results. Embolization has also been produced in bronchial arteries (Ellis et al. 1953) by the injection of vinyl-acetate and in rabbit ear vessels (Stehbens and Florey, 1960) by the injection of Pelikan ink, Gurr's carbon suspension, Hydrokollag 300 A, carmine, and mercuric sulphide. Platelet adherence to these foreign particles was a common finding.

Pieces of polyethylene tubing suspended intravascularly by Friedman and Byers (1961) was used as an attempt to develop a standard experimental method for thrombus inducement. Pearse (1940) employed metalic tubes, tubular coiled springs and flat springs for gradual arterial occlusion in dogs. This method was later used by Stone and Lord (1951) who suggested that the metalic wires specifically be magnesium or magnesium-aluminum. Such wires containing 98% magnesium and 2% aluminum were used by Gage et al. (1956) to induce experimental coronary thrombosis in the dog. These techniques stem from the use of metal electrolysis for the clotting of blood in saccule areas of dissecting aneurysms. Friedman et al. (1960) enhanced the electrolysis by pretreating magnesium-aluminum alloy wires with zinc chloride before inserting the wires into arteries and veins of rabbits and rats for a method of experimental thrombus production.

The least complicated, and perhaps the most useful and versatile, use of foreign bodies for experimental thrombus production are those methods utilizing threads inserted intravascularly. Bizzozero (1882) made use of this technique by placing cotton threads into the flowing blood stream of rabbit jugular veins. Zurhelle (1910) used silk threads in a similar manner except that care was taken not to strip the adventitia from the blood vessels during the procedure. Yatsushiro (1913) combined silk thread insertion with silver nitrate corrosion of the experimental vascular segment and Moses (1945) pretreated wool threads with defibrinated dog's blood before intravascular placement in external jugular veins of rabbits to study the effects of heparin and Dicumarol on thrombi produced. Smith (1945) studied the geometric positioning and fixation of threads imposed in the flowing blood stream of arteries in dogs on developing thrombi.

Threads inserted intravascularly offers a method to produce experimental thrombosis with possibilities to adapt the method for various purposes. Murray et al. (1937) combined mechanical injury to experimental vascular segments containing silk threads imposed in the path of blood flow or, in addition, injected sclerosing agents into the vascular segment. They were studying the effects of heparin on thrombi produce. The following method outline describes the basic procedure. Adaptations are detailed immediately thereafter.

2. Intravascular Placement of Thread with Superimposed Mechanical Vascular Injury to Induce Experimental Thrombosis

a. Method. Jacques and Ashwin (1964) recommend barbiturate anesthesia and aseptic techniques. The saphenous or brachial vein of the dog is exposed for a distance of 35 mm. A plain, straight needle (noncutting), is passed up the vein for 20 mm and a linen or silk thread (000) is pulled into the experimental segment. Hemostat clamps are used to close the puncture holes. The vein segment is crushed over the thread in several planes with an artery forcep. The clamps are removed and digital pressure is used to control any bleeding from the puncture holes. Heparin is injected into a superficial vein upstream of the experimental segment so that the drug will pass the damaged area. The exposure can be covered with saline gauze for short term experiments or the incision can be closed for long term observations. The vein segment can be removed following a selected period of time and gross appearances as well as microscopic appearances can be recorded. If desired, fixation, cutting and staining techniques can be performed.

Jacques and Ashwin (1964) suggest that if drugs are to be tested for prevention of thrombus formation that they be allowed to act for several hours before vein damage and that the vein segments be examined after six hours. To test for prevention and healing, drugs should be allowed to act over 48 hours and the vessels examined at 72 hours. To test for resolution of thrombi, drugs can be given for at least six hours and the veins can be examined up to three weeks or longer after thrombus inducement.

b. Precautions and Modifications. The general method described originally by Murray et al. (1937) produces isolated thrombosis of veins following tissue damage. The use of heparin is optional and when used reduces the clotting of blood in the experimental segment and allows thrombi formed to be composed chiefly of platelets and white blood cells. This procedure can be carried further by complete anticoagulation of the dog with heparin, Dicumarol or others. In addition, I have observed platelet thrombi adhered to the vein endothelium but not to the thread following trypsin infusion to render the dog's blood noncoagulable as measured by thrombelastography. I used Ethicon® size No. 1 silk thread[2]. The choice of thread is variable but should be used consistently in any given series of studies. Selection of at least four venous segments, two femoral and two external jugular, provides the advantage of using one of the selected veins for a control in the same animal. For example, a control can be run for several hours and removed. A drug to be tested can then be injected and further vein segments can be isolated, thrombi induced, and removed for study one hour, three hours, and six hours after injury or any other time periods selected.

This method has the advantage that no exogenous clotting factors (thrombin, etc.) sclerosing agents, or fixing agents are added. The animal is allowed to respond to the injury with his own thrombogenic or thrombolytic mechanisms under conditions of blood flow. Furthermore, blood samples can be taken from the dog at any given time for coagulation studies and blood cell counts. Other surgical procedures, such as splenectomy or sympathectomy can be performed if desired. The thrombotic materials can be harvested for chemical analyses, cytocomposition or histochemical studies. In addition, smears of the thrombus material can be made by dragging microdissected pieces across clean microslides. Fluorescent antibody studies of the protein composition or cellular inclusions can be performed.

F. Electric Currents

1. Preliminary Comments

Lutz et al. (1951) noticed that injurious faradic stimulation applied to blood vessels of the hamster cheek pouch by microelectrodes resulted in thrombosis of these vessels. Sawyer and Pate (1953) investigated bioelectric phenomena as an etiologic factor in intravascular thrombosis. These investigators later correlated abnormal electrical potential differences with thrombosis of fresh and freeze-dried aortic grafts in dogs. To visualize developing thrombi following application of current to blood vessels Sawyer et al. (1960) adapted their methods to the mesoappendix of the rat. Eisner et al. (1957) could not confirm the observations of Sawyer and Pate; however, Schwartz (1959) utilized the method to produce or prevent thrombosis in dogs by altering the electrical environment used and Callahan et al. (1960) measured thrombus thresholds for various sizes of arteries and veins in the hamster cheek pouch. Williams and Elliot (1958) utilized electric current on external jugular veins of dogs to study the effects of heparin and coumarin derivatives on the standardized intravenous thrombi developed. These studies were extended to study thrombus propagation by Carey and Williams (1960). Strutz et al. (1960) studied the effects of muscle stimulation on blood flow changes in dog hind limbs following femoral vein thrombosis induced by electric current application. Bradham and Lee (1961) and Lee et al. (1961) evaluated the dissolution effects of fibrinolysin on macro and microthrombi of blood vessels in dogs.

Two methods are presented here differing in the means of electrode application and current magnitude.

2. Application of Electric Current to Induce Experimental Thrombosis. Example Method 1

a. Method. Sawyer and Pate (1953) originally developed this method to induce intravascular thrombosis in the aorta, inferior vena cava, femoral arteries, or femoral veins of dogs. Following anesthesia the selected blood vessel is freed from surrounding tissues by sharp dissection believed to minimize trauma to the vessel. Side branches are not disturbed. A rubber dam is used to separate an experimental vascular segment in order to reduce electrical leak. Platinum electrodes are used to measure current output in control and injured blood vessels. These electrodes are made of platinum foil attached to copper leads and insulated by a cellulose bonder and an external polyethylene tube. Sawyer and Pate indi-

[2] Ethicon, Inc., Somerville, N. J., U.S.A.

cate that platinum electrodes are superior to silver electrodes since exposure to saline and passage of current disintegrate the silver electrodes to form silver chloride. Currents applied are from 2 to 4 milliamperes and are comparable to those measured by Sawyer and Pate in spontaneously thrombosing aortic grafts.

Electrodes may be arranged so that one wire electrode is inserted into the lumen of the vascular segment through a vessel branch. An external electrode (approximately 45 mm² in area) is positioned on the vessel adventitia. The internal electrode can be made positive or negative. Blood cells are precipitated at the positive electrode.

Two flat external electrodes (approximately 45 mm² in area) may be applied to the adventitia of blood vessel walls opposite each other. In this case, one electrode is positive and the other negative. Thrombosis occurs on the inner aspect of the vessel wall directly under the positive electrode.

The voltage source consists of six $1^1/_2$ volt dry cells (or equivalent) attached in series to a milliammeter (accurate to .05 milliampere) or a microammeter (accurate to 0.2 microamperes), and a series resistance (accurate to 0.1 ohm), and currents are applied from $1^1/_2$ to 5 hours.

b. Precautions and Modifications. Care must be taken to avoid excessive current application. Sawyer and Pate (1953) found that currents of 50 microamperes can produced occlusive thrombi in dog aortas providing the current was applied at least $4^1/_2$ hours. The current density measured in this case was less than 0.4 microampere/mm² and is of the same magnitude actually measured (0.6 microampere/mm²) across the wall of a segment of injured blood vessel. Femoral arteries and the inferior vena cava thrombosed with less current and femoral veins thrombosed with even less current. In the range of injury current blood cells are allowed to accumulate in time under conditions of flowing blood. Larger currents to reduce the time of thrombosis may involve protein denaturation.

Methods utilizing electric currents assume that the etiology of thrombosis is based on attraction of negatively charged blood cells and protein molecules to areas of positivity undoubtedly present in injured tissues. Even though fibrin strands are found in such accumulations in vivo or in vitro, blood coagulation is considered to be of secondary importance. That similar blood cell accumulation will occur in citrated or heparinized blood in vitro indicates that these methods certainly would not be useful if the investigator wishes to stress the efficacy of anticoagulants or fibrinolysins in the treatment of thrombosis. That thrombosis occurs clinically under conditions of proper anticoagulation and in the face of fibrinolysins may indicate that methods to induce thrombosis utilizing electric currents may be useful for the study of mechanisms involved in thrombus formation in addition to or not related to blood coagulation.

3. Application of Electric Current to Induce Experimental Thrombosis. Example Method 2

a. Method. The method of experimental thrombus production developed by Williams and Carey (1959) utilizing electrical currents is presented here since the methods for electrode application and the level of current applied differs from method No. 1 above.

External jugular veins of dogs anesthetized with sodium pentobarbital are exposed through a 10 to 12 cm incision. Three to 5 cm of each vein is isolated with incision or ligation of side branches. A small lucite cuff 2 mm in thickness and 2 cm in length is placed around the vein. The lucite cuff is made in two longitudinal halves and each half contains a 4 cm by 10 cm platinum plate made from sheet platinum .001 inch thick. The two halves of the cuff are hinged on one side by two 4–0 silk sutures at each end to allow spreading open of the cylinder to meet the size of individual veins measuring 5 mm to 7 mm in diameter.

A fine copper wire insulated with polyethylene tubing (PE-100) is soldered to each platinum sheet. Insulation is continued to 8 inches from the platinum sheet where a small knob is attached for subsequent connection to an electrical source. The entire mechanism is sterilized in 1:1000 Zephiran solution before use.

The wound is covered with a surgical sponge kept moist with 0.9% sodium chloride solution. A small hemostat is positioned over the vein downstream from the lucite cuff to develop a slight slowing of the blood flow and to prevent fluctuations in vein size due to heart beats. Clots do not always form unless the vein walls are made to maintain good contact with the electrodes.

Thrombosis can be produced by varying either the current or the time of current application. Williams and Carey (1959) found 100% thrombosed veins after application of 5 milliamperes delivered over a period of one hour. Thrombi were of rather consistent size. Less time of application resulted in a reduction of incidence. However, 2.5 milliamperes for two hours or 1.25 milliamperes for four hours resulted in 100% thrombosis.

b. Precautions and Modifications. Williams and Carey (1959) arranged an apparatus to deliver 48 to 50 millivolts and less than 1 microampere for two to three weeks without thrombotic accumulations at the electrodes. Electric currents of 1 milliampere or more produced slight bubbling and marked tissue damage at the positive electrode. No change in temperature were measured at the electrodes. Occurrence of thrombosis was related to tissue damage. This is an important consideration since Sawyer and Pate (1953) assumed that there is an attraction of platelets and other blood elements to the positive electrode. If damage to the blood vessel wall is occurring, clot formation may result from procoagulant release. Evaluation of preventive or lytic drugs such as heparin or fibrinolysin must be made in view of involvement of the clotting mechanisms as the basis for development of thrombi in these experiments. To test for formation of platelet thrombi at the site of current application experiments can be performed following the destruction of clotting mechanisms by enzymatic means, such as infusion of trypsin. Drugs can then be tested for their effects on platelet aggregation in response to electrical current changes in such experiments designed to isolate one set of mechanisms known to function in thrombus formation.

G. Dietary Regimen

1. Preliminary Comments

Thomas and Hartroft (1959, 1960) found that diets containing high fat, cholesterol, thiouricil, and sodium cholate produced thrombi in blood vessels of rats before lipid placques could be found. Gresham and Howard (1960) utilized these methods to produce independent atherosclerosis and thrombosis in rats. Bilateral ligations of femoral veins in rats and rabbits were performed by Bergentz et al. (1961) to increase the incidence of thrombosis produced by high fat diets. Davidson et al. (1961) studied blood coagulation changes following thrombus producing diets in rats. Kudrjashov et al. (1961) used fat-cholesterol diets to induce prethrombic states believed to result from dysfunction of the physiological anticoagulating system. These investigators found massive multiple thrombosis following thrombus production by the injection of thromboplastin or thrombin into jugular veins of rats fed high fat diets. Rats fed normal diets responded less severely to the thrombin or thromboplastin injections.

Many diets have been proposed to induce spontaneous intravascular thrombosis and atherosclerosis in various animals. It appears that rats and rabbits respond more readily in developing thrombi from such diets. One method is presented here as an example to indicate that experimental thrombosis can be induced by diets.

2. Experimental Thrombosis from Special Diets

a. Method. The method of Thomas and Hartroft (1959) presented here, has been developed to induce thrombotic conditions in rats. Rats weighing about 120 gm are selected and allowed water *ad libitum*. A measure of the daily food consumption is recorded although the animals are allowed all they can eat each day. Animals are followed for 18 weeks before sacrificing. Some animals may die prior to that time. Thomas and Hartroft prepared seven different diets and the three presented here were the more successful in production of thromboembolic conditions, particularly renal and coronary thrombosis with infarction.

Dry ingredients of each diet are thoroughly blended in a food mixer. Fats are added last and if solid are warmed at room temperature before adding. Blended diets are kept in a tightly stoppered plastic container at 4° C for no longer than two weeks to insure that a rancid diet is not used. The following diet ingredients are listed on a percent by weight basis.

	Diet 1	Diet 2	Diet 3
Casein	20.0	6.0	6.0
Alpha soya protein	0	6.0	6.0
Sucrose	20.5	27.7	28.7
Salt mix (Osborne, 1932)	4.0	4.0	4.0
Alphancel	6.0	6.0	6.0
Vitamin mix[3]	2.0	2.0	2.0
Propylthiouracil	0.3	0.3	0.3
Choline chloride	0.2	0.1	0
Sodium cholate	2.0	2.0	2.0
Butter	40.0	0	0
Lard	0	40.0	40.0
Cholesterol	5.0	5.0	5.0

b. Precautions and Modifications. In a later article Thomas et al. (1960) indicate that high levels of butter or margarine markedly increase the yield of thromboembolism in rabbits and that this increase is due in part to interference with the fibrinolytic system and is a general haematological effect which can be demonstrated in vitro. Corn oil or cholesterol do not have similar effects. In some rats, 1 % choline chloride was used and no differences were noted from 0.2 % used in previous studies.

The effects of diets on the tendency to develop thrombosis may be magnified by combining a diet regimen similar to those described here with other methods to induce thrombosis described elsewhere in this section. Since diets may affect the clotting or natural anticoagulant systems, care must be taken in the evaluation of exogenous anticoagulants or fibrinolysins. Thrombotic mechanisms underlying other methods described elsewhere in this section may be overlooked.

[3] Vitamin A concentrate (200,000 units/gm), 4.5 gm; Vitamin D concentrate (400,000 units/gm), 0.25 gm; Alpha tocopherol, 5.0 gm; Ascorbic acid, 45.0 gm; Inositol, 5.0 gm; Menadione, 2.25 gm; P aminobenzoic acid, 5.0 gm; Niacin, 4.5 gm; Riboflavin, 1.0 gm; Pyridoxine (hydrochloride), 1.0 gm; thiamine (hydrochloride), 1.0 gm; calcium panthothenate, 3.0 gm; Biotin, 0.02 gm; and Folic acid, 0.09 gm.

H. In Vitro Artificial Thrombi

1. Preliminary Comments

Coagulation of blood within a rotating circular length of polyethylene was introduced by Chandler (1958) to produce thrombi in vitro. Poole (1959, 1960) modified the technique slightly for the study of artificial thrombi from various animal species. Conner and Poole (1961) utilized this method to study the effects of fatty acids on the formation of thrombi in vitro. Although these methods may be useful to develop ideas for the study of thrombosis in vivo it must be remembered that data obtained concerning artificial thrombi produced in vitro refer only to artificial thrombi produced in vitro. Applications and criticisms of Chandler's method follow the detailed description.

2. Artificial Thrombosis in the Thrombogenerator (Chandler, 1958)

a. Method. One ml of blood is drawn directly into a polyvinyl tube[4] through an attached 18 gage needle. The tube is 25 cm in length and 0.375 cm in diameter. One ml of blood fills 9.9 cm of tubing. The two ends of the tube are then approximated and joined by an outside plastic collar. The circular tube is placed and centered on a turntable, tilted to an angle of 23 degrees. In vitro thrombi occur in 10 to 23 minutes for normal blood when the turntable is rotated at 17 rpm at room temperature (24 to 26° C). The calculated linear velocity is approximately 425 cm/minute. The endpoint is considered to be when the thrombus occludes the lumen of the tube and the column of blood rotates simultaneously with the tubing.

b. Precautions and Modifications. This method of in vitro artificial thrombus formation

[4] Chandler (1958) recommends tubing from a standard nonpyrogenic sterile blood donor set, List No. 563, supplied by Mead Johnson and Co., Evansville. Ind.

may be a useful tool for diagnosing impending thrombotic conditions similar to whole blood clotting times. Certain modifications to separate mechanisms such as platelet aggregation or blood clotting may be helpful. Responses of blood cells or blood proteins in the tubing should not be considered identical to events occurring in vivo. Variability of end points remains a deterrent for establishing the method for diagnostic use. Nevertheless, modifications of the method should be tested.

Chandler (1958) indicated the appearance of artificial in vitro thrombi were similar to thrombi formed in vivo when velocity in the tubing was calculated to be 425 cm/minute or about 7.1 cm/second. Variations in tube size, turntable angle, and flow velocities from 340 to 1200 cm/minute were tested by Chandler with the conclusion that flow velocity was an important factor in the production of typical thrombi. Blood flow velocity of 7.1 cm/second is found in a very limited segment of the circulation in vivo. In the aorta, flow velocity ranges from 33 cm/second in a basal state to about 231 cm/second during exercise and is pulsatile. Velocities range from 8 cm/second to 50 cm/second in the great veins and is said to be near 0.5 cm/second in capillaries. Furthermore, forces creating flow in vivo are applied to the blood resulting in velocities decreasing in magnitude from the center of the axial stream to the vessel wall. In Chandler's thrombogenerator force is imparted to the tubing containing the blood with decreasing velocities from the tubing toward the axial stream where the slowest velocity should be occurring. Cellular laminations are dragging one over the other as apposed to being pushed one over the other in the living animal. Certainly this reversal in pattern of flow needs further evaluation. Centrifugal forces are also occurring in the thrombogenerator.

Cellular and protein constituents of artificial in vitro thrombi are limited to the numbers of these elements in the blood sample collected. In vivo accumulations are not so limited since blood flow can continue to bring these elements to the site of thrombus formation and a more selective cellular or protein composition can result. Thrombolytic as well as thrombogenic mechanisms are operating in vivo simultaneously from the time of thrombus inducement. Events often referred to as "thrombus organization" have their beginnings early in thrombogenesis and continue until the thrombus is resolved by dissolution or by collagen formation, recanalization, and free surface endothelialization. Many of these mechanisms are virtually eliminated by the development of artificial thrombi in the thrombogenerator.

References

Ambrus, J. L., Back, N., Mihayli, E., and Ambrus, C. M. (1956). *Circulation Res. 4,* 430.

Ambrus, J. L., Ambrus, C. M., Back, W., Sokal, J. E., and Collins, C. L. (1957). *Ann. N. Y. Acad. Sci. 68,* 97.

Ashwin, J. G., and Jaques, L. B. (1961). *Thromb. Diath. Haemorrhag. 5,* 543.

Back, N., Ambrus, J. L., Simpson, C. L., and Shulman, S. (1958). *J. Clin. Invest. 37,* 864.

Barnard, P. J. (1953). *J. Pathol. Bacteriol. 65,* 129.

Bergentz, S. E., Gelin, L. E., and Rudenstam, C. M. (1961). *Thromb. Diath. Haemorrhag. 5,* 474.

Berman, H. J., Lutz, B. R., and Fulton, G. P. (1954). *Federation Proc. 13,* 12.

Berman, H. J., Fulton, G. P., Lutz, B. R., and Pierce, D. L. (1955). *Blood 10,* 831.

Berman, J. K., Fields, D. C., Judy, H., Mori, V., and Parker, R. J. (1956). *Surgery 39,* 399.

Bingham, J. B., Meyer, O. O., and Pohle, F. J. (1941). *Am. J. Med. Sci. 202,* 563.

Bizzozero, J. (1882). *Arch. Pathol. Anat. 90,* 261.

Blake, O. R., Ashwin, J. G., and Jaques, L. B. (1959). *J. Clin. Pathol. 12,* 118.

Borgström, S., and Gelin, L. E. (1957). *Nord. Med. 57,* 896.

Boyles, P. W. (1958). *Am. J. Clin. Pathol. 30,* 423.

Bradham, R. R., and Lee, W. H., Jr. (1961). *Surg. Gynecol. Obstet. 112,* 295.

Callahan, A. B., Lutz, B. R., Fulton, G. P., and Degelman, J. (1960). *Angiology 2,* 35.

Carey, L. C., and Williams, R. D. (1960). *Ann. Surg. 152,* 919.

Chandler, A. B. (1958). *Lab. Invest. 7,* 110.

Cliffton, E. E., Grossi, C. E., and Cannamela, D. (1954). *Ann. Surg. 139,* 52.

Conner, W. E., and Poole, J. C. (1961). *Quart. J. Exptl. Physiol. 46,* 1.

Copley, A. L., and Stefko, P. L. (1947). *Surg. Gynecol. Obstet. 84,* 451.

Dale, D. U., and Jaques, L. B. (1942). *Can. Med. Assoc. J. 46,* 546.

Davidson, E., Howard, A. N., and Gresham, G. A. (1961). *Brit. J. Exptl. Pathol. 42,* 195.

Deaton, H. L., and Anlyan, W. G. (1960). *Surg. Gynecol. Obstet. 111,* 131.

Dietrich, A. (1941). *Arch. Pathol. Anat. 307,* 281.

Duffy, P. E., and Furth, F. W. (1959). *Clin. Res. 7,* 21.

Dunn, J. S. (1920). *Quart. J. Med. 13,* 129.

Eagle, H., and Harris, T. N. (1937). *J. Gen. Physiol. 20,* 543.

Eberth, J. C., and Schimmelbusch, C. (1888). "Die Thrombose nach Versuchen und Leichenbefunden". Ferdinand Enke, Stuttgart.

Eisner, G. M., Berrian, J. H., Carter, E. L. Huggins, C. E., and Sewell, W. H. (1957). *Am. J. Physiol. 189,* 587.

Ellis, F. H., Grindlay, J. H., and Edwards, J. E. (1953). *J. Thoracic Surg. 25,* 358.

Feissly, R. (1925). *Soc. Biol. 92,* 319.

Flexner, S. (1902). *J. Med. Res. 8,* 316.

Friedman, M., Byers, S. O., and Pearl, F. (1960). *Am. J. Physiol. 199,* 770.

Friedman, M., and Byers, S. O. (1961). *Proc. Soc. Exptl. Biol. Med. 106,* 796.

Freiman, A. H., Bang, N. U., and Cliffton, E. E. (1960). *Circulation Res. 8,* 409.

Gage, A. A., Olson, K. C., and Chardack, W. M. (1956). *Ann. Surg. 143,* 535.

Grossi, C. E., Cliffton, E. E., and Cannamela, D. A. (1954). *Blood 9,* 310.

Henry, R. L. (1962). *Angiology 13,* 554.

Hirsch, E., and Loewe, L. (1946). *Proc. Soc. Exptl. Biol. Med. 63,* 569.

Holden, W. D., Cameron, D. B., Shea, P. C., Jr., and Shaw, B. W. (1949). *Surg. Gynecol. Obstet. 88,* 635.

Innerfield, I., Schwarz, A., and Angrist, A. (1952). *J. Clin. Invest. 31,* 1049.

Jaques, L. B., and Ashwin, J. (1964). *In* "Blood Coagulation, Hemorrhage and Thrombosis" (L. M. Tocantins and L. A. Kazal, eds.), pp. 436—437. Grune and Stratton, New York.

Jacques, W. E., and Hyman, A. L. (1957). *A. M. A. Arch. Pathol. 64,* 487.

Jansen, K. F., and Tage-Hansen, E. (1949). *Acta Chir. Scand. 98,* 152.

Jewell, P., Pilkington, T., and Robinson, B. (1954). *Brit. Med. J. 1,* 1013.

Johnson, A. J., and McCarty, W. R. (1959). *J. Clin. Invest. 38,* 1627.

Johnson, A. J., and Tillet, W. E. (1952). *J. Exptl. Med. 95,* 449.

Jones, W. T. (1851). *Guy's Hosp. Rep. 7,* 1.

Kamiya, K., and Fukuta, K. (1960). *Angiology 12,* 105.

Kiesewetter, W. B., and Shumaker, H. B., Jr. (1948). *Surg. Gynecol. Obstet. 86,* 687.

Knisely, M. H., Warner, L., and Harding, F. (1960). *Angiology 11,* 535.

Kojima, S. (1933). *Arch. Klin. Chir. 174,* 216.

Kristenson, A. (1921). *Acta Med. Scand. 70,* 167.

Kudrjashov, B. A., Bazasian, G. G., Sytina, N. P., and Andreenko, G. V. (1961). *Nature 189,* 67.

Lee, W. H., Jr., Bradham, R. R., Threatt, B., and Davenport, C. (1961). *Surgery 50,* 812.

Litvak, J., and Vineberg, A. (1959). *Surgery 46,* 953.

Loeb, L., and Meyers, M. K. (1910). *Arch. Pathol. Anat. 201,* 78.

Loeb, L., Strickler, A., and Tuttle, L. (1910). *Arch. Pathol. Anat. 201,* 5.

Loewe, L., Hirsch, E., and Grayzel, D. M. (1947). *Surgery 22,* 746.

Loewe, L., Hirsch, E., Grayzel, D. M., and Kashdan, F. (1948). *J. Lab. Clin. Med. 33,* 721

Lutz, B. R., Fulton, G. P., and Akers, R. P. (1951). *Circulation 3,* 339.

Mann, F. C., Herrick, J. F., Essex, H. E., and Baldes, E. J. (1938). *Surgery 4,* 249.

Marin, H. M., Stefanini, M., Soardi, F., and Mueller, L. (1961). *J. Lab. Clin. Med. 58,* 47.

McLetchie, N. G. B. (1952). *Am. J. Pathol. 28,* 413.

Mehrotra, R. M. L. (1953). *J. Pathol. Bacteriol. 65,* 307.

Mihalyi, E., and Laki, K. (1952). *Arch. Biochem. Biophys. 38,* 97.

Moses, C. (1945). *Proc. Soc. Exptl. Biol. Med. 59,* 25.

Murray, G. W. D., Jaques, L. B., Perrett, T. S., and Best, C. H. (1937). *Surgery 2,* 163.

Mustard, J. F., Murphy, E. A., Rowsell, H. C., and Downie, H. G. (1964). *J. Atheroscler. Res. 4,* 1.

Nahum, L. H., Kline, D., and Fishbein, R. (1960). *Connecticut Med. 24,* 139.

Nelson, K. O. (1952). *S. Forum (1951),* pp. 316—322.

O'Neill, J. F. (1947). *Ann. Surg. 126,* 270.

Osborne, T. B., and Mendal, L. B. (1932). *Science 75,* 339.

Pearse, H. E. (1940). *Ann. Surg. 112,* 923.

Pfitzer, R. (1879). *Arch. Pathol. Anat. 77,* 397.

Poole, J. C. (1959). *Quart. J. Exptl. Physiol. 44,* 372.

Poole, J. C. (1960). *Proc. Roy. Soc. Med. 53,* 22.

Potts, W. J., and Smith, S. (1943). *Arch. Surg. 46,* 27.

Pryce, D. M., Pike, C., and Gorrill, R. H. (1950). *J. Pathol. Bacteriol. 62,* 452.

Rabinovitch, J. (1929). *Arch. Pathol. 7,* 615.

Rabinovitch, J., and Pines, B. (1943). *Surgery 14,* 669.

Rabinovitch, J., and Pines, B. (1949). *Arch. Surg. 58,* 163.

Reimann-Hunziker, G. (1944). *Schweiz. Med. Wochschr. 74,* 66.

Richards, R. K., and Cortell, R. (1942). *Proc. Soc. Exptl. Biol. Med. 50,* 237.

Robertson, H. R., Perett, T. S., Colbeck, J. C., and Moyes, P. D. (1954). *Surg. Gynecol. Obstet. 98,* 705.

Rosenberg, N., Moolten, S. E., and Vroman, L. (1959). *Surgery 46,* 764.

Samuel, S. (1867). *Arch. Pathol. Anat. 40,* 213.

Samuels, P. B., and Webster, D. R. (1952). *Ann. Surg. 136,* 422.

Sawyer, P. N., and Pate, J. W. (1953). *Am. J. Physiol. 175,* 103.

Sawyer, P. N., Suckling, E. E., and Wesolowski, S. A. (1960). *Am. J. Physiol. 198,* 1006.

Schwartz, S. I. (1959). *Surg. Gynecol. Obstet. 108,* 533.

Senftleben. (1879). *Arch. Pathol. Anat. 77,* 421.

Sherry, S., Titchener, A., Gottesman, L., Wasserman, P., and Troll, W. (1954). *J. Clin. Invest. 33,* 1303.

Smith, S. (1945). *Surgery 18,* 627.

Solandt, D. Y., and Best, C. H. (1938). *Lancet 2,* 130.

Solandt, D. Y., Nassim, R., and Best, C. H. (1939). *Lancet 2,* 592.

Stehbens, W. E., and Florey, H. W. (1960). *Quart. J. Exptl. Physiol. 45,* 252.

Stone, P., and Lord, W. J., Jr. (1951). *Surgery 30,* 987.

Strutz, W. A., Couves, C. M., Bondar, G. F., and MacKenzie, W. C. (1960). *S. Forum 10,* 428.

Thomas, W. A., and Hartroft, W. S. (1959). *Circulation 19,* 65.

Thomas, W. A., Hartroft, S., and O'Neal, R. M. (1960). *A. M. A. Arch. Pathol. 69,* 104.

Warner, E. D., Brinkhous, K. M., Seegers, W. H., and Smith, H. P. (1939). *Proc. Soc. Exptl. Biol. Med. 41,* 655.

Wartman, W. B., Hudson, B., and Jennings, R. B. (1951). *Circulation 4,* 756.

Welch, W. H. (1887). *Trans. Path. Soc. Phila. 13,* 281.

Wessler, S. (1952). *J. Clin. Invest. 31,* 1011.

Wessler, S. (1953). *J. Clin. Invest. 32,* 610.

Wessler, S. (1953). *Federation Proc. 12,* 152.

Williams, R. D., and Carey, L. C. (1959). *Ann. Surg. 149,* 381.

Williams, R. D., and Elliot, D. W. (1958). *S. Forum 9,* 138.

Wilson, J. S. (1960). *Surgery 48,* 469.

Wright, H. P., Kubik, M. M., and Hayden, M. (1952). *Brit. J. Surg. 40,* 163.

Yatsushiro, T. (1913). *Deutsche Ztschr. Chir. 125,* 559.

Zahn, F. W. (1875). *Arch. Pathol. Anat. 62,* 81.

Zahn, F. W. (1884). *Arch. Pathol. Anat. 96,* 1.

Zielonko, J. (1873). *Arch. Pathol. Anat. 57,* 436.

Zurhelle, E. (1910). *Z. Pathol. Anat. Allg. Path. 47,* 539.

Zweifach, B. W. (1961). *Federation Proc. 20, Suppl. 8,* 18.

Experimental Animal Models for the Production of Disseminated Intravascular Coagulation

Fritz K. Beller

I. Introduction

The potential role of disseminated intravascular coagulation (DIC) in a number of clinical disease states has recently received recognition. McKay and Müller-Berghaus (1967) summarized the major categories of etiologic factors causing intravascular coagulation: 1) intravascular hemolysis, 2) release of tissue thromboplastin, 3) bacterial endotoxins, 4) proteolytic enzymes, 5) particulate or colloidal matter, 6) anoxia, 7) endothelial damage, and 8) ingestion of certain lipid substance.

The lack of a commonly accepted terminology has led to the description of this phenomenon in terms of morphological characterization or pathophysiological mechanism. Consumption coagulopathy, disseminated intravascular coagulation (DIC), defibrination syndrome, Sanarelli Shwartzman phenomenon (SSP), Generalized Shwartzman Reaction (GSR), Shwartzman equivalents and Thrombohemorrhagic Phenomena are only a few of many designations employed.

II. Pathophysiology

A. Definition

DIC may be defined as a syndrome resulting from an activation of the coagulation system in vivo. It can be present in acute, subacute, or chronic forms. The syndrome encompasses mild forms with slight activation of the clotting system and no demonstrable morphologic findings, or more severe forms with massive formation of fibrin deposits or microthrombi in multiple organ systems throughout the organism.

Present evidence indicates that the activation of the coagulation system is the primary event in DIC and that fibrinolysis, if it occurs, is a secondary protective phenomenon.

B. Development of DIC

The coagulation system can be activated in vivo by a variety of non specific mechanisms of which the most extensively studied is bacterial endotoxins. Lee (1963) has shown that the formation of antigen-antibody complexes can activate coagulation. In addition, release of thromboplastin or thrombin into the circulation is considered an important mechanism in many disease states. Certain drugs alone or in combination may also produce DIC.

When blood or plasma clots in a test tube, the "plasma" coagulation factors (prothrombin, fibrinogen, factors V and VIII) are consumed, and are therefore absent in serum. Also platelets are consumed. The activation of the coagulation system in vivo follows the same pattern and the phenomenon has therefore been termed "consumption coagulopathy" (Lasch et al. 1961a). This designation is preferable to "defibrination" (Schneider, 1951), since fibrinogen is only *one* of several factors involved in this process.

"Serum" factors (VII, IX and X) are usually found in a normal range. It is not understood why in some patients with DIC, low levels of factors VII and X have been observed (McKehee et al. 1967; Blombäck et al. 1968c; Beller et al. 1968c).

Thrombin will enzymatically attack and cleave specific peptide bonds to yield fibrin monomer and fibrinopeptides A and B. The resulting fibrin monomers are considered by many authors (Jaeger 1962; Kalbfleisch and Bird, 1960; Shainoff and Page, 1960; Smith, 1957) to be identical with cryofibrinogen or "heparin precipitable fibrinogen" (Thomas et al. 1954). Cryofibrinogen has been found in a number of disease states, but its real significance is not understood.

The further development of DIC depends on the release, potency and quantity of the clot promoting agents, balanced by the protective mechanisms of inhibition and inactivation.

1. Trigger system

The investigation of the trigger system is difficult since authors have applied different criteria to establish the presence of DIC. In most instances morphologic criteria, such as renal glomerular fibrin deposition have been used. This, however, may be inadequate since Gerber (1936) has shown that one injection of a sublethal dose of endotoxin injected into rabbits produces thrombi in multiple organ systems without necessarily involving the kidney. Later, McKay et al. (1966) and DePalma et al. (1967) demonstrated the presence of platelet and fibrin thrombi in the capillary bed of the lungs following endotoxin infusion, employing electronmicroscopy. Furthermore, endotoxin injection can result in a decrease of prothrombin, fibrinogen, factor V, factor VIII and platelets (Kliman and McKay, 1958; Kleinmeier et al. 1959) without development of glomerular fibrin depositions. Any decrease of plasma coagulation factors by consumption is therefore considered by many investigators to be indicative of the presence of DIC, provided that a major fibrinolytic component can be ruled out. Three theories are discussed at present: a) Platelet aggregation with damage of the platelet membrane and release of platelet factor 3. b) Surface activation of factor XII or interaction between factor XI and XII. c) Damage to endothelial surfaces with subsequent release of tissue thromboplastin.

The concept of platelet aggregation as a trigger is based on the observation that endotoxin induces aggregation of platelets in vitro (DePrez et al. 1961). Endotoxin as well as antigen-antibody complexes accelerate coagulation in platelet rich but not in platelet poor plasma (McKay et al. 1958; Robbins and Stetson, 1959) and endotoxin causes release of platelet factor III (Horowitz et al. 1962).

However, other experimental results seem not to support this concept. Evenson and Jerimic (1968) were able to produce glomerular fibrin deposition by injecting Liquoid in rabbits which were made thrombocytopenic by Busulphan (Myleran). This sulfonic acid ester acts as an alkylating agent producing an isolated drop in platelets through bone marrow suppression without interfering with other coagulation constituents (Evensen et al. 1968). Similar results have been obtained with rabbits in whom thrombocytopenia was first induced by injecting an antiplatelet serum. A drop in platelets per se does not necessarily indicate DIC, since an infusion of a detoxified endotoxin in small doses resulted in a decrease in platelet count without a significant change in coagulation factors and without demonstrable glomerular fibrin depositions (Beller et al. 1969). Rodriguez-Erdman (1965) injected phospholipids (platelet factor III) into rabbits and induced functional and morphological changes typical for DIC and thereby reemphasizing the central role of platelets as a trigger mechanism. These results could not be confirmed by Müller-Berghaus et al. (1967) but were recently reproduced by Rodriguez-Erdmann and Mammen (personal communication). b) The surface activation concept was evaluated by McKay and Müller-Berghaus (1968), using an in vivo model in which glomerular fibrin deposition served as the "indicator". The combination of the following substances were necessary to induce glomerular fibrin deposition: 1) norepinephrine (stimulation of adrenergic receptor sites), 2) EACA (inhibition of fibrinolysis), 3) inosithin (platelet factor III substitute and 4) ellagic acid (surface activation). When either EACA or ellagic acid were excluded, the kidney lesion failed to appear. They concluded that surface activation is an essential component of the development of GSR. Activated factor XII infused into dogs and rats, on the other hand, did not produce intravascular coagulation (Mammen, personal communication). c) Endothelial damage with release of tissue thromboplastin were considered as trigger systems by Lasch et al. (1967). A decrease of "vasculokinase" was found in rabbit aortas after injection of endotoxin (Müller-Berghaus and Lasch, 1963). However, it is not known at present whether the structural endothelial damage developing after endotoxin injection is a primary or secondary phenomenon.

2. Defense Mechanism

Four inhibitors pathways have been demonstrated: a) the interaction with plasma proteins, which act as inhibitors, e. g. the antithrombin reactions; b) clearance function of the reticuloendothelial system (RES), c) the phagocytic capacity of formed elements of the blood and d) the fibrinolytic mechanism.

As indicated in Chapter VII, p. 268, thrombin is inactivated by antithrombin II and III. The significance of the antithrombin action as a defense mechanism was considered extensively by Quick (1957). The observation of a decrease in antithrombin III activity during DIC was reported by Lasch et al. (1961b) and by von Kaulla and von Kaulla (1968).

Spaet et al. (1961) and Spaet (1962) have shown that activation product I (presumably factor X) infused in rats is cleared by the RES.

Gans et al. (1968) studied the turnover of radioactive thrombin and found that the rapid breakdown of thrombin does not seem to be antithrombin induced. Their data indicate that the injected thrombin was cleared by the Kupffer cells of the liver. When dogs were hepatectomized, these animals were not well protected against tissue thromboplastin or endotoxin. Even better studied is the reticuloendothelial clearance of fibrin monomers or polymers from the circulation. Spaet et al. (1961) and Lee (1962) observed a complete defibrination when activation products or thrombin were infused into the aorta instead of the venous system; in contrast, fibrinogen decreased only slightly following intravenous administration. Studer and Lorenz (1965) observed fibrin deposition lining the aorta when thrombin was infused intraarterially but not when intravenously administered. Similarly, Vasalli et al. (1963) observed that glomerular fibrin deposition did not develop when thrombin was infused intravenously, but did appear when thrombin was intraaortically infused. This may not necessarily be related to RES clearance. Lee and McCluskey (1962) presented immunochemical evidence for removal of fibrin particles by the liver, and Prose et al. (1965) identified fibrin in the liver by electronmicroscopy.

According to Boler and Bibighaus (1967), material with a periodicity of 175 Å to 215 Å appears in the liver as early as 15 minutes after endotoxin injection. The clearance function of the RES was also shown by perfusion experiments in the isolated liver (Gans and Lowman, 1967). Less clear is the phagocytic function of the formed blood elements. Barnhart (1964) has demonstrated a neutrophilic response after thrombin infusion. These neutrophils were able to phagocitize fibrin related material. Immature neutrophils were released from the bone marrow. Further evidence was presented by Riddle and Barnhart (1964) who found altered fibrin in ultrastructural studies of neutrophils at sites of experimental inflamation in dogs.

III. Experimental Approach to DIC

A. History and Definition

Manasse (1892) observed hyalin material and thrombi appearing in various organ systems when two injections of heat killed typhoid bacilli were injected at 24 hour intervals. A similar observation was made by Kusama (1913) who found "fibrin knots" after a spaced injection of heat destroyed bacilli. In these experiments the kidneys were not examined. Sanarelli, in 1894, observed that after two injections of typhoid toxin spaced 24 hours apart, a generalized purpura preceeded the demise of the monkeys, and this phenomenon was subsequently referred to as "epithalaxis" (Sanarelli, 1935).

According to Zdrodowsky and Brenn (1926), two injections of endotoxin, 24 hours apart, resulted in fibrin depositions in various organ systems. These authors presented the first exact pathological description, and indicated that a variety of endotoxins could produce the same results. They attributed the discovery of this phenomenon to Sanarelli (Sanarelli Phenomenon).

Shwartzman (1927, 1928) discovered what is now called the Localized Shwartzman Reaction (LSR) (see below). It is now recognized that the generalized and localized Shwartzman Reactions are two different phenomena, although the older literature does not take this into account. Only the two injections of endotoxin, spaced 24 hours apart, are identical for both.

More controversial than the historical aspect is the definition of the phenomenon. Apitz (1935) was the first to attempt to define what he termed the Generalized Shwartzman Reaction (GSR). The criteria he employed were hemorrhagic diathesis with renal cortical necrosis after two injections of endotoxin within 24 hours. They resulted in shock and death within 48 hours after the second injection. Many authors have used only the renal lesions as a criteria for DIC.

This has led to confusion since the use of terms, such as the Shwartzman equivalents or others, for pathological findings in human disease do not include the entire spectrum of changes in this phenomenon. Lesions identical to those observed in the generalized form, especially fibrin deposition in the kidney, could be produced without endotoxin and without any time lag. It was, however, the observation of the necessary time lag which resulted in the feud between Sanarelli and Shwartzman over who should be credited for describing this phenomenon. Lindberg and Riggins (1963) found that in nephrectomized animals fibrin depositions developed in other organs, such as spleen and lungs. Therefore, it seems better to use the term "disseminated intravascular coagulation "for this phenomenon, and reserve the other eponyms for experimental models as suggested by Selye (1966).

B. Experimental Models

The half-life of endotoxin after its injection is not known. A single small intravenous injection of any type of endotoxin, as shown by ^{51}Cr labelled endotoxin, disappears from the circulation within minutes. It is removed by the RES (Herring et al. 1963; Wiznitzer et al. 1960) and by phagocytosis by platelets (Braude et al. 1955). Utilizing a rabbit bioassay for endotoxin (see later), it would appear that endotoxin injected into a dog remains active for as long as 360 minutes (Spink and Starzecki, 1968). The survival time of endotoxin in the circulation, therefore, requires further study.

1. Lethal dose of endotoxin

The intravenous injection of 200 μ mg or more of a commercial endotoxin into a rabbit results in shock and death within 4–24 hours. Autopsy usually reveals little information as to the cause of irreversible shock and death under these circumstances. Fibrin thrombi can be demonstrated in lungs or spleen (Gerber, 1936) but there is no regular pattern for the formation of thrombosis, and the morphological findings are not dose related. Glomerular fibrin deposition in the kidneys occurs in less than 10% of the animals (Thomas and Good, 1952b). Heparinization offers no protection in rabbits but may do so in rats (Margaretten et al. 1967a). The lethal effect of a single injection of endotoxin can be potentiated in the rabbit by the injection of heterologous plasma (Beller et al. 1963).

2. The generalized form (Sanarelli-Shwartzman phenomenon)

Two intravenous injections of a sublethal dose of endotoxin into a rabbit, spaced 24 hours apart, result in a generalized pattern of fibrin deposition in the lungs, liver, spleen and other organs, and particularly in the glomerular capillaries of the kidneys, as first noted by Apitz (1935).

Pappas et al. (1958) used an injection schedule to produce the GSR with one part of endotoxin for the first injection and 2.5 parts for the second; Friscay et al. (1957) used 1 part to 3.5 parts.

Krecke (1964) noted that 0.05 μg/kg is sufficient for the initial dose, if the challenging dose is increased to 500–2000 μg/kg.

The kidneys are markedly swollen and multiple small infarcted and hemorrhagic areas are seen on the surface. Histologically, tubular necrosis is found and glomerular capillaries are plugged with fibrin. The obstruction of the circulation leads to ischemic necrosis and subsequently to bilateral focal or total renal cortical necrosis.

Lee and Stetson (1965) stressed the point that this type of thrombic occlusion should not be confused with bilateral ischemic necrosis due to a primary ischemia resulting from vasoconstricting drugs like epinephrine (Penner and Bernheim, 1940; Whitacker and McKay, 1962), pitressin (Byron, 1937), serotonin (Page and Glendening, 1955) and staphylococcal toxin (Thal and Enger, 1961).

It is now recognized that glomerular fibrin deposition is the result of intravascular activation of the coagulation system. The role of blood coagulation in this phenomenon became evident when it was noted by Thomas and Good (1952b) that the deposition of "fibrinoid" material could be prevented by heparin. By electronmicroscopy, Bohle et al. (1958) observed the characteristic periodicity of fibrin in the kidneys. This observation was confirmed by McKay et al. (1959) employing immunofluorescent staining.

After the first injection platelets drop (Horowitz et al. 1962) and decrease even further after the second challenging dose (McKay and Shapiro, 1958). The fibrinogen levels decrease after the first injection, but subsequently return to hypernormal values in a few hours. The second injection usually produces a significant decline in fibrinogen levels amounting to 80–100 mg% on the average (McKay and Shapiro, 1958). The possible reasons why the second injection of endotoxin results in a greater reduction of fibrinogen levels were recently enumerated by Lerner et al. (1968). The reduction of factors V and VIII is of a similar order of magnitude as the fibrinogen reduction.

The injection of endotoxin is associated with the release of a variety of other substances such as plasma kinins, serotonin from platelets (Shimamoto et al. 1958; Davis et al. 1961) histamine and catecholamines. However, the precise role of any of these substances is yet to be defined (Back, 1966). Erdoes and Miwa (1968) propose that factor XII in the very early minutes after endotoxin injection activates the kallekrein system, but formed kinin does not contribute much to the initial phase of circulatory shock in rabbits. Jacobsen et al. (1964) expressed doubt that the initial hypotension after endotoxin injection is due to epinephrine and serotonin release. However, Nies et al. (1968) relate the initial vascular effects as found in primates to the kinin system.

All of the characteristics of the Sanarelli-Shwartzman Phenomenon, especially the kidney lesions, can be produced in the rabbit by a *single continous* infusion of endotoxin in a quantity of 20—60 μg/kg/hour for a period of 6–10 hours (Beller and Graeff, 1967). These experiments suggest that in humans disseminated intravascular coagulation may occur as the end result of a continues release of endotoxin. Platelets drop continuously in a linear fashion, while fibrinogen and coagulation factors V and VIII subsequently decrease (Graeff and Beller, 1968). Plasminogen also decreases but plasmin inhibitors remain unchanged. This seems to indicate that the fibrinolytic enzyme system in the circulation is not activated. Glomerular fibrin deposition and focal renal cortical necrosis were already observed within six hours after the initiation of endotoxin infusion; thus much earlier than they were observed in the original GSR experiments (Krecke, 1964). The infusion experiments also demonstrated that local lysis of deposited fibrin is of significance and may be one defense mechanism for the protection against renal cortical necrosis.

Glomerular fibrin deposition can be produced with one injection of endotoxin in pregnant rabbits (Apitz, 1935; Rodriguez-Erdman, 1964) and in pregnant rats (Kaley et al. 1962; Wong, 1962). This reaction occurs at term or in the third trimester of pregnancy. The mechanism by which pregnancy prepares the organism for endotoxin is obscure. McKay and Müller-Berghaus (1967) have theorized that a reduction in activity of the fibrinolytic enzyme system during pregnancy might be of significance. In accordance with this concept is the findings of Epstein et al. (1968) who observed a decrease in kidney tissue activator of plasminogen in pregnant guinea pigs and rats.

3. Similar models

Many different experimental models exist for the production of the DIC. All of these models aim at the production of the kidney lesions and some of these are listed in Table 1.

Table 1. Some Methods for the Production of Glomerular Fibrin Deposition

Sensitizing Injection	Route	Challenging Injection	Route	Animal	Author	Remark
Endotoxin	i.v.	Endotoxin	i.v.	rabbit	Kusama, 1913 Sanarelli, 1925 Zdrodowski and Brenn, 1926	24 hrs. apart
Pregnancy	–	Endotoxin	i.v.	rabbit	Apitz, 1935	
Cortisone	i.v.	Endotoxin	i.v.	rabbit	Thomas and Good, 1952b	
Thorotrast or Trypan blue	i.v.	Endotoxin	i.v.	rabbit	Good and Thomas, 1952	3–12 hrs. apart
Carbon particles	i.v.	Endotoxin	i.v.	abbit	Smith et al. 1953	
Endotoxin	i.v.	certain polymers	i.v.	rabbit	Thomas et al. 1955 Brunson et al. 1955	
Endotoxin	i.v.	fat	i.v.	rabbit	Huth et al. 1967	
Liquoid Roche	i.v.	–	–	rabbit	Thomas et al. 1955	2–4 hrs. apart
Fat	i.v.	Endotoxin	i.v.	rabbit	Huth et al. 1967	
Endotoxin	i.v.	EACA	i.v.	rabbit	Lee, 1963	
Thrombin	infus.	EACA	infus.	rabbit	Lee, 1963	
Thrombin	infus.	EACA	infus.	rat	Margaretten et al. 1964	no interval
Thrombin	infus.	Protease inhibitors	infus.	rabbit	Beller et al. 1967	no interval
Thrombin	infus.	intraaortic	–	rabbit	Collins et al. 1968	
Plasma from RES depressed mice into normal mice					Blickens and Diluzio, 1965	
Colchicin	intraper.	Pregnancy	–	hamster	Galton, 1964	
Vit. E deficiency and fat rich diet			–	guinea pig	Kaunitz et al. 1962, 1963	
Endotoxin infusion for 6–14 hours				rabbit	Beller and Graeff, 1967, 1969	
Cortison or iron oxyd-saccharat	i.v.	Lysates of β hemolytic A-streptococci	–	–	Stetson, 1956	
Cholera vibriones	i.v.	staphylo-cocci	–	–	Zdrodowski, 1928	
A streptococci	i.v.	streptolysin O containing A Streptococci filtrates	i.v.		Schwab et al. 1953	short interval
A streptococci	i.v.	meningococci toxin	i.v.	rabbit	Thomas et al. 1952–1953	interval 48 hrs.

As a possible explanation for the development of the kidney lesion, Lee (1963) proposed that fibrin and partially polymerized fibrin are removed from the systemic circulation by the RES; the RES becoming subsequently saturated when a second episode of intravascular coagulation and fibrin formation is triggered by a provocative injection. Substances used to decrease RES function, for example, Thorotrast and fat have been shown to trigger the coagulation system as well (Hjort et al. 1966; Kommerell et al. 1966). Furthermore, Thorotrast produces a dose related adrenal hemorrhage (Mosley and Cluff,

1965). The fact that pregnancy can substitute for the priming endotoxin dose is not in agreement with this concept, since pregnancy does not depress the RES (Wexler and Kantor, 1966; Margaretten et al. 1967b). It is also not certain whether fibrin develops primarily in the glomerulus or is secondarily embolic in nature.

There is evidence that the development of glomerular fibrin deposition requires additional etiological factors of which one might be vasoconstriction and stasis. Trueta et al. (1947) discussed the possibility of cortico-medullary shunt mechanisms which could make the kidney vulnerable to the vasoactive effects of endotoxin (Hjort and Rapaport, 1965). Fine et al. (1959). Recently Müller-Berghaus et al. (1967) prevented the kidney lesion by injection of vasodilators, and Fine et al. (1959) and Palmiero et al. (1962) by denervation of the kidney. The reduced local fibrinolytic activity found in some animal species may be an additional factor for the development of GSR (Epstein et al. 1968).

In some species kidney glomerular fibrin deposition may be produced by intravenous injection of thrombin alone, or by infusion of thromboplastin (Vasalli et al. 1963). The lesion can be produced in the hamster with colchicine (Galton, 1964), but not with endotoxin, to which this animal is resistent. Polymyxin B prevents the GSR produced by endotoxin, when given either with the preparing or challenging dose, although the increase in cryofibrinogen after endotoxin is not prevented (Rifkind and Hill, 1967).

4. The role of leukocytes

Thomas and Good (1952b) observed a complete inhibition of the GSR in rabbits which were made leucopenic by treatment with nitrogen mustard. They also noted that when a portion of the bone marrow was protected during the injection, granulocytopenia was prevented and the GSR developed. Horn and Collins (1968) demonstrated that the GSR developed in rabbits following a granulocyte transfusion which effectively substituted for the preparatory endotoxin injection.

However, other reports have been conflicting. Wendt et al. (1967) did not find a threshold dose of granulocytes for the elucidation of the GSR. They stressed the importance of a time relationship based on the observation that rabbits were protected against the GSR only three days after the injection of nitrogen mustard but not on day four and five, at which time the leucocytes were still low.

Collins et al. (1968) could produce the GSR with an intraaortic infusion of thrombin in leucocytopenic rabbits, whereas McKay et al. (1967) were unable to produce the lesions with an infusion of watery leucocyte lysates in rats and rabbits, prepared by pregnancy, EACA, Thorotrast, cortisone and endotoxin. They concluded that leucocytes or their products do not contain a procoagulant active enough to provoke the GSR. Hjort et al. (1964) found little evidence for procoagulant material in granulocytes. However, they noted that rabbits were protected when prepared for the GSR with Thorotrast and with endotoxin as a trigger, but not with thrombin.

Thomas et al. (1954) speculated that leucocytes may provide a substance, a large acid polymer, which could form an insoluble complex with partially polymerized fibrinogen. The demonstration of sulfated mucopolysaccharides by histochemical staining in the azurophil granules (Horn and Spicer, 1964), as well as in deposited fibrin (Horn and Spicer, 1965) seem to support this concept.

5. Calciphylaxis

Selye (1962) noted in his work of calciphylaxis and calcergy that the combined injection (without a lag phase) of two simple, chemically well characterized compounds, as for example ferric chloride, lanthanum chloride or tannic acid, could produce both general and hemorrhagic thrombosis. The injections of these substances resulted in selective changes termed by Selye (1966) "The Thrombohemorrhagic Phenomenon" which were present in the kidneys, heart, blood vessels, duodenum, jejunum, spleen, salivary and lacrimary glands, adrenals, uterus and transplantable tumors. However, it is not certain whether these thrombo-hemorrhagic lesions resemble activation of the coagulation system.

6. The fibrinolytic enzyme system

The role of the fibrinolytic enzyme system in DIC is not clear. Endotoxin activates the coagulation system in the rabbit, but does not activate the fibrinolytic enzyme system in the systemic circulation (Beller et al. 1969). Fibrinolysis, however, of varying degree is frequently observed in human disease.

Glomerular fibrin deposition in some experimental conditions is not constant. The rat, infused with thrombin, does develop glomerular fibrin only for a short period (Margaretten et al. 1964). However, glomerular fibrin *persisted* in the rat under identical experimental conditions when EACA was administered. Lee (1963) observed in the rabbit, and Gans (1964) in the dog that fibrin could be produced by an infusion of thrombin and EACA, but not by thrombin alone. Lee (1963) concluded that this is due to a blockade of the RES by EACA. Beller et al. (1967) confirmed this data but demonstrated that the renal lesion was produced when thrombin was infused with a variety of protease inhibitors of different molecular structure. This does not support blockade of the RES as a likely mechanism. Glomerular fibrin deposition was related to the concentration and duration of the protease inhibitor present in the kidney, Beller and Graeff (1967) and Beller et al. (1969) demonstrated that massive glomerular fibrin resulting from endotoxin infusion underwent lysis without an apparent activation of the circulating enzyme systems. This was taken to indicate that local lysis of fibrin had occured.

Abnormal levels of fibrinolytic split products in sera from a majority of patients with DIC with little or no increase in systemic fibrinolysis was used as evidence that these split products probably result from the digestion of fibrin rather than fibrinogen (Merskey et al. 1968).

7. DIC in human disease

McKay (1964) described the presence of DIC in human disease as a disorder accompanied by shock and by alterations in certain blood coagulation factors, occasionally leading to massive hemorrhage with the presence of thrombi in the microscopic vessels of a variety of viscera. It is apparent from the definition on p. 514, that any of these findings alone would indicate the syndrome. The presence or absence of kidney lesions cannot be considered pathognonomic, and might resemble pathological lesions in man only under certain circumstances. Occasionally, the renal lesion can be produced with gram positive toxins (Nakai and Margaretten, 1963). The clinical considerations were recently reviewed by Hjort and Rapaport (1965), McKay (1964), Hardaway (1966), Merskey et al. (1967) and Beller (1968a, b) Mammen et al. (1969).

One extreme variant is the acute form, where platelets and plasma coagulation factors drop in a very short time. A more subacute form is associated with different types of cancer, whereby only slightly abnormal platelet counts and a more severe reduction of coagulation factors I, II, V and VIII were observed. The chronic form is another extreme on the scale with low platelets, normal coagulation factors, and the presence of a plasma cryofibrinogen. The entire spectrum of DIC with glomerular fibrin deposition can be encountered in some patients with endotoxin shock and also quite classically after renal homotransplantation (Starzl et al. 1968). It must be realized that DIC may be an intermittant phenomenon.

8. Summary

The effects of endotoxin on the blood and vascular system can be divided into effects on the peripheral vascular system and effects on the coagulation system and the formed elements of the blood. Still to be fully defined are:

1. The role of the reticulo-endothelial system.
2. The immune status of the host organism.
3. The role of the white blood cells, particularly the sulfated mucopolysaccharide variety.
4. The significance of the fibrinolytic enzyme system.
5. The trigger system and the inhibitory mechanisms.

Activation of the coagulation system can be produced by a wide variety of experimental models which are not all related to bacterial endotoxins. DIC can occur without glomerular fibrin deposition, the landmark of the GSR, and the present evidence suggests that the renal lesion need some specific mediatory mechanism which is not precisely determined.

IV. Localized Schwartzmann Phenomenon

Injection of one sublethal injection of endotoxin intracutaneously in the rabbit, followed by an intravenous injection, results in a hemorrhagic necrosis at the site of the intradermal injection. This was described by Shwartzman (1927, 1929) and Hanger (1927, 1928) independently in the same volume of the Proceedings of the Society for Experimental Biology and Medicine. For the preparing dose a range of 5–5000 μg was used. Higher doses can occasionally produce hemorrhagic necrosis without a challenging dose (Stetson, 1955). The challenging dose is given 6–48 hours later in a dose range of 100 μg (Lee and Stetson, 1965).

The hemorrhagic skin lesion can be produced by different substances other than endotoxin, as a preparing dose, for instance, endotoxin and BCG (Stetson, 1955). The localized reaction is considered the experimental model for the production of severe tissue damage by endotoxin (Lee and Stetson, 1965). Schmidt-Weyland (1932) produced what is now called the "catecholamine reaction" by injecting epinephrine in the skin of the rabbit ear and endotoxin intravenously. A lag time was not required to produce a hemorrhagic necrosis around the site of epinephrine skin injection. This phenomenon was used for a bioassay of endotoxemia (Douglas et al. 1963; Porter et al. 1964). The epinephrine dose should not exceed 100 μg since in a higher dose range a non-specific ischemic skin necrosis may occur.

The possible role of a diffuse intravascular coagulation in the production of the local reaction is not clear. Although the phenomenon is prevented by heparin (Good and Thomas, 1953), the main feature is the early presence of platelet and leucocyte aggregates in small blood vessels, creating a stasis in the local circulation (Stetson, 1957). Depletion of circulating leucocytes by prior total body irradiation or systematic treatment with benzene or nitrogen mustard prevents the appearance of gross and microscopic changes (Becker, 1948). Aggregation of leucocytes is considered necessary to prepare the skin. Since the experimental model is most likely not related to DIC, the interested reader is referred for further details to Lee and Stetson (1965) and Selye (1966).

References

Apitz, K. (1935). *J. Immunol. 29,* 255.

Back, N. (1966). *Federation Proc. 25,* 77.

Barnhart, M. I. (1964). *Thromb. Diath. Haemorrhag. Suppl. 13,* 157.

Becker, R. N. (1948). *Proc. Soc. Exptl. Biol. Med. 86,* 806.

Beller, F. K. (1968a). *Geburtshilfe & Frauenheilk. 28,* 113.

Beller, F. K. (1968b). *Thromb. Diath. Haemorrh. Suppl. 34,* 125.

Beller, F. K., and Graeff, H. (1967). *Nature 215,* 295.

Beller, F. K., Debrovner, C. H., and Douglas, G. W. (1963). *J. Exptl. Med. 118,* 245.

Beller, F. K., Mitchell, P., and Gorstein, F. (1967). *Thromb. Diath. Haemorrhag. 17,* 427.

Beller, F. K., Douglas, G. W., and Graeff, H. (1968a). *Geburtshilfe & Frauenheilk.* In press.

Beller, F. K., Douglas, G. W., Morris, R. H., and Johnson, A. J. (1968b). *Amer. J. Obstet. Gynecol. 101,* 587.

Beller, F. K., Maki, M., and Epstein, M. D. (1968c). *Amer. J. Obstet. Gynecol. 92,* 1121.

Beller, F. K., Graeff, H., and Gorstein, F. (1969). *Amer. J. Obstet. Gynecol. 103,* 544.

Blickens, D. A., and Di Luzio, N. R. (1965). *J. Reticuloendothel. Soc. 2,* 187.

Blombäck, M., Johansson, St. A., and Sjoeberg, H. E. (1967). *Acta Physiol. Scand. 69,* 313.

Bohle, A., Krecke, H. J., Miller, F., and Sitte, H. (1958). *1st Internat. Sympos. Immunopathology, p. 339,* Schwabe, Basel.

Boler, R. K., and Bibighaus, A. J. (1967). *Lab. Invest. 17,* 537.

Braude, A. I., Cavey, F. J., and Zalesky, M. (1955). *J. Clin. Invest. 34,* 858.

Brunson, J. G., Davis, R. L., and Thomas, L. (1955). *Amer. J. Pathol. 31,* 669.

Byron, F. B. (1937). *J. Pathol. Bacteriol. 45,* 1.

Collins, R. D., Robbins, B. H., and Mayes, Ch. E. (1968). *Johns Hopkins Med. J. 122,* 373.

Davis, R. B., Meeker, W. R., and Baily, W. L. (1961). *Federation Proc. 20,* 261.

DePalma, R. G., Coil, J., Davis, J. H., and Holden, W. D. (1967). *Surgery 62,* 505.

DePrez, R. M., Horowitz, H. I., and Cook, E. W. (1961). *J. Exptl. Med. 114,* 857.

Douglas, G. W., Beller, F. K., and Debrovner, C. H. (1963). *Amer. J. Obstet. Gynecol. 87,* 780.

Epstein, M. D., Beller, F. K., and Douglas, G. W. (1968). *Obstet. Gynecol. 32,* 494.

Erdoes, E. G., and Miwa, I. (1968). *Federation Proc. 27,* 92.

Evensen, S. A., and Jerimic, M. (1968). *Thromb. Diath. Haemorrhag. 19,* 557.

Evensen, S. A., Jerimic, M., and Hjort, P. F. (1968). *Thromb. Diath. Haemorrhag. 19,* 570.

Fine, J., Rutenburg, S., and Schweinburg, F. B. (1959). *J. Exptl. Med. 110,* 547.

Friscay, M., Eichenberger, E., and Schoenholzer, G. (1957). *Schweiz. Med. Wochschr. 87,* 631.

Galton, M. (1964). *Amer. J. Pathol. 44,* 613.

Gans, H. (1964). *Surgery 55,* 544.

Gans, H. (1966). *Ann. Surg. 163,* 175.

Gans, H., and Lowman, J. T. (1967). *Blood 29,* 526.

Gans, H., Subramanian, V., and Tan, B. H. (1968). *Thromb. Diath. Haemorrhag. 19,* 605.

Gerber, I. E. (1936). *Arch. Pathol. 21,* 776.

Good, R. A., and Thomas, L. (1952). *J. Exptl. Med. 96,* 625.

Good, R. A., and Thomas, L. (1953). *J. Exptl. Med. 97,* 871.

Graeff, H., and Beller, F. K. (1968). *Thromb. Diath. Haemorrhag. 27,* 427.

Hanger, F. M. (1927/28). *Proc. Soc. Exptl. Biol. Med. 25,* 775.

Hardaway, R. M. (1966). Syndromes of Disseminated Intravascular Coagulation. Thomas, Springfield, Ill.

Herring, W. B., Herion, J. C., Walker, R. I., and Palmer, J. G. (1963). *J. Clin. Invest. 42,* 79.

Hjort, P. F., McGehee, W. G., and Rapaport, S. I. (1964). Abstracts of the 10th Congress of the International Society of Hematology, Stockholm.

Hjort, P. F., and Rapaport, S. I. (1965). *Ann. Rev. 16,* 135.

Hjort, P. F., McGehee, W. G., and Rapaport, S. I. (1966). *Thromb. Diath. Haemorrhag. 16,* 333.

Horn, R. G., adn Spicer, S. S. (1964). *Amer. J. Pathol. 44,* 905.

Horn, R. G., and Spicer, S. S. (1964). *Amer. J. Pathol. 44,* 197.

Horn, R. G., and Collins, R. D. (1968). *Lab. Invest. 18,* 101.

Horowitz, H. I., DePrez, R. M., and Hook, E. W. (1962). *J. Exptl. Med. 116,* 619.

Huth, K., Schoenborn, W., and Knorp, K. (1967). *Thromb. Diath. Haemorrhrag. 17,* 129.

Jacobson, E. D., Mehlman, B., and Kalas, J. P, (1964). *J. Clin. Invest. 43,* 1000.

Jaeger, B. V. (1962). *New Engl. J. Med. 266,* 1962.

Kalbfleisch, J. M., and Bird, L. M. (1960). *New Engl. J. Med. 263,* 881.

Kaley, G., Demopoulos, H., and Zweifach, B. W. (1962). *Proc. Soc. Exptl. Biol. Med. 109,* 456.

Kaunitz, H., Malins, D. C., and McKay, D. G. (1962). *J Exptl. Med. 115,* 1127.

Kaunitz, H., Ganglitz, E. Jr., and McKay, D. G. (1963). *Metabolism 12,* 371.

Kleinmeier, H., Goergen, K., Lasch, H. G., Krecke, H. J., and Bohle, A. (1959). *Z. ges. exptl. Med. 132,* 275.

Kliman, A., and McKay, D. G. (1958). *Arch. Pathol. 66,* 715.

Kommerell, B., Barth, P., and Pfleiderer, M. (1966), *Thromb. Diath. Haemorrhag. 15,* 381.

Krecke, H. J. (1964). "Zum generalisierten Shwartzman-Phänomen". Gustav Fischer, Stuttgart. Veröffentlichungen aus der morphologischen Pathologie.

Kusama, S. (1913). *Beitr. Pathol. Anat. 55,* 459.

Lasch, H. G., Krecke, H. J., Rodriguez-Erdmann, F., and Schuetterle, G. (1961a). *Folia haemat. N. F. 6,* 325.

Lasch, H. G., Rodriguez-Erdman, F., and Schimpf, K. (1961b). *Klin. Wochschr. 39,* 645.

Lasch, H. G., Heene, D. L., Huth, K., and Sandritter, W. (1967). *Amer. J. Cardiol. 20,* 381.

Lee, L. (1962). *J. Exptl. Med. 115,* 1065.

Lee, L. (1963). *J. Exptl. Med. 117,* 365.

Lee, L., and McCluskey, R. T. (1962). *J. Exptl. Med. 116,* 611.

Lee, L., and Stetson, Ch. A. (1965). *In:* "The Inflammatory Process", (B. W. Zweifach, L. Grant, and R. T. McCluskey, Eds.). Academic Press, New York, London.

Lerner, R. G., Rapaport, S. I., Siemsen, J. K., and Spitzer, J. M. (1968). *Amer. J. Physiol. 214,* 532.

Lindberg, D. A. Z., and Riggins, C. K. (1963). *Exptl. Molec. Pathol. 2,* 114.

McKay, D. G. (1964). Disseminated Intravascular Coagulation. Hoeber (Harper and Row). New York and London.

McKay, D. G., and Shapiro, S. S. (1958). *J. Exptl. Med. 107,* 353.

McKay, D. G., and Müller-Berghaus, G. (1967). *Amer. J. Cardiol. 20,* 392.

McKay, D. G., and Müller-Berghaus, G. (1968). *Federation Proc. 27,* 1229.

McKay, D. G., Shapiro, S. S., and Shanberge, J. N. (1958). *J. Exptl. Med. 107,* 369.

McKay, D. G., Gitlin, D., and Craig, J. M. (1959). *Arch. Pathol. 67,* 270.

McKay, D. G., Margaretten, W., and Csavossy, I. (1966). *Lab. Invest. 15,* 1815.

McKay, D. G., Margaretten, W., and Phillips, L. L. (1967). *Lab. Invest. 16,* 511.

McKehee, S., Rapaport, S. I., and Hjort, P. F. (1967). *Amer. J. Internat. Med. 67,* 250.

Manasse, P. (1892). *Virchows Arch. Pathol. Anatomie. 30,* 217.

Mammen, E. F., Anderson, G., and Barnhart, M. (1969). Disseminated Intravascular Coagulation. *Thromb. Diath. Haemorrh. Suppl. 34.*

Margaretten, W., Zunker, H. O., and McKay, D. G. (1964). *Lab. Invest. 13,* 552.

Margaretten, W., McKay, D. G., and Phillips, L. L. (1967a). *Amer. J. Pathol. 51,* 61.

Margaretten, W., Csavossy, I., and McKay, D. G. (1967b). *Blood 2,* 169.

Merskey, C., Johnson, A. J., Kleiner, G. J., and Woil, H. (1967). *Brit. J. Haematol. 13,* 528.

Merskey, C., Johnson, A. J., and Kleiner, G. J. (1968). Abstr. XII Congress Internat. Soc. Hematology p. 209. New York.

Mosley, W. H., and Cluff, L. E. (1965). *Proc. Soc. Exptl. Biol. Med. 120,* 774.

Müller-Berghaus, G., and Lasch, H. G. (1963). *Thromb. Diath. Haemorrhag. 9,* 335.

Müller-Berghaus, G., Goldfinger, D., Margaretten, W., and McKay, D. G. (1967). *Thromb. Diath. Haemorrhag. 18,* 726.

Nakei, H., and Margaretten, W. (1963). *Pathology 76,* 38.

Nies, A., Forsyth, R. P., Williams, H. E., and Melmon, K. L. (1968). *Circul. Res. 22,* 155.

Page, E. W., and Glendening, M. B. (1955). *Obstet. Gynecol. 5,* 781.

Palminero, C., Ming, S. C., Frank, E., and Fine, J. (1962). *J. Exptl. Med. 115,* 609.

Pappas, G. D., Ross, M. H., and Thomas, L. (1958). *J. Exptl. Med. 107,* 333.

Penner, A., and Bernheim, A. L. (1940). *A. M. A. Arch. Pathol. 30,* 465.

Porter, P. J., Spierack, A. R., and Kass, E. H. (1964). *New Engl. J. Med. 271,* 445.

Prose, P. H., Lee, L., and Bulk, S. D. (1965). *Amer. J. Pathol. 47,* 403.

Quick, A. J. (1957). Hemorrhagic Diseases. Lea and Febiger, Philadelphia.

Riddle, J. M., and Barnhart, M. I. (1964). *Amer. J. Pathol. 45,* 805.

Rifkind, D., and Hill, R. B. (1967). *J. Immunol. 99,* 564.

Robbins, J., and Stetson, C. A. (1959). *J. Exptl. Med. 109,* 1.

Rodriguez-Erdman, F., (1964). *Thromb. Diath. Haemorrhag. 12,* 452.

Rodriguez-Erdmann, F. (1965). *Blood 26,* 541.

Sanarelli, G. (1894). Quoted in Sanarelli, G. (1916). *Presse Med. 24,* 505.

Sanarelli, G. (1935). *Schweiz. Med. Wochschr. 16,* 904.

Schmidt-Weyland, P. (1932). *Klin. Wochschr. 11,* 2148.

Schneider, C. L. (1951). *Surg. Gynecol. Obstet. 92,* 27.

Schwab, J. H., Watson, D. W., and Cromartie, W. J. (1953). *Proc. Soc. Exptl. Biol. Med. 82,* 754.

Selye, H. (1962). Calciphylaxis. University of Chicago Press, Chicago.

Selye, H. (1966). Thrombohemorrhagic Phenomena. Thomas, Springfield, Ill.

Shainoff, J. R., and Page, H. J. (1960). *Circulation Res. 8,* 1013.

Shimamoto, T., Yamazaki, H., Ohno, K., Uchida, H., Konoshi, T., and Iwahara, N. (1958). *Proc. Japan Acad. 34,* 444.

Shwartzman, G. (1927/28). *Proc. Soc. Exptl. Biol. Med. 25,* 560.

Smith, R. T. (1957). *J. Clin. Invest. 35,* 605.

Smith, R. T., Thomas, L., and Good, R. A. (1953). *Proc. Soc. Exptl. Biol. Med. 82,* 712.

Spaet, T. H. (1962). *Thromb. Diath. Haemorrhag. 8,* 276.

Spaet, T. H., Horowitz, H. I., Zucker-Franklin, D., Cintron, J., and Biezinsky, J. J. (1961). *Blood 17,* 196.
Spink, W. W., and Starzecki, B. (1968). *Proc. Soc. Exptl. Biol. Med. 126,* 574.
Starzl, T. E., Lerner, R. A., Dixon, F. J., Groth, C. G., Brettschneider, L., and Terasaki, P. (1968). *New Engl. J. Med. 278,* 642.
Stetson, Ch. A. (1955), *J. Exptl. Med. 101,* 431.
Stetson, Ch. A. (1957). *J. Exptl. Med. 103,* 489.
Studer, A., and Lorenz, H. P. (1965). *Pathol. Microbiol. 28,* 738.
Thal, A. P., and Enger, W. (1961). *J. Exptl. Med. 113,* 67.
Thomas, L., and Good, R. A. (1952a). *J. Exptl. Med. 95,* 409.
Thomas, L., and Good, R. A. (1952b). *J. Exptl. Med. 96,* 605.
Thomas, L., Smith, R. T., and v. Korff, R. (1954). *Proc. Soc. Exptl. Biol. Med. 86,* 813.
Thomas, L., Brunson, J., and Smith, R. T. (1955). *J. Exptl. Med. 102,* 249.
Trueta, J., Barclay, A. E., Franklin, K. J., Daniel, P. M., and Pritchard, J. (1947). Studies on Renal Circulation. Thomas, Springfield, Ill.
Vassalli, P., Simon, G., and Roullier, C. (1963). *Amer. J. Pathol. 43,* 579.
v. Kaulla, K. N., and v. Kaulla, E. (1968). *Abstr. XII Congress Internat. Soc. Hemat.,* New York, p. 184.
Wendt, F., Kapper, C., Burkhard, K., and Bohle, A. (1967). *Proc. Soc. Exptl. Biol. Med. 125,* 486.
Wexler, W. M., and Kantor, F. S. (1966). *Yale J. Biol. Med. 38,* 321.
Whitaker, A. N., and McKay, D. C. (1962). *Federation Proc. 21,* 1987.
Wiznitzer, T., Better, N., Rachlin, W., Atkins, N., Frank, E. D., and Fine, J. (1960). *J. Exptl. Med. 112,* 1157.
Wong, T. C. (1962). *Amer. J. Obstet. Gynecol. 84,* 786.
Zdrodowsky, P., and Brenn, E. (1926). *Zentralbl. Bakt. 99,* 159.

Demonstration of Plasma Proteins in Microscopic Sections with Emphasis on the Identification of Fibrin

G. Beneke

I. Introduction

Like other proteins in tissue sections, fibrin is demonstrable by methods which are based on its submicroscopic structure, staining characteristics, amino acid composition and sequence, and its serological properties.

II. Demonstration of Fibrin Based on Its Ultrastructure

Principle: Fibrin has a characteristic submicroscopic structure. It is fibrous and cross striated with a periodicity of 220 Å (Wolpers and Ruska, 1939; Hawn and Porter, 1947; Porter and Hawn, 1949; Hall, 1949; Köppel, 1962). It differs from other plasma proteins and similarly structured tissue proteins (Table 1). The crystallized structure of the fibrin fiber permits its identification in polarized light. Fibrin fibers posses birefringence in polarized light (Dungern, 1937). It can only be differentiated unequivocally from collagen by a combination of techniques such as electronmicroscopy, histochemistry, or polarizing microscopy in combination with the histochemical demonstration of tyrosine or tryptophane (Beneke, 1963).

Table 1: Structure of Various Extracellular Proteins in the electron microscope.

Protein	Structure in Electron Microscope	
	Structure	Periodicity (Å)
Albumin	Amorphous	No
Globulin	Amorphous	No
Fibrin	Fibrous	220
Basement membrane proteins	Granular	No
Amyloid	Fibrous	40
Collagen fibers	Fibrous	640
Elastic fibers	Fibrous	No

Technique: Paraffin sections containing fibrin are first stained using a histochemical reaction, e. g. the reaction for tryptophane utilizing the p-dimethylamino-benzaldehyde method of Adams (1957).
In a second step, the stained section is observed in the polarization optics microscope by use of a plate which yields a phase difference of 1 λ.

Comments: The collagen fibers appear yellow with the polarizing in the substraction position, or blue in the addition position (Table 2, Fig. 1). Fibrin and/or plasma proteins are

Table 2: Differentiation of Plasma Proteins and Connective Tissue Fibers using Combined Histochemical Amino Acid Reaction and Polarization Microscopy.

Optical Conditions	non polarized light		Polarized light and phase difference of 1 λ			
			addition position		subtraction position	
Histochemical reactions	plasma protein	collagen fibers	plasma protein	collagen fibers	plasma protein	collagen fibers
Unstained section	not visible	not visible	not visible	blue	not visible	yellow
Reaction for tyrosin	brown	not visible	brown	blue	brown	yellow
Reaction for tryptophane	dark blue	not visible	dark blue	blue	dark blue	yellow
	see Fig. 1a				see Fig. 1b	

stained blue with the histochemical tryptophane reaction. Therefore, a differentiation between collagen fibers and plasma proteins is easily achieved. However, the tryptophane reaction is not specific for fibrin, as other plasma proteins are also stained blue.

III. Demonstration of Fibrin By Specific - Histologic Stains

Principle: The principle of staining methods for fibrin involves a sequence in which nearly all tissue structures are stained. In a decolorizing (differentiation) solution the bound dye is removed from those tissue structures which do not possess specific binding characteristics. The staining methods for fibrin summarized in Table 3 are modifications of three basic techniques. The fibrin staining technique according to Weigert (1887) is mainly quoted in the German literature.
The fibrin staining method according to Mallory (1900), primarily quoted in the English literature refers to the trichome type staining technique.
Roulet (1948), Romeis (1948), Lillie (1954), Mallory (1961) have described modifications of Weigert's technique. The Mallory phosphotungstic acid hematoxylin staining was modified by Schueninoff (1908), Pearse (1960) and MacManus and Mowry (1960). According to our own experience the best modification for both staining methods is that of MacManus and Mowry (1960).

In the trichrome staining techniques, the tissue sections are stained successively or simultaneously with two or three differently colored

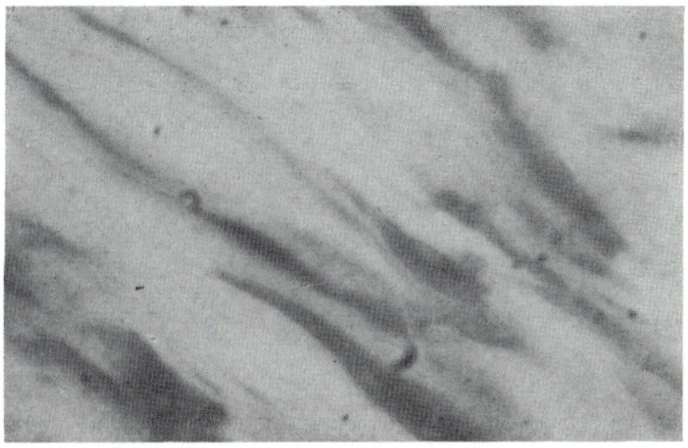

Fig. 1a. Tryptophane reaction demonstrated in non-polarized light (83/46).

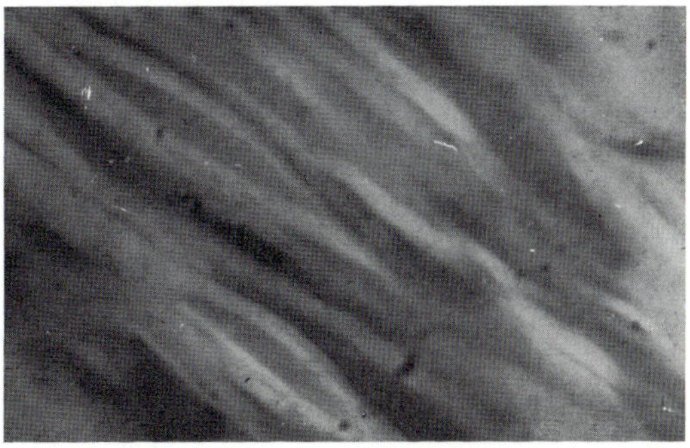

Fig. 1b. Tryptophane reaction demonstrated in polarized light by use of 1 λ phase difference in subtraction position of the polarization microscope (83/42). Magnification: 600×.

Fig. 1. Simultaneous demonstration of plasma proteins (tryptophane-reaction) and collagen fibers (polarization microscope) in tissue section.

Table 3: Survey of Various Fibrin Staining Methods.

Staining method	Class of dye	Dye	Author	Results of staining: platelet aggregates	fibrin	erythrocytes	collagen fibers	elastic fibers
So-called fibrin staining methods	Triphenyl methane dyes	Crystal violet	Weigert (1887)	–	violet	– or violet	–	–
		Polychrome methylene blue	Unna (1893)					
	Anthrachinone dye	Alizarin	Herxheimer (1909)					
	Natural dyes	Phosphotungstic acid hematoxylin	Mallory (1900)	–	violet	– or violet	–	–
		Iron hematoxylin	Mallory (1900)					
		Carmine	Fraenkel (1911)					
Trichrome staining methods	Triphenyl methane dyes	Fuchsin S Orange G Anilin blue	Mallory (1900)	blue	orange	red	blue	blue
	Quinone-imine dyes	Fuchsin S Anilin blue	Masson (1929)	blue	red	red	blue	blue
	Azo dyes	Fuchsin S Ponceau 2 R Orange G Light green S	Goldner (1938)	green	orange	red	green	green
		Azocarmine G Orange G Anilin blue	Heidenhain (1915)	blue	orange	red	blue	blue
		Various dyes (see original literature)	Lendrum et al. (1962)	Depending on the used dyes				

acid dyes. These dyes differ in molecular structure, molecular weight and position of the polar groups but not in the intensity of the total charge. In the staining process the dyes are bound to the basic groups of the proteins.

These staining methods (see Table 2) are more effective than Weigert's or Mallory's technique.

Technique: Phosphotungstic acid hematoxylin staining method: Paraffin sections are brought to water through xylol and alcohol (100%, 90%, 70%, 50%) and then placed in an iodine solution (0.5% iodine in 1.0% aqueous potassium iodide) until the sections are yellowish brown. Excess iodine is washed off in water and then in 0.5% aqueous solution of sodium thiosulfate until the sections are colorless. Next they are washed for several minutes under running tap water after which they are placed in a freshly prepared 0.25% aqueous solution of potassium permanganate for 5 minutes and washed again in water. In the next step the sections are placed in a 5% aqueous solution of oxalic acid for 1 minute followed by washing in running tap water for several minutes. The prepared sections are then stained in phosphotungstic acid hematoxylin for 15 hours.

Hematoxylin	1.0 g
Phosphotungstic acid	20.0 g
Distilled water	1000.0 ml

After the staining procedure the sections should be dried with filter paper and passed rapidly through 95% and absolute alcohol (note: extended alcohol extraction removes the red component of the stain), cleared in xylol and mounted with a conventional mounting medium (e.g. synthetic resin).

Trichrome staining method (Heidenhain, 1915):

Paraffin sections (5 μ thick) are deparaffinized by xylol and subsequently brought through alcohol (100%, 90%, 70%, 50%) into water. Then the sections are stained in azocarmine (Azocarmine B: 0.5 g, distilled water: 100.0 ml, Glacial acetic acid: 1.0 ml) at 56° C for 60 minutes. After cooling the sections to room temperature (10 minutes) they are washed in distilled water and differentiated in aniline alcohol (Aniline: 1.0 ml, Alcohol [95%]: 1000 ml) until clouds of stain no longer appear. Then the sections are rinsed in acetic alcohol (Glacial acetic acid: 1.0 ml, Alcohol [95%]: 100 ml) for 1 minute. The sections are then placed in phosphotungstic acid (Phosphotungstic acid: 5.0 g, distilled water: 100 ml) for 3 hours. They are washed quickly in distilled water and stained in aniline blue-orange G solution for 2 hours.

Stock solutions:

Aniline blue:	0.5 g
Orange G:	2.0 g
Distilled water:	100.0 ml
Glacial acetic acid:	8.0 ml

(before use dilute this stock solution 1:3 with distilled water).

The sections are then rinsed quickly in distilled water, dehydrated in 95% alcohol and absolute alcohol, cleared in xylol and mounted in conventional mounting media.

Examples: Fig. 2 demonstrates a part of a white thrombus, stained by the method of Weigert. In the center of the section, platelet aggregates can be seen. They are confined by lamellar fibrin (-----> 1). Erythrocytes are often stained (----->2) concomitantly. As a result the fine network of fibrin between the platelet aggregates does not show up.

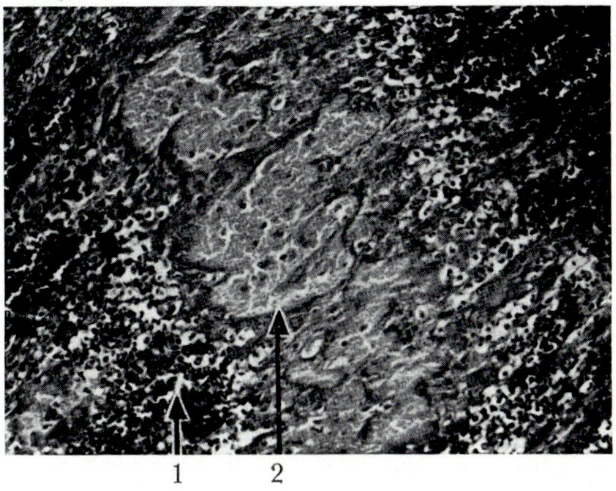

Fig. 2. Part of a white thrombus. Section is stained by the Weigert fibrin staining method.
1 Lamellar fibrin around the platelet aggregates.
2 Erythrocytes in the meshwork of the fibrin.
Magnification: 160×.

An example of a thrombus stained with Azan according to Heidenhain (1915) is shown in Fig. 3. Upon proper differentiation following staining, the platelet aggregates are demonstrable by a delicate blue color. They are surrounded by fibrin fibers which exhibit a dense orange color. Fibrin fibers are woven in a network between the platelet aggregates. Erythrocytes can be found in the meshwork of fibrin and are colored deep red.

Comments: These methods are relatively simple to perform and result in a very colorful picture. They are not primarily specific for fibrin.

The fibrin specificity depends on the following factors: 1. The diffusion velocity of the dye in the tissue (Zeiger, 1938). 2. The local concentration of the dye at specific sites of the tissue. The concentration of the dye is dependent on the amount of opposite (to the dye) charged groups in the tissue structure (Rohde, 1917; Pischinger, 1927; Singer, 1952). 3. The coincidence of the proper steric configuration of dye and the specific sites of the tissue structures. The distance between dye and substrate determines the kind of chemical binding (Otto, 1935). 4. A primarily bound dye may be displaced by a second dye due to an ion exchange effect. This takes place if the second dye has an affinity to the tissue structure which is greater than the original one.

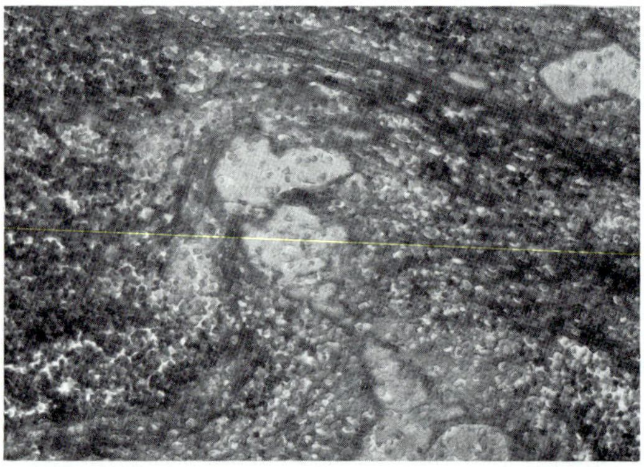

a

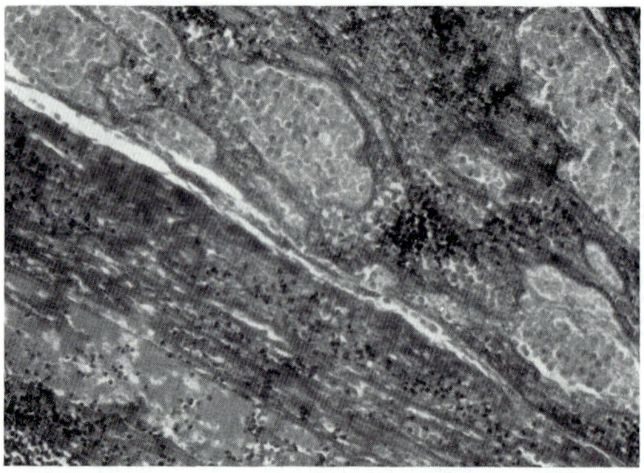

b

Fig. 3. a. Part of a white thrombus stained with trichome stain according to Heidenhain. Note the platelet aggregates (center of the picture) in light blue color. The platelet aggregates are surrounded by fiibrin (orange color). The erythrocytes are collered red. Magnification: 160×.
b. Part of a white thrombus stained with trichome stain according to Heidenhain. The older (upper right) and the freshly formed (lower left) platelet aggregates are stained blue. The fibrin network is orange or light red. Magnification: 160×.

Furthermore, the structure and composition of fibrin is an important factor (Gitlin and Craig, 1957; Gitlin et al. 1957; Beneke, 1963). Therefore, the specificity of the staining methods depends on the differentiation used after the staining procedure.

Modifications of the trichrome staining technique which also give very colorful pictures were described by Lendrum et al. (1962). The advantage of this modification is the possibility of varying the different components of the stain in the procedure. Thus, a higher differentiation in staining of the various parts of the tissue is obtained. Nevertheless, the same principle difficulties of specificity of trichrome staining methods apply.

IV. Demonstration of Fibrin and Other Proteins by their Amino Acid Composition

These methods may be used to discern plasma proteins from other tissue proteins (e. g. collagen or elastic fibers). The plasma proteins contain relatively large amounts of tyrosine and trytophane. In collagen fibers, these two amino acids are not present, while elastic fibers contain only small amounts of tyrosine. These differences in amino acid composition allow a distinction of these proteins by means of UV photometry or histochemical reactions for polymerized amino acids in polypeptide chains (Sandritter, 1958; Pearse, 1960).

A. UV Microphotometric Methods

Principle: In monochromatic ultraviolet light the amino acids tyrosine and tryptophane absorb light at the wave length 280 mμ. Proteins containing these two amino acids therefore show a maximum of absorption at this wave length. Absorption measurements in microscopic tissue sections are possible on 1μ^2 areas using suitable microspectrophotometers (Zeiss, Oberkochen, Germany; Leitz, Wetzlar, Germany).

Comments: The UV method is useful for exact differentiation of hemoglobin, plasma proteins and collagen fibers (Sandritter, 1958; Sandritter et al. 1966).
The absorption curves of plasma proteins, as well as fibrin (Fig. 4) show only one maximum at the wave length of 280 mμ (tyrosine and tryptophane). Other extracellular components such as amyloid or basement membrane proteins also yield an absorption peak at 280 mμ. For this reason these proteins cannot be differentiated from normal plasma proteins. On the other hand plasma proteins are well marked off from collagen fibers (Fig. 5).

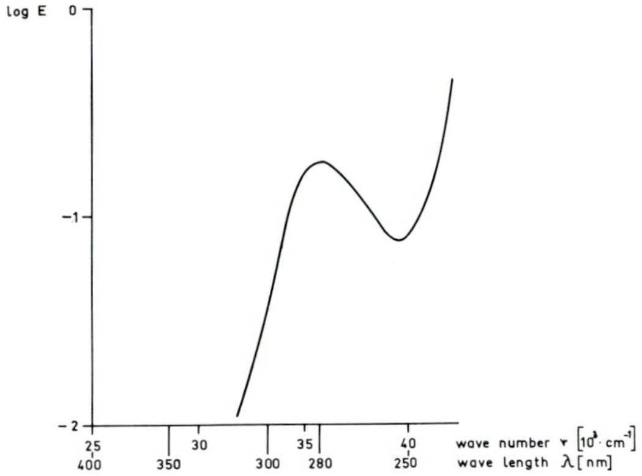

Fig. 4: Absorption curve of fibrin in tissue section measured with universal microspectrophotometer (UMSP I, Zeiss).
Maximum at 280 mμ: tyrosin and tryptophane.

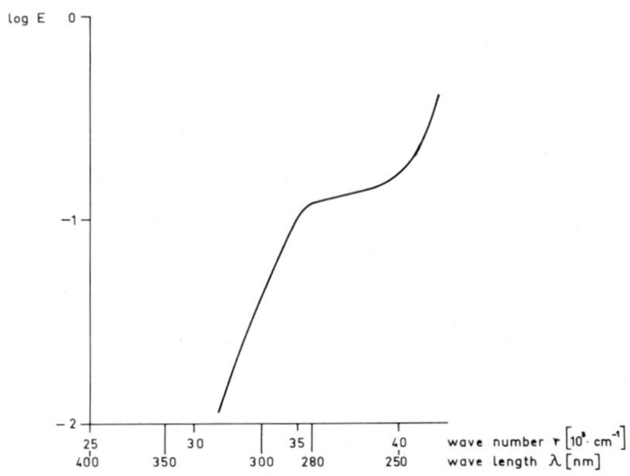

Fig. 5: Absorption curve of collagen fibers in tissue sections measured with universal microspectrophotometer (UMSP I, Zeiss).
No maximum in UV-light. The absorption curve occurs only with so called structure absorption, caused by peptid chains.

B. Histochemical Reactions

Principle: These methods are also dependent on the presence of the amino acids tyrosine, tryptophane, histidine and arginine. The advantage of these methods in contrast to the staining methods is that a specific chemical reaction is performed on the tissue sections and colored products occur as a result of this reaction.
The following methods are suitable for these investigations:

1) Reaction for tyrosine (Millon-reaction, 1849) modified according to Rash and Swift (1960).

2) Reaction for tyrosine with the nitrosophenol reaction according to Glenner (1959).

3) Reaction for tryptophane with the p-dimethylaminobenzaldehyde method according to Adams (1957).

4) Reaction for tryptophane with the ronsidole method according to Glenner, 1957).

5) Reaction for histidine with the method of Landing and Hall (1956), modified according to Bachmann and Seitz (1961).

6) Reaction for arginine (Sakaguchi-reaction, 1925) modified according to Deitch (1961).

The method for the demonstration of fibrin preferred by the author is the reaction for tryptophane according to Adams (1957) or according to Glenner (1957). Tissue fixation: Formalin (4% buffered at pH 7.0 according to Lillie (1954) or acid-alcohol solutions, e. g. Carnoy solution.

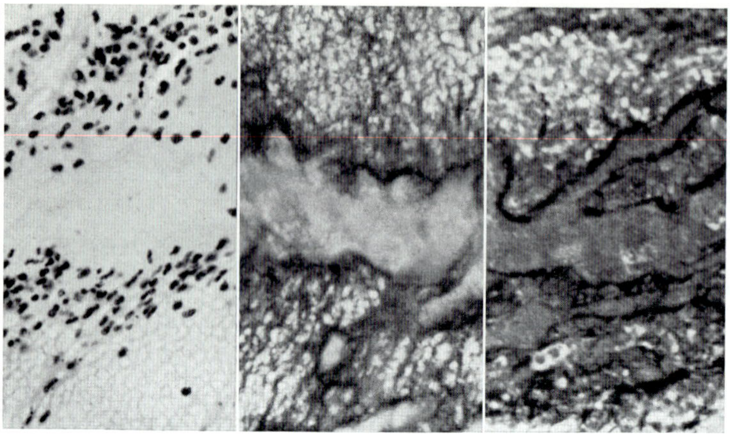

Fig. 6. Part of a white thrombus. a. Hematoxylin eosin staining (80/53). b. Tryptophane reaction (80/62). c. Arginine reaction (83/62). Magnification: 250×.

Technique: Tryptophane Reaction According to Adams (1957): Paraffin sections (5 μ thick) are brought through xylol into absolute alcohol, rinsed in alcohol and then air dried (1 minute). When the sections are dry, they are coated with celloidin. The sections are then placed in a solution of 5% p-dimethylaminobenzaldehyde in concentrated hydrochloric acid for 1 minute and after this, treated in 1% sodium nitrite (in concentrated HCL) for 1 minute.

The sections are then rinsed in absolute alcohol, tap water (30 seconds), dehydrated in ethanol, cleared in xylol and mounted in conventional mounting media.

Tryptophane Reaction According to Glenner (1957): Deparaffinized 5 μ thick sections are rinsed in absolute alcohol and air dried (1 minute). The sections are then immersed for 3 minutes at room temperature in the following solutions:

p-dimethylaminobenzaldehyde	1.0 g
perchloric acid (60%)	5.0 ml
concentrated HCl	1.0 ml
glacial acetic acid	35.0 ml

Next they are directly transferred for 1 minute into the following solutions:

Sodium nitrite	0.5 g
concentrated HCl	5.0 ml
glacial acetic acid	35.0 ml

The sections are then washed in two changes of 50% glacial acetic acid (1 minute each) cleared in 50% glacial acetic acid in xylol, 20% glacial acetic acid in xylol and in three changes of xylol and mounted in a conventional mounting medium.

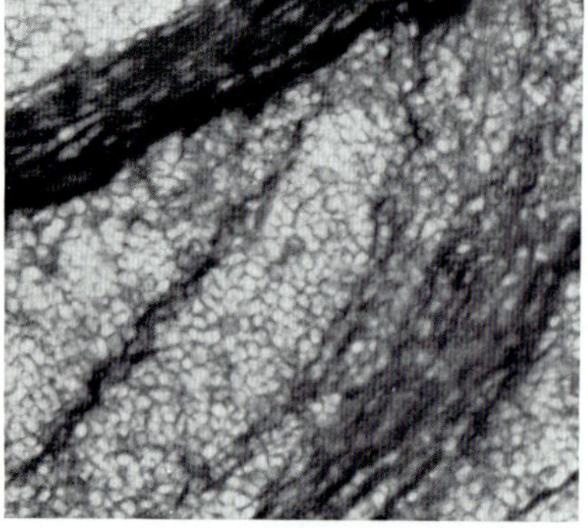

Fig. 7. Part of a red thrombus. Tryptophane reaction (80/47). Magnification: 250×.

Comments: The methods allow differentiation of plasma proteins in thrombi or other tissues. Fig. 6 shows part of a white thrombus in an H & E section. In the center of Fig. 6 platelet aggregates are demonstrated. These platelet aggregates are surrounded by leukocytes and in the lower part of the picture erythrocytes are seen. A differentiation however, between platelets and fibrin is not possible. By using tryptophane and arginine reaction (Fig. 6b), the demonstration of the network of fibrin fibers is very clearly detectable. Fig. 6c shows no reaction inside the platelet aggregates which means that no tryptophane containing proteins are present in the platelet aggregates. The very close network of fibrin fibers in the

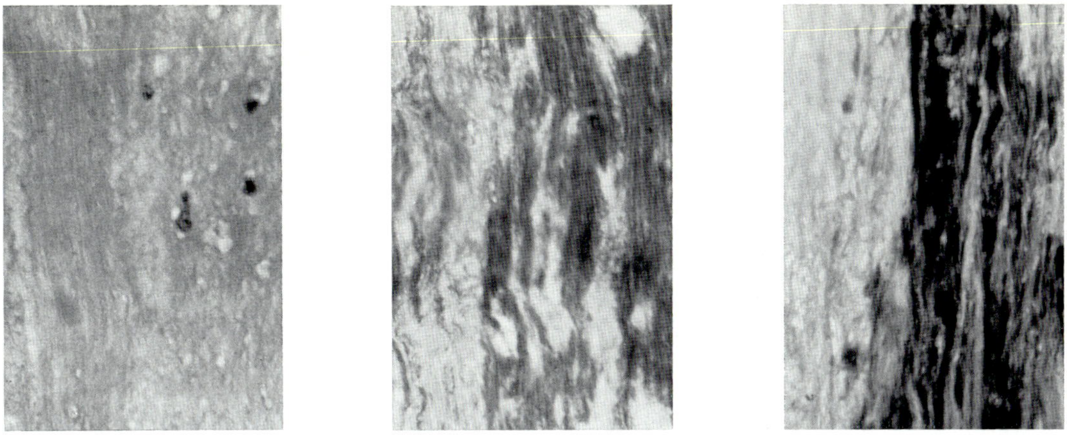

a b c

Fig. 8. Intima in arteriosclerosis. a. Hematoxylin eosin staining (79/16). b. Histidine reaction (79/2). c. Tryptophane reaction (78/50). Magnification: 250×.

red part of a thrombus may be demonstrated by the use of the tryptophane reaction (Fig. 7). The histochemical methods are relatively easy to handle. Small amounts of plasma proteins are detectable (Fig. 8) and can be differentiated from collagen and elastic fibers (Movat and More, 1957; Puchtler et al. 1961; Beneke, 1963). But, as with the UV microspectrophotometric methods, plasma proteins, basement membrane and amyloid proteins cannot be differentiated.

Table 4: Proteolytic Digestion of Fibrin, Collagen and Elastic Fibers in Tissue Sections (Unfixed, Frozen Sections).

Enzymes	Fibrin	Collagen Fibers	Elastic Fibers
Plasmin	+	—	—
Trypsin	+	—	—
Chymotrypsin	+	—	—
Papain	+	—	—
Pepsin	+	+	+
Collagenase	—	+	—
Elastase	—	—	+

V. Demonstration of Specific Proteins As Substrates for Specific Proteases

A. Proteases as Chemical Reagents

Principle: The use of proteases as chemical reagents allow the identification of a protein in tissue sections. The action of the enzymes is based on a specific sequence of amino acids in the protein. In tissue sections fibrin is digestable with the proteases plasmin, trypsin, chymotrypsin, papain and pepsin. The enzymatic solubility of fibrin differs from platelet aggregates, collagen and elastic fibers (Table 4).

Comments: The results (Schlossmann, 1942; Wagner, 1957; Busanny-Caspari, 1957; Schallock, 1960; Matsuyama et al. 1961; Hey and Beneke, 1963) are not very reliable. We have found that the use of different batches of the enzymes are a frequent cause of errors. Furthermore, these methods are relatively difficult to handle. It is necessary to perform a staining procedure on comparable tissue sections before or after the enzyme incubation. The direct observation of the proteolytic process in phase contrast microscope (Beneke and Hey, 1965) is another method of control.

B. Fibrin Layer Method

Principle: A cryostat section 5–10 μ thick is placed on a thin fibrin layer and incubated for various times. The activator from the tissue diffuses into the fibrin and activates the contaminating plasminogen to plasmin which then in turn lyses the fibrin (Todd, 1959; Beller et al. 1962; Kwaan and Astrup, 1963).

Technique (Mitchell et al. 1967):
Preparation of fibrin film: Bovine fibrinogen highly contaminated with plasminogen (Behring Werke, Marburg, Germany) is dissolved in Michaelis Veronal buffer (pH = 7.35) to a concentration of 300 mg to 600 mg per 10 ml. 20 units of Parke, Davis Topical thrombin in 1 ml of buffer is added to a test tube containing 10 ml of fibrinogen solution. The tube is inverted gently to mix the solutions and is then poured uniformly onto an 8 cm × 14 cm piece of wettable cellophane (dialysis paper) which has been saturated with the veronal buffer and placed on a perfectly level surface. The solution is permitted to clot at room temperature and is then placed in a refrigerated (4° C) wet chamber for at least one half hour. A 2 × 3 cm piece of the film may then be cut from the 8 × 14 cm piece using a siliconized surgical scissor. These sections are inverted on clean microscope slides using care so that no bubbles form under the film. The cellophane is then pealed off leaving a 2 mm fibrin film on the slide. These film are stable, when refrigerated for three days. Activator inhibitors may be incorporated into the films prior to the addition of thrombin. If the film is to be heated to destroy the plasminogen (86° C/ 30 min), this step should be carried out in a wet chamber after the fibrin has been placed on the slide.

Tissue activator assay: The tissue used in this assay must be received fresh, and immediately quick frozen onto a cryostat block. In this state, the tissue is stable for several days if it is sealed in parafilm to prevent drying.

The tissue sections are then cut 8 μ thick and placed on the fibrin film slides with a precooled forceps. If many films are to be run, they are placed in the refrigerated wet chamber and their incubations all commense simultaneously. The incubation is carried out in a moist 37° C incubator for varying periods of time. A control slide (10 min incubation) is prepared for comparison and to aid in interpretation of the results. Incubations of relatively inactive tissues have been carried out for periods of up to 24 hours. The reaction is arrested by placing the slides into a 10% formaline-saline solution.

Staining procedure:
1) Rinse slides in tap water bath
2) Place in acid hematoxylin 90 sec (or until red-blue color results)
3) Rinse in water
4) Develop in dilute ammonia water until blue
5) Rinse in water
6) 50% ethyl alcohol × 15 min
7) 70% ethyl alcohol × 15 min
8) 95% ethyl alcohol × 30 min
9) 100% ethyl alcohol × 45 min
10) Eosin Y × 20 sec
11) Wash in 100% ethyl alcohol three times
12) 50% ethyl alcohol – 50% xylol × 20 min
13) 100% xylol × 20 min
14) Trim excess fibrin film from the slides with sharp knife and cover with synthetic mounting medium and a cover slip. The entire area under the cover slip must be filled with mounting medium to prevent drying of the film. The slides are now stable, and may be stored for further reference.

Comments: The slides are best observed with a low power stereoscopic microscope. Lysed zones will first appear as depressed areas under the tissue section. Slides incubated for longer periods will have holes through the entire fibrin film at areas under the tissue that correspond to the earlier depressions. Lysis on heated films or those containing activator inhibitors (e. g. 4×10^{-4} M, EACA) is indicative of proteolytic activity in the tissue not due to plasminogen activator.

Semi-quantitative comparisons of activator activity in different tissues may be made with reference to the time of incubation necessary to produce a certain observed amount of lysis. However, these comparisons must be made only between slides which are prepared with the same batch of fibrinogen on one film and with simultaneous incubations.

It is preferable to use one batch of fibrinogen in which the plasminogen contamination is known. The method is not a histochemical assay in the true sense of the definition since the plasmin spreads. The localization is therefore dependent on a proper incubation time. Excessive incubation of the slides results in autolysis of the entire tissue section.

VI. Immunochemical Demonstration of Specific Proteins

Principle: These methods are most specific for the identification of plasma proteins and other substances in tissue sections. The principle involves precipitating an antigen (or an antibody) with a labelled antibody (or antigen) labelled (Coons et al. 1941, 1942) with a fluorescence dye. Useful fluorescence dyes are rhodamine B or fluorescein isothiocyanate.

Technique: The following methods are suitable for the determination of plasma proteins in tissue sections:

1) Frozen sections are prepared at a thickness of approximately 10 μ.
2) These sections are fixed for a short period (10 minutes) in methanol (100%).
3) The sections are rinsed in 0.9% NaCl solution to remove the excess of methanol.
4) The sections are incubated in a solution of labelled antibodies at room temperature in a moist chamber for 5 hours.
5) The sections are rinsed again in 0.9% NaCl solution to remove the non-bound antibodies.
6) Finally the sections are embedded in glycerol which is buffered at pH 7.0. The stained sections are observed in a fluorescence microscope for localization of the bound labelled antiserum.

Comments: Source of error: Beside the specific antigen-antibody-reaction, a small non specific reaction (caused by non specific salt like linkages) frequently occurs. Proper controls are therefore mandatory. These control reactions are performed in a similar way (up to step 3). Instead of step four, the sections will be incubated with an antibody which is not labelled (5 hours at room temperature). During this time a specific reaction between the antigen and the unlabelled antibody occurs. The sections will then be rinsed in 0.9% NaCl solution. This procedure is followed by a second incubation with the identical but labelled antibody. The reaction which occurs during the second incubation is the non specific reaction.

After the second incubation the control sections are treated in the same way (see step 5 and step 6).

These methods require purified antibodies. Successful fluorescence identification of fibrin requires experience. The staining is specific for fibrinogen, fibrin monomers, fibrin polymers and fibrinogen breakdown products. This is a superior method for the identification of small quantities of the desired protein.

References

Adams, C. W. M. (1957). *J. Clin. Pathol. 10,* 56.
Bachmann, R., and Seitz, H. M. (1961). *Histochemie 2,* 307.
Beller, F. K., Herschlein, H. J., and Goessner, W. (1962). *Obstet. Gynecol. 20,* 117.
Beneke, G. (1963). *Verh. Dtsch. Ges. Pathol. 47,* 234.
Beneke, G., and Hey, D. (1965). *Histochemie 5,* 366.
Busanny-Caspari, W. (1957). *Acta Histochem. 4,* 304.
Coons, H. J., Creech, H. J., and Jones, R. N. (1941). *Proc Soc. Exptl. Biol. Med. 47,* 200.
Coons, H. J., Creech, H. J., Jones, R. N., and Berliner, R. (1942). *J. Immunol. 45,* 159.
Deitch, A. D. (1961). *J. Histochem. Cytochem. 9,* 477.
Dungern, M. V. (1937). *Z. Biol. 98,* 136.
Gitlin, D., and Craig, J. M. (1957). *Am. J. Pathol. 33,* 267
Gitlin, D., Craig, J. M., and Janeway, C. A. (1957). *Am. J. Pathol. 33,* 55.
Glenner, G. G. (1957). *J. Histochem. Cytochem. 5,* 297.
Glenner, G. G. (1959). *J. Histochem. Cytochem. 7,* 423.
Hall, C. E. (1949). *J. Biol. Chem. 179,* 857.
Hawn, C. V., and Porter, K. R. (1947). *J. Exptl. Med. 86,* 286.
Heidenhain, M. (1915). *Z. wissensch. Mikrosk. 32,* 361.
Hey, D., and Beneke, G. (1963). *Verh. Dtsch. Ges. Pathol. 47,* 232.
Köppel, G. (1962). "Die Umwandlung des Fibrinogens in Fibrin". Schattauer, Stuttgart.
Kwaan, H. C., Astrup, T. (1963). *Arch. Pathol. 76,* 595.
Landing, B. H., and Hall H. E. (1956). *Stain Technol. 31,* 197.
Lendrum, A. C., Fraser, D. S., Slidders, W., and Hendreson, R. (1962). *J. Clin. Pathol. 15,* 401.
Lillie, R. D. (1954). "Histopathologic Technic and Practical Histochemistry". McGraw, New York-Toronto-London.
Mallory, F. B. (1900). *J. Exptl. Med. 5,* 15.
Mallory, F. B. (1961). "Pathological Technique". Hafner, New York.
MacManus, J. F. A., and Mowry, R. W. (1960). "Stain Methods, Histologic and Histochemical." Hoeber, New York.
Matsuyama, K., Ooneda, G., Tanaka, S., and Takamata, M. (1961). *Gumna J. Med. Sci. 10,* 83.
Millon, M. E. (1849). *C. R. Acad. Sci. 28,* 40.
Mitchell, P., Weiss, G., and Beller, F. K. (1967). In preparation.
Movat, H. Z., and More, R. H. (1957). *Am. J. Clin. Pathol. 28,* 331.
Otto, G. (1935). *Leder 6,* 207.
Pearse, A. G. E. (1960). "Histochemistry, Theoretical and Applied." Churchill, London.
Pischinger, A. (1927). *Z. Zellforsch. 5,* 347.
Porter, K. R., and Hawn, C. V. (1949). *J. Exptl. Med. 90,* 225.
Puchtler, H., Chandler, A. B., and Sweat, F. (1961). *J. Histochem. Cytochem. 9,* 340.
Rash, E., and Swift, H. (1960). *J. Histochem. Cytochem. 8,* 4.
Rhode, K. (1917). *Pflügers Arch. 168,* 419.
Romeis, B. (1948). "Mikroskopische Technik." Leibnitz, München.
Roulet, F. (1948). "Methoden der pathologischen Histologie." Springer, Wien.
Sakaguchi, S. (1925). *J. Biochem. 5,* 25.
Sandritter, W. (1958). *In:* "Handbuch der Histochemie", pp. 220—338. Fischer, Stuttgart.
Sandritter, W., Thorell, B., Schubert, W., and Schlüter, G. (1966). *Virchows Arch. Pathol. Anat. 340,* 352.
Schallock, G. (1960). *In:* "Struktur und Stoffwechsel des Bindegewebes", pp. 161—172. Thieme, Stuttgart.
Schlossmann, N. C. (1942). *Arch. Pathol. 34,* 365.
Schueninoff, S. (1908). *Zbl. Pathol. 19,* 6.
Singer, M. (1952). *Intern. Rev. Cytol. 1,* 211.
Todd, M.: *J. Pathol. Bacteriol. 78,* 281 (1959).
Unna, P. G. (1893). *Monatsh. Prakt. Dermat. 16,* 351.
Wagner, B. M. (1957). *J. Mt. Sinai Hosp. 60,* 221.
Weigert, C. (1887). *Fortschr. Med. 5,* 228.
Wolpers, C., and Ruska, H. (1939). *Klin. Wochschr. 19,* 1111.
Zeiger, K. (1938). "Physikochemische Grundlagen der histologischen Methodik." Steinkopff, Dresden and Leipzig.

Index